Contempora

MW01528192

LIBRARY

College of Physicians and Surgeons
of British Columbia

Mark R. Harrigan • John P. Deveikis

U. Joseph Schoepf
(Series Editor)

Handbook of Cerebrovascular Disease and Neurointerventional Technique

Second Edition

Springer

Authors
Mark R. Harrigan, M.D.
Department of Surgery, Division of
Neurosurgery, and Departments of
Radiology and Neurology
University of Alabama
Birmingham, AL
USA

John P. Deveikis, M.D.
Bayfront Medical Center
St. Petersburg, FL
USA

With a chapter on ischemic stroke by:
Agnieszka Anna Ardelt, M.D., Ph.D.
Department of Neurology
University of Chicago
Chicago, IL
USA

With primers on imaging by:
Joel K. Curé, M.D.
Department of Radiology
University of Alabama
Birmingham, AL
USA

ISBN 978-1-61779-945-7   ISBN 978-1-61779-946-4   (Ebook)
DOI 10.1007/978-1-61779-946-4
Springer New York Heidelberg Dordrecht London

Library of Congress Control Number: 2012945195

Dedications and Acknowledgments

The authors wish to express their endless appreciation to Susan Deveikis for both personal support and for making things happen in the neuroendovascular suite. In addition, acknowledgments again to two great people, Jason and Sabrina Deveikis, and the authors' other family members and friends who have been tremendously indulgent and supportive during the demanding professional careers thus far, culminating in completion of this project. On the professional side, we owe a debt of gratitude to the following people who helped with this edition of the handbook: Agnieszka Anna Ardelt, Joel K. Curé, Prashant S. Kelkar, Kimberly P. Kicielinski, Martee Posey, Boyd F. Richards, George Tsivgoulis, R. Shane Tubbs, and Michael Yester.

Abbreviations

A-comm	Anterior communicating artery
ACAS	Asymptomatic Carotid Atherosclerosis Study
ACCP	American College of Chest Physicians
ACE	Angiotensin converting enzyme
ACST	Asymptomatic Carotid Surgery Trial
ACT	Activated clotting time
ACTH	Adrenocorticotropic hormone
ADC	Apparent diffusion coefficient
ADH	Antidiuretic hormone
ADPKD	Autosomal dominant polycystic kidney disease
AED	Antiepileptic drug
AF	Atrial fibrillation
AHA	American Heart Association
AICA	Anterior inferior cerebellar artery
aka	Also known as
ALT	Alanine aminotransferase
AMA	Accessory meningeal artery
ANA	Antinuclear antibody
ANP	Atrial natriuretic peptide
ARCHeR	Acculink for Revascularization of Carotids in High-Risk patients
ARR	Absolute risk reduction
ARUBA	A Randomized trial of Unruptured Brain Arteriovenous malformations
ASA	Aspirin (acetylsalicylic acid)
ASAN	Atrial septal aneurysm
ASITN	American Society of Interventional and Therapeutic Neuroradiology
ASNR	American Society of Neuroradiology
atm	Atmosphere
AV	Arteriovenous
AVF	Arteriovenous fistula
AVM	Arteriovenous malformation
BA	Basilar artery
BE	Bacterial endocarditis
BEACH	Boston Scientific EPI-A Carotid stenting trial for High risk surgical patients
bFGF	Basic fibroblast growth factor
BNP	Brain natriuretic peptide
BRANT	British Aneurysm Nimodipine Trial
BRASIL	Bleeding Risk Analysis in Stroke Imaging Before Thrombolysis Study
CAA	Cerebral amyloid angiopathy
CABERNET	Carotid Artery Revascularization Using the Boston Scientific FilterWire EX/EZ and the EndoTex NexStent
CADASIL	Cerebral autosomal dominant arteriopathy with subcortical infarcts and leukoencephalopathy
CADISS	Cervical Artery Dissection in Stroke Study
cANCA	Circulating antineutrophil cytoplasmic antibody
CAPTURE	Carotid Acculink/Accunet Post-Approval Trial to Uncover Rare Events
CARASIL	Cerebral autosomal recessive arteriopathy with subcortical infarcts and leukoencephalopathy
CaRESS	Clopidogrel and Aspirin for Reduction of Emboli in Symptomatic Carotid Stenosis
CAS	Carotid angioplasty and stenting
CASANOVA	Carotid Artery Stenosis with Asymptomatic Narrowing: Operation versus Aspirin

CASES-PMS	Carotid Artery Stenting with Emboli Protection Surveillance-Post-Marketing Study
CBC	Complete blood count
CBF	Cerebral blood flow
CBV	Cerebral blood volume
CCA	Common carotid artery
CCF	Carotid cavernous fistula
CCM	Cerebral cavernous malformation
CCSVI	Chronic cerebrospinal venous insufficiency
CEA	Carotid endarterectomy
CI	Confidence interval
CK	Creatine kinase
CK-MB	Creatine kinase – MB isoenzyme (cardiac-specific CK)
CM	Cardiomyopathy; centimeter
CMS	Centers for Medicare and Medicaid Services
CN	Cranial nerve
CNS	Central nervous system
COSS	Carotid Occlusion Surgery Study
CPA	Cerebral proliferative angiopathy
CPAP	Continuous positive airway pressure
CPK	Creatine phosphokinase
CPP	Cerebral perfusion pressure
Cr	Creatinine
CREATE	Carotid Revascularization with ev3 Arterial Technology Evolution
CREST	Calcinosis, Raynauds phenomenon, esophageal dysmotility, sclerodactyly and telangiectasia; Carotid Revascularization, Endarterectomy versus Stenting Trial
CRH	Corticotropin releasing hormone
CRP	C-reactive protein
CRT	Cathode ray tube
CSC	Comprehensive stroke center
CSF	Cerebrospinal fluid
CSW	Cerebral salt wasting
CTA	CT angiography
CVP	Central venous pressure
CVT	Cerebral venous thrombosis
DAC	Distal access catheter
dAVF	Dural arteriovenous fistula
DMSO	Dimethy sulfoxide
DPD	Distal protection device
DSA	Digital subtraction angiography
DSPA	*Desmodus rotundus* salivary plasminogen activator
DVA	Developmental venous anomaly
DVT	Deep venous thrombosis
DWI	Diffusion weighted imaging
EBV	Epstein Barr Virus
EC-IC	Extracranial to intracranial
ECA	External carotid artery
ECST	European Carotid Surgery Trial
EDAMS	Encephalo-duro-arterio-myo-synangiosis
EDAS	Encephalo-duro-arterio-synangiosis
EDS	Ehlers-Danlos Syndrome
EEG	Electroencephalogram
EEL	External elastic lamina
EJ	External jugular vein
EKG	Electrocardiogram
EMG	Electromyography
EMS	Encephalo-myo-synagiosis
EPD	Embolic protection device
ESPS	European Stroke Prevention Study
ESR	Erythrocyte sedimentation rate
EVA-3S	Endarterectomy vs. Angioplasty in Patients with Symptomatic Severe Carotid Stenosis
EXACT	Emboshield and Xact Post Approval Carotid Stent Trial
F	French
FDA	Food and Drug Administration
FLAIR	Fluid attenuated inversion recovery

FMD	Fibromuscular dysplasia
fps	Frames per second
GCS	Glasgow coma scale
GESICA	Groupe d'Etude des Sténoses Intra-Crâniennes Athéromateuses symptomatiques
GIST-UK	United Kingdom Glucose Insulin in Stroke Trial
GP	Glycoprotein
Gy	Gray
HbF	Faetal haemoglobin
HbS	Haemoglobin S
HbSS	Haemoglobin S homozygosity
HDL	High density lipoprotein
HERS	Heart and Estrogen/Progestin Study
HIPAA	Health Insurance Portability and Accountability Act
HIT	Heparin-induced thrombocytopenia
HMG CoA	3-Hydroxy-3-methylglutaryl coenzyme A
HRT	Hormone replacement therapy
IA	Intra-arterial
ICA	Internal carotid artery
ICE	Intentional Cerebral Embolism
ICG	Indocyanine green
ICH	Intracerebral hemorrhage
ICP	Intracranial pressure
ICSS	International carotid Stenting Study
ICU	Intensive care unit
IEL	Internal elastic lamina
IEP	Intracranial embolization procedure
II	Image intensifier
IIH	Idiopathic intracranial hypertension
IJ	Internal jugular vein
IMA	Internal maxillary artery
IMT	Intima media thickness
INR	International Normalized Ratio
IPS	Inferior petrosal sinus
IPSS	Inferior petrosal sinus sampling
IRB	Institutional Review Board
ISAT	International Subarachnoid Aneurysm Trial
IV	Intravenous
IVH	Intraventricular hemorrhage
KSS	Kearns-Sayre syndrome
KTS	Klippel Trenaunay syndrome
LDL	Low density lipoprotein
LINAC	Linear accelerator (radiosurgery)
LMWH	Low molecular weight heparin
LOC	Level of consciousness; loss of consciousness
LV	Left ventricle
MAC	Mitral annular calcification
MACE	Major adverse cerebrovascular events
MATCH	Management of AtheroThrombosis with Clopidogrel in High-risk patients
MAVEriC	Medtronic AVE Self-Expanding Carotid Stent system with Distal Protection in the Treatment of Carotid Stenosis
MCA	Middle cerebral artery
MELAS	Mitochondrial encephalomyopathy, lactic acidosis, stroke-like episodes
MERFF	Myoclonic epilepsy and ragged red fibers
MI	Myocardial infarction
mm	Millimeter
MRA	Magnetic resonance angiography
MRI	Magnetic resonance imaging
mRS	Modified Rankin Score
MRV	Magnetic resonance venography
MTT	Mean transit time
MVP	Mitral valve prolapse; most valuable player
NA	Not available
NASCET	North American Symptomatic Carotid Endarterectomy Trial
n-BCA	N-butyl-2-cyanoacrylate
NBTE	Nonbacterial thrombotic endocarditis

NCRP	National Council on Radiation Protection and Measurements
NCS	Nerve conduction study
NEMC-PCR	New England medical Center Posterior Circulation Registry
Newt	Newton
NG	Nasogastric
NICU	Neurological intensive care unit
NIH-SS	National Institutes of Health Stroke Scale
NNH	Number needed to harm
NNT	Number needed to treat
NPH	Neutral Protamine Hagedorn insulin
NPO	Nil per os (no feeding)
NS	Not significant
NSAID	Nonsteroidal antiinflammatory drug
OA-MCA	Occipital artery to middle cerebral artery
OA-PCA	Occipital artery to posterior cerebral artery
OCP	Oral contraceptive
OEF	Oxygen extraction fraction
OSA	Obstructive sleep apnea
OTW	Over-the-wire
P-comm	Posterior communicating artery
PA	Postero-anterior
PAC	Partial anterior circulation stroke
PAN	Polyarteritis nodosa
PASCAL	Performance And Safety of the Medtronic AVE Self-Expandable Stent in the treatment of Carotid Artery Lesions
PCA	Posterior cerebral artery
PCR	Polymerase chain reaction
PCWP	Pulmonary capillary wedge pressure
PCXR	Portable chest x-ray
PEEP	Positive end-expiratory pressure
PFO	Patent foramen ovale
PICA	Posterior inferior cerebellar artery
PKD	Polycystic kidney disease
PNS	Peripheral nervous system
POC	Posterior circulation stroke
PPRF	Paramedian pontine reticular formation
Pro-UK	Prourokinase
PROACT	Prolyse in Acute Cerebral Thromboembolism
PSA	Posterolateral spinal arteries
PSV	Peak systolic velocity
PT	Prothrombin time
PTA	Percutaneous transluminal angioplasty
PTE	Pulmonary thromboembolism
PTT	Partial thromboplastin time
PVA	Polyvinyl alcohol
RA	Rheumatoid arthritis
rem	roentgen-equivalent-man
RHV	Rotating hemostatic valve (aka Y-adapter, aka Touey-Borst Valve)
RIND	Reversible ischemic neurological deficit
RPR	Rapid plasma reagin
RR	Risk reduction
RRR	Relative risk reduction
RVAS	Rotational vertebral artery syndrome
RX	Rapid exchange
SAMMPRIS	Stenting vs. Aggressive Medical Management for Preventing Recurrent Stroke in Intracranial Stenosis
SAPPHIRE	Stenting and Angioplasty with Protection in Patients at High Risk for Endarterectomy
SBP	Systolic blood pressure
SCA	Superior cerebellar artery
SCD	Sickle cell disease
SCIWORA	Spinal cord injury without radiographic abnormality
SDH	Subdural haematoma
SECURITY	Study to Evaluate the Neuroshield Bare Wire Cerebral Protection System and XAct Stent in Patients at High Risk for Endarterectomy
SIADH	Syndrome of inappropriate antidiuretic hormone secretion
SIM	Simmons catheter

Abbreviations

SIR	Society of Interventional Radiology
SLE	Systemic lupus erythematosis
SOV	Superior ophthalmic vein
SPACE	Stent-Protected Percutaneous Angioplasty of the Carotid versus Endarterectomy
SPARCL	Stroke Prevention by Aggressive Reduction in Cholesterol Levels
SPECT	Single photon emission computed tomography
SSS	Superior sagittal sinus
SSYLVIA	Stenting of Symptomatic Atherosclerotic Lesions in the Vertebral or Intracranial Arteries
STA	Superficial temporal artery
STA-MCA	Superficial temporal artery to middle cerebral artery
TAC	Total anterior circulation stroke
TASS	Ticlopidine Aspirin Stroke Study
TCD	Transcranial doppler ultrasonography
TEE	Transesophageal echocardiography
TGA	Transient global amnesia
TIA	Transient ischemic attack
TOAST	Trial of ORG 10172 in Acute Stroke Treatment
tPA	Tissue plasminogen activator
TTE	Transthoracic echocardiography
TTP	Time to peak; thrombotic thrombocytopenic purpura
U	Unit
UOP	Urinary output
USA	United States of America
VACS	Veterans Affairs Cooperative Study on Symptomatic Stenosis
VAST	Vertebral Artery Stenting Trial
VBI	Vertebrobasilar insufficiency
VDRL	Venereal Disease Research Laboratory
VERiTAS	Vertebrobasilar Flow Evaluation and Risk of Transient Ischemic Attack and Stroke.
VERT	Vertebral
VIVA	ViVEXX Carotid Revascularization Trial
VOGM	Vein of Galen malformation
VZV	Varicella zoster virus
WASID	Warfarin versus Aspirin for Symptomatic Intracranial Disease
WEST	Women Estrogen Stroke Trial
WHI	Women's Health Initiative

Introduction

To the astonishment of the authors of this handbook, the publisher agreed to a second edition. This edition permits the authors to correct many of the embarrassing *gaffes* (a.k.a. *howlers, screamers, booboos*) that saturated the first edition. More importantly, however, this edition allows for a much-needed update, as the fields of cerebrovascular disease and neurointervention are evolving at a dizzying pace. Many of the landmark trials that we based clinical decision making on in the past have been superseded by more recent, better-done studies. Wonderful new devices are coming on the market at breakneck speed; for instance, the authors learned about several important new devices currently available only days before the manuscript for this edition was delivered to the publisher. Also, this edition allowed the authors to broaden the scope of the handbook to be more relevant to an international audience. The field of neurointervention is global and has always been; this edition of the handbook is meant to reflect that more than before.

Neurointervention has evolved into a rarified and complex field, with a set of techniques and a knowledge base that are distinct from other fields within medicine. At the same time, clinicians from an assortment of disciplines have come to practice neurointerventional radiology, with backgrounds ranging from radiology to neurosurgery, neurology, cardiology, and vascular surgery. Presently, there are more people training to become neurointerventionalists than there ever have been before in history. These developments have resulted in a need for a practical, unified handbook of techniques and essential literature. This purpose of this handbook is to serve as a practical guide to endovascular methods and as a reference work for neurovascular anatomy and published data about cerebrovascular disease from a neurointerventionalist's perspective.

We attempted to enhance the accessibility and ease use of this handbook by arranging it in a semi-outline format. Dense narrative passages have been avoided wherever possible (who has time to read long, thick chapters, anyway?). In that spirit, the rest of this Introduction will be presented in the style of this book....

1. This book is divided into three parts.
   a. Fundamentals
      i. Essential neurovascular anatomy and basic angiographic techniques provide the foundation of the first section.
         1. The focus of Chapter 1 remains on vascular anatomy that is pertinent to day to day clinical practice. Embryology and discussions of angiographic shift, which is less pertinent these days because of widely available noninvasive intracranial imaging, are left out. Discussions of anatomic variants include both normal variants and anomalies.
            a. New for the second edition are some Angio-Anatomic Correlates that illustrate anatomic structures with angiographic pictures.
         2. Chapters 2 and 3 cover diagnostic angiographic techniques.
         3. New for the second edition, Chapter 4 is an introduction to basic interventional access techniques and has a special appendix on the Neurointerventional Suite, primarily intended for newcomers to the angio suite and for experienced interventionalists planning a new suite.
   b. Techniques
      i. Endovascular methods, device information, and tips and tricks are detailed.
         1. The second edition is packed with new information on evolving technology.
   c. Specific disease states
      i. Essential, useful information about each commonly encountered condition is presented.
         1. Significant clinical studies are summarized and placed into context.
         2. Interesting and novel facts (and "factlets") are included here and there.

ii. The term "systematic review" is used to refer to useful publications that have analyzed published clinical data in an organized way. The term "meta-analysis" is avoided because it refers to a specific statistical technique that is not always present in review articles purporting to be a meta-analysis.

iii. For readers with extra time on their hands, A Brief History of... sections describe the background and evolution of various techniques.

2. Core philosophy. Within the practical information contained within this book, we hope to impart our underlying patient-oriented clinical philosophy. In our view, each patient's welfare is paramount. The clinical outcome of each case takes priority over "pushing the envelope" by trying out new devices or techniques, generating material for the next clinical series or case report, or satisfying the device company representatives standing in the control room. In practical terms, clinical decision-making should be based on sound judgment and the best available clinical data. Moreover, new medical technology and drugs should be used *within reason*, and whenever possible, based on established principles of sound practice. Thus, while we have the technology and the ability to coil aneurysms in very old patients with Hunt Hess V subarachnoid hemorrhage, embolize asymptomatic and low-risk dural AV fistulas, and perform carotid angioplasty and stenting in patients with asymptomatic stenosis, we should recognize the value of conservative management when it is called for. We hope that this cautious and common sensical outlook is reflected throughout this book.

3. Cookbook presentation. We have made every attempt to present procedures in a plainly written, how-to-do-it format. Although some readers may take issue with the reduction of a field as complex as neurointervention to a relatively simplistic how-to manual, we feel that structure and standardization of technique can only serve to benefit the field in the long run. For comparison, consider commercial air travel in the present era. Air travel fatalities are extremely rare, due to pilot training, standardization of flying techniques and meticulous aircraft maintenance. Even the most skilled and careful neurointerventionalists cannot hold a candle to the stellar safety record obtained by the airline industry.

4. Conventions used in this book:
   a. Terminology can be confusing. The authors have adopted the most current and commonly used terms; synonymous terms are listed in parentheses after "aka," for *also known as*.
   b. We have limited the use of abbreviations to those commonly used in everyday conversation, such as "ICA" and "MCA." Excessive use of abbreviations, particularly for uncommon terms, can clutter the text and make it difficult to read.
   c. The terms, *see below* and *see above*, are used to indicate other material within the same chapter.

5. Overlap and redundancy. Discussion some topics may appear to be repetitive and redundant; for instance, guide catheters are discussed in Chapters 4, 5 and 7. This is intentional, as we hoped to avoid frequent cross-referencing between sections of the book, which can be annoying for a busy reader looking for quick advice. In addition, some overlap can actually be beneficial, as some topics can be discussed from different perspectives. For example, the evaluation of a stroke patient in the emergency room is discussed in Chapter 9 from the perspective of an interventionalist seeing a patient with a firm diagnosis of acute ischemic stroke, whereas a discussion of the same topic appears in Chapter 17 from the perspective of the "Code Stroke" team answering a call from the ER. There was some paring down of redundancy compared to the first edition, to create space for new content.

6. *Also new for the second edition*:
   a. Global Gems that illuminate aspects of the field outside the United States.
   b. Angio-anatomic Correlates (and a few Angio-pathologic Correlates) are special figures that have angiographic images illustrating a particularly interesting point.
   c. Newly released study results that will influence neurointerventional practice.
   d. Information on emerging technologies in this rapidly advancing field.
   e. Fewer typographical errors than the first edition.
   f. Astute readers will also find many new pearls of wisdom and a few sparks of levity.

7. Medicolegal disclaimer. This book is meant to serve as a guide to the use of a wide variety of medical devices and drugs. However, the authors and the publisher cannot be held responsible for the use of these devices and drugs by readers, or for failure by the readers of this book to follow specific manufacturer specifications and FDA guidelines.

Contents

Part 1. Fundamentals

1. Essential Neurovascular Anatomy

1.1.   Aortic Arch and Great Vessels

Aortic arch anatomy is pertinent to neuroangiography because variations of arch anatomy can affect access to the cervicocranial circulation:

1) Branches
   a) Innominate (aka brachiocephalic) artery
   b) Left common carotid artery
   c) Left subclavian artery
2) Variants (Fig. 1.1):
   a) Bovine arch (Figs. 1.1b and 1.2). The innominate artery and left common carotid artery (CCA) share a common origin (up to 27% of cases), or the left CCA arises from the innominate artery (7% of cases).[1] The bovine variant is more common in blacks (10–25%) than whites (5–8%).[2]
   b) Aberrant right subclavian artery. The right subclavian artery arises from the left aortic arch, distal to the origin of the left subclavian artery. It usually passes posterior to the esophagus on its way to the right upper extremity. This is the most common congenital arch anomaly; incidence: 0.4 – 2.0%.[3] It is associated with Down syndrome.
   c) Origin of the left vertebral artery from the arch is seen in 0.5% of cases.[1]

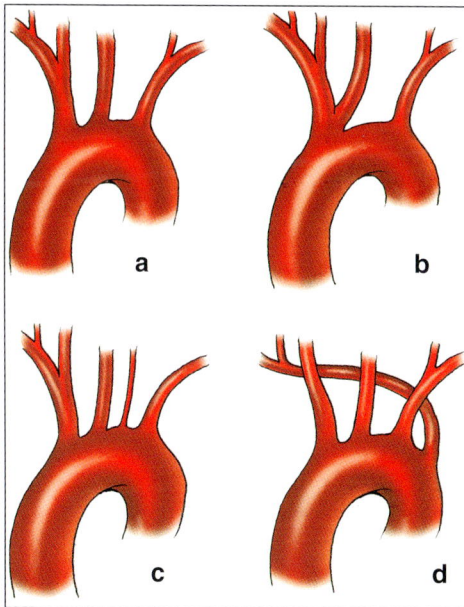

Fig. 1.1 Common aortic arch configurations. *Clockwise from upper left*: (**a**) Normal arch; (**b**) bovine arch; (**c**) aberrant right subclavian artery, and (**d**) origin of the left vertebral artery from the arch.

M.R. Harrigan, J.P. Deveikis, *Handbook of Cerebrovascular Disease and Neurointerventional Technique*, DOI 10.1007/978-1-61779-946-4_1, © Springer Science+Business Media New York 2013

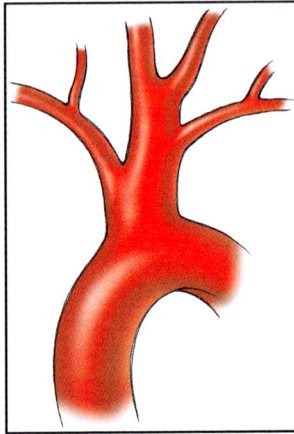

Fig. 1.2 What exactly is a "bovine arch?" Drawing of an arch from a cow. In cattle, a single great vessel originates from the aortic arch[286]. Presumably, the long brachiocephalic artery is due to the relatively long distance from the aorta to the thoracic inlet in cattle. Because humans do not have a true "bovine arch," Layton and colleagues proposed that the more precise term, "Common-Origin-of-the-Innominate-Artery-and-Left-Common-Carotid-Artery" and "Origin-of-the-Left-Common-Carotid-Artery-from-the-Innominate-Artery" supplant the term bovine arch[287]. This is akin to proposing that the universally understood term, "p-comm aneurysm" be replaced by the more accurate "aneurysm-arising-from-the-internal-carotid-artery-adjacent-to-the-origin-of-the-posterior-communicating-artery." The authors of this handbook will continue to use the well understood but anatomically imprecise terms, bovine arch and p-comm aneurysm.

    d) Less common variants (Fig. 1.3). Some of these rare anomalies can lead to formation of a vascular ring in which the trachea and esophagus are encircled by connecting segments of the aortic arch and its branches.
3) Effects of aging and atherosclerosis on the aortic arch and great vessels. The aortic arch and great vessels become elongated and tortuous with age (Fig. 1.4); this can have practical implications for neurointervention in the elderly, as a tortuous vessel can be difficult to negotiate with wires and catheters. Although atherosclerosis has been implicated in the etiology of this phenomenon, more recent data suggest that the cervical internal carotid artery (ICA) may undergo *metaplastic transformation*, in which elastic and muscular tissue in the artery wall is replaced by loose connective tissue.[4]

The most common subclavian artery configuration is shown in Fig. 1.5. Major branches are:
- Vertebral artery
- Thyrocervical trunk
  - Inferior thyroid artery
  - Ascending cervical artery (most commonly a branch of transverse cervical)
  - Transverse cervical artery
  - Suprascapular artery
- Costocervical trunk
  - Deep cervical artery
  - Superior or supreme intercostal artery
- Dorsal scapular artery (may also arise from transverse cervical)[5]
- Internal thoracic (mammary) artery

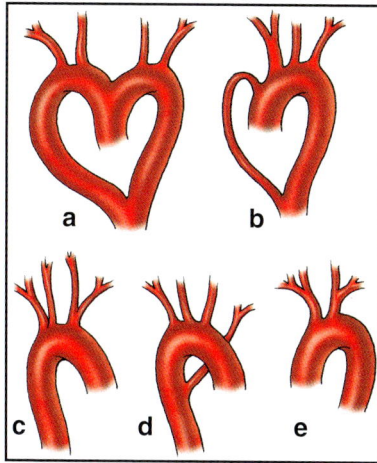

Fig. 1.3 Selected aortic arch anomalies. (**a**) Double aortic arch. The arches encircle the trachea and esophagus to form the descending aorta, which is usually on the *left*. The *right arch* is larger than the *left* in up to 75% of cases[1]. (**b**) Double aortic arch with left arch atresia. (**c**) Right aortic arch with a mirror configuration. The descending aorta is on the *right side* of the heart. This anomaly does not form a vascular ring, but is associated with other anomalies such as tetralogy of Fallot[1]. (**d**) Right aortic arch with a nonmirror configuration and an aberrant left subclavian artery. The descending aorta is on the *right side* of the heart, and the left subclavian artery arises from the proximal aorta. A common cause of a symptomatic vascular ring[288]. (**e**) Bi-innominate artery.

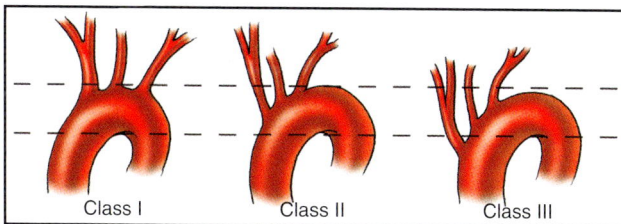

Fig. 1.4 Aortic arch elongation classification scheme.

1.2. Common Carotid Arteries

The CCAs travel within the carotid sheath, which also contains the internal jugular vein and the vagus nerve. The right CCA is usually shorter than the left. The CCAs typically bifurcate at the C3 or C4 level (upper border of the thyroid cartilage), although the bifurcation may be located anywhere between T2 and C2.[6] The CCAs do not usually have branches, although anomalous branches can include the superior thyroid, ascending pharyngeal, or occipital arteries.[1]

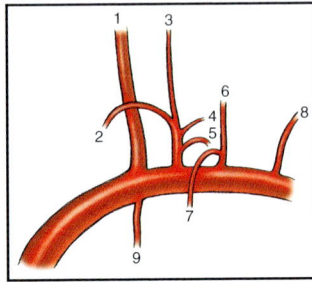

Fig. 1.5 Subclavian artery. (*1*) Vertebral artery; (*2*) inferior thyroid artery; (*3*) ascending cervical artery; (*4*) transverse cervical artery; (*5*) Suprascapular artery; (*6*) deep cervical artery; (*7*) supreme intercostal artery; (*8*) dorsal scapular artery; (*9*) internal mammary artery.

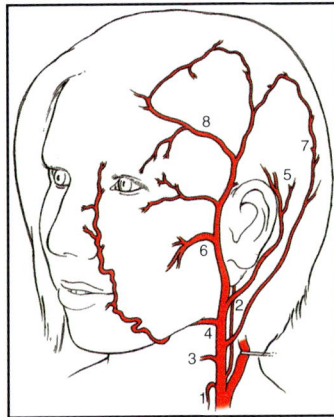

Fig. 1.6 External carotid artery. (*1*) Superior thyroid artery; (*2*) ascending pharyngeal artery; (*3*) lingual artery; (*4*) facial artery; (*5*) posterior auricular artery; (*6*) internal maxillary artery; (*7*) occipital artery; (*8*) superficial temporal artery.

1.3.   External Carotid Artery

The external carotid artery (ECA) originates at the common carotid bifurcation. From its origin, the ECA usually curves forward medial to the internal carotid, then immediately begins a cephalad ascent, curving laterally and slightly posteriorly until it ends behind the mandible in its terminal bifurcation into the internal maxillary and superficial temporal arteries.[7] Thus, on a frontal radiographic view, the external carotid begins medially and swings cephalad and laterally, and on a lateral view it begins anteriorly and then ascends, angling slightly posteriorly.

Mnemonic for the external carotid Branches
After reading this book . . .
Some **A**ngry **L**inguists **F**ind **O**ur **P**aragraphs **S**omewhat **I**rritating
    Superior thyroid
    Ascending pharyngeal
    Lingual
    Facial
    Occipital
    Posterior auricular
    Superficial temporal
    Internal maxillary
More amusing and off-color mnemonics are available to assist the novice in remembering these branches. If the readers' imaginations fail them, the authors would be more than happy to supply additional memory aids for this purpose.

1. Branches
   There are eight major branches of the ECA (Fig. 1.6). Commonly, the branches are listed in order by their point of origin from proximal to distal.[1]
   1. Superior thyroid artery
   2. Ascending pharyngeal artery
   3. Lingual artery
   4. Facial artery
   5. Occipital artery
   6. Posterior auricular artery
   7. Superficial temporal artery
   8. Internal maxillary artery

   Occasionally, these branches arise from the ECA trunk. The ventral group arises anteriorly from the ECA and the dorsal group of branches arises posteriorly from the ECA. Therefore, grouping the ECA branches based on their ventral or dorsal axis is more useful and more consistent.
   Ventral external carotid branches:
   - Superior thyroid artery
   - Lingual artery
   - Facial artery
   - Internal maxillary artery

   Dorsal external carotid branches
   - Ascending pharyngeal artery
   - Occipital artery
   - Posterior auricular artery
   - Superficial temporal artery

2. Territories
   The ECA supplies much of the soft tissue and bony structures of the head and face, the deep structures of the upper aero-digestive tract, and much of the dura of the intracranial compartment. Numerous anastamoses are present between ECA branches and the branches of the internal carotid and vertebral arteries. These anastamoses provide collateral flow to the vascular territories distal to a proximal occlusion. Anastamoses to carotid or vertebral arteries can also be considered "dangerous anastamoses" when attempting to embolize vascular lesions in the head and neck via external carotid branches. See below for discussion of individual ECA branch anastamoses and Tables 1.1, 1.2, 1.3, and 1.4.

3. Variants:
   (a) The most frequent branching pattern seen at the common carotid bifurcation (in 48.5%) is the external carotid arises anteromedially while the internal carotid arises posterolaterally. The most frequent branching pattern seen at the common carotid bifurcation finds the external carotid arising anteromedially. Occasionally, the ECA arises posterolaterally or directly laterally.[8,9]
   (b) The ECA and ICA may rarely arise as separate branches of the aortic arch.[7,10]
   (c) Some ECA branches, especially the superior thyroid artery, may arise from the CCA.
   (d) Some branches (especially the ascending pharyngeal or occipital arteries) may originate from the ICA.
   (e) A common origin of superior thyroid, occipital, and ascending pharyngeal arteries from the ICA has been reported.[11]

Table 1.1 Anastamoses to anterior circulation

Anastamosis from	Anastamosis to	Comments/reference
Ascending pharyngeal, neuromeningeal trunk	Cavernous carotid via meningohypophyseal trunk	19
Ascending pharyngeal, inferior tympanic branch	Petrous carotid via caroticotympanic	19
Ascending pharyngeal, superior pharyngeal	Cavernous carotid via inferolateral trunk	19
Ascending pharyngeal, superior pharyngeal	Petrous carotid via mandibular branch	19
Accessory meningeal (cavernous branch)	Cavernous carotid via inferolateral trunk, posterior branch	19
Middle meningeal (cavernous branch)	Cavernous carotid via inferolateral trunk, posterior branch	19
Middle meningeal (cavernous branch)	Cavernous carotid via meningohypophyseal trunk	19
Distal internal maxillary (artery of foramen rotundum)	Cavernous carotid via inferolateral trunk, anterolateral branch	19

Table 1.2 Common anastamoses to ophthalmic artery

Anastamosis from	Anastamosis to	Reference
Middle meningeal, sphenoidal branch	Ophthalmic	19
Middle meningeal, frontal branch	Ophthalmic via anterior falx artery	19
Inferolateral trunk, anteromedial branch	Ophthalmic	19
Distal internal maxillary, anterior deep temporal	Ophthalmic	19
Distal internal maxillary, infraorbital	Ophthalmic	19
Distal internal maxillary, sphenopalatine	Ophthalmic via ethmoidal branches	19
Distal facial	Ophthalmic	19
Transverse facial	Ophthalmic	19
Superficial temporal, frontal branch	Ophthalmic	19
Cavernous carotid, inferolateral trunk	Ophthalmic via recurrent meningeal branch	19

Table 1.3 Common anastamoses to posterior circulation

Anastamosis from	Anastamosis to	Comments/reference
Ascending cervical	Vertebral segmental branches	19
Deep cervical	Vertebral segmental branches	19
Occipital, muscular branches	Vertebral segmental branches	19
Ascending pharyngeal, muscular branches	Vertebral segmental branches	19
Ascending pharyngeal, neuromeningeal trunk	C3 segmental vertebral via odontoid arch	Odontoid arch connects side-to-side[19]

Table 1.4 More trouble: cranial nerve blood supply

Cranial nerve	Arterial supply	References
I: Olfactory	Anterior cerebral	19
II: Optic	Supraclinoid carotid, ophthalmic	19
III: Oculomotor	Basilar, superior cerebellar, posterior cerebral, inferolateral trunk, ophthalmic	19,73
IV: Trochlear	Inferolateral trunk, meningohypophyseal trunk	19,73
V: Trigeminal	Inferolateral trunk, meningohypophyseal trunk, middle meningeal, accessory meningeal, artery of foramen rotundum, infraorbital	19,73
VI: Abducens	Inferolateral trunk, meningohypophyseal trunk, middle meningeal, accessory meningeal, ascending pharyngeal (jugular branch)	19,24,73
VII: Facial	Stylomastoid (from post auricular or occipital), middle meningeal (petrous branch), ascending pharyngeal (inferior tympanic and odontoid arcade)	19,74
VIII: Auditory	Basilar, AICA, ascending pharyngeal jugular branch	19,75
IX: Glossopharyngeal	Ascending pharyngeal jugular branch	19,24
X: Vagus	Ascending pharyngeal jugular branch, superior and inferior thyroid, laryngeal branches	19,24
XI: Spinal Accessory	Ascending pharyngeal (jugular, inferior tympanic and musculospinal branches)	19,24
XII: Hypoglossal	Ascending pharyngeal, hypoglossal branch and proximal trunk, occipital, directly from external carotid, lingual	19,76

(f) Rarely, all external carotid branches may arise from the ICA.[12]
(g) External carotid branches may arise as common trunks with other branches including: linguofacial trunk (20% of cases), thyrolingual trunk (2.5% of cases), thyrolinguofacial trunk (2.5% of cases), and occipitoauricular trunk (12.5% of cases).[13]
(h) Persistent stapedial artery,[14] or, for the anatomic purist, the persistent hyoido-stapedial artery,[15] arises from the petrous ICA, passes through the middle ear, and forms the middle meningeal. The prevalence of persistent stapedial arteries in 1,000 temporal bones was 0.48%.[16] This anomaly can be associated with the so-called *aberrant course of the ICA in the middle ear*, which probably really represents a collateral pathway involving the inferior tympanic branch of the ascending pharyngeal artery bypassing a segmental agenesis of the true ICA.[17,18]

Superior Thyroid Artery

Whether it arises above or below the common carotid bifurcation, the superior thyroid artery originates from the anterior surface of the parent artery and immediately turns caudally to supply the anterior soft tissue structures of the neck.
1. Branches
   (a) Infrahyoid artery
   The infrahyoid (hyoid) artery travels medially from its origin, and then follows along the lower hyoid bone. It can anastamose with the submental artery, providing a collateral pathway to the facial artery.[19]
   (b) Superior laryngeal artery
   The superior laryngeal artery travels alongside the internal laryngeal nerve inferomedially from its origin and pierces the thyrohyoid membrane to supply the mucosa of the larynx superior to the vocal cords and taste buds of the epiglottis.[20]
      i. Branches
      The superior thyroid artery has two major branches and a small epiglottic branch. Its ventral branch anastomoses with the both the cricothyroid artery and superior laryngeal arcade. The dorsal branch anastamoses with the longitudinal laryngeal arcade.[19]

    ii. Territory
        The superior laryngeal artery supplies the pharyngeal and laryn-geal structures as well as the internal laryngeal nerve. It anasta-moses with its contralateral partner and with the inferior laryngeal artery from the inferior thyroid artery.
    iii. Variants
       – May arise as a separate branch from the ECA or ascending pharyngeal artery.[19]
       – In 6 of 22 anatomic specimens, the superior laryngeal artery does not pierce the thyrohyoid membrane but instead passes through a foramen in the thyroid cartilage to supply the soft tissues of the larynx.[21]
  (c) Sternocleidomastoid artery
     The sternocleidomastoid artery feeds the middle part of the sternocleido-mastoid muscle. It anastamoses superiorly with the muscular branches of the occipital and posterior auricular and inferiorly with the thyrocervi-cal trunk and suprascapular. It can also connect with the glandular branches of the superior thyroid artery.
  (d) Cricothyroid artery
     Anastamoses with the superior laryngeal artery and feeds the upper trachea.
  (e) Glandular branches
     These are a continuation of the superior thyroid trunk with superior, medial and lateral arcades to supply the thyroid gland. They freely anas-tamose with their contralateral counterparts.
2. Territories
  (a) The superior thyroid artery supplies the majority of the blood to the lar-ynx, its associated musculature, and the upper pole of the thyroid gland.[7] In a minority of cases the superior thyroid provides blood flow to the parathyroid glands.[22] The superior laryngeal branch accompanies and can supply the internal laryngeal nerve. The superior thyroid branches freely anastamose with their contralateral counterparts and the inferior thyroid artery (from the thyrocervical trunk).
3. Variants
  (a) The superior thyroid artery arises from the ECA in 46% of cases and more commonly, from the CCA in 52% of cases.[23]
  (b) The superior thyroid artery may arise in a common trunk with the lin-gual as a thyrolingual trunk.
  (c) Rarely, the superior thyroid artery may arise from the ICA.[11]

Ascending Pharyngeal Artery

    The ascending pharyngeal artery is a thin, slender branch that arises from the very proximal posterior aspect of the ECA or in the crotch of the CCA (Fig. 1.7). It travels cephalad parallel to the ICA. Its termination in the superior pharynx creates a forward and medial right angle turn.
1. Branches
  (a) Inferior pharyngeal artery
     A relatively small vessel arising from the proximal ascending pharyn-geal, the inferior pharyngeal travels anteriorly in a zigzag fashion. It sup-plies the pharyngeal muscles and mucosa. It anastamoses with its contralateral counterpart.
  (b) Musculospinal artery
     The vessel may arise from the ascending pharyngeal itself or from the neuromeningeal trunk. It extends posteriorly and superiorly for a short distance before curving inferiorly. It primarily supplies muscles, but also may supply the ipsilateral upper spinal nerve roots, the eleventh cranial nerve, and superior sympathetic ganglion. In addition, it may anasta-mose with the ascending and deep cervical and vertebral arteries.[19,24]
  (c) Neuromeningeal trunk
     This is a major branch of the ascending pharyngeal artery that continues cephalad but angles gently to the posterior. It has several important branches that pass through foramina in the skull base.

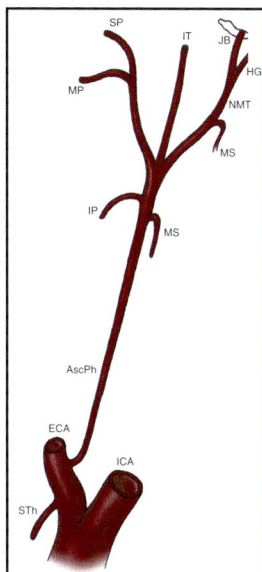

Fig. 1.7 Ascending pharyngeal artery. A common branching pattern of the ascending pharyngeal artery is shown. Note internal carotid (*ICA*), external carotid (*ECA*), superior thyroid (*STh*), ascending pharyngeal (*AscPh*), inferior pharyngeal (*IP*), middle pharyngeal (*MP*), superior pharyngeal (*SP*), inferior tympanic (*IT*), musculospinal branches (*MS*), neuromeningeal trunk (*NMT*), jugular branch (*JB*) entering the jugular foramen, hypoglossal branch (*HG*) entering the hypoglossal foramen, and prevertebral (not shown).

(i) Branches
  – *Musculospinal artery*
    This branch may variably arise from the neuromeningeal trunk instead of originating from the ascending pharyngeal artery.
  – *Jugular artery*
    Often the largest branch of the neuromeningeal trunk, this vessel heads straight cephalad to the jugular foramen. It supplies the ninth through the eleventh cranial nerves and their ganglia. A medial branch ascends on the clivus to supply the eleventh cranial nerve. Its lateral branch travels along the dura around the sigmoid sinus. It can be a major contributor to the dura of the posterior fossa. Anastamoses with the lateral clival branch of the meningohypohyseal trunk and dural branches of the vertebral artery are possible.[19]
  – *Hypoglossal artery*
    This branch enters the hypoglossal canal and supplies the twelfth cranial nerve. It also supplies the dura in the posterior cranial fossa and anastamoses with the jugular branch, medial clival branches of the meningohypophyseal trunk, the contralateral hypoglossal artery, and the odontoid arcade.[19,25]
  – *Prevertebral artery*
    It often arises from the neuromeningeal trunk and contributes to the odontoid arcade. It anastamoses with its

contralateral counterpart, the anterior meningeal branch of the vertebral and hypoglossal artery branches.[25]

    ii. Territories

The very important neuromeningeal trunk of the ascending pharyngeal artery supplies cranial nerves VI, IX, X, XI, and XII, and potentially collateralizes to the upper three spinal nerves and the superior sympathetic ganglion. Its meningeal territory includes a large portion of the posterior fossa meninges. Anastamotic channels exist to its contralateral counterpart and meningeal branches of the vertebral artery and the meningohypophyseal trunk.[24]

    iii. Variants

All branches of the neuromeningeal trunk are in vascular equilibrium with each other and with their anastamotic connecting vessels. Hypoplasia or absence of one or more vessels is accompanied by hypertrophy of the existing branches.

(d) Prevertebral artery

Occasionally, this artery arises directly from the ascending pharyngeal artery and contributes to the odontoid arcade.[25]

(e) Inferior tympanic artery

    i. Branches

There are three common branches of the inferior tympanic artery.[19]
- Ascending branch connects to petrosal branch of middle meningeal artery
- Anterior branch connects to the caroticotympanic branch
- Posterior branch connects to the stylomastoid artery, a branch of the posterior auricular artery

    ii. Territories

Supplies the middle ear cavity and associated nerves, including the twelfth nerve and tympanic branch of the ninth cranial nerve (aka *Jacobson's nerve*).

    iii. Variants

May arise from the neuromeningeal branch, the ascending pharyngeal artery, or it may appear as a trifurcation with the inferior tympanic artery arising in between neuromeningeal and pharyngeal divisions.[19]

(f) Middle pharyngeal artery

    i. Branches

No named branches.

    ii. Territories

Supplies mucosa and muscles of the naso- and oropharynx as well as the soft palate.[26] Anastamoses with contralateral middle pharyngeal artery, ipsilateral ascending palatine artery, greater palatine artery, and branches of the accessory meningeal artery.

    iii. Variants

May arise from ascending pharyngeal artery proximal or occasionally distal to the origin of neuromeningeal trunk.

(g) Superior pharyngeal artery

As the most cephalad anterior branch of the ascending pharyngeal artery, this tends to be a small vessel. The pharyngeal branches take an abrupt anterior and medial angulation from the vertical ascending pharyngeal artery.

    i. Branches

There are several common branches of the superior pharyngeal artery, but only one is named.
- The carotid branch actually traverses the cartilage filling the foramen lacerum and connects to the cavernous ICA via the inferolateral trunk.
- Anterior unnamed branches to the upper nasopharynx and adjacent tissues.

    ii. Territories

Supplies upper nasopharynx including the orifice of the Eustachian tube as well as associated muscles, including superior constrictor. Has many potential anastamoses, including accessory meningeal, pterygovaginal, and contralateral superior pharyngeal. If a Vidian branch is present, this is a potentially dangerous anastamosis during embolization procedures and it may also contribute to cavernous carotid fistulas via the petrous ICA.

iii. Variants

Pharyngeal territories of the superior pharyngeal artery may be primarily supplied by the accessory meningeal artery, Vidian artery, and other nasopharyngeal feeders.

2. Territories

Ascending pharyngeal artery supplies the mucosa and adjacent muscles of the pharynx, soft palate, odontoid process, bones, and muscles and nerve roots at C1 and C2. It also supplies the lower cranial nerves (IX–XII and potentially VI and VII); lower clivus and medial skull base; meninges of the posterior fossa; portions of the middle cranial fossa; and the middle ear. The ascending pharyngeal artery has extensive anastamoses with its contralateral counterpart, the occipital, middle and accessory meningeal and distal internal maxillary arteries. Moreover, it has particularly dangerous anastamoses with the internal carotid and vertebral arteries.[24] This is a *very busy little artery*.

Angio-Anatomic Correlate! Ascending Pharyngeal Artery Collaterals
(Fig. 1.8)

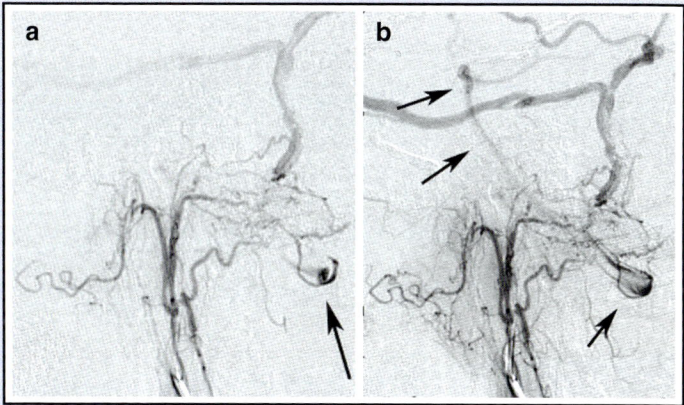

Fig. 1.8 Lateral view selective injections of the ascending pharyngeal artery in a patient with a dural arteriovenous fistula. Early arterial phase (**a**) starts to show faint anastamotic filling of the vertebral artery at the C1 level (*arrow*). Later arterial phase (**b**) shows considerable filling of the vertebral and basilar arteries (*arrows*).

3. Variants
   (a) The ascending pharyngeal artery may arise from the ICA.
   (b) Often arises as a common trunk with the occipital artery.
   (c) Ascending cervical artery may supply the territory of the ascending pharyngeal artery.[19]
   (d) Can contribute to the persistent hypoglossal artery variant.
   (e) Can reconstitute an occluded or aplastic vertebral artery.
   (f) The so-called "aberrant ICA" in the middle ear cavity is probably more appropriately termed the *ascending pharyngeal artery*, providing a collateral pathway for the territory of a segmentally occluded ICA.[17,18]

Lingual Artery

Arises from the ventral aspect of the external carotid and takes a gentle anterior-inferior path creating a characteristic "U" shaped curve on both frontal and lateral angiographic projections. It then curves upward, as the dorsal lingual branch forms an arc through the tongue with an arcade of radiating branches.

1. Branches
   - (a) Suprahyoid artery
     This small branch runs along the superior aspect of the hyoid bone and anastamoses with the contralateral suprahyoid artery.[7]
   - (b) Dorsal lingual artery
     May consist of two or three upwardly arching branches that curve up over the tongue – forming radiating branches that follow the pattern of the radiating intrinsic lingual muscle. The dorsal lingual artery anastamoses with its contralateral counterpart.[7]
   - (c) Sublingual artery
     This branch angles anteriorly to supply the sublingual gland and floor of the mouth. It anastamoses with the submental branch of the facial artery and with its contralateral counterpart. A small branch pierces the lingual foramen of the mandible and supplies the adjacent bone.[7]
   - (d) Deep lingual artery
     This is a small terminal branch to the frenulum of the tongue.[7]
2. Territories
   The lingual artery provides generous arterial supply to the tongue and floor of the mouth. There are anastamoses with the contralateral lingual and ipsilateral facial arteries via the submental branch. However, remember that branches extending to the tip of the tongue are effectively *end arteries*. Distal embolization with small particles or liquid agents can produce ischemic necrosis of the tip of the tongue, especially if the emboli are forced across the midline via the side-to-side anastamosis, or if bilateral embolization is intentionally done.
3. Variants
   - (a) The lingual artery often arises with the facial artery from a common facial-lingual trunk (20% of cases).[13]
   - (b) Occasionally, can arise with the superior thyroid artery as a common thyrolingual trunk (2.5% of cases), or thyrolinguofacial trunk (2.5% of cases).[13]
   - (c) It rarely arises from the CCA.
   - (d) The lingual artery can supply variable amounts of the submental artery's supply to the floor of the mouth.

Facial Artery

The facial artery is usually one of the larger ECA branches and arises from the anterior aspect of the ECA. It then curves in a slightly redundant fashion through the submandibular gland, under and around the angle of the mandible, and then angles forward and cephalad, as well as medially to extend up along the angle of the nose as the angular artery. The facial artery has a number of named and unnamed branches that anastamose freely from one to the other and with other vessels in the face (Fig. 1.9).

1) Branches
   - a) Ascending palatine artery
     - i) This artery ascends for a few centimeters from its origin, and then takes a right angle forward to the soft palate by making a small loop-de-loop as it curves around the tonsils. Consequently, the ascending palatine artery can be a casualty of tonsillectomy or palatal surgery,[26] and, along with the smaller tonsillar arteries, a source of post-op bleeding.
       - (1) Branches
         - (a) A cadaver study of palatine blood supply found three fairly constant and several less constant branches.[27]
           - (i) *Glossal branch*. Arises at the level of the upper border of the tongue and supplies the palato-glossus muscle.

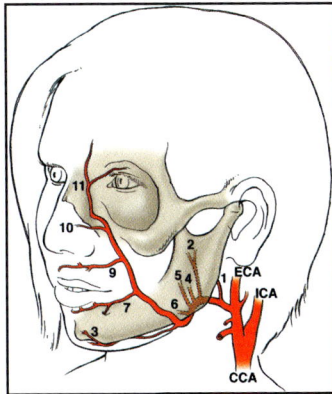

Fig. 1.9 Facial artery. (*1*) Ascending palatine artery; (*2*) tonsillar artery; (*3*) submental artery; (*4*) inferior masseteric artery; (*5*) jugal trunk; (*6*) middle mental artery; (*7*) inferior labial artery; (*8*) anterior jugal artery (not shown); (*9*) superior labial artery; (*10*) lateral nasal artery; (*11*) angular artery.

           (ii) *Tonsillar branch.* Arises at the level of the oropharyngeal tonsil and supplies the tonsil and palatopharyngeus muscle and sometimes the palatoglossal muscles.

          (iii)*Hamular branch.* Arises adjacent to the hamulus of the medial pterygoid plate and mucosa and palatoglossus muscle.

          (iv) Variable branches to uvula, levator palatini, palatoglossus, and palatopharyngeus muscles.

  ii) Territories

     (1) Supplies mucosa and muscles of the lateral oropharynx and soft palate. Anastamoses with contralateral ascending palatine artery, ipsilateral middle pharyngeal artery, the greater palatine artery, and the branches of accessory meningeal artery.

  iii) Variants

     (1) Usually arises from the proximal facial artery. May arise directly from the ECA, from a common trunk with the submandibular branch, occasionally from the middle pharyngeal artery (from the ascending pharyngeal artery) or even from the accessory meningeal artery.[19]

b) Tonsillar artery

  i) This artery is comprised of one or more small proximal facial branches to the tonsils. The tonsillar artery, along with the ascending palatine artery, pharyngeal branches of the ascending pharyngeal, dorsal lingual branch of the lingual, and greater palatine branch of the internal maxillary, provide the dominant supply to the palatine (oropharyngeal) tonsil.[7] The tonsillar artery must, therefore, be considered a culprit in postoperative bleeding after tonsillectomy, along with the ascending palatine artery. The tonsillar branches of the facial artery can also contribute to the nasopharyngeal tonsils, but most of the blood supply to that tonsil comes from the superior pharyngeal artery, ascending palatine artery, pterygo-vaginal artery, and occasionally the inferior hypophyseal branch of the meningohypophyseal trunk.[7]

c) Submandibular branches
    i) A small branch or branches to the submandibular gland region may arise from the submental artery and anastamose to the lingual and superior thyroid branches.[28]
d) Submental artery
    i) This fairly large artery travels along the inferior margin of the mandible. It supplies the floor of the mouth in conjunction with the lingual artery. The submental artery anastamoses with the lingual artery via its submandibular branch and with the superior thyroid artery via its infrahyoid branch. It also has side-to-side anastamoses with its contralateral partner.[28] Its terminal branches curve up to the chin to anastamose with the middle mental and inferior labial arteries.[7]
e) Inferior masseteric artery
    i) This anterior-superior angling branch follows and supplies the lower masseter muscle. It may have a small amount of collateral flow to the superior masseteric branch of the internal maxillary.[28]
f) Jugal trunk
    i) The name is derived from the Latin *jugālis*, and refers to the *zygoma* or cheek. The jugal trunk is one of the three main superior-to-inferior anastamoses in the soft tissues of the cheek.
        (1) Branches
        (2) Two angiographically visible branches arise from the jugal trunk:
            (a) *Bucco-masseteric (aka buccal)*. Arises from the jugal trunk at the level of the ramus of the mandible, then heads in a cephalad direction and deeply into the cheek. It gives rise to a buccal branch that supplies the mucosa and deep parts of the cheek and a masseteric branch that feeds its namesake – the masseter. The buccal artery anastomoses with the distal internal maxillary artery via its buccal branch and the superior masseteric. The masseteric branch anastomoses with the transverse facial and infraorbital arteries. It characteristically crosses the transverse facial artery at a right angle on lateral angiographic views.[28]
            (b) *Posterior jugal*. This branch travels obliquely anterior-superiorly and anastomoses with the infraorbital branch of the internal maxillary, superior alveolar, and the transverse facial.[28]
g) Middle mental artery
    i) A small horizontal branch along the body of the mandible that supplies skin and adjacent subcutaneous tissues. It anastomoses to adjacent facial artery branches and the inferior alveolar branch of the internal maxillary artery.[28]
h) Inferior labial artery
    i) This anterior and medially directed branch is the major supplier to the lower lip. It anastamoses with the contralateral inferior labial artery and the ipsilateral superior labial and submental arteries.[28] In 10% of angiograms this artery shares a common origin with the superior labial artery.[29]
i) Middle jugal artery
    i) An inconstant branch that parallels and potentially anastamoses with the anterior and posterior jugal trunks.[28]
j) Superior labial artery
    i) Anterior and medially directed branch to the upper lip. It runs parallel to the inferior labial artery and is usually larger than that artery. It has septal and alar branches to the nose. It freely anastamoses with the contralateral superior labial artery and has potentially dangerous anastamoses with nasal branches of the ophthalmic artery.[7,28]
k) Anterior jugal artery
    i) The anterior-most of the upward angulated branches in the cheek, it supplies the anterior cheek and lateral aspect of the upper lip and nose. It freely anastamoses with the infraorbital, the posterior and middle jugal arteries, the transverse facial artery, and superior alveolar artery.[28]

l) Lateral nasal (aka alar) artery
    i) This small branch extends anteriorly to supply the nostril and anastamoses with the contralateral alar artery.[7]
m) Nasal arcade
    i) These arteries are a network of anastamotic channels curving over and across the nose. They collect and connect inputs bilaterally from the facial and ophthalmic arteries.[28]
n) Angular artery
    i) Travels up along the angle lateral to the nose, hence it's name. It supplies the cheek beside the nose and the lateral aspect of the nose, contributing to the nasal arcade. It has dangerous anastamoses with inferior palpebral and nasal branches of the ophthalmic artery.[28]

2) Territories
    a) The facial artery is the major supplier to the superficial soft tissues of the face and contributes to the masseter muscle, parotid gland, palate and tonsils, floor of the mouth, and portions of the buccal mucosa. It provides vasa nervora to distal facial artery branches in the face. There are numerous anastamoses between facial branches and to virtually every other artery in the facial region, including major connections to the internal maxillary artery, transverse facial artery, and important collaterals to distal ophthalmic artery branches.

3) Variants
4) Lasjaunias proposed a theory of hemodynamic balance in the face to explain the variety of arterial configurations.[19,28] At six regions in the face (termed jugal, infraorbital, and ophthalmic superiorly, and mandibular, labial and nasal inferiorly), dominance of blood flow to the region by one or the other potential inputs determines the course and size of the facial artery. For instance, there is balance between the buccal and masseteric arteries in the posterolateral aspect of the face and balance between the infraorbital and transverse facial arteries in the mid-portion. Numerous variations are possible.
    a) The facial artery frequently arises as a common trunk with the lingual (20% of cases).[13]
    b) The proximal facial artery may have a posterolateral "jugal" course through the jugal region.[19]
    c) The facial artery may also travel anteromedially through the labial point for a "labial course."[19]
    d) The left and right facial arteries are symmetrical in 68% of autopsy cases.[30]
    e) The facial artery terminates in the:[30]
        i)   Angular artery (68%)
        ii) Lateral nasal branch (26%)
        iii) Superior labial artery (4%)

Occipital Artery

The occipital artery is a large branch of the posterior aspect of the ECA and travels posteriorly and superiorly. The initial segment is straight as it goes up through the upper neck, and the artery becomes more tortuous and redundant as it travels up the posterior scalp (Fig. 1.10).

1) Branches
    (a) Sternocleidomastoid branches (aka *muscular branches*)
         There may be multiple muscular branches. The hypoglossal nerve hooks around the lowest branch of this artery as the nerve first heads inferiorly and then anteriorly toward the tongue.[7] Each muscular branch characteristically tends to curve cephalad for a short distance before taking an abrupt turn posteroinferiorly. Each muscular branch corresponds to a vertebral level and provides segmental supply to the muscles, nerves, and bone at the corresponding levels. The occipital artery shares segmental vertebral blood supply with the vertebral artery, ascending pharyngeal artery, and deep cervical artery, which all anastomose extensively with the occipital artery muscular branches. The muscular branches that usually come from the occipital artery may also arise from the posterior auricular artery or directly from the ECA.[19]
    (b) Stylomastoid artery
         The stylomastoid artery arises from the occipital artery in 20–50% of cases.[19,31] It is a common source of blood flow to the facial nerve and

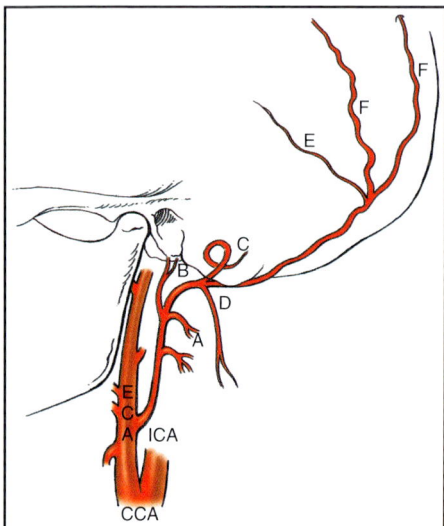

Fig. 1.10 Occipital artery. (*A*) Sternocleidomastoid branches; (*B*) stylomastoid artery; (*C*) mastoid branch; (*D*) descending branch; (*E*) lateral meningeal branch; (*F*) occipital branches.

middle ear and it has anastamoses with the inferior tympanic, anterior tympanic, and superior tympanic arteries.
(c) Mastoid artery
This vessel angles cephalad and medially from the occipital artery, giving some supply to the soft tissue in the adjacent scalp before entering the skull via the occipital foramen.
   i.   Branches
        After it enters the skull, the mastoid commonly divides into three groups of branches:[19]
        – *Descending branches.*
          These approach the jugular foramen and anastamose with the jugular branch of the ascending pharyngeal.
        – *Ascending branches.*
          These approach the internal auditory canal and can anastamose with the subarcuate branch of the anterior-inferior cerebellar artery.
        – *Posteromedial branches.*
          These spread out into the lateral dura of the posterior fossa and anastomose with branches of the hypoglossal branch of the ascending pharyngeal artery or the posterior meningeal branch arising from the vertebral (or posterior-inferior cerebellar) artery.[19]
   ii. Territories
        The mastoid artery supplies the superficial soft tissue, bone and dura in the mastoid and temporal bone region. It may supply large areas of the dura in the posterior fossa.
   iii. Variants
        The mastoid artery may be absent or hypoplastic. Its territory may be supplied by middle meningeal artery, hypoglossal artery, jugular branches, or the meningeal branches of the vertebral artery.
(d) Descending branch
The most cephalad muscular branch at the occipital-C1 junction tends to be quite prominent, usually with large anastomotic connections to the vertebral artery and a descending branch connecting to the deep cervical artery.

(e) Lateral meningeal branches

Distal to the origin of the mastoid branch, there may be one or more branches entering the skull via a small parietal foramen to supply the supratentorial dura. There are usually anastamoses with middle meningeal branches.

(f) Occipital branches

Multiple scalp vessels, with a redundant zigzag configuration, arise from the occipital to supply the scalp, muscles, and pericranium. These anastamose with the contralateral occipital branches, the scalp branches of the posterior auricular, and the superficial temporal arteries.[7]

2) Territories

The occipital artery travels 3 cm lateral to the inion. It generally supplies the posterior third of the scalp, the occipital-frontalis, trapezius, and sternocleidomastoid muscles, portions of the occipital, mastoid and temporal bones, dura, the seventh and ninth cranial nerves, and the first few spinal nerves. There are numerous anastamoses to the contralateral occipital artery, the ipsilateral ascending pharyngeal artery, vertebral artery, middle meningeal artery, superficial temporal artery, posterior auricular artery, deep cervical artery and even the anterior–inferior cerebellar artery.

3) Variants

(a) The ascending pharyngeal may arise from the occipital artery.

(b) There can be a common origin of the occipital with the posterior auricular artery as an occipitoauricular trunk (12.5% of cases).[13]

(c) The occipital artery may arise from the ICA.

(d) The occipital artery can be a part of persistent carotid-vertebral anastamoses, such as a persistent proatlantal artery.

(e) The occipital artery may originate from C1 or C2 segmental branches of the vertebral artery or from the ascending cervical artery.[19,32]

Posterior Auricular Artery

This posterior branch of the distal external carotid is fairly small and can be identified angiographically by the tortuous scalp branch curving cephalad behind the ear.

1) Branches

(a) Sternocleidomastoid (aka *muscular*) branch

Proximal branch of the posterior auricular can assist the occipital in providing blood flow to the sternocleidomastoid, digastric, and stylohyoid muscles.[7]

(b) Parotid branches

Small branches from the proximal posterior auricular to the parotid that can supply portions of the facial nerve.

(c) Stylomastoid branch

The stylomastoid artery arises from the posterior auricular in 50–70% of cases.[31,33] In order of frequency; it may also arise from the occipital or directly from the external carotid. It feeds the facial nerve and middle ear, mastoid air cells and portions of the inner ear.[7] It can anastamose with anterior tympanic artery (from middle meningeal) and inferior tympanic (from ascending pharyngeal) artery.

(d) Auricular branch

A fairly constant branch seen in 65% of cases, this vessel supplies much of the posterior aspect of the pinna.[34] Its branches from a dense arterial network in the ear.

(e) Occipital (aka retroauricular) branch

Also a fairly constant branch and is seen in 65% of cases. It supplies the scalp behind the ear.

(f) Parietal branch

A fairly inconstant branch seen only when the superficial temporal does not have a dominant parietal branch. It has the typical ascending, tortuous appearance of a scalp vessel.

2) Territories

The posterior auricular artery supplies the auricle and enters the middle part of the ear posteriorly.[35] It is the major supplier of blood flow to the ear.[36] It can supply portions of the parotid gland, facial nerve, sternocleidomastoid, digastric and stylohyoid muscles.[7] It has variable supply to the scalp posterior and superior to the ear, depending on the dominance of the superficial temporal and occipital arteries. It anastamoses with the superficial temporal and occipital arteries via the scalp and auricular branches. It also anastomoses with the middle meningeal artery (anterior tympanic branch) and ascending pharyngeal artery (inferior tympanic branch) via the stylomastoid artery.

3) Variants
    (a) Shares a common origin with the occipital artery (occipitoauricular trunk) in 12.5% of cases.[13]
    (b) The scalp territories of the posterior auricular artery are in a hemodynamic balance with the superficial temporal and occipital arteries. If one is hypoplastic, the adjacent vessels are hypertrophic, and vice versa.

Superficial Temporal Artery

One of the two terminal branches of the external carotid (the other is the internal maxillary artery), this vessel continues the general vertical course of the ECA. The superficial temporal artery arises behind the neck of the mandible within the parotid gland. It is easily palpable anterior to the ear at the tragus.[7] The superficial temporal artery typically provides two major branches that then angle cephalad in a wavy, redundant fashion typical of scalp vessels.

1) Branches
    (a) Transverse facial artery
    Originating anteriorly from the superficial temporal artery (within the parotid gland) the transverse facial artery travels anteriorly and slightly inferiorly between the parotid duct and zygomatic arch, supplying facial structures.[7] On a lateral angiogram it crosses the buccal artery at a right angle.[19] With agenesis or diminution of the facial artery, this branch may be the dominant artery of the face.
      i. Branches
      The transverse facial artery commonly has a number of branches, but only one (superior masseteric) has a well-described formal name.
        – *Parotid branches.*
        These supply the parotid gland and duct and may contribute to facial nerve branches.
        – *Superior masseteric.*
        Prominent branch to the masseter muscle that anastamoses with the buccal artery (from the facial artery).[19]
        – *Jugal branches.*
        One or more descending branches to the cheek that may anastamose with the jugal branches of the facial artery.
        – *Zygomatic branches.*
        These spread out into the face and anastamose with branches of the zygomatico-orbital branch of the superficial temporal artery.[19] Distally, these terminal branches may anastamose with the infraorbital and lacrimal arteries.[7]
      ii. Territories
      The transverse facial artery supplies the superficial soft tissues of the upper face. It anastamoses with other superficial temporal and facial branches, as well as collaterals to the infraorbital and ophthalmic arteries.
      iii. Variants
      The transverse facial artery may arise directly from the ECA.
    (b) Anterior auricular artery
    It is a proximal branch of the superficial temporal, supplying blood primarily to the anterior aspect of the ear. It has three branches, the most superior of which curves up over the helix to anastamose with posterior auricular artery. The lower two branches only provide limited supply to the anterior ear.[35]
    (c) Zygomatico-orbital artery (aka zygomaticotemporal)
    This variably prominent, anteriorly directed branch of the superficial temporal artery runs just superior to the zygomatic arch toward the lateral aspect of the orbit. It supplies the scalp and the orbicularis occuli muscles.[7] It has numerous anastamoses with the frontal branch of the superficial temporal artery, transverse facial artery, and the

supraorbital, frontal, palpebral, and lacrimal branches of the ophthalmic artery.[19]
  (d) Middle temporal artery
      Also called the posterior deep temporal by some authors, this is a relatively small branch supplying the temporalis muscle, specifically its posterior aspect.[37] It potentially anastomoses with the deep temporal branches of the internal maxillary.[7]
  (e) Frontal branch
      One of the two large terminal branches of the superficial temporal takes a tortuous course over the frontal scalp and supplies tissue from skin down to pericranium. It anastomoses with its contralateral counterpart across the midline, the ipsilateral zygomatico-orbital branch of the superficial temporal, and the supraorbital and supratrochlear branches of the ophthalmic artery.[7] The distal frontal branch over the vertex can also provide branches that pass through foramina for emissary veins to anastomose with middle meningeal branches.[19] This is why superficial temporal arteries sometimes supply intracranial lesions such as meningiomas.
  (f) Parietal branch
      The other, usually larger terminal branch of the superficial temporal, angles more posteriorly to supply the parietal scalp. It anastomoses with the contralateral parietal branch, ipsilateral frontal branch, posterior auricular, and occipital branches. It can also provide some transcranial anastomoses with the middle meningeal branches.
2) Territories
   The superficial temporal is a major contributor of blood flow to the scalp and is in a hemodynamic equilibrium with the occipital and posterior auricular arteries. There are extensive anastomoses between the superficial temporal branches and branches of the occipital, posterior auricular, middle meningeal, ophthalmic and facial arteries.
3) Variants
   The major superficial branches vary considerably in size and territory. Hemodynamic balance exists between individual superficial temporal artery branches and competing scalp arteries. Therefore, when one artery is large and covers a wide territory, adjacent arteries may be small or absent.

Internal Maxillary Artery

The internal maxillary artery (IMA) is the larger of the two terminal branches of the ECA. Inclusion of the term *internal* may seem superfluous, although in earlier days, the facial artery was referred to as the external maxillary artery. The IMA arises at a right angle from the external carotid behind the neck of the mandible and travels anteriorly.[7] Anatomically, it can be divided into three segments: (1) the proximal mandibular part that travels horizontally, first posterior and then medial to the mandible; (2) the middle pterygoid part that travels anteriorly and cephalad (in a slightly oblique fashion) adjacent to the lateral pterygoid muscle (medial or lateral to it depending on whether it is the superficial or deep variant as described below); (3) the distal pterygopalatine part that passes between the upper and lower heads of the lateral pterygoid, curves medially, and travels through the pterygomaxillary fissure into the pterygopalatine fossa.[7]
    The IMA is found in two configurations:
  1) The superficial-type IMA travels lateral to the lateral pterygoid. In this variant, the accessory meningeal artery arises from the middle meningeal artery. The inferior alveolar and the middle deep temporal arteries arise separately from the IMA (Fig. 1.11).[38,39]
  2) The deep-type IMA travels medial to the lateral pterygoid. It gives rise to a common origin of the inferior alveolar and middle deep temporal arteries. The accessory meningeal artery, in this variant, arised directly from IMA.[38,39] Hint: Remember that the *deep*-type IMA has a common origin of the inferior alveolar and middle *deep* temporal arteries (Fig. 1.12).

  1) Branches
     The mandibular part of the IMA gives rise to the deep auricular, anterior tympanic, middle meningeal, accessory meningeal, and inferior alveolar arteries (i.e., branches that traverse foramina or fissures). The pterygoid part usually has deep temporal, pterygoid, masseteric, and buccal branches (i.e., muscular

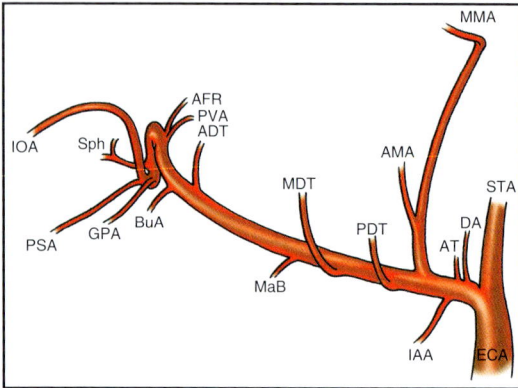

Fig. 1.11 Internal maxillary artery, superficial-type variant. The internal maxillary artery (IMA) travels lateral to the lateral pterygoid muscle, and is characterized by separate origins of the middle deep temporal (MDT) and inferior alveolar artery (IAA). The accessory meningeal (AMA) arises from the proximal middle meningeal (MMA). Other IMA branches include deep auricular (DA), anterior tympanic (AT), posterior deep temporal (PDT), pterygoid branches (not shown), masseteric branches (MaB), buccal artery (BuA), anterior deep temporal (ADT), posterior superior alveolar (PSA), infraorbital (IOA), greater palatine (GPA), pterygo-vaginal (PVA), artery of foramen rotundum (AFR), sphenopalatine (Sph).

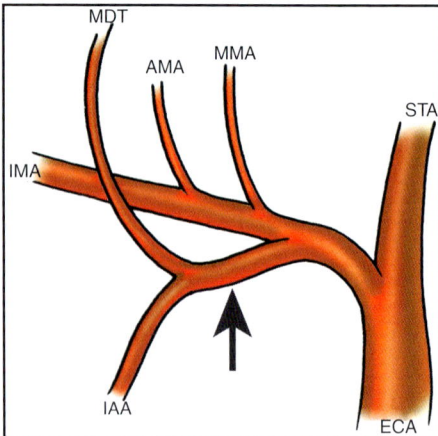

Fig. 1.12 Internal maxillary artery, deep-type variant. The deep type internal maxillary (IMA) is medial to the lateral pterygoid muscle. This variant has a common trunk (arrow) that gives rise to the middle deep temporal (MDT) and inferior alveolar artery (IAA). Also note separate origins of the accessory meningeal (AMA) and middle meningeal artery (MMA). Superficial temporal origin (STA) and distal external carotid (ECA) are also shown.

branches). The pterygopalatine part provides the posterior superior alveolar, infraorbital, artery of foramen rotundum, pterygovaginal, descending palatine, Vidian, and sphenopalatine arteries.[7]

a) Deep auricular artery
   i) Tiny branch of very proximal internal maxillary
   ii) Branches
     (1) No named branches.
   iii) Territories
     (1) Supplies external auditory meatus, tympanic membrane, and temporomandibular joint.[7]
   iv) Variants
   v) May arise in a common trunk with the anterior tympanic artery

b) Anterior tympanic artery
   i) Very small branch of very proximal internal maxillary
   ii) Branches
     (1) No named branches.
   iii) Territories
     (1) Supplies tympanic cavity and anastamoses with the stylomastoid artery, pterygovaginal branch of the IMA, and caroticotympanic artery from petrous ICA.[7]
   iv) Variants
     (1) Analysis of 104 cadaveric specimens revealed extremely variable anterior tympanic artery origins.[40]
     (2) May arise as a common trunk with deep auricular artery, middle meningeal artery, accessory meningeal artery, or posterior deep temporal artery.
     (3) The anterior tympanic artery is a branch of the right IMA in 78% of cases and a branch of the left IMA in 45% of cases.
     (4) Next most common site of origin: superficial temporal artery.
     (5) 1–4% arise directly from the ECA.
     (6) Rarely, the anterior tympanic artery may be duplicated, triplicated, or absent.[40]

c) Middle meningeal artery (Fig. 1.13)
   i) The first substantial ascending branch of the internal maxillary enters the cranial cavity through foramen spinosum. It then takes a characteristic right-angle turn. In the sagittal plane, it turns anteriorly and in the coronal plane it turns laterally.
   ii) Branches
     (1) *Accessory meningeal branch*
       (a) This may be a major extracranial branch of the middle meningeal or may arise separately from the internal maxillary. The accessory meningeal is discussed in detail below.
     (2) *Petrous branch*
       (a) The small but important petrous branch first gives a medial cavernous branch to the cavernous sinus that can anastamose with the posterior branch of the inferolateral trunk. It then gives a posterior basal tentorial branch, which anastamoses with basal tentorial branches of the petrosquamosal branch of the middle meningeal artery and cavernous branches of the ICA.[19] The artery then follows along the greater petrosal nerve and sends the superior tympanic branch to the facial nerve and geniculate ganglion. This portion of the artery anastamoses with the stylomastoid artery.[7]
     (3) *Petrosquamosal branch*
       (a) A posteriorly directed branch of the proximal intracranial middle meningeal artery, the petrosquamosal branch supplies the middle cranial fossa dura. It can have a basal tentorial branch to the dura of the posterior fossa, and it anastamoses with the jugular branch of the ascending pharyngeal.[19]
     (4) *Sphenoidal branch*
       (a) This branch supplies dura along the planum sphenoidale and then enters the orbit via the superior orbital

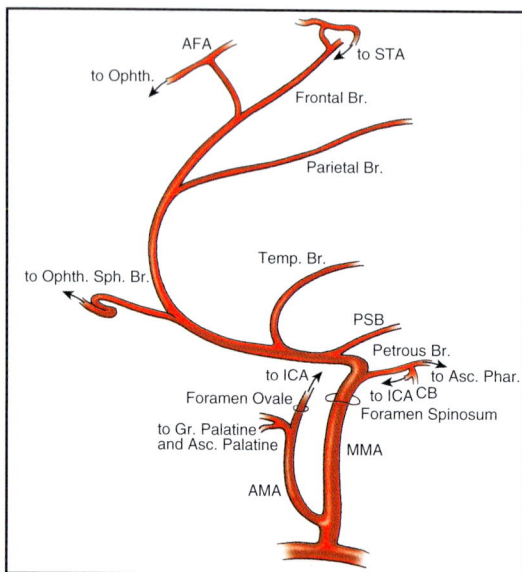

Fig. 1.13 Middle meningeal artery: branches and anastomoses. The middle meningeal artery (*MMA*) often has a large extracranial branch, the accessory meningeal artery (*AMA*), which, in turn has anastomoses with the greater palatine (*Gr. Palatine*) and ascending palatine (*Asc. Palatine*) arteries before entering the skull via the foramen ovale and anastomosing with cavernous branches of the internal carotid (*ICA*). The middle meningeal artery continues into the skull via the foramen spinosum. The petrous branch (*Petrous Br.*) is the first intracranial branch and anastomoses with ascending pharyngeal branches (*Ascending Pharyngeal*) in the temporal bone and with ICA branches via its cavernous branch (*CB*). Petrosquamosal (*PSB*), temporal (*Temporal Branch*), parietal (*Parietal Branch*), and frontal branches (*Frontal Branch*) supply the dura over the middle and anterior fossa. Transcranial anastamoses with the superficial temporal (*STA*) and midline anastamoses with the anterior falx (*AFA*) branch of the ophthalmic (*Ophth.*) are depicted. The sphenoidal branch (*Sph. Br.*) is a major collateral to the ophthalmic.

fissure to communicate with the ophthalmic artery.[41] Sphenoidal collaterals to the ophthalmic artery are present in 16% of cadaveric specimens.[42]

(5) *Meningolacrimal branch*

    (a) The orbital branch is derived from the superior branch of the primitive stapedial artery and enters the orbit through the cranio-orbital foramen (of Hyrtl) and directly fills the lacrimal artery.[41] This branch is present in 43% of cadaveric specimens.[42]

(6) *Temporo-occipital (aka temporal) branch*

    (a) This branch arises distal to the sphenoidal branch and curves posteriorly. It supplies skull and dura of the middle cranial fossa. It may extend completely around the calvaria to the midline and contribute to the posterior falx and tentorium, but this is generally seen only in pathological states. It anastomoses with the petrosquamosal and parietal branches of the middle meningeal artery and with scalp arteries via transcranial collaterals.

(7) *Parietal branch*
    (a) One of the two terminal branches of the middle meningeal artery, this vessel supplies the anterior cranial fossa dura. It can vary in size and distribution, since it anastomoses with and is in a hemodynamic balance with the frontal and temporo-occipital branches. The parietal branch reaches the vertex and contributes to the walls of the superior sagittal sinus and falx. At the midline, it anastamoses with the contralateral middle meningeal artery. Transcranial anastamoses with scalp arteries (superficial temporal and occipital) are present in nearly all cadaveric specimens.[43]
(8) *Frontal branch*
    (a) Usually the last branch of the middle meningeal artery, this branch is in hemodynamic balance with the parietal branch; therefore, it can vary in size and distribution. It is a major contributor to the anterior cranial fossa dura. It can reach the midline and frequently anastamoses with the anterior falx branch of the ophthalmic artery. Other anastamoses include the ipsilateral parietal branch, the contralateral frontal branch, and transcranial collaterals of the scalp arteries, especially the frontal branch of the superficial temporal artery.

iii) Territories
    (1) The middle meningeal artery provides extensive flow to the calvaria and meninges of the anterior and middle fossae (Table 1.5). It has important collaterals to the ICA circulation.[44] The middle meningeal artery also contributes to the cranial nerves in the cavernous sinus via the cavernous branch and also to the facial nerve via the superior tympanic branch.

iv) Variants
    (1) The middle meningeal artery develops from the fetal stapedial artery. The stapedial artery arises from the fetal hyoid artery, a branch that becomes the petrous ICA, and passes through the mesenchyma that later becomes the stapes (hence the name). The stapedial artery gives off supraorbital, maxillary, and mandibular branches, which are later incorporated into the ECA. The supraorbital artery anastamoses with the developing ophthalmic artery.[7] Persistence of portions of fetal arteries that usually regress and/or regression of segments that usually persist, results in a number of congenital variants.[45]
    (2) The distal middle meningeal artery frequently arises from the ophthalmic artery.[46]
    (3) The middle meningeal artery may arise from the ICA.[47,48]
    (4) The ophthalmic artery may arise from the middle meningeal artery.[49–52]
    (5) A number of extracranial branches may arise from the middle meningeal artery, including a palatine branch,[53] as well as the posterior superior alveolar artery.[54]
    (6) Tentorial branches (usually arising from cavernous ICA) may arise from the middle meningeal artery.[55]
    (7) Occasionally, the middle meningeal artery may arise from the basilar artery.[56–58]
    (8) The size and direction of the distal middle meningeal branches is extremely variable.
    (9) Dural-to-pial collateral flow from middle meningeal artery branches to anterior or middle cerebral branches can occur. However, these variants are usually seen in the presence of occlusive disease (such as carotid occlusion with impaired collateral flow)[59] or with high-flow lesions (such as brain arteriovenous malformations). These are likely acquired connections due to high flow demand and release of angiogenic factors, rather than true congenital variants.

Table 1.5 Intracranial dural vascular supply

Dural structure/ region	Feeding arteries	...Which usually arise from	Reference
Posterior fossa	Petrosquamosal	Middle meningeal	
	Petrous	Middle meningeal	
	Mastoid	Occipital	6
	Jugular	Ascending pharyngeal	6
	Hypoglossal	Ascending pharyngeal	6
	Posterior meningeal	Vertebral	6
	Anterior meningeal	Vertebral	
Tentorium	Artery of Bernasconi and Cassinari (marginal tentorial)	Cavernous carotid	19
	Basal tentorial	Cavernous carotid	19
	Petrosquamosal	Middle meningeal	19
	Mastoid	Occipital	19
	Artery of Davidoff and Schechter	Posterior cerebral	63
Falx cerebri	Anterior falx artery	Ophthalmic	
	Frontal and parietal branches	Middle meningeal	
	Artery of Davidoff and Schechter	Posterior cerebral	63
Anterior cranial fossa	Ethmoidals	Ophthalmic	6
	Recurrent meningeal	Ophthalmic	
	Anterior falx	Ophthalmic	
	Sphenoidal	Middle meningeal	
	Frontal and parietal branches	Middle meningeal	
Middle cranial fossa	Inferolateral trunk	Cavernous carotid	6
	Accessory meningeal	Middle meningeal	6
	Temporo-occipital	Middle meningeal	6
	Recurrent meningeal	Ophthalmic	6
	Carotid branch	Ascending pharyngeal	6

These vessels should be considered when evaluating vascular lesions in or around the dura.

d) Accessory meningeal artery
   i) This small branch arising either from the proximal middle menin-
      geal or, less commonly, from the IMA just distal to the middle men-
      ingeal artery takes a characteristic gently curving antero-superior
      course. Ironically, in spite of its name, only about 10% (range
      0–40%) of its blood supply is intracranial.[60]
   ii) Branches
       (1) Terminal branches of the accessory meningeal vary in size
           and configuration and are variably named in the litera-
           ture.[61] The major branches, ascending, descending, and
           recurrent rami, are named for the direction they take after
           arising from the accessory meningeal artery.[60]
       (2) Lateral territory ascending ramus (aka posterior branch)
       (3) Medial territory ascending ramus (aka inferomedial
           branch)
       (4) Intracranial ascending ramus (aka intracranial branch)
       (5) Small branch usually enters the skull via foramen ovale
       (6) Descending companion ramus to the medial pterygoid nerve
           (aka arteria pterygoida medialis)
       (7) Anterior descending ramus (aka inferopalatine branch).
           This is the continuation of the main accessory meningeal
           artery and supplies the soft palate and the nasal cavity.
       (8) Variable recurrent rami to mandibular nerve and otic
           ganglion

iii) Territories
  (1) There are lateral, medial, and intracranial territories. Most of the blood supply is extracranial supplying lateral and medial pterygoid, the levator veli palatine muscles, the pteryoid plates, the greater wing of the sphenoid bone, the mandibular nerve, and otic ganglion. The artery also supplies the posterior nasal cavity and can be a source of nasal bleeding.[62] The intracranial contribution is usually small and enters the skull through foramen ovale (most commonly) or the sphenoidal emissary foramen of Vesalius (in 22% of cases).[60] The intracranial rami supply the meninges of variable portions of the middle cranial fossa, portions of the cavernous sinus and the trigeminal nerve and its ganglion. It can anastamose with the posterior limb of the infero-rolateral trunk of the cavernous ICA.[63]

iv) Variants
  (1) The origin of the accessory meningeal artery is from the middle meningeal artery when the internal maxillary artery is lateral to the lateral pterygoid muscle (superficial type IMA).
  (2) The origin is from the internal maxillary artery when IMA is medial to the lateral pterygoid (deep type IMA).
  (3) There can be multiple accessory meningeal arteries (25% of cases), but the artery is rarely absent (4% of cases).[60]
  (4) The rare persistent trigeminal variant consists of an anastamosis from the accessory meningeal artery to the superior cerebellar artery.[64]

e) Inferior alveolar artery (aka dental artery)
  i) This branch takes an anterior-inferior angulation from its origin from the proximal internal maxillary artery. It then enters the mandibular foramen, following along the mandibular canal.
  ii) Branches
    (1) *Mylohyoid branch.* This is a small branch to the mylohoid muscle arising from the inferior alveolar artery before entering the mandibular canal. It anastamoses with the submental branch of the facial artery.[7]
    (2) *Incisive branch.* One of two terminal branches of the inferior alveolar. Under the incisor teeth, the incisive branch reaches the midline, anastomosing with the contralateral incisive branch.[7]
    (3) *Mental branch.* This branch travels out through the mental foramen of the mandible to anastamose with the submental and inferior labial branches of the facial artery.[7]
  iii) Territories
    (1) The inferior alveolar supplies the mylohyoid muscle, the mandible, mandibular teeth, inferior alveolar nerve, and the soft tissues of the chin.
  iv) Variants
    (1) The inferior alveolar artery arises as a common trunk with the middle deep temporal artery in the deep type internal maxillary artery variant.
    (2) The inferior alveolar artery may arise directly from the ECA.[65]

f) Middle deep temporal artery
  i) Complicating things further, some authors refer to this branch as the *posterior deep temporal artery*, but most authorities refer to it as the *middle deep temporal artery*. The deep temporal arteries ascend in a relatively straight course unlike the redundant superficial temporal branches. The middle deep temporal artery provides approximately one-half of the blood flow to the temporalis muscle.[37] It anastamoses with the superficial temporal artery and occasionally the transcranial collaterals from this vessel can anastamose with the middle meningeal artery branches. A component of the deep-type internal maxillary variant is a common origin of the inferior and middle deep temporal arteries.[38,39]

g) Pterygoid branches
   i) Small inferiorly directed branches of the distal pterygoid part to the pterygoid muscles that are not often visualized angiographically.
h) Masseteric artery
   i) Small, inferiorly directed branch to the masseter that anastamoses with masseteric branches of the facial and the transverse facial arteries.
i) Buccal artery
   i) Inferiorly directed branch that connects to the jugal trunk of the facial artery and supplies the soft tissues of the cheek from mucosa to skin. It provides collateral flow between the distal internal maxillary and facial arteries and has a connection to the transverse facial artery.
j) Anterior deep temporal artery
   i) This artery angles cephalad in a fairly straight course to provide approximately 30% of the blood supply to the temporalis muscle.[37] This artery has important anastamoses to the lacrimal branch of the ophthalmic artery.
k) Posterior superior alveolar artery
   i) This artery descends behind the maxilla before sending branches to bone, teeth, and gingiva in the posterior aspect of the maxilla.
l) Infraorbital artery
   i) Anterior-most branch of the IMA that passes through the inferior orbital fissure, then enters the infraorbital canal to outline the roof of the maxillary sinus.[7]
   ii) Branches
      (1) *Middle superior alveolar branch*. Contributes to the alveolar process of the mandible.
      (2) *Anterior superior alveolar branch*. Also contributes to the supply of the maxillary teeth.
      (3) *Orbital branch*. This artery primarily supplies the adipose tissue in the inferior aspect of the orbit and can anastamose with the ophthalmic artery.[66]
      (4) *Palpebral branch*. Distal branch to the lower eyelid. It anastamoses with the dorsal nasal branch of the ophthalmic artery.
      (5) *Naso-orbital branch*. Small branches to the anterior-inferior orbit and side of the nose that anastamose with the ophthalmic artery.
      (6) *Zygomatic branches*. Lateral branch (or branches) supplying the cheek and connecting to the transverse facial artery and jugal trunk of the facial artery.
   iii) Territories
      (1) The infraorbital artery supplies the adjacent infraorbital (maxillary) nerve, mucosa, and bony margin of the maxillary sinus.[67] Distal branches contribute to the lower eyelid and pre-maxillary cheek soft tissue.[7] Both the orbital branch and the distal infraorbital branch (palpebral branch) anastamose with the ophthalmic artery, putting vision at risk when anything toxic is injected in the infraorbital artery.[68] The infraorbital artery connects to the posterior superior alveolar, sphenopalatine, and facial arteries.
   iv) Variants
      (1) May be hypoplastic or hypertrophic, depending on the size of the facial artery.
      (2) Can arise in a common trunk with the posterior superior alveolar artery.
m) Pterygovaginal artery
   i) This is a small branch running posteriorly from the IMA into the pterygoid canal. It anastamoses with the accessory meningeal artery and ascending pharyngeal artery branches to the Eustachian tube region, and may connect with the petrous ICA.
n) Vidian artery (aka artery of the pterygoid canal)[69,70]
   i) This artery may arise from the pterygovaginal artery, or separately from the IMA. It enters the Vidian canal and may anastamose with a Vidian branch of the petrous ICA.

o) Artery of foramen rotundum
   i) Small, posteriorly directed branch with a characteristic wavy appearance as it passes through the foramen rotundum. Supplies the maxillary nerve and adjacent skull base. It is an important collateral to the anterolateral branch of the inferolateral trunk of the cavernous ICA.
p) Descending palatine artery
   i) This large artery descends obliquely from its origin, travels in the pterygopalatine (aka greater palatine) canal, turns abruptly forward horizontally and travels medial to the maxillary teeth to supply the palate. When it emerges from the greater palatine foramen, it then becomes the *Greater palatine artery*.
   ii) Branches
       (1) *Lesser palatine artery*. Smaller branch or branches running parallel to the greater palatine artery in a separate bony canal, usually without a distal horizontal segment. May arise independently from the IMA.[27]
       (2) *Palatine branch*. It is a small branch turning posteriorly to supply the soft palate and anastamoses with the middle pharyngeal and/or the ascending palatine.
       (3) *Septal branch*. It is the terminal branch of the greater palatine at the incisive canal. It supplies the nasal septum and anastamoses with sphenopalatine and ethmoidal arteries.
   iii) Territories
       (1) A major contributor to the blood supply of the hard palate, it also contributes to the mucosa, gingiva, soft palate, and tonsils.[7] Anastamotic connections exist with the contralateral greater palatine artery, ipsilateral middle pharyngeal artery, ascending palatine artery, sphenopalatine artery, and ethmoidal branches of the ophthalmic.[19]
   iv) Variants
       (1) The greater palatine artery may be hypoplastic or absent on one or both sides.
       (2) Bilateral hypolasia of the greater palatine artery is seen in cleft palate syndrome.[71]
q) Sphenopalatine artery
   i) This is a major branch of the terminal IMA that enters the sphenopalatine foramen to supply the nasal cavity. This artery can be a major source of bleeding in epistaxis cases. The sphenopalatine artery can also supply vascular lesions in the nasal cavity such as juvenile nasopharyngeal angiofibromas.
   ii) Branches
       (1) *Septal branch*
           This is a small branch that first goes straight medially, takes a right angle cephalad and another right angle medially before spreading out into the nasal septum. It also supplies the superior turbinate in 72% of cases.[72]
       (2) *Lateral nasal branch* (aka posterior lateral nasal branch). This branch travels inferiorly before ramifying along the nasal turbinates to supply the nasal cavity mucosa.
   iii) Territories
       (1) Sphenopalatine arteries supply the mucosa of nasal cavity and are a very common source of bleeding in idiopathic epistaxis. They anastamose with ethmoidal branches of the ophthalmic artery, the greater palatine artery, and the septal branch of the superior labial artery.[7]
   iv) Variants
       (1) None described.
2) Territories (IMA)
   (a) The IMA supplies bones in the mid and lower face, muscles of mastication mucosa in the nasal cavity, the palate, numerous cranial nerves (III–VII) and large areas of dura.[7] There are multiple potential anastamoses with the internal carotid directly, the ophthalmic and numerous other vessels in the face and head.
3) Variants (IMA)
   (a) Superficial-type versus deep-type IMA (see beginning of IMA section, above).
   (b) Rarely, the IMA shares a common origin with the facial artery.[73]

Other ECA Branches

Variable unnamed branches of the ECA are present. They are usually small and not well seen on angiography unless they are involved with a vascular malformation or neoplasm. The named branches that occasionally arise from the ECA usually arise from one of its major branches:

(a) Tiny carotid body branches arise from the proximal ECA itself or from the proximal branches of the ECA.

(b) The sternocleidomastoid branch (or branches) can arise from the ECA, but usually arises from the superior thyroid, occipital, or posterior auricular artery.

(c) The superior laryngeal artery usually originates from the superior thyroid artery, but can arise separately from the ECA.

(d) A recurrent pharyngeal branch to the upper oropharynx and palate can arise directly from the ECA.[27]

(e) A small branch to the stylomastoid muscle arises from the distal ECA.

(f) A small masseteric branch originates from the distal ECA.

(g) The ascending palatine artery usually arises from the facial artery, but may originate directly from the proximal ECA.

(h) The transverse facial artery frequently arises separately from the distal ECA, although it is more often a branch of the superficial temporal artery.

1.4.   Internal Carotid Artery

Several classification schemes exist for the segments of the ICA, including various numbering systems (Fig. 1.14). The numbering systems can be confusing and needlessly arcane for the purposes of everyday clinical work. The authors of this handbook favor the following simple system (corresponding to the description by Gibo and colleagues):[74]

1. Cervical
2. Petrous
3. Cavernous
4. Supraclinoid

The segmental nomenclature used by Bouthillier and coworkers will be used in this chapter for the purpose of anatomic description.[75]

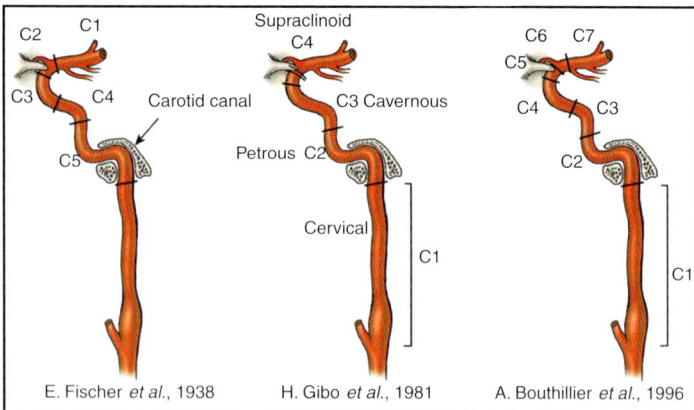

Fig. 1.14 Selected segmental classification schemes of the internal carotid artery.[74–76]

The system established by Fischer in 1938 was intended to describe angiographic patterns of arterial displacement by intracranial tumors, numbered the ICA segments against the flow of blood, and excluded the extracranial ICA.[76] Subsequent systems have included the cervical segment and have numbered the segments with the flow of blood.

Angio-Anatomic Correlate! Carotid Bifurcation (Fig. 1.15)

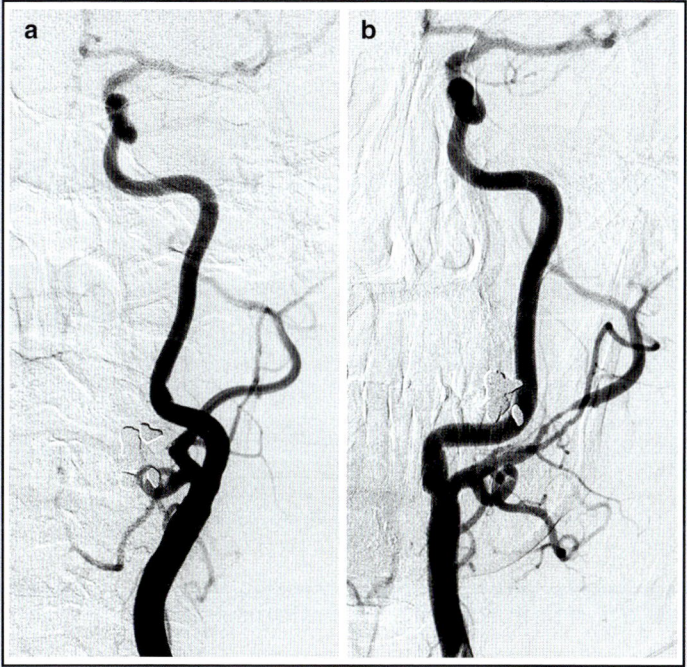

Fig. 1.15 The ICA usually arises lateral to the ECA, and is thought to be fixed at birth. Exceptions can occur, however. In this patient with lupus, the ICA changed from a lateral position (**a**) to a medial position (**b**) after 4 months on high dose steroids.

Cervical Segment (C1)

This segment begins at the carotid bifurcation and ends at the skull base and usually has no branches. The carotid bifurcation is usually at the level of C3. The ICA receives approximately 80% of the flow from the CCA. The ICA is encircled by sympathetic fibers, and travels in the carotid sheath, which also contains the internal jugular vein and the vagus nerve. The uppermost portion of the carotid sheath (superior to the nasopharynx) also contains cranial nerves IX, XI, and XII.

1) Divisions
    (a) *Carotid bulb*. Focal dilation of the ICA at the origin, measuring 7.4 mm in diameter on average, compared to 7.0 mm for the CCA and 4.7 mm for the ICA distal to the carotid bulb.[77]
    (b) *Ascending cervical segment*. The diameter remains relatively constant throughout its course. Coiling or complete looping of the vessel is seen in up to 15% of angiograms.[1]
2) Branches: None.
3) Variants
    (a) Position of origin. The carotid bifurcation can be found as low as T2 or as high as C1.[1] Rarely, the ICA may arise directly from the aortic arch; in these cases the non-bifurcating carotid artery gives rise to all of the branches normally supplied by the ECA and then continues as the ICA.[78]
    (b) Agenesis and hypoplasia
        i. Congenital absence or hypoplasia of the ICA may occur sporadically in a association with other congenital anomalies, such as anencephaly or basal telangectasia.[79] Intracranial aneurysms are associated in 67% of cases.[80]
        ii. Agenesis of the ICA has a prevalence of 0.01%[81] and can be distinguished from ICA occlusion by imaging of the skull base; in patients with agenesis, the carotid canal is absent.[82] Agenesis is more frequent on the left.[83]
        iii. Bilateral ICA agenesis is seen in <10% of ICA agenesis cases[83] and is associated with intracranial aneurysms in some 25% of cases.[84]
        iv. *ICA Hypoplasia* has an incidence of 0.079%,[83] and should not be confused with diffuse narrowing of the ICA, which is most commonly seen with fibromuscular dysplasia, dissection, or secondary to high-grade atherosclerotic stenosis. Congenital hypoplasia can be distinguished from acquired stenosis by the presence of a small petrous carotid canal.[82]
    (c) Anomalous branches are rare but can include:[85]
        i. Ascending pharyngeal artery
        ii. Superior thyroid artery
        iii. Occipital artery
        iv. Posterior meningeal artery
        v. Persistent stapedial artery
        vi. Vidian artery
    (d) Duplication and fenestration of the cervical ICA has been reported.[86,87]
    (e) Carotid-vertebrobasilar anastamoses.

Carotid–Vertebrobasilar Anastomoses

Transient connections appear during development between the carotid and hindbrain circulations. These anastomoses usually disappear as the posterior communicating arteries develop and rarely persist into adulthood. The most common of these is the persistent fetal origin of the posterior cerebral artery, which has a prevalence of some 18–22% in the general population (see below).[88] Three of the four other embryonic arteries are named for the cranial nerves they parallel. From superior to inferior, these persistent fetal vessels (excepting the fetal PCA) include: *trigeminal*, *otic*, *hypoglossal*, and *proatlantal intersegmental* arteries (Fig. 1.16). A mnemonic for this uses the acronym *TO(h)P*: The primitive anastomotic vessels appear near the *TO(h)P* of the craniospinal axis.
    1. Persistent trigeminal artery
        (a) Most common carotid-basilar anastomosis, seen in some 0.1–0.2% of angiograms.[33,85]
        (b) Extends from the cavernous ICA to the upper part of the basilar artery and often perforates the dorsum sella.
            i. The vertebrobasilar system proximal to the upper basilar artery may be hypoplastic, with the primitive trigeminal artery supplying most of the flow to the PCAs and the SCAs.

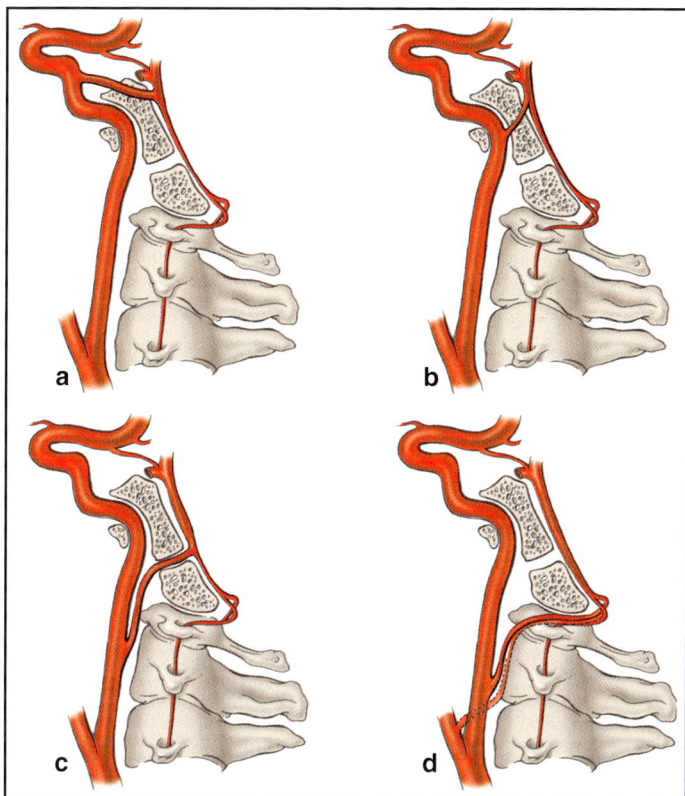

Fig. 1.16 Carotid–vertebrobasilar anastomoses. The most common configuration of each type of persistent embryologic connection between the carotid and vertebrobasilar system are shown. The persistent fetal origin of the PCA is illustrated in Fig. 1.20. (**a**) Persistent trigeminal artery; (**b**) persistent otic artery; (**c**) persistent hypoglossal artery; (**d**) Proatlantal intersegmental artery, Type I (*solid*) and Type II (*dashed*).

      (c) Two main variants.[89] The relative prevalence of the two types is almost equal.[90]
          i. *Saltzman Type I*. The persistent trigeminal artery supplies the PCA and SCA territories. The posterior communicating arteries and the basilar artery proximal to the anastomosis are hypoplastic.
          ii. *Saltzman Type II*. The PCAs are supplied by the posterior communicating arteries and the persistent trigeminal artery joins the basilar artery at the level of the SCAs.
      (d) A less common trigeminal artery variant consists of the superior cerebellar artery arising from the internal carotid.[91]
      (e) Associated with intracranial aneurysms.
      (f) May have an intrasellar component and should not be mistaken for a pituitary mass.[92]

2. Persistent otic artery
   (a) Most rare carotid-basilar anastomosis.
   (b) Extends from the petrous ICA to the basilar system via the internal auditory canal.[93,94]
   (c) The existence of this variant is controversial. Some authors argue that the otic artery does not exist as a separate entity.[95]
3. Persistent hypoglossal artery
   (a) Second most common carotid-basilar anastomosis, seen in 0.03–0.26% of angiograms.[96]
   (b) Extends from the cervical ICA to the basilar artery via the hypoglossal canal.
      i. Arises from the ICA between the carotid bifurcation and C1.
      ii. The posterior communicating arteries may be absent.[97]
      iii. The ipsilateral vertebral artery is usually hypoplastic.
   (c) May be associated with an aneurysm.[98]
4. Proatlantal intersegmental artery
   (a) Extends from the cervical ICA or ECA to the vertebrobasilar system via the foramen magnum. Extremely rare.
   (b) Associated with aplasia or hypoplasia of the vertebral arteries in 50% of cases.[99]
   (c) Type I
      i. Arises from the ICA at C2-3, courses horizontally above the atlas, and gives rise to the ipsilateral vertebral artery.
      ii. More common than Type II.
   (d) Type II
      i. Arises from ECA and joins the vertebral artery at C1.
      ii. May have a common origin with the occipital artery.[100]

Petrous Segment (C2)

The petrous segment extends from the opening of the carotid canal in the skull base to the posterior edge of the foramen lacerum. The vertical subsegment transitions into the horizontal subsegment via the genu of the petrous ICA, which is a 90° bend in the vessel. At the entrance into the carotid canal, the carotid sheath splits into two layers; the inner layer continues as the periosteum of the carotid canal, and the outer layer is continuous with the periosteum of the inferior surface of the skull base. Postganglionic sympathetic fibers (internal carotid nerve) continue to travel with the ICA. A venous plexus (internal carotid artery plexus of Rektorzik) also surrounds the petrous ICA;[101] the existence of this venous plexus has been proposed to effectively dampen the pulsation of the carotid, making it less perceptible by the adjacent hearing apparatus.[102] In fact, anatomic specimens have shown that the venous plexus seems to be most prominent on the side of the vessel facing the cochlea, a finding that lends support to the theory (Fig. 1.17).

1) Subsegments
   (a) Vertical
      i. Average length is 10.5 mm.[103]
   (b) Horizontal
      i. Approximately twice the length of the vertical subsegment; average length is 20.5 mm.[103]
      ii. A 1-cm length of this segment may be exposed in the floor of the middle fossa lateral to the trigeminal nerve, and covered by dura only or a thin layer of cartilage.
2) Branches
   (a) Normal petrous ICA branches are visible on angiography in only 23% of cases.[104] In a cadaver dissection series, the petrous ICA was found to have branches in only 38% of the specimens (a Vidian branch in was found in 30%, and a periosteal branch was present in 8%); the "caroticotympanic artery," was not found in single case.[103]
   (b) Periosteal branch
      i. Arises at the entrance of the ICA into the carotid canal. Found in 8% of the dissections.[103]

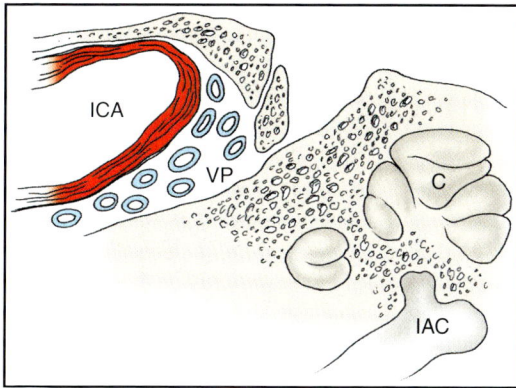

Fig. 1.17 Relationship between the pericarotid venous plexus and the cochlea. Drawing of a histological section through the temporal bone showing that the pericarotid venous plexus (*VP*) is most developed on the side of the ICA facing the cochlea (*C*) IAC, internal auditory canal.

    (c) Caroticotympanic artery
        i. Commonly described branch of the petrous ICA, although its existence has been disputed by some authors.[103]
        ii. Arises from the petrous ICA near the genu and travels superiorly and posteriorly to the middle ear cavity.
        iii. Anastomoses with the ascending pharyngeal artery via the inferior tympanic artery.[104]
    (d) Vidian artery (aka artery of the pterygoid canal)
        i. Small branch that may arise from the horizontal petrous ICA and travels anteriorly within the Vidian (pterygoid) canal to the pterygo-palatine fossa. The Vidian canal is in the floor of the sphenoid sinus and also contains the Vidian nerve.
           – The Vidian nerve is formed by the combination of the deep petrosal nerve (containing sympathetic fibers from the plexus surrounding the ICA) and the greater superficial petrosal nerve (containing parasympathetic and sensory fibers).
        ii. The Vidian artery anastomoses with branches of the IMA.
  3) Variants
    (a) Aberrant ICA.
        i. The ICA enters the temporal bone posterior to the external auditory meatus, ascends between the facial canal and the jugular bulb and passes within the middle ear cavity.
           – May present as a pulsatile mass within the middle ear or with hearing loss; this variant must be kept in mind to avoid a potentially disastrous biopsy procedure.
           – Predilection for woman (67% of patients are female); 15% are bilateral.[105]
           – As discussed above, the so-called "aberrant ICA" is more appropriately termed *ascending pharyngeal artery*, and supplies collateral flow to a segmentally atretic internal carotid.[18]
    (b) Persistent stapedial artery
        i. A rare, persistent embryonic vessel that appears as a branch of the vertical segment of the petrous ICA, travels through the middle ear, and gives rise to the middle meningeal artery.[106]
    (c) Persistent otic artery (described with the other carotid-vertebrobasilar anastomoses, above).

Lacerum Segment (C3)

The lacerum segment is a short part of the artery that extends from the petrous ICA to the cavernous segment, over the foramen lacerum. The foramen lacerum is approximately 1 cm long and is filled with fibrocartilage, amounting to a "closed floor" over which the ICA passes.[103] The foramen lacerum is not a true foramen, as no significant structures (other than the Vidian nerve) travel through it. The lacerum segment is separated from the cavernous segment by the petrolingual ligament. The petrolingual ligament is a small fold of periosteum that extends from the lingula of the sphenoid bone to the petrous apex,[107] and represents a continuation of the periosteum of the carotid canal.[75] The lacerum segment lies inferior to the trigeminal ganglion, and has thus been termed the "trigeminal segment" by some authors.[108] The foramen lacerum is vulnerable to wayward placement of needles or electrodes during percutaneous procedures, such as foramen ovale instrumentation for trigeminal neuralgia.[109] Among patients with basilar skull fractures, the junction between the lacerum and cavernous segments is the most frequently fractured segment of the carotid canal (62% of all carotid canal fractures occur at that site).[110]

1. Subsegments: None.
2. Branches: None.
3. Variants: None.

Cavernous Segment (C4)

The cavernous segment is S-shaped and extends from the superior margin of the petrolingual ligament, through the cavernous sinus, to the proximal dural ring (Fig. 1.18). This portion of the ICA is surrounded by areolar tissue, fat, postganglionic sympathetic fibers, and the interconnecting venous chambers of the cavernous sinus. The ICA rests directly against the lateral surface of the body of the sphenoid bone in a groove called the carotid suclus, which defines the course of the cavernous segment of the ICA.[111] The cavernous ICA also travels directly adjacent to the wall of the sphenoid sinus; a layer of bone less than 0.5-mm thick separates the artery from the sinus in almost 90% of cases, and a complete absence of bone between the artery and the sinus is present in nearly 10%.[111] In some cases, the ICA may actually extend into the sphenoid sinus, an anatomic variant that should be kept in mind during surgery of the sphenoid sinus. The cavernous segment of the ICA forms the greater part of the carotid siphon (Fig. 1.19).

1. Subsegments:[112]
   (a) Posterior vertical
   (b) Posterior bend
   (c) Horizontal
       i. Longest part of the cavernous ICA.
   (d) Anterior bend
   (e) Anterior vertical
2. Branches:
   (a) The most prominent branches of the cavernous ICA can be divided into three groups.[113] These branches are highly variable; the most consistent branches are the posterior and lateral trunks.[112]
       i. Posterior trunk (meningohypophyseal artery) arises from the posterior bend of the cavernous ICA approximately 10 mm distal to the foramen lacerum.[112] All three of the following branches are found in some 70% of dissections:[112]
           – Tentorial artery. This vessel is the most consistent branch of the posterior trunk, being present in 100% of dissections.[114] It has two branches:
               (a) Marginal artery of the tentorium (aka artery of *Bernasconi and Cassinari*).[115] Travels posteriorly along the medial edge of the tentorium. This artery may arise directly from the ICA.

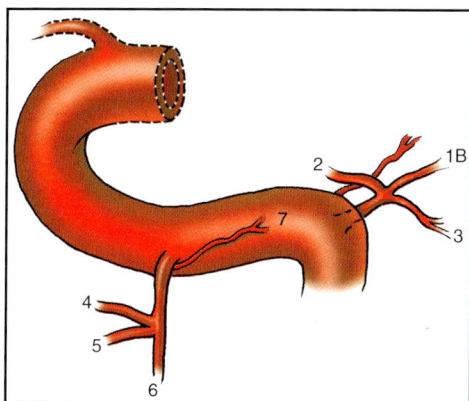

Fig. 1.18 Cavernous internal carotid artery. Lateral view of the cavernous segment of the ICA. Major branches: Posterior trunk: (a) Tentorial artery (*1*), (b) Inferior hypophyseal artery (*2*), and (c) Dorsal meningeal artery (*3*). Lateral trunk: (a) Anteromedial branch (*4*), (b) Anterolateral branch (*5*), and (c) Posterior branch (*6*). Tentorial branch (*7*) may sometimes arise from this part of the cavernous carotid. Medial branch group is not shown here because they arise from the opposite side of the ICA from that shown.

                (b) Basal tentorial artery. Travels laterally along the border between the tentorium and the petrous ridge. Anastomoses with the middle meningeal artery and the dural arteries of the posterior fossa.[6]

        – Inferior hypophyseal artery

                (a) Travels in a superior and medial direction to supply the posterior lobe of the pituitary gland.[116] It anastomoses with the superior hypophyseal artery, the medial branch group, and the contralateral inferior hypophyseal artery.

        – Dorsal meningeal artery. Found traversing Dorello's canal in 75% of dissections.[117] Two branches that supply dura of the skull base:

                (a) Lateral clival artery: supplies dura around Durello's canal and abducens nerve.

                (b) Dorsal (aka medial) clival artery: supplies superior clival dura.

        – Recurrent artery of foramen lacerum: Tiny vessel that may anastamose with the carotid branch of the ascending pharyngeal.[19]

      ii. Lateral trunk (aka the inferolateral trunk, artery of the inferior cavernous sinus, or lateral main stem) arises from the lateral aspect of the horizontal segment and travels superior to the abducens nerve to supply cranial nerves within the cavernous sinus. It is found in about 66% of dissections.[113]

        – *Anteromedial branch.* May anastomose with the ophthalmic artery via its recurrent meningeal branch.

        – *Anterolateral branch.* May anastomose with the artery of the foramen rotundum.

        – *Posterior branch.* May anastomose with the cavernous branches of the middle and accessory meningeal arteries.

        – *Superior branch.* Very small vessel that may anastomose with ophthalmic.[19]

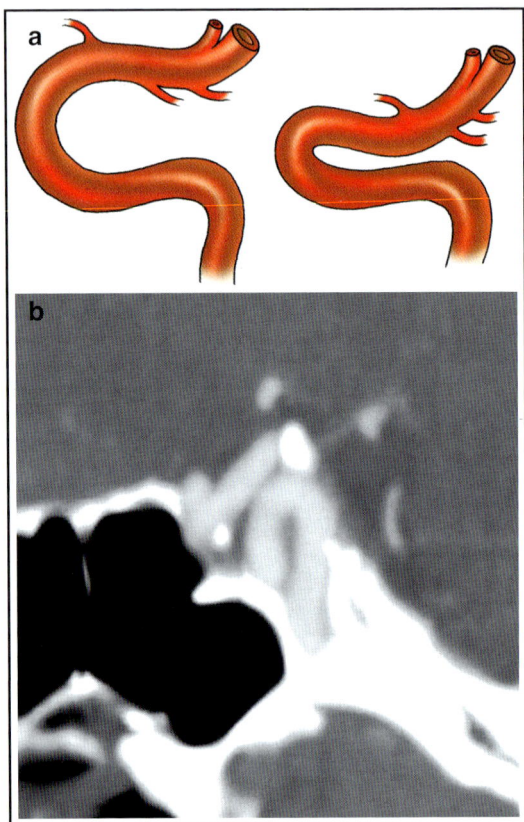

Fig. 1.19 Carotid siphon. The *carotid siphon* is an S-shaped part to the ICA; it begins at the posterior bend of the cavernous ICA and ends at the ICA bifurcation. It can have an open configuration (**a**) or a closed one (**b**), with obvious implications for the ease of endovascular navigation in this region. A closed siphon anatomy can be attributed in some cases to exaggerated tortuosity of the ICA, as can be seen in patients with advanced age or fibromuscular dysplasia[122]. A CTA image of a closed siphon in a patient with an ophthalmic segment aneurysm (*below*).

      iii. Medial branch group (aka capsular arteries of McConnell) arises from the most superior portion of the cavernous segment, and supplies the pituitary gland. They are found in only about 28% of dissections.[113]
      iv. Other cavernous ICA branches:
         – Ophthalmic artery (found to arise from the cavernous segment, instead of the ophthalmic segment), in about 8% of cases.[118]
         – Recurrent artery of the foramen lacerum.
         – Artery of the Gasserian ganglion.
3. Variants:
    (a) Kissing intrasellar ICAs
      i. The cavernous ICA may extend beyond the medial wall of the cavernous sinus and run medially in the sella turcica. The ICAs

Angio-Anatomic Correlate! Lateral Trunk Collaterals (Fig. 1.20)

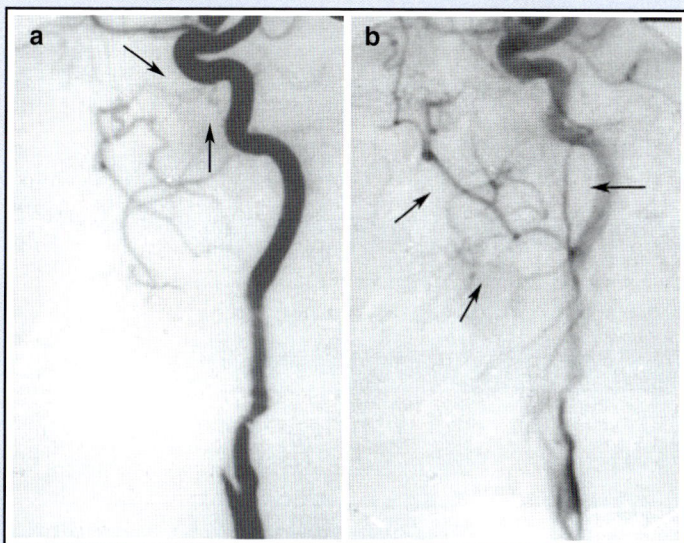

Fig. 1.20 The lateral trunk provides potential collateral flow between the cavernous segment of the internal carotid artery and external carotid artery branches. Carotid artery injection (**a**) in this patient with prior external carotid ligation shows filling of anterolateral and posterior branches of the lateral trunk (*arrows*). Later phase of arteriogram (**b**) shows these branches reconstitute multiple external carotid branches (*arrows*).

approach within 4 mm of each other within the sella in some 10% of cases.[119] This variant is associated with acromegaly.[120]

   (b) Intercavernous ICA anastomoses
      i. Hypoplasia or agenesis of the ICA can be associated with an intercavernous ICA anastomosis, in which a large collateral vessel connects the cavernous carotid arteries.[81,82,121,122]
   (c) Persistent trigeminal artery (described with the other carotid–vertebrobasilar anastomoses, above).

Clinoidal Segment (C5)

The clinoidal segment comprises a tiny wedge-shaped part of the ICA between the proximal and distal dural rings (Fig. 1.21). The anterior clinoid process lies superior and lateral to the clinoidal ICA, over the part of widest separation between the dural rings. Although this segment is described as "interdural," the ICA is surrounded in this region by a dural collar that contains venous tributaries of the cavernous sinus, known as the clinoid venous plexus.[114] These venous channels extend to the distal dural ring and have implications for surgery in this region.

   1. Subsegments: None
   2. Branches: The ophthalmic artery may arise from the clinoidal segment in rare cases.[1]
   3. Variants: None.

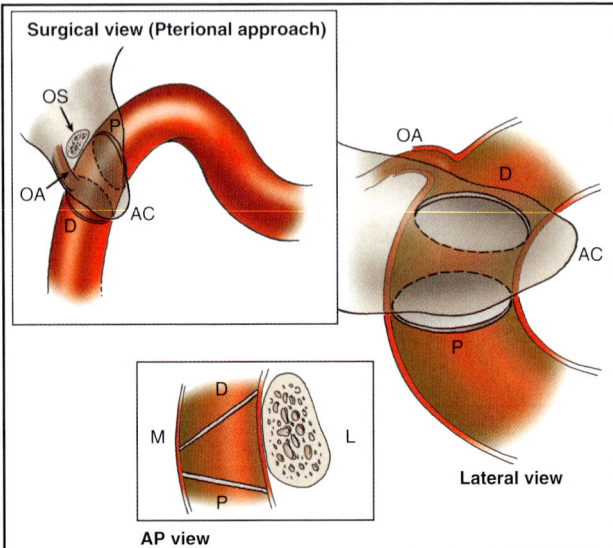

Fig. 1.21 Clinoidal segment. The clinoidal segment is defined by the proximal (*P*) and distal (*D*) *dural rings*, which are related to one another at an angle, like two dinner plates nearly touching on one edge. The space between the dural rings is wide on the lateral aspect of the ICA and small on the medial aspect, where the dural rings come closest together. The medial part of the distal dural ring is incomplete; this region, which includes the proximal portion of the ophthalmic segment, is known as the "carotid cave" and is a site for aneurysm formation.[108,289] The anterior clinoid process (*AC*) extends like a thumb over the clinoidal segment; the relationships between the dural rings and the anterior clinoid are variable. *OA* ophthalmic artery, *OS* optic strut, *M* medial, *L* lateral.

Ophthalmic Segment (C6)

The ophthalmic segment is the most proximal intradural part of the ICA and extends from the distal dural ring to the origin of the posterior communicating artery. The average length is 9.6 mm.[74] The optic nerve travels superior and medial to the ICA in this region, and the sphenoid sinus is anterior and inferior. The optic strut is a bony process that extends between the base of the anterior clinoid to the body of the sphenoid bone. The optic strut separates the optic canal from the superior orbital fissure, and the identification of the optic strut on CT can help distinguish cavernous segment aneurysms from ophthalmic segment aneurysms.[123]

1. Subsegments: None.
2. Branches:
   (a) *Ophthalmic artery* (Fig. 1.22)
      i. The ophthalmic artery arises from the anterior aspect of the ICA medial to the anterior clinoid process. The vessel originates distal to or at the distal dural ring in ≥90% of cases; in about 8% of cases, the vessel arises from the cavernous segment.[118] The artery then usually travels inferior and lateral to the optic nerve in the optic canal. Within the orbit, the ophthalmic artery loops inferior and lateral to the optic nerve in 83% of cases, and then approaches the globe along

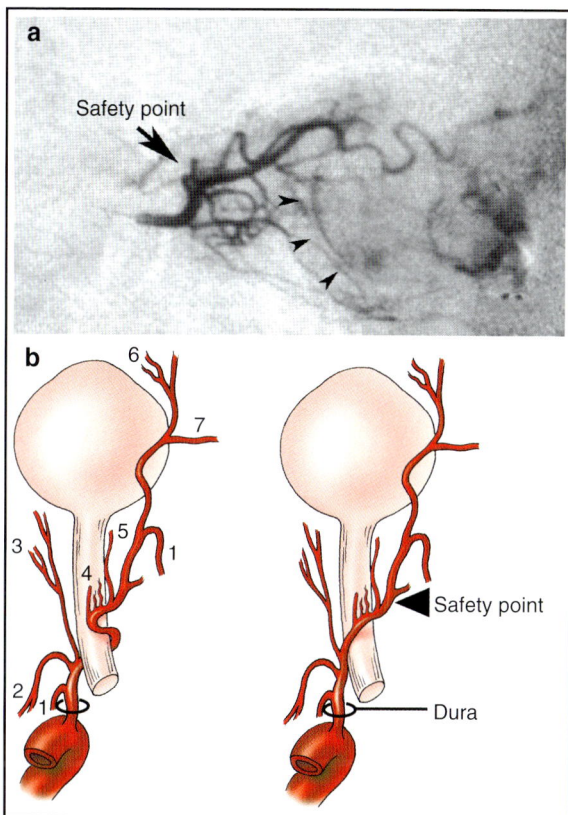

Fig. 1.22 Ophthalmic artery. Lateral view of a selective ophthalmic artery angiogram (*above*) and superior views of the ophthalmic artery (OA, **a**). On the angiogram, note the typical upward course of the OA as it crosses over the optic nerve (*arrow*) and the choroidal blush (*arrowheads*). In 83% of cases, the OA passes around the lateral aspect of the optic nerve (**b**, *left*); in the remaining cases the OA stays medial to the optic nerve (**b**, *right*). Significant branches include: (*1*) Recurrent meningeal arteries, (*2*) posterior ethmoidal artery, (*3*) muscular branches, (*4*) central retinal artery, (*5*) ciliary arteries (anterior and posterior), (*6*) lacrimal artery, and (*7*) anterior falx artery. The OA can be divided into three segments:[290] (*1*) Segment 1. Extends from the entrance of the OA into the orbit to the point where the vessel changes direction to cross over or under the optic nerve. (*2*) Segment 2. Short part of the vessel as it passes over or under the nerve. (*3*) Segment 3. Extends from the bend in the vessel on the medial aspect of the optic nerve, to the edge of the orbit. The *safety point*, beyond which embolization can be done with minimal risk of embolization of the retina, is generally thought to be anywhere beyond Segment 2.[291]

> its medial aspect. In 17% of cases, the ophthalmic artery stays medial and inferior to the optic nerve throughout its course.[118]
>
> ii. The diameter of the ophthalmic artery at the origin averages 1.4 mm (range, 0.9–2.1 mm).[124]
>
> iii. Ophthalmic artery branches. The ophthalmic artery branches are highly variable, and anastomoses with the branches of the external

carotid artery are extensive. Ophthalmic artery branches can be divided into three groups:

1. Ocular group
   (a) Central retinal artery
      i. Arises from the ophthalmic artery as a single trunk or in common with a posterior ciliary artery, then penetrates the optic nerve sheath to supply the retina.[124] The central retinal artery is a terminal branch of the ophthalmic artery and a true end-artery, with no appreciable collateral circulation. Occlusion of the central retinal artery usually results in loss of vision.
      ii. The inner diameter averages 400 μm (range, 300–600 μm).[124]
   (b) Ciliary arteries
      i. Divided into posterior and anterior ciliary arteries, these vessels produce the *choroidal blush* seen on lateral angiography.
2. Orbital group
   (a) Lacrimal artery
      i. The lacrimal artery arises from the ophthalmic artery adjacent to the optic nerve and passes along the lateral rectus muscle to irrigate the lacrimal gland and conjunctiva. It anastomoses anteriorly with branches of the superficial temporal artery and with multiple branches of the internal maxillary artery.[125]
      ii. A significant branch of the lacrimal artery is the recurrent meningeal artery, which travels back and out of the orbit through the superior orbital fissure, and anastomoses with the middle meningeal artery.[126]
      iii. Zygomaticofacial branches anastamose with deep temporal and transverse facial branches.[126]
   (b) Muscular branches
      i. Arteries that irrigate the extraocular muscles and periosteum of the orbit; each branch is named for the structure it irrigates (e.g., muscular branch to the medial rectus).
3. Extraorbital group
   (a) Ethmoidal arteries
      i. These vessels supply the upper nasal mucosa and anastomose with branches of the sphenopalatine branches of the internal maxillary artery. They also perforate the cribriform plate to irrigate the dura of the anterior fossa.
      ii. Anterior ethmoidal artery
         1. Gives rise to the anterior falx artery, which enters the intracranial space via the foramen caecum.
      iii. Posterior ethmoidal artery
         1. Anastomoses with branches of the sphenopalatine artery.
   (b) Palpebral artery
      i. Divides into medial, inferior medial, and superior medial palpebral branches.[118] These branches anastomose with the frontal branch of the superficial temporal artery and the infraorbital branch of the internal maxillary artery.
   (c) Terminal portion of the ophthalmic artery
      i. The ophthalmic artery terminates by dividing into the
         1. Supratrochlear branch
            a. Anastomoses with branches of the superficial temporal artery.
         2. Dorsal nasal branch
            a. Anastomoses with branches of the facial artery.

iv. Ophthalmic artery variants
Several anomalous origins of the ophthalmic artery have been described. The most common is a middle meningeal artery origin, seen in nearly 16% of cases in a dissection series[127] (conversely, an ophthalmic origin of the middle meningeal artery is seen in about 0.5% of the angiograms.).[46] Other reported anomalous origins include the cavernous ICA, the MCA, ACA, PCA, and the basilar artery.[118]

(b) *Superior hypophyseal artery*

i. There is an average of 1.8 superior hypophyseal arteries arising from the ICA, and most originate within 5 mm of the ophthalmic artery origin.[128] Superior hypophyseal arteries appear in two forms: in 42% of cases, a single large artery branches like a candelabra into smaller branches, and in the remaining cases, two or three hypophyseal arteries are present.[128] The vessels then travel toward the origin of the pituitary stalk and connect with the branches of the contralateral superior hypophyseal artery and the posterior communicating arteries to form a circuminfundibular anastomosis.[128] The superior hypophyseal arteries and the circuminfundibular plexus are distributed to the pituitary stalk and the anterior lobe of the pituitary (the inferior hypophyseal branch of the meningohypophyseal artery irrigates the posterior lobe).[74]

(c) *Perforating branches*

i. Several perforating branches arising from the ophthalmic segment are not properly included with the superior hypophyseal arteries. They arise from the posterior or medial aspect of the ICA and primarily irrigate the optic chiasm, the optic nerve, the floor of the third ventricle, and the optic tract.[74]

3. Variants: Most anatomic variants of the ophthalmic segment of the ICA amount to anomalous origins of the ophthalmic artery (see above). A fenestration of the ophthalmic segment of the ICA has been reported.[129]

Communicating Segment (C7)

The communicating segment begins just proximal to the origin of the posterior communicating artery and ends with the bifurcation of the ICA into the ACA and the MCA. The average length is 10.6 mm.[74]

1. Branches

(a) *Posterior communicating artery*

i. The posterior communicating artery arises from the ICA an average of 9.6 mm distal to the ophthalmic artery and 9.7 mm proximal to the ICA bifurcation.[74] It travels posteromedially an average distance of 12 mm to join the PCA at the junction between the P1 and P2 segments.

ii. Branches. The number of perforating arteries ranges from four to 14, with an average of 7.8.[74] These branches terminate in the floor of the third ventricle, the posterior perforated substance, optic tract, pituitary stalk, and optic chiasm.[130] These perforators reach the thalamus, hypothalamus, and internal capsule. These arteries are called anterior thalamoperforators to distinguish them from the thalamoperforators that arise from the P1 segment. The largest and the most constant of these is the premamillary artery.[88]

iii. Variants

1. Persistent fetal origin. A "fetal configuration" is defined as a prominent P-comm artery that gives rise to, and has the same diameter of, the P2 segment of the PCA (Fig. 1.23). This anatomy is present in 18–22% of cases.[88] The ipsilateral P1 segment is usually hypoplastic.

2. Infundibulum. A funnel-shaped origin of the P-comm artery (see below).

3. Hypoplasia. Although a "hypoplastic" P-comm artery is present in up to 34% of the dissections, the complete absence of the vessel is very rare.[88]

4. Absence. Complete absence of the P-comm artery is found in 0.6% of the dissections.[131]

5. Fenestration of the P-comm artery has been reported.[132]

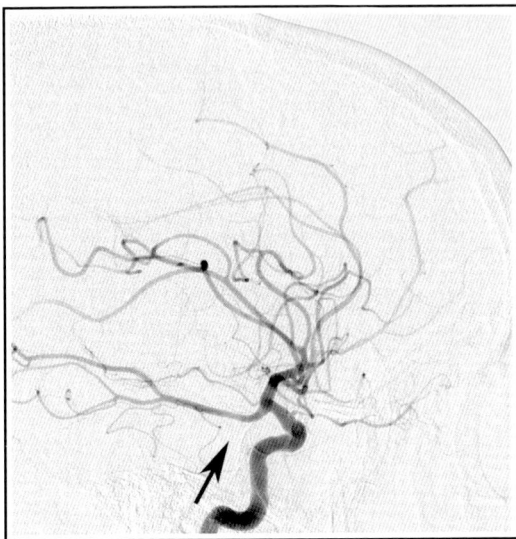

Fig. 1.23 Persistent fetal configuration of the posterior communicating artery. A posterior communicating artery is a "fetal" variant (*arrow*) when the diameter of the vessel is equal to the diameter of the P2 segment it connects to.

(b) *Anterior choroidal artery*

    i. The anterior choroidal artery (Fig. 1.24) arises from the posterolateral aspect of the ICA, 2–4 mm distal to the posterior communicating artery, and an average of 5.6 mm proximal to the ICA bifurcation.[74] The diameter of the vessel averages 1.0 mm,[74] and is duplicated in 4% of cases.[133] The anterior choroidal artery has two segments:

        1. *Cisternal segment.* From the ICA, the vessel travels in a posterior direction, sweeping first medially, then laterally to pass around the cerebral peduncle. The anterior choroidal artery then angles upward as it passes through the choroidal fissure to enter the temporal horn of the lateral ventricle. The cisternal segment averages 24 mm in length and gives rise to an average of eight perforating branches;[133] these are the branches of the anterior choroidal artery that irrigate most of the vital structures that are vulnerable to ischemic injury with anterior choroidal artery occlusion.

        2. *Intraventricular segment.* Within the ventricle, the anterior choroidal artery travels with the choroid plexus, anastomosing with branches of the lateral posterior choroidal artery in this region. The artery then arcs up and around the thalamus, and in some cases it reaches as far as the Foramen of Monro and anastomoses with branches of the medial posterior choroidal artery (from the posterior cerebral). Branches from the intraventricular segment supply to the optic tract, lateral geniculate body and thalamus.[134]

    ii. Territories

        1. The anterior choroidal artery sends branches, in decreasing order of frequency, to the optic tract, cerebral peduncle, lateral geniculate body, uncus, and temporal lobe.[74] The brain structures irrigated by these branches include the optic radiation, globus pallidus, midbrain, thalamus, and posterior limb of the internal capsule. Occlusion of the anterior choroidal artery can produce contralateral hemiplegia, hemianesthesia, hemianopia,

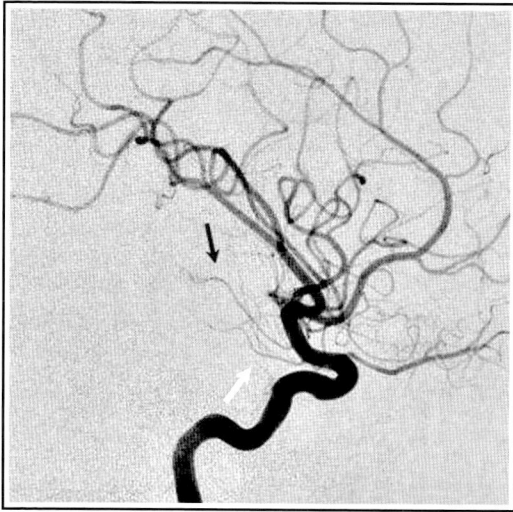

Fig. 1.24 Anterior choroidal artery. On a lateral angiogram, the cisternal segment of the anterior choroidal artery has a characteristic gentle, undulating appearance as it passes around the cerebral peduncle. A kink appears in the vessel (the plexal point, (*black arrow*)) where it enters the temporal horn. The posterior communicating artery (*white arrow*) travels inferior and parallel to the anterior choroidal artery.

memory loss, and somnolence. Regions of the brain affected by the anterior choroidal artery occlusion on CT include the posterior limb of the internal capsule, the retrolenticular portion of the internal capsule, the internal portion of the globus pallidus, and the lateral thalamus.[135] The severity of neurologic change after occlusion of the vessel is highly variable, however, presumably because of varying anastomoses with the posterior choroidal arteries as well as the PCA (and less commonly, the ACA and MCA). Irving S. Cooper, M.D., a functional neurosurgeon, demonstrated this variability.[136] During a subtemporal approach for a cerebral pedunculotomy to treat a patient with Parkinson's disease, Cooper occluded the anterior choroidal artery because of an inadvertent injury to the vessel. The patient awoke after surgery with complete resolution of his tremor and rigidity and without any persistent hemiparesis. Deliberate occlusion of the anterior choroidal artery was done for the treatment of Parkinson's disease in the 1950s.[137]

    iii. Variants
       1. Ectopic origin. Seen in 4% of the dissections.[134]
         (a) The anterior choroidal artery may originate from the MCA or PCA.
         (b) Rarely, the anterior choroidal artery may originate from the ICA proximal to the posterior communicating artery.[138]
       2. Absence of the anterior choroidal artery is seen in 3% of angiograms.[139]
       3. Hyperplasia, in which the anterior choroidal artery supplies part of the PCA territory, is seen in 2.3% of angiograms.[139]
  (c) *Perforating branches*
    i. Perforators arising from the communicating segment extend to the optic tract, floor of the third ventricle, and the anterior perforated substance.[74]

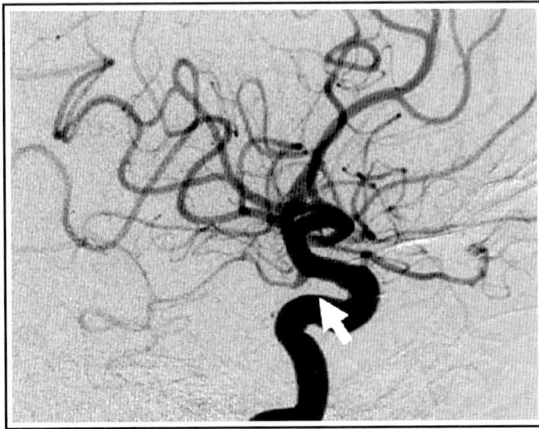

Fig. 1.25 Posterior communicating artery infundibulum (*arrow*).

The Infundibulum: A Normal Variant

An infundibulum is a conical, triangular, or funnel-shaped dilatation at the origin of an artery, and is found most commonly at the junction of the posterior communication artery and ICA (Fig. 1.25). At this location, an infundibulum is defined as a symmetric bulge at the origin of the P-comm, with a maximum diameter of 3 mm.[140,141] The authors of this handbook have also found infundibula at the P-comm-PCA junction, the P2 segment, in the anterior communicating artery complex, the ophthalmic artery origin, and at the origin of the anterior choroidal artery. The reported prevalence of infundibula on otherwise normal angiograms is 7–15%.[142–144] Bilateral P-comm infundibula are present in 25% of cases. Angiographic criteria for infundibular dilation include round or conical in shape, ≤3 mm in the maximum diameter, without aneurysmal neck, and with a posterior communicating artery arising from its apex.[140]

1.5.   Circle of Willis

The circle of Willis is the ring of interconnecting vessels encircling the pituitary infundibulum providing important collateral circulation between the carotid territories and the vertebrobasilar system (Fig. 1.26). It is actually a nonagon, a nine-sided structure, rather than a circle. Although it bears the name of Thomas Willis (named in honor of Willis by his student Lower), who described the structure in 1664 in a publication illustrated by Sir Christopher Wren,[145] earlier anatomists had recognized an arterial circle at the base of the brain.[146] Although a complete circle of Willis is present in some 90% of individuals, a well-developed and symmetric circle is found in ≤50% of cases.[147] In most 60% of cases, at least one component of the circle is relatively hypoplastic and diminished in its capacity to provide collateral flow.[1] Asymmetry of the circle of Willis results in significant asymmetric flow[148] and is an important factor in the development of intracranial aneurysms and in ischemic stroke. Patients with aneurysms are more likely to have asymmetry or an anomaly of the circle.[149] The

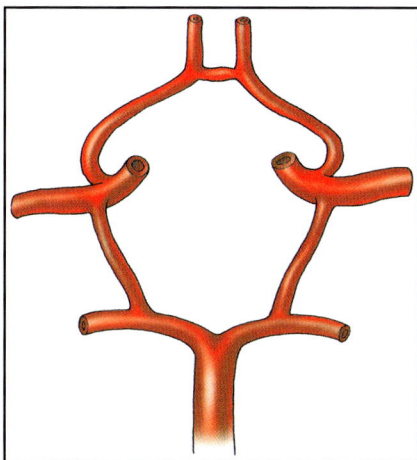

Fig. 1.26 Circle of Willis.

Table 1.6 Sources of asymmetry in the circle of Willis

Vessel	Variant	Incidence
A1 segment	Hypoplastic	10%[152]
	Absent	1–2%[1]
A-comm artery	Absent	5%[171]
P-comm artery	Hyperplastic (Fetal)	18–22%[88]
	Hypoplastic	34%[88]
	Absent	0.6%[131]
ICA	Hypoplastic	0.079%[83]
	Absent	0.01%[81]
P1 segment	Hypoplastic	15–22%
	Absent	Rare[131]

presence of a nonfunctional anterior collateral pathway in the circle of Willis in patients with ICA occlusive disease is strongly associated with ischemic stroke.[150] The individual components of the circle are discussed separately in this handbook. Anatomic variations causing asymmetry of the circle are listed in Table 1.6.

Anterior Cerebral Artery

Several classification schemes for the ACA have been described. The simplest and most common system includes three segments (Fig. 1.27):

1. A1. From ICA to anterior communicating artery
2. A2. From anterior communicating artery to the origins of the pericallosal and supramarginal arteries
3. A3. Distal branches

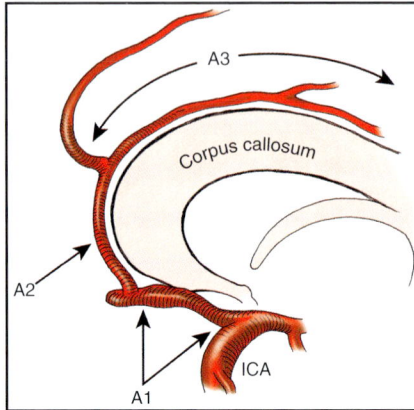

Fig. 1.27 Anterior cerebral artery. Left lateral oblique view of the left ACA.

A1 Segment and Anterior Communicating Artery Complex

The A1 segment (aka the precommunicating segment)[1] extends from the ICA bifurcation in a medial and superior direction to its junction with the anterior communicating artery within or just inferior to the interhemispheric fissure. It travels superior to the optic chiasm or optic nerves and inferior to the anterior perforated substance. The A-comm complex is highly variable and may take one of the four main patterns (Fig. 1.28). The A-comm artery averages 4.0 mm in length and 1.7 mm in diameter.[151]

1. Branches
   (a) A1 perforating branches can be divided into superior and inferior branches
       i. Some 2–15 superior branches are medial lenticulostriate arteries that travel superiorly and posteriorly into the anterior perforated substance and supply the anterior hypothalamus, septum pellucidum, anterior commissure, fornix, and the anterior striatum.[152]
       ii. Inferior branches supply the optic chiasm and optic nerves.
   (b) A-comm artery branches
       i. Perforating branches of the A-comm artery can be divided into subcallosal, hypothalamic, and chiasmatic branches, according to their vascular territories.[151] The subcallosal branch is usually single and the largest branch of the A-comm artery; it supplies the septum pellucidum, columns of the fornix, corpus callosum and lamina terminalis.[153] The hypothalamic branches are smaller and multiple. A chiasmatic branch is present in only 20% of cases.[151]
   (c) The recurrent artery of Heubner, most often an A2 branch, may arise from the A1 segment in up to 17% of cases and from the ACA-A-comm junction in 35% of cases.[154,155] (See below for further discussion of Heubner).
2. Variants
   (a) A1 variants
       i. Asymmetry. The left and right A1 segments are asymmetric in size in up to 80% of cases.[6] Right A1 segments tend to be longer, more tortuous, deviated and narrow than left A1 segments.[156] About 10% of the A1 vessels are hypoplastic (defined as having a diameter of ≤1.5 mm).[152]
       ii. Absence. Absence of one A1 segment is seen in 1–2% of cases.[1]

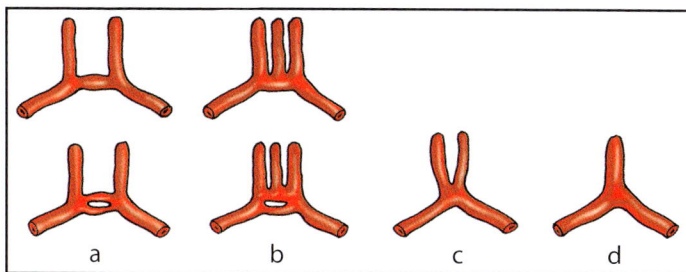

Fig. 1.28 Anterior communicating artery complex. In most cases, the A-comm complex assumes one of the four configurations[151]. (**a**) A single or duplicated A-comm forms a bridge between the ACAs. (**b**) A single large branch arises from the A-comm. (**c**) The A-comm vessel is not present, and the two ACAs join together directly. (**d**) Azygos ACA.

      iii. Persistent olfactory artery. Rare anomaly in which a persistent primitive olfactory artery travels from the ICA, along the olfactory tract, to supply the distal ACA territory.[157] May be associated with an aneurysm.[158]

      iv. Infraoptic ACA. In rare cases the A1 segment may travel inferior to or through the optic nerve.[159–161] Associated with aneurysms (Fig. 1.29).

      v. Fenestration of the A1 segment is rare and is associated with aneurysms.[162–164]

      vi. Accessory ACA. An atypical branch of the ICA courses under the optic nerve and ACA to give rise to the orbitofrontal and frontopolar arteries.[165]

      vii. Anomalous origins of the A1 from the cavernous ICA,[166] from the ICA at or proximal to the ophthalmic artery,[167] and from the contralateral ICA[168] have been reported.

(b) A-comm artery variants. Some 227 A-comm artery complex variations have been described.[169] A "normal" A-comm artery, in which single vessel forms a link between two non-anomalous ACAs, is present in only about 40% of cases.[151,154,169,170] Anomalous A-comm anatomy is present in the remaining 60% of cases. These patterns included the plexiform (i.e., multiple complex vascular channels, 33%), dimple (i.e., incomplete fenestration, 33%), fenestration (21%), duplication (18%), string (18%), fusion (12%), median artery of the corpus callosum (6%), and azygos ACA (3%).[151] The A-comm artery is absent in some 5% of cases.[171]

A2 Segment

The A2 segment travels in a vertical direction from the A-comm artery to its division into the pericallosal and callosomarginal arteries, adjacent to the genu of the corpus callosum. Defined in this way, the A2 segment is analogous to the M1 segment of the MCA, which is defined in this handbook as ending with its bifurcation into the superior and inferior divisions. Although the authors of this handbook prefer this definition of the A2 segment, it is somewhat problematic, as some 18% of the hemispheres do not have a definite callosomarginal branch.[172] Other authors have defined the A2–A3 junction as the part of the ACA immediately anterior to the corpus callosum genu[i] or at the junction between the rostrum and genu of the corpus callosum.[6]

The length of the A2 segment averages 43 mm when it is defined as extending from the A-comm to the origin of the callosomarginal artery.[172] The left and right A2 segments usually travel together in the interhemispheric fissure, although the right A2 is more often (72% of cases) anterior to the left A2 in the sagittal plane.[172]

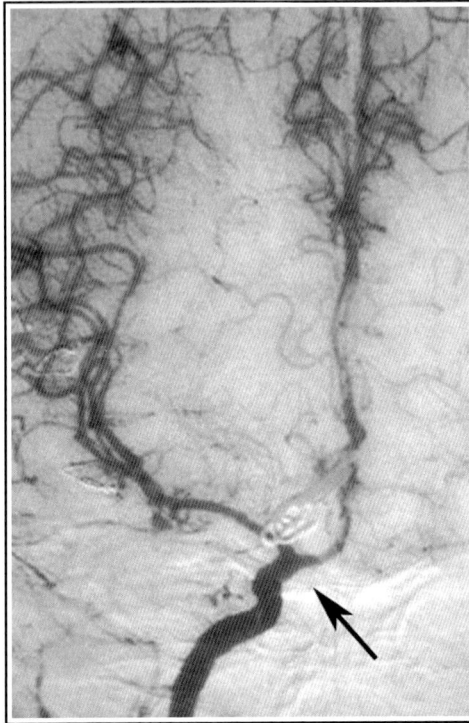

Fig. 1.29 Infraoptic anterior cerebral artery. The infraoptic ACA originates in an unusually proximal location from the ICA (*arrow*).

1. Branches
    (a) *Perforators*. Perforating branches of the A2 segment are located along the first 5 mm of the segment, and penetrate the brain at the gyrus rectus and olfactory sulcus.[154]
    (b) *Recurrent artery of Heubner*. This artery, which is a large lenticulostriate artery, arises from the A2 segment in most (57–78%) cases.[152,154] It doubles back and runs in the opposite direction to the A1 segment to enter the lateral anterior perforated substance lateral to the ICA bifurcation.[155] The artery supplies the head of the caudate nucleus, anterior limb of the internal capsule, and the anterior third of the putamen.[173] Although it is often not large enough to be seen on angiography (Fig. 1.30), it is regularly identified during surgery of the A-comm complex; inadvertent occlusion of the vessel can occur by pinching the vessel during retraction of the frontal lobe. Isolated infarction of the territory of this vessel can be clinically silent, or produce a hemiparesis that is most prominent in the face and upper extremity.[6]
    (c) *Orbitofrontal artery*. This artery is the first cortical branch of the A2 segment, and may appear as two or three vessels rather than single branch.[172] The artery runs close to the midline in an anterior direction to the gyrus rectus, olfactory bulb, and medial aspect of the inferior frontal lobe.
    (d) *Frontopolar artery*. This artery may also appear as a group of vessels and usually arises from the distal A2 segment, below the corpus callosum. It travels anteriorly and superiorly towards the frontal pole.

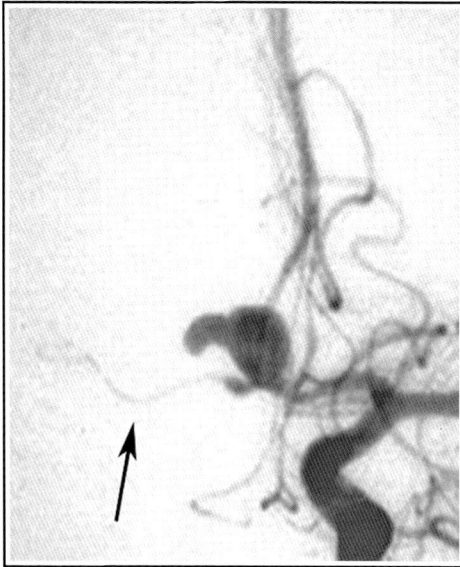

Fig. 1.30 Recurrent artery of Heubner. Left carotid injection with filling of contralateral A2 segment via the A-comm artery. The recurrent artery of Heubner is visible (*arrow*) because it is not obscured by other arteries. Clipping of the aneurysm could put the recurrent artery of Heubner at risk.

2. Variants
   (a) *Bihemispheric ACA.* In this variant, one A2 segment is hypoplastic and the other A2 vessel irrigates both the hemispheres. Present in up to 7% of cases.[172]
   (b) *Azygos ACA.* This is defined as a single unpaired A2 segment that arises from the junction of the A1s (Fig. 1.31). It is present in ≤1% of the general population;[174] as many as 41% of patients with an azygos ACA have a terminal aneurysm.[175,176] This anomaly is also associated with holoprosencephaly.[177]
   (c) *Duplicated A2.* More than one A2 segment has been reported in up to 13% of cases.[1] In some cases, this may represent persistence of the primitive median artery of the corpus callosum,[1] which is found in 6% of cases.[151]
   (d) *Superior anterior communicating artery.* An anomalous communicating vessel between the ACAs near the corpus callosum has been described and is associated with aneurysms.[178]

A3 Branches

The "A3 branches" include all the ACA branches distal to the origin of the pericallosal and callosomarginal arteries (Fig. 1.32). The distal ACA may be further subdivided into A4 and A5 segments;[76,172] the A3 segment is defined as the part of the ACA that extends around the genu of the corpus callosum, and the A4 and A5 segments comprise the part of the ACA that travels posteriorly over the corpus callosum. The A4 and A5 segments are separated by the coronal suture.[172] The distal ACA branches have extensive anastomoses with distal branches of the MCA and PCA. These connecting arteries, in the furthest reaches of the intracranial circulation, comprise the watershed zones; the corresponding territories of the brain are the most vulnerable to ischemia during hemodynamic failure.

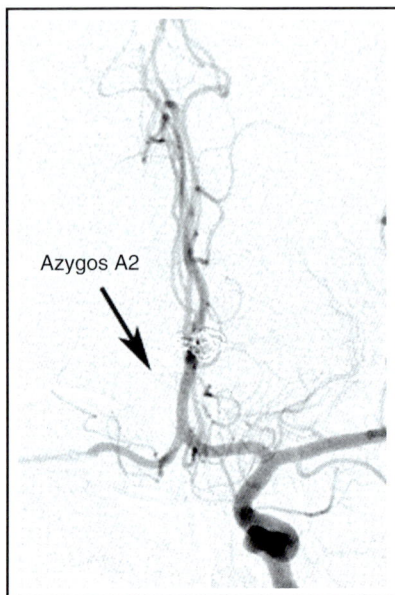

Fig. 1.31 Azygos anterior cerebral artery. In an azygos anterior cerebral artery, both A1 segments join to form single A2 segment.

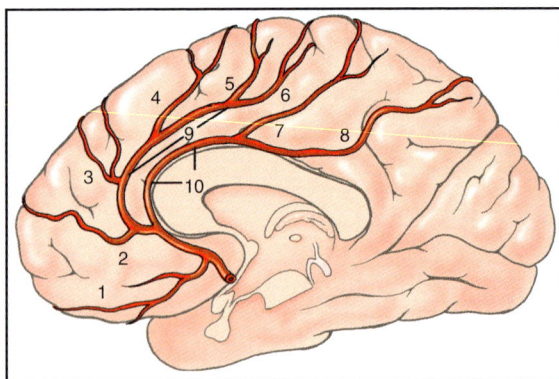

Fig. 1.32 Distal ACA branches. (*1*) Orbitofrontal artery; (*2*) frontopolar artery; (*3*) anterior internal frontal artery; (*4*) middle internal frontal artery; (*5*) posterior internal frontal artery; (*6*) paracentral artery; (*7*) superior parietal artery; (*8*) inferior parietal artery; (*9*) callosomarginal artery; (*10*) pericallosal artery.

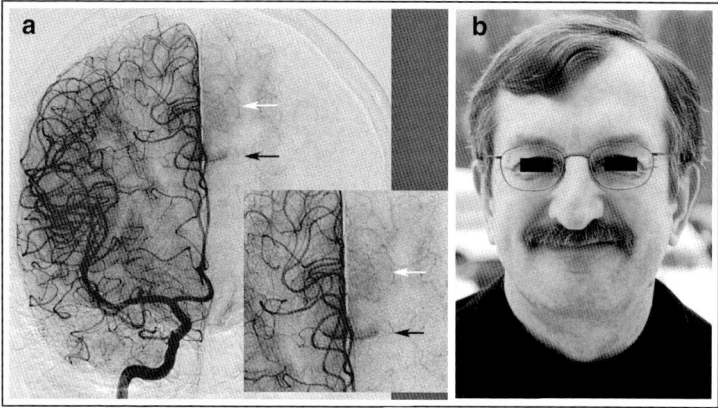

Fig. 1.33 The smile and the mustache. During the late arterial phase of an AP angiogram (high magnification, *inset*), the branches of the pericallosal artery curve upward along the surface of the corpus callosum, forming a smile (**a**, *black arrows*). Branches of the callosomarginal artery curve downward, forming a mustache (**a**, *white arrows*). This pattern is nicely demonstrated in a photograph of someone looking quite a bit like the senior author of this handbook (**b**). *Black bars* have been placed across his eyes to protect his privacy and to comply with HIPAA regulations.

1. Branches
    (a) *Pericallosal artery*. The pericallosal artery is the main trunk of the ACA as it passes posteriorly over the corpus callosum. It gives off multiple small branches ("short callosal arteries")[172] that travel laterally along the corpus callosum (Fig. 1.33) and anastomose with the splenial artery (the "posterior pericallosal branch"), a branch of the PCA. Infrequently, a "long callosal artery" may be present, which is a branch of and runs parallel to the pericallosal artery.[172]
    (b) *Callosomarginal artery*. The callosomarginal artery is the second largest distal branch of the ACA, after the pericallosal artery. It travels superiorly over the cingulate gyrus to run in a posterior direction within the cingulate sulcus. It is absent in 18% of hemispheres.[172]
    (c) *Internal frontal branches*. These branches are identified according to which part of the superior frontal gyrus they supply. They may arise from the pericallosal or callosomarginal artery.
        i. Anterior internal frontal arteries
        ii. Middle internal frontal arteries
        iii. Posterior internal frontal arteries
    (d) *Paracentral artery*. This vessel arises from the pericallosal or callosomarginal artery midway between the genu and splenium of the corpus callosum, to supply the paracentral lobule.
    (e) *Parietal arteries*. These are the final and most distal branches of the ACA. They supply the medial aspect of the hemisphere above the corpus callosum and most of the precuneus.[179] They anastomose with the parietooccipital branch of the PCA. They can be divided into:
        i. Superior parietal artery
        ii. Inferior parietal artery
2. Variants
    (a) Branches to the contralateral hemisphere are found in 64% of brains.[172]
    (b) Although the anatomy of the distal ACA branches are highly variable, true developmental anomalies in this region are uncommon.[1]

1.6.   Middle Cerebral Artery

Most classification schemes divide the MCA into four segments. The authors of this handbook favor the following system (Fig. 1.34):

1. M1 From ICA to the bifurcation (or trifurcation)
2. M2 From the MCA bifurcation to the circular sulcus of the insula
3. M3 From the circular sulcus to the superficial aspect of the sylvian fissure
4. M4 Cortical branches

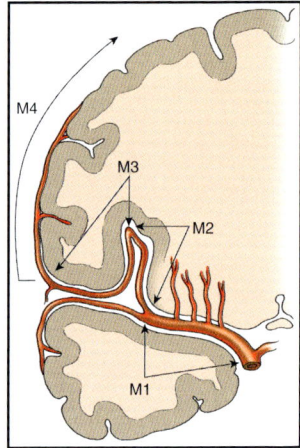

Fig. 1.34 Middle cerebral artery.

M1 Segment

The M1 segment (aka horizontal segment or sphenoidal segment)[180] arises from the ICA and travels in a lateral direction, parallel to the sphenoid wing, and terminates by dividing into the M2 segments. The M1 origin is usually twice the size of the A1 origin.[1] Although most anatomic studies define the M1 segment as the ending where the MCA branches take a 90° turn within the sylvian fissure[76,180] (and thus having both *pre*bifurcation and *post*bifurcation subsegments), the division point of the main MCA trunk is considered by most clinicians to be the M1/M2 junction.[6] The MCA bifurcates in 71% of cases, trifurcates in 20% of cases, and divides into four branches in 9% of cases.[181] The M1 segment averages about 16 mm in length.[181]

1. Branches
    (a) *Lateral lenticulostriate branches*. Approximately 80% of the lenticulostriates that arise from the MCA arise from the M1 segment. These branches average 10 in number,[181,182] and most arise from the superior aspect of the M1 segment. They enter the anterior perforated substance to supply the anterior commissure, internal capsule, caudate nucleus, putamen, globus pallidus, and substantia innominata.
    (b) *Anterior temporal artery*. The anterior temporal artery typically arises near the midpoint of the M1 segment. Less commonly, it arises from the inferior division (an M2 segment) or as part of an M1 trifurcation. It travels in an anterior and inferior direction over the temporal tip and does not usually enter the sylvian fissure itself.[1] It supplies the anterior temporal lobe.

2. Variants
   (a) *MCA duplication*. This anomaly consists of a large MCA branch arising from the ICA proximal to the ICA bifurcation, and has a frequency of 0.2–2.9%.[183] This vessel travels parallel and inferior to the main M1 segment and primarily supplies the anterior temporal lobe.[183,184] It is associated with aneurysms.[185,186]
   (b) *Accessory MCA*. An accessory MCA arises from the ACA and runs parallel to the M1 segment, and has a prevalance of 0.3–4.0%.[183,187] There is a classification scheme for accessory MCAs:[188] Type 1 arises from the ICA (i.e., MCA duplication), type 2 from the A1 segment, and type 3 from the A2 segment. The accessory MCA primarily supplies the orbitofrontal area,[189] and is also associated with aneurysms.[185,190] This anomaly should not be confused with a large recurrent artery of Heubner.[191]
   (c) *Aplasia*. Aplasia of the MCA is rare and is associated with aneurysms.[192]
   (d) *Fenestration*. Fenestration of the M1 segment has been reported.[184]

M2 Segments

The M2 segments (aka insular segments) extend from the main division point of the M1 segment, over the insula within the sylvian fissure, and terminate at the circular sulcus of the insula. The MCA divisions are equal in diameter and size in 18% of the hemispheres; the superior division is larger (dominant) in 28% of the hemispheres and the inferior division is larger in 32% of the hemispheres.[180] The cortical area supplied by the superior division extends from the orbitofrontal area to the posterior parietal area. The cortical area supplied by the inferior division extends from the temporal pole to the angular area. The M2 segments number from six to eight arteries at the point of transition into the M3 segments.

M3 Segments

The M3 segments (opercular segments) begin at the circular sulcus of the insula and end at the surface of the sylvian fissure. These vessels travel over the surface of the frontal and temporal opercula to reach the external surface of the sylvian fissure. The M3 branches, together with the M2 vessels, give rise to the *stem arteries*, which in turn give off the cortical branches. There are usually eight stem arteries per hemisphere, and each one typically gives rise to one to five cortical branches.[180]

M4 Branches

The M4 branches (aka cortical branches) begin at the surface of the sylvian fissure and extend over the surface of the cerebral hemisphere (Figs. 1.35 and 1.36). The smallest cortical branches arise from the anterior sylvian fissure and the largest ones emerge from the posterior sylvian fissure.[180] The cortical branches can be grouped according to the region of the cortex that they supply; any given region may have a single artery or several arteries supplying it. The following 12-subdivision system is in common usage.[1,180,193] Although each branch is discussed as a single artery, any given cortical artery may actually exist as several branches (up to five) from a single stem artery.
   1. *Orbitofrontal artery* May arise from the M1 or M2 segment, and may share a common origin with the prefrontal artery. Travels within the anterior horizontal ramus of the sylvian fissure to supply orbital surface of the frontal lobe.
   2. *Prefrontal artery* May share a common origin with the orbitofrontal artery. Supplies the opercular part of the inferior frontal gyrus and most of the middle frontal gyrus.
   3. *Precentral artery* Travels in the precentral sulcus. Supplies part of the inferior frontal gyrus and the inferior part of the precentral gyrus.
   4. *Central artery* (aka Rolandic artery) Travels within the central sulcus. May share a common origin with the anterior parietal artery. Largest MCA branch

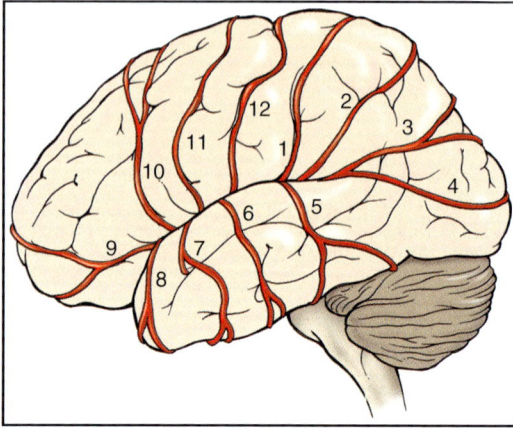

Fig. 1.35 MCA cortical branches. The most common branching pattern of the MCA is shown: (*1*) anterior parietal artery, (*2*) posterior parietal artery, (*3*) angular artery, (*4*) temporo-occipital artery, (*5*) posterior temporal artery, (*6*) middle temporal artery, (*7*) anterior temporal artery, (*8*) temporopolar artery, (*9*) orbitofrontal artery, (*10*) prefrontal artery, (*11*) precentral artery, and (*12*) Central artery.

to the frontal lobe.[180] Supplies the superior part of the precentral gyrus and the inferior half of the postcentral gyrus.

5. *Anterior parietal artery* May arise with the central artery or the posterior parietal artery. Travels in the postcentral sulcus. Supplies the superior part of the postcentral gyrus, the upper part of the central sulcus, the anterior part of the inferior parietal lobule, and the anteroinferior part of the superior parietal lobule.

6. *Posterior parietal artery* The most posterior ascending branch of the MCA. May share a common trunk with the anterior parietal artery or the angular artery. Supplies the posterior part of the superior and inferior parietal lobules, including the supramarginal gyrus.

7. *Angular artery* The terminal and largest branch of the MCA. It emerges from the posterior end of the sylvian fissure to travel over the superior temporal gyrus and terminate over the superior half of the occipital lobe. Supplies the posterior part of the superior temporal gyrus, and parts of the supramarginal and angular gyri, and superior parts of the lateral occipital lobe.

8. *Temporo-occipital artery* May share an origin with the angular artery. Supplies the posterior half of the superior temporal gyrus, the posterior extent of the middle and inferior gyri, and the inferior parts of the lateral occipital lobe.

9. *Posterior temporal artery* Leaves the posterior sylvian fissure and crosses over the superior and middle temporal gyri. Supplies the middle and posterior parts of the superior temporal gyrus, the posterior third of the middle temporal gyrus, and the posterior extent of the inferior temporal gyrus.

10. *Middle temporal artery* Emerges from the middle of the sylvian fissure. Supplies the middle parts of the temporal gyri.

11. *Anterior temporal artery* Passes inferiorly and posteriorly over the temporal lobe, and terminates in the middle temporal sulcus. Supplies the anterior parts of the superior, middle, and inferior temporal gyri.

12. *Temporopolar artery* Supplies the anterior pole of the temporal lobe.

The cortical branches can be grouped according to which lobe they supply:[193]

1. *Frontal lobe* Orbitofrontal, prefrontal, precentral, and central arteries

2. *Parietal lobe* Anterior and posterior parietal arteries and angular artery

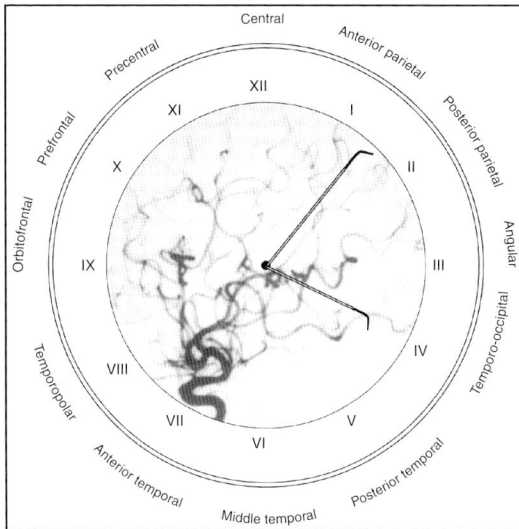

Fig. 1.36 Mnemonic for the cortical MCA branches. Because of the astonishing coincidence that there are 12 cortical branches and 12 h on the clock, the cortical branches can be remembered by assigning each one to an hour of the day. The *central* artery occupies the *central* position on the clock, that of high noon. The position of the angular artery at 3 o'clock, reflects the importance of that vital artery, because, as we all know, 3 o'clock was the time that school let out when we were kids. The *middle* temporal artery is at 6 o'clock, which is in the *middle* position at the bottom of the clock. The orbitofrontal artery is at the extreme left position, at 9 o'clock, which is appropriate because the orbitofrontal artery is the most extreme anterior branch of the MCA.

    3. *Temporal lobe* Temporopolar, anterior, middle and posterior temporal arteries, and temporo-occipital artery
    4. *Occipital lobe* Temporo-occipital artery
The cortical branches can also be grouped according to which M2 segment they arise from:[180]
    1. *Superior division* Orbitofrontal, prefrontal, precentral, and central arteries.
    2. *Inferior division* Temporopolar, temporo-occipital, angular, and anterior, middle, and posterior temporal arteries.
    3. *Dominant division* (these branches may arise from either division, and usually come off of the larger of the MCA divisions). Anterior and posterior parietal arteries.

Leptomeningeal collaterals

These are a network of anastamotic channels up to 1 mm in diameter connecting distal cortical arterial branches.[194] Otto Heubner first described their existence in 1874.[195] Since then there has been increasing recognition of their importance in cases of ischemic stroke.[196] They are quite variable in size and distribution[197] and this may explain variable outcomes in situations of arterial occlusions. These collaterals may also be the target of therapeutic maneuvers such as blood pressure modification in cases of cerebral vasospasm or other causes of ischemia.

Angio-Anatomic Correlate! Leptomeningeal Collaterals (Fig. 1.37)

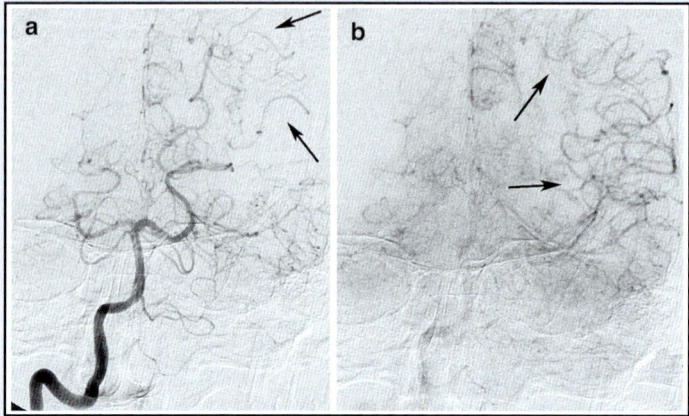

Fig. 1.37 Leptomeningeal collaterals. Leptomeningeal collaterals can be difficult to see on an angiogram unless occlusive disease is present. In this patient with severe left middle cerebral stenosis, early arterial phase vertebral arteriography (**a**) shows leptomeningeal collateral flow from the posterior cerebral branches (*arrows*). Later arterial phase (**b**) shows flow from these collaterals into the middle cerebral artery territory (*arrows*).

1.7.   Posterior Cerebral Artery

Most classification schemes for the PCA include three or four segments. The following system is the most common (Fig. 1.38):
1. P1 From the basilar artery bifurcation to the junction with the P-comm artery.
2. P2 From the P-comm artery to the posterior aspect of the midbrain.
3. P3 From the posterior aspect of the midbrain to the calcarine fissure.
4. P4 The terminal branches of the PCA distal to the anterior limit of the calcarine fissure.

PCA Branches

The PCA branches (Fig. 1.39) can be divided into three categories:
1. Perforating branches, to the brainstem and thalamus
2. Ventricular branches
3. Cortical branches

Perforating branches arise from the P1 and P2 segments. Ventricular branches originate mostly from the P2 segment. Cortical branches arise from the P2, P3, and P4 segments. Perforating arteries are divided into direct branches, which pass directly into the brain, and circumflex vessels, which travel around the brainstem for various distances before entering the brain.

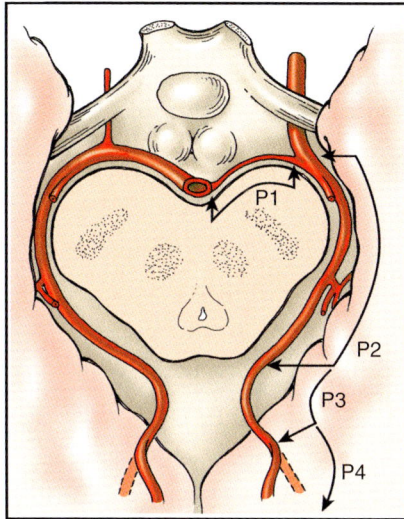

Fig. 1.38 Posterior cerebral artery. The most common PCA configuration is on the *left*, and the persistent fetal origin of the PCA is on the *right*.

P1 Segment

The P1 segment (aka precommunicating, mesencephalic or horizontal segment) lies immediately superior to the oculomotor and trochlear nerves. The average length is 6.6 mm; when a fetal PCA is present, the vessel averages 8.6 mm in length.[198]

1. Branches
    (a) Perforators
        i. Direct perforating branches (posterior thalamoperforating arteries) from the P1 segment pass directly into the brainstem. These are termed the posterior thalamoperforators to distinguish them from the anterior thalamoperforators, which arise from the P-comm artery. These arteries average 2.7 in number,[198] and arise from the posterior and superior aspects of the P1 segment, although, rarely, they may arise from the anterior aspect of the vessel.[130] The direct perforators enter the brain medial cerebral peduncles and posterior perforated substance to supply parts of the thalamus, brainstem, and posterior internal capsule.
        ii. Circumflex arteries. The circumflex arteries (aka peduncular, mesencephalic, or tegmental thalamoperforating arteries) arise from the P1 and P2 segments and encircle the midbrain parallel and medial to the PCA. They are subdivided into short and long circumflex arteries. The short and long circumflex arteries number 0.8 and 1.3 per hemisphere, respectively.[198]
            1. *Short circumflex arteries* One or more short circumflex arteries travel a short distance around the brainstem before entering the brain, and reach only as far as the geniculate bodies. Most short circumflex arteries arising from P1 terminate at the posterolateral border of the peduncle.[198]

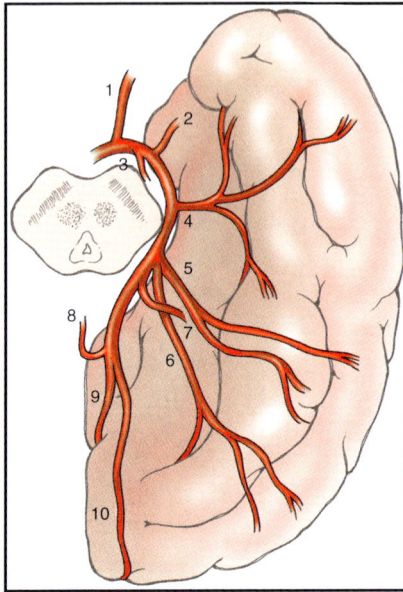

Fig. 1.39 Major branches of the posterior cerebral artery. (*1*) Posterior communicating artery; (*2*) hippocampal artery; (*3*) posteromedial choroidal artery; (*4*) anterior temporal artery; (*5*) middle temporal artery; (*6*) posterior temporal artery; (*7*) posterolateral choroidal artery; (*8*) splenial artery; (*9*) parieto-occipital artery; (*10*) Calcarine artery.

    2. *Long circumflex arteries* Up to three long circumflex arteries (aka quadrigeminal arteries) pass around the brainstem, to supply the geniculate bodies and superior colliculi. They arise from the PCA distal to the origin of the short circumflex arteries; in 80% of cases they arise from P1 and in the remaining cases they arise from P2.[198] The long circumflex artery anastomoses with the branches of the superior cerebellar arteries.

(b) Posteromedial choroidal artery This vessel usually arises from the P2 segment (see below), but arises from the P1 segment in 12% of cases.[198]

(c) Meningeal branch (aka artery of Davidoff and Schecter). A small branch from the P1 segment to supply a midline strip of the inferior surface of the tentorium may be enlarged by pathological processes.[199]

2. Variants

(a) Side-to-side asymmetry of the P1 segments common is present in 52% of angiograms.[200] When a fetal P-comm artery is present, the ipsilateral P1 is typically hypoplastic, and may not fill noticeably on angiography, making it appear to be absent or occluded.

(b) In some persistent carotid–vertebrobasilar anastomoses, the PCA may be supplied by branches from the carotid system (see above).

(c) True anomalies of the P1 segment are uncommon, accounting for 3% of cases in an autopsy series.[201] These include duplication, fenestration, and a bilateral shared origin of the PCA and SCA.

(d) Congenital absence of the P1 is rare.[130]

(e) There may be a prominent perforating branch that supplies portions of both the ipsilateral and contralateral thalamus and potentially midbrain.[202] This perforator has been called the artery of Percheron.[203,204]

P2 Segment

The P2 segment (aka ambient segment) is relatively long, averaging 50 mm in length.[198] It is subdivided by some authors into an anterior half and a posterior half for discussion of surgical approaches.[198] The P2 segment begins at the P-comm artery junction and travels around the lateral aspect of the midbrain within the ambient cistern, parallel and inferior to the basal vein of Rosenthal. Other adjacent structures are the trochlear nerve, the free edge of the tentorium, and the superior cerebellar artery.

1. Branches
    (a) Perforators
        i. Direct perforators
            1. Thalamogeniculate arteries originate from the midportion of the P2 segment, and arise in a superior and lateral direction to perforate the inferior surface of the geniculate bodies. They number 1–3 per hemisphere,[198,205] and supply the posterior half of the lateral thalamus, the posterior limb of the internal capsule, and the optic tract.
            2. Peduncular perforating arteries pass directly into the cerebral peduncle and supply multiple structures within the brainstem as well as parts of the oculomotor nerve. They average 2.8 per hemisphere.[198]
        ii. Circumflex arteries. The circumflex arteries usually arise from the P1 segment. In 20% of cases the long circumflex artery arises from the P2 segment.[198]
    (b) Posteromedial choroidal artery (Fig. 1.40). This artery (aka medial posterior choroidal artery) is single in 54% of the hemispheres and may be duplicated or triplicated.[198] The vessel arises from the P2 segment in most cases. Other sites of origin of the posteromedial choroidal artery are the P1 segment (12%), P3 segment (4%), parieto-occipital artery (10%), and calcarine artery (3%),[198] or, rarely, the basilar artery.[206] The posteromedial choroidal artery has two segments:
        i. *Cisternal segment.* This segment averages 42 mm in length.[207] From its origin, the vessel curves around the brainstem medial to the main trunk of the PCA and gives off small tegmental branches before it turns forward adjacent to the pineal gland to enter the roof of the third ventricle. The tegmental branches irrigate portions of the midbrain, tectal plate, pineal gland, thalamus, and medial geniculate body.
        ii. *Plexal segment.* This segment travels anteriorly within the velum interpositum between the thalami, adjacent to the internal cerebral vein and the contralateral medical posterior choroidal artery. It travels through the foramen of Monro to enter the choroid plexus of the lateral ventricle and anastomose with the terminal branches of the lateral posterior choroidal artery. Branches from the plexal segment irrigate the choroid plexus of the third ventricle, as well as the thalamus and the stria medullaris.[207]
    (c) Posterolateral choroidal arteries. Unlike the posteromedial choroidal artery, the posterolateral choroidal arteries are multiple in the majority (84%) of cases[207] and number up to nine (average: 4).[198] They arise from the P2 segment in 51% of cases; other sites of origin include the

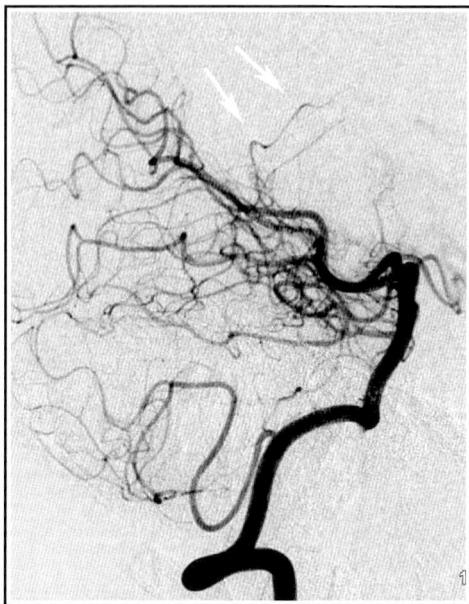

Fig. 1.40 Posteromedial choroidal artery. The undulating course of the posteromedial choroidal artery as it passes over the quadrigeminal plate, gives it a characteristic undulating "3" pattern (*arrows*).

parieto-occipital (13%), anterior temporal (10%), hippocampal (8%), posterior temporal (9%), posteromedial choroidal (4%), calcarine (2%), or middle temporal artery (2%).[198] The sizes of these arteries are inversely proportional to the size of the anterior choroidal artery.[208] The posterolateral choroidal arteries travel laterally to enter the choroidal fissure, and have two segments:

  i. *Cisternal segment.* The cisternal segment averages 23 mm in length and sends branches to the thalamus, geniculate bodies, fornix, cerebral peduncle, pineal body, corpus callosum, tegmentum, and temporal occipital cortex.[207]

  ii. *Plexal segment.* This segment begins with the passage of the lateral posterior choroidal arteries through the choroidal fissure lateral to the ambient cistern at the level of the temporal horn or atrium. They travel along the medial border of the choroid plexus in the lateral ventricle, eventually intermingling with branches of the medial posterior choroidal artery in the body of the ventricle and at the foramen of Monro.[207] Branches from plexal segment vessels irrigate the choroid plexus and penetrate the ventricular surfaces of the thalamus and fornix.

(d) Hippocampal artery. A hippocampal artery arises from the P2 segment in 64% of cases; when present, it is the first cortical branch of the PCA.[198] This artery supplies the uncus, hippocampal gyrus, hippocampal formation, and dentate gyrus. Some authors include the hippocampal artery with the inferior temporal arteries.[198]

(e) Inferior temporal arteries. The inferior temporal arteries are distinguished from the temporal arteries, which are branches of the MCA. The inferior

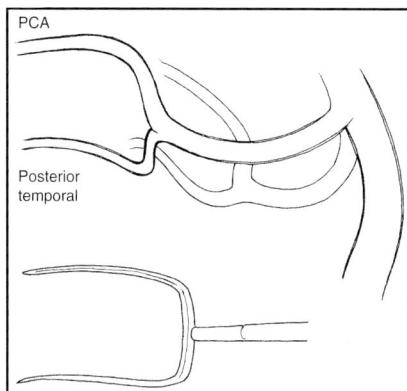

Fig. 1.41 The PCA pitchhfork. A distinctive identifying landmark of the PCA on a lateral view is the "pitchhfork" appearance of the take-off of the posterior temporal artery from the main trunk of the PCA. Visualization of this feature can help distinguish the PCA from other arteries on a cluttered angiogram.

temporal arteries are variable and may appear as a single initial branch of the P2 segment, called a common temporal artery (aka lateral division of the PCA or lateral occipital artery), which is seen in 16% of cases.[198]

    i. *Anterior inferior temporal artery*. The anterior temporal artery is usually the second cortical branch of the PCA. It may be duplicated. It travels anteriorly and laterally inferior to the hippocampal gyrus, and anastomoses with anterior temporal branches of the MCA.[200]

    ii. *Middle inferior temporal artery*. A middle temporal artery is present in 38% of hemispheres and supplies the inferior surface of the temporal lobe.[198]

    iii. *Posterior inferior temporal artery* (Fig. 1.41). The posterior temporal artery is a prominent branch of the PCA and usually arises from the inferior and lateral aspect of the P2 segment and travels obliquely toward the occipital pole. It supplies the inferior temporal and occipital surfaces. This vessel arises from the P3 segment in 6% of cases.

(f) Parieto-occipital artery. The parieto-occipital artery arises as a single trunk from the P2 segment slightly more often than from the P3 segment.[198] It travels posteriorly and laterally within the parieto-occipital fissure, which separates the parietal lobe from the occipital lobe, to supply the posterior parasagittal region, cuneus, precuneus, and lateral occipital gyrus. In 24% of cases it sends branches through the choroidal fissure into the lateral ventricle.

(g) Calcarine artery. The calcarine artery arises from the P2 segment slightly less commonly than from the P3 segment (see below).

(h) Splenial artery. The splenial artery originates from the P2 segment in 4% of cases (see below).[198]

(i) Artery of Davidoff and Schechter (dural branch). Generally only seen in pathological conditions, this artery supplies the apex of the tentorium, walls of the vein of Galen, and then curves forward along the free edge of the falx cerebri.[209] It can also provide some collateral supply to the superior vermis and inferior colliculi.[210] The artery of Davidoff and Schechter is often difficult to see angiographically, even when enlarged, due to superimposition with other PCA branches. It is more commonly found on the left.[211]

2. Variants
    (a) Anomalous origin of cortical branches. In rare cases, the parieto-occipital, posterior temporal, or calcarine artery may arise directly from the ICA.[1,212] Similarly, anomalous anterior choroidal artery supply to temporal, parietal and occipital cortical regions normally supplied by branches of the PCA has been reported.[213]

Angio-Anatomic Correlate! Accessory Posterior Cerebral Artery
(Fig. 1.42)

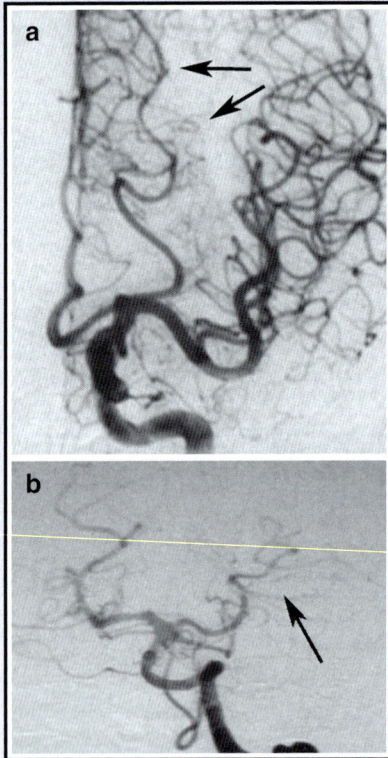

Fig. 1.42 Carotid artery injection (**a**) shows an accessory PCA that looks like a fetal origin posterior cerebral artery supplying the posterior parietal and occipital territories of the PCA (*arrows*). Vertebral artery injection (**b**) shows the native PCA that mainly fills the posterior temporal branch of the PCA (*arrow*).

P3 Segment

The P3 segment (aka quadrigeminal segment) extends in a medial and posterior direction from the quadrigeminal plate to the anterior limit of the calcarine fissure, and averages 20 mm in length. The P3 segments from each side approach each other. The point where the two PCAs are nearest to each other is referred to as the collicular, or quadrigeminal point; this separation averages 8.9 mm.[198] The PCA often divides into its two terminal branches (the calcarine and parieto-occipital arteries) between the quadrigeminal plate and the calcarine fissure.

1. Branches
    (a) Parieto-occipital artery. The parieto-occipital artery arises from the P3 segment in 46% of the hemispheres (see above).
    (b) Posterolateral choroidal artery. This artery arises from the P3 segment in 11% of cases (see above).[207]

P4 Segment

The P4 segment begins at the anterior limit of the calcarine fissure, and includes one of the two main terminal branches of the PCA, the calcarine artery. The other main terminal branch of the PCA, the parieto-occipital artery, frequently arises from the P2 or P3 segment.

1. Branches
    (a) Calcarine artery. The calcarine artery travels posteriorly and medially within the calcarine fissure to reach the occipital pole. It is duplicated in 10% of cases and arises from the parieto-occipital artery in 10% of cases.[198] The calcarine artery sends branches to the lingual gyrus and inferior cuneus; it primarily supplies the visual cortex.
    (b) Splenial artery. The splenial artery (aka posterior pericallosal artery) arises from the parieto-occipital artery in 62% of cases, but may arise from the calcarine artery (12%), posteromedial choroidal artery (8%), posterior temporal artery (6%), P2 or P3 segments (4% each) or the posterolateral choroidal artery (4%).[198] The splenial artery is relatively constant and travels superiorly around the splenium of the corpus callosum to anastomose with the pericallosal artery.

1.8.   Vertebral Artery

The vertebral artery has four segments (Fig. 1.43):
1. V1 From the subclavian artery to the foramen transversarium of C6.
2. V2 From C6 to the foramen transversarium of C1.
3. V3 From the C1 to the dura.
4. V4 Intradural part of the vertebral artery.

V1 Segment

The V1 segment (extraosseous segment) arises from the posterosuperior wall of the subclavian artery (Fig. 1.44) and travels in a superior and posterior direction. It passes posterior to the anterior scalene muscles and enters the transverse foramen of the C6 (90% of most cases), C5 (7%) or C7 (3%). Supplies the stellate ganglion.[214]

1. Variants
    (a) *Anomalous origin.* The left vertebral artery arises directly from the aortic arch in about 0.5% of cases.[1] Anomalous origins of the right vertebral artery from the arch,[215] of both vertebral arteries from the arch,[216] and of the right vertebral artery from the right common carotid artery[217] have been reported.
    (b) *Duplication and fenestration.* Duplication[218] or fenestration of the vertebral artery is found in ≤1% of dissections.[113]

V2 Segment

The V2 segment (foramenal segment) travels in a vertical direction within the foramen transversaria, usually from C6 to C2. It is surrounded by sympathetic fibers (although this is now debatable)[219] from the stellate ganglion and by a venous plexus that covers the entire V2 segment and drains through the vertebral vein into the subclavian or internal jugular veins.[220] The vertebral vein (or veins) is usually large and is directly anterior to the vertebral artery.[221]

1. Branches
    (a) *Spinal branches.* These branches (aka radiculomedullary branches) arise from the vertebral artery from C1 to C5 and may vary in the number and side of origin.[220,221] They supply the spinal cord as well as the periosteum and bone of the vertebrae.
    (b) *Muscular branches.* Multiple small muscular branches arise from the V2 segment to supply the cervical muscles.

Artery of the cervical enlargement. The artery of the cervical enlargement usually arises from both vertebral arteries in the region of C4 to C6 and anastomoses with the anterior spinal artery to supply the ventral spinal cord. This artery may also arise from the thyrocervical trunk (see General Principles of Spinal Arterial Anatomy, below).[6]

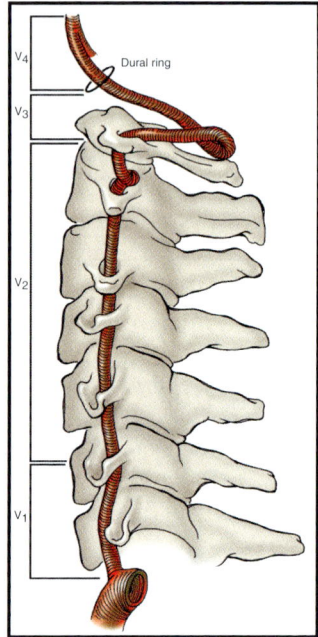

Fig. 1.43 Vertebral artery.

    (c) *Anterior meningeal artery.* Originates from the distal V2 segment and supplies the dura around the foramen magnum and extends up the clivus. Forms collaterals with the ascending pharyngeal artery via the odontoid arcade and the dural branches of the ascending pharyngeal artery, and with the ICA via the meningohypophyseal trunk branches.
    (d) *Posterior meningeal artery.* Arises near the foramen magnum and supplies the medial occipital dura and the falx cerebelli (Fig. 1.45).
    (e) *PICA.* Occasionally the PICA originates at the C1 level.[222]

V3 Segment

The V3 segment (aka extraspinal segment) begins as the vertebral artery exits the transverse foramen of C1 on the medial side of the lateral rectus muscle of the head. It then travels in a horizontal and medial direction superior to the posterior arch of C1 and runs inferior to the posterior atlanto-occipital membrane before turning superiorly and anteriorly to penetrate the dura.

1. Branches
    (a) *PICA.* In some 5–20% of cases, the PICA has an extradural origin, usually from the V3 segment.[222] In these cases the PICA may originate at any point along the V3 segment.
    (b) *Suboccipital artery of Salmon.* One, or up to three muscular branches supplying the suboccipital muscles is seen in 67% of cases.[223]

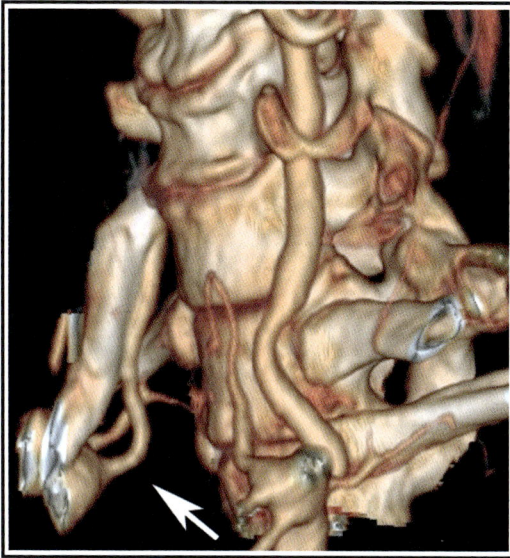

Fig. 1.44 Vertebral artery origin. Anterolateral view of a cervical spine CT angiogram showing the right vertebral artery (*arrow*) arising from the posterior wall of the subclavian artery. The optimal angiographic projection is usually an AP view with 20–30° of Townes.

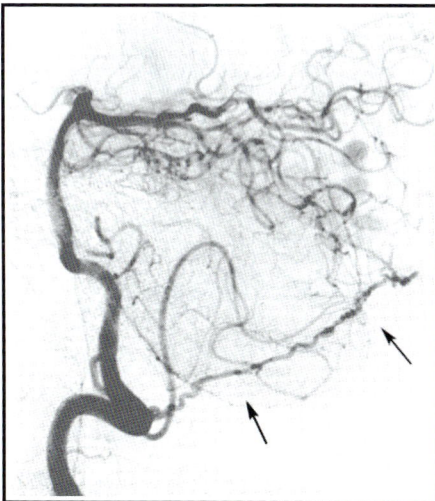

Fig. 1.45 Posterior meningeal artery. Posterior meningeal artery (*arrows*) arises from the vertebral artery at C1 and supplies the falx cerebelli. The posterior meningeal artery in this particular case is enlarged due to the presence of a dural arteriovenous fistula.

V4 Segment

The V4 segment is the intradural part of the vertebral artery and extends from its entrance through the dura to the junction with the opposite vertebral artery. The dura is thickened and it forms a fibrous dural ring around the vertebral artery.[224] The length of the V4 segment averages 22 mm.[225] The left and right V4 segments usually come together at the level of the pontomedullary junction. The branches of the intradural vertebral artery can be separated into medial branches (including the anterior spinal artery and branches of the foramen caecum) and lateral branches, the most prominent of which is the PICA.[225] A wide anastomotic net usually interconnects the branches of V4.[225]

1. Branches
    (a) *Posterior inferior cerebellar artery (PICA)*. The PICA is the largest and most complex of the cerebellar arteries (Fig. 1.46). It originates approximately 16–17 mm proximal to the vertebrobasilar junction, an average of 8.6 mm superior to the foramen magnum.[226] The territory supplied by the PICA includes the lower medulla and inferior aspects of the fourth ventricle, cerebellar tonsils, vermis, and inferolateral cerebellar hemisphere. The PICA arises from the vertebral artery and travels posterolaterally around the medulla. Over the dorsal aspect of the brainstem, the vessel travels inferiorly for a variable distance – sometimes as far south as C2 – then forms a loop (the *caudal loop*) and turns 180° to travel superiorly adjacent to the cerebellar tonsil. The vessel then reaches its superior extent and forms another loop (the *cranial loop*) and then travels inferiorly and laterally to emerge over the cerebellar hemisphere (Fig. 1.47). The PICA can be divided into five segments, detailed below. The first four segments can be remembered by using the acronym, *ALPS*.
        i. Anterior medullary segment. Extends from the origin to the inferior olivary prominence. In some 40% of cases, there is no anterior medullary segment, because the PICA arises lateral, rather than anterior to the medulla.[226] This segment averages one perforator.[226]
        ii. Lateral medullary segment. Extends from the inferior olivary prominence to the origins of the ninth, tenth, and eleventh cranial nerves, and averages 1.8 perforators.[226]
        iii. Posterior medullary segment. This segment (aka tonsillomedullary segment) begins where the PICA passes posterior to the lower cranial nerves and ends where the ascending vessel reaches the midlevel of the medial surface of the tonsil. It passes immediately posterior to the roof of the lower half of the fourth ventricle, and averages 3.3 perforators.[226]
        iv. Supratonsillar segment. This segment, the telovelotonsillar segment, begins midway up the tonsil, includes the cranial loop, and ends where the PICA exits the fissures between the vermis, tonsil, and cerebellar hemisphere to reach the cortical surface. On a lateral angiogram, the supratonsillar segment outlines the tonsil along its anterior, superior, and posterior aspects.[6]
        v. Cortical segments. These segments are also known as hemispheric branches. The PICA often bifurcates into medial and lateral trunks where the vessel emerges onto the inferior cortical surface. The medial trunk gives rise to the vermian and tonsillar branches, and the lateral trunk produces the hemispheric branches.
        vi. PICA branches
            1. Perforators
                (a) Direct perforators. These branches travel directly into the brainstem, and are found in all three medullary segments.
                (b) Circumflex perforators. These perforators travel around the brainstem for some distance before entering it. These vessels arise mostly from the lateral and posterior medullary segments.
            2. Choroidal arteries. Branches to the choroid plexus of the fourth ventricle arise from the posterior and supratonsillar segments.

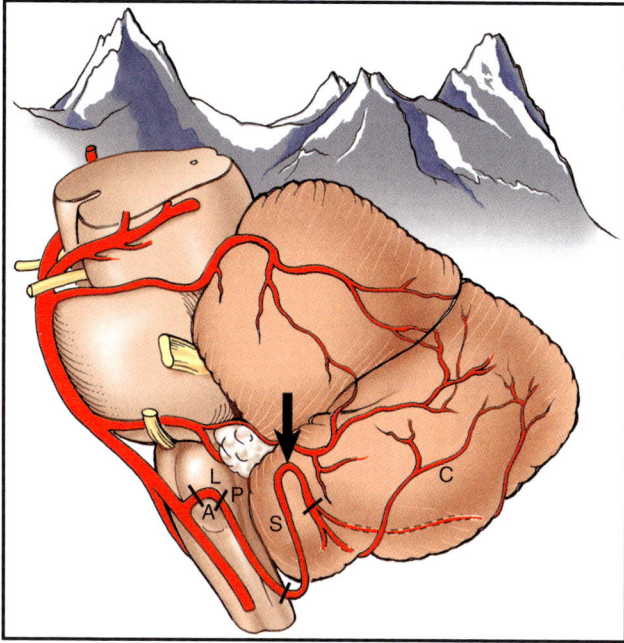

Fig. 1.46 Posterior inferior cerebellar artery. Lateral view of the brainstem and cerebellum. The segments of the PICA include the anterior medullary (*A*), lateral medullary (*L*), posterior medullary (*P*), supratonsillar (*S*), and cortical (*C*) segments. *Arrow* indicates the choroidal point. The artist was inspired to depict the Swiss Alps in the background.

3. Cortical arteries
    (a) Vermian branches
    (b) Tonsillar branches
    (c) Hemispheric branches
4. Meningeal branches. The posterior meningeal artery and the artery of the falx cerebelli may arise from the PICA.
vii. PICA variants
  1. Anomalous origin. Extradural origin of the PICA is found in 5–20% of cases (see above). Origination of the PICA from the ICA,[227] the posterior meningeal artery,[228] a hypoglossal artery,[229] and a proatlantal artery[229] have been reported.
  2. Duplication. The PICA is duplicated in some 2.5–6% of cases.[226]
  3. Hypoplasia. The PICA is hypoplastic in 5–16% of the hemispheres.[229,230]
  4. Absence. The PICA is absent on one side in 15–26% of cases and on both sides in 2% of cases.[3,229,230]
  5. A shared AICA-PICA trunk is a normal variant.[1]
  6. The vertebral artery terminates in PICA in 0.2% of cases.[1]
(b) *Perforators*. An average of 4.2 perforators arise directly from each vertebral artery and supply lateral medulla, inferior cerebellar peduncle, and the medullary surface of the cerebellum.[225]

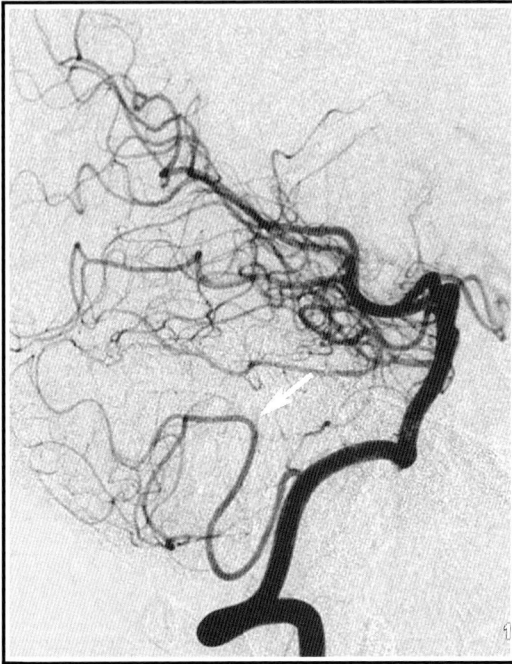

Fig. 1.47 The choroidal point. The single most important anatomical fact about the PICA for neurointerventionalists has to do with the cranial loop (*arrow*), aka the *choroidal point*. The choroidal point is the superior-most point of the PICA. The PICA gives off branches to the brainstem proximal to the choroidal point but not distal to it. Occlusion of the PICA at or distal to the choroidal point does not usually result in a functionally significant ischemic injury, because of anastomotic connections with AICA and SCA.[292,293]

(c) *Anterior spinal artery*. The anterior spinal artery arises from the vertebral artery 6.5 mm proximal to the vertebrobasilar junction[225] and travels in an inferior direction to supply the anterior surface of the medulla and spinal cord. In about 50% of cases a small communicating artery (the anterior spinal communicating artery) connects the left and right anterior spinal arteries on the anterior surface of the medulla.[225]

(d) *Branches of the foramen caecum*. In about one third of cases branches of the vertebral artery travel superiorly to supply the foramen caecum at the base of the pons.[225]

(e) *Lateral spinal artery*. The lateral spinal artery may arise from the V4 segment or from the PICA,[231] and may be difficult to see on angiography.[6] It originates lateral to the medulla and travels in a caudal direction, anterior to the posterior spinal nerve roots and posterior to the dentate ligament. It supplies the eleventh cranial nerve and the lateral and posterior surfaces of the cord via branches to the C1–C4 spinal nerves.

(f) *Meningeal branches*. The posterior meningeal artery and the artery of the falx cerebelli may arise from the PICA.

1.9.   Basilar Artery

The basilar artery originates at the pontomedullary junction, travels anterior to the pons, and terminates near pontomesencephalic junction. The artery averages 32 mm in length[130] and travels in the midline, or at least medial to the lateral margins of the clivus, in 98% of cases.[232] The course of the artery is straight in 45% of cases, curved in 35%, and tortuous in 20%.[233] The outer diameter is typically constant, averaging 4.1 mm in adults,[234] except for a widening at the basilar bifurcation, giving it a "cobra-like appearance," in 16% of cases.[130]

1. Branches
   (a) *Anterior inferior cerebellar artery (AICA).* The AICA arises from the basilar artery an average of 9.6 mm distal to the vertebrobasilar junction.[233] It travels in a posterior, inferior and lateral direction across the pons toward the cerebellopontine angle. It terminates by passing over and sending branches to the anterolateral surface of the cerebellar hemisphere.[235] Usually the smallest of the three cerebellar arteries, the AICA has reciprocal relationships and extensive anastomoses with the SCA and the PICA. It also has anastomoses with the SCA. The sixth cranial nerve crosses the AICA 6–7 mm distal to the origin of the artery,[234] and the vessel lies adjacent to the seventh and eighth cranial nerves in the cerebellopontine angle.[236] The AICA has three segments:
       i. Premeatal segment. Extends from the origin of the vessel to the seventh and eighth cranial nerves.
       ii. Meatal segment. The part of the AICA that is related to the internal auditory canal.
       iii. Postmeatal segments. The AICA typically divides into rostral and caudal trunks in the cerebellopontine angle.[237,238] After crossing the seventh and eighth cranial nerves, the rostral trunk travels laterally over the flocculus to reach the middle cerebellar peduncle and the superior part of the anterolateral (petrosal) surface of the cerebellar hemisphere. The caudal trunk supplies the inferior part of the anterolateral surface.
       iv. AICA branches
           1. Perforators. The brainstem receives small perforating branches from the premeatal segment and recurrent perforating branches from the meatal segment.
           2. Internal auditory artery (labyrinthine artery). This vessel arises from the AICA in 45% of cases.[1] The vessel may arise from the premeatal or meatal segment, or from the lateral branch of the postmeatal segment. The internal auditory artery travels with the seventh and eighth cranial nerves into the internal auditory meatus and is distributed to the inner ear.[239]
           3. Subarcuate artery. The subarcuate artery arises from the AICA medial to the internal auditory meatus and penetrates the dura covering the subarcuate fossa on the posterior surface of the temporal bone and supplies the bone in the region of the semicircular canals.[240]
           4. Cerebellar cortical branches.
       v. AICA variants
           1. Duplication. The origin of the artery is single in 72% of cases, duplicate in 26%, and triplicate in 2%.[240]
           2. Anomalous origin. Origination of the AICA from the ICA has been reported.[241]
   (b) *Basilar artery perforators.* An average of 17 perforators arises from the basilar artery from its origin to the SCAs.[233] In addition, on average, another 2.5 average small horizontal brainstem perforators arise from the posterior surface of the basilar artery distal to the origin of the SCAs.[242] Significantly, no perforators arise directly from the tip of the basilar artery.[242,243] Basilar perforators supply the posterior perforated

substance and brainstem structures such as the corticospinal and corticobulbar tracts, pontine nuclei, and the lemnisci, fasciculi, and motor nuclei of the midbrain and pons.

    i. Medial perforators. Medial perforators average 5.8 mm in length and enter the pons in the basilar suclus or within a few mm of it.[233]

    ii. Circumflex perforators. Circumflex perforators average 16 mm in length and travel around the brainstem for various distances before entering.

(c) *Superior cerebellar artery (SCA)*. The SCA is the most constant cerebellar artery and arises from the basilar artery immediately prior to the basilar bifurcation. The SCA travels posterolaterally around the brainstem, inferior to the third and fourth cranial nerves and superior to the fifth cranial nerve. The SCA comes into contact with the fifth cranial nerve in 50% of cases,[244] and is usually the target of surgical microvascular decompression for trigeminal neuralgia (the AICA and adjacent veins may also come into contact with the fifth nerve). At an average distance of 18.5 mm from the origin, the SCA bifurcates into a rostral and a caudal trunk.[245] The rostral trunk continues around the brainstem, gives off direct and circumflex perforators, sends branches to the inferior colliculi, and supplies the superior surface of the vermis and the paramedian aspect of the cerebellar hemisphere. The caudal trunk supplies the superior lateral surface of the cerebellar hemisphere, the superior cerebellar peduncle and dentate nucleus, and part of the brachium pontis. The SCA can be divided into four segments:[245]

    i. Anterior pontomesencephalic segment. This segment (aka anterior pontine segment) extends from the SCA origin to the anterolateral margin of the brainstem.

    ii. Lateral pontomesencephalic segment. This segment (aka ambient segment) extends from the anterolateral margin of the brainstem to the anterior margin of the cerebellomesencephalic groove. This segment is parallel to the PCA and basal vein of Rosenthal. The fourth cranial nerve crosses the midportion of this segment.

    iii. Cerebellomesencephalic segment. This segment (aka quadrigeminal segment) travels within a groove between the cerebellum, the midbrain, and the superior cerebellar peduncles.

    iv. Cortical segments. The cortical segments include branches to the vermis and superior cerebellar hemisphere cortical surface.

    v. SCA branches

        1. Perforators. An average of two perforators arises from the main SCA trunk, five from the rostral trunk, and two from the caudal trunk.[245] Direct perforators from the SCA are less common than circumflex perforators.

        2. Precerebellar arteries. The precerebellar arteries arise from the hemispheric branches (average: four) and the vermian branches (average: two), and supply the deep cerebellar nuclei, the inferior colliculi, and the superior medullary velum.[245]

        3. Cortical arteries.
            (a) Hemispheric branches
            (b) Vermian branches
            (c) Marginal artery

        4. Internal auditory artery. This vessel is most often a branch of the AICA (see above) but arises from the SCA in 25% of cases.[1]

    vi. SCA variants
        1. Duplication. The SCA is duplicated in 14% of hemispheres;[245] in these cases, the duplicate vessels correspond to the rostral and caudal trunks.

        2. Absence. Although rare, absence of the SCA has been reported.[246]

        3. May arise from the cavernous ICA in a persistent trigeminal artery variant.[91]

(d) *Internal auditory artery*. This vessel is most often a branch of the AICA (see above) but arises directly from the basilar artery in 16% of cases.[1]

Table 1.7 Intracranial arterial fenestrations

Vessel	References
ICA	244
A1 segment	245
Azyos anterior cerebral artery	246
M1 segment	184
P-comm artery	133
P1 segment	196
Vertebral artery	247,248
Basilar artery	219,249

2. Variants
   (a) Fenestration of the basilar artery is found in 1.33% of dissection and 0.12% of angiograms.[1,247]
      i. Fenestration or segmental duplication is a rare congenital anomaly. In a review of 5,190 cerebral- angiograms, arterial fenestration was observed in 37 (0.7%).[248] Considering all fenestrations, the prevalence of an associated aneurysm is 7%.[248] Table 1.7 is an inventory of reported intracranial fenestrations.

1.10.   Venous System

The most important facts about the craniocervical venous system are:
1. Venous anatomy is highly variable.
2. The venous structures of the head and neck are widely interconnected.
3. Valves are not present in the intracranial venous system.
4. Valves are typically present at several predictable locations in the cervical region.

Two other useful generalizations can be made:
1. Many veins have reciprocal relationships with other veins. For instance, if the vein of Labbé is large, the vein of Trolard is usually small.
2. In addition to anatomical variation, the size and flow direction of any given vein can vary greatly with the patient's head and neck position and in the presence of pathology.

As the venous system is so variable, the following discussion details the most common venous anatomic patterns and selected clinically relevant variants. An exhaustive inventory of known variations would be mind-numbingly tedious to read and not particularly useful.

Extracranial Veins

Scalp Veins

The scalp veins have extensive connections with the emissary veins of the skull, although these connections are not normally seen on angiography.
1. *Frontal vein.* Drains the anterior part of the skull and forehead and communicates with the supratrochlear and supraorbital veins.
2. *Supratrochlear vein.* Drains the frontal scalp and forehead and descends over the forehead medial to the supraorbital vein.
3. *Supraorbital vein.* Drains the frontal scalp and forehead and travels over the superior orbital rim lateral to the supratrochlear vein to anastomose with the orbital veins and the angular vein.

4. *Medial temporal vein*. Drains the anterior temporal region and joins the superficial temporal vein.
5. *Superficial temporal vein*. Usually runs together with the corresponding superficial temporal artery. It descends in front of the ear and penetrates the parotid glands, where it is joined by the maxillary vein to form the retromandibular vein, which drains into the internal jugular (IJ) or external jugular (EJ) vein.
6. *Posterior auricular vein*. Drains the retroauricular area and connects to the IJ or EJ.
7. *Occipital vein*. Drains the occipital and posterior cervical areas and anastomoses with the deep cervical and vertebral veins and the transverse sinus via the mastoid emissary vein. It drains into the IJ or EJ (Fig. 1.48).

Orbital Veins

The orbital veins comprise an important anastomoses between the intracranial and extracranial venous systems, and are typically enlarged in the presence of a carotid-cavernous fistula.

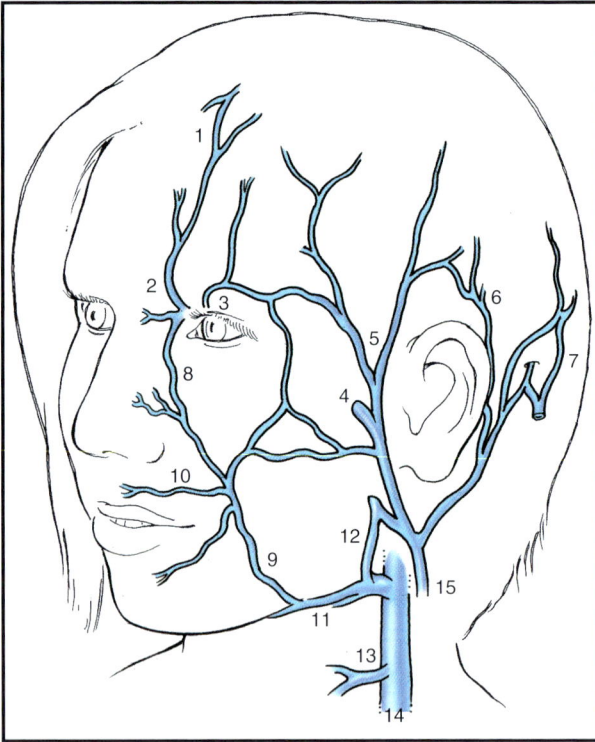

Fig. 1.48 Superficial extracranial veins. (*1*) frontal vein; (*2*) supratrochlear vein; (*3*) supraorbital vein; (*4*) medial temporal vein; (*5*) superficial temporal vein; (*6*) posterior auricular vein; (*7*) occipital vein; (*8*) angular vein; (*9*) facial vein; (*10*) labial veins; (*11*) submental vein; (*12*) retromandibular vein; (*13*) thyroid veins; (*14*) internal jugular vein; (*15*) external jugular vein.

1. *Superior ophthalmic vein (SOV)*. The largest and the most constant orbital vein.[249] It originates near the trochlea below the medial orbital roof and travels posteriorly and medially to enter the cavernous sinus. The common direction of flow in the ophthalmic veins is from extracranial to intracranial;[250] reversal of flow in the SOV should raise suspicion of intracranial venous hypertension. The SOV anastomoses with the supraorbital vein and the angular vein.
2. *Inferior ophthalmic vein*. Much smaller than the SOV, it is connected to the SOV via several anastomotic vessels (anterior, medial, and posterior anastomosing veins), and drains into the cavernous sinus or directly into the superior ophthalmic vein.
3. *Medial ophthalmic vein*. Present in some cases.

Facial Veins (Figs. 1.48 and 1.49)

1. *Angular vein*. The angular vein is formed by the junction of the supratrochlear and supraorbital veins. It travels in an inferior direction at an angle next to the nose (thus the name) and medial to the orbit. The angular vein communicates with orbital veins and continues inferiorly as the facial vein.
2. *Facial vein*. The facial vein (aka anterior facial vein) is the continuation of the angular vein, and it begins at the medial palpebral angle. The facial vein descends obliquely across the face and curves around the inferior edge of the mandible to merge with the submental and retromandibular veins to drain into the IJ. Along its course, the facial vein receives tributaries from the orbit, facial muscles, and submental region.[1] It has extensive connections with deep facial vein, pterygoid plexus, and cavernous sinus.[250]
3. *Pterygoid plexus*. The pterygoid plexus is a network of venous channels that is nestled between the temporalis and lateral pterygoid muscles. It is connected to the facial vein via the deep facial vein, and it receives a wide array of tributaries from deep facial and oropharyngeal structures. It connects to the cavernous sinus via emissary veins that travel through the foramen ovale and spinosum, and to the IJ via the maxillary vein.
4. *Deep facial vein*. Connection between the facial vein and the pterygoid plexus.
5. *Maxillary vein*. This vein connects to the pterygoid plexus and travels posteriorly to join the superficial temporal vein to form the retromandibular vein.
6. *Labial veins*. The superior and inferior labial veins drain the upper and lower lips, respectively, and drain into the facial vein.
7. *Retromandibular vein*. This vein (aka temporo-maxillary vein) is formed by the confluence of the maxillary and superficial temporal veins, and passes within the parotid gland to join the facial vein.
8. *Common facial vein*. Formed by the junction of the facial, lingual anterior division of the retromandibular and communicating veins. It receives submental, lingual and thyroid tributaries, and drains into the IJ.[1]
9. *Submental vein*. Drains the floor of the mouth and runs under the mandible. It drains into the facial vein.

Cervical Veins

1. *Internal jugular vein (IJ)*. The IJ begins in the jugular fossa and is the continuation of the sigmoid sinus. The jugular bulb is the enlargement of the IJ at its origin. The IJ travels within the carotid sheath posterior and lateral to the common carotid artery, and connects with the subclavian vein on each side to form the branchiocephalic vein. A valve is usually present where the IJ meets the subclavian vein. The right IJ is usually dominant.
2. *External jugular vein (EJ)*. The EJ is formed by the junction of the posterior division of the retromandibular and posterior auricular veins. It originates inferior to the angle of the mandible and travels across the sternocleidomastoid muscle to drain into the subclavian vein. A valve may be present where the EJ meets the subclavian vein.

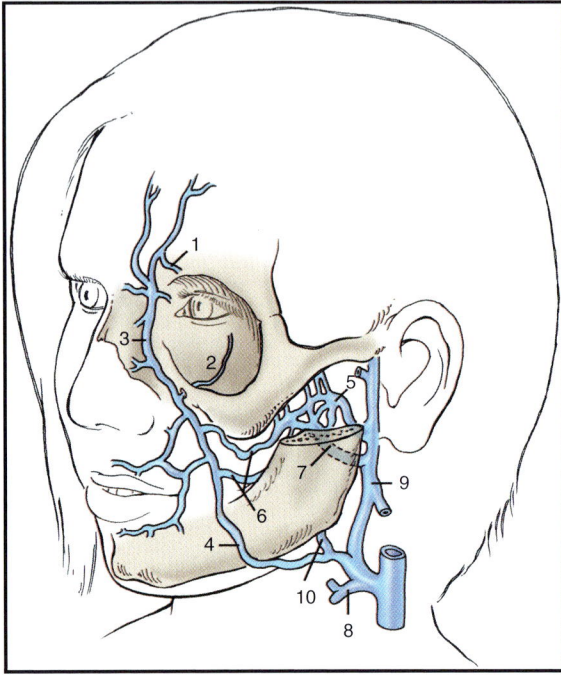

Fig. 1.49 Deep extracranial veins. (*1*) superior orbital vein; (*2*) inferior orbital vein; (*3*) angular vein; (*4*) facial vein; (*5*) pterygoid plexus; (*6*) deep facial veins; (*7*) maxillary vein; (*8*) common facial vein; (*9*) suboccipital veins; (*10*) pharyngeal vein.

3. *Suboccipital veins.* These veins drain the suboccipital region and communicate with the vertebral venous plexus.
4. *Thyroid veins.* Superior and inferior thyroid veins drain the thyroid gland and connect to IJ.
5. *Pharyngeal vein.* Drains the posterior pharyngeal region and connects to the IJ.
6. *Anterior condylar confluence (of Trolard).* Present in essentially 100% of cases, it is possibly the dominant outflow of the venous drainage of the brain in the upright position.[101] It lies adjacent to the hypoglossal canal and connects the jugular bulb to the anterior, posterior, and lateral condylar veins.
7. *Anterior condylar vein.* The anterior condylar vein travels through the hypoglossal canal and connects the inferior petrosal sinus with the vertebral venous plexus and suboccipital veins. It is the rostral equivalent of a spinal radicular vein.[251]
8. *Posterior condylar vein (aka condylar emissary vein).* Connection between the sigmoid sinus and vertebral venous plexus.[1]
9. *Lateral condylar vein.* Also drains to the vertebral venous plexus. Seen on 76% of sides of cadaveric specimens.[101]
10. *Spinal radicular veins.* Each spinal radicular vein corresponds to a spinal artery. These veins travel within the neural foramena and connect the epidural venous plexus to the vertebral venous plexus.
11. *Vertebral venous plexus.* The vertebral venous plexus begins in the suboccipital region and extends inferiorly along the vertebral column to drain into the brachiocephalic vein. It surrounds the V2 segment of the vertebral artery and has

numerous connections with the occipital veins, epidural venous plexus, and other cervical and facial veins.

12. *Vertebral vein*. The vertebral vein (aka anterior vertebral vein)[252] is anterior to the vertebral artery[221] and drains into the vertebral venous plexus.

Venous Structures of the Skull

A rich network of veins connects the intracranial venous system to the extracranial venous system.

1. *Diploic veins*. The cancellous bone between the inner and outer tables of the skull contains an extensive network of veins that do not cross suture lines and are not normally seen on angiography.[6] They communicate widely with meningeal and pericranial veins, and with the dural sinuses.

2. *Emissary veins*. These veins connect the extracranial veins to the intracranial venous sinuses.

   (a) *Parietal emissary veins*. Communicate between the scalp veins and the superior sagittal sinus.

   (b) *Mastoid emissary veins*. Communicate between the occipital and posterior auricular veins and the sigmoid sinus.

Meningeal Veins

Meningeal veins lie on the outer surface of the dura and each corresponds to its respective meningeal artery.[6] The anterior meningeal vein joins the superficial Sylvian vein to form the sphenoparietal sinus.

Intracranial Venous Sinuses

The dural sinuses are venous channels that are located between the meningeal and endosteal layers of dura. They are rigid and do not have valves. They may be trabeculated and contain bands, chords, and bridges.[126] They also contain arachnoid granulations; *Pacchionian granulations* are macroscopic arachnoid granulations that project directly into the venous sinuses. Pacchionian granulations may measure up to 1 cm in diameter[253] and should not be mistaken on angiography for intraluminal thrombus (Fig. 1.50). Dural sinuses are also present within the falx cerebri and tentorium. There are two main groups of dural venous sinuses: the superior group and the inferior group.[253]

Superior Group

The superior group primarily drains the majority of the brain and skull (Fig. 1.51).

1. *Superior sagittal sinus (SSS)*. The SSS lies in a shallow midsagittal groove at the junction of the falx cerebri and the dura lining the inner table of the calvaria. It originates near the crista galli and terminates in the torcular Herophili. The transverse diameter of the SSS ranges from 4 mm in the frontal area to 10 mm in the occipital region.[126] The "1/3rd Rule" states that it is generally safe to therapeutically occlude the SSS in the anterior third of the structure, without a significant risk of venous infarction.[254] Cortical venous tributaries are most prominent in the middle third of the SSS, and relatively few in number and caliber in the posterior third.

   (a) Venous connections

      i. Facial and nasal veins: Although there have been denials of its existence,[255,256] there can be a vein of the foramen caecum draining the nasal veins to the superior sagittal sinus, more commonly seen in infants[257]

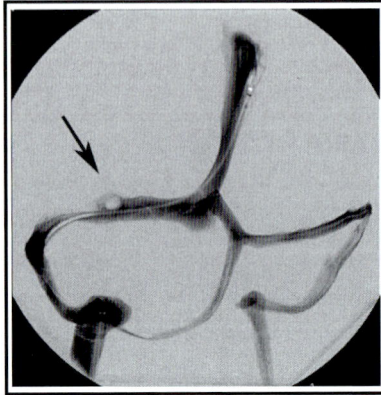

Fig. 1.50 Arachnoid granulation. Venogram of the inferior venous sinuses, showing an arachnoid granulation in the transverse sinus (*arrow*). Arachnoid granulations can have a "punched out" appearance on angiography that can mimic a flow void due to intraluminal thrombus.

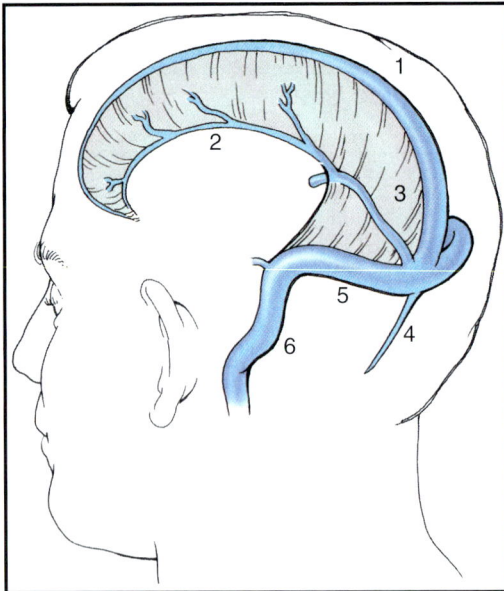

Fig. 1.51 Superior group of dural venous sinuses. (*1*) Superior sagittal sinus; (*2*) inferior sagittal sinus; (*3*) straight sinus; (*4*) occipital sinus; (*5*) transverse sinus; (*6*) sigmoid sinus.

  ii. Scalp veins

  iii. Cortical veins

  iv. "Intermediate veins":[253] Diploic, meningeal, and emissary veins. These structures provide important collateral pathways in the event of venous sinus occlusion

2. *Inferior sagittal sinus.* The inferior sagittal sinus is relatively small and travels in or slightly superior to the falx. It begins at the junction of the anterior and middle thirds of the falx, runs above the corpus callosum, and terminates at the falcotentorial apex by connecting with the vein of Galen to form the straight sinus. It is more prominent in infants and young children, than adults.[253]

  (a) Venous connections

   i. Tributaries from the falx, corpus callosum, medial cerebral hemispheres, and SSS via falcine veins.

3. *Straight sinus.* The straight sinus is formed by the confluence of the inferior sagittal sinus and vein of Galen. It travels posteriorly and inferiorly beneath the splenium of the corpus callosum toward the internal occipital protuberance. The straight sinus averages 5 cm in length[258] and drains into the confluence of the sinuses, or predominantly into one transverse sinus, usually the left.[253] The straight sinus is single channel in most cases, but is doubled or tripled in some 15% of cases.[259]

  (a) Venous connections

   i. Vermian veins

   ii. Tentorial sinuses

   iii. Cerebellar hemispheric veins.

4. *Occipital sinus.* The occipital sinus is present in 65% of cases, and travels in the midline, within the attached margin of the falx cerebelli, between the confluence of the sinuses and the marginal sinus.[260]

5. *Torcular Herophili.* The confluence of the sinuses (Fig. 1.52) is formed by the junction of the SSS, straight sinus, transverse sinuses, and occipital sinus. The torcular Herophili is typically asymmetric and widely variable in its configuration. In 10–15% of cases, the superior sagittal sinus drains into one transverse sinus and there is no direct connection between the left and right transverse sinuses.[261]

6. *Transverse sinus.* The transverse sinuses (aka lateral sinus) travel within the peripheral margins of the tentorium and extend from the internal occipital protuberances to the bases of the petrous temporal bones. The right and left transverse sinuses are asymmetric in about half of cases, and the right transverse sinus is usually larger.[261] In some 20% of cases, there is partial or total agenesis of one of the transverse sinuses, usually the left, and in these cases the sigmoid sinus may fill via the vein of Labbé.[261]

  (a) Venous connections

   i. SSS and contralateral transverse sinus

   ii. Veins from the inferior and lateral surfaces of the temporal and occipital lobes, including the vein of Labbé.

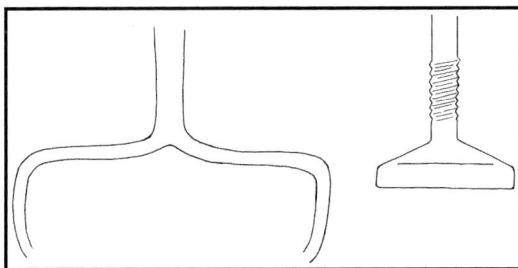

Fig. 1.52 Torcular herophili. The confluence of the sinuses carries the eponym, *Torcular Herophili*, after the anatomist, Herophilus of Chalcedon. The term "torcular" is commonly thought to be translated from the ancient Greek as "wine press," as the four-limbed confluence (*left*) bears some resemblance to a wine press (*right*)[294]. An alternative school of thought holds that this is a mistranslation, and that Torcular Herophili actually refers to the concavity on the interior of the occipital bone that houses the confluence.[295]

iii. Cerebellar veins.
iv. Veins of the scalp via mastoid emissary veins.
v. Superior petrosal sinus

7. *Sigmoid sinus*. The sigmoid sinus originates where the transverse sinus leaves the tentorial margin. It forms a gentle S-shape and terminates at jugular bulb, where the internal jugular vein begins.
   (a) Venous connections
       i. Transverse sinus and internal jugular vein.
       ii. Suboccipital muscular and scalp veins and the vertebral venous plexus via the mastoid and condylar emissary veins.

Inferior Group

The inferior group primarily drains the sylvian veins, the inferior surface of the brain, and the orbits (Fig. 1.53).

1. *Cavernous sinus*. Each cavernous sinus lies lateral to the body of the sphenoid bone and extends from the superior orbital fissure to the petrous apex. The anterior and posterior part of the cavernous sinuses are connected to each other via the *intercavernous sinus* (aka "circular sinus") around the sella turcica and

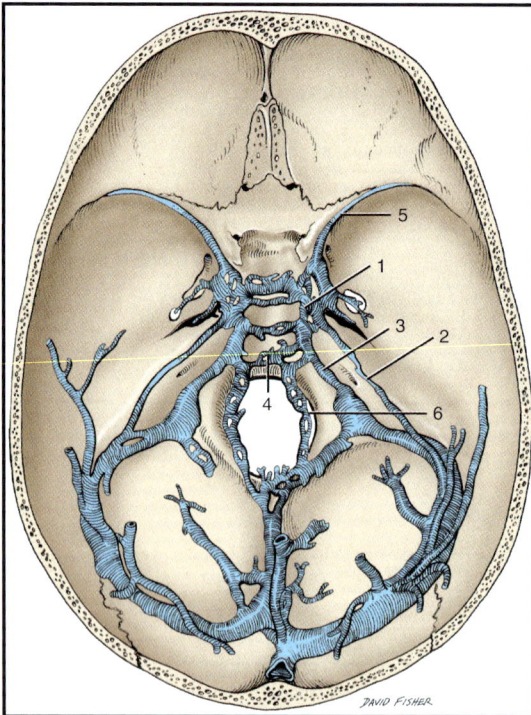

Fig. 1.53 Inferior group of dural venous sinuses. (*1*) Cavernous sinus. (*2*) Superior petrosal sinus. (*3*) Inferior petrosal sinus. (*4*) Basilar venous plexus. (*5*) Sphenoparietal sinus. (*6*) Marginal sinus.

the basilar venous plexus. This consists of an anterior intercavernous sinus in front of the sella, a posterior intercavernous sinus behind the sella, and in some cases an inferior intercavernous sinus as well.[262] Cranial nerves III, IV, V1, and V2 travel in the lateral wall of the cavernous sinus, and the ICA, sympathetic plexus, and cranial nerve VI are suspended by fibrous trabeculae within the lumen of the cavernous sinus.[253]

    (a) Venous connections
        i.   Superior and inferior ophthalmic veins
        ii. Sphenoparietal sinus
        iii. Superior petrosal vein
        iv. Inferior petrosal sinus
        v.   Pterygoid plexus via emissary veins of the foramen ovale, foramen lacerum, and foramen Vesalius.

2. *Inferior petrosal sinus.* The inferior petrosal sinus travels in groove between the petrous apex and the clivus (Dorello's canal), extending from the posterior part of the cavernous sinus to the anterior superior aspect of the jugular bulb. In 39% of cases the left and right inferior petrosal sinuses are markedly asymmetric, and in 8% of cases the sinus is absent on at least one side.[263]

    (a) Venous connections
        i.   Cavernous sinus
        ii. Basilar venous plexus
        iii. Internal auditory veins
        iv. Cerebellar and brainstem veins
        v.   Internal jugular vein

3. *Superior petrosal sinus.* The superior petrosal sinus extends from the transverse sinus to the cavernous sinus, and travels along the attachment of the tentorium to the superior margin of the petrous temporal bone. The direction of flow is presumably from posterior to anterior.[264]

    (a) Venous connections
        i.   Transverse sinus
        ii. Petrosal vein
        iii. Lateral mesencephalic vein
        iv. Cerebellar veins
        v.   Veins draining the tympanic cavity
        vi. Cavernous sinus

4. *Sphenoparietal sinus.* The sphenoparietal sinus (aka sinus of Breschet) is the medial extension of the Sylvian veins.[253] It travels beneath the lesser wing of the sphenoid bone and drains into the cavernous sinus, pterygoid plexus, or into the inferior petrosal sinus or transverse sinus.[264] A "true" sphenoparietal sinus exists when the structure anastomoses with other venous structures at both ends.[249]

5. *Basilar venous plexus.* The basilar venous plexus (aka clival venous plexus) is a network of dural veins that extends over the dorsal surface of the clivus.

    (a) Venous connections
        i.   Cavernous sinus
        ii. Inferior petrosal sinus
        iii. Marginal sinus

6. *Marginal sinus.* The marginal sinus lies in the margin of the foramen magnum and drains into the jugular bulbs. It anastomoses with the occipital sinus and vertebral venous plexuses.

7. *Vertebral venous plexus.* The venous plexus is the extensive network of veins associated with the spine. It can be subdivided into internal and external components.

Supratentorial Cortical Veins

The cortical veins drain the outer 1–2 cm of the cortex and the subcortical white matter, and travel centrifugally (Fig. 1.54). They have no valves. They exhibit reciprocal prominence, i.e., when one vein is large on a given side, others are usually small.[253] Cerebral cortical drainage occurs via three principle routes:

1. *Sylvian veins.* The Sylvian veins (aka superficial middle cerebral veins) originate in the posterior third of the lateral Sylvian fissure and travel through the lateral aspect of the sylvian fissure and drain parts of the frontal and temporal lobes into the cavernous sinus and pterygoid plexus.[253,265]

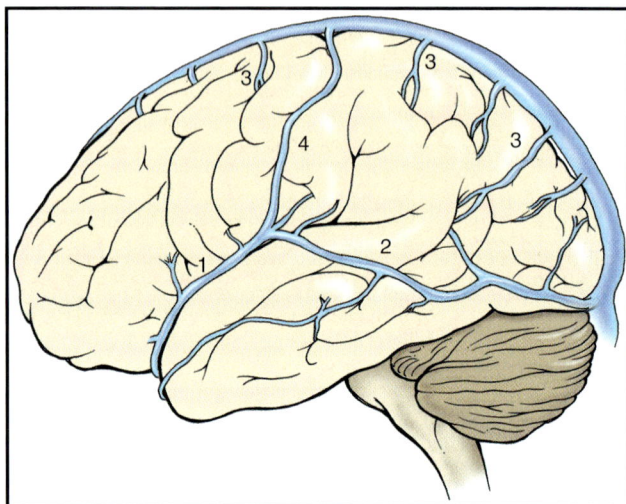

Fig. 1.54 Superficial cortical veins. (*1*) Sylvian vein; (*2*) vein of Labbé; (*3*) superior convexity veins; (*4*) vein of Trolard.

2. *Temporo-occipital veins*. These veins drain temporal, occipital and parts of the parietal cortex into the transverse sinus.
    (a) *Vein of Labbé* (aka occipito-temporal vein) is defined as the largest cortical vein crossing the temporal lobe convexity from the Sylvian vein to the transverse sinus.[6] It can be identified on one or both hemispheres in 75% of dissections,[266] and is most commonly larger in the dominant hemisphere.[267] It travels in the occipitotemporal sulcus and may have important anastomotic connections with tentorial dural sinuses.
3. *Superior convexity veins*. These veins, which average 14 per hemisphere,[126] drain the superolateral and superomedial cortex into the superior sagittal sinus. The veins enter the superior sagittal sinus perpendicularly in the anterior frontal region; the angle becomes progressively more acute (i.e., opposite to the direction of flow in the superior sagittal sinus) in the parietal and occipital regions. Occipital region veins may pass for a considerable distance before connecting to the superior sagittal sinus, and may be confused with venous anomalies.[253] The vein of Rolando travels in the central sulcus.
    (a) *Vein of Trolard* (aka frontoparietal vein) is defined as the largest anastomotic channel connecting the Sylvian vein to the superior sagittal sinus.[6] It is most commonly larger in the non-dominant hemisphere.[267]

Deep Venous System

The deep venous system drains the periventricular white matter, basal ganglia, and thalamic regions (Fig. 1.55). In contrast to the cortical venous system, which runs centrifugally, the deep venous system runs centripetally. The deep veins can be divided into a *ventricular group* (which includes the subependymal veins and internal cerebral vein) and a *cisternal group* (primarily consisting of the basal vein of Rosenthal and its tributaries).
1. *Medullary veins*. The medullary veins are an array of veins that drain the cerebral white matter. They originate 1–2-cm deep to the cortical mantle and join the subependymal veins. They are typically straight and perpendicular to the subependymal veins.

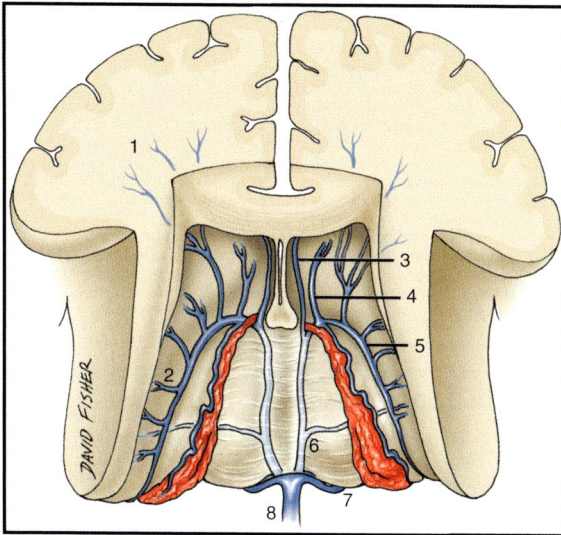

Fig. 1.55 Deep venous system. (*1*) Medullary veins; (*2*) subependymal veins; (*3*) septal vein; (*4*) anterior caudate vein; (*5*) thalamostriate vein; (*6*) internal cerebral vein; (*7*) basal vein of Rosenthal; (*8*) vein of Galen (aka great cerebral vein).

2. Subependymal veins

   (a) *Septal veins.* The septal veins originate at the lateral aspect of the frontal horns and travel posteriorly and medially to run along the septum pelucidum. In the majority of cases, the septal veins join the thalamostriate veins to form the internal cerebral vein. The venous angle is the junction of the septal vein with the thalamostriate vein. Although the venous angle is generally considered to approximate the location of the foramen of Monro on angiography, in 47.5% of hemispheres the septal vein joins the internal cerebral vein an average of 6 mm posterior to the foramen of Monro.[268] The septal veins drain the deep frontal white matter and anterior corpus callosum.

   (b) *Anterior caudate veins.* The anterior caudate veins (aka longitudinal caudate veins or anteroinferior caudate veins) are a group of tributaries from the medial surface of the caudate nucleus that drain into the thalamostriate vein.

   (c) *Thalamostriate vein.* The thalamostriate vein arises from tributaries that converge on the sulcus between the caudate nucleus and the thalamus, and travels in a medial direction towards the Foramen of Monro to join the septal veins and form the internal cerebral vein. It drains the posterior frontal lobe, anterior parietal lobe, caudate nucleus, and internal capsule. Despite its name, the thalamostriate vein does not receive significant tributaries from the thalamus.

   (d) *Medial and lateral atrial veins.* These veins drain the walls of the atrium, and may drain directly into the internal cerebral vein, basal vein of Rosenthal, or the vein of Galen.[269]

3. *Internal cerebral vein.* The internal cerebral vein is formed by the junction of the septal veins and the thalamostriate vein posterior to the foramen of Monro. It travels posteriorly to join the contralateral internal cerebral vein to form the vein of Galen. The internal cerebral vein receives subependymal tributaries and, just anterior to the vein of Galen, the ipsilateral basal vein of Rosenthal. It averages 30.2 mm in length[269] and drains the posterior

frontal lobe, anterior parietal lobe, caudate nucleus, lentiform nucleus, and internal capsule.

4. *Basal vein of Rosenthal*. The basal vein of Rosenthal (aka basal vein) is the most prominent cisternal vein and is formed below the anterior perforated substance by the junction of the *anterior cerebral* and *deep middle cerebral veins*. The anterior cerebral vein originates near the optic chiasm and is connected to its contralateral counterpart by the anterior communicating vein. The deep middle cerebral vein is formed near the limen insula by the confluence of the insular veins. The basal vein of Rosenthal travels posteriorly between the midbrain and the temporal lobe and terminates by joining the internal cerebral vein or the vein of Galen. It receives extensive tributaries from the temporal lobe, thalamus, and midbrain.

5. *Vein of Galen*. The vein of Galen (aka great cerebral vein) originates in the quadrigeminal cistern by the union of the internal cerebral veins. It curves in a posterosuperior direction towards the apex of the tentorium, where it joins the straight sinus. It is 5–20 mm in length[6] and its tributaries include the posterior pericallosal, superior cerebellar, and precentral cerebellar veins.

Infratentorial Venous System

The veins of the posterior fossa can be grouped according to the principle route of drainage (Fig. 1.56).

1. *Superior (vein of Galen) group*. These veins drain the upper part of the cerebellar hemispheres, vermis, and midbrain.

   (a) *Precentral cerebellar vein*. The unpaired midline precentral cerebellar vein receives the superior hemispheric and vermian tributaries, and

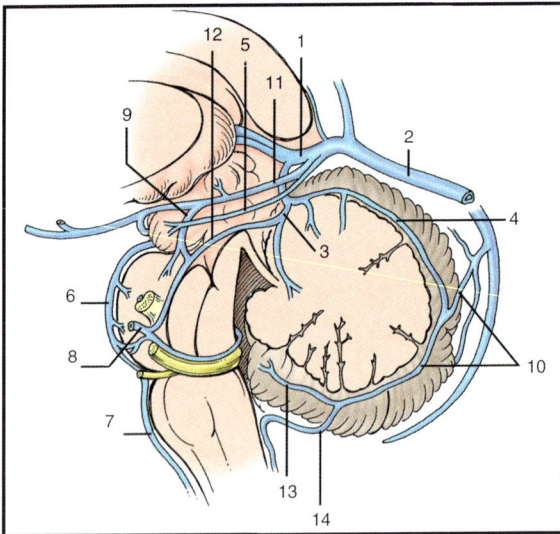

Fig. 1.56 Infratentorial venous system. (*1*) Vein of Galen; (*2*) straight sinus; (*3*) precentral cerebellar vein; (*4*) superior vermian vein; (*5*) basal vein of Rosenthal; (*6*) anterior pontomesencephalic vein; (*7*) anterior medullary vein; (*8*) petrosal vein; (*9*) lateral mesencephalic vein; (*10*) inferior vermian vein; (*11*) posterior mesencephalic vein; (*12*) brachial vein; (*13*) superior retrotonsillar vein; (*14*) inferior retrotonsillar vein.

travels superiorly and posteriorly parallel to the roof of the forth ventricle. It enters the vein of Galen posterior to the inferior colliculi.

(b) *Superior vermian vein*. The paired superior vermian veins originate from tributaries in the culman, posterior to the precentral cerebellar vein. They travel superiorly to drain into the vein of Galen, with or anterior to the precentral cerebellar vein.

(c) *Posterior mesencephalic vein*. This vein originates in the interpeduncular fossa and curves around the midbrain to enter the vein of Galen or internal cerebral vein.[249]

2. *Anterior (petrosal vein) group*. These veins drain the anterior part of the brainstem and cerebellum, and empty primarily into the superior and inferior petrosal sinuses.

(a) *Anterior pontomesencephalic vein*. The unpaired midline pontomesencephalic vein travels along the anterior belly of the pons, connecting the midline *anterior medullary vein* inferiorly (which, in turn, connects to the *anterior spinal vein*) to the *peduncular vein*, in the interpeduncular cistern. It may also communicate with the petrosal vein and the basal vein of Rosenthal.

(b) *Petrosal vein (aka Dandy's vein)*. The petrosal vein is formed by numerous tributaries from the pons, medulla, and cerebellum. It is 2–2.5 cm long,[249] and travels anterior and lateral to the trigeminal nerve to enter the superior petrosal sinus above the internal auditory meatus.

(c) *Lateral mesencephalic vein*. This vein runs in the lateral mesencephalic sulcus and anastomoses with the posterior mesencephalic and petrosal veins.

3. *Posterior (tentorial) group*. These veins drain toward the tentorium.

(a) *Inferior vermian veins*. The paired inferior vermian veins are formed by the superior and inferior retrotonsillar veins. The inferior vermian veins receive tributaries from the vermis and cerebellar hemispheres, and travel posteriorly and superiorly along the inferior vermis to drain into the tentorial, straight, or transverse sinus.

Intracranial Venous System Variants

The intracranial venous system is widely variable. Selected variants and anomalies are detailed below:

1. *Developmental venous anomaly (DVA)*. A DVA (aka venous angioma or cerebral venous malformation) is a normal variant in which a network of small medullary veins converges into single large central venous channel (see also Chap. 16). They are found in some 2% of autopsies.[270] They have a characteristic stellate appearance on imaging, and have been hypothesized to occur when medullary veins become hypertrophic to compensate for the occlusion or absence of some other adjacent venous structure. They are frequently found adjacent to cavernous malformations; among patients with cavernous malformations, and up to 29% have an associated developmental venous anomaly.[271,272] In fact, focal venous congestion within developmental venous anomalies are thought to contribute to the formation of cavernous malformations.[273]

2. *Vein of Galen malformation*. This anomaly consists of a dramatically enlarged persistent median vein of the prosencephalon, which is the embryonic precursor to the vein of Galen (see also Chap. 14).[274] Multiple feeding arteries typically flow directly into the varix and usually arise from the anterior and posterior choroidal arteries and the anterior cerebral artery. The malformation develops prior to the formation of the vein of Galen and the straight sinus, and the venous pouch drains via the falcine sinus to the superior sagittal sinus. The straight sinus may be hypoplastic or absent. The deep venous system, as a rule, does not appear to communicate with the malformation, although there is a well-documented case of visualization of a communication to normal deep veins after treatment of a vein of Galen malformation.[275]

3. *Chiari II malformation*. In the Chiari II malformation (Fig. 1.57), the posterior fossa is very small and the straight sinus is angled sharply downward. The confluence of sinuses may be at or below the level of the foramen magnum.

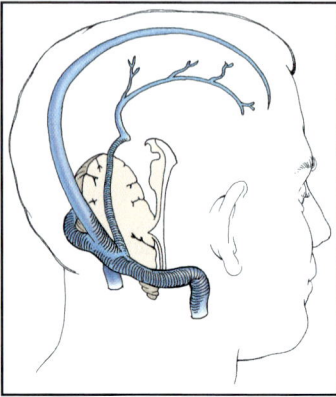

Fig. 1.57 Chiari II malformation. The Chiari II malformation is characterized by an abnormally small posterior fossa, with downward angulation of the straight sinus and low-lying transverse sinuses.

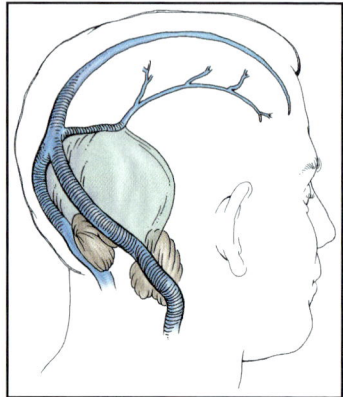

Fig. 1.58 Dandy–walker complex. The tentorium, straight sinus, and torcular Herophili are displaced superiorly by cystic dilatation of the fourth ventricle and enlargement of the posterior fossa.

4. *Dandy–Walker complex*. The Dandy-Walker complex is a congenital syndrome that includes cystic dilatation of the forth ventricle and enlargement of the posterior fossa (Fig. 1.58). The straight sinus and torcular Herophili are often elevated and the transverse sinuses angle inferiorly.

1.11. Spinal Neurovascular Anatomy

The spine, and in particular, the spinal cord, is supplied by a number of relatively small and variable arteries with similarly small and variable veins. There is a general organization of spinal blood supply that is constant: Segmental arteries contribute to the segmental levels of the spine and may contribute to the extrinsic arteries of the spinal cord, which then contribute to the intrinsic arteries within the substance of the cord. Similarly, the intrinsic veins of the spinal cord drain into the extrinsic veins on the surface of the cord, which then drains to epidural and paraspinal venous structures.

These vessels should be considered when evaluating vascular lesions in the spine (Table 1.8).

Spinal Cord Blood Supply: General Principles

- Segmental arteries are the source of blood flow to longitudinal arteries within the spine.
- Longitudinal intraspinal veins drain via segmental veins into the longitudinal epidural and paraspinal venous systems.
- Inter-segmental and side-to-side anastamoses are *common* (Table 1.9).
- Variability of segmental connections to longitudinal arterial and venous systems is *very common*.

Table 1.8 Arteries supplying the spine

Vertebral level(s)	Feeding arteries	…Which usually arise from:
C1–C2	Ascending pharyngeal Occipital Vertebral Ascending cervical Deep cervical	External carotid External carotid Subclavian Thyrocervical trunk Costocervical trunk
C3–C7	Vertebral Ascending cervical Deep cervical	Subclavian Thyrocervical trunk Costocervical trunk
T1–T3	Supreme intercostal	Costocervical trunk
T3–T4	T4 ("Superior") intercostal	Aorta
T5–T12	T5–T12 intercostal	Aorta
L1–L4	Lumbar arteries	Aorta
L5	Median sacral iliolumbar	Aortic bifurcation Internal iliac
Sacrum	Median sacral Lateral sacral	Aortic bifurcation Internal iliac

Table 1.9 Spinal vascular anastomoses

Anastamosis from	Anastamosis to	Comments
Lumbar and intercostals arteries	Radiculomedullary or radiculopial branches	Side-to-side and interseg-mental anastamoses are common
Costocervical trunk	Artery of cervical enlargement	Spinal cord artery may arise from costocervical trunk or from subclavian as a separate vessel
Ascending cervical artery	Anterior spinal artery	
Deep cervical artery	Posterolateral spinal artery	
Segmental vertebral branches	Anterior or posterolateral spinal arteries	
Occipital and muscular branches	Spinal arteries via segmental vertebral branches	
Ascending pharyngeal artery and muscular branches	Spinal arteries via segmental vertebral branches	

General Principles of Spinal Arterial Anatomy

1. Vertebral artery contributions to the spine (Fig. 1.59)
   (a) Anterior spinal artery
       The anterior spinal artery has two, very short paired branches from the extreme distal vertebral arteries creating a V-like configuration that merges to a single midline artery that descends from the vertebrobasilar junction inferiorly in the ventral sulcus of the cord. Sometimes one limb of the V is hypoplastic and the anterior spinal arises from only one of the distal vertebral arteries.
   (b) Posterolateral spinal artery
       The posterolateral spinal artery arises from the distal vertebral artery or proximal posterior inferior cerebellar artery (PICA), and travels inferi-orly along the posterior cord. There is one on each side. There are two

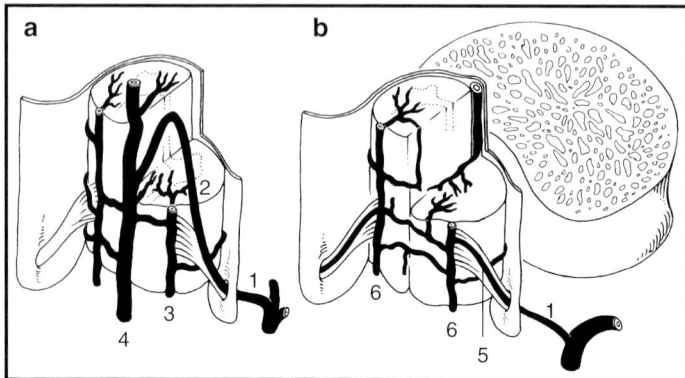

Fig. 1.59 Normal spinal arterial anatomy. (**a**) Anterior view. Radicular artery (*1*),
radiculomedullary artery (*2*), pial arterial plexus (*3*), anterior spinal artery (*4*); (**b**)
Posterior view. Radicular artery (*1*), radiculopial artery (*5*), posterolateral arteries (*6*).

major variants of this artery. Each is associated with variations in the
size and course of the distal vertebral artery and level of origin of the
PICA.[231,276]

    i. Posterior spinal artery

       This artery arises from either the distal extracranial portion of the
vertebral or commonly also from the proximal part of an extracranial origin of PICA. Each posterior spinal artery then travels inferiorly along the posterior cord dorsal to the posterior spinal nerve
roots.[276]

    ii. Lateral spinal artery

       This artery arises from the distal vertebral artery or proximal
PICA. However, the lateral spinal artery travels along the posterolateral cord ventral to the posterior roots of C1 through C4.[231] The
lateral spinal artery joins the ipsilateral posterior spinal artery at
the C4 or C5 level.[276]

(c) Segmental branches

    These small paired arteries provide muscular and osseous blood flow in
the cervical region. They are variable and can supply anterior and posterior radicular branches that follow the spinal nerve roots. These radicular branches can connect to either the anterior spinal artery or to the
posterolateral spinal artery to provide segmental input to these longitudinal spinal arteries, usually below C3.[277]

(d) A particularly large radicular input into the cervical anterior spinal
artery is sometimes termed the *artery of the cervical enlargement*. This
artery often is a branch of the vertebral artery, although it may arise
from the costocervical trunk (Fig. 1.60) or even directly from the subclavian artery.

2. Deep cervical artery

    The deep cervical artery arises from the costocervical trunk or directly from
the second part of the subclavian artery. The left and right deep cervical
arteries paired longitudinal arterial systems that are posterior to the transverse processes. They have considerable muscular territories, anastomose
with the vertebral arteries, and can provide flow to the radicular arteries
along the C7 and C8 roots.[277] They variably contribute to the lower cervical
cord.

3. Ascending cervical artery

    The ascending cervical artery is a branch of the thyrocervical trunk and ascends
in the neck anterior to the transverse processes. This artery supplies cervical
muscles, anastomoses with the vertebral artery, and can provide radicular
branches.

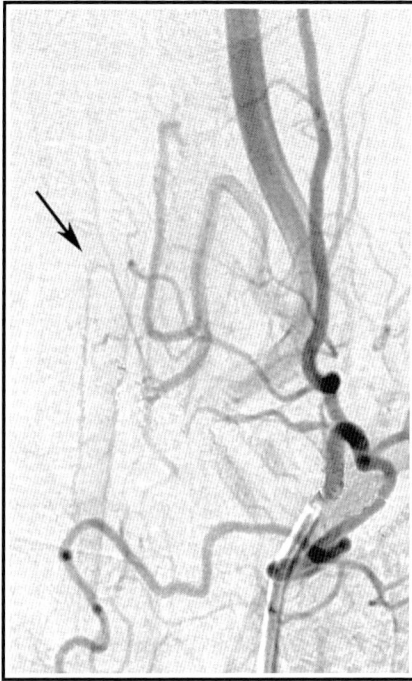

Fig. 1.60 Artery of cervical enlargement. A dominant branch to the cervical portion of the anterior spinal artery often arises from the segmental branches of the vertebral artery, but in this case can be seen to fill on an injection of the costocervical trunk. This is a frontal view with injection into the left thyrocervical trunk. Note the hair-pin turn of the artery as it joins the anterior spinal artery (*arrow*).

4. Supreme intercostal artery
   This artery arises from the costocervical trunk or directly from the subclavian artery and descends to supply several spinal levels, generally providing radicular arteries to the C7 and C8 levels[277] and sometimes one or two levels below. Branches contribute to bone, connective tissue and muscle at the cervicothoracic junction usually at T1 and T2 and collateralizing to T3. The supreme intercostal arteries occasionally arise directly from the aorta.[7]

5. Intercostal (aka posterior intercostal) artery
   Usually nine pairs of intercostal arteries arise from the aorta. Occasionally, adjacent intercostal arteries arise as a common trunk. Intercostal arteries provide branches to the spine and paraspinal tissues before traveling laterally under the rib in the costal groove. Adjacent intercostal arteries share numerous collaterals. The intercostal arteries have several branches:[7]
   (a) Dorsal branch
       The dorsal branch divides into a spinal branch that supplies bone and dura, which in turn provides a radicular branch that supplies the nerves and possibly the spinal cord. The dorsal branch also has medial and lateral musculocutaneous branches that supply posterior muscles and overlying skin.
   (b) Collateral intercostal branch
       This branch anastamoses to adjacent intercostal arteries.

(c) Muscular branches
This branch supplies lateral and anterior chest wall muscles and anastamose with lateral thoracic branches of the axillary artery.
(d) Lateral cutaneous
This branch supplies intercostal nerves and lateral chest wall skin.
(e) Multiple small branches to ribs and deep chest wall tissues.
6. Lumbar arteries
Usually four pairs of lumbar arteries arise from the aorta. There are collaterals between ipsilateral lumbar arteries and from side-to-side. The lumbar arteries have branches that are similar to the intercostal arteries:[7]
(a) Dorsal branch
The dorsal branch gives osseous branches to the vertebral body, and then provides a spinal branch that supplies bone and dura via a post-central branch in the anterior region of the spinal canal, and a prelaminar branch to the posterior region of the canal. In between those two branches, the spinal artery provides a radicular branch to supply the nerves and the spinal cord. The dorsal branch also has medial and lateral musculo-cutaneous branches that supply the posterior muscles and the overlying skin of the lumbar region.
(b) Collateral lumbar branches
These branches anastamose with adjacent lumbar arteries.
(c) Muscular branches
These branches supply lateral and posterior muscles and anastamose with lower intercostal arteries, adjacent lumbar, iliolumbar, inferior epigastric, and deep circumflex iliac arteries.[7]
7. Iliolumbar artery
This branch of the posterior division of the internal iliac artery has branches to the psoas muscle, collaterals to the fourth lumbar artery, an L5 radicular artery, and supplies the gluteal and abdominal wall muscles.[7]
8. Lateral sacral artery
The paired lateral sacral arteries are branches of the internal iliac arteries. They supply upper sacral radicular arteries and can anastamose with median sacral artery branches.
9. Median sacral artery
A single descending median sacral artery arises at the aortic bifurcation and supplies multiple levels of the sacrum. It anastamoses with the lateral sacral and iliolumbar arteries.[7] This artery is the remnant of the caudal aorta prior to the development of the limb buds.

Segmental Contributions to Neural Territories

Radicular Arteries (Anterior and Posterior)

The radicular arteries enter the spine along the spinal nerves and include an anterior radicular artery along the ventral root and a posterior radicular artery along the dorsal root. They may or may not be present at each level and do not necessarily contribute to the spinal cord at every level. In the cervical spine there is an average of 2–3 radicular artery connections to the spinal cord, including 2–3 anteriorly and 1 or 2 posteriorly.[277] In the thoracolumbar region, 80% of spinal cord blood flow comes from two radicular contributions.[278] Throughout the cord, anterior radicular contributions to the cord number 3–15, and posterior radicular artery contributions number 14–25.[279] There are two commonly mentioned types of radicular artery contributions to the spinal cord: the radiculomedullary and radiculopial arteries.
1) *Radiculomedullary* arteries. These radicular branches connect the anterior radicular artery to the anterior spinal artery.
a) The artery of Adamkiewicz (aka "arteria radicularis magna" or "artery of the lumbar enlargement") is the dominant radiculomedullary contribution to anterior spinal artery in thoracolumbar spine. It supplies an average of 68% of blood flow to the lower cord, with an average diameter of 0.7 mm.[278] It has a classic "hairpin turn" appearance. It travels sharply cephalad from a radicular artery, and then takes a sharp caudal turn as it joins the anterior spinal artery.
b) The origin of the artery of Adamkiewicz is variable. In nearly all cases it arises from the intercostal and lumbar arteries from T8–L2 and is on the

left in 80% of cases.[33] In 70% of cases the artery of Adamkiewicz arises from a lumbar artery.[280] A dominant radiculomedullary artery below L3 was found in only 3 of 4,000 spine angiograms.[281] When it arises from above T8 or below L2 there may be a second dominant radiculomedullary contributor above or below.

2) *Radiculopial* arteries. These radicular branches connect the posterior radicular branches to a pial network and the posterolateral spinal arteries.[282] In 63% of cases a radiculomedullary feeder also has a posterior radiculopial contribution to posterior spinal artery.[95]

Strange, but True

Albert Wojciek Adamkiewicz's study of the vascular anatomy of the spinal cord was the result of his interest in syphilis. He wanted to determine how the bacteria responsible for syphilis made their way to the spinal cord. This originated with his idea that tabes dorsalis was a blood-borne disease.[277,283,284] The rest is history.

Extrinsic Spinal Cord Arteries

These intradural arteries run along the surface of the spinal cord (Fig. 1.59).
1) Anterior spinal artery
   a) The anterior spinal artery is a longitudinal artery that originates from the distal vertebral arteries and runs continuously down the cord in the anterior median sulcus with variable contributions from radiculomedullary inputs.[280] Occasionally, it may split into two channels, but almost never below C5–6.[277]
2) Posterolateral spinal arteries
   a) These paired longitudinal arteries originate from the vertebral arteries proximal to the PICA origins (or from the PICA itself) and run more or less discontinuously along the posterolateral cord, with sporadic contributions from radiculopial arteries. In the cervical region there may be two pairs of longitudinal vessels posteriorly, including the lateral spinal ventral to the dorsal root and posterior spinal dorsal to that dorsal root; these two systems merge at C4 or C5.[276] A single pair of posterior longitudinal arteries exist throughout the majority of the extent of the cord.
3) Pial network
   a) This is a variable network of longitudinal and interconnecting axial vessels, that primarily anastamose to the posterior spinal arteries with only very small connections to anterior spinal artery.[279]
4) Conus basket
   a) The anterior spinal artery and posterior spinal arteries join together in a "basket" of arteries around the lower part of the conus medularis.
   b) An important arterial source for the conus is the artery of Deproges–Gotteron (aka the cone artery).[285] This artery is inconstant and may arise from the internal iliac artery or its branches. It courses along the L-5 or S-1 nerve roots to anastomos with the conus basket.

Intrinsic Cord Arteries

1) Sulcal commissural arteries
   a) These arteries arise from ASA, dive into the median sulcus, and feed the grey matter structures.
2) Radial perforating arteries
   a) These arteries originate from the pial network, penetrate deeply, and primarily supply white matter tracts.
3) Intrinsic anastamoses
   a) Axial and longitudinal precapillary connections interconnect the intrinsic arteries in all planes from one to another at the same axial level, and to the vessels cranial and caudal to that level.[282]

Spinal Venous System

Spinal venous anatomy is many ways similar to and in other ways different from the corresponding arterial organization. They are "the same, but different." Lasjaunias provided an exhaustive description of spinal venous anatomy.[282]

1) Intrinsic spinal cord veins
   a) Intrinsic cord veins are radially oriented venules with axial and longitudinal anastomoses. They are uniformly distributed throughout the cord. They drain into ventral and dorsal sulcal veins.
2) Extrinsic spinal cord veins
   a) Ventromedial and dorsomedial veins
      i) These are continuous longitudinal craniocaudal channels of more or less equal size. Unlike spinal cord arteries, ventral and dorsal veins do not differ significantly in size.[282] Transmedullary anastomoses are present between ventral and dorsal sulcal veins.
   b) Ventral and dorsal pial network
      i) Small interconnected veins connecting radial intrinsic veins with longitudinal veins.
   c) Dorsal and ventral radicular veins
      i) Variable veins connecting cord veins to epidural veins. Levels without a patent radicular vein may have a fibrotic remnant. Transdural portion of the vein has a relative narrowing.
   d) In thoracic region: Longitudinal ventromedial and dorsomedial veins often split up into three channels. Many more patent radicular veins are usually present, compared to the cervical and lumbar regions. The upper thoracic cord drains cephalad, and the lower thoracic cord drains in a caudal direction, producing a potential "watershed zone" at variable levels in the thoracic spinal cord.[282]
3) Epidural and extra-spinal veins
   a) Epidural venous plexus
      i) Dense, multichannel network from skull-base to sacrum. There are lateral longitudinal channels and side-to-side connections without valves at each vertebral level. The ventral channels are more prominent.
   b) Dorsal and ventral emissary radicular veins
      i) These veins connect the epidural plexus to the longitudinal spinal veins (vertebral, azygos/hemiazygos, lumbar, and sacral veins).
   c) Cervical region: Vertebral veins connect with the suboccipital plexus above and the jugular veins and deep cervical veins below.
   d) Thoracic region: On the right drainage is into the azygos vein; on the left drainage is into the superior (aka accessory) and inferior hemiazygos veins.
   e) Lumbar region: Drainage is into the azygos vein and directly into the inferior vena cava and left renal vein.
   f) Sacrum: Drainage is into the internal iliac veins.

References

1. Osborn AG. Diagnostic cerebral angiography. 2nd ed. Philadelphia: Lippincott Williams & Wilkins; 1999.
2. De Garis CF, Black IB, Riemenschneider EA. Patterns of the aortic arch in American white and Negro stocks, with comparative notes on certain other mammals. J Anat. 1933; 67:599–618.
3. Freed K, Low VH. The aberrant subclavian artery. AJR Am J Roentgenol 1997;168:481–4.
4. La Barbera G, La Marca G, Martino A, et al. Kinking, coiling, and tortuosity of extracranial internal carotid artery: is it the effect of a metaplasia? Surg Radiol Anat. 2006;28:573–80.
5. Reiner A, Kasser R. Relative frequency of a subclavian vs. a transverse cervical origin for the dorsal scapular artery in humans. Anat Rec. 1996;244:265–8.
6. Morris P. Practical neuroangiography. Baltimore: Williams & Wilkins; 1997.
7. Standring S. Gray's anatomy. 39th ed. New York: Elsevier; 2005.
8. Handa J, Matsuda M, Handa H. Lateral position of the external carotid artery. Report of a case. Radiology. 1972;102: 361–2.
9. Teal JS, Rumbaugh CL, Bergeron RT, Segall HD. Lateral position of the external carotid artery: a rare anomaly? Radiology. 1973;108:77–81.
10. Dahn MS, Kaurich JD, Brown FR. Independent origins of the internal and external carotid arteries – a case report. Angiology. 1999;50:755–60.
11. Aggarwal NR, Krishnamoorthy T, Devasia B, Menon G, Chandrasekhar K. Variant origin of superior thyroid artery, occipital artery and ascending pharyngeal artery from a common trunk from the cervical segment of internal carotid artery. Surg Radiol Anat. 2006;28:650–3.
12. Kaneko K, Akita M, Murata E, Imai M, Sowa K. Unilateral anomalous left common carotid artery; a case report. Ann Anat. 1996;178:477–80.
13. Zumre O, Salbacak A, Cicekcibasi AE, Tuncer I, Seker M. Investigation of the bifurcation level of the common carotid artery and variations of the branches of the external carotid artery in human fetuses. Ann Anat. 2005;187:361–9.
14. Silbergleit R, Quint DJ, Mehta BA, Patel SC, Metes JJ, Noujaim SE. The persistent stapedial artery. AJNR Am J Neuroradiol. 2000;21:572–7.
15. Rodesch G, Choi IS, Lasjaunias P. Complete persistence of the hyoido-stapedial artery in man. Case report. Intra-petrous origin of the maxillary artery from ICA. Surg Radiol Anat. 1991;13:63–5.
16. Moreano EH, Paparella MM, Zelterman D, Goycoolea MV. Prevalence of facial canal dehiscence and of persistent stapedial artery in the human middle ear: a report of 1000 temporal bones. Laryngoscope. 1994;104:309–20.
17. Lasjaunias P, Moret J. Normal and non-pathological variations in the angiographic aspects of the arteries of the middle ear. Neuroradiology. 1978;15:213–9.
18. Lasjaunias P, Santoyo-Vazquez A. Segmental agenesis of the internal carotid artery: angiographic aspects with embryological discussion. Anat Clin. 1984;6:133–41.
19. Lasjaunias P, Berenstein A. Functional anatomy of craniofacial arteries. New York: Springer; 1987.
20. Monfared A, Kim D, Jaikumar S, Gorti G, Kam A. Microsurgical anatomy of the superior and recurrent laryngeal nerves. Neurosurgery. 2001;49:925–32; discussion 32–3.
21. Liu JL, Liang CY, Xiang T, et al. Aberrant branch of the superior laryngeal artery passing through the thyroid foramen. Clin Anat. 2007;20:256–9.
22. Delattre JF, Flament JB, Palot JP, Pluot M. Variations in the parathyroid glands. Number, situation and arterial vascularization. Anatomical study and surgical application. J Chir (Paris). 1982;119:633–41.
23. Lo A, Oehley M, Bartlett A, Adams D, Blyth P, Al-Ali S. Anatomical variations of the common carotid artery bifurcation. ANZ J Surg. 2006;76:970–2.
24. Hacein-Bey L, Daniels DL, Ulmer JL, et al. The ascending pharyngeal artery: branches, anastomoses, and clinical significance. AJNR Am J Neuroradiol. 2002;23:1246–56.
25. Haffajee MR. A contribution by the ascending pharyngeal artery to the arterial supply of the odontoid process of the axis vertebra. Clin Anat. 1997;10:14–8.
26. Mercer NS, MacCarthy P. The arterial supply of the palate: implications for closure of cleft palates. Plast Reconstr Surg. 1995;96:1038–44.
27. Huang MH, Lee ST, Rajendran K. Clinical implications of the velopharyngeal blood supply: a fresh cadaveric study. Plast Reconstr Surg. 1998;102:655–67.
28. Lasjaunias P, Berenstein A, Doyon D. Normal functional anatomy of the facial artery. Radiology. 1979;133:631–8.
29. Djindjian R, Merland J. Superselective arteriography of the external carotid artery. New York: Springer; 1978.
30. Niranjan NS. An anatomical study of the facial artery. Ann Plast Surg. 1988;21:14–22.
31. Moreau S, Bourdon N, Salame E, et al. Facial nerve: vascular-related anatomy at the stylomastoid foramen. Ann Otol Rhinol Laryngol. 2000;109:849–52.
32. Tubbs RS, Salter G, Oakes WJ. Continuation of the ascending cervical artery as the occipital artery in man. Anat Sci Int. 2004;79:43–5.
33. Lasjaunias P, Berenstein A, ter Brugge KG. Surgical neuroangiography, volume 1: clinical vascular anatomy and variations. Berlin: Springer; 2001.
34. McKinnon BJ, Wall MP, Karakla DW. The vascular anatomy and angiosome of the posterior auricular artery. A cadaver study. Arch Facial Plast Surg. 1999;1:101–4.
35. Pinar YA, Ikiz ZA, Bilge O. Arterial anatomy of the auricle: its importance for reconstructive surgery. Surg Radiol Anat. 2003;25:175–9.
36. Imanishi N, Nakajima H, Aiso S. Arterial anatomy of the ear. Okajimas Folia Anat Jpn. 1997;73:313–23.
37. Burggasser G, Happak W, Gruber H, Freilinger G. The temporalis: blood supply and innervation. Plast Reconstr Surg. 2002;109:1862–9.
38. Lauber H. Ueber einige varietaeten im verlaufe der arteria maxillaris interna. Anat Anz. 1901;19:444–8.
39. Lurje A. On the topographical anatomy of the internal maxillary artery. Acta Anat. 1947;2:219–31.
40. Wasicky R, Pretterklieber ML. The human anterior tympanic artery. A nutrient artery of the middle ear with highly variable origin. Cells Tissues Organs. 2000;166:388–94.
41. Diamond MK. Homologies of the meningeal-orbital arteries of humans: a reappraisal. J Anat. 1991;178:223–41.
42. Erturk M, Kayalioglu G, Govsa F, Varol T, Ozgur T. The cranio-orbital foramen, the groove on the lateral wall of the human orbit, and the orbital branch of the middle meningeal artery. Clin Anat. 2005;18:10–4.
43. Yoshioka N, Rhoton Jr AL, Abe H. Scalp to meningeal arterial anastomosis in the parietal foramen. Neurosurgery. 2006;58:ONS123–6; discussion ONS-6.
44. Tolosa E. Collateral circulation in occlusive vascular lesions of the brain. The role of the middle meningeal artery in the collateral circulation in compensating for occlusions of the internal carotid artery or its branches. Prog Brain Res. 1968;30:247–54.
45. Dilenge D, Ascherl Jr GF. Variations of the ophthalmic and middle meningeal arteries: relation to the embryonic stapedial artery. AJNR Am J Neuroradiol. 1980;1:45–54.
46. Gabriele OF, Bell D. Ophthalmic origin of the middle meningeal artery. Radiology. 1967;89:841–4.
47. McLennan JE, Rosenbaum AE, Haughton VM. Internal carotid origins of the middle meningeal artery. The ophthalmic-middle meningeal and stapedial-middle meningeal arteries. Neuroradiology. 1974;7:265–75.
48. Kawai K, Yoshinaga K, Koizumi M, Honma S, Tokiyoshi A, Kodama K. A middle meningeal artery which arises from the internal carotid artery in which the first branchial artery participates. Ann Anat. 2006;188:33–8.

49. Brucher J. Origin of the ophthalmic artery from the middle meningeal artery. Radiology. 1969;93:51–2.

50. Hiura A. An anomalous ophthalmic artery arising from the middle meningeal artery. Anat Anz. 1980;147:473–6.

51. Watanabe A, Hirano K, Ishii R. Dural caroticocavernous fistula with both ophthalmic arteries arising from middle meningeal arteries. Neuroradiology. 1996;38:806–8.

52. Liu Q, Rhoton Jr AL. Middle meningeal origin of the ophthalmic artery. Neurosurgery. 2001;49:401–6; discussion 6–7.

53. Anderson RJ. A palatine branch from the middle meningeal artery. J Anat Physiol. 1880;15:136–8.

54. Kresimir Lukic I, Gluncic V, Marusic A. Extracranial branches of the middle meningeal artery. Clin Anat. 2001;14:292–4.

55. Silvela J, Zamarron MA. Tentorial arteries arising from the external carotid artery. Neuroradiology. 1978;14:267–9.

56. Seeger JF, Hemmer JF. Persistent basilar/middle meningeal artery anastomosis. Radiology. 1976;118:367–70.

57. Lasjaunias P, Moret J, Manelfe C, Theron J, Hasso T, Seeger J. Arterial anomalies at the base of the skull. Neuroradiology. 1977;13:267–72.

58. Waga S, Okada M, Yamamoto Y. Basilar-middle meningeal arterial anastomosis. Case report. J Neurosurg. 1978;49:450–2.

59. Hofmeijer J, Klijn CJ, Kappelle LJ, Van Huffelen AC, Van Gijn J. Collateral circulation via the ophthalmic artery or leptomeningeal vessels is associated with impaired cerebral vasoreactivity in patients with symptomatic carotid artery occlusion. Cerebrovasc Dis. 2002;14:22–6.

60. Baumel JJ, Beard DY. The accessory meningeal artery of man. J Anat. 1961;95:386–402.

61. Vitek JJ. Accessory meningeal artery: an anatomic misnomer. AJNR Am J Neuroradiol. 1989;10:569–73.

62. Duncan IC, Dos Santos C. Accessory meningeal arterial supply to the posterior nasal cavity: another reason for failed endovascular treatment of epistaxis. Cardiovasc Intervent Radiol. 2003;26:488–91.

63. Lasjaunias P, Theron J. Radiographic anatomy of the accessory meningeal artery. Radiology. 1976;121:99–104.

64. Komiyama M, Kitano S, Sakamoto H, Shiomi M. An additional variant of the persistent primitive trigeminal artery: accessory meningeal artery–antero-superior cerebellar artery anastomosis associated with moyamoya disease. Acta Neurochir (Wien). 1998;140:1037–42.

65. Khaki AA, Tubbs RS, Shoja MM, Shokouhi G, Farahani RM. A rare variation of the inferior alveolar artery with potential clinical consequences. Folia Morphol (Warsz). 2005;64:345–6.

66. Chien HF, Wu CH, Wen CY, Shieh JY. Cadaveric study of blood supply to the lower intraorbital fat: etiologic relevance to the complication of anaerobic cellulitis in orbital floor fracture. J Formos Med Assoc. 2001;100:192–7.

67. Traxler H, Windisch A, Geyerhofer U, Surd R, Solar P, Firbas W. Arterial blood supply of the maxillary sinus. Clin Anat. 1999;12:417–21.

68. Markham JW. Sudden loss of vision following alcohol block of the infraorbital nerve. Case report. J Neurosurg. 1973;38:655–7.

69. Osborn AG. The vidian artery: normal and pathologic anatomy. Radiology. 1980;136:373–8.

70. Tubbs RS, Salter EG. Vidius vidius (guido guidi): 1509–1569. Neurosurgery. 2006;59:201–3; discussion 201–3.

71. Amin N, Ohashi Y, Chiba J, Yoshida S, Takano Y. Alterations in vascular pattern of the developing palate in normal and spontaneous cleft palate mouse embryos. Cleft Palate Craniofac J. 1994;31:332–44.

72. Lee HY, Kim HU, Kim SS, et al. Surgical anatomy of the sphenopalatine artery in lateral nasal wall. Laryngoscope. 2002;112:1813–8.

73. Pretterklieber ML, Krammer EB, Mayr R. A bilateral maxillofacial trunk in man: an extraordinary anomaly of the carotid system of arteries. Acta Anat (Basel). 1991;141:206–11.

74. Gibo H, Lenkey C, Rhoton Jr AL. Microsurgical anatomy of the supraclinoid portion of the internal carotid artery. J Neurosurg. 1981;55:560–74.

75. Bouthillier A, van Loveren HR, Keller JT. Segments of the internal carotid artery: a new classification. Neurosurgery. 1996;38:425–32; discussion 32–3.

76. Fischer E. Die Lageabweichungen der vorderen Hirnarterie im Gefässbild. Zentralbl Neurochir. 1938;3:300–13.

77. Kerber CW, Know K, Hecht ST, Buxton RB. Flow dynamics in the human carotid bulb. Int J Neuroradiol. 1996;2:422–9.

78. Morimoto T, Nitta K, Kazekawa K, Hashizume K. The anomaly of a non-bifurcating cervical carotid artery. Case report. J Neurosurg. 1990;72:130–2.

79. Pascual-Castroviejo I, Viano J, Pascual-Pascual SI, Martinez V. Facial haemangioma, agenesis of the internal carotid artery and dysplasia of cerebral cortex: case report. Neuroradiology. 1995;37:692–5.

80. Lee JH, Oh CW, Lee SH, Han DH. Aplasia of the internal carotid artery. Acta Neurochir (Wien). 2003;145:117–25; discussion 25.

81. Chen CJ, Chen ST, Hsieh FY, Wang LJ, Wong YC. Hypoplasia of the internal carotid artery with intercavernous anastomosis. Neuroradiology. 1998;40:252–4.

82. Quint DJ, Boulos RS, Spera TD. Congenital absence of the cervical and petrous internal carotid artery with intercavernous anastomosis. AJNR Am J Neuroradiol. 1989;10:435–9.

83. Tasar M, Yetiser S, Tasar A, Ugurel S, Gonul E, Saglam M. Congenital absence or hypoplasia of the carotid artery: radioclinical issues. Am J Otolaryngol. 2004;25:339–49.

84. Cali RL, Berg R, Rama K. Bilateral internal carotid artery agenesis: a case study and review of the literature. Surgery. 1993;113:227–33.

85. Teal JS, Rumbaugh CL, Segall HD, Bergeron RT. Anomalous branches of the internal cartoid artery. Radiology. 1973;106: 567–73.

86. Glasscock 3rd ME, Seshul M, Seshul Sr MB. Bilateral aberrant internal carotid artery case presentation. Arch Otolaryngol Head Neck Surg. 1993;119:335–9.

87. Chess MA, Barsotti JB, Chang JK, Ketonen LM, Westesson PL. Duplication of the extracranial internal carotid artery. AJNR Am J Neuroradiol. 1995;16:1545–7.

88. Pedroza A, Dujovny M, Artero JC, et al. Microanatomy of the posterior communicating artery. Neurosurgery. 1987;20:228–35.

89. Saltzman GF. Patent primitive trigeminal artery studied by cerebral angiography. Acta Radiol. 1959;51:329–36.

90. McKenzie JD, Dean BL, Flom RA. Trigeminal-cavernous fistula: Saltzman anatomy revisited. AJNR Am J Neuroradiol. 1996;17:280–2.

91. Uchino A, Sawada A, Takase Y, Kudo S. MR angiography of anomalous branches of the internal carotid artery. AJR Am J Roentgenol. 2003;181:1409–14.

92. Richardson DN, Elster AD, Ball MR. Intrasellar trigeminal artery. AJNR Am J Neuroradiol. 1989;10:205.

93. Lie AA. Congenital anomolies of the carotid arteries. Amsterdam: Excerpta Medica Foundation; 1968.

94. Patel AB, Gandhi CD, Bederson JB. Angiographic documentation of a persistent otic artery. AJNR Am J Neuroradiol. 2003;24:124–6.

95. Lasjaunias PL, Berenstein A. Surgical neuroangiography: functional vascular anatomy of brain, spinal cord and spine. New York: Springer; 1991.

96. De Caro R, Parenti A, Munari PF. The persistent primitive hypoglossal artery: a rare anatomic variation with frequent clinical implications. Ann Anat. 1995;177:193–8.

97. Brismar J. Persistent hypoglossal artery, diagnostic criteria. Report of a case. Acta Radiol Diagn (Stockh). 1976;17:160–6.

98. Kanai H, Nagai H, Wakabayashi S, Hashimoto N. A large aneurysm of the persistent primitive hypoglossal artery. Neurosurgery. 1992;30:794–7.

99. Kolbinger R, Heindel W, Pawlik G, Erasmi-Korber H. Right proatlantal artery type I, right internal carotid occlusion, and left internal carotid stenosis: case report and review of the literature. J Neurol Sci. 1993;117:232–9.

100. Suzuki S, Nobechi T, Itoh I, Yakura M, Iwashita A. Persistent proatlantal intersegmental artery and occipital artery originating from internal carotid artery. Neuroradiology. 1979;17:105–9.

101. San Millan Ruiz D, Gailloud P, Rufenacht DA, Delavelle J, Henry F, Fasel JH. The craniocervical venous system in relation to cerebral venous drainage. AJNR Am J Neuroradiol. 2002;23:1500–8.

102. De Ridder D, De Ridder L, Nowe V, Thierens H, Van de Heyning P, Moller A. Pulsatile tinnitus and the intrameatal vascular loop: why do we not hear our carotids? Neurosurgery. 2005;57:1213–7.

103. Paullus WS, Pait TG, Rhoton Jr AL. Microsurgical exposure of the petrous portion of the carotid artery. J Neurosurg. 1977;47:713–26.

104. Quisling RG, Rhoton Jr AL. Intrapetrous carotid artery branches: radioanatomic analysis. Radiology. 1979;131:133–6.
105. Windfuhr JP. Aberrant internal carotid artery in the middle ear. Ann Otol Rhinol Laryngol Suppl. 2004;192:1–16.
106. Pahor AL, Hussain SS. Persistent stapedial artery. J Laryngol Otol. 1992;106:254–7.
107. Tauber M, van Loveren HR, Jallo G, Romano A, Keller JT. The enigmatic foramen lacerum. Neurosurgery. 1999;44: 386–91; discussion 91–3.
108. Ziyal IM, Salas E, Wright DC, Sekhar LN. The petrolingual ligament: the anatomy and surgical exposure of the postero-lateral landmark of the cavernous sinus. Acta Neurochir (Wien). 1998;140:201–4; discussion 4–5.
109. Ziyal IM, Ozgen T, Sekhar LN, Ozcan OE, Cekirge S. Proposed classification of segments of the internal carotid artery: anatomical study with angiographical interpretation. Neurol Med Chir (Tokyo). 2005;45:184–90; discussion 90–1.
110. Marshman LA, Connor S, Polkey CE. Internal carotid-inferior petrosal sinus fistula complicating foramen ovale telemetry: successful treatment with detachable coils: case report and review. Neurosurgery. 2002;50:209–12.
111. Resnick DK, Subach BR, Marion DW. The significance of carotid canal involvement in basilar cranial fracture. Neurosurgery. 1997;40:1177–81.
112. Rhoton Jr AL. The sellar region. Neurosurgery. 2002;51: S335–74.
113. Inoue T, Rhoton Jr AL, Theele D, Barry ME. Surgical approaches to the cavernous sinus: a microsurgical study. Neurosurgery. 1990;26:903–32.
114. Tran-Dinh H. Cavernous branches of the internal carotid artery: anatomy and nomenclature. Neurosurgery. 1987;20: 205–10.
115. Rhoton Jr AL. The cavernous sinus, the cavernous venous plexus, and the carotid collar. Neurosurgery. 2002;51: S375–410.
116. Bernasconi V, Cassinari V. Angiographical characteristics of meningiomas of tentorium. Radiol Med (Torino). 1957;43:1015–26.
117. Tsitsopoulos PD, Tsonidis CA, Petsas GP, Hadjiioannou PN, Njau SN, Anagnostopoulos IV. Microsurgical study of the Dorello's canal. Skull Base Surg. 1996;6:181–5.
118. Parkinson D. Collateral circulation of cavernous carotid artery: anatomy. Can J Surg. 1964;7:251–68.
119. Hayreh SS. Orbital vascular anatomy. Eye. 2006;20: 1130–44.
120. Renn WH, Rhoton Jr AL. Microsurgical anatomy of the sellar region. J Neurosurg. 1975;43:288–98.
121. Sacher M, Som PM, Shugar JM, Leeds NE. Kissing intra-sellar carotid arteries in acromegaly: CT demonstration. J Comput Assist Tomogr. 1986;10:1033–5.
122. Midkiff RB, Boykin MW, McFarland DR, Bauman JA. Agenesis of the internal carotid artery with intercavernous anastomosis. AJNR Am J Neuroradiol. 1995;16:1356–9.
123. Kobayashi S, Kyoshima K, Gibo H, Hegde SA, Takemae T, Sugita K. Carotid cave aneurysms of the internal carotid artery. J Neurosurg. 1989;70:216–21.
124. Gonzalez LF, Walker MT, Zabramski JM, Partovi S, Wallace RC, Spetzler RF. Distinction between paraclinoid and cavernous sinus aneurysms with computed tomo-graphic angiography. Neurosurgery. 2003;52:1131–7; discussion 8–9.
125. Tsutsumi S, Rhoton Jr AL. Microsurgical anatomy of the central retinal artery. Neurosurgery. 2006;59:870–8; discus-sion 8–9.
126. Gray H. Gray's anatomy. 1901st ed. Philadelphia: Running Press; 1901.
127. Hayreh SS. Arteries of the orbit in the human being. Br J Surg. 1963;50:938–53.
128. Lang J, Kageyama I. The ophthalmic artery and its branches, measurements and clinical importance. Surg Radiol Anat. 1990;12:83–90.
129. Krisht AF, Barrow DL, Barnett DW, Bonner GD, Shengalaia G. The microsurgical anatomy of the superior hypophyseal artery. Neurosurgery. 1994;35:899–903; discussion 903.
130. Alvarez H, Rodesch G, Garcia-Monaco R, Lasjaunias P. Embolisation of the ophthalmic artery branches distal to its visual supply. Surg Radiol Anat. 1990;12:293–7.
131. Saeki N, Rhoton Jr AL. Microsurgical anatomy of the upper basilar artery and the posterior circle of Willis. J Neurosurg. 1977;46:563–78.
132. Alpers BJ, Berry RG, Paddison RM. Anatomical studies of the circle of Willis in normal brain. AMA Arch Neurol Psychiatry. 1959;81:409–18.
133. Tripathi M, Goel V, Padma MV, et al. Fenestration of the posterior communicating artery. Neurol India. 2003;51: 75–6.
134. Rhoton Jr AL, Fujii K, Fradd B. Microsurgical anatomy of the anterior choroidal artery. Surg Neurol. 1979;12:171–87.
135. Morandi X, Brassier G, Darnault P, Mercier P, Scarabin JM, Duval JM. Microsurgical anatomy of the anterior choroidal artery. Surg Radiol Anat. 1996;18:275–80.
136. Paroni Sterbini GL, Agatiello LM, Stocchi A, Solivetti FM. CT of ischemic infarctions in the territory of the anterior chor-oidal artery: a review of 28 cases. AJNR Am J Neuroradiol. 1987;8:229–32.
137. Das K, Benzil DL, Rovit RL, Murali R, Couldwell WT. Irving S. Cooper (1922–1985): a pioneer in functional neu-rosurgery. J Neurosurg. 1998;89:865–73.
138. Cooper IS. Surgical occlusion of the anterior choroidal artery in parkinsonism. Surg Gynecol Obstet. 1954;92:207–19.
139. Moyer DJ, Flamm ES. Anomalous arrangement of the ori-gins of the anterior choroidal and posterior communicating arteries. Case report. J Neurosurg. 1992;76:1017–8.
140. Takahashi S, Suga T, Kawata Y, Sakamoto K. Anterior choroidal artery: angiographic analysis of variations and anomalies. AJNR Am J Neuroradiol. 1990;11:719–29.
141. Taveras JM, Wood EH. Diagnostic neuroradiology. 2nd ed. Baltimore: Williams & Wilkins; 1976. p. 584–7.
142. Waga S, Morikawa A. Aneurysm developing on the infundibular widening of the posterior communicating artery. Surg Neurol. 1979;11:125–7.
143. Ohyama T, Ohara S, Momma F. Fatal subarachnoid hemor-rhage due to ruptured infundibular widening of the poste-rior communicating artery–case report. Neurol Med Chir (Tokyo). 1994;34:172–5.
144. Saltzman GF. Infundibular widening of the posterior com-municating artery studied by carotid angiography. Acta Radiol. 1959;51:415–21.
145. Wollschlaeger G, Wollschlaeger PB, Lucas FV, Lopez VF. Experience and result with postmortem cerebral angiogra-phy performed as routine procedure of the autopsy. Am J Roentgenol Radium Ther Nucl Med. 1967;101:68–87.
146. Willis T. Cerebri anatome; cui accessit nervorum descriptio et usus. London: J. Flesher; 1664.
147. Wolpert SM. The circle of Willis. AJNR Am J Neuroradiol. 1997;18:1033–4.
148. Krabbe-Hartkamp MJ, van der Grond J, de Leeuw FE, et al. Circle of Willis: morphologic variation on three-dimensional time-of-flight MR angiograms. Radiology. 1998;207:103–11.
149. Hendrikse J, van Raamt AF, van der Graaf Y, Mali WPTM, van der Grond J. Distribution of cerebral blood flow in the circle of Willis. Radiology. 2005;235:184–9.
150. Alpers BJ, Berry RG. Circle of Willis in cerebral vascular disorders. The anatomical structure. Arch Neurol. 1963;8: 398–402.
151. Rhoton Jr AL, Saeki N, Perlmutter D, Zeal A. Microsurgical anatomy of common aneurysm sites. Clin Neurosurg. 1979;26:248–306.
152. Hoksbergen AW, Legemate DA, Csiba L, Csati G, Siro P, Fulesdi B. Absent collateral function of the circle of Willis as risk factor for ischemic stroke. Cerebrovasc Dis. 2003;16: 191–8.
153. Serizawa T, Saeki N, Yamaura A. Microsurgical anatomy and clinical significance of the anterior communicating artery and its perforating branches. Neurosurgery. 1997; 40:1211–6; discussion 6–8.
154. Dunker RO, Harris AB. Surgical anatomy of the proximal anterior cerebral artery. J Neurosurg. 1976;44:359–67.
155. Gomes FB, Dujovny M, Umansky F, et al. Microanatomy of the anterior cerebral artery. Surg Neurol. 1986;26:129–41.
156. Zurada A, St Gielecki J, Tubbs RS, et al. Three-dimensional morphometry of the A1 segment of the anterior cerebral artery with neurosurgical relevance. Neurosurgery. 2010;67:1768–82.
157. Marinkovic S, Milisavljevic M, Kovacevic M. Anatomical bases for surgical approach to the initial segment of the

anterior cerebral artery. Microanatomy of Heubner's artery and perforating branches of the anterior cerebral artery. Surg Radiol Anat. 1986;8:7–18.

158. Moffat DB. A case of peristence of the primitive olfactory artery. Anat Anz. 1967;121:477–9.

159. Nozaki K, Taki W, Kawakami O, Hashimoto N. Cerebral aneurysm associated with persistent primitive olfactory artery aneurysm. Acta Neurochir (Wien). 1998;140:397–401; discussion 401–2.

160. Bollar A, Martinez R, Gelabert M, Garcia A. Anomalous origin of the anterior cerebral artery associated with aneurysm–embryological considerations. Neuroradiology. 1988; 30:86.

161. Maurer J, Maurer E, Perneczky A. Surgically verified variations in the A1 segment of the anterior cerebral artery. Report of two cases. J Neurosurg. 1991;75:950–3.

162. Given 2nd CA, Morris PP. Recognition and importance of an infraoptic anterior cerebral artery: case report. AJNR Am J Neuroradiol. 2002;23:452–4.

163. Minakawa T, Kawamata M, Hayano M, Kawakami K. Aneurysms associated with fenestrated anterior cerebral arteries. Report of four cases and review of the literature. Surg Neurol. 1985;24:284–8.

164. Suzuki K, Onuma T, Sakurai Y, Mizoi K, Ogawa A, Yoshimoto T. Aneurysms arising from the proximal (A1) segment of the anterior cerebral artery. A study of 38 cases. J Neurosurg. 1992;76:455–8.

165. Choudhari KA. Fenestrated anterior cerebral artery. Br J Neurosurg. 2002;16:525–9.

166. Ladzinski P, Maliszewski M, Majchrzak H. The accessory anterior cerebral artery: case report and anatomic analysis of vascular anomaly. Surg Neurol. 1997;48:171–4.

167. Singer RJ, Abe T, Taylor WH, Marks MP, Norbash AM. Intracavernous anterior cerebral artery origin with associated arteriovenous malformations: a developmental analysis: case report. Neurosurgery. 1997;40:829–31; discussion 831.

168. Spinnato S, Pasqualin A, Chioffi F, Da Pian R. Infraoptic course of the anterior cerebral artery associated with an anterior communicating artery aneurysm: anatomic case report and embryological considerations. Neurosurgery. 1999;44:1315–9.

169. Burbank NS, Morris PP. Unique anomalous origin of the left anterior cerebral artery. AJNR Am J Neuroradiol. 2005; 26:2533–5.

170. Busse O. Aneurysmen und Bildungsfehler der A. Communicans Anterior. Virchows Arch Pathol Anat. 1927;229:178–89.

171. Perlmutter D, Rhoton Jr AL. Microsurgical anatomy of the anterior cerebral-anterior communicating-recurrent artery complex. J Neurosurg. 1976;45:259–72.

172. Marinkovic S, Milisavljevic M, Marinkovic Z. Branches of the anterior communicating artery. Microsurgical anatomy. Acta Neurochir (Wien). 1990;106:78–85.

173. Perlmutter D, Rhoton Jr AL. Microsurgical anatomy of the distal anterior cerebral artery. J Neurosurg. 1978;49:204–28.

174. Ostrowski AZ, Webster JE, Gurdjian ES. The proximal anterior cerebral artery: an anatomic study. Arch Neurol. 1960;3:661–4.

175. Baptista AG. Studies on the arteries of the brain. Ii. The anterior cerebral artery: some anatomic features and their clinical implications. Neurology. 1963;13:825–35.

176. Huber P, Braun J, Hirschmann D, Agyeman JF. Incidence of berry aneurysms of the unpaired pericallosal artery: angiographic study. Neuroradiology. 1980;19:143–7.

177. Cinnamon J, Zito J, Chalif DJ, et al. Aneurysm of the azygos pericallosal artery: diagnosis by MR imaging and MR angiography. AJNR Am J Neuroradiol. 1992;13:280–2.

178. Osaka K, Matsumoto S. Holoprosencephaly in neurosurgical practice. J Neurosurg. 1978;48:787–803.

179. Yasargil MG, Carter LP. Saccular aneurysms of the distal anterior cerebral artery. J Neurosurg. 1974;40:218–23.

180. Gloger S, Gloger A, Vogt H, Kretschmann HJ. Computerassisted 3D reconstruction of the terminal branches of the cerebral arteries. I. Anterior cerebral artery. Neuroradiology. 1994;36:173–80.

181. Gibo H, Carver CC, Rhoton Jr AL, Lenkey C, Mitchell RJ. Microsurgical anatomy of the middle cerebral artery. J Neurosurg. 1981;54:151–69.

182. Umansky F, Gomes FB, Dujovny M, et al. The perforating branches of the middle cerebral artery. A microanatomical study. J Neurosurg. 1985;62:261–8.

183. Grand W. Microsurgical anatomy of the proximal middle cerebral artery and the internal carotid artery bifurcation. Neurosurgery. 1980;7:215–8.

184. Komiyama M, Nakajima H, Nishikawa M, Yasui T. Middle cerebral artery variations: duplicated and accessory arteries. AJNR Am J Neuroradiol. 1998;19:45–9.

185. Umansky F, Dujovny M, Ausman JI, Diaz FG, Mirchandani HG. Anomalies and variations of the middle cerebral artery: a microanatomical study. Neurosurgery. 1988;22:1023–7.

186. Uchino M, Kitajima S, Sakata Y, Honda M, Shibata I. Ruptured aneurysm at a duplicated middle cerebral artery with accessory middle cerebral artery. Acta Neurochir (Wien). 2004;146:1373–4; discussion 5.

187. Takahashi T, Suzuki S, Ohkuma H, Iwabuchi T. Aneurysm at a duplication of the middle cerebral artery. AJNR Am J Neuroradiol. 1994;15:1166–8.

188. Jain KK. Some observations on the anatomy of the middle cerebral artery. Can J Surg. 1964;7:134–9.

189. Gloger S, Gloger A, Vogt H, Kretschmann HJ. Computerassisted 3D reconstruction of the terminal branches of the cerebral arteries. II. Middle cerebral artery. Neuroradiology. 1994;36:181–7.

190. Abanou A, Lasjaunias P, Manelfe C, Lopez-Ibor L. The accessory middle cerebral artery (AMCA). Diagnostic and therapeutic consequences. Anat Clin. 1984;6:305–9.

191. Morioka M, Fujioka S, Itoyama Y, Ushio Y. Ruptured distal accessory anterior cerebral artery aneurysm: case report. Neurosurgery. 1997;40:399–401; discussion 401–2.

192. Takahashi S, Hoshino F, Uemura K, Takahashi A, Sakamoto K. Accessory middle cerebral artery: is it a variant form of the recurrent artery of Heubner? AJNR Am J Neuroradiol. 1989;10:563–8.

193. Han DH, Gwak HS, Chung CK. Aneurysm at the origin of accessory middle cerebral artery associated with middle cerebral artery aplasia: case report. Surg Neurol. 1994;42:388–91.

194. Van Der Zwan A, Hillen B. Araldite F as injection material for quantitative morphology of cerebral vascularization. Anat Rec. 1990;228:230–6.

195. Heubner O. Die luetischen Erkrankungen der Hirnarterien. Leipzig: FC Vogel; 1874. p. 170–214.

196. Vander Eecken HM, Adams RD. The anatomy and functional significance of the meningeal arterial anastomoses of the human brain. J Neuropathol Exp Neurol. 1953;12:132–57.

197. Brozici M, van der Zwan A, Hillen B. Anatomy and functionality of leptomeningeal anastomoses: a review. Stroke. 2003;34:2750–62.

198. Michotey P, Moscow NP, Salamon G. Anatomy of the cortical branches of the middle cerebral artery. In: Newton TH, Potts DG, editors. Radiology of the skull and brain. St. Louis: C.V. Mosby; 1974. p. 1471–8.

199. Hart JL, Davagnanam I, Chandrashekar HS, Brew S. Angiography and selective microcatheter embolization of a falcine meningioma supplied by the artery of Davidoff and Schechter. J Neurosurg. 2011;114:710–3.

200. Margolis MT, Newton TH, Hoyt WF. Gross and roentgenologic anatomy of the posterior cerebral artery. In: Newton TH, Potts PC, editors. Radiology of the skull and brain. St. Louis: C.V. Mosby; 1974. p. 1551–76.

201. Margolis MT, Newton TH, Hoyt WF. Cortical branches of the posterior cerebral artery. Anatomic-radiologic correlation. Neuroradiology. 1971;2:127–35.

202. Caruso G, Vincentelli F, Rabehanta P, Giudicelli G, Grisoli F. Anomalies of the P1 segment of the posterior cerebral artery: early bifurcation or duplication, fenestration, common trunk with the superior cerebellar artery. Acta Neurochir (Wien). 1991;109:66–71.

203. Percheron G. Arteries of the human thalamus. II. Arteries and paramedian thalamic territory of the communicating basilar artery. Rev Neurol (Paris). 1976;132:309–24.

204. Raphaeli G, Liberman A, Gomori JM, Steiner I. Acute bilateral paramedian thalamic infarcts after occlusion of the artery of Percheron. Neurology. 2006;66:E7.

205. Matheus MG, Castillo M. Imaging of acute bilateral paramedian thalamic and mesencephalic infarcts. AJNR Am J Neuroradiol. 2003;24:2005–8.

206. Milisavljevic MM, Marinkovic SV, Gibo H, Puskas LF. The thalamogeniculate perforators of the posterior cerebral artery: the microsurgical anatomy. Neurosurgery. 1991;28: 523–9; discussion 9–30.

207. Berland LL, Haughton VM. Anomalous origin of posterior choroidal artery from basilar artery. AJR Am J Roentgenol. 1979;132:674–5.

208. Fujii K, Lenkey C, Rhoton Jr AL. Microsurgical anatomy of the choroidal arteries: lateral and third ventricles. J Neurosurg. 1980;52:165–88.

209. Galloway JR, Greitz T. The medial and lateral choroid arteries. An anatomic and roentgenographic study. Acta Radiol. 1960;53:353–66.

210. Wollschlaeger PB, Wollschlaeger G. An infratentorial meningeal artery. Radiologe. 1965;5:451–2.

211. Ono M, Ono M, Rhoton Jr AL, Barry M. Microsurgical anatomy of the region of the tentorial incisura. J Neurosurg. 1984;60:365–99.

212. Bojanowski WM, Rigamonti D, Spetzler RF, Flom R. Angiographic demonstration of the meningeal branch of the posterior cerebral artery. AJNR Am J Neuroradiol. 1988;9:808.

213. Furuno M, Yamakawa N, Okada M, Waga S. Anomalous origin of the calcarine artery. Neuroradiology. 1995; 37:658.

214. Abrahams JM, Hurst RW, Bagley LJ, Zager EL. Anterior choroidal artery supply to the posterior cerebral artery distribution: embryological basis and clinical implications. Neurosurgery. 1999;44:1308–14.

215. Tubbs RS, Salter G, Wellons 3rd JC, Oakes WJ. Blood supply of the human cervical sympathetic chain and ganglia. Eur J Morphol. 2002;40:283–8.

216. Lemke AJ, Benndorf G, Liebig T, Felix R. Anomalous origin of the right vertebral artery: review of the literature and case report of right vertebral artery origin distal to the left subclavian artery. AJNR Am J Neuroradiol. 1999;20: 1318–21.

217. Goray VB, Joshi AR, Garg A, Merchant S, Yadav B, Maheshwari P. Aortic arch variation: a unique case with anomalous origin of both vertebral arteries as additional branches of the aortic arch distal to left subclavian artery. AJNR Am J Neuroradiol. 2005;26:93–5.

218. Palmer FJ. Origin of the right vertebral artery from the right common carotid artery: angiographic demonstration of three cases. Br J Radiol. 1977;50:185–7.

219. Goddard AJ, Annesley-Williams D, Guthrie JA, Weston M. Duplication of the vertebral artery: report of two cases and review of the literature. Neuroradiology. 2001;43:477–80.

220. Tubbs RS, Loukas M, Remy AC, Shoja MM, Salter EG, Oakes WJ. The vertebral nerve revisited. Clin Anat. 2007; 20:644–7.

221. Brink B. Approaches to the second segment of the vertebral artery. In: Berguer R, Bauer R, editors. Vertebrobasilar arterial occlusive disease. New York: Raven; 1984. p. 257–64.

222. Diaz FG, Ausman JI, Shrontz C, et al. Surgical correction of lesions affecting the second portion of the vertebral artery. Neurosurgery. 1986;19:93–100.

223. D'Antoni AV, Battaglia F, Dilandro AC, Moore GD. Anatomic study of the suboccipital artery of Salmon with surgical significance. Clin Anat. 2010;23(7):798–802.

224. Fine AD, Cardoso A, Rhoton Jr AL. Microsurgical anatomy of the extracranial-extradural origin of the posterior inferior cerebellar artery. J Neurosurg. 1999;91:645–52.

225. de Oliveira E, Rhoton Jr AL, Peace D. Microsurgical anatomy of the region of the foramen magnum. Surg Neurol. 1985;24:293–352.

226. Akar ZC, Dujovny M, Slavin KV, Gomez-Tortosa E, Ausman JI. Microsurgical anatomy of the intracranial part of the vertebral artery. Neurol Res. 1994;16:171–80.

227. Lister JR, Rhoton Jr AL, Matsushima T, Peace DA. Microsurgical anatomy of the posterior inferior cerebellar artery. Neurosurgery. 1982;10:170–99.

228. Ahuja A, Graves VB, Crosby DL, Strother CM. Anomalous origin of the posterior inferior cerebellar artery from the internal carotid artery. AJNR Am J Neuroradiol. 1992;13: 1625–6.

229. Ogawa T, Fujita H, Inugami A, Shishido F, Higano S, Uemura K. Anomalous origin of the posterior inferior

230. Margolis MT, Newton TH. The posterior inferior cerebellar artery. In: Newton TH, Potts DG, editors. Radiology of the skull and brain. St. Louis: C.V. Mosby; 1974. p. 1710–74.

231. Salamon G, Huang YP. Radiologic anatomy of the brain. Berlin: Springer; 1976. p. 305–6.

232. Lewis SB, Chang DJ, Peace DA, Lafrentz PJ, Day AL. Distal posterior inferior cerebellar artery aneurysms: clinical features and management. J Neurosurg. 2002;97:756–66.

233. Smoker WR, Price MJ, Keyes WD, Corbett JJ, Gentry LR. High-resolution computed tomography of the basilar artery: 1. Normal size and position. AJNR Am J Neuroradiol. 1986;7:55–60.

234. Torche M, Mahmood A, Araujo R, Dujovny M, Dragovic L, Ausman JI. Microsurgical anatomy of the lower basilar artery. Neurol Res. 1992;14:259–62.

235. Shrontz C, Dujovny M, Ausman JI, et al. Surgical anatomy of the arteries of the posterior fossa. J Neurosurg. 1986; 65:540–4.

236. Amarenco P, Rosengart A, DeWitt LD, Pessin MS, Caplan LR. Anterior inferior cerebellar artery territory infarcts. Mechanisms and clinical features. Arch Neurol. 1993;50: 154–61.

237. Naidich TP, Kricheff II, George AE, Lin JP. The normal anterior inferior cerebellar artery. Anatomic-radiographic correlation with emphasis on the lateral projection. Radiology. 1976;119:355–73.

238. Atkinson WJ. The anterior inferior cerebellar artery: it's variation, pontine distribution and significance in surgery of cerebello-pontine angle tumors. J Neurol Neurosurg Psychiatry. 1949;12:137–51.

239. Rhoton Jr AL. Microsurgery of the internal acoustic meatus. Surg Neurol. 1974;2:311–8.

240. Brunsteins DB, Ferreri AJ. Microsurgical anatomy of VII and VIII cranial nerves and related arteries in the cerebellopontine angle. Surg Radiol Anat. 1990;12:259–65.

241. Martin RG, Grant JL, Peace D, Theiss C, Rhoton Jr AL. Microsurgical relationships of the anterior inferior cerebellar artery and the facial-vestibulocochlear nerve complex. Neurosurgery. 1980;6:483–507.

242. Ito J, Takeda N, Suzuki Y, Tekeuchi S, Osugi S, Yoshida Y. Anomalous origin of the anterior inferior cerebellar arteries from the internal carotid artery. Neuroradiology. 1980;19: 105–9.

243. Caruso G, Vincentelli F, Giudicelli G, Grisoli F, Xu T, Gouaze A. Perforating branches of the basilar bifurcation. J Neurosurg. 1990;73:259–65.

244. Pedroza A, Dujovny M, Ausman JI, et al. Microvascular anatomy of the interpeduncular fossa. J Neurosurg. 1986; 64:484–93.

245. Hardy DG, Rhoton Jr AL. Microsurgical relationships of the superior cerebellar artery and the trigeminal nerve. J Neurosurg. 1978;49:669–78.

246. Hardy DG, Peace DA, Rhoton Jr AL. Microsurgical anatomy of the superior cerebellar artery. Neurosurgery. 1980;6: 10–28.

247. Stopford JSB. The arteries of the pons and medulla oblongata. J Anat. 1916;50:131–64.

248. De Caro R, Serafini MT, Galli S, Parenti A, Guidolin D, Munari PF. Anatomy of segmental duplication in the human basilar artery. Possible site of aneurysm formation. Clin Neuropathol. 1995;14:303–9.

249. Sanders WP, Sorek PA, Mehta BA. Fenestration of intracranial arteries with special attention to associated aneurysms and other anomalies. AJNR Am J Neuroradiol. 1993;14:675–80.

250. Huber P. Cerebral angiography. 2nd ed. New York: Thieme; 1982.

251. Osborn AG. Craniofacial venous plexuses: angiographic study. AJR Am J Roentgenol. 1981;136:139–43.

252. Braun JP, Tournade A. Venous drainage in the craniocervical region. Neuroradiology. 1977;13:155–8.

253. Andrews BT, Dujovny M, Mirchandani HG, Ausman JI. Microsurgical anatomy of the venous drainage into the superior sagittal sinus. Neurosurgery. 1989;24:514–20.

254. Curé JK, Van Tassel P, Smith MT. Normal and variant anatomy of the dural venous sinuses. Semin Ultrasound CT MR. 1994;15:499–519.

255. Boyd GI. The emissary foramina of the cranium in man and the anthropoids. J Anat. 1930;65:108–21.

256. Thewissen JG. Mammalian frontal diploic vein and the human foramen caecum. Anat Rec. 1989;223:242–4.

257. San Millan Ruiz D, Gailloud P, Rufenacht DA, Yilmaz H, Fasel JH. Anomalous intracranial drainage of the nasal mucosa: a vein of the foramen caecum? AJNR Am J Neuroradiol. 2006;27:129–31.

258. Jaeger R. Observations on resection of the superior longitudinal sinus at and posterior to the rolandic venous inflow. J Neurosurg. 1951;8:103–9.

259. Hasegawa M, Yamashita J, Yamashima T. Anatomical variations of the straight sinus on magnetic resonance imaging in the infratentorial supracerebellar approach to pineal region tumors. Surg Neurol. 1991;36:354–9.

260. Browder J, Kaplan HA, Krieger AJ. Anatomical features of the straight sinus and its tributaries. J Neurosurg. 1976;44: 55–61.

261. Das AC, Hasan M. The occipital sinus. J Neurosurg. 1970;33:307–11.

262. Green HT. The venous drainage of the human hypophysis cerebri. Am J Anat. 1957;100:435–69.

263. Tubbs RS. Herophilus of Chalcedon: a pioneer in neuroscience. Neurosurgery. 2006;58:E590; discussion E.

264. Gebarski SS, Gebarski KS. Inferior petrosal sinus: imaging-anatomic correlation. Radiology. 1995;194:239–47.

265. Hacker H. Superficial supratentorial veins and dural sinues. In: Newton TH, Potts DG, editors. Radiology of the skull and brain: veins. St. Louis: C.V. Mosby; 1974. p. 1851–902.

266. Galligioni F, Bernardi R, Pellone M, Iraci G. The superficial sylvian vein in normal and pathologic cerebral angiography. Am J Roentgenol Radium Ther Nucl Med. 1969;107: 565–78.

267. Sener RN. The occipitotemporal vein: a cadaver, MRI and CT study. Neuroradiology. 1994;36:117–20.

268. Di Chiro G. Angiographic patterns of cerebral convexity veins and superficial dural sinuses. Am J Roentgenol Radium Ther Nucl Med. 1962;87:308–21.

269. Ture U, Yasargil MG, Al-Mefty O. The transcallosal-transforaminal approach to the third ventricle with regard to the venous variations in this region. J Neurosurg. 1997;87:706–15.

270. Ono M, Rhoton Jr AL, Peace D, Rodriguez RJ. Microsurgical anatomy of the deep venous system of the brain. Neurosurgery. 1984;15:621–57.

271. Garner TB, Del Curling Jr O, Kelly Jr DL, Laster DW. The natural history of intracranial venous angiomas. J Neurosurg. 1991;75:715–22.

272. Wilms G, Bleus E, Demaerel P, et al. Simultaneous occurrence of developmental venous anomalies and cavernous angiomas. AJNR Am J Neuroradiol. 1994;15:1247–54; discussion 55–7.

273. Abe T, Singer RJ, Marks MP, Norbash AM, Crowley RS, Steinberg GK. Coexistence of occult vascular malformations and developmental venous anomalies in the central nervous system: MR evaluation. AJNR Am J Neuroradiol. 1998;19:51–7.

274. Mullan S, Mojtahedi S, Johnson DL, Macdonald RL. Embryological basis of some aspects of cerebral vascular fistulas and malformations. J Neurosurg. 1996;85:1–8.

275. Raybaud CA, Strother CM, Hald JK. Aneurysms of the vein of Galen: embryonic considerations and anatomical features relating to the pathogenesis of the malformation. Neuroradiology. 1989;31:109–28.

276. Gailloud P, O'Riordan DP, Burger I, Lehmann CU. Confirmation of communication between deep venous drainage and the vein of galen after treatment of a vein of Galen aneurysmal malformation in an infant presenting with severe pulmonary hypertension. AJNR Am J Neuroradiol. 2006;27:317–20.

277. Siclari F, Burger IM, Fasel JH, Gailloud P. Developmental anatomy of the distal vertebral artery in relationship to variants of the posterior and lateral spinal arterial systems. AJNR Am J Neuroradiol. 2007;28:1185–90.

278. Chakravorty BG. Arterial supply of the cervical spinal cord (with special reference to the radicular arteries). Anat Rec. 1971;170:311–29.

279. Schalow G. Feeder arteries, longitudinal arterial trunks and arterial anastomoses of the lower human spinal cord. Zentralbl Neurochir. 1990;51:181–4.

280. Rodriguez-Baeza A, Muset-Lara A, Rodriguez-Pazos M, Domenech-Mateu JM. The arterial supply of the human spinal cord: a new approach to the arteria radicularis magna of Adamkiewicz. Acta Neurochir (Wien). 1991;109:57–62.

281. Biglioli P, Roberto M, Cannata A, et al. Upper and lower spinal cord blood supply: the continuity of the anterior spinal artery and the relevance of the lumbar arteries. J Thorac Cardiovasc Surg. 2004;127:1188–92.

282. Tveten L. Spinal cord vascularity. III. The spinal cord arteries in man. Acta Radiol Diagn (Stockh). 1976;17:257–73.

283. Lo D, Vallee JN, Spelle L, et al. Unusual origin of the artery of Adamkiewicz from the fourth lumbar artery. Neuroradiology. 2002;44:153–7.

284. Adamkiewicz A. Die Blutgefasse desmenschlichen Ruckenmarkes. I. Theil. Die Gefasse der Ruckenmarkssubstanz. Sitzungsberichte der Kaiserlichen Akademie der Wissenschaften, mathematisch-naturwissenschaftliche Classe. 1881;84:469–502.

285. Desproges-Gotteron R. Contribution á l'étude de la sciatque paralysante (thése). Paris; 1955.

286. Habel RE, Budras KD. Bovine anatomy: an illustrated text. Hanover: Schlütersche GmbH & Co.; 2003.

287. Layton KF, Kallmes DF, Cloft HJ, Lindell EP, Cox VS. Bovine aortic arch variant in humans: clarification of a common misnomer. AJNR Am J Neuroradiol. 2006;27: 1541–2.

288. Pickhardt PJ, Siegel MJ, Gutierrez FR. Vascular rings in symptomatic children: frequency of chest radiographic findings. Radiology. 1997;203:423–6.

289. Gottfried ON, Soleau SW, Couldwell WT. Suprasellar displacement of intracavernous internal carotid artery: case report. Neurosurgery. 2003;53:1433–4; discussion 4–5.

290. Fujimura M, Seki H, Sugawara T, Tomichi N, Oku T, Higuchi H. Anomalous internal carotid artery-anterior cerebral artery anastomosis associated with fenestration and cerebral aneurysm. Neurol Med Chir (Tokyo). 1996;36: 229–33.

291. Hayreh SS, Dass R. The ophthalmic artery. II. Origin and intracranial and intra-canalicular course. Br J Ophthalmol. 1962;46:165–85.

292. Lasjaunias P, Vallee B, Person H, Ter Brugge K, Chiu M. The lateral spinal artery of the upper cervical spinal cord. Anatomy, normal variations, and angiographic aspects. J Neurosurg. 1985;63:235–41.

293. Barr JD, Lemley TJ. Endovascular arterial occlusion accomplished using microcoils deployed with and without proximal flow arrest: results in 19 patients. AJNR Am J Neuroradiol. 1999;20:1452–6.

294. Zouaoui A, Hidden G. Cerebral venous sinuses: anatomical variants or thrombosis? Acta Anat (Basel). 1988;133: 318–24.

295. Acar F, Naderi S, Guvencer M, Ture U, Arda MN. Herophilus of Chalcedon: a pioneer in neuroscience. Neurosurgery. 2005;56:861–7; discussion 861–7.

2. Diagnostic Cerebral Angiography

Catheter angiography is still considered the gold standard for imaging cerebral vasculature. Diagnostic angiography is also typically done as the first step during neurointerventional procedures. Mastery of diagnostic angiography is a prerequisite for neurointerventional training. Training standards formulated by the American Society of Interventional and Therapeutic Neuroradiology (ASITN), the Joint Section of Cerebrovascular Neurosurgery, and the American Society of Neuroradiology (ASNR) recommend the performance of at least 100 diagnostic angiograms before entering neuroendovascular training.[1] This handbook authors' preference, however, is for a neurointerventionalist-in-training to perform at least 250 diagnostic cerebral angiograms prior to becoming the lead operator in neurointerventional cases.

2.1.   Indications

1. Diagnosis of primary neurovascular disease (e.g., intracranial aneurysms, arteriovenous malformations, dural arteriovenous fistulas, atherosclerotic stenosis, vasculopathy, cerebral vasospasm, acute ischemic stroke)
2. Planning for neurointerventional procedures
3. Intra-operative assistance with aneurysm surgery
4. Follow-up imaging after treatment (e.g., after aneurysm coiling or clipping, treatment of arteriovenous fistulas)

2.2.   A Brief History of Cerebral Angiography

The first report of X-ray angiography of blood vessels was in 1896. In Vienna, E. Haschek and O.T. Lindenthal obtained x-rays of blood vessels by injecting a mixture of petroleum, quicklime, and mercuric sulfide into the hand of a cadaver.[2] António de Egas Moniz, a Portuguese neurologist, is credited with the introduction of cerebral angiography. Moniz was interested in developing "arterial encephalography" as a means to localize brain tumors. He obtained cerebral angiograms in cadavers using a solution of strontium bromide and sodium iodide. These early studies demonstrated universal branching patterns among the intracranial arteries, which were contrary to popular theories based on cadaver dissection. After studies in dogs and monkeys, Moniz and his pupil Almeida Lima, performed the first angiogram on living human patients in 1927.[3] The initial attempts were done using percutaneous injections of strontium bromide and failed to show any opacified vessels.[4] In later attempts, cervical internal carotid artery was surgically exposed and temporarily occluded with a ligature while a total of 5 mL of a solution of 25% sodium iodide was injected into the vessel. Flow was restored in the artery while simultaneously obtaining an X-ray. After the ninth attempt, successful visualization of the vessels was obtained. Monitz reportedly declared: "*Nous avons realise notre desideratum.*"[4] (Very loosely translated: "Now *that's* what I needed.") Although no complications were noted during the procedure, one patient died 2 days later in status epilepticus.[5] Moniz went on to obtain successful angiograms in other patients with epilepsy, brain tumors, and postencephalitic Parkinsonism.[6,7] The first cerebral venogram was accomplished in 1931 when an inadvertent delay in photographing an angiographic plate led to an image of the venous angiographic phase, which Moniz termed a "cerebral phlebogram."

The technique became fully developed in the 1930s. By then, cerebral angiography involved direct percutaneous puncture of the carotid artery and injection of iodinated organic contrast media.[8] Despite a flurry of publications about cerebral

M.R. Harrigan, J.P. Deveikis, *Handbook of Cerebrovascular Disease and Neurointerventional Technique*, DOI 10.1007/978-1-61779-946-4_2, © Springer Science+Business Media New York 2013

angiography over the ensuing decade, many by Moniz himself, ventriculography and encephalography remained more popular as methods to image intracranial pathology.[9] Moniz was awarded the Nobel Prize in Physiology and Medicine in 1949 for his work on frontal leukotomy for psychiatric disorders, which, unlike cerebral angiography, gained early and widespread acceptance by the medical community.[10] The popularity of cerebral angiography did rise significantly by the 1950s, becoming the premier method to image the intracranial space. The neurosurgeon Gazi Yasargil performed some 10,000 angiograms between 1953 and 1964.[9]

Direct percutaneous puncture of the cervical carotid artery remained the primary technique for cerebral angiography in the 1950s and 1960s. Direct puncture of the vertebral artery was reported in 1956;[11] the posterior circulation was also imaged by puncture of the right brachial artery and retrograde injection of the contrast into the vertebral artery.[12,13] The movie *The Exorcist* (1973) featured a graphic (and realistic) depiction of a direct carotid stick. The transition from direct puncture of the cervical vessels to transfemoral artery arteriography began in the late 1960s[14] and became widespread in the 1970s.

The introduction of computed tomography (CT) in the early 1970s sharply reduced the demand for diagnostic angiography, although the field continued to develop because of the advent of interventional cardiology and other interventional fields. Metrizamide, introduced in the 1970s, was the first nonionic isosmolar iodinated contrast medium. Nonionic contrast media improved the safety and comfort of angiographic procedures considerably.

Digital subtraction angiography (DSA) was introduced in the 1980s as a method for intravenous injection of contrast for imaging the arterial system, as the contrast in the arterial system following intravenous injection was too dilute to be imaged with standard X-rays. Over the ensuing decade, the spatial resolution of DSA imaging improved to the extent that it began to rival the resolution of unsubtracted X-ray images. Further technical refinements in recent years include rotational angiography, 3D angiography, and flat panel detectors for imaging.

Global Gem

Europe was the cradle of cerebral angiography. After Moniz introduced cerebral angiography in Portugal, numerous other Old World pioneers contributed to the early development of the technique, including Herbert Olivecrona, Erik Lysholm, Georg Schönander, and Sven-Ivar Seldinger (Sweden); Norman Dott (Scotland); Arne Torkildsen (Norway); Sigurd Wende (Germany); Fedor Serbinenko (Russia); Georg Salamon and René Djindjian (France); and George Ziedses des Plantes (the Netherlands).

2.3. Complications of Diagnostic Cerebral Angiography

Informed consent prior to an angiogram should include an estimate of the risk of complications.

Neurological Complications

Neurological complications in cerebral angiography are most commonly cerebral ischemic events that occur as a result of thromboembolism or air emboli from catheters and wires. Other causes include disruption of atherosclerotic plaques and vessel dissection. Less common neurological complications include transient cortical blindness[15,16] and amnesia.[17]

In a prospective analysis of 2,899 diagnostic cerebral angiograms, the largest recent series published to date, Willinsky and colleagues reported an overall rate of neurological complications of 1.3%.[18] Of these, 0.9% were transient or reversible, and

Table 2.1 Quality improvement guidelines for adult diagnostic neuroangiography

		Suggested complication – specific threshold (%)
Neurological complications	Reversible neurologic deficit	2.5
	Permanent neurologic deficit	1
Non-neurologic complications	Renal failure	0.2
	Arterial occlusion requiring surgical thrombectomy or thrombolysis	0.2
	Arteriovenous fistula/pseudoaneurysm	0.2
	Hematoma requiring transfusion or surgical evacuation	0.5
All major complications		2

Adapted from Citron et al.,[26] with permission

0.5% were permanent. The Asymptomatic Carotid Atherosclerosis Study (ACAS) reported an often quoted neurological complication rate of 1.2% with angiography.[19]

The risk of complications appears to be related to the underlying disease process. Patients with atherosclerotic carotid disease have been reported to be at elevated risk of neurological complications with cerebral angiography.[20] Other risk factors for neurological complications include a recent cerebral ischemic event,[21,22] advanced age,[18,20] a long angiography procedure time,[20,23,24] and a diagnosis of hypertension,[24] diabetes[24] or renal insufficiency.[25]

The risk of neurological complications in patients with subarachnoid hemorrhage, intracranial aneurysms, and arteriovenous malformations was found to be relatively low in a meta-analysis of prospective studies of angiography.[22] For these patients, the overall rate of neurological complications was 0.8%, and the rate of permanent neurological complications was 0.07%. The Joint Standards of Practice Task Force of the Society of Interventional Radiology, the American Society of Interventional and Therapeutic Neuroradiology, and the American Society of Neuroradiology reviewed the complications reported in clinical series and produced guidelines for expected complication rates in neuroangiography (Table 2.1).[26] The figures in these guidelines can be quoted to patients during informed consent.

Nonneurological Complications

Nonneurological complications of cerebral angiography via the femoral artery include groin and retroperitoneal hematoma, allergic reactions, femoral artery pseudoaneurysm, thromboembolism of the lower extremity, nephropathy, and pulmonary embolism.[27] In a review of 2,899 cerebral angiograms, hematomas occurred in 0.4% of procedures, allergic cutaneous reactions occurred in 0.1%, and a pseudoaneurysm occurred after one (0.03%) procedure.[18]

2.4.   Cerebral Angiography: Basic Concepts

Preprocedure Evaluation

1. A brief neurological exam must be conducted to establish a baseline, should a neurologic change occur during or after the procedure.
2. The patient should be asked if he or she has had a history of iodinated contrast reactions.

3. The femoral pulse, as well as the dorsalis pedis and posterior tibialis pulses, should be examined.
4. Blood work, including a serum creatinine level and coagulation parameters, should be reviewed.

Pre-angiogram Orders

1. NPO except medications for 6 h prior to the procedure.
2. Place 1 peripheral IV (2 if an intervention is anticipated).
3. Place foley catheter (only if an intervention is anticipated).

Contrast Agents

Nonionic contrast agents are safer and less allergenic than ionic preparations.[28–31] Iohexol (Omnipaque®, GE Healthcare, Princeton, NJ), a low osmolality, nonionic contrast agent, is relatively inexpensive and probably the most commonly used agent in cerebral angiography.
1. Diagnostic angiogram: Omnipaque®, 300 mg I/mL
2. Neurointerventional procedure: Omnipaque®, 240 mg I/mL
Patients with normal renal function can tolerate as much as 400–800 mL of Omnipaque®, 300 mg I/mL without adverse effects.[32]

Femoral Artery Sheath (vs. No Sheath)

Trans-femoral angiography can be done with or without a sheath.

Sheath

1. Allows for the rapid exchange of catheters and less potential for trauma to the arteriotomy site.
2. Shown in a randomized trial to lessen the frequency of intraprocedural bleeding at the puncture site, and to ease catheter manipulation.[33]
3. Short sheath (10–13-cm arterial sheath) is used most commonly.
4. Longer sheath (25 cm) is useful when ileofemoral artery tortuosity or atherosclerosis might impair catheter navigation.
5. Technique: A 5F sheath (Check-Flo® Performer® Introducer set; Cook, Bloomington, IN) is slowly and continuously perfused with heparinized saline (10,000 U heparin per liter of saline) under arterial pressure.
6. Sheaths come in sizes 4F up to 10F or larger. The size refers to the inner diameter. The outer diameter is 1.5–2.0F larger than the stated size.

No Sheath

1. Slightly smaller arteriotomy and permitting earlier ambulation.
2. Use a 4F, 5F, or 3.3F catheter.[34]
3. Technique: After the Potts needle enters the femoral artery, a 145 cm 0.035 in. J-tipped wire (for most 4F catheters) or a 145 cm 0.038 in. J-tipped wire (for most 5F catheters) is introduced instead of a short J-wire. The Potts needle is then exchanged for an appropriately sized dilator, which is then exchanged for the diagnostic catheter.
4. Note: If a 4F or smaller catheter is going to be used without a sheath, use an appropriately sized micropuncture set, because a standard 18 gauge Potts needle creates an arteriotomy larger than the catheter, resulting in bleeding around the catheter.

Sedation/Analgesia

1. Midazolam (Versed®) 1–2 mg IV for sedation; lasts approximately 2 h
2. Fentanyl (Sublimaze®) 25–50 μg IV for analgesia; lasts 20–30 min

The use of sedation should be minimized, as over-sedation makes it hard to detect subtle neurological changes during the procedure. Paradoxical agitation has been reported in up to 10.2% of patients[35], particularly elderly patients and patients with a history of alcohol abuse or psychological problems.[36] Flumazenil (Romazicon®) 0.2–0.3 mg IV can reverse this effect.[37]

Suggested Wires and Catheters for Diagnostic Cerebral Angiography

Hydrophilic Wires

1. The 0.035 in. angled Glidewire® (Terumo Medical, Somerset, NJ) is soft, flexible, and steerable.
2. The 0.038 in. angled Glidewire® (Terumo Medical, Somerset, NJ) is slightly stiffer than the 0.035 in., making it helpful when added wire support is needed.
3. Extra-stiff versions of these wires are available for even more support, but they should be used with extreme caution because of the tendency of the tip to dissect vessels.

Catheters

Many catheters are suitable for cerebral angiography (Fig. 2.1). As a general rule, use 100 cm long catheters that have a curve that allows selection of the vessels from the arch. Simpler curves (e.g. Berenstein curve) are adaptable to many anatomic situations and are most appropriate for young patients with straighter vessels.

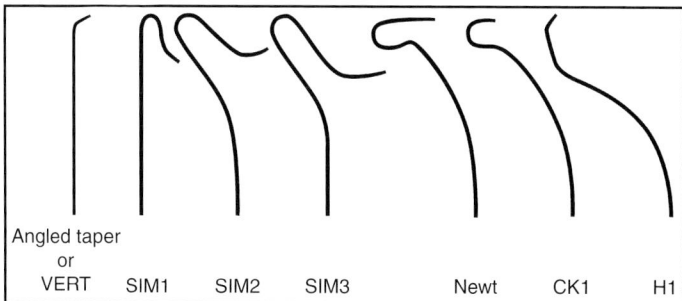

Fig. 2.1 Recommended diagnostic catheters: 5F Angled Taper, Good all-purpose diagnostic catheter. 4 or 5F Vertebral, Good all-purpose diagnostic catheter, slightly stiffer than the Angled Taper but similar in shape. 4 or 5F Simmons 1, Spinal angiography. 4 or 5F Simmons 2 or 3, Left common carotid artery; bovine configuration; tortuous aortic arch; patient's age > 50. 5F CK-1 (aka HN-5), Left common carotid or right vertebral artery. 5F H1 (aka Headhunter), Right subclavian artery; right vertebral artery. 4 or 5F Newton, Tortuous anatomy, patients >65.

More complicated curves (e.g. Simmons curve) help deal with more difficult aortic arch anatomy.

Measurement systems
Needles: Gauge, which is a measurement system too obscure for the human mind to grasp. The larger the gauge, the smaller the needle
Catheters: French (F), defined as the outer diameter of a catheter measured as a multiple of thirds of a millimeter (French number/3 = outer diameter in mm)
Wires: Measured in thousandths of an inch. (a 0.035 wire is 0.035 in. thick)

Global Gem! The French System
The French system comes from Joseph-Frédéric-Benoît Charrière, a nineteenth-century Parisian maker of surgical instruments.[38] A urinary catheter 5 mm in diameter was made by rolling a 15 mm wide strip of rubber into a tube. The diameter (circumference/π, or ~15 mm/3.14) was roughly equal to three times the width of the strip plus the glue to hold it together. The incomprehensible gauge system was developed by the British.

2.5.   Catheter Navigation

Diagnostic catheters should usually be advanced over a hydrophilic wire. The wire keeps the catheter tip from rubbing against the wall of the vessel and causing a dissection. When advancing the wire and catheter toward the aortic arch from the femoral artery, the tip of the wire should be followed by direct fluoroscopic visualization. The catheter/wire assembly should never be advanced with <8–10 cm of wire extending from the tip, as a short length of leading wire can act as a spear and cause injury to the intima. A catheter/wire assembly with only a few cm of wire sticking out can resemble a Roman short sword (Fig. 2.2).

2.6.   Roadmapping

Roadmapping should be used when engaging the vertebral arteries, and the internal and external carotid arteries. Roadmapping is essential during intracranial navigation. In some angiography suites, a "false roadmap" can be created using a regular digital subtraction angiogram; a frame from an angiographic run is selected, then inverted (i.e., vessels are turned white against a black background). This technique conserves contrast and reduces radiation exposure.

2.7.   Double Flushing

Double flushing consists of aspiration of the contents of the catheter with one 10-mL syringe of heparinized saline, followed by partial aspiration and irrigation with a second syringe of saline. This maneuver clears clots and air bubbles from the catheter, and should be done every time a wire is removed from the catheter, prior to the injection of contrast. Meticulous attention to detail is required to prevent blood from sitting in the catheter lumen, where it can coagulate into potential emboli. Any air bubbles in the system can also occlude small vessels if injected intravascularly.

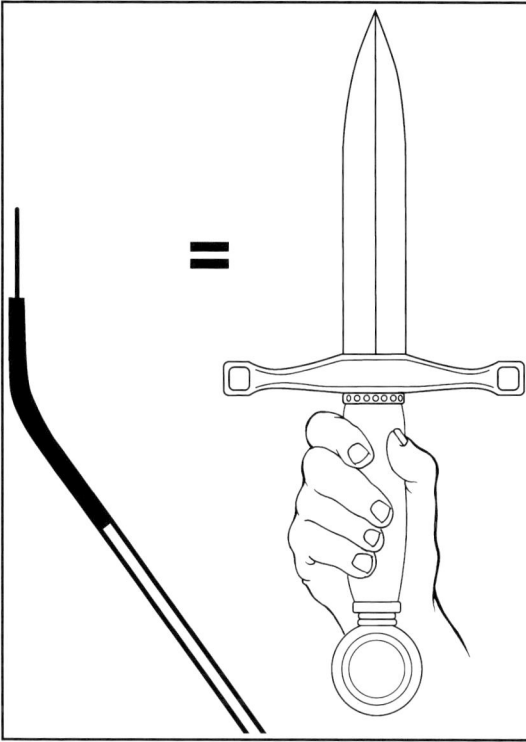

Fig. 2.2 Roman short sword.

2.8.   Continuous Saline Infusion

A three-way stopcock or manifold can be used to provide a heparinized saline drip through the catheter. This continuous drip is particularly useful if there is any delay between injections of contrast, because it keeps the catheter lumen free of blood products. Careful double flushing is still required if a wire is inserted and removed or if any blood is present in the lumen. Use of stopcocks and continuous infusion is mandatory for any therapeutic intervention.

2.9.   Hand Injection

A 10-mL syringe containing contrast should be attached to the catheter, and the syringe should be snapped with the middle finger several times to release bubbles stuck to the inside surface. The syringe should be held in a vertical position, with the plunger directed upward, to allow bubbles to rise away from the catheter (Fig. 2.3). For larger

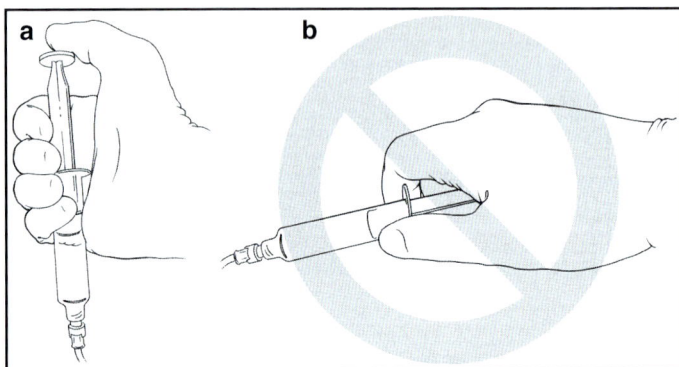

Fig. 2.3 Syringe holding method for hand injections. Correct method (**a**): the syringe is grasped in the palm of the hand when it is attached to the catheter; this position places the plunger in an upright position to allow bubbles to rise away from the attachment to the catheter. Incorrect method (**b**): the syringe is held in a horizontal position, like a weapon. Bubbles can go any which way.

vessels, like the common carotid artery, the plunger on the syringe can be depressed with the palm of the hand in order to generate enough force; for smaller vessels, like the vertebral arteries, thumb-depression of the plunger is sufficient. An adequate angiographic run can be done with a single swift injection of 4–6 mL of contrast (70%) mixed with saline (30%). The patient should be instructed to stop breathing ("Don't move, don't breath, don't swallow") for several seconds during the angiogram, then told to start breathing again.

> *A Poetic Interlude*
> *Bubbles*
> *I love 'em in my lager.*
> *I love 'em in my stout.*
> *But when they get inside my head*
> *I want to get them out!*
> *I hate them in carotids.*
> *I hate them in the "verts."*
> *They end up doing something bad.*
> *Oh yes, it really hurts!*
> *The small ones make me stupid.*
> *The big ones make me dead.*
> *'Cause when they get inside me*
> *They dance around my head!*
> *The little doctors search and search*
> *And shake out all they find.*
> *The ones they missed*
> *(It makes me pissed!)*
> *Will make me lose my mind!*
> *They find them in my saline.*
> *They find them everywhere!*
> *And superficial temporal ones*
> *Will make me lose my hair!*

Prevention of Cerebral Air Emboli
- Use meticulous technique for flushing and contrast injections (see above).
- Whenever possible, flush the catheter in the descending aorta to keep bubbles away from the cerebral circulation.

- After filling a syringe, allowing it to sit for a few minutes before injection will allow bubbles to come out of suspension and become visible.[39]
- A slower flush is less likely to cause bubbles than a rapid flush.[39]
- 1.2 μm Intrapur® filter (B. Braun Medical, Bethlehem, PA) or Posidyne® filter (Pall Medical, Port Washington, NY) in the tubing for contrast or saline injections can reduce the risk of air emboli.[40]

Management of Cerebral Air Emboli
- *Prevention is best, but if air emboli are suspected, urgent treatment is required to prevent stroke caused by occlusion of flow in vessels due to the surface tension produced by the interface between air and blood.*
- If the gas embolus is large enough to be detected fluoroscopically, and the vessel is easily accessible, a microcatheter may be used to aspirate the gas embolus and flush the vessel with heparinized saline to break up the remaining bubbles.
- Quick and readily available (though unproven) methods include the use of transcranial Doppler (to agitate and break up bubbles), heparinization (to prevent clot from forming in vessels stagnating from the air), and administration of oxygen and induction of hypertension (as in vasospasm therapy).
- If available, hyperbaric oxygen chambers have been shown (anecdotally and in small series) to result in good outcomes.[41–44] One report indicated a benefit even after a delay in initiated hyperbaric therapy.[45]
- However, a larger series showed 67% good outcome when hyperbaric treatment was started within 6 h after the onset of symptoms, versus only 35% good outcomes when treatment began later.[46]
- Induction of retrograde cerebral flow by infusing arterial blood under pressure in the jugular vein has been shown to limit ischemic damage to the brain.[47]
- When in doubt, a variety of methods can be used simultaneously, including hyperbaric oxygen *plus* retrograde cerebral flow *plus* induction of barbiturate coma to attempt to protect the brain.[48]
- The most important thing is to recognize that air emboli have occurred and then use whatever treatment modalities that are available.

2.10. Mechanical Injection

A power contrast injector is necessary for aortic arch angiograms, and some operators prefer to use an injector routinely for other vessels as well. Mechanical injection can lower radiation exposure to the operator's hands and body.[49] The pressure (pounds per square inch, psi) and flow rate during the injection should not exceed the rated pressure or flow rate of the catheter. Likewise, if a stopcock is used, the psi during injection should not exceed the rated pressure and flow rate. Common power injector settings for selective catheter digital subtraction diagnostic angiograms using a 5F catheter are listed in Table 2.2. The term "rate rise" refers to a setting on the mechanical injector that causes it to gradually increase the rate of contrast flow during the injection, to prevent the catheter tip from being kicked out of the vessel it is in. Rate rise is defined as the time required

Table 2.2 Standard power injector settings

Vessel	Power injector settings
Aortic arch	20 mL/s; total of 25 mL
Common carotid artery	8 mL/s; total of 12 mL
Subclavian artery	6 mL/s; total of 15 mL
Internal carotid artery	6 mL/s; total of 8 mL
External carotid artery	3 mL/s; total of 6 mL
Vertebral artery	6 mL/s; total of 8 mL

For digital subtraction angiography using a 5F catheter

during the injection to reach the maximum flow rate. If the vessel is smaller than average, occluded, or if the catheter is in an unstable position within the vessel, a rate rise of 0.3–0.5 s should be used. Power injector settings are different (longer) when a 3D angiogram is done; typical settings for 3D images are 3 mL/s, total of 18 mL or 4 mL/s; total of 24 mL.

2.11.   Vessel Selection

A cerebral angiogram should begin with the vessel of interest first, so that the most important vessels can be imaged in case problems with the equipment or the patient prevent completion of the entire angiogram. Following catheterization of the vessel of interest, it is usually easiest to navigate from right to left (i.e., the right vertebral artery, followed by the right common carotid artery, etc.).

Angiographic Images and Standard Views

1) Biplane angiography is the standard of care for cerebral angiography. It allows for orthogonal images to be simultaneously obtained with a single contrast injection, limiting the time and amount of contrast needed to adequately visualize the cerebral vasculature. Monoplanar cerebral angiography is acceptable only when biplane equipment is not available; the use of monoplane imaging is limited by its inability to perform automatic optical calibration and to image from orthogonal views simultaneously.
2) When viewing the angiographic images, the contrast and brightness of the image should be adjusted so that vessels are semitransparent; this can allow visualization of aneurysms, branches, or filling defects (e.g., intraluminal thrombus), which may otherwise not be visible.
3) Other imaging features worthy of attention during the performance of a cerebral angiogram:
   a) Vessel contour and size ("angioarchitecture")
   b) Contrast flow patterns
   c) Presence or absence of a vascular blush
   d) Venous phase (i.e., do not forget to examine the venous phase)
   e) Bony anatomy

Standard skull views are illustrated in Fig. 2.4. The "standard" postero-anterior (PA) projection angulates the X-ray tube usually 15–20° in a cranial direction to superimpose the roof of the orbits and top of the petrous ridges. This has been the traditional angiographic view for the carotid injections since it gives good overview of the arterial structures and allows a standard projection regardless of how much the patient's head is angulated on the table. A straight PA view may place the petrous ridges at variable relationships with the roof of the orbits, with resultant variable appearance of the intracranial vessels depending on how the patient is positioned. This view is frequently used since it requires no angulation of the X-ray C-arm. The Caldwell projection is usually done with approximately 25° caudal angulation of the X-ray tube. It aligns the petrous ridges with the bottom third of the orbits to provide a view of orbital and supratentorial structures unobstructed by the petrous ridges. The Towne's view, with 30–40° cranial angulation aligns the petrous ridges below the superior rim of the orbits and is the standard PA view for imaging the posterior fossa, since it elongates the posterior cerebral arteries. The patient can be asked to tuck his or her chin to the chest to optimize the cranial angulation. The Water's view is inclined 45° caudal and positions the petrous ridges some distance below the orbits; this is a good view for imaging the maxillary sinuses, and is an excellent view to show the full length of the basilar artery. Sub-mentovertex (aka basal or axial) view requires very steep caudal angulation such that the image intensifier is often touching the patient's chest. It helps to tilt the patient's head back to obtain this view. This is a very useful view for the middle cerebral bifurcation and Acomm. Lateral views should line up the floor of the anterior fossa and external auditory canals bilaterally to ensure a true lateral view.

The Haughton projection is a lateral view and is helpful for imaging the carotid siphon and the middle cerebral bifurcation (Fig. 2.5). The patient's head is inclined

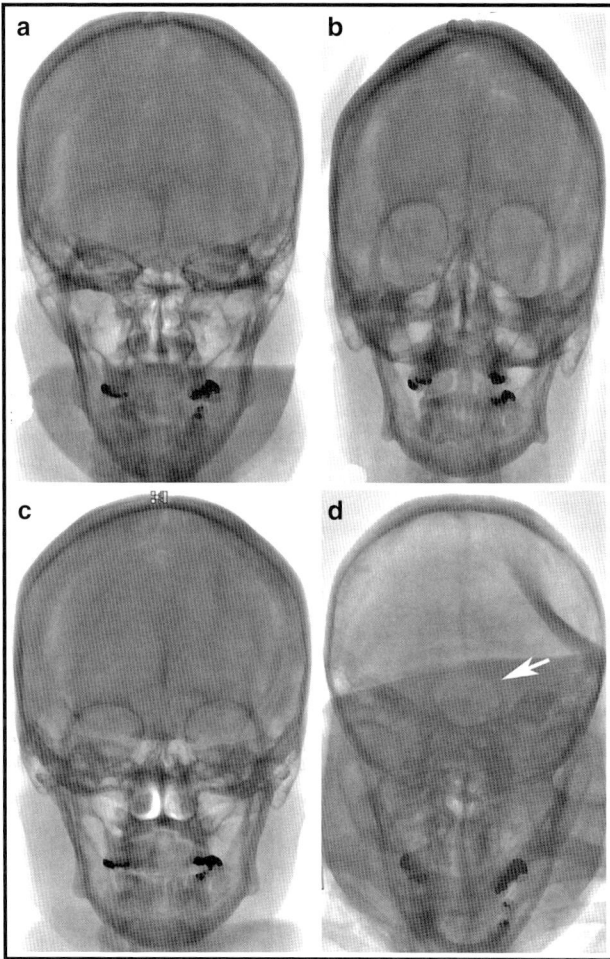

Fig. 2.4 Standard PA and lateral projections. (**a**) Standard PA. The petrous bones line up with the *upper margin* of the orbits. Elderly angiographers prefer this traditional view for intracranial anterior circulation angiography. (**b**) Straight PA. No cranial, or caudal angulation is done. In this case, the petrous bones are at the lower edge of the orbits. Younger angiographers prefer this view to the "standard PA" view. (**c**) Caldwell. 25° caudal angulation. The petrous bones are about one third of the way up the orbits. (**d**) Towne. 35° cranial angulation. The foramen magnum (*arrow*) can be seen through the calvarium.

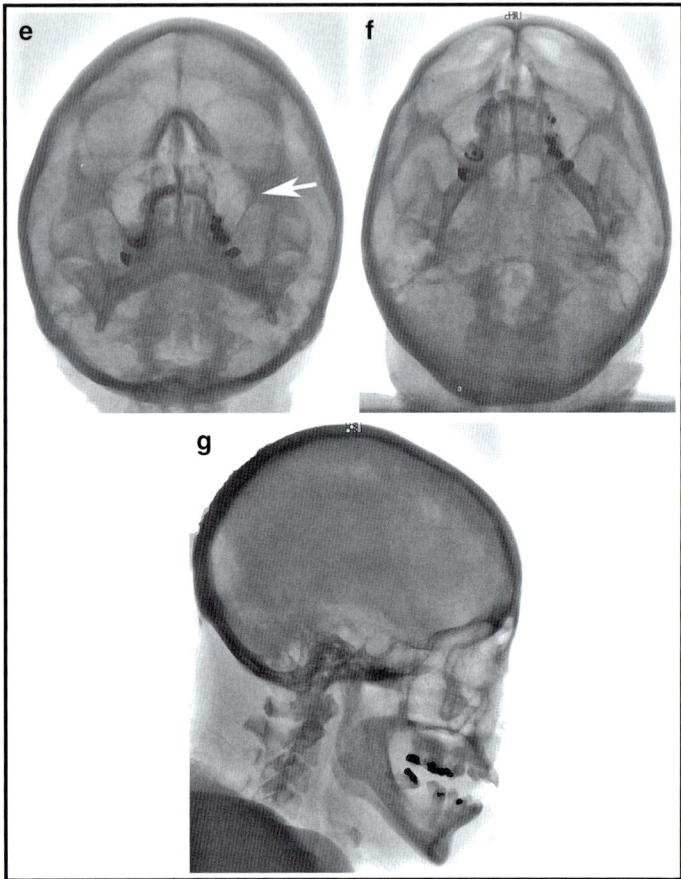

Fig. 2.4 (continued) (**e**) Water. The view is from below with 45° caudal angulation; the maxillary sinuses (*arrow*) can be seen clearly. (**f**) Submentovertex. The view is from way below, with as much caudal angulation as possible; the vertex of the skull should be framed by the mandible. (**g**) Lateral. On a straight lateral view, the floor of the left and right anterior fossa directly overlap.

away from the side of the injected carotid artery;[50] this view opens up the carotid siphon. Specific views commonly used to optimize display of certain anatomic structures are listed in Table 2.3. All of these views should be done with tight collimation of the X-ray source over the area of interest to limit scatter radiation and with the imaging detector as close to the head as possible to minimize image degradation from geometric magnification.

Pearl
Mnemonic for remembering the relative positions of the standard PA projections: The *Water(s)* runs beneath the *Town(e)*. *Caldwell* is in between.

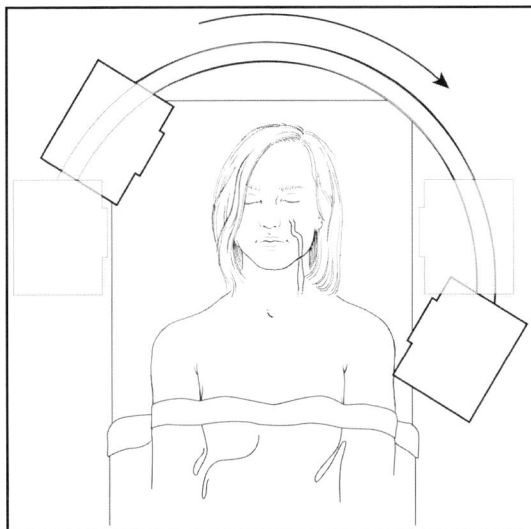

Fig. 2.5 Haughton view for imaging the left carotid siphon and MCA candelabra. The carotid siphon and MCA candelabra can often be seen most clearly by positioning the lateral arc as if the patient's head is tilted *away* from the side of injection. A mnemonic to remember this is: "The X-ray tube should *touch the shoulder* on the side of interest".

Frame Rates for Digital Subtraction Angiography

Most cerebral angiography can be done with 3–5 fps. Higher rates (e.g., 8–20 fps) are useful for imaging arteriovenous malformations and other high-flow lesions. Usually, a variable frame rate may be used to limit radiation dose, since a higher frame rate (3/s) is needed in the arterial phase, whereas a lower rate (0.5–1/s) can be used in the venous phase. For standard cerebral arteriography, a 10–12 s imaging sequence allows for visualization of arterial, capillary, and venous phases.

Calibration and Measurement

Biplanar angiography units are capable of auto-calibration by analysis of simultaneous orthogonal images. Monoplanar angiography requires placement of a marker on or in the patient. A United States dime is 18 mm in diameter and can be taped to the patient's face or head; however a marker on the surface of the patient's body can be inaccurate in the measurement of internal structures because of magnification. Magnification error can lead to errors in linear measurement of up to 13%.[51] Markers on intravascular catheters and wires, placed close to the angiographic target, are more accurate. The ATW™ Marker Wire (Cordis, Miami Lakes, FL) has radio-opaque markers that are 1-mm wide and spaced 10 mm apart. "Two-tipped" microcatheters for detachable coil deployment have markers that are spaced 3 cm apart. To maximize accuracy, the calibration marker and the structure being measured should be as close to the center of the image as possible to minimize the effect of X-ray beam divergence.

Table 2.3 Standard views

Target	Optimal views	Additional views/comments
Carotid bifurcation	Standard PA	Ipsilateral oblique
	Lateral	
Anterior intracranial circulation	Standard PA	
	Lateral	
ICA cavernous segment	Caldwell	Haughton
	Lateral	
ICA ophthalmic segment	Caldwell	Transorbital oblique
	Lateral	
Posterior communicating artery aneurysms	Haughton	Lateral
	Transorbital oblique	
ICA bifurcation	Transorbital oblique	
Anterior communicating artery aneurysms	Transorbital oblique	Sometimes submentovertex
Middle cerebral artery aneurysms	Transorbital oblique	
	Submentovertex	
Middle cerebral artery candelabra	Lateral with Haughton	
	Waters with oblique	
Vertebral artery origin	Towne	The vertebral artery arises from the posterior aspect of the subclavian artery
Posterior circulation	Water	Ipsilateral oblique
	Lateral	
Basilar artery	Water	Ipsilateral oblique
	Lateral	Water will "elongate" the basilar artery trunk
PCA, SCA, AICA, PICA	Towne	Towne elongates PCA. Ipsilateral oblique helps
	Lateral	Caveat: Paired vessels overlap
Basilar apex aneurysms	Water	Ipsilateral oblique
	Lateral	

Angiographic positions for common anatomical targets. *ICA* internal carotid artery, *PCA* posterior cerebral artery, *SCA* superior cerebellar artery, *AICA* anterior inferior cerebellar artery, *PICA* posterior inferior cerebellar artery

2.12. Procedures

Femoral Artery Puncture

1) Prepare and drape the groin area.
2) Palpate the femoral pulse at the inguinal crease, and infiltrate local anesthesia (2% lidocaine), first by raising a wheal and then injecting deeply toward the artery.
   Caveat: Do not inject anesthesia too laterally: Injecting directly in the nerve can cause a femoral neuropathy that persists for hours.
3) Make a 5 mm incision parallel to the inguinal crease with an 11-blade scalpel.
4) Insert a Potts needle with the bevel facing upward. Advance it at a 45° angle to the skin, pointing toward the patient's opposite shoulder.
5) Attempt a single-wall puncture especially if heparin or antiplatelet agents are used. Do it by looking for blood return from the hollow stylet of the Potts needle. Advance the needle 1–2 mm after the first blood return since the stylet protrudes that far beyond the tip of the needle.

6) Make a two-wall puncture by advancing the needle through-and-through both vessel walls, remove the stylet, and slowly withdraw the needle until pulsatile blood return is obtained.
7) When bright red, pulsatile arterial blood is encountered, gently advance a J-wire through the needle for 8–10 cm.
8) Exchange the needle for a 5F sheath, and secured it with a silk stitch.

Pearls
If the artery is difficult to locate, try the following tricks:
- After inserting the Potts needle, let go of it. If the needle pulsates medially or laterally, the artery is usually located to the side that the needle is pulsating toward.
- Fluoroscopic bony landmarks. On PA fluoroscopy, the femoral artery is located 1 cm medial to the center of the femoral head (Fig. 2.6).

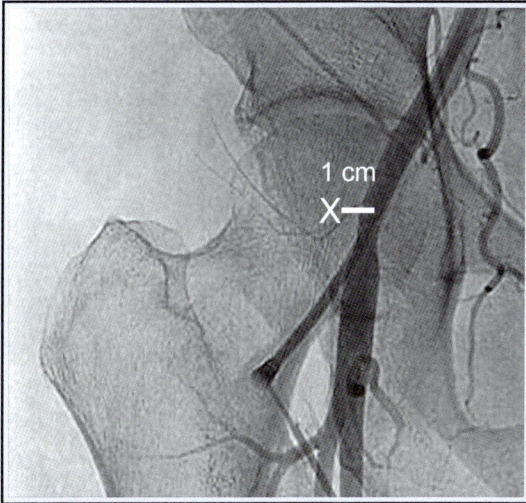

Fig. 2.6 Fluoroscopic landmarks for femoral artery puncture. The femoral artery is located approximately 1 cm medial to the center of the femoral head. The *X* indicates the center of the femoral head.

- Use a micropuncture set (see instructions below). An atherosclerotic femoral artery can be heavily calcified and deflect larger needles; a smaller needle can sometimes be helpful.
- Use a needle with a Doppler ultrasound stylet (Smart-needle®, Vascular Solutions, Minneapolis, MN) (20 gauge or smaller) to allow puncture of a non-palpable vessel.
- Try the opposite groin or the upper extremity approach.
- Puncturing vascular grafts can be difficult due to extensive scar tissue. This may require use of a stiff Amplatz guidewire, use of dilators one size larger than the inserted catheter or sheath, and certain soft catheters should not be used because they may fracture. In general, it is best to use a sheath in Gore Tex® grafts (W.L. Gore, Flagstaff, AZ).

Micropuncture Technique
1. Obtain micropuncture set appropriately sized (4 or 5F).
2. Insert the 21 gauge needle in same fashion as a Potts needle.
3. Insert 0.018 in. microwire.
4. Exchange 21 gauge needle for the dilator.
5. Exchange dilator for the sheath.

The Buffalo Scale for Procedural Blood Loss Estimation*
A Novel Method
A Number One: We're having fun.
A Number Two: It's on the shoe.
A Number Three: It's on your knee.
A Number Four: It's on the floor.
A Number Five: It's in the sky.
A Number Six: Can't be fixed.
A Number Seven: Patient's going to heaven.
A Number Eight: Call for a crate.
**Developed and validated during the fellowship of one this handbook's authors.*

Aortic Arch Imaging

1) Guide a 4F or 5F pigtail catheter over a hydrophilic wire into the ascending part of the aortic arch.
2) Place the image intensifier (II) on low magnification and rotate 30° to the left.
3) The patient's head is thus rotated to the left, so that his or her face is facing the II (this position will permit visualization of the cervical vessels).
4) Use a power injector to administer contrast.
5) Supplement standard left anterior oblique (LAO) view with a lateral view by rotating the II 30° to the right.

Carotid Artery Catheterization

1) Advance an angled diagnostic catheter over a hydrophilic wire over the aortic arch to a position proximal to the innominate artery.
2) Bring back the wire into the catheter, and gently pull the catheter back, with the tip of the catheter facing superiorly, until the innominate artery is engaged. Advance the wire superiorly in the right common carotid artery, followed by the catheter.
3) To engage the left common carotid artery, pull the catheter gently and slowly out of the innominate artery, with the wire inside the catheter and the tip facing to the patient's left, until the catheter "clicks" into the left common carotid. Then advance the wire superiorly, followed by the catheter.
4) For older patients (>50 years), and those with a bovine arch configuration, the Simmons II catheter is helpful for accessing the left common carotid.
5) If selective internal carotid artery catheterization is planned, first do angiography of the cervical carotid system to check for internal carotid artery stenosis in any patient at risk of atherosclerosis. Catheterization of the internal carotid artery should be done under roadmap guidance.
6) Turning the patient's head away from the carotid being catheterized may allow the wire and/or catheter to enter the vessel more easily.
7) Once the common carotid is catheterized, turning the head away from the side being catheterized facilitates internal carotid artery catheterization, and turning toward the ipsilateral side facilitates external carotid catheterization.
8) When the wire or catheter does not advance easily into the vessel of interest, ask the patient to cough. It often bounces the catheter into position.

Vertebral Artery Catheterization

1) Place an angled diagnostic catheter over a hydrophilic wire and into the subclavian artery. Intermittent "puffing" of contrast will allow identification of the vertebral artery origin.
2) Make a road map and pass the wire into the vertebral artery until the tip of the wire is in the upper third of the cervical portion of the vessel. Placing the wire relatively high in the vertebral artery provides adequate purchase for advancement of the catheter, will help straighten out any kinks in the artery that may be present near the origin, and will also facilitate smooth passage of the catheter past the entrance of the of artery into the foramen transversarium at C6. The C6 foramen transversarium is where the vertebral artery makes a transition from free-floating to fixed, and is a region at risk for iatrogenic dissection if the catheter is allowed to scrape against the wall of the vessel.
3) Remember that the vertebral artery makes a right angle turn laterally at C2, so be careful not to injure the vessel at that point with the wire.
4) After removal of the wire, and double flushing, do an angiogram with the tip of the catheter in view, to check for dissection of the vessel during catheterization.
5) For patients at risk of atherosclerosis, do an angiogram of the vertebral artery origin prior to accessing the vessel to check for stenosis.
6) Uncommonly, the left vertebral artery arises directly from the aorta, which should be kept in mind when the origin of the vessel cannot be found on the left subclavian artery.
7) When kinks or loops in the vessel prevent catheterization, ask the patient to tilt their head away from the vertebral artery being catheterized.

Several options exist for patients in whom vessel tortuosity (usually of the innominate artery) makes catheterization of the vertebral artery difficult.

1. Do a roadmap with an ipsilateral oblique Towne view; this will show the vertebral artery origin, and separate the vertebral artery from the common carotid artery.
2. Try a Headhunter catheter. It is well suited for navigation through a tortuous innominate artery.
3. Other catheters that can be helpful in negotiating a difficult right vertebral artery are the Vertebral catheter and the DAV catheter.
4. When catheterization of the vertebral artery is not possible because of tortuosity of the great vessels or atherosclerotic stenosis, inflate a blood pressure cuff on the ipsilateral upper extremity and inject 100% contrast into the subclavian artery with a power injector. The inflated cuff will direct flow away from the arm and toward the vertebral artery. Be careful not to place the catheter with its tip in the thyrocervical or costocervical trunks. A large volume contrast injection in these small vessels can be painful, and can cause spinal cord injury in cases where large spinal cord feeders arise from these branches, or even directly from the subclavian artery. If the catheter tip cannot be placed in a stable position in the subclavian artery proximal to the origin of the vertebral artery, place the tip distal to the origin of the vertebral artery.
5. Set the power injector to allow a good injection without kicking the catheter out: 6 mL/s; total of 25 mL, linear rate rise: 0.5 s.

Reconstituting a Simmons 2 Catheter

The Simmons 2 catheter is useful in the catheterization of the left common carotid artery, particularly when there is a bovine configuration, when the aortic arch is tortuous, and in patients aged >50. The catheter can be reconstituted in the left subclavian artery, the aortic arch, or the aortic bifurcation (Figs. 2.7 and 2.8). Reconstitution in the left subclavian or aortic bifurcation is preferred to the aortic arch, to minimize risk of dislodging atherosclerotic plaque material and subsequent embolization into the intracranial circulation.

Remember that the tip of the Simmons catheter advances into the vessel when the catheter is pulled back at the groin and pulls out of the vessel when the catheter is pushed forward at the groin. This effect is the reverse of the behavior of more simple-curved or angled catheters. The Simmons catheter can also be advanced antegrade over a wire, allowing for selective catheterization of the internal or external carotid arteries.

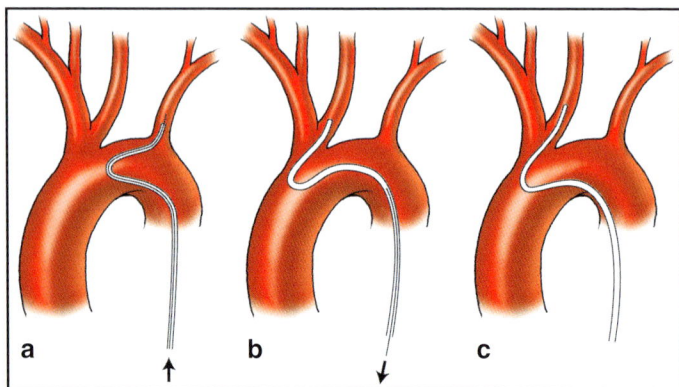

Fig. 2.7 Reconstituting a Simmons 2 catheter in the left subclavian artery. The catheter is advanced over a hydrophilic wire into the left subclavian artery so that the tip is in the subclavian artery (**a**), and the primary bend in the catheter (the "elbow") is in the aortic arch. The wire is then withdrawn until the tip is proximal to the elbow (**b**), and the catheter is then pushed forward, until the elbow moves into the proximal part of the aortic arch (**c**), and the tip of the catheter is out of the subclavian artery, directed backward toward the shaft of the catheter.

Femoral Artery Puncture Site Management

The "gold standard" for management of the arteriotomy after an angiogram is manual compression.

1. Remove the sheath and apply pressure to the groin 1–2 cm superior to the skin incision.
2. Apply pressure for 15 min: usually 5 min of occlusive pressure, followed by 10 min of lesser pressure.
    (a) For patients on aspirin and/or clopidogrel, a longer time is required, usually 40 min. At the end of the time period, slowly release pressure on the groin.
3. At the end of the time period, release pressure on the groin slowly and apply a pressure dressing.
4. The Chito-seal™ pad (Abbott Laboratories, Abbott Park, IL) and the Syvek® NT Patch (Marine Polymer Technologies, Inc., Danvers, MA) are topical hemostatic agents that can be applied to the incision after sheath removal to accelerate hemostasis.
    (a) In an animal model the Syvek® Patch was found to control bleeding better than Chito-seal™.[52]
    (b) These topical agents cannot be expected to produce the same security of hemostasis as the closure devices described below, especially if the sheath size is greater than 5F.
5. A balloon compression dressing (FemoStop®plus Femoral Compression System, Radi Medical Systems, Wilmington, MA) compresses the site with a balloon, but the balloon must be deflated after 1 h to prevent pressure injury to the skin. The dressing is then left in place and the balloon can be reinflated if oozing from the site occurs.
6. After compression, the patient should remain supine for 5 h, then be allowed to ambulate but remain under nursing observation for one more h prior to discharge.
7. Of note: A study of coronary angiographic procedures showed no difference in vascular complications between 2, 4, or 6 h bedrest after hemostasis, even when using abciximab.[53]

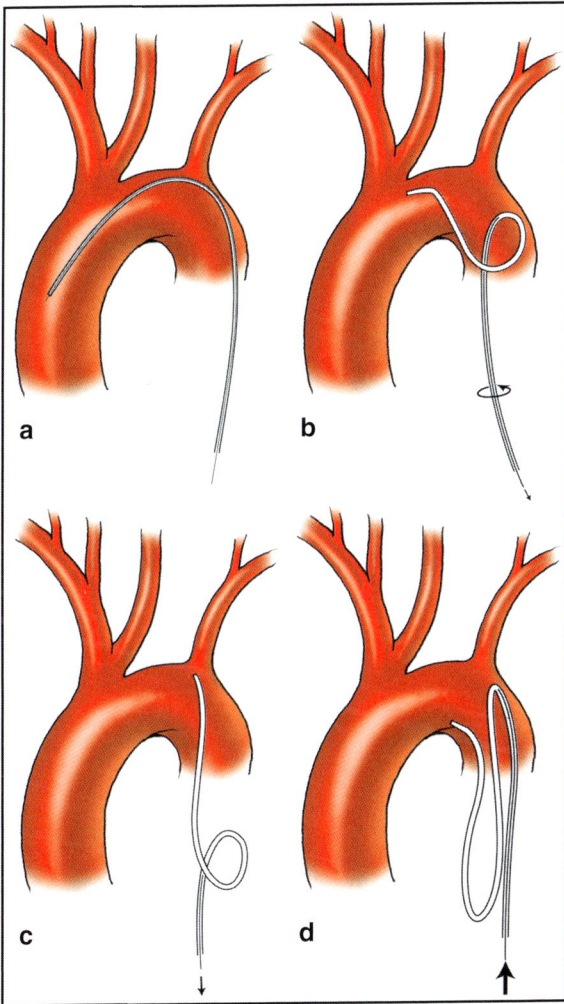

Fig. 2.8 Alternative method for reconstituting a Simmons 2 catheter. The catheter is advanced over a hydrophilic wire so the tip of the catheter is in the ascending aorta (**a**). The wire is then withdrawn until the wire tip is proximal to the elbow, and the catheter is rotated clockwise as it is simultaneously withdrawn so that the loop is in the descending aorta (**b**, **c**). The wire is then advanced swiftly (**d**), to reconstitute the catheter.

8. Early mobilization even as early as 1.5 h after hemostasis does not significantly increase the incidence of hematomas but definitely reduces complaints of back pain.[54]

9. Using topical hemostatics, the patient should generally remain flat in bed for 2 h, and can ambulate in 3 h.

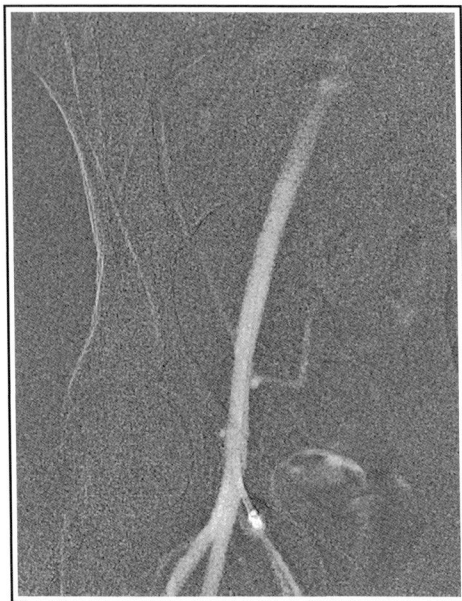

Fig. 2.9 Femoral artery angiogram done prior to the use of a closure device. Injection of contrast through the sheath shows that the sheath enters the femoral artery proximal to the bifurcation. Optimal visualization of the femoral bifurcation is usually obtained with an ipsilateral or contralateral oblique angiogram.

Closure Devices

Percutaneous femoral artery closure devices can allow the patient to ambulate sooner than with compression techniques, and can be helpful when the patient is on antiplatelet or anticoagulant medications. Most closure device instructions recommend puncture site arteriograms (Fig. 2.9) since use of these devices may be contraindicated if a bifurcation or excessive plaque is at the puncture site. When a closure device is used, the patient should remain supine for 1 h. However, there is a greater risk of complications with the use of closure devices. In a meta-analysis to assess the safety of closure devices in patients undergoing percutaneous coronary procedures, an overall analysis favored mechanical compression over closure devices.[55]

Selected Femoral Artery Closure Devices

1) Perclose® Pro-glide™ (Abbott Vascular, Abbott Park, IL, Inc.).
    a) Closure method: A proline stitch is placed in the arteriotomy.
    b) Requires a femoral artery angiogram; the puncture site must be at least 1 cm away from major branches of the vessel, such as the femoral artery bifurcation (Fig. 2.8).
    c) Advantage: The same artery can be re-punctured immediately if necessary.
2) Angio-Seal™ (St. Jude Medical, St. Paul, MN).
    a) Closure method: The device creates a mechanical seal by sandwiching the arteriotomy between a bioabsorbable anchor and a collagen sponge, which dissolves within 60–90 days.

b) May be used at femoral artery branch points.

c) If re-puncture of the same femoral artery is necessary within 90 days, then the reentry site should be 1 cm proximal to the previous site.[56,57]

3) Mynx™ Cadence (AccessClosure, Mountain View, CA).

a) Closure method: The device places an expanding glycolic sealant over the arteriotomy.

b) In a series of 146 devices deployed in 135 patients, 18% were found to have intravascular Mynx sealant on follow-up vascular imaging, and 11% were found to have pseudoaneurysms.[58] Another study comparing Mynx to Angio-Seal found a higher rate of device failure with Mynx.[59]

Post-angiogram Orders

1) Bed rest with the accessed leg extended, head of bed ≤30°, for 5 h, then out of bed for 1 h. (If a closure device is used, bed rest, with head of bed ≤30°, for 1 h, then out of bed for 1 h).

2) Vital signs: Check on arrival in recovery room, then Q 1 h until discharge. Call physician for SBP <90 mmHg or decrease 25 mmHg; pulse >120.

3) Check the puncture site and distal pulses upon arrival in recovery room, then Q 15 min × 4, Q 30 min × 2, then Q 1 h until discharge. Call physician if:

a) Bleeding or hematoma develops at puncture site.

b) Distal pulse is not palpable beyond the puncture site.

c) Extremity is blue or cold.

4) Check puncture site after ambulation.

5) IVF: 0.9N.S. at a maintenance rate until patient is ambulatory.

6) Resume pre-angiogram diet.

7) Resume routine medications.

8) PO fluids 400 mL.

9) D/C IV prior to discharge.

2.13.   Special Techniques and Situations

Brachial and Radial Artery Puncture

The arteries of the upper extremity are a useful alternative to the femoral artery for both diagnostic cerebral angiography and some neurointerventional procedures. Access via the brachial artery[60] or radial artery[61] eliminates the risk of retroperitoneal hemorrhage and the need for several hours of bed rest that are associated with femoral artery puncture. In addition, an upper extremity approach can be advantageous when vessel tortuosity makes access to the vertebral artery difficult from a femoral approach. The authors prefer the brachial artery approach to the radial artery approach because an Allen test is not needed for the brachial artery approach and the threat of hand ischemia – and the potential loss of the patient's dominant hand – is less.

Approaches to the Great Vessels from the Arm

The upper extremity approach is nicely suitable for access to the ipsilateral vertebral artery. The common carotid arteries and left subclavian artery can be reached from the right arm by reflecting a 5F Simmons 2 catheter off of the aortic valve (Fig. 2.10).

Brachial Artery Access

Position the patient's upper extremity on an arm board, extending away from the angiography table. The table is rotated about 20° to permit fluoroscopy of the upper extremity. Palpate the brachial artery just proximal to the elbow, then map out the

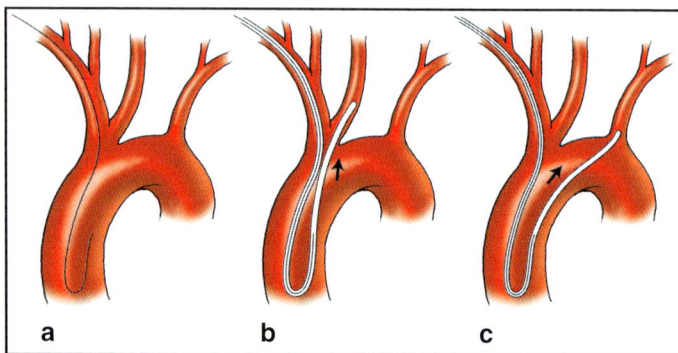

Fig. 2.10 Access to the great vessels from the *right* arm. A 0.035-in. hydrophilic wire is advanced into the ascending aorta and reflected off of the aortic valve (**a**). A Simmons 2 catheter is then advanced over the wire and into the right or left common carotid artery (**b**), or the left subclavian artery (**c**).

vessel with a hand-held Doppler device. Prep the area is prepped and place a sterile "hole drape" over the puncture site. Inject local anesthetic, and use a micropuncture set to place a 4F or 5F sheath in the brachial artery. Connect a heparinized saline pressure bag to the sheath. Do a gentle angiogram immediately after placement of the sheath to rule out a dissection and to confirm that antegrade flow in the artery is preserved after placement of the sheath. If significant vasospasm is present, consider injecting the radial artery cocktail (see below).

Radial Artery Access

Prior to the radial artery puncture, an Allen test is necessary to ensure adequate collateral circulation to the hand from the ulnar artery. Place a pulse oximeter on the patient's thumb, and instruct the patient to repeatedly clench the fist. Compress both the radial artery and the ulnar artery until the pulse oximetry tracing flattens, then take pressure off the ulnar artery. Normal capillary refill time is 5 s or less; a refill time of greater than 10 s is abnormal and an evidence of poor collateral circulation to the hand from the ulnar artery via the palmar arch. In a series of patients undergoing coronary catheterization, an Allen test finding indicating poor collateral circulation was found in 27% of patients.[62]

Once adequate circulation is confirmed by the Allen test, prep and drape the forearm. Inject local anesthetic, and use a micropuncture set to place a 4F or 5F sheath in the radial artery. If the radial artery is difficult to locate, map the vessel out with a Doppler probe. Also, a nitrate patch applied to the wrist will produce a 10% increase in the diameter of the radial artery.[63] Once the sheath is inserted, open the stopcock on the sheath briefly and pulsatile arterial backflow will confirm adequate positioning of the sheath within the artery. Infuse 10 mL "radial artery cocktail" into the sheath as a measure to minimize the risk of vasospasm and thrombosis of the radial artery. Unlike sheaths in the femoral artery, a continuous heparinized saline pressure bag is not used with a radial sheath, due to the pressure and pain it can produce. An alternative to using a sheath is to use a 3F Angioptic™ catheter (AngioDynamics, Queensbury, NY) directly in the radial artery. After completion of the angiogram, remove the sheath and/or catheter and apply a pressure dressing to the wrist. The patient can sit up immediately.

Radial Artery Cocktail
Ten mL of saline containing heparin (5,000 IU), verapamil (2.5 mg), cardiac lidocaine (2%, 1.0 mL), and nitroglycerin (0.1 mg). (Enjoy responsibly.)

Selected Patient-Specific Considerations

1. **Patients receiving heparin**: The heparin infusion should be stopped 6 h prior to the angiogram.
   (a) If the need is urgent, an angiogram can still be done in patients on heparin or who are coagulopathic with minimal risk. The initial puncture should be made with a micropuncture set to minimize potential bleeding.
2. **Patients receiving warfarin**: Hold Warfarin (and place the patient should be placed on a heparin infusion or low-molecular weight heparin if necessary) until the INR ≤1.4.
3. **Patients receiving metformin**. See below.
4. **Thrombocytopenia**: Minimum platelet count for angiography is 75,000/μL.
5. **Diabetic patients**:
   (a) Patients taking insulin: Reduce the insulin dose to half of the usual dose on the morning of the procedure, when the patient is NPO. Do the procedure as early in the day as possible, and the patient's usual diet and insulin should then be resumed.
   (b) Patients taking metformin-containing oral anti-hyperglycemic medications: See below.
   (c) Protamine should not be used to reverse heparin if the patient has received neutral protamine Hagedorn.NPH insulin.[64,65]
6. **Pregnant patients**: Every effort should be made to study pregnant patients noninvasively. Occasionally, a catheter angiogram is necessary (e.g., head and neck trauma with possible vascular injury, spontaneous epistaxis, intracranial AVM). Cerebral angiography can be performed safely during pregnancy.
   (a) Informed consent of the patient or guardian should include a theoretical risk of injury to the fetus.
   (b) Current recommendations for radiation exposure of the fetus include a maximum dose of 0.5 rem (roentgen-equivalent-man).[66]
      • By shielding the uterus with a lead apron, the maximum dose to the fetus is less than 0.1 rem during cerebral angiography.[67]
      • In general, fetal malformations only occur above a threshold dose of 100–200 mGy (~10–20 rem).[68]
   (c) Iodinated contrast agents are physiologically inert and pose little risk to the fetus.[69]
   (d) Provide adequate hydration to avoid fetal dehydration.[70]
   (e) Fluoroscopy: Minimize time and pulse/s during the procedure.
   (f) Decrease fps during diagnostic runs to a minimum.
7. **Pediatric patients**. See below.

Contrast-Induced Nephropathy

Iodinated contrast-induced nephropathy usually appears as an acute worsening in renal function within 3–4 days of the procedure.[71] Contrast-induced nephropathy is usually defined as an increase in serum creatinine of 25–50% over baseline, or an absolute rise in serum creatinine of 0.5–1 mg/dL.[72,73] Patients with renal insufficiency are up to ten times more likely to develop contrast-induced renal failure with administration of iodinated contrast than patients in the general population.[74] Patients with renal insufficiency (creatinine ≥1.5 mg/dL)[75] require measures to minimize the risk of contrast-induced injury nephropathy during angiography. Nonionic, low-osmolality contrast agents, such as iodixanol (Visipaque™, GE Healthcare, Princeton, NJ) and iopromide (Ultravist®, Schering, Berlin) have been shown to be less renal-toxic when compared to iohexol (Omnipaque®).[76] The smallest possible amount of contrast should be used during the procedure. One of the authors was able to do a carotid angioplasty and stent procedure using a total of 27 mL of Visique™ by diluting the contrast with saline and using it sparingly. Forty-eight hours should be allowed to elapse between procedures utilizing iodinated contrast when possible.[77] The antioxidant, N-acetylcysteine (Mucomyst®, Bristol-Myers Squibb, New York) is thought to function as a free-radical scavenger and to stimulate intrarenal vasodilation. Acetylcisteine was shown in a randomized trial to reduce serum creatinine elevation in patients undergoing radiological procedures using non-ionic, low osmolality contrast material.[78] Prophylactic administration of acetylcysteine (600 mg PO BID) and 0.45% saline IV, before and after administration of the contrast agent, leads to a significant decrease in serum creatinine compared to patients receiving saline only. Subsequently, isotonic IV fluid was found to be superior to half-isotonic IV fluid in reducing the incidence of contrast-induced nephropathy in patients undergoing coronary angioplasty.[79] Gadolinium contrast has also been used as a non-iodinated contrast agent in cerebral angiography,[80,81] but extensive testing has not been done to ensure the safety of gadolinium compounds in the cerebral arteries. Hemofiltration has been shown to reduce creatinine elevations after angiography.[82] For patients with dialysis-dependent renal failure, arrangements should be made with the patient's neph-rologist to schedule dialysis after the angiogram.

Risk Factors for Contrast-Induced Nephropathy

- Serum creatinine level ≥1.5 mg/dL
- Diabetes mellitus
- Dehydration
- Cardiovascular disease and the use of diuretics
- Age ≥60 years
- Paraproteinemia (e.g., multiple myeloma)
- Hypertension
- Hyperuricemia

The patients at greatest risk for contrast nephrotoxicity are those with both diabetes and renal insufficiency.[83,84]

Methods to Reduce Risk of Contrast-Induced Nephropathy

- Minimize the use of contrast
- Use Visipaque™ (270 mL I/mL) instead of Omnipaque™[76]
- PO hydration (water, 500 mL prior to the procedure and 2,000 mL after the procedure)
- IV hydration with 0.9% sodium chloride[79]
- Acetylcisteine 600 mg (3 mL) PO BID on the day before and the day of the procedure[78]

Metformin

Metformin is an oral anti-hyperglycemic and is used in several preparations (listed below). Metformin-associated lactic acidosis is rare but has been reported to have a mortality rate as high as 50%.[85] Metformin use should be held for 48 h after the procedure, and restarted only after serum creatinine has been checked and found to be unchanged. The procedure may be done even if the patient has taken metformin earlier on the same day of the procedure.[86] Although metformin use seems to be associated with lactic acidosis, a systematic review article has questioned whether there is a causal relationship.[87]

Metformin-Containing Medications

- Metformin (generic)
- Glucophage®
- Avandamet®
- Glucovance®
- Metaglip®

Anaphylactic Contrast Reactions: Prevention and Management

Although the overall rate of anaphylactic iodinated contrast reactions with IV administration is 0.7–2%,[88,89] the rate of anaphylactic reactions with cerebral angiography is much lower. This is thought to be because a passage of a bolus of contrast through the pulmonary vasculature, which occurs with IV administration, is more likely to incite an anaphylactic reaction than the relatively diluted dose given during an arteriogram. Large series of cerebral angiograms have reported the following incidences of allergic reactions: 0 out of 1,358 cases (0/1,358),[90] 0/2,154,[91] 1/2,924,[92] and 0/3,636.[93]

Risk Factors for Contrast Reactions

- History of a reaction to iodinated contrast agents (except flushing, a sensation of heat, or a single episode of nausea)
- History of serious allergic reactions to other materials
- Asthma
- Renal insufficiency
- Significant cardiac disease (e.g., patients with angina, congestive heart failure, severe aortic stenosis, primary pulmonary hypertension, severe cardiomyopathy)
- Anxiety

Previous reaction to contrast medium is the most important risk factor in the prediction of an adverse event.[94] Patients who have had a previous reaction to ionic contrast may not have a reaction to nonionic agents.[95] A history of seafood allergies, without a specific history of an iodine reaction, usually indicates a hypersensitivity to allergens in seafood, and does not indicate that the patient is unable to tolerate contrast media.[96]

Premedication with steroids can reduce the risk of a serious contrast reaction.[97] Repeat contrast reactions in patients with a history of previous reactions to iodinated contrast occur in 10–18% of cases despite premedication.[89,98]

Gadolinium has been used for cerebral angiography in patients with a sensitivity to iodinated contrast material.[81,99] However, IA gadolium produces images that are reduced in quality compared to iodinated contrast, and patients undergoing coronary angiography with gadolinium have relatively high rate (21%) of complications, such as cardiac arrhythmias and hemodynamic instability.[100]

Premedication Regimen

1. Prednisone 50 mg PO (or hydrocortisone 200 mg IV) 13, 7, and 1 h prior to contrast injection
2. Diphenhydramine (Benadryl®) 50 mg IV, IM or PO 1 h prior to contrast injection

Steroids should be given at least 6 h prior to the procedure; administration less than 3 h prior to the procedure does not reduce the risk of an adverse reaction.[86]

Acute Contrast Reactions: Signs and Symptoms

- Cutaneous signs (flushing, urticaria, pruritis)
- Mucosal oedema
- Generalized oedema
- Sudden loss of consciousness
- Hypotension + tachycardia (anaphylactic reaction)
- Hypotension + bradycardia (vasovagal reaction)
- Respiratory distress

Acute Contrast Reactions: Treatment

Effective treatment depends on prompt recognition of the problem and rapid management (Table 2.4).[101]

Intraoperative Angiography

Intraoperative angiography is employed by some neurosurgeons during surgery for intracranial aneurysms and arteriovenous malformations. In aneurysm surgery, intraoperative angiography findings, such as residual aneurysm or parent vessel compromise, have led to reexploration and clip adjustment in up to 12.4% of cases.[102,103] Factors associated with a need for revision include large aneurysm size,[102] the superior hypophyseal artery and clinoidal segment locations,[102] and the occurrence of an intraoperative

Table 2.4 Management of acute contrast reactions in adults

Urticaria
1. Discontinue procedure if not completed
2. No treatment needed in most cases
3. Give H$_1$-receptor blocker: Diphenhydramine (Benadryl®) PO/IM/IV 25–50 mg. If severe or widely disseminated: alpha agonist (arteriolar and venous constriction) Epinephrine SC (1:1,000) 0.1–0.3 mL (=0.1–0.3 mg) (if no cardiac contraindications)
Facial or laryngeal edema
1. Give alpha agonist (arteriolar and venous constriction): Epinephrine sc or IM (1:1,000) 0.1–0.3 mL (=0.1–0.3 mg) or, if hypotension evident, Epinephrine (1:10,000) slowly IV 1 mL (=0.1 mg). Repeat as needed up to a maximum of 1 mg
2. Give O$_2$ 6–10 L/min (via mask)
3. If not responsive to therapy or if there is obvious acute laryngeal edema, seek appropriate assistance (e.g., cardiopulmonary arrest response team)
Bronchospasm
1. Give O$_2$ 6–10 L/min (via mask)
2. Monitor: electrocardiogram, O$_2$ saturation (pulse oximeter), and blood pressure
3. Give inhaled beta-agonist [bronchiolar dilator, such as albuterol (Proventil® or Ventolin®)], 2 to 3 puffs from metered dose inhaler. Repeat PRN. If unresponsive to inhalers, use SC, IM, or IV epmephrine
4. Give epinephrine SC or IM (1:1,000) 0.1–0.3 mL (=0.1–0.3 mg) or, if hypotension evident, Epinephrine (1:10,000) slowly IV 1 mL (=0.1 mg)
5. Repeat as needed up to a maximum of 1 mg
Alternatively: Give aminophylline: 6 mg/kg IV in D$_5$W over 10–20 min (loading dose), then 0.4–1 mg/kg/h, as needed (caution: hypotension)
Call for assistance (e.g., cardiopulmonary arrest response team) for severe bronchospasm or if O$_2$ saturation <88% persists
Hypotension with tachycardia
1. Legs elevated 60° or more (preferred) or Trendelenburg position
2. Monitor: electrocardiogram, pulse oximeter, blood pressure
3. Give O$_2$ 6–10 L/min (via mask)
4. Rapid intravenous administration of large volumes of isotonic Ringer's lactate or normal Saline
If poorly responsive: Epinephrine (1:10,000) slowly IV 1 mL (=0.1 mg) (if no cardiac contraindications). Repeat as needed up to a maximum of 1 mg
If still poorly responsive seek appropriate assistance (e.g., cardiopulmonary arrest response team)
Hypotension with bradycardia (vagal reaction)
1. Monitor vital signs
2. Legs elevated 60° or more (preferred) or Trendelenburg position
3. Secure airway: give O$_2$ 6–10 L/min (via mask)
4. Secure IV access: rapid fluid replacement with Ringer's lactate or normal saline
5. Give atropine 0.6–1 mg IV slowly if patient does not respond quickly to steps 2–4
6. Repeat atropine up to a total dose of 0.04 mg/kg (2–3 mg) in adult
7. Ensure complete resolution of hypotension and bradycardia prior to discharge
Hypertension, severe
1. Give O$_2$ 6–10 L/min (via mask)
2. Monitor electrocardiogram, pulse oximeter, blood pressure
3. Give nitroglycerine 0.4 mg tablet, sublingual (may repeat ×3); or, topical 2% ointment, apply 1 in. strip
4. Transfer to intensive care unit or emergency department
5. For pheochromocytoma – phentolamine 5 mg IV

(continued)

Table 2.4 (continued)

Seizures or convulsions
1. Give O_2 6–10 L/min (via mask)
2. Consider diazepam (Valium®) 5 mg (or more, as appropriate) or midazolam (Versed®) 0.5–1 mg IV
3. If longer effect needed, obtain consultation; consider phenytoin (Dilantin®) infusion 15–18 mg/kg at 50 mg/min. Careful monitoring of vital signs required, particularly of pO_2 because of risk of respiratory depression with benzodiazepine administration
4. Consider using cardiopulmonary arrest response team for intubation if needed
Pulmonary edema
1. Elevate torso; rotating tourniquets (venous compression)
2. Give O_2 6–10 L/min (via mask)
3. Give diuretics – furosemide (Lasix®) 20–40 mg IV, slow push
4. Consider giving morphine (1–3 mg IV)
5. Transfer to intensive care unit or emergency department
6. Corticosteroids optional

From Manual on Contrast Media Version 10.[86] Reprinted with permission of the American College of Radiology

rupture.[104] A portable C-arm digital subtraction angiography unit is necessary for intraoperative angiography, and a radiolucent head holder (Ohio Medical Instruments, Cincinnati, OH) and radiolucent operating table (Skytron, Grand Rapids, MI) are helpful, although adequate intraoperative imaging can be done even without radiolucent hardware. A femoral artery sheath should be placed prior to the operation. Use of a braided sheath will prevent kinking if the patient is moved after sheath placement. Continuous infusion of heparinized saline (5,000 U in 500 mL saline on a pressure bag at 3 mL/h) will maintain the patency of the sheath without a perceptible effect on systemic coagulation. A technique for intraoperative angiography for anterior circulation aneurysms by injection of contrast into the superficial temporal artery has also been described.[105]

Paediatric Cerebral Angiography

Use noninvasive imaging modalities whenever possible. Although neurological complications are rare, children have higher rates of femoral artery access complications than adults do. In a series of 176 paediatric cerebral angiograms, no neurological complications occurred but puncture site complications (groin hematoma, bleeding, or reduced pedal pulse) occurred in 4.5%.[106]

Access

1. Draping: use small aperture drape for the groin, and a regular femoral angiography drape for the rest of the angio table.
2. Newborns: the umbilical artery and vein can be used to access both arterial and venous circulations which allow for fairly easy catheterization.
3. The femoral artery is surprisingly superficial.
4. The femoral artery in children is prone to catheter-induced vasospasm, so minimize the amount of manipulation and the size of devices (e.g., use a micropuncture kit and small catheters).
5. Work without a sheath if possible.
6. Caveat: Initial catheterization of the femoral artery is sometimes surprisingly difficult because of the integrity of the connective tissue around the femoral artery; be sure that the wire that is used to introduce the diagnostic catheter is size-matched to the catheter to facilitate entry.
7. A twisting action can be helpful as the catheter is passed into the femoral artery.
8. A 20 or 22 gauge butterfly needle is useful for the initial femoral artery puncture (hint: cut clear the plastic tubing off the butterfly needle hub).
9. Sometimes an ultrasound-guided needle (e.g., Smart-needle®, Vascular Solutions, Minneapolis, MN) (20 gauge or smaller) is helpful.[107]

10. Femoral artery puncture site management:
    (a) When compressing the artery after removal of the catheter, pay close attention to the distal lower extremity to ensure adequate perfusion. Overly aggressive manual compression or trauma to the femoral artery can result in long-standing femoral artery stenosis or occlusion, leading to limb atrophy.
    (b) After compression, the hip and lower extremity can be immobilized by taping or strapping it to an IV board.

Catheters

1. Catheters should be small in calibre and short in length (to minimize dead space in the catheter) (≤60 cm).
2. Newborns and young infants:
    (a) 3F Harwood-Nash.
        • Very peculiar curve makes it easy to access the left subclavian artery but difficult to navigate into the aortic arch
        • Requires a small guidewire (e.g., 0.018–0.025 in. steerable hydrophilic wire)
3. Older infants and young children:
    (a) 4F Pediatric Berenstein
    (b) 4F Harwood-Nash
4. All paediatric patients:
    (a) 3F Angioptic™ (AngioDynamics, Queensbury, NY).
        • Comes in steam-shapeable straight or curved configurations
        • Use a 21 gauge needle and a small guidewire (e.g., 0.018–0.021 in. steerable hydrophilic wire)

Saline, Contrast Dose, and Volume Considerations

1. Use less heparin in the flush: Saline with 1 units of heparin per mL
2. Double flushing with heparinized saline: Be careful to aspirate the minimum amount of blood to minimize blood loss and heparin dose
3. Use small syringes (3 mL or 5 mL) to limit the amount of volume
4. Limit contrast to 4 mL of Omnipaque® 300 per kg body weight
5. Limiting volume is particularly critical in children with Vein of Galen malformations, as these patients often have some degree of high-output congestive heart failure

Imaging Parameters and Radiation Exposure

1. Image intensifier:
    (a) Use a small field of view.
    (b) Remove the filter if possible.
    (c) Lower the X-ray dose as much as possible.
2. Limit fluoroscopy time.
3. Lower the pulse rate during fluoroscopy (e.g., 3–6 fps).
4. Maximize collimation to minimize scatter.
5. Use "low-dose fluoro option" if available as a part of the imaging equipment.
6. Place a lead shield under the gonads if possible.

2.14. Tips for Imaging Specific Vascular Structures and Lesions

Atherosclerotic Carotid and Vertebrobasilar Disease

• Aortic arch angiogram: identifies aortic atheromas and common carotid artery lesions, and helps planning for potential carotid angioplasty and stenting procedures.

- To image the carotid bifurcation, on the PA and lateral views, place the angle of the mandible in the center of the image.
- Oblique views are sometimes necessary to obtain the optimal view of an atherosclerotic plaque.
- When high grade stenosis prevents passage of enough contrast to image the internal carotid artery (ICA), the degree of stenosis can be estimated using the diameter of the contralateral ICA.[108]
- The vertebral artery origin is best seen with an AP Townes view, because the vertebral artery arises from the posterior wall of the subclavian artery (see Fig. 1.37).
- The intracranial vertebral arteries and basilar artery are best seen with an AP Waters view, because the basilar artery travels parallel to the clivus, which is tilted anteriorly in the sagittal plane.

Intracranial Aneurysms

- A complete four-vessel angiogram should be done in the setting of subarachnoid haemorrhage, as two or more aneurysms will be found in 15–20% of patients.[109]
- Selective catheterization of the ICA will prevent branches of the ECA from obscuring the intracranial images.
- External carotid angiography may be needed in aneurysm cases if an extracranial to intracranial arterial bypass is anticipated for surgical treatment, in order to visualize possible donor vessels.
- If a study is done in the setting of subarachnoid haemorrhage, and no aneurysm is found on internal carotid arteriography, external carotid angiography may be useful to rule out an arteriovenous fistula (see below).
- Aneurysm dome, neck, parent vessel, and adjacent vessels should be discerned.
- 3-D angiography is very helpful in determining configuration of the aneurysm neck.
- Selective microcatheter angiography may be helpful in imaging large and giant aneurysms.

Cerebral Arteriovenous Malformations

- All feeding arteries and draining veins should be identified; this usually requires a complete bilateral internal carotid, external carotid, and vertebral angiogram.
- High-speed runs (>5 fps) can help clarify anatomy of AVMs, as they are typically high-flow lesions. High-speed runs may also permit more precise measurements of arteriovenous transit times.
- Intranidal aneurysms can be identified and distinguished from enlarged veins by their location on the *arterial side* of the nidus.[110] In contrast, nidal "pseudoaneurysms" have been described in the arterial or venous side of the nidus; they can be recognized when they appear as a new finding on subsequent angiography.[111]
- Small, obscure AVMs may sometimes be made to be more apparent on angiography by having the patient deliberately hyperventilate for several minutes. Normal vessels will constrict and AVM vessels will be unchanged (Cure, 2007, personal communication).

Cerebral Proliferative Angiopathy
(see Chap. 14)

- A complete 6-vessel angiogram should be done (bilateral internal and external carotid and vertebral arteries), to identify meningeal feeders, which are frequently present.[112]
- Feeding vessels (such as the ICAs and M1 segments) should be imaged well to look for the presence of arterial stenosis.

Dural Arteriovenous Fistulas

- All feeding vessels should be identified; selective catheterization of branches of the external carotid artery is usually necessary.
- After each injection, the angiogram should be allowed to continue until the draining vein (or venous sinus) is imaged.
- On internal carotid and vertebral injections, the venous drainage pathways of the normal brain must be determined to see how it relates to the drainage pathways of the fistula.

Direct (High-Flow) Carotid-Cavernous Fistulas

- High-speed runs (>5 fps) are usually helpful.
- Huber maneuver: Injection of contrast into the ipsilateral vertebral artery with manual compression of the carotid artery; reflux of contrast into the carotid artery can demonstrate the defect in the cavernous carotid artery.[113]
- Slow injection into the internal carotid artery with a compression of the carotid artery below the catheter tip in the neck can also demonstrate the defect in the vessel.[114]
- Special attention should be given to venous drainage and determining whether there is a retrograde cortical venous flow.

Aortic Arch

- Angiography of the aortic arch is best done with a power injector and a pigtail catheter positioned in the ascending aorta. The optimal projection is left anterior oblique, 30°, with the patient's head rotated to the left to face the image intensifier. Power injector settings are 20 mL/s; total of 25 mL.
- For these high-volume injections care should be taken that the injection pressure does not exceed the nominal rating for the catheter and any stopcock.

Assessment of the Circle of Willis

- Patency and calibre of the posterior communicating artery can be assessed with the Huber (or Allcock) manoeuvre: Injection of contrast into the ipsilateral vertebral artery with manual compression of the carotid artery; reflux of contrast into the carotid artery can demonstrate posterior communicating artery.
- The anterior communicating artery can be demonstrated by "cross compression" of the carotid artery. Manual compression of the contralateral common carotid artery while wearing a lead glove during injection of contrast into the ipsilateral internal carotid artery will help visualize the anterior communicating artery.

Carotid Siphon and MCA Candelabra

- The "Haughton view" can be used to open up the carotid siphon (useful for imaging the origins of the P-comm and anterior choroidal arteries) and to unfurl the branches of the MCA within the Sylvian fissure.[50] This view is also helpful for imaging ICA and MCA aneurysms. The lateral arc is positioned as if the patient's head is tilted away from the side of the injection and away from the X-ray tube (see Fig. 2.5).

References

1. Higashida RT, Hopkins LN, Berenstein A, Halbach VV, Kerber C. Program requirements for residency/fellowship education in neuroendovascular surgery/interventional neuroradiology: a special report on graduate medical education. AJNR Am J Neuroradiol. 2000;21:1153–9.

2. Haschek E, Lindenthal OT. Ein Beitrag zur praktischen Verwerthung der Photographie nach Röntgen. Wien Klin Wochenschr. 1896;9:63–4.

3. Krayenbühl H. History of cerebral angiography and its development since Egaz Moniz. In: Egas Moniz centenary: scientific reports. Lisbon: Comissao Executiva das Comemoracoes do Centenario do Nascimento do Prof. Egas Moniz; 1977. p. 63–74.

4. Bull JW. The history of neuroradiology. Proc R Soc Med. 1970;63:637–43.

5. Norlén E. Importance of angiography in surgery of intracranial vascular lesions. In: Egas Moniz centenary: scientific reports. Lisbon: Comissao Executiva das Comemoracoes do Centenario do Nascimento do Prof. Egas Moniz; 1977. p. 31–9.

6. Lima A. Egas Moniz 1874–1955. Surg Neurol. 1973;1:247–8.

7. Dámasio AR. Egas Moniz, pioneer of angiography and leucotomy. Mt Sinai J Med. 1975;42:502–13.

8. Moniz EL. L'angiographie cérébrale. Paris: Masson & Cie; 1934.

9. Dagi TF. Neurosurgery and the introduction of cerebral angiography. Neurosurg Clin N Am. 2001;12:145–53, ix.

10. Ligon BL. The mystery of angiography and the "unawarded" Nobel Prize: Egas Moniz and Hans Christian Jacobaeus. Neurosurgery. 1998;43:602–11.

11. Sheldon P. A special needle for percutaneous vertebral angiography. Br J Radiol. 1956;29:231–2.

12. Gould PL, Peyton WT, French LA. Vertebral angiography by retrograde injection of the brachial artery. J Neurosurg. 1955;12:369–74.

13. Kuhn RA. Brachial cerebral angiography. J Neurosurg. 1960;17:955–71.

14. Hinck VC, Judkins MP, Paxton HD. Simplified selective femorocerebral angiography. Radiology. 1967;89:1048–52.

15. Mentzel H-J, Blume J, Malich A, Fitzek C, Reichenbach JR, Kaiser WA. Cortical blindness after contrast-enhanced CT: complication in a patient with diabetes insipidus. AJNR Am J Neuroradiol. 2003;24:1114–6.

16. Saigal G, Bhatia R, Bhatia S, Wakhloo AK. MR findings of cortical blindness following cerebral angiography: is this entity related to posterior reversible leukoencephalopathy? AJNR Am J Neuroradiol. 2004;25:252–6.

17. Yildiz A, Yencilek E, Apaydin FD, Duce MN, Ozer C, Atalay A. Transient partial amnesia complicating cardiac and peripheral arteriography with nonionic contrast medium. Eur Radiol. 2003;13 Suppl 4:L113–5.

18. Willinsky RA, Taylor SM, TerBrugge K, Farb RI, Tomlinson G, Montanera W. Neurologic complications of cerebral angiography: prospective analysis of 2,899 procedures and review of the literature. Radiology. 2003;227:522–8.

19. Young B, Moore WS, Robertson JT, et al. An analysis of perioperative surgical mortality and morbidity in the asymptomatic carotid atherosclerosis study. ACAS Investigators. Asymptomatic Carotid Artheriosclerosis Study. Stroke. 1996;27:2216–24.

20. Heiserman JE, Dean BL, Hodak JA, et al. Neurologic complications of cerebral angiography. AJNR Am J Neuroradiol. 1994;15:1401–7; discussion 8–11.

21. Hankey GJ, Warlow CP, Molyneux AJ. Complications of cerebral angiography for patients with mild carotid territory ischaemia being considered for carotid endarterectomy. J Neurol Neurosurg Psychiatry. 1990;53:542–8.

22. Cloft HJ, Joseph GJ, Dion JE. Risk of cerebral angiography in patients with subarachnoid hemorrhage, cerebral aneurysm, and arteriovenous malformation: a meta-analysis. Stroke. 1999;30:317–20.

23. Mani RL, Eisenberg RL. Complications of catheter cerebral arteriography: analysis of 5,000 procedures. III. Assessment of arteries injected, contrast medium used, duration of procedure, and age of patient. AJR Am J Roentgenol. 1978;131:871–4.

24. Dion JE, Gates PC, Fox AJ, Barnett HJ, Blom RJ. Clinical events following neuroangiography: a prospective study. Stroke. 1987;18:997–1004.

25. Earnest FT, Forbes G, Sandok BA, et al. Complications of cerebral angiography: prospective assessment of risk. AJR Am J Roentgenol. 1984;142:247–53.

26. Citron SJ, Wallace RC, Lewis CA, et al. Quality improvement guidelines for adult diagnostic neuroangiography: cooperative study between ASITN, ASNR, and SIR. J Vasc Interv Radiol. 2003;14:S257–62.

27. Kurokawa Y, Abiko S, Okamura T, et al. Pulmonary embolism after cerebral angiography – three case reports. Neurol Med Chir (Tokyo). 1995;35:305–9.

28. Katholi RE, Taylor GJ, Woods WT, et al. Nephrotoxicity of nonionic low-osmolality versus ionic high-osmolality contrast media: a prospective double-blind randomized comparison in human beings. Radiology. 1993;186:183–7.

29. Barrett BJ, Carlisle EJ. Metaanalysis of the relative nephrotoxicity of high- and low-osmolality iodinated contrast media. Radiology. 1993;188:171–8.

30. Barrett BJ, Parfrey PS, McDonald JR, Hefferton DM, Reddy ER, McManamon PJ. Nonionic low-osmolality versus ionic high-osmolality contrast material for intravenous use in patients perceived to be at high risk: randomized trial. Radiology. 1992;183:105–10.

31. Barrett BJ, Parfrey PS, Vavasour HM, O'Dea F, Kent G, Stone E. A comparison of nonionic, low-osmolality radiocontrast agents with ionic, high-osmolality agents during cardiac catheterization. N Engl J Med. 1992;326:431–6.

32. Rosovsky MA, Rusinek H, Berenstein A, Basak S, Setton A, Nelson PK. High-dose administration of nonionic contrast media: a retrospective review. Radiology. 1996;200:119–22.

33. Moran CJ, Milburn JM, Cross III DT, Derdeyn CP, Dobbie TK, Littenberg B. Randomized controlled trial of sheaths in diagnostic neuroangiography. Radiology. 2001;218:183–7.

34. Kiyosue H, Okahara M, Nagatomi H, Nakamura T, Tanoue S, Mori H. 3.3F catheter/sheath system for use in diagnostic neuroangiography. AJNR Am J Neuroradiol. 2002;23:711–5.

35. Weinbroum AA, Szold O, Ogorek D, Flaishon R. The midazolam-induced paradox phenomenon is reversible by flumazenil. Epidemiology, patient characteristics and review of the literature. Eur J Anaesthesiol. 2001;18:789–97.

36. Mancuso CE, Tanzi MG, Gabay M. Paradoxical reactions to benzodiazepines: literature review and treatment options. Pharmacotherapy. 2004;24:1177–85.

37. Thurston TA, Williams CG, Foshee SL. Reversal of a paradoxical reaction to midazolam with flumazenil. Anesth Analg. 1996;83:192.

38. Iserson KV. The origins of the gauge system for medical equipment. J Emerg Med. 1987;5:45–8.

39. Markus H, Loh A, Israel D, Buckenham T, Clifton A, Brown MM. Microscopic air embolism during cerebral angiography and strategies for its avoidance. Lancet. 1993;341:784–7.

40. Bendszus M, Koltzenburg M, Bartsch AJ, et al. Heparin and air filters reduce embolic events caused by intra-arterial cerebral angiography: a prospective, randomized trial. Circulation. 2004;110:2210–5.

41. Dexter F, Hindman BJ. Recommendations for hyperbaric oxygen therapy of cerebral air embolism based on a mathematical model of bubble absorption. Anesth Analg. 1997;84:1203–7.

42. Branger AB, Lambertsen CJ, Eckmann DM. Cerebral gas embolism absorption during hyperbaric therapy: theory. J Appl Physiol. 2001;90:593–600.

43. Calvert JW, Cahill J, Zhang JH. Hyperbaric oxygen and cerebral physiology. Neurol Res. 2007;29:132–41.

44. LeDez KM, Zbitnew G. Hyperbaric treatment of cerebral air embolism in an infant with cyanotic congenital heart disease. Can J Anaesth. 2005;52:403–8.

45. Bitterman H, Melamed Y. Delayed hyperbaric treatment of cerebral air embolism. Isr J Med Sci. 1993;29:22–6.

46. Blanc P, Boussuges A, Henriette K, Sainty JM, Deleflie M. Iatrogenic cerebral air embolism: importance of an early hyperbaric oxygenation. Intensive Care Med. 2002;28:559–63.

47. Shrinivas VG, Sankarkumar R, Rupa S. Retrograde cerebral perfusion for treatment of air embolism after valve surgery. Asian Cardiovasc Thorac Ann. 2004;12:81–2.

48. Gregoric ID, Myers TJ, Kar B, et al. Management of air embolism during HeartMate XVE exchange. Tex Heart Inst J. 2007;34:19–22.

49. Hughes DG, Patel U, Forbes WS, Jones AP. Comparison of hand injection with mechanical injection for digital subtraction selective cerebral angiography. Br J Radiol. 1994;67: 786–9.

50. Haughton VM, Rosenbaum AE, Baker RA, Plaistowe RL. Lateral projections with inclined head for angiography of basal cerebral aneurysms. Radiology. 1975;116:220–2.

51. Elisevich K, Cunningham IA, Assis L. Size estimation and magnification error in radiographic imaging: implications for classification of arteriovenous malformations. AJNR Am J Neuroradiol. 1995;16:531–8.

52. Fischer TH, Connolly R, Thatte HS, Schwaitzberg SS. Comparison of structural and hemostatic properties of the poly-N-acetyl glucosamine Syvek Patch with products containing chitosan. Microsc Res Tech. 2004;63:168–74.

53. Vlasic W, Almond D, Massel D. Reducing bedrest following arterial puncture for coronary interventional procedures – impact on vascular complications: the BAC Trial. J Invasive Cardiol. 2001;13:788–92.

54. Hoglund J, Stenestrand U, Todt T, Johansson I. The effect of early mobilisation for patient undergoing coronary angiography; a pilot study with focus on vascular complications and back pain. Eur J Cardiovasc Nurs. 2011;10:130–6.

55. Nikolsky E, Mehran R, Halkin A, et al. Vascular complications associated with arteriotomy closure devices in patients undergoing percutaneous coronary procedures: a meta-analysis. J Am Coll Cardiol. 2004;44:1200–9.

56. Applegate RJ, Rankin KM, Little WC, Kahl FR, Kutcher MA. Restick following initial Angioseal use. Catheter Cardiovasc Interv. 2003;58:181–4.

57. St. Jude Medical. Restick Following Initial Angio-Seal Device Use Shown to be Safe. Press release. Minnetonka: 2008.

58. Fields JD, Liu KC, Lee DS, et al. Femoral artery complications associated with the mynx closure device. AJNR Am J Neuroradiol. 2010;31:1737–40.

59. Azmoon S, Pucillo AL, Aronow WS, et al. Vascular complications after percutaneous coronary intervention following hemostasis with the Mynx vascular closure device versus the AngioSeal vascular closure device. J Invasive Cardiol. 2010;22:175–8.

60. Uchino A. Selective catheterization of the brachiocephalic arteries via the right brachial artery. Neuroradiology. 1988;30:524–7.

61. Levy EI, Boulos AS, Fessler RD, et al. Transradial cerebral angiography: an alternative route. Neurosurgery. 2002;51: 335–40; discussion 40–2.

62. Benit E, Vranckx P, Jaspers L, Jackmaert R, Poelmans C, Coninx R. Frequency of a positive modified Allen's test in 1,000 consecutive patients undergoing cardiac catheterization. Cathet Cardiovasc Diagn. 1996;38:352–4.

63. Hildick-Smith DJ, Ludman PF, Lowe MD, et al. Comparison of radial versus brachial approaches for diagnostic coronary angiography when the femoral approach is contraindicated. Am J Cardiol. 1998;81:770–2.

64. Stewart WJ, McSweeney SM, Kellett MA, Faxon DP, Ryan TJ. Increased risk of severe protamine reactions in NPH insulin-dependent diabetics undergoing cardiac catheterization. Circulation. 1984;70:788–92.

65. Cobb 3rd CA, Fung DL. Shock due to protamine hypersensitivity. Surg Neurol. 1982;17:245–6.

66. Measurements NCoRPa. Recommendations on limits for exposure to ionizing radiation. NCRP Report No. 91. 1987.

67. Piper J. Fetal toxicity of common neurosurgical drugs. In: Loftus C, editor. Neurosurgical aspects of pregancy. Park Ridge: American Association of Neurological Surgeons; 1996. p. 1–20.

68. Kal HB, Struikmans H. Pregnancy and medical irradiation; summary and conclusions from the International Commission on Radiological Protection, Publication 84. Ned Tijdschr Geneeskd. 2002;146:299–303.

69. Dalessio D. Neurologic diseases. In: Burrow G, Ferris T, editors. Medical complications during pregnancy. Philadelphia: WB Saunders; 1982. p. 435–47.

70. Dias MS, Sekhar LN. Intracranial hemorrhage from aneurysms and arteriovenous malformations during pregnancy and the puerperium. Neurosurgery. 1990;27:855–65; discussion 65–6.

71. Morcos SK. Contrast media-induced nephrotoxicity – questions and answers. Br J Radiol. 1998;71:357–65.

72. Barrett BJ, Parfrey PS, editors. Clinical aspects of acute renal failure following use of radiocontrast agents. New York: Marcel Dekker; 1992.

73. Solomon R. Contrast-medium-induced acute renal failure. Kidney Int. 1998;53:230–42.

74. Rudnick MR, Goldfarb S, Wexler L, et al. Nephrotoxicity of ionic and nonionic contrast media in 1196 patients: a randomized trial. The Iohexol Cooperative Study. Kidney Int. 1995; 47:254–61.

75. Porter GA. Radiocontrast-induced nephropathy. Nephrol Dial Transplant. 1994;9 Suppl 4:146–56.

76. Sharma S, Kimi A. Effect of nonionic radiocontrast agents on the occurrence of contrast-induced nephropathy in patients with mild-moderate chronic renal insufficiency: pooled analysis of the randomized trials. Catheter Cardiovasc Interv. 2005;65:386–93.

77. Cohan RH, Ellis JH. Iodinated contrast material in uroradiology. Choice of agent and management of complications. Urol Clin North Am. 1997;24:471–91.

78. Tepel M, van der Giet M, Schwarzfeld C, Laufer U, Liermann D, Zidek W. Prevention of radiographic-contrast-agent-induced reductions in renal function by acetylcysteine. N Engl J Med. 2000;343:180–4.

79. Mueller C, Buerkle G, Buettner HJ, et al. Prevention of contrast media-associated nephropathy: randomized comparison of 2 hydration regimens in 1620 patients undergoing coronary angioplasty. Arch Intern Med. 2002;162: 329–36.

80. Nussbaum ES, Casey SO, Sebring LA, Madison MT. Use of gadolinium as an intraarterial contrast agent in digital subtraction angiography of the cervical carotid arteries and intracranial circulation. Technical note. J Neurosurg. 2000;92:881–3.

81. Arat A, Cekirge HS, Saatci I. Gadodiamide as an alternative contrast medium in cerebral angiography in a patient with sensitivity to iodinated contrast medium. Neuroradiology. 2000;42:34–7; discussion 7–9.

82. Marenzi G, Marana I, Lauri G, et al. The prevention of radiocontrast-agent-induced nephropathy by hemofiltration. N Engl J Med. 2003;349:1333–40.

83. Parfrey PS, Griffiths SM, Barrett BJ, et al. Contrast material-induced renal failure in patients with diabetes mellitus, renal insufficiency, or both. A prospective controlled study. N Engl J Med. 1989;320:143–9.

84. Schwab SJ, Hlatky MA, Pieper KS, et al. Contrast nephrotoxicity: a randomized controlled trial of a nonionic and an ionic radiographic contrast agent. N Engl J Med. 1989;320: 149–53.

85. Wiholm BE, Myrhed M. Metformin-associated lactic acidosis in Sweden 1977–1991. Eur J Clin Pharmacol. 1993;44:589–91.

86. Manual on Contrast Media, Version 7. Reston: American College of Radiology; 2010.

87. Lalau JD, Race JM. Lactic acidosis in metformin therapy: searching for a link with metformin in reports of 'metformin-associated lactic acidosis'. Diabetes Obes Metab. 2001;3: 195–201.

88. Thomsen HS, Bush Jr WH. Adverse effects of contrast media: incidence, prevention and management. Drug Saf. 1998;19: 313–24.

89. Davenport MS, Cohan RH, Caoili EM, Ellis JH. Repeat contrast medium reactions in premedicated patients: frequency and severity. Radiology. 2009;253:372–9.

90. Horowitz MB, Dutton K, Purdy PD. Assessment of complication types and rates related to diagnostic angiography and interventional N euroradiologic procedures. A four year review (1993–1996). Interv Neuroradiol. 1998;4:27–37.

91. Leonardi M, Cenni P, Simonetti L, Raffi L, Battaglia S. Retrospective study of complications arising during cerebral and spinal diagnostic angiography from 1998 to 2003. Interv Neuroradiol. 2005;11:213–21.

92. Dawkins AA, Evans AL, Wattam J, et al. Complications of cerebral angiography: a prospective analysis of 2,924 consecutive procedures. Neuroradiology. 2007;49:753–9.

93. Fifi JT, Meyers PM, Lavine SD, et al. Complications of modern diagnostic cerebral angiography in an academic medical center. J Vasc Interv Radiol. 2009;20:442–7.

94. Bettmann MA, Heeren T, Greenfield A, Goudey C. Adverse events with radiographic contrast agents: results of the SCVIR Contrast Agent Registry. Radiology. 1997;203: 611–20.

95. Osborn AG. Diagnostic cerebral angiography. 2nd ed. Philadelphia: Lippincott Williams & Wilkins; 1999.

96. Dewachter P, Trechot P, Mouton-Faivre C. "Iodine allergy": point of view. Ann Fr Anesth Reanim. 2005;24:40–52.

97. Lasser EC, Berry CC, Mishkin MM, Williamson B, Zheutlin N, Silverman JM. Pretreatment with corticosteroids to prevent adverse reactions to nonionic contrast media. AJR Am J Roentgenol. 1994;162:523–6.

98. Freed KS, Leder RA, Alexander C, DeLong DM, Kliewer MA. Breakthrough adverse reactions to low-osmolar contrast media after steroid premedication. AJR Am J Roentgenol. 2001;176:1389–92.

99. Sakamoto S, Eguchi K, Shibukawa M, et al. Cerebral angiography using gadolinium as an alternative contrast medium in a patient with severe allergy to iodinated contrast medium. Hiroshima J Med Sci. 2010;59:15–6.

100. Kalsch H, Kalsch T, Eggebrecht H, Konorza T, Kahlert P, Erbel R. Gadolinium-based coronary angiography in patients with contraindication for iodinated x-ray contrast medium: a word of caution. J Interv Cardiol. 2008;21: 167–74.

101. Cohan RH, Leder RA, Ellis JH. Treatment of adverse reactions to radiographic contrast media in adults. Radiol Clin North Am. 1996;34:1055–76.

102. Tang G, Cawley CM, Dion JE, Barrow DL. Intraoperative angiography during aneurysm surgery: a prospective evaluation of efficacy. J Neurosurg. 2002;96:993–9.

103. Chiang VL, Gailloud P, Murphy KJ, Rigamonti D, Tamargo RJ. Routine intraoperative angiography during aneurysm surgery. J Neurosurg. 2002;96:988–92.

104. Nanda A, Willis BK, Vannemreddy PS. Selective intraoperative angiography in intracranial aneurysm surgery: intraoperative factors associated with aneurysmal remnants and vessel occlusions. Surg Neurol. 2002;58:309–14; discussion 14–5.

105. Lee MC, Macdonald RL. Intraoperative cerebral angiography: superficial temporal artery method and results. Neurosurgery. 2003;53:1067–74; discussion 74–5.

106. Fung E, Ganesan V, Cox TS, Chong WK, Saunders DE. Complication rates of diagnostic cerebral arteriography in children. Pediatr Radiol. 2005;35:1174–7.

107. Vucevic M, Tehan B, Gamlin F, Berridge JC, Boylan M. The SMART needle. A new Doppler ultrasound-guided vascular access needle. Anaesthesia. 1994;49:889–91.

108. Dix JE, McNulty BJ, Kallmes DF. Frequency and significance of a small distal ICA in carotid artery stenosis. AJNR Am J Neuroradiol. 1998;19:1215–8.

109. Bjorkesten G, Halonen V. Incidence of intracranial vascular lesions in patients with subarachnoid hemorrhage investigated by four-vessel angiography. J Neurosurg. 1965;23: 29–32.

110. Marks MP, Lane B, Steinberg GK, Snipes GJ. Intranidal aneurysms in cerebral arteriovenous malformations: evaluation and endovascular treatment. Radiology. 1992;183:355–60.

111. Garcia-Monaco R, Rodesch G, Alvarez H, Iizuka Y, Hui F, Lasjaunias P. Pseudoaneurysms within ruptured intracranial arteriovenous malformations: diagnosis and early endovascular management. AJNR Am J Neuroradiol. 1993;14:315–21.

112. Lasjaunias PL, Landrieu P, Rodesch G, et al. Cerebral proliferative angiopathy: clinical and angiographic description of an entity different from cerebral AVMs. Stroke. 2008;39: 878–85.

113. Huber P. A technical contribution of the exact angiographic localization of carotid cavernous fistulas. Neuroradiology. 1976;10:239–41.

114. Mehringer CM, Hieshima GB, Grinnell VS, Tsai F, Pribram HF. Improved localization of carotid cavernous fistula during angiography. AJNR Am J Neuroradiol. 1982;3:82–4.

3. Spinal Angiography

Catheter angiography of the spine is much less common than cerebral angiography, but it remains the gold standard for imaging spinal vasculature. Non-invasive imaging of spinal vasculature, including high resolution MRA or CTA, can sometimes be helpful to screen for larger vascular abnormalities, but fails to provide precise information regarding flow patterns and collateral flow; many times the vessels of interest are below the spatial resolution of these non-invasive modalities. Diagnostic spinal angiography is also typically done as the first step during neurointerventional procedures involving the spine and spinal cord. The techniques and skills required for spinal angiography can overlap those required for cerebral angiography, since the upper cervical spine and spinal cord are supplied by the vertebral arteries. However, the spine extends from the base of the skull to the sacrum, and imaging the vasculature is a procedure entirely different from cerebral angiography.

3.1.   Indications

1. Evaluation of patients with myelopathy, suspected to have spinal dural arteriovenous fistulas (most common indication).
2. Evaluation of patients with known or suspected spinal arteriovenous malformations or vascular neoplasms (e.g., with spinal intramedullary or subarachnoid haemorrhages).
3. Rarely for evaluation of suspected spinal cord ischemia ischaemia (since cord blood supply is so variable, and treatment options for cord ischaemia are so limited, angiography is mainly done to rule out a fistula as the cause of symptoms).
4. Planning for neurointerventional procedures on spine or spinal cord.
5. Pre-op mapping of cord vasculature prior to spinal or aortic procedures that risk occlusion of the spinal vessels.
6. Intra-operative assistance with surgery on spinal vascular lesions.
7. Follow-up imaging after treatment (e.g., after treatment of arteriovenous fistulas or malformations).

3.2.   Complications of Diagnostic Spinal Angiography

Informed consent prior to an angiogram should include a discussion of the risk of complications.

Neurological Complications

Neurological complications in spinal angiography may include the same risk of cerebral ischaemic events that may occur during cerebral angiography when the cervical region is being studied (see Chap. 2). In addition, there is the risk of vessel dissection, embolic occlusion with thrombus, atherosclerotic plaque, or air emboli occluding the spinal cord vessels and producing myelopathy. Forbes et al. reported that a series of 134 spinal angiograms had three (2.2%) neurological complications, all transient.[1] Two more recent series, with over 300 cases, have *zero* neurological complications from diagnostic spinal angiography.[2,3] High-volume contrast injection in vessels feeding the

M.R. Harrigan, J.P. Deveikis, *Handbook of Cerebrovascular Disease and Neurointerventional Technique*, DOI 10.1007/978-1-61779-946-4_3,
© Springer Science+Business Media New York 2013

spinal cord (although not necessarily performed as part of spinal angiography) has also been shown to produce temporary or permanent injury to the spinal cord.[4-6]

Non-neurological Complications

Non-neurological complications of spinal angiography via the femoral artery include the same local and systemic complications seen in cerebral angiography (as seen in Chap. 2). Forbes reported 8.2% puncture-site complications and 3.7% systemic complications from spinal angiography.[1] More recently, 1% puncture site complications and 0.7% systemic complications were reported.[3]

3.3. Selective Spinal Angiography: Basic Concepts

Pre-procedure Evaluation

1. Brief neurological exam should be done to establish a baseline, should a neurologic change occur during or after the procedure.
2. The patient should be asked if he or she has had a history of iodinated contrast reactions.
3. The femoral pulse, as well as the dorsalis pedis and posterior tibialis pulses should be examined.
4. Blood work, including a serum creatinine level and coagulation parameters, should be reviewed.

Pre-angiogram Orders

1. NPO except medications for 6 h prior to the procedure.
2. Place peripheral IV (two if an intervention is anticipated).
3. Place Foley catheter (almost always, unlike cerebral angiography).

Sedation/Analgesia/Anesthesia

The choice between general anesthesia and conscious sedation for spinal angiography depends upon the circumstances. General anesthesia allows for patient immobility including prolonged interruption of respiration while imaging tiny spinal vessels that are present in the thoracic and lumbar region. General anesthesia also spares the patient the potential discomfort of a long, involved angiographic procedure. Using nonionic, iso-osmolar contrast, procedures can be done under local anesthesia with minimal sedation, and adequate image quality is possible in cooperative patients. The advantage of local anesthesia is the avoidance of any of the potential complications of general anesthesia and the ability to monitor the neurological status of the patient during the procedure. The limited ability to monitor the neurological status of the patient during general anesthesia may be partially mitigated by the use of neurophysiological monitoring, such as somatosensory and/or motor evoked potentials.[2] However, neurophysiological monitoring adds to the cost and complexity of the procedure, and may not be readily available or reliable, depending on the institution.

Contrast Agents

Non-ionic contrast agents are almost always used due to their lower osmolality and better tolerance when injected into the small vessels feeding the spine. Iodixanol (Visipaque™, GE Healthcare, Princeton, NJ), an iso-osmolar and a nonionic contrast agent, is more expensive and more viscous than other contrast agents commonly used but is the best tolerated agent for spinal angiography.

1. Diagnostic angiogram: Omnipaque®, 300 mg I/mL, or Visipaque™, 320 mg I/mL.
2. Neurointerventional procedure: Omnipaque®, 240 mg I/mL or Visipaque™, 270 mg I/mL.

Patients with normal renal function can tolerate up to 400–800 mL of Omnipaque®, and 300 mg I/mL without adverse effects.[7] Contrast volumes in spinal angiography can routinely approach these limits, given the large number of injections required.

Femoral Artery Sheath

Trans-femoral spinal angiography is almost always done with a sheath.

Sheath:

1. Advantages: allows the rapid exchange of catheters and less potential for trauma to the arteriotomy site. Spinal angiography frequently requires several different catheters per case.
2. Unlike cerebral angiography, catheter position is often tenuous in the vessels being selected, and the sheath allows for more precise manipulation and positioning of the catheter.
3. Short sheath (10–13-cm arterial sheath) is used most commonly.
4. Longer sheath (25 cm) is useful when iliac or femoral artery tortuosity or atherosclerosis can impair catheter navigation. Longer sheaths may need to be pulled back, partially out of the iliac artery, when selective catheterization of the ipsilateral internal iliac artery is needed.
5. Technique: Standard arterial puncture techniques are used. Most commonly, a 5F or 6F sheath (Pinnacle® Sheath; Terumo Medical, Somerset, NJ) is used. The lumen of the sheath (and the angiographic catheter) is continuously perfused with heparinized saline (5,000 U heparin per liter of saline) under arterial pressure.

No Sheath:

1. Spinal angiography without a sheath offers the advantage of a slightly smaller arteriotomy, but is rarely done.
2. Situations in which a sheath may not be needed include paediatric cases in which a smaller arteriotomy is desired and very limited follow-up angiograms in which only one catheter may be used for a quick procedure.

Suggested Wires and Catheters for Diagnostic Spinal Angiography

Guidewires

- 0.035' or 0.038' J-tip wire for sheath insertion.
- The 0.035' angled Glidewire® (Terumo Medical, Somerset, NJ) is soft, flexible, and steerable.
- The 0.038' angled Glidewire® (Terumo Medical, Somerset, NJ) is slightly stiffer than the 0.035 in. may be helpful when added wire support is needed.

Catheters for Diagnostic Spinal Arteriography

In general, catheters for spinal angiography (Table 3.1 and Fig. 3.1) are the same shapes typically used for visceral angiography, although cerebral-type catheters may be used for catheterization of brachiocephalic vessels. Occasionally, straight catheters may be steam-shaped to an appropriate curve for a particular application. Straight catheters may also be used as-is for retrograde flush aortic injections (see below).

Table 3.1 Catheters for spinal angiography

Catheter	Use
5F Angled Taper	Good all-purpose diagnostic catheter for supra-aortic vessels
5F Mikaelsson	Good all-purpose catheter for intercostal and lumbar arteries
5F Simmons 1	Alternative to Mikaelsson
4 or 5F Cobra	Intercostal and lumbar arteries in younger patients
5.5F RDC	Very stable and torquable, but stiff
5F Straight	For retrograde flush aortic runs

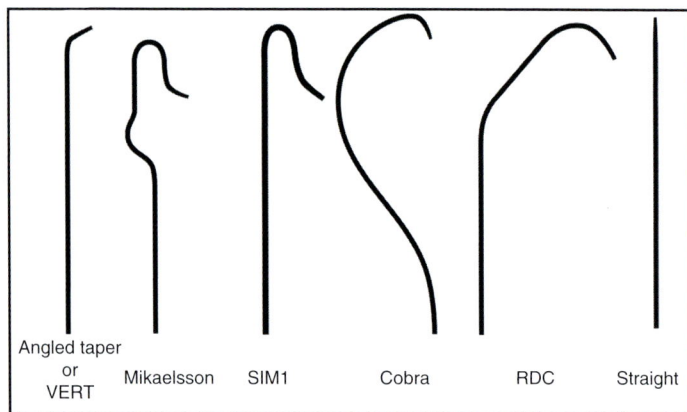

Angled taper or VERT | Mikaelsson | SIM1 | Cobra | RDC | Straight

Fig. 3.1 Recommended diagnostic catheters used for spinal arteriography.

Vessel Catheterization

Selective spinal angiography may be either complete spinal angiography, or a partial, focused study for a specific lesion. Complete spinal angiography is a major undertaking, in which all vessels that may relate to the spinal canal are selectively catheterized and studied. This is most often used in the evaluation of a patient with a suspected dural arteriovenous fistula causing myelopathy. The vascular lesion can be anywhere from the head to the sacrum, and evaluation of all vessels supplying these structures may be required (Table 3.2). When the lesion is obviously confined to a specific region of the spine, a more focused study may be more appropriate. This should include all the vessels that supply the area of interest, and the levels above and below the lesion, given the possibility of collateral flow from adjacent spinal vessels. Another useful rule of thumb is to visualize normal spinal cord vessels above and below any lesion affecting the cord. Assessing spinal cord blood supply may require selective angiography of the vertebral arteries (Fig. 3.2), thyrocervical and costocervical trunks, subclavian arteries, intercostal arteries (Fig. 3.3), lumbar arteries (Fig. 3.4), and lateral and medial sacral arteries.

Roadmapping

Roadmapping can be used to aid catheterization of the supra-aortic vessels, such as vertebral arteries, and the thyrocervical and costocervical trunks. Roadmapping is less helpful in catheterizing the intercostal and lumbar arteries, since respiratory motion degrades the image.

Table 3.2 Blood supply to various spinal regions

Level	Feeding arteries
Upper cervical	Vertebral, ascending pharyngeal, occipital, deep cervical
Lower cervical	Vertebral, deep cervical, ascending cervical
Upper thoracic	Supreme intercostal, superior intercostal
Mid-lower thoracic	Intercostal
Upper-to-mid lumbar	Lumbar
Lower lumbar	Iliolumbar
Sacrum	Anterior and lateral sacral

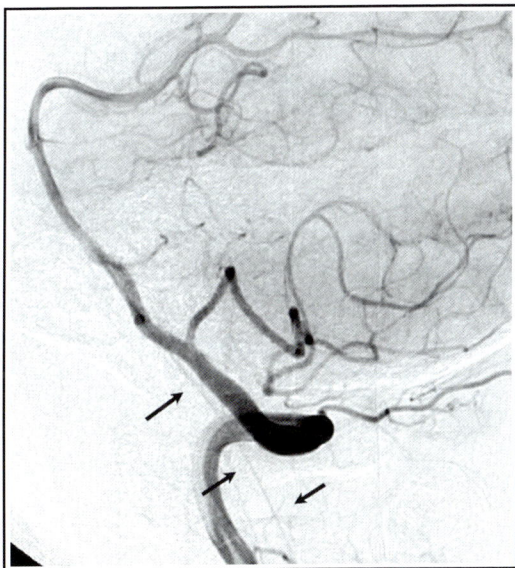

Fig. 3.2 Lateral vertebral artery angiogram showing anterior spinal artery (*arrows*).

Double Flushing

Catheter flushing technique is discussed in Chap. 2. Although some practitioners advocate double flushing of catheters only in the supra-aortic vessels, it makes more sense to use a meticulous flushing technique anywhere in the vascular system. This ensures that one will not forget to use good technique when it is most needed. Moreover, thrombus or air emboli in spinal cord vessels can be just as disabling as cerebral ischemia.

Continuous Saline Infusion

Three-way stopcock or manifolds can be used to provide a heparinized saline drip through the catheter. This is particularly useful for long spinal angiographic

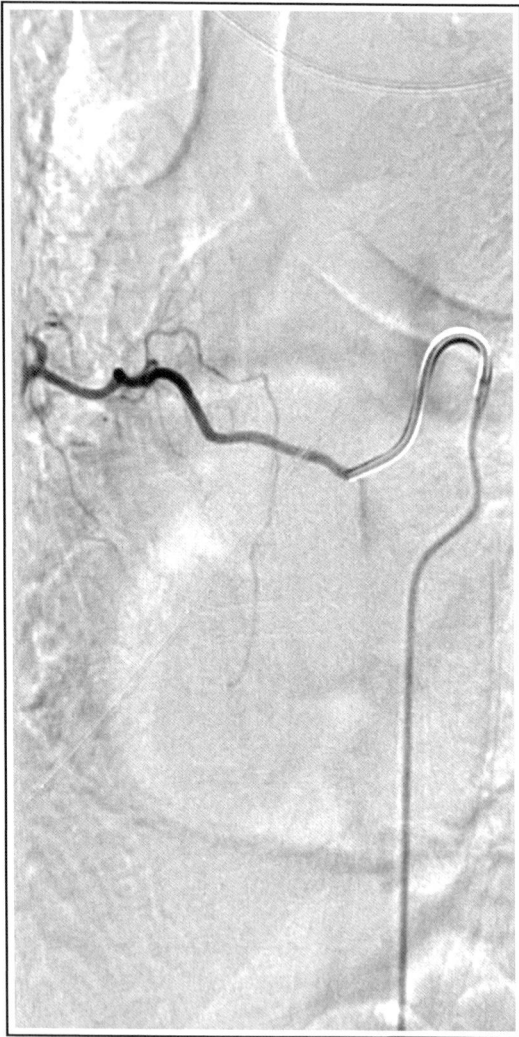

Fig. 3.3 Typical intercostal artery.

procedures. In-line air filters (B. Braun, Bethlehem, PA) on the saline drip tubing provide added protection from bubbles (as discussed in Chap. 4). A rotating adapter on the stopcock is needed to prevent the stopcock from being a drag on free manipulation of the catheter. Using both a rotating three-way stopcock and a rotating hemostatic valve on the catheter allows for two pivot points to allow free rotation of the catheter. This is important, as the catheter may not be in a stable position in the small lumbar and intercostal arteries.

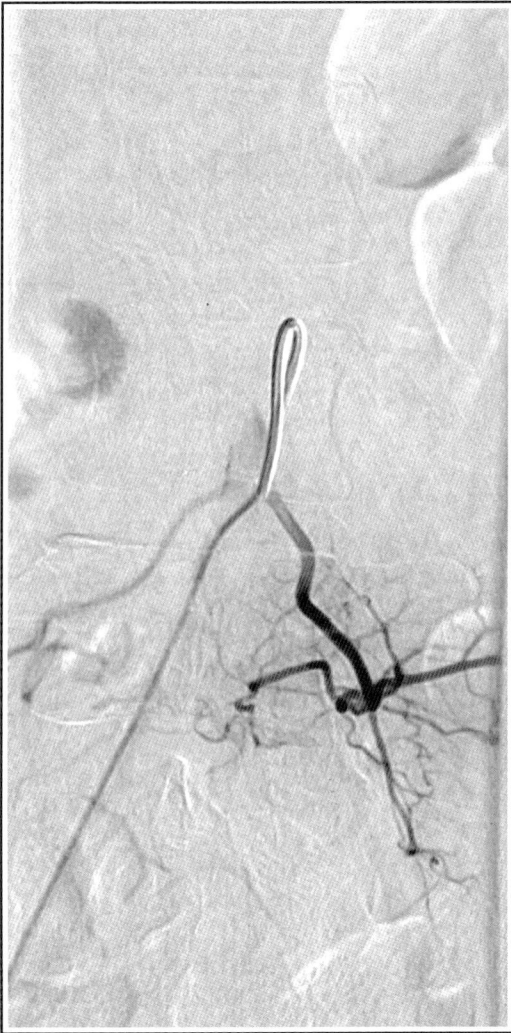

Fig. 3.4 Typical lumbar artery.

Hand Injection

Frequent small injections ("puffing") of contrast can be used to help manipulate the catheter into the desired lumbar and intercostal arteries. A 20 mL syringe containing contrast can be left attached to the catheter for these injections, and then used immediately for hand injections of contrast for angiographic runs. As is done in the cerebral vasculature, the syringe is held vertically and care is taken not to allow bubbles to enter the catheter. Most spinal vessels are best imaged with hand injections of contrast, to allow for modulation of the injection rate and volume, depending on the size of the vessel and stability of the catheter. An adequate angiographic run can be usually done with a single 2–3 s injection of 4–6 mL (100% contrast) of contrast. The goal is to adequately opacify the vessel of interest without displacing the catheter or refluxing too much into the aorta or into the ever-present collaterals to other spinal vessels. Patients should be warned that they will experience warmth and/or cramping in the territory of the injected vessel, and breathing should be suspended during the angiographic run, but the phase of respiration at which the breath-holding should occur depends on the spinal level being imaged (see below).

Mechanical Injection

A power contrast injector is necessary for thoracic or lumbar aortic angiograms, and for large vessels such as subclavian or iliac arteries. As stated in Chap. 2, the pressure and flow rate settings should not exceed the ratings of the stopcock or catheter. Common power injector settings for vessels studied in spinal angiograms using a 5F catheter are listed in Table 3.3. Note that one may need to increase or decrease these rates and volumes, depending on the size of the vessels, the stability of the catheter, and the quickness of the runoff of the contrast on a test injection. Use *extreme* caution if the catheter is wedged in the vessel and be especially careful if there is a possibility that a spinal cord vessel is arising from the branch one is injecting, since high-pressure power injections can damage the cord. *When in doubt, use careful hand-injections of contrast.*

Vessel Selection

If the exact level of the lesion is known from non-invasive imaging, the spinal angiogram should begin with those vessels supplying that area. Following catheterization of the vessel of interest, it is then customary to work systematically above and below the lesion to include normal territory adjacent to the lesion. Lesions of the cord itself usually require mapping of the spinal cord supply above and below the lesion. For complete spinal angiography, it is particularly important to image the intercostal and lumbar arteries in a systematic fashion so that one does not inadvertently miss or repeat a level. It is helpful to maintain a worksheet during the procedure, and list the sides and vessels injected during each angiographic run. Radio-opaque marker rulers can be placed under the patient on the table or marker tapes can be affixed to the patient's back, slightly off midline to have a reference available on each film to help confirm the levels studied. Additionally, bony landmarks, such as the 12th rib, can also help with keeping track of the vessels being studied.

Table 3.3 Standard power injector settings[a]

Vessel	Power injector settings
Aortic arch	20 mL/s; total of 25 mL
Retrograde aortic flush	10 mL/s; total of 30 mL
Iliac artery	10 mL/s; total of 20 mL
Subclavian artery	6 mL/s; total of 15 mL
Vertebral artery	6 mL/s; total of 8 mL
Lumbar or intercostal artery	2 mL/s; total of 6 mL
For 3D imaging	0.5–2 mL/s; total 7–30 mL (higher doses for high flow AVF)

[a]For digital subtraction angiography using a 5F catheter

Angiographic Images and Standard Views

Spinal angiography has a number of features that make it less desirable to use biplane imaging routinely. The vascular anatomy is usually quite simple compared to cerebral vessels. Moreover, when one images the spine in lateral view, higher doses of x-rays are required to adequately penetrate the thoracic or lumbar region to give good visualization of the structures. Consequently, to limit the radiation dose to the patient and operator, and to prevent over-heating the X-ray tube, usually only single plane, frontal images of the thoracic, lumbar, and sacral spine are usually performed. Lateral views are taken when the vessels supplying the lesion are found. Additionally, when a complex vascular lesion is found, 3D rotational imaging can be done when the proper imaging equipment is available. Prestigiacomo and colleagues found that 3D imaging was better than conventional angiography for spinal AVMs in determining the relationship of lesions to the spinal cord and detecting intranidal aneurysms.[8] Three-dimensional imaging requires general anesthesia to ensure immobility during the 15 s imaging acquisition and contrast must be slowly injected in the vessel of interest for approximately 15–17 s beginning 1 s prior to starting the acquisition to ensure that the vessels are opacified throughout the full rotation of the gantry.

1. When viewing the spinal angiographic images, the normal anatomic features should be recognized. Segmental spinal vessels have osseous branches that supply the vertebra at that level, radicular branches, variable radiculomedullary branches that connect to the anterior spinal artery, variable radiculopial branches that feed the posterolateral spinal arteries, muscular branches, and anastamoses to the contralateral and cephalad and caudal adjacent segmental branches.

2. Other imaging features worthy of attention during the performance of a spinal angiogram:
   (a) Vessel contour and size (angioarchitecture).
   (b) Presence or absence of evident contribution to spinal cord. Look for the hair-pin turn of the artery of Adamkiewicz (Fig. 3.5) and fairly straight ascending and/or descending vessels in the spinal canal.
   (c) Presence of abnormal or unexpected vascular channels (neovascularity).
   (d) Presence or absence of an abnormal vascular blush. Note that normal muscle and bone normally display a vascular blush.
   (e) Early venous filling indicative of an AV shunt.
   (f) When there is a shunt, where do the veins drain to?
   (g) Injection of intercostal or lumbar arteries that fill the anterior spinal artery should be examined for the appearance of the coronal venous plexus of the spinal cord within about 15 s after contrast injection. Lack of visualization or delayed visualization of the veins along the cord and the radicular veins that anastamose with the epidural veins can be evidence of severe spinal venous hypertension.

Pearl
Remember, the anterior spinal artery is in the midline. The posterolateral spinal arteries are slightly off midline.

Frame Rates for Digital Subtraction Angiography

Most spinal angiography can be done with relatively slow frame rates of one or two frames per second (fps). Most arteriovenous fistulas in the spine are relatively slow filling. Only very high flow arteriovenous shunts would require 3 fps or faster imaging. Routine use of fast frame rate while imaging the spine below the cervical region will soon overheat the X-ray tube and may not even be possible with lower quality imaging chains. For most spinal arteriography, a 10–12 s imaging sequence allows for visualization of arterial, capillary, and venous phases. However, when screening for causes of spinal venous hypertension, such as a spinal dural AVF, injection of the segmental vessel supplying the artery of Adamkiewicz may require imaging for 20–25 s to visualize the venous phase of the spinal cord vasculature.

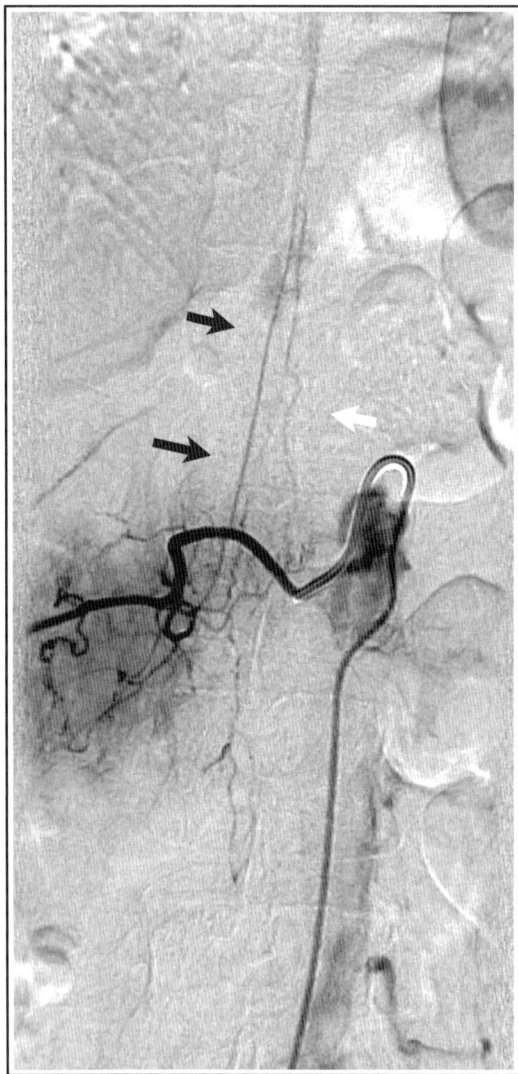

Fig. 3.5 L1 lumbar artery injection showing the artery of Adamkiewicz (*black arrows*), with the characteristic hairpin turn, followed by the anterior spinal artery (*white arrow*).

Calibration and Measurement

Size measurements and calibration can be done as described in Chap. 2. In spinal angiography, radio-opaque rulers may be placed under the patient for reference and utilized for calibration.

3.4.   Spinal Angiographic Procedures

Femoral Artery Puncture

1. Standard arterial access is obtained (see Chap. 2).
2. A femoral arterial sheath is placed (5F or 6F).

Brachial/Axillary/Radial Artery Catheterization

1. Very rarely, spinal angiography may require access from the arm if there are femoral, iliac, or aortic occlusions.
2. If lower lumbar arteries must be imaged using an upper extremity artery for access, use an axillary approach, since even 100 cm catheters may not reach from a radial or even brachial approach.

Aortic Imaging

1. Screening aortic injections by pigtail catheter are a way to get a rough idea of vascular anatomy in the thoracic and lumbar region.
2. It is most helpful in elderly patients with aortic atherosclerosis or aortic aneurysms to see which segmental vessels may be occluded.
3. As a rule, aortic injections provide poor visualization of small spinal vessels, so they do not eliminate the need for selective spinal angiography.
4. In the lumbar region, pigtail catheter injections fill all the visceral vessels as well as the lumbar arteries. This can obscure even fairly extensive vascular abnormalities in the spine.
5. For most cases, it is not worth wasting the time or contrast on aortic injections.

Retrograde Aortic Flush

1. Better visualization of the segmental spinal arteries can be obtained with a retrograde aortic flush, as opposed to standard pigtail injections.[9,10]
2. Bilateral femoral arterial sheaths are required (five or six F).
3. A straight catheter (five or six F) is positioned in each common iliac artery.
4. Simultaneous power injection of contrast in each catheter is needed. A sterile Y-connector that is rated for high pressure can connect the tubing from the injector to both catheters. Alternatively, two separate injector machines may be used.
5. 20 mL/s for a total of 50 mL distributed equally between the two catheters is injected.
6. Contrast usually streams up the posterior wall or the aorta, providing visualization of the lumbar, and lower intercostal arteries, with less obscuration of the anterior visceral arteries.

7. More viscous contrast, such as Omnipaque 350 or Visipaque 320 works best with this technique.
8. Usually no more than five vertebral levels are well imaged by this technique. The catheters may need to be positioned in the upper lumbar aorta to visualize the higher thoracic levels.
9. This technique is still not a replacement for selective spinal angiography.
10. Retrograde aortic flush is *contraindicated* in very tortuous aorta or iliac vessels, in the presence of extensive atherosclerosis, or aortic or iliac aneurysmal disease, due to a risk of dissection or plaque disruption.

Intercostal and Lumbar Artery Catheterization

1. For complete spinal angiography, these segmental vessels constitute the majority of the vessels to be studied.
2. Unless the exact site of a lesion is known from other imaging studies, the segmental spinal vessels should be studied in a systematic fashion to ensure that all are being visualized.
3. Using a Mikaelsson or Simmons catheter, it is often most efficient to go from caudal to cranial, to avoid un-forming the curve of the catheter.
4. Using most other catheters, such as Cobra catheters, it works best to go from cranial to caudal.
5. From one level to the next, the segmental vessels come off at similar positions along the wall of the aorta, so it is best to go from one level to the next and do all on one side before going back and doing all on the other side. This is much quicker than rotating the catheter from one side to the other at each level.
6. The catheter is slowly rotated and moved forward or backward while puffing small amounts of contrast until the desired vessel is engaged.
7. The catheter is gently pulled back to ensure it is seated in the vessel.
8. The catheter should be held in position with one hand to prevent it from rotating out of the vessel, and contrast injected for an angiographic run, during transient arrest of respiration.
9. Keeping the catheter at the same angle of rotation, it is then gently pushed forward (for Mikaelsson or Simmons) or withdrawn (for Cobra) to disengage from the vessel.
10. Again keeping the same angle of rotation, the catheter is moved to the next vertebral level and it should just pop into the lumbar or intercostal branch.
11. Alternatively, the catheter can be left in the branch, then slowly rotated toward the right or left until it enters the contralateral segmental branch at the same vertebral level.
12. Continue the process in a systematic fashion until all the desired vessels are studied.

Optimizing Images by Reducing Respiratory or Other Motion

General anesthesia can be used to prevent patient motion. With or without general anesthesia, imaging the intercostal and lumbar arteries should be done during breath-holding. For lower lumbar imaging, the patients can hold their breath in either inspiration or expiration, whichever moves aerated bowel away from the area of interest. Upper lumbar and lower thoracic imaging is best if the patients hold in expiration, to keep the interface of lung and diaphragm out of the imaging field. In the mid thoracic region above the diaphragm, the patients should hold their breath in inspiration, to keep the diaphragm below the area of interest. In the upper thoracic region, catheter positioning is frequently very tenuous, and deep respirations in anticipation of breath holding can displace the catheter. In this region, it is best to have the patient suspend respiration without deep inspiration or expiration.

In the lumbar region, bowel peristalsis can sometimes degrade subtraction images. Bowel movement can be temporarily slowed by injecting 1 mg of glucagon or 40 mg of hyoscine-N-butylbromide (Buscopan®; Boehringer Ingelheim GmbH, Germany) IV just prior to acquiring the images.[11]

Pearls

To facilitate catheterization of the intercostal and lumbar arteries, remember the following facts:

1. The more caudal, the more posterior the origins of the segmental vessels are.[12], and the more symmetrical the origin of the right and left segmental vessels.

2. Upper thoracic right-sided intercostal arteries arise from the lateral wall of the aorta; the left are more posterior. Right and left lower lumbar arteries both arise from the posterior wall of the aorta (Fig. 3.6).

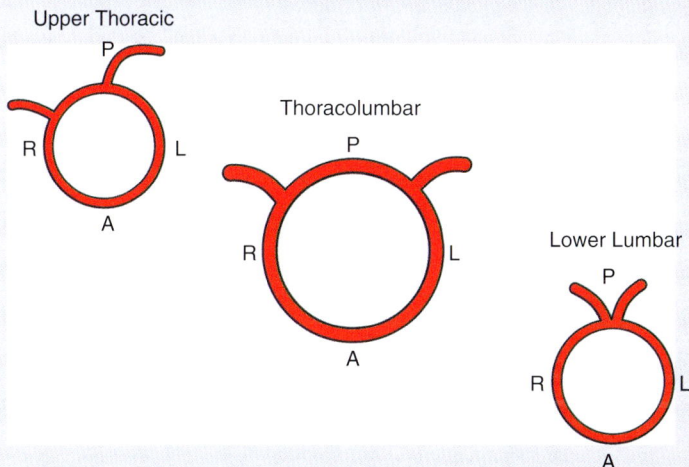

Fig. 3.6 Orientation of segmental arteries. *Upper thoracic*: Right intercostal arises from lateral aspect of aorta, the right from posterior surface. *Thoracolumbar*: both intercostal/lumbar arteries arise from lateral aspect of aorta. *Lower lumbar*: Both lumbar arteries arise from posterior wall of aorta. *A* anterior, *P* posterior.

3. The right and left lower lumbar arteries may have a common origin from the aorta.

4. In lumbar and lower thoracic regions, segmental branches usually arise just below the level of the pedicle.

5. In the more cephalad levels in the thoracic region, the intercostal arteries are closer together, and slope cephalad to supply vertebral levels above the level of the aorta from which they arise.

6. The highest intercostal arteries are close together, and their angulation often makes it difficult to keep the catheter in a stable position in the vessel.
7. Just below the aortic arch, the superior intercostals ascend and variably supply two or three thoracic vertebral levels above the origins of the vessels (Fig. 3.7).
8. Do not forget that the supreme intercostals are at the costocervical trunks (hence, the name "costo-"cervical) and supply the most cranial two or three thoracic levels.

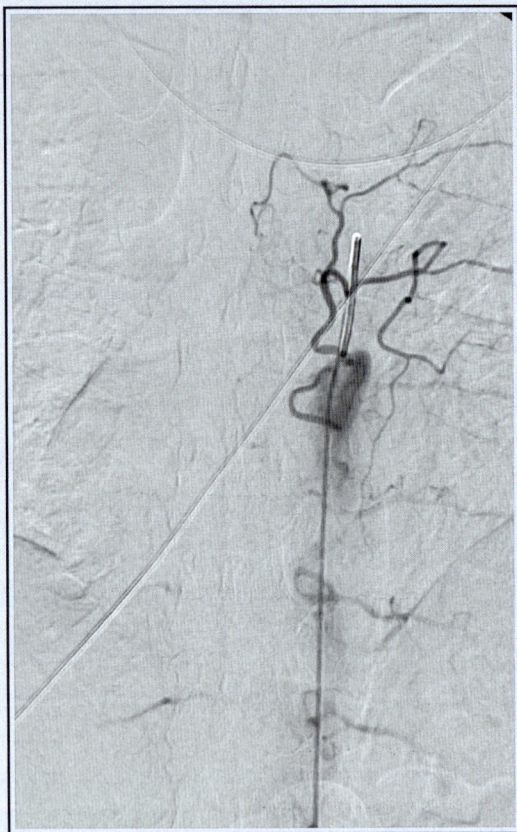

Fig. 3.7 Superior intercostal artery. This is the most cephalad intercostal artery arising from the aorta, ascending to supply several vertebral levels. Not to be confused with supreme intercostal arising from the costocervical trunk.

Sacral and Ileolumbar Artery Catheterization

1. The anterior sacral artery starts at the aortic bifurcation, and is usually catheterized with any reverse-curve catheter (like Mikaelsson or Simmons).
2. Ileolumbar and lateral sacral arteries come off the internal iliac arteries.
3. Common iliac injections can be done to locate the spinal vessels to be selected.
4. Iliac arteries and their branches contralateral to the femoral puncture site are catheterized by engaging the iliac with the catheter, then advancing a hydrophilic wire well down into the contralateral femoral artery. The catheter is then advanced antegrade over the wire into the external iliac. While injecting small amounts of contrast, it is slowly pulled back and rotated until the desired vessel is catheterized.
5. Iliac arteries ipsilateral to the femoral puncture require a fully formed Mikaelsson or Simmons in the aorta, which is slowly withdrawn and rotated so that it points back into the ipsilateral iliac. As small amounts of contrast are injected, it is withdrawn and rotated into the vessel of interest.
6. The ipsilateral iliac vessels can often be well imaged from a retrograde injection of a catheter or sheath with its tip in the distal external iliac artery.
7. If a sheath is used, it may have to be pulled back into the external iliac to allow catheterization of the iliac branches.
8. Truly selective injections of the ileolumbar and lateral sacral arteries may require the use of a microcatheter/micro-guidewire assembly placed coaxially through the 5F catheter positioned with its tip at the origin of the internal iliac artery.
9. Ileolumbar arteries are at the very proximal internal iliac and the lateral sacral a little more distally off the posterior division of the internal iliac.
10. Warn patients that they will feel the heat of the contrast in very private places when injected in the iliac arteries and their branches.

Vertebral Artery Catheterization

1. For complete spinal angiography, the vertebral arteries must be studied.
2. Vertebral artery catheterization is discussed in detail in Chap. 2.
3. The vertebral arteries fill the anterior spinal arteries at the vertebrobasilar junction and the posterolateral spinal arteries proximal to, or directly from, PICA.
4. Remember that segmental branches of the vertebral may contribute also to the spinal cord. If the catheter tip is positioned too high up in the vertebral artery, lower segmental feeders to the cord may be overlooked.

Thyrocervical/Costocervical Trunk Catheterization

1. For complete spinal angiography, these subclavian artery branches must be studied.
2. For most cases, a simple curve on the catheter (Angled Taper, Vertebral, or Berenstein curve) works best.
3. Advance the catheter over a wire into the subclavian artery well beyond the origin of the vertebral artery.
4. Double flush the catheter, then slowly withdraw the catheter, keeping the tip pointed cephalad, while gently injecting small quantities of contrast until the catheter engages the desired vessel.
5. The costocervical trunk is just distal to the thyrocervical trunk, which is just distal to the vertebral artery.
6. There may be an anomalous artery of the cervical enlargement, supplying the cord directly from the subclavian.
7. With tortuous vessels or confusing anatomy, a subclavian injection, using a slight ipsilateral oblique view can help.

Carotid Artery Catheterization

1. For complete spinal angiography, branches of the carotid arteries must be studied.
2. Carotid artery catheterization is discussed in detail in Chap. 2.
3. External and internal carotid injections, and preferably, selective injections of ascending pharyngeal and occipital arteries are needed. The middle meningeal artery may also contribute to AV fistulas that drain to the spinal cord veins.

Reconstituting a Mikaelsson Catheter

The Mikaelsson catheter has a reverse curve that must be reconstituted after the catheter is introduced into the aorta, similar to the Simmons catheter. The Simmons 2 catheter is discussed in detail in Chap. 2. The Mikaelsson can be reconstituted if a wire is advanced into the contralateral iliac artery or a renal artery. The catheter is then advanced over the wire until the primary curve is just into the iliac or renal artery. Then the wire is pulled back and the catheter gently advanced, reforming the shape of the reverse curve. As the catheter continues to advance, it will pull out of the engaged renal or iliac artery and be fully formed in the aorta. Sometimes the catheter will spontaneously reform its shape if it is advanced up to the aortic arch distal to the left subclavian artery, and then rotated. Reconstitution in the left subclavian or the aortic valve is usually not an option due to the short length of the catheter.

Remember that pulling back on the Mikaelsson can engage intercostal arteries, lumbar arteries, and those pesky visceral vessels, which can un-form the catheter curve if it is pulled back further. The catheter should always be pulled back slowly under fluoroscopic visualization, as the catheter is constantly rotated to avoid snagging vessels along the way.

Femoral Artery Puncture Site Management

Arterial puncture site management and closure techniques and devices are discussed in Chap. 2.

Post-angiogram Orders

1. Bed rest with accessed leg extended, head of bed ≤30°, for 6 h, then out of bed for 1 h. (If a closure device is used, bed rest, with head of bed ≤30°, for 1 h, then out of bed for 1 h).
2. Vital signs: Check on arrival in recovery room, then Q 1 h until discharge. Call physician for SBP ≤90 mmHg or decrease 25 mmHg; pulse ≥120.
3. Check puncture site and distal pulses upon arrival in recovery room, then Q 15 min × 4, Q30 min × 2, then Q 1 h until discharge. Call physician if:
   (a) Bleeding or haematoma develops at puncture site.
   (b) Distal pulse is not palpable beyond the puncture site.
   (c) Extremity is blue or cold.
4. Check puncture site after ambulation.
5. IVF: 0.9N. S. at 100 mL/h until patient is ambulatory.
6. Resume pre-angiogram diet.
7. Resume routine medications.
8. PO fluids at least 500 mL.
9. D/C Foley catheter and IV prior to discharge.
10. Check BUN and creatinine 24–48 h post procedure if very large volumes of contrast were used.

3.5.   Special Techniques and Situations

Intraoperative Spinal Angiography

Intraoperative spinal angiography is employed by some neurosurgeons during surgery for spinal AV fistulas and arteriovenous malformations.[13] It can be helpful to localize small lesions and to confirm complete removal of lesions. It correlates well with post-operative angiography in the angiography suite, and can show an unexpected residual AV shunt in up to 33% of cases.[14] Intraoperative spinal angiography poses technical challenges compared to intraoperative cerebral angiography. First, the patient is usually prone during the operation. This requires that a long (at least 25 cm) sheath be placed in the femoral artery prior to the patient being positioned prone. The sheath is only inserted a short distance, and is positioned so that its hub is along the lateral aspect of the hip, so it can be accessed after the patient is turned prone. An alternative for arterial access is a transradial approach.[15] Another challenge is the fact that most operating room tables are not radiolucent, which can make it a challenge getting the right C-arm angle to visualize the catheter and the desired vessels. A Jackson frame should be used instead of an operating table if possible. Prone positioning can also confuse the angiographer and make catheterization of the desired vessels difficult.[16] An easy aid to catheterization is to reverse the fluoroscopic image side-to-side when working the catheter on a prone patient. These challenges may be overcome, but are one reason why intraoperative spinal angiography is not more commonly practiced.

Tips for Imaging Specific Lesions

Spinal Intramedullary or Perimedullary Arteriovenous Malformations

- All feeding arteries and draining veins should be identified; this requires visualization of the spinal cord vessels at the level of the lesion, and several segmental levels above and below the lesion.
- Normal spinal arteries should be seen above and below the lesion to ensure all feeders have been seen.
- Biplane, magnified runs are useful to evaluate the architecture and relationship to the cord.
- Rapid imaging rates of 3–5 fps can sometimes provide a better visualization of the angioarchitecture of the lesion.
- Images should be carefully evaluated to determine how the lesion relates to the anterior and posterolateral spinal arteries.
- Look for intranidal aneurysms and pseudo-aneurysms.
- 3D imaging may be useful.

Type IV Spinal Perimedullary Arteriovenous Fistulas

- These are uncommon, congenital fistulas that are usually obvious on noninvasive imaging.
- Like other vascular malformations, normal spinal arteries should be seen above and below the lesion to ensure all feeders have been seen.
- Biplane, magnified runs are useful to evaluate the architecture and relationship to the cord.
- These are high flow lesions, requiring rapid imaging rates of 3–15 fps.
- 3D imaging may be useful.

Type I Spinal Dural Arteriovenous Fistulas

- By far the most common indication for spinal angiography.
- Non-invasive imaging such as MRI may suggest the diagnosis, but the sensitivity of MR in detecting fistulae is only 51% [3]
- Even if the area of myelopathy is known from clinical symptoms and non-invasive imaging, the site of the arteriovenous fistula may be remote from the area affected, so be prepared to do complete spinal angiography.
- Look for an enlarged vein filling from a radicular of a lumbar or intercostal artery in most cases.
- Occasionally, the fistula may be found at the craniocervical junction,[17] intracranially,[18] or in the paraspinal region.[15]
- Seek out, and carefully study the injection of the vessel supplying the artery of Adamkiewicz (Fig. 3.5).
- In cases of thoracic myelopathy from a dural AV fistula, lack of visualization of the coronal venous plexus and radicular veins after injection of the artery of Adamkiewicz provides convincing evidence for venous hypertension and confirms the diagnosis of an AV fistula.[19]
- Conversely, good visualization of normal spinal cord veins within 15 s after seeing the artery of Adamkiewicz makes the diagnosis of AV a fistula much less likely.
- An exception of this rule is the cranial dAVF draining into cord veins. Injection of the artery of Adamkiewicz may look normal.[20]

Spinal Intramedullary Vascular Tumors

- The most common indication is spinal hemangioblastoma, usually preoperative and/or pre-embolization.
- All feeding arteries and draining veins should be identified; this requires visualization of the spinal cord vessels at the level of the lesion, and several segmental levels above and below the lesion.
- Biplane, magnified runs are useful to evaluate the architecture and relationship to the cord.

Spinal Extradural Vascular Tumors

- Usual indications are in cases of pre-operative evaluation of patients with aneurysmal bone cyst or vascular metastases such as renal or thyroid cancer.
- All feeding arteries should be identified; this requires visualization of the segmental spinal vessels bilaterally at the level of the lesion, and several segmental levels above and below the lesion.
- Normal spinal arteries at the level of the lesion or at nearby levels should be identified so that they can be carefully spared during any anticipated embolization procedure or at the time of surgery.

Preoperative Angiography for Surgery That May Risk Occlusion of the Spinal Cord Blood Supply

- Major spinal surgery, aortic aneurysm repair, or stent-grafts may carry a risk of myelopathy if radiculomedullary contributors to the anterior spinal artery and adjacent segmental collateral vessels are all occluded.
- Preoperative spinal angiography can locate the variable spinal cord vessels. If a dominant spinal cord feeder is at risk in the surgical field it could be spared, or the feeding intercostal or lumbar artery could be reimplanted into the aorta.
- On the other hand, one study of over 100 cases in which preoperative spinal angiography was done showed no impact on neurological outcome when vessels were preserved or reimplanted based on angiographic findings.[21]

References

1. Forbes G, Nichols DA, Jack Jr CR, et al. Complications of spinal cord arteriography: prospective assessment of risk for diagnostic procedures. Radiology. 1988;169:479–84.
2. Niimi Y, Sala F, Deletis V, Setton A, de Camargo AB, Berenstein A. Neurophysiologic monitoring and pharmacologic provocative testing for embolization of spinal cord arteriovenous malformations. AJNR Am J Neuroradiol. 2004;25:1131–8.
3. Chen J, Gailloud P. Safety of spinal angiography: complication rate analysis in 302 diagnostic angiograms. Neurology. 2011;77:1235–40.
4. Moseley IF, Tress BM. Extravasation of contrast medium during spinal angiography: a case of paraplegia. Neuroradiology. 1977;13:55–7.
5. Ramirez-Lassepas M, McClelland RR, Snyder BD, Marsh DG. Cervical myelopathy complicating cerebral angiography. Report of a case and review of the literature. Neurology. 1977;27:834–7.
6. Miller DL. Direct origin of the artery of the cervical enlargement from the left subclavian artery. AJNR Am J Neuroradiol. 1993;14:242–4.
7. Rosovsky MA, Rusinek H, Berenstein A, Basak S, Setton A, Nelson PK. High-dose administration of nonionic contrast media: a retrospective review. Radiology. 1996;200:119–22.
8. Prestigiacomo CJ, Niimi Y, Setton A, Berenstein A. Three-dimensional rotational spinal angiography in the evaluation and treatment of vascular malformations. AJNR Am J Neuroradiol. 2003;24:1429–35.
9. Rauste J, Somer K. Semiselective renal angiography, a useful method for evaluating the vascular supply in both kidneys. Radiol Clin (Basel). 1977;46:281–8.
10. Ogawa R. Semiselective renal and lumbar angiography: experimental and clinical evaluation of this new angiographic method. Nippon Igaku Hoshasen Gakkai Zasshi. 1995;55:20–33.
11. Kozak RI, Bennett JD, Brown TC, Lee TY. Reduction of bowel motion artifact during digital subtraction angiography: a comparison of hyoscine butylbromide and glucagon. Can Assoc Radiol J. 1994;45:209–11.
12. Shimizu S, Tanaka R, Kan S, Suzuki S, Kurata A, Fujii K. Origins of the segmental arteries in the aorta: an anatomic study for selective catheterization with spinal arteriography. AJNR Am J Neuroradiol. 2005;26:922–8.
13. Barrow DL, Colohan AR, Dawson R. Intradural perimedullary arteriovenous fistulas (type IV spinal cord arteriovenous malformations). J Neurosurg. 1994;81:221–9.
14. Schievink WI, Vishteh AG, McDougall CG, Spetzler RF. Intraoperative spinal angiography. J Neurosurg. 1999;90:48–51.
15. Lang SS, Eskioglu E, A Mericle A. Intraoperative angiography for neurovascular disease in the prone or three-quarter prone position. Surg Neurol. 2006;65:283–9; discussion 289.
16. Benes L, Wakat JP, Sure U, Bien S, Bertalanffy H. Intraoperative spinal digital subtraction angiography: technique and results. Neurosurgery. 2003;52:603–9; discussion 608–9.
17. Pulido Rivas P, Villoria Medina F, Fortea Gil F, Sola RG. Dural fistula in the craniocervical junction. A case report and review of the literature. Rev Neurol. 2004;38:438–42.
18. Li J, Ezura M, Takahashi A, Yoshimoto T. Intracranial dural arteriovenous fistula with venous reflux to the brainstem and spinal cord mimicking brainstem infarction–case report. Neurol Med Chir (Tokyo). 2004;44:24–8.
19. Willinsky R, Lasjaunias P, Terbrugge K, Hurth M. Angiography in the investigation of spinal dural arteriovenous fistula. A protocol with application of the venous phase. Neuroradiology. 1990;32:114–6.
20. Trop I, Roy D, Raymond J, Roux A, Bourgouin P, Lesage J. Craniocervical dural fistula associated with cervical myelopathy: angiographic demonstration of normal venous drainage of the thoracolumbar cord does not rule out diagnosis. AJNR Am J Neuroradiol. 1998;19:583–6.
21. Minatoya K, Karck M, Hagl C, et al. The impact of spinal angiography on the neurological outcome after surgery on the descending thoracic and thoracoabdominal aorta. Ann Thorac Surg. 2002;74:S1870–2; discussion S1892–8.

4. General Considerations
for Neurointerventional Procedures

This chapters covers fundamental aspects of neurointerventional procedures, including preprocedural preparation, vascular access, antithrombotic management, post-procedural care, and complication management and avoidance. The Appendix discusses the neurointerventional suite.

4.1.   A Series of Unfortunate Events

One overriding principle should be kept in mind by every neurointerventionalist: Adverse outcomes always occur because of a series of minor deviations from standard practice, and rarely from only a single event.[1,2] This simple truism has been noted in a wide range of human endeavors, from mountaineering[3] to computer networks[4] to aviation and space flight. A series of errors must occur in the correct order, and at just the right time, for a catas. For instance, a patient will never die *only* of an intracerebral hematoma after a neurointerventional procedure. That patient will have died because of: A) a failure to handle the exchange-length microwire properly, followed by B) failure to visualize the tip the of wire closely enough on fluoroscopy during the exchange, followed by C) a failure to recognize the immediate blood pressure and heart rate changes due to a wire perforation, followed by D) a failure to recognize a small area of contrast extravasation from a distal middle cerebral artery branch on the follow-up angiogram, followed by E) a failure to reverse the anticoagulation in a timely manner, and so on. Bad outcomes always result from a cascade of failures, never a single failure. Conversely, disaster may be avoided by recognizing components of this cascade early on, and avoiding making those decisions that compound the problem.

Tips for Preventing and Stopping a Cascade of Errors

1. Always make sure that the planned procedure is truly indicated, and that the benefits outweigh the risks.
   Example: Is coiling of a tiny unruptured asymptomatic aneurysm prudent? For a young patient with a previous history of subarachnoid haemorrhage, it may be; for an elderly patient with no other risk factors for haemorrhage, it may not be.
2. Planning and preparation are mandatory.
   Example: Airline pilots must submit a written checklist before each flight. If neurointerventionalists were required to do the same, then they might be safer.
3. Always have a Plan B. And sometimes a Plan C.
   Example: If Plan A is to coil an aneurysm that is also clippable, have a reasonable threshold to change to Plan B (surgery) if significant obstacles to coiling begin to appear.
4. To avoid making mistakes, one should constantly assume one is going to make one.[3] Approach every procedure with a humble mindset and the knowledge that whatever can go wrong, may well go wrong.
   Example: During coiling of a ruptured basilar tip aneurysm, a routine guide catheter angiogram was done with injection of contrast into the RHV. Due to

M.R. Harrigan, J.P. Deveikis, *Handbook of Cerebrovascular Disease and Neurointerventional Technique*, DOI 10.1007/978-1-61779-946-4_4, © Springer Science+Business Media New York 2013

some excessive redundancy in the microcather, and because the RHV was not cinched down tightly (two small errors), the microcatheter tip was launched with the contrast injection through the dome of the aneurysm, and in spite of rapid coiling of the aneurysm and placement of a ventriculostomy, the patient died.

5. Have a low threshold to **STOP**! when things begin to go wrong, particularly for non-emergent procedures. Regroup and recover from the first thing that went wrong.

   Example: A sizable groin haematoma develops soon after the femoral artery puncture in a high-risk carotid stenting case. Solution: Stop, deal with the haematoma, and reattempt the stenting procedure another time.

6. Encourage and accept input from everybody during procedures, including nurses, technologists, anesthesiologists, residents, fellows, and when appropriate, device company representatives.

   Example: A visitor during a coiling case, observing from the control room, was the first to notice a clot forming at the tip of the guide catheter, which helped the operators during the case tremendously.

4.2. Preprocedure Preparation

General preparations for most neurointerventional procedures:

1. Routine pre-procedure work-up:
   a. History and physical
   b. Neurological exam
   c. Imaging
   d. Blood work (CBC, Cr, PT, PTT)
   e. EKG
   f. Anesthesia evaluation, if needed
2. Informed consent
3. One or two peripheral IVs
4. Foley catheter
   a. In the patient's private room or pre-op area for awake patients
   b. In the angio suite, after induction of anesthesia, for asleep patients
5. NPO after midnight or 6 h prior to the procedure except for medications.
6. Make sure that all devices that may be needed are available in the angio suite prior to the procedure.
7. Premedication:
   a. Dual antiplatelet therapy. Necessary for any stenting case, and an option for other interventions such as intracranial aneurysm coiling and liquid embolic procedures. See below (*Antiplatelet therapy*) for dosing.
   b. Protection against nephrotoxicity for patients with renal insufficiency (creatinine $\geq$1.5 mg/dL):
      i. PO hydration (water, 500 mL prior to the procedure and 2,000 mL after the procedure)
      ii. IV hydration with 0.9% sodium chloride.[5]
      iii. Acetylcysteine 600 mg (3 mL) PO BID on the day before and the day of the procedure.[6]
   c. Protection against anaphylaxis for patients with history of contrast allergy:
      i. Prednisone 50 mg PO (or hydrocortisone 200 mg IV) 13, 7, and 1 h prior to contrast injection.
      ii. Diphenhydramine (Benadryl®) 50 mg IV, IM or PO 1 h prior to contrast injection.
         1. Steroids should be given at least 6 h prior to the procedure; administration less than 3 h prior to the procedure does not reduce the risk of an adverse reaction.[7]
8. Make sure that all devices that may be needed are available in the angio suite prior to the procedure.

4.3.   Awake or Asleep?

Some operators prefer to use general anesthesia for most neurointerventional cases whereas others prefer to do them with the patient awake. Each approach has advantages and disadvantages. General anesthesia eliminates procedural discomfort, which can be substantial during some procedures, such as liquid embolic embolization and intracranial angioplasty. It also helps patients endure lengthy procedures, keeps them still for precise intracranial maneuvering, and simplifies the procedure for the operators somewhat, eliminating the need for constant coaching and neurological assessment of an awake patient. General anesthesia makes it possible to pause respirations intermittently, to obtain highly precise angiograms and roadmaps. However, general anesthesia makes it difficult to detect neurological changes in the patient, although electroencephalography and monitoring of somatosensory and/or motor evoked potentials can help remedy this. On the other hand, physiological monitoring during general anesthesia can cause crowding of the angio suite during procedures, and the reliability of monitoring is less than certain.

Doing neurointerventional procedures awake eliminates the risks associated with general anesthesia, permits constant monitoring of the patient's neurological status, and reduces procedure time and room turnover time. Occasional patients simply cannot tolerate general anesthesia, most often because of cardiac or pulmonary disease. Shepherding an awake patient through a complex intracranial intervention, however, takes patience and skill on the part of the operator, and the judicious use of sedation and analgesia. Whatever the institutional practice is at any given center, it behooves the operator – and particularly those in training – to do cases awake occasionally to maintain the skills and comfort level necessary to do awake cases.

Awake

1. Obtain IV access and a Foley catheter placement before the patient is brought to the angio suite.
2. An abbreviated neurological exam is rehearsed with the patient prior to draping (e.g., patient is asked to say "Methodist Episcopal," show their teeth and gums, wiggle their toes, and squeeze a rubber duckie (Fig. 4.1) with the hand contralateral to the side being treated).
3. Throughout the case, the patient is reminded to stay completely still. The patient's head can be lightly taped to the head holder with a piece of plastic tape across the forehead, to remind him or her to stay still. Place a piece of non-adherent Telfa™ dressing (Kendall/Covidien, Mansfield, MA) between the tape and the forehead to ensure that the skin is not injured.
4. Warn the patient prior to contrast injections or potentially uncomfortable catheter movements so there are no surprises.
5. Check on the patient with gentle questions and reminders constantly throughout the procedure.
6. Keep sedation and analgesia to a minimum to facilitate the patient's full cooperation.

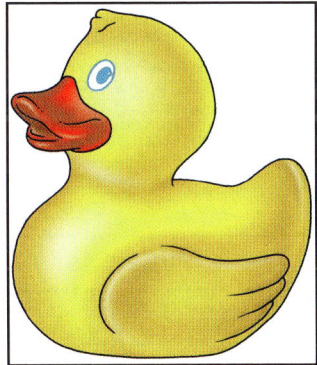

Fig. 4.1 Rubber duckie. Other squeaky toys may be substituted if a duck is not available.

Options for sedation:
    i.   Midazolam (Versed®) 1–2 mg IV for sedation; lasts approximately 2 h
   ii.   Fentanyl (Sublimaze®) 25–50 μg IV for analgesia; lasts 20–30 min

Asleep

1. Patient is placed under general anesthesia on the angiography table.
    a.   Endotracheal anesthesia is most commonly used. Laryngeal mask anesthesia is also feasible, although the patient cannot be chemically paralyzed, and will move with respiration.
    b.   If arterial blood pressure monitoring is needed during induction (e.g., when intubating patients with a ruptured aneurysm), then several options exist:
        i.   Radial arterial line (SAH patients usually arrive in the angio suite with an A-line)
       ii.   Femoral artery sheath. The sheath may be placed prior to induction and used to transduce blood pressure. A femoral artery sheath is less uncomfortable than a radial A-line.
2. Strict attention to blood pressure is important during induction.
3. If neurophysiological monitoring is used, baseline evoked potentials are obtained prior to the intervention. Depending on the anatomic location of the lesion, electroencephalography or monitoring of somatosensory, motor, visual or auditory evoked potentials may be useful. The authors of this handbook routinely use monitoring for procedures involving the spinal cord.
4. The anesthesiologist is asked to report any abrupt changes in blood pressure or heart rate during the case, which can indicate intracranial haemorrhage.
5. Following anesthesia, the patient's neurological status is assessed.

4.4.   Contrast Agents

1. For most cases: Iohexol (Omnipaque®, GE Healthcare, Princeton, NJ) 240 mg I/mL. Patients with normal renal function can tolerate as much as 400–800 mL of Omnipaque®, 300 mg I/mL without adverse effects.[8]
2. For patients with renal insufficiency: Iodixanol (Visipaque™, GE Healthcare, Princeton, NJ) 270 mg I/mL.
3. See Chap. 2 for more detail about contrast agents, renal insufficiency, and iodinated contrast agent anaphylaxis.

4.5.   Vascular Access

    All neurointerventional procedures consist of 1) an access phase and 2) an intervention phase. The access phase usually consists of placement of a guide catheter in the carotid or vertebral artery via the femoral artery.
1. The patient is placed on the angiography table.
2. Dorsalis paedis and posterior tibialis pulses are assessed and marked.
3. The right and left groins are clipped, prepped, and draped.
    a.   Clipping is preferred to shaving since it creates less skin irritation.[9]
    b.   Both groins are always prepped in case femoral artery access cannot be obtained on one side, or if a second sheath needs to be inserted.
    c.   For sensitive patients, EMLA® (AstraZeneca, Wilmington, DE), a topical anesthetic cream, is applied over the expected puncture site 30 min prior to the procedure, and an occlusive dressing is placed.
4. The PA C-arm is brought into position to enable fluoroscopy of the femoral artery, if needed for puncture of the vessel.
5. Using Seldinger technique (see Chap 2).

6. A sheath is placed in the femoral artery.
   a. The size of the sheath depends on the intervention. For most intracranial cases, a 6F is suitable. A 7F sheath has the advantage of being large enough to accommodate a 6F guide catheter and still permit A-line transduction through the sheath.
   b. Sheaths are available in various lengths, most commonly 10 or 25 cm. The 25-cm version has the advantage that it bypasses any tortuosity in the iliac arteries. Having the distal end of the sheath in the aorta prevents any danger of injuring the iliac artery during catheter introduction through the sheath.
   c. Use a 0.038 J-tip wires ("Safety wires") for sheath placement.
7. If the use of a femoral artery closure device is planned, do a femoral artery angiogram at the beginning of the case right after insertion of the sheath, because the C-arm is positioned over the groin.
8. If needed, do a diagnostic angiogram prior to the intervention.
   Prior to the intervention, do intracranial PA and lateral angiograms, to serve as a baseline for later comparison, to check for the possibility of thromboembolism or haemorrhage in the intracranial circulation during or after the procedure.
9. Obtain angiographic images of the access vessel (carotid or vertebral artery). Biplane imaging is best.
10. Guide catheter selection. The authors prefer to use one of four guide catheters, depending on the situation:
    a. **6F 0.053 in. Neuron**™ Intracranial Access System (Penumbra, Inc., San Leandro, CA).
       i. Distal end: 5F OD, 3.9F ID. Comes in straight and angled shapes.
       ii. Advantages: Extremely soft and flexible; able to be positioned within the very distal intracranial ICA or vertebral artery.
       iii. Disadvantages: Less stable than other catheters, very slippery. Can be pushed out of the access vessel if the catheter is not in a distal-enough position. Only the distal tip is radio-opaque; the radiolucent shaft can be difficult to see on fluoroscopy. Narrow lumen makes for limited-quality angiograms with a microcatheter in position.
       iv. Technique and tips:
          1. Usually must be exchanged into position.
          2. Two lengths are available: 105 cm (for most patients) and 115 cm (for patients >6 ft in height).
          3. Two distal flexible zone lengths are available: 6 cm (for most cases) and 12 cm (for cases in which a very tortuous ICA or vertebral artery must be traversed, e.g., a cervical ICA with a 360° loop).
          4. A standard hydrophilic wire is used for initial positioning of the Neuron™.
          5. Coaxial microcatheter technique for final positioning of the Neuron™ 0.053 catheter:
             Advance a microcatheter over a microwire through the Neuron™ into the target vessel distal to the desired final position of the guide catheter. Then advance the Neuron™ over the microcatheter to its final position. A more substantial microcatheter such as a Renegade® (Stryker Neurovascular, Fremont, CA) or Prowler® Plus (Codman Neurovascular, Raynham, MA) with a substantial 0.016 in. guidewire can provide good support to facilitate distal placement of the Neuron™.
          6. The more distal the tip, the more stable the Neuron will be; e.g., position the tip in the horizontal segment of the petrous ICA or the V4 segment of the vertebral artery for maximum stability. Optimal positioning is distal to at least two 90° turns in the vessel to provide sufficient support for the coaxial placement of a microcatheter.
          7. Guide catheter angiograms may be of marginal quality when a microcatheter is inside the guide catheter, because of the relatively narrow lumen. Injection of 100% contrast in a 3 mL syringe, rather than a 10 mL syringe, will produce better angiograms.
          8. The Neuron™ 053 will accept most microcatheters, but it may be difficult to inject contrast around 18-system microcatheters

like the Renegade® (Stryker Neurovascular, Fremont, CA) or Prowler® Plus (Codman Neurovascular, Raynham, MA).

9. *Warning*: When the Neuron™ is in its final intracranial position, use caution when flushing or injecting contrast. Use smaller volumes and lower pressures since the pressure is transmitted directly to the intracranial vessels. This can be particularly dangerous if there is an aneurysm nearby the catheter tip. *Avoid using a power-injector while a micro-catheter is in the Neuron™*

b. **6F 0.70 in. Neuron**™ Intracranial Access System (Penumbra, Inc., San Leandro, CA).
   i. Distal end: 6F OD, 0.70 in. (~5.4F) ID. Comes in straight and angled shapes.
   ii. Advantages: Large lumen, able to accommodate two microcatheters (e.g., useful for balloon-remodeling). Permits good angiograms with a microcatheter in position.
   iii. Disadvantage: Relatively stiff, less navigable than the smaller Neuron. Straight tip means it usually has to be exchanged into position.
   iv. Technique and tips:
       1. Usually must be exchanged into position.
       2. Two distal flexible zone lengths are available: 6 and 8 cm.
       3. Can be advanced into a distal position by placing a Distal Access Catheter (DAC®, Concentric Medical, Mountain View, CA), inside the Neuron, which eliminates the large step-off between the tip of the Neuron and the guide wire.

c. **Guider Softip**™ XF guide catheter (Stryker Neurovascular, Fremont, CA):
   i. Advantages: Soft, atraumatic tip. Minimizes risk of vasospasm and dissection in narrow, tortuous vessels. Angled tip allows it to be navigated into position primarily, without an exchange.
   ii. Disadvantages: Relatively flimsy, prone to fall into the arch when the vasculature is tortuous.

d. **Envoy**® (Codman Neurovascular, Raynham, MA):
   i. Advantages: Relatively rigid, provides a good platform in tortuous vessels, large internal lumen. Nice for working in the external carotid artery. Angled tip allows it to be navigated primarily.
   ii. Disadvantages: Stiff, sharp-edged tip.

11. Alternative guide catheters:
a. **6 Fr 90 cm Cook Shuttle**® (Cook, Inc., Bloomington, IN):
   i. Very large, stable platform.
   ii. Technique:
       1. Requires either an 8F sheath, or an exchange for a smaller sheath (e.g., for carotid stent cases). If a smaller sheath (e.g. 5F sheath) is placed first, a diagnostic catheter is then placed in the access artery. The diagnostic catheter is then exchanged over an exchange-length hydrophilic wire for the Cook Shuttle®, with the obturator still in place. When the Cook is ~2 cm proximal to the desired final position, the obturator is removed and several mL of blood are allowed to spill backwards out of the sheath, to remove any bubbles or clot. *Note: the obturator is not radio-opaque*.
       2. Tip: if the Cook winds up in the aortic arch, access to the great vessels can be obtained by advancing a hydrophilic wire and a 125 cm 5F Vitek catheter within the Cook. The Vitek has a shape similar to a Simmons 2 catheter, and can be used to navigate the Cook back into the carotid or subclavian arteries.

b. **Merci**® **Balloon Guide catheter** (Concentric Medical, Mountain View, CA)
   i. Capable of temporarily occluding flow in the carotid or vertebral artery during thrombectomy procedures using the Merci® Retrieval system or the Solitaire™ stent.
       1. Available in 7, 8 and 9F sizes; the 7F is recommended for a small vertebral artery and the 9F is for a large carotid artery.
       2. It is packaged with an obturator for smooth vessel access. The proximal end of the guide catheter includes a straight hub for device insertion and an angled hub for distal balloon inflation.

3. The compliant silicone balloon at the distal end of the guide catheter inflates to a 10 mm diameter with the maximum inflation volume of 0.8 mL is used. A 3 mL syringe, prepared with 50% contrast in saline, is used for balloon inflation.
4. Caution: This guide catheter is flimsy and is prone to fall into the aortic arch when significant counter-force is generated by the microcatheter.

c. **Neuron™ MAX 088 Large Lumen Catheter** (Penumbra, Inc., San Leandro, CA)
   i. Large catheter, available either as a long sheath (for use like the Cook Shuttle) or a guide catheter. Four cm distal tip is more flexible than the Cook.
   ii. Available in 80 and 90 cm lengths.
   iii. Technique:
       1. Obtain access to the target vessel (carotid or vertebral artery) with a diagnostic catheter first, then exchange the MAX 088 into position over an exchange-length hydrophilic wire.
       2. The MAX 088 comes with an inner dilator. A larger Neuron Select catheter can also be used within it.

d. **ReFlex™** (Reverse Medical Corporation, Irvine, CA)
   i. 2 sizes are available, 0.58 in. and 0.72 in.
   ii. Very similar to the Neuron™ Intracranial Access System.

e. **Berenstein Large Lumen Balloon Guide Catheter** (Boston Scientific, Natick, MA)
   i. Advantages: 11.5 mm diameter balloon allows for proximal flow control, to prevent distal migration of embolic agent in high flow states.
   ii. Disadvantages: Relatively small lumen (despite it's name). Short length (80 cm) limits the use to short patients and a very proximal catheter position.

f. **Pinnacle® Destination®** (Terumo Medical, Somerset, NJ)
   i. Advantages: Designed as a long sheath to also act as a guide catheter. Inner dilator provides a smooth transition to guidewire as it is advanced. Relatively rigid to provides a very stable platform. Large lumen. An inner guide catheter can be placed to provide added stability ("Tower of Power").
   ii. Disadvantages: Rigid sheath should not be placed too distally or in small vessels to prevent vessel injury. Somewhat less rigid and less stable than other systems.

g. **6F Northstar® Lumax® Flex Catheter** (Cook, Inc., Bloomington, IN):
   i. Device contour consists of a smooth, tapered transition between the guidewire, inner dilator, and catheter, which minimizes trauma to vessel walls. The dilator also allows introduction without the use of a groin sheath. Relatively rigid, providing a stable platform.
   ii. Disadvantages:
       1. Relatively stiff.
       2. Extremely lubricious (may cause the catheter to slide out of vessels).

12. Guide catheter size:
   a. The guide catheter should be 90 cm long (and not longer) for use with the Wingspan stent system.
   b. 6F for most cases.
   c. 5F if the vessel caliber is small and collateral circulation is limited:
       i. e.g., for use in a small vertebral artery when the contralateral vessel is hypoplastic.
       ii. Disadvantage: Angiograms with a microcatheter or balloon in place are more difficult to obtain because of limited space within the guide catheter.

13. Straight or angled?
   a. Straight guide catheter is useful in relatively straight vessels, or in situations where the guide catheter is gently navigated through a convoluted vessel:
       i. Usually requires exchanging (see below).
       ii. Preferred for the vertebral artery.
   b. Angled guide catheter is useful when the final position of the catheter tip is in a vessel curve:
   c. Angled catheters are easier to navigate through the aortic arch than straight catheters.

14. Guide catheter placement technique:
    a. The guide catheter is typically placed in the ICA or vertebral artery only after the heparinization is therapeutic (usually 5 min or more after the IV loading dose is given).
    b. Exchange method:
        i. Usually necessary for the Neuron™ guide catheters and other straight guide catheters, because the absence of an angle at the tip make it difficult to navigate the catheter primarily. It is also useful in patients with tortuous anatomy, atherosclerosis, or fibromuscular dysplasia. This technique minimizes risk of injury to the carotid or vertebral artery, particularly at the vessel origin.
        ii. Guide a 5F diagnostic catheter into the CCA or vertebral artery over an exchange-length (300 cm) 0.035 in. or 0.038 in. hydrophilic wire.
        iii. The tip of the hydrophilic wire is advanced into a distal branch of the ECA or the distal extracranial vertebral artery (usually the first 90° turn of the vessel at C2) using road mapping technique.
        iv. The diagnostic catheter is then gently removed while the tip of the hydrophilic wire is continuously visualized on fluoroscopy.
        v. The hydrophilic wire is wiped down with a dripping-wet Telfa™ (Kendall/Covidien, Mansfield, MA) sponge.
            1. Avoid wiping hydrophilic wires with dry cotton sponges. It leaves numerous thrombogenic cotton fibers on the wire.
        vi. The guide catheter is advanced over the wire while continuously visualizing the tip of the wire.
    c. Direct navigation method:
        i. Possible in patients with nontortuous, nonatherosclerotic vessels.
        ii. Navigate an angled guide catheter gently into the carotid or vertebral artery over a 0.035 or 0.038 in. hydrophilic wire.
15. Guide catheter position
    a. Carotid artery
        i. Using a roadmap, advance the guide catheter over a hydrophilic wire into the ICA as distally as possible. A "high position" of the guide catheter will maximize the stability of the guide and improves control over the microcatheter and microwire. In a non-tortuous, healthy carotid system, the authors of this handbook prefer to position the tip of the guide catheter in the vertical segment of the petrous ICA. In a cervical ICA with a significant curve in the vessel, the guide can be adequately positioned immediately proximal to the curve. Moderate curves in the vessel can be straightened out by guiding a relatively stiff hydrophilic wire (e.g., an 0.038 in. wire) through the affected segment, followed by the catheter, but this may compromise flow in the vessel due to kinking or spasm.
    b. Vertebral artery
        i. Using a roadmap, position the guide catheter in the distal extracranial vertebral artery, usually at the first curve (at C2).
    c. Once the guide catheter is in position, do a gentle injection of contrast through the guide catheter under fluoroscopy, to examine the configuration of the vessel around the tip and to check for the presence of vasospasm or vessel dissection around the tip. If catheter tip-induced vasospasm is present and flow-limiting, withdrawal of the catheter tip by several millimeters is often sufficient to restore flow.
16. Keep the tip of the guide catheter in view on one or both biplane fluoroscopic views for the duration of the case. Correct displacement of the guide catheter tip, and, if the catheter appears to unstable, consider replacement with a more stable guide catheter system.
17. Guide catheter care and maintenance
    a. Guide catheter irrigation
        i. Continuous irrigation of the guide with heparinized saline (10,000 units of heparin per liter of saline) is important.
        ii. Meticulous attention to the RHV and the guide catheter is necessary throughout the procedure is necessary to identify thrombus or bubbles, should they appear.
    b. Tips to minimize or treat guide catheter-induced vasospasm:
        i. Withdraw the catheter into a lower segment of the vessel when significant catheter-induced vasospasm appears.
        ii. Keep the catheter tip away from kinks and bends in the vessel if possible.

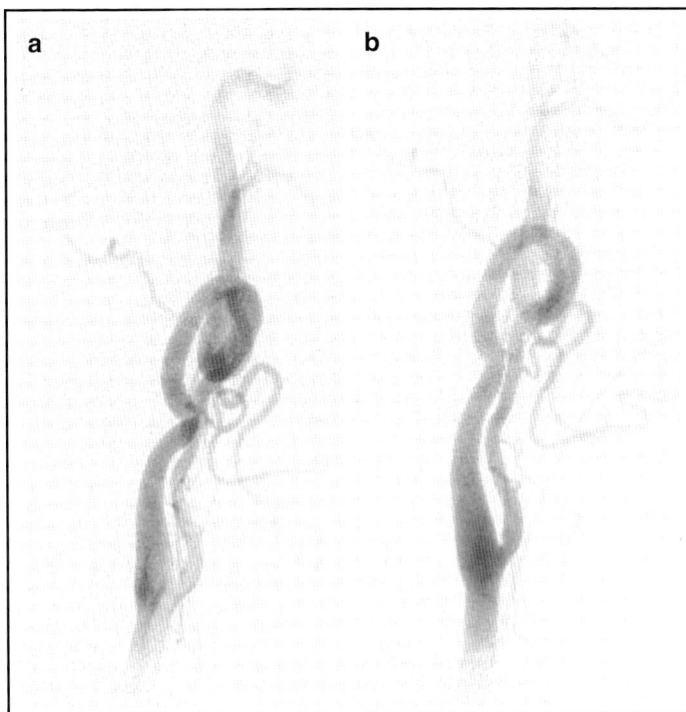

Fig. 4.2 Head tilt technique. Lateral angiogram of left carotid system in a neutral position (*left*) and with the head tilted toward the opposite shoulder (*right*).

       1. A curvaceous carotid or proximal vertebral artery can some-
          times be straightened out by tilting the patient's head
          toward the opposite shoulder (Fig. 4.2).
    iii. Selective injection of IA nitroglycerin (30 µg per injection)
       1. This can also help distinguish vasospasm from vessel dis-
          section, if a dissection is suspected
    iv. Use Visipaque™ (GE Healthcare, Princeton, NJ) contrast instead
       of Omnipaque; according to the manufacturer, this contrast mate-
       rial is less spasmogenic than Omnipaque®.
    v. Use a soft-tipped guide catheter.
    vi. Use a guide catheter with an inner obturator (e.g., Northstar®
       Lumax® Flex Catheter.Cook, Inc., Bloomington, IN).

Tips for Difficult Access Cases

1. Femoral artery is not accessible.
   a. Use an alternative route (see below)
2. Aortic arch or great vessels are tortuous
   a. Use the ECA to anchor the wire.
   b. During the initial placement of the diagnostic catheter in the CCA, use a
      0.035-in. hydrophilic wire to advance the diagnostic catheter into a
      branch of the ECA.

      c. Then remove the wire and replace it with a stiffer exchange-length wire, such as a 0.038-in. hydrophilic wire or an Amplatz stiff wire.

      d. Then exchange the diagnostic catheter for the 90-cm sheath.

      e. This technique works well in the left CCA using a Simmons 2 catheter as the diagnostic catheter.

3. "Tower of power" technique to add stability to the 90-cm sheath:

      a. Advance a 6F guide catheter, e.g., 6F Envoy (Codman Neurovascular, Raynham, MA), inside of an 6F 90-cm sheath.

      b. Larger diameter 90-cm sheath (e.g., 7 or 8F) will add stability.

      c. Use an intermediate catheter (e.g. DAC®, Stryker Neurovascular, Fremont, CA) inside a guide catheter inside a 90 cm sheath to create the ultimate "Tower of power".

4. Buddy wire technique.

      a. Use a larger diameter 90-cm sheath (e.g., 8F sheath) and a 0.014 or 0.018-in. wire anchored into the subclavian artery or a branch of the ECA.

Alternative Access Routes

If the femoral artery cannot be accessed (e.g., because of high grade iliac or femoral artery stenosis or occlusion, innominate or subclavian artery tortuosity, patients unable to tolerate laying flat, morbid obesity, or aortic disease) several other options exist. The arm approach is nicely suited for access to the ipsilateral vertebral artery. For access to the great vessels from the arm, use a 5F Simmons 2 catheter to access the target vessel (see Fig. 2.7), then exchange a guide catheter into position over an exchange-length 0.035 in. or 0.038 in. hydrophilic wire. See Chap. 2 for further details about techniques.

1. Brachial artery.[10]

      a. Advantages:

          i. Large enough for 6 and 7F sheaths.

         ii. Hand ischemia is usually not a threat.

        iii. Large enough to use a closure device.

             1. Off-label use of the Perclose® Pro-glide™ (Abbott Vascular, Abbott Park, IL, Inc.) in the brachial artery is feasible.

      b. Disadvantages:

          i. Median nerve injury is a potential complication, because of the proximity of the nerve to the brachial artery.

2. Radial artery.[11]

      a. Advantages:

          i. Easier to get haemostasis after the sheath is removed, compared to the brachial artery approach.

         ii. Less potential for nerve injury.

      b. Disadavantages:

          i. Smaller vessel compared to the brachial artery. Usually limited to a 5F sheath.[12,13]

         ii. Has the potential for hand ischemia.

        iii. Radial artery cocktail is usually necessary (see Chap. 2).

3. Axillary artery.

      a. An option,[14] but the axillary artery approach is generally obsolete presently.

4. Carotid artery.

      a. Cut-down and direct puncture of the common carotid artery.[15]

      b. Direct percutaneous puncture can be done for embolization procedures with few complications.[16]

      c. Stent-assisted coiling was done with a direct carotid puncture and closed successfully with the Angio-Seal™ closure device(St. Jude Medical, Minnetonka, MN).[17]

4.6.   Antithrombotic Therapy During Neurointerventional Procedures

The overall risk of thromboembolic complications during neurointerventional procedures is significant. Aneurysm coiling, for example, carries a 2–8% risk of symptomatic thromboembolic complications.[18-21] Strategies for antithrombotic medication management vary widely. Anticoagulation with heparin, to some degree or another, is standard for most procedures. Dual antiplatelet therapy is standard for all stenting procedures. Some operators also advocate routine antiplatelet therapy (e.g., aspirin) for many neurointerventional procedures, such as aneurysm coiling.

Anticoagulation

1. Heparin for flushes and irrigation.
   a. Use heparinized saline 10,000 units of heparin per liter of saline, (except in paediatric patients < 6 years of age, then use 1,000 units of heparin per liter of saline)
2. Systemic anticoagulation:
   a. Loading dose of IV heparin (5,000 units or 70 units/kg) prior to placement of the guide catheter in the access vessel. Additional heparin is given during the procedure, if necessary, 1,000 units IV every hour.
   b. Monitoring of activated clotting time (ACT): 5 min after giving IV heparin, draw a 5 mL specimen of blood for an activated clotting time (ACT) from the sheath. The target ACT range is 250–300 s. If the first ACT is not within the target range, additional heparin may be given and the ACT resent. The guide catheter is placed in the ICA or vertebral artery only after the heparinization is therapeutic (usually 5 min or more after the IV loading dose is given, or after the ACT has been found to be in the target range). Additional doses of heparin (1,000 units/h) may be given for longer cases.
      i. Most literature about ACT in neurointervention comes from carotid stenting. One CAS study reported an optimal range of ACT to be 250–299 s.[22] ACT was also reported to be inversely correlated with amount of debris found during CAS.[23]
   c. *ACT monitoring is a neurointerventional tradition with little scientific foundation, and some operators do not routinely check the ACT.*
3. Alternatives to heparin
   a. Argatroban (Novastan®, Abbott, North Chicago, IL) is an antithrombotic suitable for use in patients with heparin induced thrombocytopaenia.[24,25] Coronary interventional doses of 350 µg/kg bolus over 3–5 min have been used for neurointerventional procedures, and adequacy of antithrombotic effect is monitored by ACT values around 250–300 s. A continuous drip of 10–25 µg/kg/ min can be used for longer procedures, or, alternatively, 150 µg/kg boluses at hourly intervals if the ACT falls below 250. The saline infusions through the catheter or sheath lumen must obviously not contain any heparin. Argatroban has no specific antidote, and the only course of action to employ in the case of active bleeding is to stop the infusion and wait for the effect to wear off. Therefore this agent must be used with caution.
   b. Bivalirudin (Angiomax™, The Medicines Company, Cambridge, MA) is a synthetic direct thrombin inhibitor that is popular in interventional cardiology and has been used in neuro-endovascular procedures in select cases.[26] It can also be used in patients who cannot tolerate heparin, as in cases of heparin-induced thrombocytopaenia.[27] However, like argatroban, there is no rapid reversal agent for bivalirudin, and its routine use in patients for intracranial procedures is not recommended.
   c. Other designer antithrombotics that can be used in patients with heparin contra-indications include lepirudin and danaparoid.[28]
   In some hospitals these unusual antithrombotic medications may have restrictions on their use and may require a Haematology consult in order to obtain the drug from the pharmacy.

Antiplatelet Therapy

Thrombosis in the arterial system is of the platelet-rich "white clot" variety; therefore, antiplatelet therapy during neurointerventional procedures makes sense. Dual antiplatelet therapy helps prevent stent thrombosis in patient undergoing endovascular stenting procedures,[29] and treatment with aspirin and clopidogrel is commonly used for any patient undergoing a neurointerventional stenting procedure. Recent evidence suggests that oral antiplatelet therapy may reduce thromboembolic complications in patients undergoing coiling of intracranial aneurysms,[30–33] although it may carry an increased risk of haemorrhage.[34]

1. Aspirin
   Standard loading and maintenance dose: 325 mg PO QD. Available as a suppository.
2. Clopidogrel (Plavix®, Sanofi-Aventis, Bridgewater, NJ)
   Standard loading dose: 300 or 600 mg, followed by 75 mg QD.[35–38]
3. Dual antiplatelet therapy
   a. Aspirin 325-mg PO QD for ≥3 days prior to the procedure *and*
   b. Clopidogrel 75-mg PO QD for ≥3 days prior to the procedure.[39]
   Or
   c. Aspirin 325-mg PO QD for ≥3 days prior to the procedure *and*
   d. Ticlopidine (Ticlid® Lilly, Indianapolis, IN) for ≥3 days prior to the procedure.[40]
      1. Adverse reactions include rash, gastrointestinal side effects, neutropaenia (2.4%), thrombocytopaenia, aplastic anemia, and thrombotic thrombocytopaenic purpura.[41]
      2. Neutropaenia occurs in 2.4% of patients and may appear within a few days.
         i. Monitoring for neutropaenia: CBC with absolute neutrophil count and peripheral smear should be done prior to initiation of therapy and every 2 weeks through the third month of therapy
   e. Alternatively, a loading dose of Aspirin 325 mg PO and clopidogrel 600 mg PO can be given the day before or at least 5 h before the procedure.
4. Glycoprotein IIB/IIIA inhibitors.
   a. Treatment with IV or IA GP IIB/IIIA inhibitors are useful in two situations:
      i. Rapid protection against platelet aggregation when a stent must be used and the patient has not been pretreated with dual antiplatelet drugs.
      ii. Treatment of thromboembolic complications of endovascular procedures.[42–44]
   b. Abciximab (ReoPro® Merck & Co., Whitehouse Station, NJ)
      i. Dose: 0.25 mg/kg IV rapid bolus followed by 125 μg kg/min infusion (to a maximum of 10 mg/min) for 12 h.
      ii. *Caution: Partial dosing of Abciximab should be avoided, unless point of care testing confirms adequate receptor blockade.*[45] The authors recommend the use of a full loading dose followed by IV infusion for 12 h, unless the threat of haemorrhagic complications is prohibitive. The authors of this handbook have personally witnessed paradoxical drug-induced platelet activation effect with lower levels of platelet inhibition with abciximab, and a corresponding increase in thrombotic complications.
      iii. The effect of Abciximab can be reversed, if needed, with platelet transfusion. The drug is a monoclonal antibody, with high affinity to the GP IIB/IIIA receptor on platelets.
   c. Eptifibitide (Integrilin® Lilly, Indianapolis, IN)
      i. Dose: 180 μg/kg IV bolus.[42]
      Coronary stenting regimen: 180 μg/kg IV bolus, then a second 180 μg/kg IV bolus 10 min after the first bolus, followed by 2 μg/kg infusion for 12 h.[46]
      ii. Eptifibitide cannot be reversed with platelet transfusions. It is a small-molecule drug with low affinity for the GP IIB/IIIA receptor.

Clopidogrel Resistance and Platelet Function Testing

Clopidogrel is a thienopyridine antiplatelet agent. It acts by irreversibly inhibiting the platelet surface $P2Y_{12}$ adenosine diphosphate (ADP) receptor. Blockade of the $P2Y_{12}$ receptor prevents aggregation of platelets and cross-linking by fibrin by preventing activation of the GP IIb/IIIa receptor.[47] Clopidogrel is a prodrug; after absorption by the duodenum, it is metabolized by the cytochrome P450 system in the liver to the active metabolite, R-130964. Some 5–10% of ingested clopidogrel is converted to the active metabolite.[48] Polymorphisms of at least two genes involved with clopidogrel have been found to influence either the bioavailability of the drug or it's effect on platelets. Polymorphisms in the ABCB1 gene, which codes for a glycoprotein involved with the passage of clopidogrel across the duodenal wall, have been found to influence the bioavailability of clopidogrel.[49,50] The CYP2C19 gene codes for a hepatic esterase responsible for converting clopidogrel to the active metabolite; >33 different alleles of the CYP2C19 gene have been identified. Each allele is defined by variations in the DNA sequence, which may result in functional differences in the CYP2C19 enzyme.[51] The CYP2C19*1 allele is common in people of European origin and the CYP2C19*2 allele is present in 30%, 15% and 17% of Asian, Caucasian, and black patients, respectively.[52] Carriers of CYP2C19*2 have reduced effectiveness of clopidogrel[53,54] and have an elevated risk of cardiovascular events and coronary stent thrombosis.[55] Because of these findings the FDA issued a safety warning in May, 2009 that clopidogrel has reduced effectiveness in patients who are poor metabolizers of the drug.[52,56] Aside from genetic tendencies, other causes of poor responsiveness to clopidogrel include noncompliance, drug interactions,[57] inadequate absorption,[58] body mass index,[37,59] and increased platelet activity related to an acute thrombotic event.[60] Platelet activation is a significant threat in neurointervention, contributing to overall rates of acute thromboembolic events up to 8%.[18,21,61,62]

Several techniques are available for so-called point-of-care detection of poor responsiveness to antiplatelet therapy.[63] Among the most commonly used are the VerifyNow™ Rapid Platelet Function Assay (Accumetrics, San Diego, CA), Innovance® Platelet Function Analyzer (Siemens Healthcare Diagnostics, Inc., Deerfield, IL) and the Multiplate® Multiple electrode aggregometry device (Dynabyte Medical, Munich).[63] Point-of-care testing is meant to identify patients who are at higher risk of thromboembolic complications during percutaneous interventional procedures. Point-of-care testing has become *de rigueur* in some cardiac cath labs and neuroangio suites, but the vast majority of published experience with point-of-care testing has been from cardiology.[64,65]

Several studies of point-of-care platelet function testing in neurointerventional procedures have been published. In a series of 50 patients undergoing cerebrovascular stenting procedures, 28% were classified as clopidogrel nonresponders, and there was a significant correlation between clopidogrel nonresponse (as assessed by the Multiplate® device) and procedural adverse events.[66] In another study of 76 patients undergoing cerebrovascular stenting procedures, clopidogrel resistance (as assessed by the VerifyNow™ assay) was reported in 51.9%.[67] A study of 186 aneurysm coiling patients found that diminished clopidogrel responsiveness (by VerifyNow™) correlated with thromboembolic events.[62] Another study of 216 neurointerventional patients found that inadequate platelet inhibition (by VerifyNow™) was found in 13% of patients on aspirin and 66% of patients on clopidogrel.[68] Yet another study of 106 neurointerventional patients found that 42.9% were poor responders to clopidogrel (by VerifyNow™), and that all cases of intraprocedural thrombosis occurred in the poor-response group.[37]

Should Routine Platelet Function Testing Be Done Prior to Neurointerventional Procedures?

Point-of-care platelet function testing is controversial. In the medical management of ischemic stroke, recent editorials have argued for and against platelet function testing.[69–71] A number of publications have concluded that routine platelet function testing is not justified.[51,63] No standards, guidelines, or randomized trial data exist for the use of platelet function testing for neurointervential procedures, yet some operators use it routinely while others do not. This practice remains an option until more definitive data on the question is available.

1. *Arguments in favour of routine point-of-care platelet function testing*:
   a. A significant percentage of patients (28–66%) are poor responders to clopidogrel.[37,66–68]
   b. Acute thrombosis due to platelet activation is a significant source of morbidity.
   c. Point-of-care testing is relatively easy and feasible.
   d. Identification of poor responders serves to heighten awareness of the possibility of acute thrombosis during neurointerventional procedures.
   e. A contingency plan may be activated for these patients; e.g., an additional antiplatelet drug, such as abciximab, can be made available for quick use should a thromboembolic complication occur.

f. Alternative treatment strategies can be formulated for poor responders (e.g., if stent-assisted coiling was planned, then a balloon remodeling procedure might be done instead, or a patient might have a carotid endarterectomy instead of a stent).

g. Poor responders may be pre-treated with dual antiplatelet therapy for a prolonged period of time, if feasible.

h. Longer periods of treatment with antiplatelet agents (e.g., >7 days) are associated with heightened antiplatelet activity.[68,72]

2. *Arguments against routine point-of-care platelet function testing*:

a. Point-of-care testing is not universally available.

b. There is no consensus on the definition of "poor responsiveness" to antiplatelet medication.[63]

c. Optimal management based on point-of-care testing has not been defined.

d. There is no evidence that management based on point-of-care testing improves outcome.

e. Point-of-care testing techniques vary widely.

f. The results of studies using the VerifyNow device, for instance, cannot be extrapolated to centers were other platelet function tests are used.

g. Other medications with better effectiveness than clopidogrel (possibly, such as prasugril) may gain popularity in neurointervention.

Clopidogrel and Proton Pump Inhibitors

Current American Heart Association guidelines recommend that in order to minimize gastrointestinal complications all patients on dual antiplatelet therapy be prescribed a proton pump inhibitor (PPI).[73] PPIs suppress CYP2C19 activity, and omeprazole (Prilosec®, AstraZeneca, Wilmington, DE) has shown more of this effect than newer PPIs such as pantoprazole (Protonix®, Pfizer, New York, NY).[74] For patients taking omeprazole and clopidogrel, there is a significant increase in residual platelet activity compared to patients taking clopidogrel alone.[75] In 2009, the FDA issued an announcement recommending against the concomitant use of clopidogrel and omeprazole. However, studies of interactions between other PPIs and clopidogrel have been inconsistent. Although a number of retrospective studies have linked concomitant use of PPIs and clopidgrel with an increased risk of cardiovascular adverse events and death,[76,77] other studies have found no evidence of increased risk.[77,78] A recent case-control study of clopidogrel in 2,765 stroke patients found no association between proton pump inhibitors and an increased risk of recurrent stroke.[79] Furthermore, alternatives to PPIs, such as H2 blockers, have not been found to be as beneficial as PPIs in reducing GI bleeding risk with used in combination with aspirin or clopidogral.[80] Therefore, considering the conflicting evidence, it seems reasonable to use PPIs in patients who are on a dual antiplatelet regimen.[51]

4.7.   Air Emboli Prevention

Any air introduced into the arterial system can cause ischemic complications. The surface tension between blood and air can be enough to stop flow in distal branches. The largest component of air, namely nitrogen is poorly soluble in water, so the bubbles can persist long enough to cause permanent ischemia. Meticulous technique is required to ensure there are no bubble in syringes, in the contrast injector and its tubing, and in any heparinized saline flushes.

There were significantly fewer diffusion weighted lesions on MRI in cerebral angiography patients in whom air filters (B.Braun, Meslungen AG, Germany) were installed in the saline infusion lines.[81] These are cheap, and easy to install. One of the authors of this handbook uses an air filtration system, Posidyne® filter (Pall Medical, Port Washington, NY) routinely.

4.8.   Intervention Phase

The intervention phase usually consists of microcatheter access to the lesion, followed by treatment that is specific to the type and location of the lesion. This section will cover general microcatheter selection and techniques.

Devices

1. Microcatheter selection
   a. Microcatheters vary in size and design. All available microcatheters have a hydrophilic coating, which reduces thrombogenicity.[82] Most microcatheters are either fiber-braided or metal coil-braided, which serves to preserve the inner lumen when the catheter is curved, and enhances pushability.
   b. Smaller microcatheters permit better guide catheter angiograms, particularly when smaller guide catheters (e.g., 5F) are employed.
   c. Some situations call for larger and/or stiffer microcatheters.
   d. When the catheter access to the lesion is tenuous because of vascular anatomy, and increased microcatheter stiffness will add stability.
   e. Single-tip versus two-tipped microcatheters. Obviously, two-tipped microcatheters, rather than single-tipped catheters, are necessary for aneurysm coiling. The two tips in microcatheters used in aneurysm coiling are always 3 cm apart – this feature can be used for calibration and measurements.
   f. Preferred microcatheters for most cases:
      i. Excelsior® SL-10 (Stryker, Fremont, CA)
         1. Can be used for 10-system and 18-system coils.
         2. Retains its shape better after steam-shaping than other microcatheters of the same size.[83]
      ii. Echelon™ 10 (ev3, Irvine, CA).
         1. The relatively small proximal outer diameter of 2.1F (versus 2.4F for the Excelsior® SL-10), permits better guide catheter angiograms when a 5F guide catheter is used.
         2. Compatible with Onyx®.
      iii. Ultraflow™ (ev3, Irvine, CA)
         1. Flow directed, very small catheter single-tipped microcatheter.
         2. Useful for NBCA embolization
      iv. Magic® microcatheter (AIT-Balt, Miami, FL).
         1. By far, the most flow-directed microcatheter of them all.
         2. The catheter is only compatible with nBCA.
         3. Comes in 1.8F and 1.2F sizes and also the Olive version, which has an olive-shaped tip and is even more flow-directed.
      v. Marksman™ (ev3, Irvine, CA)
         1. Robust microcatheter, resistant to ovalization.
         2. Useful for Neuroform® EZ (Stryker, Fremont, CA) stent deployment.
         3. Should be soaked in heparinized saline for 10 min prior to use, when possible, to enhance lubricity.
      vi. Excelsior® 1018® (Stryker, Fremont, CA)
         1. Large microcatheter, can accommodate 10- and 18-system coils.
         2. Good for PVA embolization – large inner diameter minimizes risk of clogging.
      vii. Prowler® Select™ Plus (Codman, Raynham, MA)
         Large microcatheter, intended for use with the Enterprise™ Vascular Reconstruction System (Codman, Raynham, MA)
   g. Steerable microcatheters
      As of this writing, no steerable microcatheters are available in the U.S. The Pivot™ (Stryker, Fremont, CA) and the Enzo™ (Micrus Endovascular,

San Jose, CA) steerable microcatheters have both been taken off of the market by their manufacturers. The Plato™ Microcath steerable microcatheter (Scientia Vascular, Reno, NV) is currently available in Europe. See below for steerable microcatheter technique.

2. Microcatheter shape: *Pre-shaped* vs. *straight* vs. *steam-shaped*
   a. A shaped microcatheter can be advantageous in accessing aneurysms that arise from the parent vessel at an acute angle, and in stabilizing the microcatheter during coiling.
   b. Pre-shaped microcatheters retain their shape better than steam-shaped microcatheters.[84] Steam-shaping is reserved for obtaining catheter shapes that are not available in pre-shaped devices.
   Steam shaping technique:
       i. Shape the wire mandrel into the desired shape, with an exaggerated degree of curvature (as the microcatheter will recoil to some degree after steam-shaping).
       ii. Hold over steam for 10 s.
       iii. Cool in sterile water and remove mandrel.
   c. Non-braided (e.g., Tracker and FasTracker) and fiber-braided (e.g., Excelsior®) microcatheters are more likely to retain their shape after steam shaping, than metal coil-braided (e.g., Prowler and Echelon™) microcatheters.[84]

3. Microwires
   a. A variety of microwires are available, with differing properties such as size, softness, visibility on fluoroscopy, shapeability, and steerability, trackability, and torque control.
   b. Preferred microwires for most cases:
       i. Synchro®-14 0.014 in. (Stryker Neurovascular, Fremont, CA)
           1. Very soft, flexible distal tip, good for navigation into small aneurysms or through difficult anatomy.
           2. "Supreme torque control."
       ii. Transend™ EX 0.014 in. Floppy tip (Stryker Neurovascular, Fremont, CA)
           1. Smooth, non-abrasive tip, similar to the Synchro®.
       iii. Transend™ EX 0.014 in. Platinum (Stryker Neurovascular, Fremont, CA)
           1. Superior torque control, compared to other microwires.
           2. Heightened radio-opacity makes the tip easy to see on fluoroscopy.
       iv. Neuroscout™ 14 Steerable Guidewire (Codman Neurovascular, Raynham, MA)
           1. Very, very good torque control.
           2. Tip tends to maintain shape better than other wires.
       v. Headliner™ J-tip 0.012 in. (Terumo Medical Corporation, Somerset, NJ)
           1. J-tip is atraumatic to the vessel walls.
           2. Best suited for uncomplicated vessel anatomy (tends to follow the straightest vessel).

Microcatheter Technique

1. Angiograms are done with the guide catheter in optimal position and working views are selected.
2. The guide catheter must be visible on at least one view for the duration of the case.
3. Find optimal working views for both PA and lateral detectors. Sometimes the orthogonal views can provide critical complementary information. For instance, even if an ideal working view is present on the PA view, don't let the lateral view "go to waste."
4. Using a roadmap, advance the microcatheter over the microwire into position. Grasp the microwire with the palm facing up (Fig. 4.3).
5. Any redundancy (i.e., slack) in the microcatheter should be removed by gently pulling back on the microcatheter to straighten it out.
6. Once the microcatheter tip is positioned at the target, the microwire should be withdrawn and advanced several times for most of the distance between the guide catheter and tip of the microcatheter. This maneuver helps to straighten out any

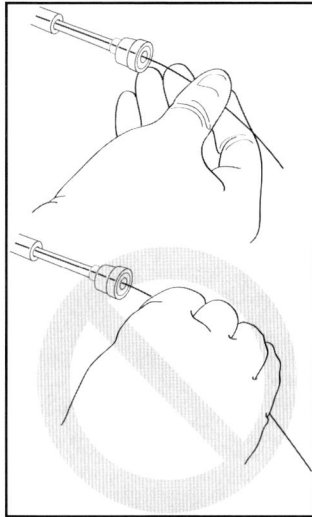

Fig. 4.3 Proper microwire technique. Grasp the microwire with your palm facing up (*top*). This permits fine finger control of the microwire; with the palm facing down (*below*), operating the microwire becomes more of a wrist action than a fine motion.

remaining redundancy in the microcatheter, eliminating "potential energy" in the microcatheter that may cause it to leap forward unexpectedly.

7. When guide catheter angiograms are done, the RHV should be tightened around the microcatheter, securing it to prevent the microcatheter from being carried forward by the contrast as it is injected.

8. A 3 mL syringe should be used for guide catheter angiograms when a microcatheter is within the 6F 0.053 in. Neuron™. A 3 mL syringe will provide better results than a 10 mL syringe.

Steerable Microcatheter Technique

1. Although no steerable microcatheter is currently commercially available in the U.S., the Plato™ Microcath steerable microcatheter (Scientia Vascular, Reno, NV) is CE mark approved and currently available in Europe. Steerable microcatheters tend to be stiffer than regular ones. The following is a general technique for steerable microcatheters:

2. Preload and shape an appropriate microwire into the microcatheter, such as a 0.014 in. Transend™ or Synchro™ wire (Stryker Neurovascular, Fremont, CA)

3. Use a fairly robust guide catheter that is placed as high as safely possible in the cervical carotid or vertebral artery.

4. Use the peel-away introducer to insert the microcatheter into the guide catheter.

5. Carefully advance the microcatheter under roadmap guidance over the guide-wire. When encountering a sharp turn in the vessel, rotate the catheter during advancement, to make the turn.

6. Keep the tip of the guide catheter on the roadmap working view, and remember that the steerable microcatheter will try to push the guiding catheter back, as it is advanced.

7. When rotating the microcatheter, hold the flange at the microcatheter hub. Ensure that any slack in the microcatheter or guiding catheter is removed and that the RHV on the guide catheter is not too tight, as these factors can limit the transmission of torque to the tip of the microcatheter.

8. If the microcatheter tip is not moving forward as it is advanced at the groin, rotate it slightly, and it may move forward again.
9. Beware that the microcatheter can jump forward abruptly as it is being rotated, especially if pushing it forward results in little response at the tip. All that pushing has stored energy into the system and it releases quickly when the catheter is rotated.
10. If the microcatheter will not advance and the guide catheter pushes back, pull back on the microcatheter to release tension, and try again, using various combinations of forward pushing and rotating of the microcatheter, as well as gentle rotation of the guidewire.
11. The stiffness of the microcatheter can straighten small, sharply curved vessels, so it may be advisable to use a smaller catheter system for very distal catheterization of small vessels.

Specific Interventional Techniques

1. Aneurysm treatment: Chap. 5
    a. Includes coiling, stent-assisted coiling, balloon-remodelling, Onyx embolization, and flow diversion.
2. Provocative testing: Chap. 6
3. Intracranial embolization: Chap. 7
    a. Includes liquid embolic and coil embolization of tumors and vascular lesions.
4. Extracranial embolization: Chap. 8
    a. Includes transarterial embolization of head and neck lesions and spinal lesions, and percutaneous injection procedures.
5. Thrombectomy and thrombolysis for acute ischemic stroke: Chap. 9
6. Extracranial angioplasty and stenting: Chap. 10
7. Intracranial angioplasty and stenting: Chap. 11
    a. Includes treatment of atherosclerotic stenosis and cerebral vasospasm.
8. Venous procedures: Chap. 12

Intermediate Catheter Technique

The introduction of the Distal Access Catheter (DAC®, Stryker Neurovascular, Fremont, CA), which is intermediate in size between a guide catheter and a microcatheter, inspired the development of the so-called "intermediate" (or triaxial) catheter technique. The DAC was originally developed for buttressing access for the MERCI devices (Stryker Neurovascular, Fremont, CA), but it quickly became clear that the DAC can provide stable access to the intracranial target by functioning as a bridge and support between the guide catheter and the microcatheter (Fig. 4.4). By softening the curves of the microcatheter within it, the DAC reduces the ovalization forces in the microcatheter that add friction and resistance to the microcatheter and microwire. The DAC is also advantageous because it has a relatively large lumen, but it is as navigable as many microcatheters. It has been used in a number of off-label settings, including aneurysm and AVM embolization and treatment of acute ischemic stroke and intracranial stenosis.[85,86] Other catheters can be used besides the DAC in a triaxial arrangement.
    Technique:
1. Case selection
    a. Intermediate catheter technique is helpful in certain situations:
    a. Tortuous and redundant proximal anatomy
    b. Tortuous intracranial anatomy
    c. Need for remote intracranial access (e.g., a distal MCA AVM paedicle)
    d. Need for a large microcatheter (e.g., when a larger microcatheter cannot be guided through the carotid siphon, placing it within a DAC might help)
    e. Acute ischemic stroke cases in which the operating microcatheter must be advanced and withdrawn repeatedly, such as in Penumbra cases
    f. Intracranial venous sinus thrombosis aspiration
2. DAC selection
    a. Be careful to choose a DAC that will be small enough to fit inside the guide catheter and large enough to accommodate the microcatheter. Generally, a larger guide catheter is necessary. DACs come in four different sizes and 2–3 lengths for each size. The Excelsior® SL-10 is small enough fit inside all of the DACs.

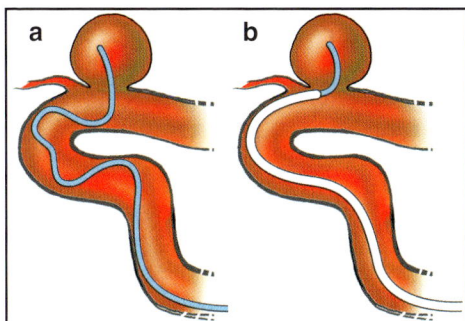

Fig. 4.4 Intermediate catheter technique. Microcatheter positioning in an ophthalmic segment ICA aneurysm without (**a**) and with (**b**) a Distal Access Catheter (DAC). Without a DAC, some redundancy is present in the microcatheter throughout the caroid siphon, which diminishes microcatheter stability, ovalizes the microcatheter in the sharp turns, and lengthens the amount of microcatheter subject to movement during the coiling. With the microcatheter positioned within the DAC, the curviness of the microcatheter is reduced and the unconstrained length of microcatheter is minimized, improving stability and control.

      b. DAC sizes:
      c. DAC 038 (2.9F ID, 3.9F OD)
          i. This DAC will fit inside a <u>Neuron</u>™ 6F 053 guide catheter, but with difficulty.
      d. DAC 044 (3.3F ID, 4.3F OD)
          i. Largest DAC to fit inside a <u>Neuron</u>™ 6F 070 guide catheter.
      e. DAC 057 (4.3F ID, 5.2F OD)
          i. Largest DAC to fit inside a 6F Envoy® guide catheter
          ii. Smallest DAC to accommodate a Marksman™ microcatheter.
      f. DAC 070 (5.3F ID, 6.3F OD)
          i. Requires a large guide catheter, such as a 6F Cook Shuttle®.
      g. Also choose the length of the DAC very carefully. It must be long enough to extend out of the guide catheter and reach distal enough to provide support for the catheter. However it must not be so long that there is not enough length of the microcatheter to extend the desired length beyond the tip of the DAC.
      h. Ideally one should use the shortest length necessary to do the job.
   3. Triaxial technique
      a. Prepare three heparinized flushes with RHVs.
      b. Position the guide catheter.
      c. Advance the microwire, microcatheter, and DAC within the guide catheter as a single unit. Maintain the microcatheter and DAC on continuous heparin saline flush throughout the procedure.
   4. DAC tips
      a. Be sure the microcatheter is long enough to extend out of the DAC by a meaningful distance.
      b. Use a 3 or 1 mL syringe for guide catheter angiograms.
      c. Attempt to make a roadmap with the guide catheter before the DAC is introduced that will be useable throughout the procedure. Because of crowding within the guide catheter, later guide catheter angiograms are of limited quality.
   5. At-a-glance triaxial combinations:
      The most challenging part of using the intermediate catheter technique can be simply figuring out which catheters will fit within which other catheters. Here are some triaxial combinations that work:
          i. 6F Cook shuttle/Penumbra 054/Penumbra 032
          ii. Neuron 088 MAXX/Penumbra 054/Penumbra 032
          iii. Neuron 088 MAXX/Penumbra 041/SL-10
          iv. Neuron 070/DAC 044/any microcatheter

Other Intermediate Catheters

Other manufactures have entered the intermediate catheter game.
1. Revive™ Intermediate Catheter (Codman Neurovascular, San Jose, CA)
   a. Sizes
   b. REVIVE 044 (3.3F ID, 4.1F OD)
      i. Available in 115 and 130 cm (usable) lengths.
      ii. Will fit in a Neuron™ 6F 070 guide catheter.
   c. REVIVE 056 (4.3F ID, 5.0F OD)
      i. Available in 115 and 125 cm (usable) lengths.
      ii. May barely fit in an 070 Neuron™
2. Fargo and FargoMAX (Balt Extrusion, Montmorency, France). These are CE mark approved, but not available in the United States.
   a. Sizes
   b. Fargo 6F (4.2F ID, 6.0F OD)
      i. Available in 105, 115, 125, and 135 cm lengths.
      ii. Available in straight or pre-shaped multi-purpose curve.
   c. Fargo MAX (5.3F ID, 6.0F OD)
      i. Available in 105, 115 and 125 cm lengths.
      ii. Available in straight or pre-shaped multi-purpose curve.

Additional Imaging Techniques for Neurointervention

Flat panel angiography technology lead to the development of rapid 3-dimensional rotational angiography and road mapping, and rotational flat panel computed tomography.
1. 3-D angiography
   a. Rotational flat panel 3-dimensional angiography creates a 3-D image on a workstation that can be rotated, edited, and measured. Particularly helpful for finding the optimal working view for treatment of intracranial lesions.
   b. Technique
      i. Park the lateral C-arm out of the way.
      ii. Adjust to the narrowest possible field of view, centered on the target.
      iii. Position the patient at isocenter.
      iv. Connect the power injector.
          Settings: 3 mL/s for 15 mL total.
      v. All personnel should step out of the angio suite and into the control room during acquisition of the images, if possible, because of the large amount of radiation scatter.
      vi. Post-processing is automatic. Adjusting windowing, magnification, and view of the image on the workstation as needed.
   c. Some angiographic suites allow a 3-D angio to be a mask for roadmapping, as in the *syngo* iPilot from Siemens and Dynamic 3D Roadmap from Philips.
2. Cone beam CT
   a. Rotational flat panel CT (aka "cone beam" CT) generates a fine-cut head CT with less contrast resolution compared to conventional multidetector CT.[87–89] Useful in neurointervention for identifying new intracranial haemorrhage, hydrocephalus, ventriculostomy catheter position and other anatomic information.[90,91]
      i. Siemens' version: DynaCT.[92]
      ii. Philips' version: XperCT.[93]
      iii. GE, Toshiba and Shimadzu have similar cone beam CT protocols.
   b. Technique:
      i. Park the lateral C-arm.
      ii. Adjust to a wide field of view.
      iii. Position the patient at the isocenter.
      iv. Program the workstation to acquire "low definition" images. The low definition setting provides faster image acquisition with a lower radiation dose compared to "high definition."

v. All personnel should step out of the angio suite and into the control room during acquisition of the images, if possible, because of the large amount of radiation scatter. Image acquisition takes only several seconds.

vi. Post-processing of the CT images is automatic and takes several minutes.

4.9. Puncture Site Management

Because most patients are anticoagulated and/or on antiplatelet agents after neurointerventional procedures, a closure device is usually more practical than manual compression. See Chap. 2 for details about femoral artery puncture site management.

4.10. Postprocedure Care

The first priority after any neurointerventional procedure is to assess the patient's neurological status. For awake cases, a brief neurological exam after the procedure is sufficient. If general anesthesia was used, work with anesthesia to make sure the patient has a smooth emergence, and then assess the patient when they are awake.

It is conventional to admit patients to the hospital for observation after neurointerventional procedures. Urgent and emergent cases, (e.g., acute stroke and ruptured aneurysm cases) and elective procedures in which a complication occurs, require admission to a Neurological Intensive Care Unit (NICU). Patients undergoing uncomplicated elective procedures may be admitted to a Step-down Unit for observation. Step-down Unit admission for these patients saves time and is more cost-effective than NICU admission.[94]

Post-procedure Orders

1. Admit to NICU or Step-down unit
2. Neuro checks Q1 h. Call physician for any change.
3. Bed rest with the accessed leg extended, head of bed ≤30°, for 5 h. (If a closure device is used, bed rest, with head of bed ≤30°, for 1 h).
4. Vital signs: Check on arrival in recovery room, then Q 1 h until discharge. Call physician for SBP <90 mmHg or decrease 25 mmHg; pulse >120.
5. Check the puncture site and distal pulses upon arrival, then Q 15 min × 4, Q 30 min × 2, then Q 1 h until discharge. Call physician if:
   a. Bleeding or hematoma develops at puncture site.
   b. Distal pulse is not palpable beyond the puncture site.
   c. Extremity is blue or cold.
6. IVF: 0.9 N.S. at a maintenance rate.
7. Resume routine medications.
8. Sequential compression devices for DVT prophylaxis.

4.11. Appendix: The Neuroendovascular Suite

This appendix addresses the design and staffing of the endovascular suite, as well as monitoring and pharmacological considerations. The objectives are to provide an introduction to residents and fellows new to the angio suite, and serve as guidelines for the fortunate experienced operators planning a new suite.

Organization and Essential Equipment

The neurointerventional suite should be dedicated to the neurointerventional service. The AHA Intercouncil Report on Peripheral and Visceral Angiographic and Interventional Laboratories produced detailed recommendations for the design and equipment needed for an interventional suite.[95] Although these guidelines were not designed specifically for neurointerventional suites, they are a useful resource for planning and equipment selection. Once new equipment is installed, a medical physicist should be contracted to check out the equipment to ensure that all the specifications are met and that the image quality is adequate. In addition, annual checks by the physicist are necessary to maintain image quality and minimize radiation dose.

1. Size. The procedure room should be large enough to accommodate anesthesia personnel and their equipment, as well as additional personnel and equipment that may be needed for particular procedures. For example, electroencephalography and other electrophysiology monitoring devices are required during Wada testing. The size of a typical interventional suite is at least 30×25 ft, or 750 square feet, with a ceiling height of 10–12 ft.[95,96]

2. Entrances. Separate entrances for patient transportation and for personnel, usually from the control room, facilitate rapid room turnover and reduce crowding.

3. Standard equipment.
   a. High-resolution computer monitors with PACS access to allow viewing of imaging studies.
   b. Usually at least two monitors should display the patient's haemodynamic data.
   c. Several other computer stations should be available for anesthesia, nursing and other personnel to access medical records, protocols, electronic copies of this handbook, etc.
   d. Sinks for waste and for cleaning
   e. Telephones
   f. Glass-fronted storage cabinets for equipment and devices.

4. Anesthesia requirements.
   The room should be equipped with oxygen, suction, gas evacuation lines, and a separate telephone for anesthesia personnel.

5. Lighting.
   a. Overhead lights should be controlled with a rheostat to allow dimming of the room lights.
   b. Foot pedals to control the lights and an overhead spotlight to illuminate procedures (such as during wire and catheter shaping and arterial access site closure) are helpful.

6. Tables
   a. Patient table. The patient's table should be capable of four-way motion, permitting wide excursion and pivot rotation. The table should also be able to be angled up to 30° from horizontal, to facilitate myelographic procedures and Trendelenburg position in cardiovascular emergencies. Weight capacity should be at least 500 pounds with a higher peak capacity for performing chest compression in emergency situations.
   b. Second table. A second table, within easy reach of the operator, is used for device preparation and placement of devices and materials for use during procedures.
   c. Third table. A third table is needed for procedures in which some materials, such as glue or particles for embolization, must be kept separate from the other devices.

7. Power contrast injector.
   a. The power injector should be capable of delivering rates up to 50 mL/s.
   b. Ceiling-mounted or table-mounted injectors are preferred over floor models.

8. Control room.
   a. Contains the console for operating the angiographic equipment.
   b. The control room should be spacious enough to accommodate ancillary personnel, as well as medical students and visitors (at least 130 square feet).[95]
   c. The control room window should be expansive (≥4 ft by 8 ft) should be equipped with a Venetian blind to provide patient privacy during procedures such as groin prepping and Foley catheter placement.

d. The control room should also contain an image processing workstation to permit viewing, storage, and analysis of images.
e. One or more computers for looking up electronic medial records, scheduling programs, protocols, the latest football scores, etc.
9. Storage space – Often not considered during room planning. There should be enough space to store plenty of device stock, both within the angiography suite and in other rooms close by. Glass-fronted storage cabinets in the suite facilitate rapid device selection during procedures. A separate, out-of-room storage space should be at least 250 square feet.[95]
10. Power requirements
a. Three-phase 220 and 440 V AC power with a minimum of 100 A per phase.[95]
b. Emergency room power (sufficient to keep the room running for at least several minutes in a power outage).
11. Temperature and humidity must be kept within narrow limits:[96]
a. Temperature: $72 \pm 10°$
b. Humidity: $45\% \pm 15\%$
12. Equipment room. A separate, cooled and ventilated room traditionally contained transformers, power modules, and related equipment. The recommended size for the equipment room is 100 square feet.[95]
a. Modern systems have much more compact generators and electronics.
b. An alternative to a separate room is an alcove for electronics that can be partially closed off by sliding or swinging doors. Air supply and return vents are positioned over the electronics cabinets, with a separate thermostat for the area.
13. Data management
a. Data storage. The system should be able to store at least several weeks worth of imaging data to allow for rapid comparison of studies on patients that return for urgent follow-up, including patients who have suspected vasospasm, in whom subtle caliber changes are easier to detect if prior studies are available real-time.
b. A picture archiving and communication system (PACS) is a computer system that manages the acquisition, transmission, storage, distribution, display, and interpretation of medical images. Multiframe studies such as angiography will require extensive storage capacity, especially if the raw DICOM data is stored. The advantage of storing the data as it comes out of the angio suite is that it could later be processed to better see a specific lesion. The data is also embedded with positioning information that would allow for repeating specific views at a later date. A cheap solution is to only store selected subtracted images of each study, saving each like a screen-save that cannot be later processed. PACS display systems are reviewed by Badano,[97] and guidelines for the acquisition of and test of PACS are discussed in depth by Samei and colleagues.[98]

Angiography Equipment

Isocentric biplane digital subtraction angiographic equipment is much preferable to a single plane system. Biplane technique decreases time necessary for procedures, reduces radiation exposure, minimizes contrast dose, and offers a definite technical advantage by permitting simultaneous imaging of the anteroposterior and lateral planes. Rotational 3D angiography is also useful in defining tortuous and intricate neurovascular anatomy. Ceiling-mounted equipment, such as video monitors and power-contrast injectors, are easier to manage and are less obtrusive than floor- or table-mounted devices.

Technical Specifications

1. Generator
a. Rating should be a minimum of 80 kW, kV(p) ≥125, 800 mA at 100 kV(p), or 1,000 mA at 80 kV(P), with a minimum switching time of 1 ms.
b. Should be a high-frequency inverter generator with a power rating of 80–100 kW.[95]

      c. Should automatically compensate for voltage fluctuation.

      d. Should be spatially and electrically isolated, and high-voltage cables need to be shielded.

2. X-ray tube

      a. Focal spot indicates the size of the x-ray source. The smaller the source, the greater the resolution. Although some vendors only offer two, three focal spot sizes are preferred:

         i.   Small, 0.3 mm, kilowatt rating 20–30 kW.

         ii. Medium, 0.8 mm, kilowatt rating 40–60 kW.

         iii. Large, 1.3 mm kilowatt rating 80–100 kW.

      b. Heat capacity should be at least 800,000 to 1 million units.[95]

         Anode heat unit capacity of 2.4 million heat units is typical at the present time; a unit with too few heat units will cause a lengthy procedure to be intermittently placed on standby.

3. The target angle should be ≤12°.

4. The anode disk typically consists of graphite, with a surface coating of tungsten/rhenium alloy, and a minimum diameter of 150 mm.

5. Image intensifier (II) size should range from 9 to 12 in. The smaller the II, the higher the resolution at high magnification (drawback: the smaller the II, the smaller the field of view). The field-of-view size can be electronically adjusted using tableside controls. The II should be selected for high resolution and high contrast ratio

      a. The conversion efficiency factor should be greater than 250 candelas per meter squared per milliroentgen per second (cd/m^2)/mR/s measured at 80 kW.[95]

      b. Spatial resolution is measured at the II tube and should be at least 2.2 line-pairs/mm in the 9 in. field of view, and 3.3 line-pairs/mm for a 6 in. field of view.

      c. Contrast ratio should be at least 20:1.

6. Flat panel technology can replace the imaging intensifier. With the appropriate software, it allows for rotational cone-beam 3-D CT, allowing visualization of soft tissues just like a standard CT scan.

      a. Advantages: No need for correction for magnetic field distortion; radiation exposure can be reduced with acceptable image quality; larger and more variable field of view; improved image quality because flat panel detectors have a higher contrast resolution. Spatial resolution is primarily limited by the matrix size; maintains image quality longer in the life of the equipment, unlike II technology in which image quality inevitably degrades.

      b. Drawbacks: In the fluoroscopy mode, the displayed image is noisier than II images, which takes getting used to. More expensive to purchase. Flat panel detectors can fail and are more expensive to replace.

7. Monitors

      a. Five angiography video monitors are necessary and should be mounted on the ceiling. Two monitors are used to view digital subtraction angiograms or roadmaps; the other two are used for live fluoroscopic imaging during procedures. The fifth is a monitor for 3D reconstructions. Yet another monitor to display haemodynamic parameters should be positioned next to the angiography monitors. The monitors should measure at least 17 in. in the diagonal and have an antiglare coating. Large monitors are available and software can combine the equivalent of multiple displays on a single screen. Two kinds of monitors are available: CRTs and flat panels.

      b. Flat panel monitors

         i.   Advantages: Good contrast and brightness. Lighter and less bulky than old cathode ray tubes.

         ii. Disadvantages: More expensive, may have viewing angle and noise texture limitations.

         iii. Minimum specs: $1,600 \times 1,200$ resolution, brightness ≥700 nit (cd/m^2), 700:1 contrast ratio, 170° viewing angle.

      c. The monitors should be able to display at least $1,024 \times 1,024$ resolution.[99]

      d. Spatial resolution should be at least 1.8 line pairs/mm in the 9 in. mode.

      e. Color display is needed for 3D imaging display, but grey-scale is used to display fluoroscopy and DSA images.

8. Vendors. All five angiography equipment manufacturers make equipment that features biplane DSA, flat panel technology, and 3-D imaging. Some advantages or disadvantages with each company are listed below:
   a. Toshiba
      Biplane imaging equipment features a variable isocenter – allows for easier adjustments in c-arm positioning. Toshiba equipment also has a unique direct x-ray-to-electronic flat panel system, which theoretically lowers noise in the system.
   b. Siemens
      Probably the most common biplane system worldwide. Nice 3-D imaging algorithm. Siemens x-ray tubes have a relatively high x-ray heat capacity, which makes for fewer interruptions during procedures due to over-heating. Siemens has "Dynavision," which produces soft tissue imaging similar to CT scanning.
   c. Philips
      Good all-around functionality. Philips' rapid tube rotation, for 3-D imaging, produces a faster acquisition than other systems. The "default x-ray settings" on Philips equipment can produce a lower x-ray exposure for the patient, at the cost of lower imaging quality (however, these settings can be adjusted if needed).
   d. General Electric
      Decent all-around functionality. In the past, GE has tended to have a less dense imaging matrix compared to other vendors and focal spots have been larger.
   e. Shimadzu
      Also features a variable isocenter, and has the direct-conversion flat panel detector design. Shimadzu equipment has a unique motion-artifact correction feature. Shimadzu 3-D imaging is not as advanced as the other vendors, but is improving.

Radiation Safety

Patient Radiation Exposure

1. The overall radiation exposure with most neurointerventional procedures is variable, depending on the procedure.
   a. In a published series of eight neurointerventional cases, the mean effective radiation dose was 1.67 mSv (range, 0.44–3.44 mSv).[100]
   b. The estimated risk of death by radiation-induced cancer with the highest effective dose was approximately one for every 6,000 procedures.
   c. However, doses ten times that or higher can easily be reached in complicated interventional cases, with resultant hair loss.[101]
2. Another concern is that dose can be cumulative, and patients having multiple interventional procedures plus CT studies will be at a greater risk of skin injury or other adverse effects.[102]
3. Although there is no defined maximum radiation exposure for patients, as the medical benefits are assumed to outweigh the presumed risks,[103] radiation exposure to patients should be minimized.[104]
4. Cornerstones of minimizing radiation dose to the patient:[95]
   a. Minimizing exposure time.
      i. Limit fluoroscopy time. Use the last image hold feature to study an image rather than standing on the fluoroscopy pedal.
      ii. Limit the pulse rate for fluoroscopy.
   b. Dynamic acquisition (i.e. angio runs) gives more dose than simple fluoroscopy. Do only the angiographic runs that are needed. (e.g. use one 3D acquisition instead of six different oblique runs)
      i. Use as low a frame rate as necessary to see the findings.
      ii. Use the fluoro-fade (aka mask overlay) function instead of standard roadmapping. It uses lower dose.[105]
   c. Collimate. It improves image quality and only exposes the area of interest.
      Modern suites feature virtual collimation that allows positioning and collimation without using fluoroscopy.

d. Use overhead and table-side shielding to protect body parts not being studied.

e. Maximize distance from the x-ray source.

5. The National Council on Radiation Protection and Measurements (NCRP) has made recommendations for the design of structural shielding[8] and x-ray equipment.[106]

6. Have up-to-date imaging equipment. Vendors are constantly improving efficiency of their products and radiation protection protocols. A study showed maximum skin dose reduced from 4.1 to 1.0 Gy after installing a new neurointerventional suite.[107]

a. Modern suites make use of robotic positioning that allows positioning based on position sense in the system rather than fluoroscopic positioning.

b. Information on positioning and acquisition parameters is stored with each image, allowing later reproduction of views without fluoroscopic positioning.

c. Advanced systems may allow spatial information imported from prior CT or MR studies guiding navigation with minimal additional radiation.

d. Electronic zoom functions allow electronic magnification without additional X-ray dosage.

Staff Radiation Exposure

1. The National Council on Radiation Protection and Measurements has published guidelines for radiation exposure for medical personnel that are defined as "as low as reasonably achievable".[104,108]

2. Fluoroscopy is the major source of occupational radiation exposure.[109]

3. The operating physician is at the greatest risk of receiving the maximum occupational dose.[95]

a. Positioning of the x-ray tube under the table minimizes scatter radiation to the operator's head and neck.[110]

b. In biplane systems, keep the lateral tube on the side away from the operator.

4. Moveable, ceiling-mounted clear lead glass shields can be draped with sterile plastic and positioned over the patient, protecting the patient's lower body and the operator from radiation exposure.

5. Rolling floor mounted x-ray shields should be available to shield anesthesia or other personnel.

6. Lead aprons

a. Should provide at least 0.5 mm lead equivalent thickness.

b. All full-time physicians, technologists, and nurses should wear custom-fitted aprons to ensure optimal coverage and comfort (Fig. 4.5).

c. Extra aprons should be available for anesthesia staff and visitors.

7. Pregnant staff members.

a. The NCRP-recommended maximum gestational radiation exposure is 5 mSv per gestational period, or 0.5 mSv per month.[103]

b. Options to minimize fetal radiation exposure:

i. Wear an apron with 1.0 mm lead equivalent thickness (essentially double apron coverage but they are very heavy).

ii. Use draped free-standing or ceiling-mounted shields.

iii. Wear wrap-around aprons to cover front and back.

iv. Pregnant staff members should wear two radiation badges, with one under the apron to monitor fetal dose.

8. Other personal radiation protection, including thyroid shields, lead glasses, should be available to all staff members.

Physiological Monitoring

Meticulous monitoring of the patient's condition during a neurointerventional procedure is critical.

1. When possible, procedures should be performed with the patient awake to permit continuous assessment of neurological status.

2. Monitoring of vital signs and pulse oximetry is routine; continuous arterial line and intracranial pressure (ICP) monitoring is done as needed.

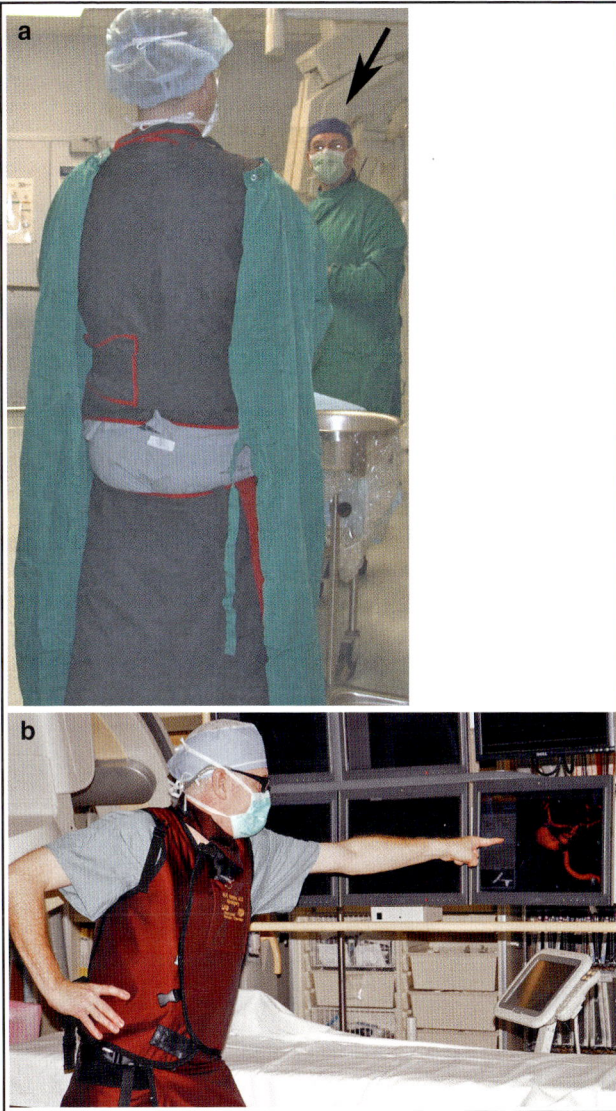

Fig. 4.5 Lead apron technique. Improperly worn lead apron, as demonstrated by the junior author of this handbook early in his career (**a**), unfortunately witnessed by the senior author (*arrow*). Proper lead apron wearing technique is demonstrated by the junior author in a typically heroic pose in a more recent photograph (**b**).

3. Equipment
   a. Transducers should have a linear response from −10 to 400 mmHg.[95]
   b. Two or more pressure channels and two ECG channels should be available.
   c. An overhead monitor that projects the clinical data, including colour-coded tracings, should be positioned next to the angiography monitors.
   d. Arterial line monitoring. Patients with subarachnoid haemorrhage or intracranial haemorrhage should undergo continuous arterial line monitoring of their vital signs by means of a radial artery line placed before the procedure. Alternatively, monitoring may be done via the arterial sheath in patients undergoing elective procedures, such as endovascular treatment of intracranial aneurysms. To obtain an adequate tracing, the sheath must be larger than the guide catheter; monitoring can be done through a 7F femoral artery sheath when a 6F guide catheter is used.
   e. Intracranial pressure monitoring. Continuous monitoring of ICP should be performed in patients with a ventriculostomy. An ICP tracing on one of the overhead angiography monitors provides immediate feedback, should an abrupt change in ICP occur during the procedure, such as during an aneurysm rupture.

Personnel

The neurointerventional team is a multidisciplinary group with expertise in neurointervention, radiology techniques, and radiation safety. At the center of this group are the interventionists, technologists, and nurses. The team is supplemented by anesthesiologists and anesthesia monitoring staff. It is important that the individuals in the team are experienced, highly motivated, and flexible. The rapidly evolving field of neurointervention, combined with the complexity of the disorders and the procedures requires that the team functions as a cohesive, adaptable unit. Moreover, the team should be large enough to allow organization of a call schedule that will provide continuous 24-h availability, without risking "burn-out" of key members.

Neurointerventionists

The neurointerventionist is a neurosurgeon, neuroradiologist, or neurologist who has completed a dedicated fellowship in neurointerventional radiology. Detailed knowledge of the pathophysiology of neurovascular disease must be combined with a comprehensive understanding of neuroanatomy as well as fundamentals of neurocritical care and interventional techniques.

Neurointerventional Technologists

Technologists in the neurointerventional suite have a background in basic radiology techniques and further expertise in computerized digital subtraction imaging. They are responsible for setting up the equipment for procedures, processing of the images, trouble-shooting during procedures, and ordering and stocking of devices. They also are responsible for alerting specialized service technicians when needed; technologists are not usually responsible for maintaining and repairing imaging equipment. At some centers, technologists may also be responsible for patient positioning and the establishment and maintenance of irrigation lines.

Nursing Staff

Neurointerventional nurses should be registered nurses with a background in neurointensive care. Neurointerventional nurses are responsible for patient preparation before the procedure, the establishment of intravenous access, the administration of sedation and analgesia, monitoring the patient's condition, and maintenance of irrigation lines. Additional specific duties of the nursing staff include evaluation of the preprocedure laboratory tests, checking for allergies or drug reactions, verifying and witnessing informed consent for the procedure, placement of a Foley catheter, ven-

Table 4.1   Medications that should be easily available for prompt access or emergent use

Medication	Use
Atropine	Treatment of bradycardia or asystole during carotid angioplasty and stenting
Epinephrine	Vasopressor
Fentanyl	Analgesia
Glycoprotein (GP) IIb–IIIa inhibitor (e.g., eptifibitide or abciximab)	Rescue treatment when platelet-rich thrombosis occurs
Heparin	Anticoagulation
Labetalol hydrochoride	Blood pressure control
Lidocaine	Local anesthesia
Midazolam	Sedation
Nitroglycerin	Treatment of catheter-induced vasospasm
Protamine	Reversal of systemic heparin anticoagulation
tPA or other thrombolytic	Acute stroke treatment

triculostomy and lumbar drain management, performance of an Allen test before radial artery procedures, monitoring peripheral pulses, and management of the arterial access site at the completion of the procedure. At some centers, a second nurse acts as the first assistant to the neurointerventionist during procedures.

Pharmacologic Considerations

Certain medications should be available for prompt access (Table 4.1). During procedures in which intravenous heparin is administered, protamine should be drawn up in a sterile syringe and placed on the back table in preparation for rapid administration in the event of a haemorrhage during the procedure. Medications used on a routine basis are listed in Table 4.2.

Future Developments

Numerous technological advances are currently in progress that offer promise in the continued evolution of the neurointerventional suite. Ultra-high resolution digital subtraction angiography has the potential to improve visualization during neurointerventional procedures. This technique has pixels sizes of 35 μm and is capable of imaging up to 30 frames per second, compared to traditional flat panel detectors, which have pixel sizes of 194 μm or larger.[111,112] Magnetically guided angiography, currently available at some centers, uses extracranial magnets to help catheter and wire navigation.[113,114] This technology offers the potential to permit more precise intravascular navigation while shortening fluoroscopy and procedure times. MRI-guided angiography, with the potential advantages of detailed tissue imaging as well as the elimination of radiation exposure, is another innovation under development.[115–117]

Table 4.2 Routine medications

Medication	Use
Acetylcysteine	Treatment of patients with renal insufficiency
Aspirin (oral and suppository preparations)	Antiplatelet therapy
Benadryl	Treatment of allergic reactions
Clopidogrel	Antiplatelet therapy
Dobutamine	Blood pressure and heart rate support
Dopamine	Blood pressure and heart rate support
Flumazenil	Reversal of benzodiazepines
Furosemide	Management of elevated intracranial pressure
Glucagon	Control of gastric motility during spinal angiography; may be useful for treatment of anaphylaxis in patients on beta blockers
Lidocaine (preservative-free, for provocative testing)	Provocative testing of the retina or peripheral nervous system before embolization
Mannitol	Management of elevated intracranial pressure
Naloxone	Reversal of narcotics
Norepinephrine	Vasopressor
Ondansetron	Antiemetic
Phenylephrine	Blood pressure and heart rate support
Propofol	Sedation and analgesia
Sodium amobarbital (Amytal)	Provocative testing before embolization of the central nervous system or for Wada testing
Sodium methohexital (Brevital)	Provocative testing before embolization of the central nervous system
Sodium nitroprusside	Blood pressure control
Vasopressin	Vasopressor

References

1. Mold JW, Stein HF. The cascade effect in the clinical care of patients. N Engl J Med. 1986;314:512–4.
2. Woolf SH, Kuzel AJ, Dovey SM, Phillips Jr RL. A string of mistakes: the importance of cascade analysis in describing, counting, and preventing medical errors. Ann Fam Med. 2004;2:317–26.
3. Schulz K. Being wrong: adventures in the margin of error. New York: Harper Collins; 2010.
4. Schwartz J. Who needs hackers? New York Times 2007 Sept 12, 2007.
5. Mueller C, Buerkle G, Buettner HJ, et al. Prevention of contrast media-associated nephropathy: randomized comparison of 2 hydration regimens in 1620 patients undergoing coronary angioplasty. Arch Intern Med. 2002;162:329–36.
6. Tepel M, van der Giet M, Schwarzfeld C, Laufer U, Liermann D, Zidek W. Prevention of radiographic-contrast-agent-induced reductions in renal function by acetylcysteine. N Engl J Med. 2000;343:180–4.
7. Manual on Contrast Media, Version 7. Reston: American College of Radiology; 2010.
8. Rosovsky MA, Rusinek H, Berenstein A, Basak S, Setton A, Nelson PK. High-dose administration of nonionic contrast media: a retrospective review. Radiology. 1996;200:119–22.
9. Kjonniksen I, Andersen BM, Sondenaa VG, Segadal L. Preoperative hair removal–a systematic literature review. AORN J. 2002;75:928–38, 40.
10. Al-Mubarak N, Vitek JJ, Iyer SS, New G, Roubin GS. Carotid stenting with distal-balloon protection via the transbrachial approach. J Endovasc Ther. 2001;8:571–5.
11. Bendok BR, Przybylo JH, Parkinson R, Hu Y, Awad IA, Batjer HH. Neuroendovascular interventions for intracranial posterior circulation disease via the transradial approach: technical case report. Neurosurgery. 2005;56:E626; discussion E.
12. Kim JY, Yoon J, Jung HS, et al. Feasibility of the radial artery as a vascular access route in performing primary percutaneous coronary intervention. Yonsei Med J. 2005;46:503–10.
13. Yoo BS, Yoon J, Ko JY, et al. Anatomical consideration of the radial artery for transradial coronary procedures: arterial diameter, branching anomaly and vessel tortuosity. Int J Cardiol. 2005;101:421–7.
14. McIvor J, Rhymer JC. 245 transaxillary arteriograms in arteriopathic patients: success rate and complications. Clin Radiol. 1992;45:390–4.
15. Ross IB, Luzardo GD. Direct access to the carotid circulation by cut down for endovascular neuro-interventions. Surg Neurol. 2006;65:207–11; discussion 11.
16. Nii K, Kazekawa K, Onizuka M, et al. Direct carotid puncture for the endovascular treatment of anterior circulation aneurysms. AJNR Am J Neuroradiol. 2006;27:1502–4.
17. Blanc R, Mounayer C, Piotin M, Sadik JC, Spelle L, Moret J. Hemostatic closure device after carotid puncture for stent and coil placement in an intracranial aneurysm: technical note. AJNR Am J Neuroradiol. 2002;23:978–81.
18. Qureshi AI, Luft AR, Sharma M, Guterman LR, Hopkins LN. Prevention and treatment of thromboembolic and ischemic complications associated with endovascular procedures: part II–clinical aspects and recommendations. Neurosurgery. 2000;46:1360–75; discussion 75–6.
19. Derdeyn CP, Cross 3rd DT, Moran CJ, et al. Postprocedure ischemic events after treatment of intracranial aneurysms with guglielmi detachable coils. J Neurosurg. 2002;96:837–43.
20. Friedman JA, Nichols DA, Meyer FB, et al. Guglielmi detachable coil treatment of ruptured saccular cerebral aneurysms: retrospective review of a 10-year single-center experience. AJNR Am J Neuroradiol. 2003;24:526–33.
21. Ross IB, Dhillon GS. Complications of endovascular treatment of cerebral aneurysms. Surg Neurol. 2005;64:12–8.
22. Saw J, Bajzer C, Casserly IP, et al. Evaluating the optimal activated clotting time during carotid artery stenting. Am J Cardiol. 2006;97:1657–60.
23. Castellan L, Causin F, Danieli D, Perini S. Carotid stenting with filter protection. Correlation of ACT values with angiographic and histopathologic findings. J Neuroradiol. 2003;30:103–8.
24. Lewis BE, Ferguson JJ, Grassman ED, et al. Successful coronary interventions performed with argatroban anticoagulation in patients with heparin-induced thrombocytopenia and thrombosis syndrome. J Invasive Cardiol. 1996;8:410–7.
25. Matthai Jr WH. Use of argatroban during percutaneous coronary interventions in patients with heparin-induced thrombocytopenia. Semin Thromb Hemost. 1999;25 Suppl 1:57–60.
26. Harrigan MR, Levy EI, Bendok BR, Hopkins LN. Bivalirudin for endovascular interventions in acute ischemic stroke: case report. Neurosurgery. 2004;54:218–22; discussion 22–3.
27. Clayton SB, Acsell JR, Crumbley 3rd AJ, Uber WE. Cardiopulmonary bypass with bivalirudin in type II heparin-induced thrombocytopenia. Ann Thorac Surg. 2004;78: 2167–9.
28. Keeling D, Davidson S, Watson H. The management of heparin-induced thrombocytopenia. Br J Haematol. 2006;133: 259–69.
29. Steinhubl SR, Berger PB, Mann 3rd JT, et al. Early and sustained dual oral antiplatelet therapy following percutaneous coronary intervention: a randomized controlled trial. JAMA. 2002;288:2411–20.
30. Ries T, Grzyska U, Fiehler J. Antiaggregation before, during, and after coiling of unruptured aneurysms: growing evidence between scylla and charybdis. AJNR Am J Neuroradiol. 2008;29:e33.
31. Hwang G, Jung C, Park SQ, et al. Thromboembolic complications of elective coil embolization of unruptured aneurysms: the effect of oral antiplatelet preparation on periprocedural thromboembolic complication. Neurosurgery. 2010;67:743–8; discussion 8.
32. Kang HS, Han MH, Kwon BJ, et al. Is clopidogrel premedication useful to reduce thromboembolic events during coil embolization for unruptured intracranial aneurysms? Neurosurgery. 2010;67:1371–6; discussion 6.
33. Yamada NK, Cross 3rd DT, Pilgram TK, Moran CJ, Derdeyn CP, Dacey Jr RG. Effect of antiplatelet therapy on thromboembolic complications of elective coil embolization of cerebral aneurysms. AJNR Am J Neuroradiol. 2007;28:1778–82.
34. Zhang XD, Wu HT, Zhu J, He ZH, Chai WN, Sun XC. Delayed intracranial hemorrhage associated with antiplatelet therapy in stent-assisted coil embolized cerebral aneurysms. Acta Neurochir Suppl. 2011;110:133–9.
35. Yan BP, Clark DJ, Ajani AE. Oral antiplatelet therapy and percutaneous coronary intervention. Expert Opin Pharmacother. 2005;6:3–12.
36. Siller-Matula JM, Huber K, Christ G, et al. Impact of clopidogrel loading dose on clinical outcome in patients undergoing percutaneous coronary intervention: a systematic review and meta-analysis. Heart. 2011;97:98–105.
37. Lee DH, Arat A, Morsi H, Shaltoni H, Harris JR, Mawad ME. Dual antiplatelet therapy monitoring for neurointerventional procedures using a point-of-care platelet function test: a single-center experience. AJNR Am J Neuroradiol. 2008;29:1389–94.
38. Mangiacapra F, Muller O, Ntalianis A, et al. Comparison of 600 versus 300-mg clopidogrel loading dose in patients with ST-segment elevation myocardial infarction undergoing primary coronary angioplasty. Am J Cardiol. 2010;106:1208–11.
39. Gruberg L, Beyar R. Optimized combination of antiplatelet treatment and anticoagulation for percutaneous coronary intervention: the final word is not out yet! letter; comment. J Invasive Cardiol. 2002;14:251–3.
40. Schleinitz MD, Olkin I, Heidenreich PA. Cilostazol, clopidogrel or ticlopidine to prevent sub-acute stent thrombosis: a meta-analysis of randomized trials. Am Heart J. 2004;148:990–7.

41. Bennett CL, Weinberg PD, Rozenberg-Ben-Dror K, Yarnold PR, Kwaan HC, Green D. Thrombotic thrombocytopenic purpura associated with ticlopidine. A review of 60 cases. Ann Intern Med. 1998;128:541–4.

42. Yi HJ, Gupta R, Jovin TG, et al. Initial experience with the use of intravenous eptifibatide bolus during endovascular treatment of intracranial aneurysms. AJNR Am J Neuroradiol. 2006;27:1856–60.

43. Ries T, Siemonsen S, Grzyska U, Zeumer H, Fiehler J. Abciximab is a safe rescue therapy in thromboembolic events complicating cerebral aneurysm coil embolization: single center experience in 42 cases and review of the literature. Stroke. 2009;40:1750–7.

44. Song JK, Niimi Y, Fernandez PM, et al. Thrombus formation during intracranial aneurysm coil placement: treatment with intra-arterial abciximab. AJNR Am J Neuroradiol. 2004;25:1147–53.

45. Steinhubl SR, Talley JD, Braden GA, et al. Point-of-care measured platelet inhibition correlates with a reduced risk of an adverse cardiac event after percutaneous coronary intervention: results of the GOLD (AU-assessing ultegra) multi-center study. Circulation. 2001;103:2572–8.

46. Merck & Co. Inc. Integrilin prescribing information. Whitehouse Station; 2011.

47. Fontana P, Dupont A, Gandrille S, et al. Adenosine diphos-phate-induced platelet aggregation is associated with P2Y12 gene sequence variations in healthy subjects. Circulation. 2003;108:989–95.

48. Farid NA, Kurihara A, Wrighton SA. Metabolism and disposition of the thienopyridine antiplatelet drugs ticlopidine, clopidogrel, and prasugrel in humans. J Clin Pharmacol. 2010;50:126–42.

49. Simon T, Verstuyft C, Mary-Krause M, et al. Genetic determinants of response to clopidogrel and cardiovascular events. N Engl J Med. 2009;360:363–75.

50. Taubert D, von Beckerath N, Grimberg G, et al. Impact of P-glycoprotein on clopidogrel absorption. Clin Pharmacol Ther. 2006;80:486–501.

51. Anderson CD, Biffi A, Greenberg SM, Rosand J. Personalized approaches to clopidogrel therapy: are we there yet? Stroke. 2010;41:2997–3002.

52. Ellis KJ, Stouffer GA, McLeod HL, Lee CR. Clopidogrel pharmacogenomics and risk of inadequate platelet inhibition: US FDA recommendations. Pharmacogenomics. 2009;10:1799–817.

53. Hulot JS, Bura A, Villard E, et al. Cytochrome P450 2 C19 loss-of-function polymorphism is a major determinant of clopidogrel responsiveness in healthy subjects. Blood. 2006;108:2244–7.

54. Mega JL, Close SL, Wiviott SD, et al. Cytochrome p-450 polymorphisms and response to clopidogrel. N Engl J Med. 2009;360:354–62.

55. Sofi F, Giusti B, Marcucci R, Gori AM, Abbate R, Gensini GF. Cytochrome P450 2 C19*2 polymorphism and cardio-vascular recurrences in patients taking clopidogrel: a meta-analysis. Pharmacogenomics J. 2011;11:199–206.

56. Administration USFaD. FDA drug safety communication: reduced effectiveness of plavix (clopidogrel) in patients who are poor metabolizers of the drug. Rockville: Administration USFaD; 2010.

57. Lau WC, Waskell LA, Watkins PB, et al. Atorvastatin reduces the ability of clopidogrel to inhibit platelet aggregation: a new drug-drug interaction. Circulation. 2003;107:32–7.

58. Nguyen T, Frishman WH, Nawarskas J, Lerner RG. Variability of response to clopidogrel: possible mechanisms and clinical implications. Cardiol Rev. 2006;14:136–42.

59. Feher G, Koltai K, Alkonyi B, et al. Clopidogrel resistance: role of body mass and concomitant medications. Int J Cardiol. 2007;120:188–92.

60. Soffer D, Moussa I, Harjai KJ, et al. Impact of angina class on inhibition of platelet aggregation following clopidogrel loading in patients undergoing coronary intervention: do we need more aggressive dosing regimens in unstable angina? Catheter Cardiovasc Interv. 2003;59:21–5.

61. Kanaan H, Jankowitz B, Aleu A, et al. In-stent thrombosis and stenosis after neck-remodeling device-assisted coil embolization of intracranial aneurysms. Neurosurgery. 2010;67:1523–33.

62. Kang H-S, Kwon BJ, Kim JE, Han MH. Preinterventional clopidogrel response variability for coil embolization of intracranial aneurysms: clinical implications. AJNR Am J Neuroradiol. 2010;31:1206–10.

63. Seidel H, Rahman MM, Scharf RE. Monitoring of antiplatelet therapy. Current limitations, challenges, and perspectives. Hamostaseologie. 2011;31:41–51.

64. Bonello L, Tantry US, Marcucci R, et al. Consensus and future directions on the definition of high on-treatment plate-let reactivity to adenosine diphosphate. J Am Coll Cardiol. 2010;56:919–33.

65. Price MJ, Berger PB, Teirstein PS, et al. Standard- vs high-dose clopidogrel based on platelet function testing after per-cutaneous coronary intervention: the GRAVITAS randomized trial. JAMA. 2011;305:1097–105.

66. Müller-Schunk S, Linn J, Peters N, et al. Monitoring of clopidogrel-related platelet inhibition: correlation of nonre-sponse with clinical outcome in supra-aortic stenting. AJNR Am J Neuroradiol. 2008;29:786–91.

67. Prabhakaran S, Wells KR, Lee VH, Flaherty CA, Lopes DK. Prevalence and risk factors for aspirin and clopidogrel resis-tance in cerebrovascular stenting. AJNR Am J Neuroradiol. 2008;29:281–5.

68. Pandya DJ, Fitzsimmons BF, Wolfe TJ, et al. Measurement of antiplatelet inhibition during neurointerventional procedures: the effect of antithrombotic duration and loading dose. J Neuroimaging. 2010;20:64–9.

69. Alberts MJ. Platelet function testing for aspirin resistance is reasonable to do: yes! Stroke. 2010;41:2400–1.

70. Eikelboom JW, Emery J, Hankey GJ. The use of platelet func-tion assays may help to determine appropriate antiplatelet treatment options in a patient with recurrent stroke on baby aspirin: against. Stroke. 2010;41:2398–9.

71. Selim MH, Molina CA. Platelet function assays in stroke man-agement: more study is needed. Stroke. 2010;41:2396–7.

72. Järemo P, Lindahl TL, Fransson SG, Richter A. Individual variations of platelet inhibition after loading doses of clopi-dogrel. J Intern Med. 2002;252:233–8.

73. Bhatt DL, Scheiman J, Abraham NS, et al. ACCF/ACG/AHA 2008 expert consensus document on reducing the gastrointes-tinal risks of antiplatelet therapy and NSAID use: a report of the American College of Cardiology foundation task force on clinical expert consensus documents. Circulation. 2008;118:1894–909.

74. Ogilvie BW, Yerino P, Kazmi F, et al. The proton pump inhibitor, omeprazole, but not lansoprazole or pantoprazole, is a metabolism-dependent inhibitor of CYP2C19: implica-tions for coadministration with clopidogrel. Drug Metab Dispos. 2011;39:2020–33.

75. O'Donoghue ML, Braunwald E, Antman EM, et al. Pharmacodynamic effect and clinical efficacy of clopidogrel and prasugrel with or without a proton-pump inhibitor: an analysis of two randomised trials. Lancet. 2009;374:989–97.

76. Ho PM, Maddox TM, Wang L, et al. Risk of adverse out-comes associated with concomitant use of clopidogrel and proton pump inhibitors following acute coronary syndrome. JAMA. 2009;301:937–44.

77. Kwok CS, Loke YK. Meta-analysis: the effects of proton pump inhibitors on cardiovascular events and mortality in patients receiving clopidogrel. Aliment Pharmacol Ther. 2010;31:810–23.

78. Bhatt DL, Cryer BL, Contant CF, et al. Clopidogrel with or without omeprazole in coronary artery disease. N Engl J Med. 2010;363:1909–17.

79. Juurlink DN, Gomes TM, Mamdani MM, Gladstone DJ, Kapral MK. The safety of proton pump inhibitors and clopi-dogrel in patients after stroke. Stroke. 2011;42:128–32.

80. Lanas A, Garcia-Rodriguez LA, Arroyo MT, et al. Effect of anti-secretory drugs and nitrates on the risk of ulcer bleeding associated with nonsteroidal anti-inflammatory drugs, antiplatelet agents, and anticoagulants. Am J Gastroenterol. 2007;102:507–15.

81. Bendszus M, Koltzenburg M, Bartsch AJ, et al. Heparin and air filters reduce embolic events caused by intra-arterial cere-bral angiography: a prospective, randomized trial. Circulation. 2004;110:2210–5.

82. Kallmes DF, McGraw JK, Evans AJ, et al. Thrombogenicity of hydrophilic and nonhydrophilic microcatheters and guid-ing catheters. AJNR Am J Neuroradiol. 1997;18:1243–51.

83. Abe T, Hirohata M, Tanaka N, et al. Distal-tip shape-consistency testing of steam-shaped microcatheters suitable for cerebral aneurysm coil placement. AJNR Am J Neuroradiol. 2004;25:1058–61.
84. Kiyosue H, Hori Y, Matsumoto S, et al. Shapability, memory, and luminal changes in microcatheters after steam shaping: a comparison of 11 different microcatheters. AJNR Am J Neuroradiol. 2005;26:2610–6.
85. Spiotta AM, Hussain MS, Sivapatham T, et al. The versatile distal access catheter: the cleveland clinic experience. Neurosurgery. 2011;68:1677–86.
86. Binning MJ, Yashar P, Orion D, et al. Use of the outreach distal access catheter for microcatheter stabilization during intracranial arteriovenous malformation embolization. AJNR Am J Neuroradiol. 2011. Epub ahead of print.
87. Engelhorn T, Struffert T, Richter G, et al. Flat panel detector angiographic CT in the management of aneurysmal rupture during coil embolization. AJNR Am J Neuroradiol. 2008;29:1581–4.
88. Struffert T, Richter G, Engelhorn T, et al. Visualisation of intracerebral haemorrhage with flat-detector CT compared to multislice CT: results in 44 cases. Eur Radiol. 2009;19:619–25.
89. Doelken M, Struffert T, Richter G, et al. Flat-panel detector volumetric CT for visualization of subarachnoid hemorrhage and ventricles: preliminary results compared to conventional CT. Neuroradiology. 2008;50:517–23.
90. Struffert T, Eyupoglu IY, Huttner HB, et al. Clinical evaluation of flat-panel detector compared with multislice computed tomography in 65 patients with acute intracranial hemorrhage: initial results. Clinical article. J Neurosurg. 2010;113:901–7.
91. Sato K, Matsumoto Y, Kondo R, Tominaga T. Usefulness of C-arm cone-beam computed tomography in endovascular treatment of traumatic carotid cavernous fistulas: a technical case report. Neurosurgery. 2010;67:467–9; discussion 9–70.
92. Namba K, Niimi Y, Song JK, Berenstein A. Use of dyna-CT angiography in neuroendovascular decision-making. A case report. Interv Neuroradiol. 2009;15:67–72.
93. Söderman M, Babic D, Holmin S, Andersson T. Brain imaging with a flat detector C-arm: technique and clinical interest of XperCT. Neuroradiology. 2008;50:863–8.
94. Richards BF, Fleming JB, Shannon CN, Walters BC, Harrigan MR. Safety and cost effectiveness of step-down unit admission following elective neurointerventional procedures. J NeuroInterv Surg. 2011. Epub ahead of prin.
95. Cardella JF, Casarella WJ, DeWeese JA, et al. Optimal resources for the examination and endovascular treatment of the peripheral and visceral vascular systems: AHA intercouncil report on peripheral and visceral angiographic and interventional laboratories. J Vasc Interv Radiol. 2003;14:517S–30.
96. Larson TCI, Creasy JL, Price RR, Maciunas RJ. Angiography suite specifications. In: Maciunas RJ, editor. Endovascular neurological intervention. Park Ridge: American Association of Neurological Surgeons; 1995.
97. Badano A. AAPM/RSNA tutorial on equipment selection: PACS equipment overview: display systems. Radiographics. 2004;24:879–89.
98. Samei E, Seibert JA, Andriole K, et al. AAPM/RSNA tutorial on equipment selection: PACS equipment overview: general guidelines for purchasing and acceptance testing of PACS equipment. Radiographics. 2004;24:313–34.
99. American Society of Interventional and Therapeutic Neuroradiology. General considerations for endovascular surgical neuroradiologic procedures. AJNR Am J Neuroradiol. 2001;22:1S–3.
100. Bergeron P, Carrier R, Roy D, Blais N, Raymond J. Radiation doses to patients in neurointerventional procedures. AJNR Am J Neuroradiol. 1994;15:1809–12.
101. Hayakawa M, Moritake T, Kataoka F, et al. Direct measurement of patient's entrance skin dose during neurointerventional procedure to avoid further radiation-induced skin injuries. Clin Neurol Neurosurg. 2010;112:530–6.
102. Moskowitz SI, Davros WJ, Kelly ME, Fiorella D, Rasmussen PA, Masaryk TJ. Cumulative radiation dose during hospitalization for aneurysmal subarachnoid hemorrhage. AJNR Am J Neuroradiol. 2010;31:1377–82.
103. National Council on Radiation Protection and Measurements. Limitation of exposure to Ionizing radiation: recommendations of the National Council on Radiation Protection and Measurements. Bethesda; 1993. Report No.: 116.
104. National Council on Radiation Protection and Measurements. Radiation dose management for fluoroscopy-guided interventional medical procedures. Bethesda: 2010. Report No.: 168.
105. Given CA, Thacker IC, Baker MD, Morris PP. Fluoroscopy fade for embolization of vein of Galen malformation. AJNR Am J Neuroradiol. 2003;24:267–70.
106. National Council on Radiation Protection and Measurements. Medical x-ray, electron beam, and gamma-ray protection for energies up to 50 MeV/G (equipment design, performance, and use): recommendations of the national council on radiation protection and measurements. Bethesda; 1989. Report No.: NCRP report 102.
107. Mooney RB, Flynn PA. A comparison of patient skin doses before and after replacement of a neurointerventional fluoroscopy unit. Clin Radiol. 2006;61:436–41.
108. National Council on Radiation Protection and Measurements. Implementation of the principle of as low as reasonable achievable (ALARA) for medical and dental personnel: recommendations of the National Council on Radiation Protection and Measurements. Bethesda: The Council; 1990. Report No.: NCRP report 107.
109. Edwards M. Development of radiation protection standards. Radiographics. 1991;11:699–712.
110. Boone JM, Levin DC. Radiation exposure to angiographers under different fluoroscopic imaging conditions. Radiology. 1991;180:861–5.
111. Wang W, Ionita CN, Keleshis C, et al. Progress in the development of a new angiography suite including the high resolution micro-angiographic fluoroscope (MAF), a control, acquisition, processing, and image display system (CAPIDS), and a new detector changer integrated into a commercial C-arm angiography unit to enable clinical use. Proc SPIE. 2010;7622:762251.
112. Binning MJ, Orion D, Yashar P, et al. Use of the micro-angiographic fluoroscope for coiling of intracranial aneurysms. Neurosurgery. 2011;69:1131–8.
113. Schiemann M, Killmann R, Kleen M, Abolmaali N, Finney J, Vogl TJ. Vascular guide wire navigation with a magnetic guidance system: experimental results in a phantom. Radiology. 2004;232:475–81.
114. Chu JC, Hsi WC, Hubbard L, et al. Performance of magnetic field-guided navigation system for interventional neurosurgical and cardiac procedures. J Appl Clin Med Phys. 2005;6:143–9.
115. Seppenwoolde JH, Bartels LW, van der Weide R, Nijsen JF, van Het Schip AD, Bakker CJ. Fully MR-guided hepatic artery catheterization for selective drug delivery: a feasibility study in pigs. J Magn Reson Imaging. 2006;23:123–9.
116. Wacker FK, Hillenbrand C, Elgort DR, Zhang S, Duerk JL, Lewin JS. MR imaging-guided percutaneous angioplasty and stent placement in a swine model comparison of open- and closed-bore scanners. Acad Radiol. 2005;12:1085–8.
117. Wacker FK, Hillenbrand CM, Duerk JL, Lewin JS. MR-guided endovascular interventions: device visualization, tracking, navigation, clinical applications, and safety aspects. Magn Reson Imaging Clin N Am. 2005;13:431–9.

Part 2. Interventional Techniques

5. Intracranial Aneurysm Treatment

5.1.   Intracranial Aneurysm Embolization

Indications and Contraindications

Indications for the endovascular treatment of intracranial aneurysms are discussed in depth in Chap. 13.

General indications:
1) Aneurysmal subarachnoid haemorrhage.
2) Unruptured intracranial aneurysms
3) Size ≥2 mm
4) Poor surgical candidates
   i)   Elderly patients
   ii) Patients with significant medical problems
   iii) Patients requiring chronic systemic anticoagulation (i.e., patients with atrial fibrillation)
5) Posterior circulation aneurysms
6) Cavernous segment ICA aneurysms

Relative contraindications:
1) Vascular anatomy that is prohibitive (e.g., some giant, wide-necked aneurysms, exaggerated vessel tortuosity).
2) Significant atherosclerotic disease or other abnormalities affecting the parent vessel (e.g., significant atherosclerotic stenosis of the carotid bifurcation).
3) Coagulation disorders or heparin hypersensitivity.
4) Active bacterial infection (i.e., bacteremia at time of endovascular treatment).

Patient Preparation

Evaluation

1. History and physical.
2. Neurological exam.
3. Imaging
   1) Head CT and
   2) CTA, MRA, or catheter angiogram
      a) The authors of this handbook obtain a CTA in nearly every case, even if a catheter angiogram has already been done. A CTA can provide information that is complimentary to an angiogram, such as precise measurements, three dimensional views, imaging of intraluminal thrombus, and skull base imaging that can be useful, should the patient undergo craniotomy.
   3) Imaging considerations
      i)   Aneurysm location, size, shape, and neck size.
      ii) Parent vessel anatomy.
      iii) Presence or absence of intraluminal thrombus
      iv) Access vessel anatomy (e.g., dominant vs. hypoplastic vertebral artery or ACA, degree of tortuosity).
      v)   Presence or absence of atherosclerosis or fibromuscular dysplasia in the access vessel.

M.R. Harrigan, J.P. Deveikis, *Handbook of Cerebrovascular Disease*
and Neurointerventional Technique, DOI 10.1007/978-1-61779-946-4_5,
© Springer Science+Business Media New York 2013

Treatment Strategy

Prior to the case, preferably the previous day, the patient should be assessed and all the available imaging reviewed in preparation for the case. Decisions about overall strategy should be made ahead of time, to permit accurate device selection and smooth and efficient performance during the case. Plans should include:

1. Choice of access vessel
2. Endovascular technique (i.e., primary embolization vs. stent-assisted or balloon-assisted coiling vs. flow diversion)
3. Device types and sizes

Pre-procedure Preparation

1) Informed consent.
2) Two peripheral IVs.
3) Foley catheter.
4) NPO after midnight or 6 h prior to the procedure except for medications
5) Make sure that all devices that may be needed are available in the angio suite prior to the procedure.
6) Antiplatelet therapy.
   a) If stent-assisted coiling is planned, dual antiplatelet therapy is necessary. Antiplatelet therapy is also an option for balloon remodeling cases, and is recommended by some for all endovascular aneurysm treatment procedures.
   b) Do platelet function testing if desired (see Chap. 4).
7) Patients with subarachnoid haemorrhage:
8) Arterial line and central venous access are established prior to the procedure
9) If a ventriculostomy is present, the catheter must be attached to a monitor, to permit continuous ICP monitoring during the case.
   a) The ICP is an "early warning system" for aneurysm rupture or re-rupture during embolization.
   b) The ventriculostomy should be "on monitor" (and not "to drain"), if possible, during the entire procedure, to permit continuous monitoring. Open the drain only intermittently, if CSF drainage during the procedure is necessary.

Endovascular Technique

The technique of endovascular aneurysm treatment varies from case to case. The following is a general outline of the procedure used by the authors of this handbook for most patients. The case is divided into a vascular *access* phase, and an *intervention* phase. Access consists of placing a guide catheter in the internal carotid artery or vertebral artery. The intervention phase involves microcatheter treatment of the aneurysm.

Awake or Asleep?

Some operators prefer to use general anesthesia for aneurysm cases, whereas others prefer to do them with the patient awake. Each approach has advantages. Endovascular treatment with the patient awake permits continuous neurological monitoring, eliminates the risks of general anesthesia, can shorten the length of the case, and has been shown to be safe and feasible.[1,2] Doing the procedure with the patient awake is less practical in patients with reduced mental status and in those with small aneurysms (in which a small amount of patient motion can lead to aneurysm perforation). General anesthesia can eliminate patient mobility, allow the operator to focus on the procedure rather than on coaching and assessing the patient, be more palatable for anxious patients, and permit tight blood pressure control. The authors of this handbook prefer to use general anesthesia, except for cases in which medical issues place the patient at elevated risk with anesthesia (e.g., severe heart disease).

AWAKE
1. Throughout the case, the patient is reminded to stay completely still. The patient's head can be lightly taped to the head holder with a piece of plastic tape

across the forehead, to remind him or her to stay still. Place a piece of non-adherent Telfa™ dressing (Covidien, Mansfield, MA) between tape and skin to prevent skin irritation from the adhesive tape.

2. Sedation and analgesia are kept to a minimum to facilitate the patient's full cooperation.

ASLEEP

1) Strict attention to blood pressure control during anesthesia induction is necessary to minimize the risk of aneurysm rupture.

2) A radial arterial line is not necessary for blood pressure monitoring prior to induction in patients with unruptured aneurysms.

3) If arterial monitoring is felt to be necessary prior to induction, place a 7F femoral sheath while the patient is still awake. Placement of a femoral artery sheath is less uncomfortable than a radial artery line. A 7F sheath is large enough to permit passage of a 6F guide catheter, and still allow arterial line monitoring.

4) The anesthesiologist should report any abrupt changes in blood pressure or heart rate during the case, which can indicate intracranial haemorrhage.

Vascular Access Phase

See Chap. 4 for a general discussion of access techniques.

1) Place a 7F sheath in the femoral artery. A 7F sheath is large enough to permit transduction of an arterial line tracing when a 6F guide catheter is in place. Use an 8F sheath if use of 6F Cook Shuttle is anticipated.

2) Guide catheter selection
   a) The authors of this handbook prefer to use the Neuron™ Intracranial Access System (Penumbra, Inc., San Leandro, CA) for nearly all cases.
      (1) Neuron™ 0.053 in. guide catheter.
         (a) Use this catheter for most straightforward primary coiling cases.
      (2) Neuron™ 0.070 in. guide catheter
         (a) Use this catheter when balloon-remodeling is anticipated, or when high quality angiograms are necessary when the microcatheter is in position, since the larger lumen allows for easier injections of contrast.
      (3) Neuron™ MAX 0.088 in. guide catheter
         (a) The big lumen and availability of an inner dilator makes it essentially a long sheath (similar to a Shuttle® (Cook Inc., Bloomington, IN)). Ample lumen for use of multiple micro-catheters/balloons of almost any size.

3) Guide catheter access is obtained in the usual fashion (see Chap. 4).

4) Antithrombotic medication. Thromboembolic complications can occur during coiling, particularly when there is a slowing of flow in the parent vessel caused by the guide catheter. Prevention and management of these complications are reviewed extensively by Qureshi and colleagues.[3,4] The importance of routine prophylactic systemic anticoagulation during aneurysm coiling, however, is unclear. Systemic anticoagulation with IV heparin appears to carry relatively low risk in patients with unruptured aneurysms, and judicious use of heparin in patients with ruptured aneurysms also appears to be relatively low-risk, particularly as the drug can be rapidly reversed with IV or IA protamine.
   a) Unruptured aneurysms
      i) Use a loading dose of IV heparin (5,000 units or 70 units/kg)
   b) Ruptured aneurysms
      i) Controversial
      ii) Some operators withhold heparin until enough coils have been placed in the aneurysm to occlude the dome, which is where most aneurysms are thought to have ruptured, then give a full or partial loading dose of IV heparin (50–70 units/kg).
   c) Protamine on stand-by – *Critical*
      i) A syringe containing protamine, enough to reverse the total amount of heparin the patient has received, should be kept on the back table for easy access to the operator should haemorrhage occur during the case.
      ii) Dose of protamine required to reverse heparin: 10 mg protamine per 1,000 U heparin.

iii) The authors of this handbook routinely keep a sterile syringe containing 50 mg of protamine on the back table. The drug is infused into the guide catheter or sheath when intracranial haemorrhage occurs.

5) Other antithrombotic agents
   i) Antiplatelet agents. Some operators advocate routine pretreatment with aspirin and clopidogrel for patients with unruptured aneurysms. One study reported a diminished rate of thromboembolic complications in patients pretreated with antiplatelet agents.[5]

5.2. Aneurysm Treatment Phase

Preparations are made for coiling once the guide catheter is in position. A good "working view" must be obtained; several angiograms with injection of contrast through the guide catheter are usually necessary to find the optimal images. Alternatively, a 3-D angiogram can be done and the image of the aneurysm be rotated on the workstation monitor to obtain the ideal working view, and corresponding position of the x-ray tube. Ideally, the working view should be under high magnification and should demonstrate the aneurysm, parent vessels, and guide catheter clearly. It is important to keep the guide catheter in view on at least one projection (PA or lateral) during the whole case, to permit correction of the guide catheter should the catheter be pushed down (which is not uncommon) or become unstable during passage of the microcatheter. The working view should also permit the aneurysm dome and neck to be distinguished from the parent vessel (Fig. 5.1).

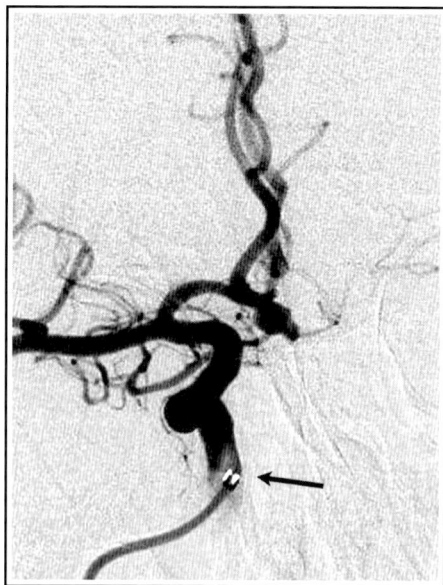

Fig. 5.1 Working view for coiling. The guide catheter (*arrow*) is in view, as are the aneurysm, aneurysm neck, and parent vessel.

Devices

1) Microcatheter selection
   a. The smallest catheter that will accommodate the coil size anticipated should be used in most cases for the following reasons:
      i) Small microcatheters are more likely to be soft and flexible near the tip, which will allow "paint-brushing," a back-and-forth movement of the tip during as the coil is inserted, permitting a more uniform distribution of the coils within the aneurysm.
      ii) Smaller microcatheters permit better guide catheter angiograms, particularly when smaller guide catheters (e.g., 5F) are employed.
      iii) The closer the match between the inner diameter of the microcatheter and the diameter of the coil, the less likely that buckling of the coil within the microcatheter will occur (e.g., a 10-system coil will work best in a 10-system microcatheter).
   b. Some situations call for larger and/or stiffer microcatheters.
      i) Large aneurysms, or aneurysms in which the use of 18-system coils, or Penumbra 400 coils, are planned.
   c. Two-tip marker microcatheters, rather than single-marker catheters, are necessary for aneurysm coiling. The two radio-opaque markers in microcatheters used in aneurysm coiling are always 3 cm apart to align with the marker on the coil pusher wire – this feature can also be used for calibration and measurements.
   d. Preferred microcatheters for most cases:
      i) Excelsior® SL-10 (Stryker Neurovascular, Fremont, CA)
         1. Accommodates both 0.010 in. and 0.014 in. microwires.
         2. Can be used for 10-system and 14-system coils.
      ii) Echelon 10 (ev3 Neurovascular, Irvine, CA).
         1. The relatively small proximal outer diameter of 2.1F (versus 2.4F for the Excelsior® SL-10), permits better guide catheter angiograms when a 5F guide catheter is used.
         2. Able to accommodate 18-system coils (although it's a tight fit).
         3. Very stable for a 10-size system.
      iii) Excelsior® 1018® (Stryker Neurovascular, Fremont, CA)
         1. Accommodates both 10-system and 18-system coils
      iv) Marksman™ (ev3 Neurovascular, Irvine, CA)
         1. Useful for Neuroform® EZ (Stryker Neurovascular, Fremont, CA) stent deployment.
      v) Headway® (Microvention/Terumo, Tustin, CA)
         1. Many options: the Headway 17 size has regular, extra-support and advanced styles for increasing stiffness and stability.
         2. The Headway® 21 version can be used for the Enterprise™ Vascular Reconstruction System (Codman Neurovascular, Raynham, MA).
         3. The Headway® 27 can be used to deploy Neuroform® EZ (Stryker Neurovascular, Fremont, CA) or Pipeline™ Embolization Device (ev3 Neurovascular, Irvine, CA)
      vi) Prowler® Select™ Plus (Codman Neurovascular, Raynham, MA)
         1. Intended for use with the Enterprise™ Vascular Reconstruction System (Codman Neurovascular, Raynham, MA)
      vii) PX 400™ (Penumbra, Inc., Alameda, CA)
         1. Has a 0.025 in. internal lumen to accommodate the larger Penumbra Coil 400™ (Penumbra, Inc., Alameda, CA)
   e. Microcatheter shaping. Microcatheters come in several prepared shapes (straight, 45°, 90°, "J" and "S"). Steam shaping permits tailoring of the microcatheter shape to fit the target. Steam shaping is particularly useful for paraclinoid aneurysms (Fig. 5.2).[6]
      i) Steam shaping technique
         1. Shape the wire mandrel into the desired shape, with an exaggerated degree of curvature (as the microcatheter will recoil to some degree after steam-shaping).
         2. Hold over steam for 10 s.
         3. Cool in sterile water and remove mandrel.
         4. Non-braided and fiber-braided (e.g., Excelsior®) microcatheters are more likely to retain their shape after steam shaping

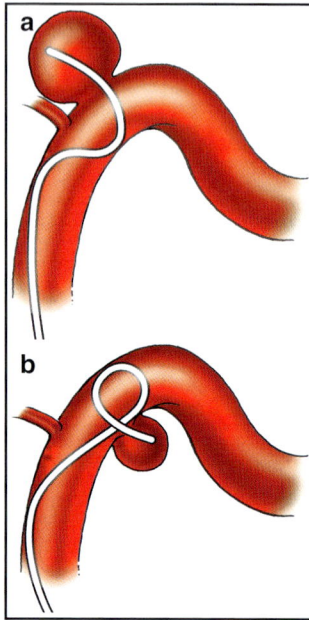

Fig. 5.2 Microcatheter shapes for paraclinoid aneurysms. An "S" shaped microcatheter often works best for superiorly directed aneurysms (**a**). A pigtail shape can be helpful with superior hypophyseal aneurysms (**b**) (From Kwon et al. [6], with permission).

than metal coil-braided (e.g., Prowler® and Echelon™) microcatheters.[7]

5. Factory preshaped catheters retain their shape better than steam-shaped catheters.

2) Microwires

    a. Preferred microwires for most cases:

        i) Synchro®-14 0.014 in. (Stryker, Fremont, CA)

            1. Very soft, flexible distal tip, good for navigation into small aneurysms or through difficult anatomy.

            2. "Supreme torque control."

        ii) Neuroscout®-14 0.014 in. (Codman, Raynham, MA)

            1. Very soft, flexible distal tip, good for navigation into small aneurysms or through difficult anatomy.

            2. "Supreme torque control." Similar to Synchro®

            3. Better tip-shape retention.

        iii) Transend™ EX 0.014 in. Floppy tip (Stryker, Fremont, CA)

            1. Smooth, non-abrasive tip.

            2. Good torque control.

        iv) Transend™ EX 0.014 in. Platinum tip (Stryker, Fremont, CA)

            1. Superior torque control, compared to other microwires.

            2. Heightened radiopacity makes the tip easy to see on fluoroscopy.

        v) Headliner™ J-tip 0.012 in. (Microvention/Terumo, Tustin, CA)

            1. J-tip is atraumatic to the vessel walls.

            2. Best suited for uncomplicated vessel anatomy (tends to follow the straightest vessel).

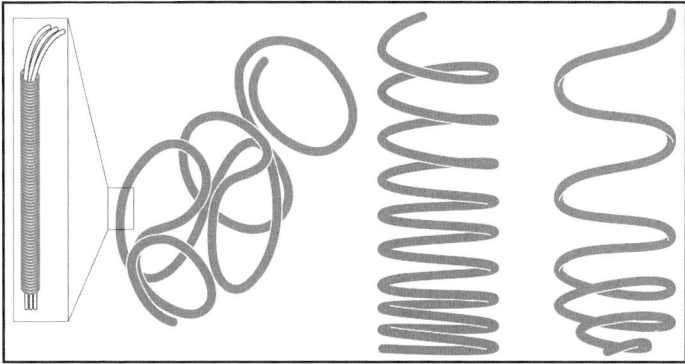

Fig. 5.3 Basic coil shapes. Three-dimensional framing coil (*left*), standard helical filling coil (*middle*), and two-diameter soft "finishing coil" (*right*). Insert demonstrates inner filament of coil surrounded by tightly wound fine platinum wire.

      vi) Traxcess™ 0.014 in. (Microvention/Terumo, Tustin, CA)
         1. Wire tapers to 0.012 in. distally.
         2. Has available docking wire that adds 100 cm to the wire to make it exchange-length.

3) Coils
   a. A dizzying array of coils is on the market, varying in size, shape, design, stiffness, presence or absence of "bioactive" material, and detachment systems. Firm, scientific data to support one coil over another is nearly nonexistent (although the device companies would prefer to have us believe otherwise). Very good results have been obtained with all the coils. The single most important principle of coil selection is for the operator to use coil system with which he or she is most experienced and comfortable.
   b. *Fundamentals of detachable coil design*
      i) A coil consists of a fine platinum thread tightly looped around a thicker platinum wire. The coil is connected to a "pusher wire;" the attachment site is the location of detachment mechanism, which may be electrolytic, thermal, mechanical, or hydraulic in design. The coil and pusher wire come from the manufacturer in a slim plastic delivery sheath; the sheath is placed within the hub of the RHV, and the coil and pusher wire are threaded together into the microcatheter. The operator controls the pusher wire and the coil together prior to detachment, which allows sequential advancement and withdrawal of the coil, as necessary, to deploy the coil within the aneurysm in the desired configuration. The coil is designed to assume one of a number of shapes as it is pushed out of the microcatheter (Fig. 5.3).
   c. *Framing* vs. *filling* vs. *finishing* coils
      i) Framing coils. These three-dimensional coils are designed to "frame" the aneurysm; that is, these coils are meant to "ovalize" or "sphericize" the aneurysm with gentle outward radial force to permit packing with two-dimensional coils. Ideally, some parts, or strands, of the three-dimensional coil will also extend across the neck of the aneurysm, helping to narrow the effective neck area and facilitate further coil deposition. The standard design consists of a large omega followed by a small omega, followed by a large omega, and so forth.
         1. Examples: Microsphere® coils; Target® 360 coils; Orbit Galaxy™ complex coils
      ii) Filling coils. Intended to occupy space within the aneurysm after framing, these coils usually have a helical shape and are of intermediate stiffness.
         1. Examples: Helipaq® coils; Target® 360 soft; Orbit Galaxy™ fill

iii) Finishing coils. The softest coils are designed for final packing of the aneurysm and "finishing off" of the neck.
  1. Examples: Deltapaq® coils and Deltaplush® coils; Target® Ultra coils; Orbit Galaxy™ Xtrasoft coils; Microplex™ HyperSoft coils.
d. 10-system vs. 18-system.
  i) The nomenclature indicating the two size categories of coils originated with the first microcatheters used for GDC coils, the Tracker-10 and the Tracker 18 from the original Target Therapeutics (now Stryker Neurovascular Fremont, CA), designed specifically to accommodate GDC-10 coils and GDC-18 coils, respectively. The actual diameter of GDC-10 coils is 0.008 in. and for GDC-18 coils is 0.016 in.. 10-system coils are adequate for most aneurysms. 18-system coils are typically thicker and stiffer than 10-system coils, reminiscent of rebar (Fig. 5.4), and are appropriate for framing larger, unruptured aneurysms. An exception is the Orbit-Galaxy system coil (Codman Neurovascular, Raynham, MA), which is 0.012 in. but with softness that is comparable to GDC-10 coils. The Cashmere® coils (Codman Neurovascular, Raynham, MA) are 0.015 in. and quite soft as well.

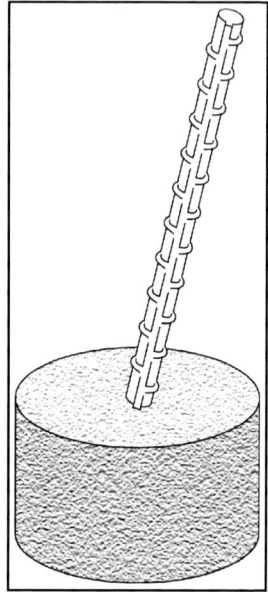

Fig. 5.4 Rebar. The astute operator will be reminded of rebar, which are reinforcing steel bars inside poured concrete, when using 18-system coils.

  ii) Even larger than an 18 coil is the Penumbra Coil 400™ (Penumbra Inc., Alameda, CA) which has a 0.020 diameter and consequently has a greater filling volume (400% of the volume of 10-system coils). These coils surprisingly have softness comparable to 10-system coils, but require a much larger microcatheter lumen (0.025 in.) for delivery.
e. Platinum vs. "augmented" coils.
  i) Continuing observations of aneurysm recanalization after treatment with bare platinum coils lead to the introduction of coils containing materials meant to enhance fibrosis within the aneurysm and decrease the chance of recanalization. Several "augmented" coil systems are on the market presently; some contain polyglycolic-polylactic acid (PGLA), a biopolymer similar to absorbable suture material. The polymer degrades by hydrolysis to glycolic acid and lactic acid, which promote fibrocellular proliferation. Matrix2™ (Stryker Neurovascular, Fremont, CA) coils consist of platinum coils covered by PGLA. Matrix coils have been found to accelerate aneurysm fibrosis and neointima formation in animals, compared to bare platinum coils.[8] Cerecyte™ (Codman Neurovascular, Raynham, MA) and Nexus (ev3, Irvine, CA) also incorporate PGLA. The HydroCoil® system (MicroVention/Terumo, Tustin, CA) consists of platinum coils coated with an expandable hydrogel (see below).
    1. *Note: Two randomized, multicenter industry-sponsored trials (the Cerecyte trial and the Matrix And Platinum Science.MAPS) failed to show a benefit with PGLA-treated coils.*

2. *The HELPS trial showed improved recanalization rates with the hydrogel coils compared to bare platinum, but differences in long term outcome are less certain.*
  f. Stretch resistance.
     i) Stretching of a coil occurs when the distal end of the coil become trapped, or entangled, in the aneurysm and the outer coil wire then unravels when the coil is withdrawn under tension. Coil stretching is problematic, because control over the coil is lost, and the entire coil can no longer be fully deployed into the aneurysm or withdrawn. A design modification to prevent this was to place a reinforcing filament (usually nylon) within the coil, to resist stretching. Most currently available coil lines have "stretch-resistant" models. *Stretch-resistance does not equal stretch-proof; stretching, although less likely, is still possible with stretch-resistant coils.*
  g. Alternative coil designs
     i) "Complex shape" (3D, spherical, or random loops) These coils produce higher packing densities with complex coil shapes in contrast to simple helical shapes.[9]
     ii) Target® and GDC®-360° (Stryker Neurovascular, Fremont, CA). Coil design with a larger number of random "breaks" than most other coils, allowing it to conform to multiple lobes in complex aneurysms.
     iii) Deltapaq™ (Codman Neurovascular, Raynham, MA). A simple helical shape but can form more random loops in a confined space. Reported to produce higher packing densities compared to other coils.[10]
     iv) HydroCoil® (MicroVention/Terumo, Tustin, CA). Platinum coil with a hydrogel coating that swells when it contacts blood. The hydrogel provides a higher filling volume than bare platinum coils by filling the interstices of the coil mass.[11] For instance, a "HydroCoil® 10" coil has five times the volume of a bare platinum 10 coil of the same length when fully expanded.
     v) Galaxy coils (Codman Neurovascular, Raynham, MA). Coils with a slightly greater platinum wire diameter (0.012 in. compared to 0.010 in.), presumably leading to a higher packing density.[12]
     vi) Presidio™ coils (Codman Neurovascular, Raynham, MA). Framing coils that are about double the length of other 3-D coils, which presumably are more stable than regular 3-D coils.
     vii) Axium™ Detachable Coil System (ev3, Irvine, CA). Detachment system is mechanical "hooking/unhooking" mechanism
     viii) Penumbra Coil 400™ (Penumbra Inc., Alameda, CA). Very large, but soft platinum coils with 0.020 in. wire diameter. This leads to quadrupling the packing density compared to standard 10-system coils. (Hence the "400")
4) Preferred coils for most cases:
  a. Codman Micrus and Orbit Galaxy™ systems
  b. ev3 Axium™ system
  c. For larger aneurysms: Penumbra Coil 400™

Electrolytic Coil Detachment and the Heart
The GDC coil detachment system employed an electrical current that creates an electrical field in the patient's body. ECG perturbations have been observed during detachment with the GDC SynerG System, both at 1 mA and 2 mA power supply settings. These changes seem to occur more frequently at 2 mA and towards the end of the procedure. These observations initially raised concern that patients with or without cardiac pacemakers might be at risk for arrhythmias, but bench testing by the manufacturers and extensive clinical experience showed that the electrical fields generated did not affect cardiac electrophysiology. However, there is a theoretical risk that automatic defibrillators implanted in patients may sense the electrical activity generated during detachment, and interpret the activity as a cardiac arrhythmia, producing inadvertent defibrillator activation. Although the authors of this handbook have used GDC coils in patients with pacemakers and defibrillators without incident, they prefer to use non-electrical coil detachment systems, such as the Codman Galaxy system in these patients.

Aneurysm Access Technique

1. Navigate the microcatheter under roadmap guidance over the microwire into position within the parent vessel adjacent to the aneurysm.
2. For an end-artery aneurysm (e.g., basilar apex aneurysms), the microwire can usually be carefully advanced directly into the aneurysm, followed by the microcatheter.
3. For sidewall aneurysms (e.g., ophthalmic segment ICA aneurysms and SCA aneurysms), the microwire and microcatheter can sometimes be advanced directly into the aneurysm. Alternatively, if a shaped microcatheter is being used, the aneurysm can be accessed by guiding the microwire and microcatheter tip beyond the aneurysm neck. The microwire is pulled into the microcatheter, and the microcatheter is slowly pulled back, allowing the tip to flip into the aneurysm (Fig. 5.5).
4. The ideal position of the catheter tip within the aneurysm depends on the phase of the procedure (Fig. 5.6). When initially framing the aneurysm using a 3D-type coil, it is often best to have the tip of the microcatheter at the neck of the aneurysm to allow the coil to assume its spherical shape, to keep the coil from protruding into the parent artery, and to maximize the number of loops across the neck. Once the aneurysm is nicely framed, the microcatheter tip is placed in the center of the aneurysm, two thirds of the way to the top of the dome for added stability during the bulk of the filling phase of the procedure. During the finishing phase, it may be necessary to reposition the microcatheter several times to fill residual pockets within the aneurysm.
5. Once the microcatheter tip is positioned within the aneurysm, advance and withdraw the microwire several times for most of the distance between the guide catheter and aneurysm. This maneuver helps to straighten out any remaining redundancy in the microcatheter, eliminating "potential energy" in the microcatheter that may cause it to leap forward unexpectedly during coiling.
6. When guide catheter angiograms are done, the RHV should be tightened around the microcatheter, securing it to prevent the microcatheter from being carried forward by the contrast as it is injected.

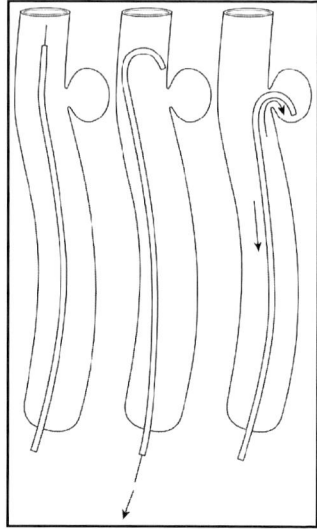

Fig. 5.5 Sidewall aneurysm technique. Technique for accessing side-wall aneurysms with a J-shaped microcatheter. Advance the microcatheter and microwire past the aneurysm neck (*left*). Withdraw the microwire several millimeters into the microcatheter (*middle*), and gently pull the microcatheter back until the tip flips into the aneurysm (*right*).

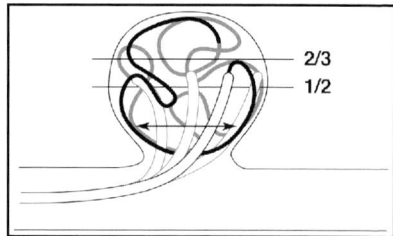

Fig. 5.6 Optimal microcatheter position for most aneurysms. Position the microcatheter tip between half-way and two-thirds of the way into the aneurysm dome. The tip of the microcatheter will "paintbrush" (i.e., sway back and forth) as the coil loops are deployed.

7. Occasionally, the anatomy of the aneurysm and the surrounding vessels (e.g., some SCA aneurysms) make it difficult to confirm that the microcatheter tip is positioned within the aneurysm. A microcatheter angiogram can clarify the position of the microcatheter and also delineate the size and configuration of the aneurysm neck.
   (a) A 1 mL syringe is filled with 100% contrast and connected directly to the microcatheter hub after removal of the RHV for the angiogram.
   (b) Obviously, "aneurysm-o-grams" should be undertaken with caution in patients with subarachnoid haemorrhage.

Coiling Technique

1. Place the framing coils once the microcatheter tip is in a stable position. The first 3-D coil should be equal or slightly larger than the diameter of the aneurysm dome. A slightly larger 3-D coil may "ovalize" the aneurysm and improve the effective dome-to-neck ratio.
2. Gentle forward and backward movement of the microcatheter during framing of the aneurysm will distribute the loops of the coil within the aneurysm in a more controlled fashion.
   (a) "Paintbrushing," i.e., the side-to-side motion of the microcatheter tip, is an indication that the microcatheter tip is in a good position, and not wedged between other coils, or between the coil mass and the dome of the aneurysm.
   (b) Care must be taken to avoid placing any parts of a new coil between the existing coil mass and the dome of the aneurysm, as this can tear the aneurysm wall.
3. After each coil is deployed, prior to detachment, a guide catheter angiogram is done to check for:
   (a) Coil position
   (b) Thrombus within the parent vessel
   (c) Perforation (i.e., contrast extravasation)
   (d) Flow in adjacent vessels and/or vessel drop-out (e.g., when coiling a basilar apex aneurysm, flow in both PCAs) should be monitored, as developing asymmetry in the filling of these vessels may be the first indication of parent artery compromise by coil or clot.
4. The coil is detached according to the manufacturer's instructions for use.
5. After detachment, the pusher wire is slowly withdrawn under fluoroscopic visualization, to ensure that the coil has successfully detached.
6. If the coil pulls back into the catheter, the coil has not detached. Carefully reinsert it and attempt to detach again until it works.
7. In larger aneurysms, several 3-D coils can be placed within the aneurysm, each one smaller than the previous one (the "Russian Doll" technique).
8. After several coils are deployed, each additional coil becomes more difficult to see among the coils already in place. A *negative roadmap* can enable visualization of a coil as it is placed among other coils.
   (a) To make a negative roadmap, the roadmap function is activated but no contrast is injected. This creates a blank white screen; during subsequent fluoroscopy, the coil being deployed will stand out as a black image.
9. Microcatheter control during coiling:
   (a) Memorize the position of the proximal marker in relation to skull landmarks on fluoroscopy (Fig. 5.7).
   When a negative roadmap is used, a "white dot" will appear on the screen when the proximal marker changes position.
   (b) When advancing the microcatheter, avoid applying enough force to cause "buckling" of the microcatheter in the parent vessel. Buckling of the microcatheter indicates that a potentially hazardous amount of force is being applied to the microcatheter that could cause the tip to jump forward and puncture the aneurysm.
10. After one or more 3-D coils are deployed to frame the aneurysm, filling coils are deployed, and then, toward the end of the procedure, finishing coils are placed.
11. Decisions about when to switch from 3-D to filling coils, and then to finishing coils, depend on several factors, such as the amount of resistance encountered when advancing each coil, the appearance of the coil mass on fluoroscopy, and the position and stability of the microcatheter. Generally, any given type of coil should be used until resistance to coil advancement begins to rise. An increase in resistance should prompt a change to a coil with smaller dimensions, or to a softer type of coil.

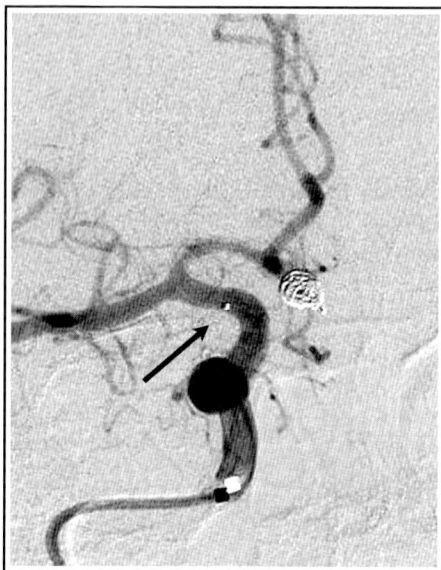

Fig. 5.7 Proximal marker position. The proximal microcatheter marker (*arrow*) is within the ICA. Attention to the proximal marker and its relationship to skull landmarks on fluoroscopy can provide information about the location of the tip of the microcatheter inside the aneurysm.

12. The goal is to maximize packing of the aneurysm, i.e., coiling of the aneurysm should proceed until the amount of resistance encountered with additional coils becomes prohibitive.
    (a) Packing density (i.e., the total length of coil material placed in the aneurysm per unit of volume) is inversely related to the risk of aneurysm recurrence.[13–15]
        i. However, a recent study has shown that differences in packing density affect hemodynamics in the aneurysm only in relatively loosely packed aneurysms.[16]
        ii. Once packing density approaches 30%, additional coils may provide little additional benefit in recurrence risk, and this is borne out in some clinical series.[17]
13. Occasionally, complex multilobed aneurysms require the use of more than one shaped microcatheter. Depending on the anatomy of the aneurysm, a microcatheter of one shape can be used to coil one lobe of the aneurysm, and a second microcatheter can be used for the other lobe.
14. When coiling is complete, high magnification PA and lateral angiograms should be obtained to confirm that the coiling is complete, prior to removal of the microcatheter.
15. Remove the microcatheter by advancing a microwire into the distal part of the microcatheter to straighten out the microcatheter and prevent it from hooking on coil loops as it is removed from the aneurysm. The wire can also ensure that a tail of the coil is not protruding into the microcatheter, which can pull the coil out of the aneurysm when the catheter is withdrawn. The microcatheter and microwire are then withdrawn from the aneurysm together.
16. Final PA and lateral intracranial angiograms are done to check for vessel dropout and other abnormalities.
17. Withdraw the guide catheter into the proximal part of the CCA or vertebral artery and do a final angiogram to check for vessel dissection.

Hydrocoil® Tips

1. Hydrocoil® technique:
   a. In many cases it is best to first frame the aneurysm with at least one 3-D coil that is bare platinum or one with thinner hydrogel coating such as the Hydroframe® then use the standard Hydrocoils® to fill in the basket.
   b. Hydrocoils® come with the self-contained electrolytic V-Trac® system, which easily attaches to the end of the pusher wire during detachment. It is quicker and more reliable than most detachment systems.
   c. These coils are stiffer and harder to insert than bare platinum, so choose a coil with a smaller diameter loop and shorter length than for a similar platinum coil.
   d. Hydrocoils® come in different wire thicknesses, so use a microcatheter with a properly sized internal lumen. A Hydrocoil® 10 requires at least 0.015 in. lumen, Hydrocoil® 14 requires 0.019 in. lumen, and Hydrocoil® 18 requires 0.021 in. lumen.
   e. The hydrogel softens with heat, so it can be helpful to briefly steam the coil immediately before insertion to soften it and allow the coil to take its helical shape.
   f. Do not allow the coil to contact blood or blood-stained saline, prior to insertion. This can start the swelling process.
   g. Insert the Hydrocoil® into the microcatheter and advance it into the aneurysm.
   h. As soon as even a small length of the coil begins to exit the microcatheter, start a timer. After about 5 min the coil will have swollen so much that it can no longer be pulled back through the microcatheter. Working time may be a little longer if the microcatheter has a big internal lumen.
   i. Even though working time is limited, be careful when advancing the relatively stiff Hydrocoil® into the aneurysm. Slow insertion can promote softening of the hydrogel due to the patient's body heat. This allows the coil to more easily conform to the available space in the aneurysm.
   j. Detach the Hydrocoil® when it is in good position, with no encroachment on the parent artery, as confirmed by an angiographic run or roadmap.
   k. If the Hydrocoil® must be removed prior to detachment, be very careful. Resistance is an indication that a significant amount of coil swelling has occurred. If the Hydrocoil® binds in the microcatheter, it may detach if pulled back against resistance.
   l. If the swollen Hydrocoil® binds in the microcatheter, the only way to remove it is to withdraw the coil and microcatheter together. Do not stretch the coil or dislodge the previously placed coils from the aneurysm.
   m. Avoid problems by not advancing the Hydrocoil® against resistance and using multiple shorter coils rather than fewer longer coils.
   n. After fairly tight packing of the aneurysm with Hydrocoils® is obtained, fill the remaining spaces with the softer Hydrosoft™ coils that have a thin hydrogel coating or bare platinum Microplex™ Hypersoft coils (MicroVention/Terumo, Tustin, CA) or other soft, stretch resistant finishing coils.
2. Consider prophylactic dexamethasone therapy and careful clinical monitoring, especially for aneurysms larger than 10 mm in diameter. Chemical meningitis[18] and hydrocephalus[19] have been reported after use of these coils.

Penumbra Coil 400™ Tips

1. Due to the larger catheter used to deliver these coils, they are useful mainly for larger aneurysms, especially those ≥6 mm.
2. The large delivery microcatheter cannot easily be advanced through stent, making stent-assisted coiling problematic. The jailing technique can be used with the Penumbra coiling system (see below).
3. Penumbra coil technique
   a) Decide on a catheter shape to optimize positioning of the microcatheter. The PX 400™ (Penumbra, Inc., Alameda, CA) comes in preshaped 45, 90, or J-shapes, or one can steam shape a more complex curve.

b) Advance the PX 400™ (Penumbra, Inc., Alameda, CA) over a microwire to the aneurysm. One must use a fairly robust wire, especially in tortuous vessels, but for most cases a 0.016 Headliner™ (Terumo/Microvention, Tustin, CA) is adequate.
c) The catheter tip *must* be placed in the center of the aneurysm.
 i) Microcatheter positioning is very important with this system since the catheter does not readily move or "paintbrush" as coils are placed, making it harder to uniformly distribute the coils throughout the aneurysm.
 ii) Avoid positioning the micocatheter tip along the wall of the aneurysm, since coil loops may compartmentalize in this region and there may be a risk of putting too much stress on that wall of the aneurysm.
d) Carefully insert the first complex-shaped coil sized to, or slightly smaller than the dimensions of the aneurysm. If it is a complex shaped aneurysm, select the size of the coils by extrapolating between the largest and smallest diameter of the aneurysm.
e) As with any coil, it should be carefully positioned in the aneurysm using biplane roadmapping, and positioning checked prior to detachment with a follow-up arteriogram to ensure there is no encroachment on the parent artery.
f) At least the first one or two coils should be the Penumbra Complex Standard (i.e. stiffer) coil design, if possible, to provide a stable basket to deposit the rest of the coils.
g) Detach the coil by attaching the Penumbra coil detachment handle and flicking the switch according to manufacturer's instructions.
 i) Ensure that the coil pusher wire is not pushed, pulled or rotated while manipulating the detachment handle.
h) Once the aneurysm has been framed with a stable basket of coils, fill it with softer Penumbra Complex Soft coils or the amorphous "J" coils.
i) The microcatheter may pull back toward the neck as the aneurysm fills with coils. Ensure it does not pull all the way out of the aneurysm, since it can be tricky to re-enter the coil mass with the big PX 400 catheter.
j) Finish the coiling with one or two helical Penumbra Curved Extrasoft coils.
 i) Do not attempt to use the PX 400 catheter to finish coiling the aneurysm using other manufacturer's coils, especially 10-sized coils. The huge lumen of the catheter will allow smaller coils to fold up on themselves and become stuck or stretched in the catheter.
k) It takes surprisingly few coils to obtain tight packing of the aneurysm because of the large diameter of the Penumbra 400 coils.
 i) The need for fewer coils per case reduces procedure time.
 ii) Whether the larger coils and potentially higher packing densities improves long-term occlusion rates remains to be seen.

Steerable Microcatheter Aneurysm Coiling Tips

Although no steerable microcatheter is currently commercially available in the U.S., the Plato™ Microcath steerable microcatheter (Scientia Vascular, Reno, NV) is presently available in Europe. Steerable microcatheters behave differently than regular ones. See Chap. 4 for a general discussion of steerable microcatheter technique. The following are tips for coiling aneurysms using steerable microcatheters:
1) When nearing the target, slow down, remove the slack in the microcatheter and microwire, and make smaller forward pushing and rotating movements to avoid jumping into (or through) the aneurysm.
2) Position the microcatheter tip in the proximal half of the aneurysm away from the dome. This minimizes the risk of puncturing dome with the catheter. Steerable microcatheters are a great deal more stable than regular microcatheters, so one deep catheter placement, to maintain position during coiling, is less important.
3) For stent-assisted coiling, the curve of the microcatheter can be used to direct a soft-tip microwire through the desired area of the stent and into the aneurysm. The microcatheter is then gently pushed and rotated back-and-forth, to wriggle it across the stent and into the aneurysm.

4) The steerable microcatheter can be gently rotated to distribute loops of coils throughout the aneurysm.
5) If the microcatheter becomes displaced from the desired location in the aneurysm, rotate it back into position without a microwire. Use gentle forward and rotating movements, and always keep an eye on what is happening to the catheter in the parent artery. Steerable microcatheters can loop backwards in the cervical region when they are manipulated without a microwire.
6) When nearing the end of coiling the aneurysm, the microcatheter can be turned to pack areas still patent with small finishing coils.

Did You Know?
Coiling of aneurysms with a branch arising from the dome may be okay. In a study of nine patients in whom an aneurysm with a branch arising from the dome underwent coiling, the branch was preserved in seven cases and no patients had any known thromboembolic complications [20]

Onyx®

Onyx® (ev3, Irvine, CA) is an embolic agent that is supplied by the manufacturer in liquid form, dissolved in the organic solvent, dimethyl sulfoxide (DMSO). Onyx®, an ethylene vinyl alcohol copolymer, is infused through a microcatheter into an aqueous environment; the DMSO diffuses outward into the surrounding tissue, allowing the material to precipitate into a spongy, space-occupying cast. The primary advantage of Onyx® over other polymer embolic agents, such as n-butyl cyanoacrylate (NBCA), is that it is non-adhesive and carries a lower risk of binding to the microcatheter or other devices. Onyx® is FDA-approved for embolization of intracranial AVMs. Onyx® HD-500 embolization for the treatment of intracranial aneurysms is under a Humanitarian Device Exemption; it can only be used under a protocol approved by each institution's Investigational Review Board (IRB). Onyx® embolization of aneurysms requires balloon-assistance technique, to permit infusion of the material into the aneurysm without embolization into the distal circulation. All devices must be compatible with DMSO. Onyx® comes in three concentrations:

1. Onyx®-18 (6%) – for AVM nidus
2. Onyx®-34 (8%) (more viscous) – for direct AV fistulas
3. Onyx® HD (20%) (the most viscous) – for aneurysms

Onyx® Technique

1. Prior to the case, the patient should be placed on a combination antiplatelet regimen (aspirin, 325 mg PO daily, and clopidogrel, 75 mg PO daily for ≥3 days).
2. The Onyx must be placed in a warmer at 70°C for 5 min then placed on an automated shaker for 20 min, then rewarmed for an additional 5 min.
3. Systemic heparinization is critical.
4. Guide catheter: Must be large enough to accommodate a balloon catheter and a microcatheter – use a 6F guide catheter or larger.
5. Place a deflated compliant DMSO-compatible balloon (Hyperglide™, ev3 Neurovascular, Irvine, CA) in the parent vessel adjacent to the aneurysm.
6. Navigate a DMSO-compatible microcatheter (Rebar®, ev3 Neurovascular, Irvine, CA) into the aneurysm.
   a. Position the tip in the upper one-third of the aneurysm dome.
   b. Avoid J-shaped catheters or looping the catheter around the dome of the aneurysm. A catheter curving back over itself may be difficult to retrieve when encased in Onyx.
7. Inflate the balloon and do a gentle microcatheter angiogram to confirm that the balloon adequately seals over the aneurysm neck.
   a. Record the inflation volume required to occlude the vessel. This volume will be used later for each balloon inflation.

8. Deflate the balloon, irrigate the microcatheter with heparinized saline and then prime it with DMSO at a rate no greater than 0.30 mL per minute with a volume to match the microcatheter dead space (Rebar-14 dead space: 0.20 mL).

9. Fill a Cadence Precision Injector syringe (ev3, Irvine, CA) with Onyx and attach it to the hub of the microcatheter. This syringe permits controlled injection of small, precise volumes. When the safety "Quick-stop" is engaged, each rotation of the threaded syringe handle creates a tactile "click" and delivers 0.015 mL. Other DMSO-compatible 1 mL syringes may be used.

10. Inject the Onyx under fluoroscopic observation at a rate of about 0.1 mL per minute or slower to fill the catheter lumen. Inject no more than the dead-space of the catheter (0.20 mL for Rebar-14).

11. Wait 1 min to allow DMSO to wash out of the aneurysm, then reinflate the balloon and begin slowly injecting Onyx into the aneurysm.

12. *Always* inject no faster than 0.1 mL per minute and *always* follow the injection on fluoroscopy.

13. The initial injections of Onyx should focus on creating a kernel of Onyx around the microcatheter tip; further injection should grow the kernel to fill the aneurysm lumen. This will develop a cohesive mass of Onyx that will not fragment and embolize when the balloon is deflated.

14. Continue the injection and pause after each incremental volume of approximately 0.2–0.3 mL. Wait 3 min to allow the material to solidify and then temporarily deflate the balloon.
    a. Intermittent deflations of the balloon are necessary to prevent too great a volume of Onyx, blood, and DMSO to accumulate in the aneurysm while the balloon is inflated, and also to permit reperfusion of affected circulation.
    b. Leave the balloon deflated for 2 min, then re-inflate and continue Onyx injection.
    c. Multiple sequential re-inflations and injections may be necessary.
    d. The routine is: inject Onyx (balloon inflated) for 2 min, wait (balloon inflated) for 3 min, wait (balloon deflated) for 2 min, then repeat.
    e. Do not adjust the microcatheter position at all during the embolization.
    f. Periodic remasking of the roadmap makes it easier to see each new Onyx injection within the developing ball of Onyx in the aneurysm.

15. *Important*: Do not pause the injections for more than about 2 min at a time to avoid polymerization of the Onyx material within the microcatheter. Polymerization of Onyx within the microcatheter can cause it to rupture with additional injections.
    a. *Stop whenever there is any question that the microcatheter is clogged.* Remove the microcatheter and try a new one.

16. Do periodic guide catheter angiograms to monitor progress.

17. Fill the aneurysm down to the neck, but take care toward the final injections around the neck to avoid injecting Onyx around the periphery of the balloon. Creating a cast of Onyx around the periphery of the parent artery can cause delayed thrombosis of the vessel.

18. When the embolization is completed, deflate the balloon and decompress the microcatheter by aspirating 0.2 mL; this prevents dribbling of Onyx material during the removal of the microcatheter.

19. Allow 10 min to elapse before removing the microcatheter to permit the Onyx to set within the aneurysm.

20. To remove the microcatheter, deflate the balloon a final time to 75% of occlusion volume to stabilize the Onyx mass as the microcatheter is withdrawn. Loosen the RHV, take up the slack in the microcatheter and apply some gentle tension to the microcatheter. A quick wrist snap can then dislodge the catheter from the aneurysm.

21. The patient should be kept on an antiplatelet regimen for at least 1 month after the procedure.

Neucrylate™ AN

Neucrylate™ AN (Valor Medical, San Diego, CA) is a liquid 1-Hexyl n-cyano-acrylate formulated for aneurysm treatment that polymerizes when it contacts blood. It comes mixed with gold particles to make it radio-opaque. Neucrylate™, is infused through a microcatheter during temporary balloon inflation at the aneurysm neck, similar to the technique for Onyx® (ev3 Neurovascular, Irvine, CA). The advantage over Onyx® embolization of aneurysms is that the injection and polymerization are much faster. Early reports indicate approximately 1 min for injection plus polymerization. An initial study of 12 patients with aneurysms that were felt to be suboptimal for either clipping or coiling were treated with Neucrylate™ and 75% achieved initial occlusion of over 90% of the aneurysm. There were 33% neurological complications and 55% recurrence at 6 months in that study, although it should be remembered that these were difficult aneurysms. The agent received CE mark approval in May 2011. As of the writing of this edition it has not yet received FDA approval.

Neucrylate™ Technique

1. Although initially used without antiplatelet agents, it may be prudent to place the patient on a combination antiplatelet regimen (aspirin 325 mg PO daily and clopidogrel, 75 mg PO daily for ≥3 days).
2. Have several vials of Neucrylate available.
3. Systemic heparinization is critical.
4. Guide catheter: Must be large enough to accommodate a balloon catheter and a microcatheter – use a 6F guide catheter or larger.
5. Place a deflated compliant balloon (Hyperglide™ or Hyperform™, ev3 Neurovascular, Irvine, CA) in the parent vessel adjacent to the aneurysm.
6. Navigate a microcatheter (Excelsior® SL-10, Stryker Neurovascular, Fremont, CA) into the aneurysm.
   a. Position the tip in the mid-portion of the aneurysm dome.
   b. Avoid J-shaped catheters or looping the catheter around the dome of the aneurysm. A catheter curving back over itself may be difficult to retrieve when encased in Neucrylate™.
7. Inflate the balloon and do a gentle microcatheter angiogram to confirm that the balloon adequately seals over the aneurysm neck.
   a. Record the inflation volume required to occlude the vessel. This volume will be used later for each balloon inflation.
8. Deflate the balloon.
9. Attach a glue-compatible one-way stopcock to the microcatheter and then flush it and the microcatheter with dextrose solution (D5W), and while injecting turn off the stopcock to trap the D5W in the microcatheter.
10. Fill a 3 ml syringe with Neucrylate™ and attach it to the hub of the one-way stopcock. Neucrylate-compatible syringes must be used.
11. Begin to inject the Neucrylate™ under fluoroscopic observation. Inject slightly less than the dead-space of the catheter (0.20 mL), and definitely stop if it becomes fluoroscopically visible near the tip of the catheter.
12. Reinflate the balloon and begin injecting Neucrylate™ into the aneurysm.
13. Inject over 1–3 min and *always* carefully follow the injection on fluoroscopy.
14. Attempt to fill the lumen and then conform to the balloon at the neck. Pause for 10 s then, with the balloon still inflated, aspirate from the microcatheter to stop continued forward movement of Neucrylate and withdraw and remove the microcatheter.
15. Wait an additional 10–20 s (longer for really large aneurysms) to allow the material to solidify and then deflate the balloon and remove it.
    a. Aspirate and flush the guide catheter.
    b. Repeat angiography to assess whether there is any filling of the aneurysm.
    c. If so, reinsert a new balloon and microcatheter and repeat the injection steps above.
    d. Do not re-use the microcatheter or balloon catheter for additional injections.
16. *Important*: Do not pause the injections for more than a few seconds at a time to avoid polymerization of the material within the microcatheter. Polymerization within the microcatheter can cause it to rupture with additional injections.
    a. *Stop whenever there is any question that the microcatheter is clogged.* Aspirate and remove the microcatheter and try a new one.
17. Fill the aneurysm down to the neck, but take care toward the final injections around the neck to avoid injecting Neucrylate™ around the periphery of the balloon and into the parent artery which can cause delayed thrombosis of the vessel.

18. Always allow 10 s to elapse before removing the microcatheter to permit the Neucrylate™ to set within the aneurysm.
19. Prior reports have not used antiplatelet therapy, but it would be helpful to keep the patient on an antiplatelet regimen for at least 1 month after the procedure.

Post-procedure Management

1. Complete neurological exam.
2. Admit to the NICU with neuro exams and groin checks Q 1 h.
3. Most patients with unruptured aneurysms can be discharged on post-procedure day 1.
4. Routine radiographic follow-up: MRA at 6 months and 18 months and annually after that. MRA is both accurate[21–23] and cost-effective[24] for routine surveillance of coiled aneurysms; catheter angiography is no longer necessary for most coiled aneurysms. Although gadolinium-enhancement is an option, is usually not needed to have good visualization of the vasculature. If the 6-month MRA shows no significant change, additional MRAs are obtained on a yearly basis indefinitely. See Appendix.
5. Note that MRA after stent-assisted coiling may be suboptimal, especially in the vicinity of the stent. There may be a better way to noninvasively image stent-assisted aneurysm coilings with gated CTA.[25]

Tips and Tricks for Coiling Small Aneurysms
Coiling of small aneurysms (<3 mm) can be surprisingly difficult and the risk of procedure failure [26] and aneurysm perforation is higher than in larger aneurysms [27] However, good outcomes are attainable with these lesions [28] A number of techniques can reduce the risk of complications:
- Rule 1. Avoid entering the aneurysm with the microwire. Wherever possible, use the microwire to get the microcatheter in the vicinity of the aneurysm, then pull the microwire back into the microcatheter and manipulate it into the aneurysm. The curved microwire in the microcatheter can be rotated and often it turns the tip of the microcatheter to the desired direction.
- Rule 2. Choose a curved tip microcatheter matched to the anatomy of the aneurysm. Ideally the shape of the curve will allow the microcatheter to point right into the aneurysm from the parent artery, without having to force it to make a turn into the aneurysm. That is sometimes easier said than done if the catheter curve wants to point away from the aneurysm. A steerable microcatheter, like the Plato™ (Scientia Vascular, Reno, NV), can be rotated in the desired direction.
- Rule 3. Whenever possible, pull the microcatheter back to engage the aneurysm rather than pushing it forward. Pushing the microcatheter forward can store kinetic energy in the catheter, and it could release suddenly and cause the catheter to jerk forward. Pulling it back releases the stored energy. Advance the microcatheter over the microwire in the parent artery distal to the aneurysm, pull the microwire back into the microcatheter, and then slowly withdraw the microcatheter. If the shape of the tip of the microcatheter is correct, it will pop into the aneurysm, and not have a tendency to continue to move forward.
- Rule 4. Do not advance the microcatheter deeply into the aneurysm. Small aneurysms can often be successfully coiled with the microcatheter tip at the neck, or even in the parent artery just pointing into the aneurysm. This prevents trauma to the aneurysm from the microcatheter and also allows the coils advanced into the aneurysm, to begin to curve before they reach the dome, pushing on the dome with a broad, curved surface, rather than the sharp point of the tip of the coil.
- Rule 5. Always remove any slack in the microcatheter and guide catheter.
- Rule 6. Advance as soft a coil as possible very, very slowly into the aneurysm.
- Rule 7. Be prepared to gently adjust the microcatheter as the coil is going in to relieve any pressure the coil is putting on the aneurysm and to ensure that it is pointing in the proper direction to deploy the coil.
- Rule 8. If the microcatheter backs up too much, consider using a softer or smaller diameter coil.
- Rule 9. If the coil prolapses into the parent artery, consider using a different design coil (3-D vs. helical configuration), a slightly firmer coil (soft vs. ultra-soft), or use a balloon remodeling technique (see below).

- Rule 10. As the coil is fully deployed, be certain that there is no forward tension on the microcatheter. (It may move forward when the coil detaches and the coil pusher wire is pulled back). Occasionally, the microcatheter may be allowed to back out of the aneurysm as long as the coil loops are all in the aneurysm. This is particularly true when only one coil is needed.
- Rule 11. Check again for slack, tighten the RHV on the guide catheter before doing a contrast injection, and do only low-pressure hand injections to prevent launching the microcatheter forward during the injection.
- Rule 12. Have a low threshold for placing a stent, even after coil detachment, if it has a wide neck.
- Rule 13. Small aneurysms may thrombose with relatively few coils. Even a single coil may provide stable occlusion in small aneurysms[29]
- Rule 14. Use an intermediate catheter to improve control of the microcatheter (see Chap. 4).

Packing Density Calculation

The degree of packing density is inversely related to the chance of recanalization.[14,15] Free software is now available that can be used to estimate packing density during coiling procedures. The idea is that real-time packing density data can help the operator reduce recanalization rates by obtaining higher packing densities. This concept is particularly attractive now that coil technology has evolved to permit higher packing densities with some devices and coiling techniques.[9,10]

1) AngioSuite (www.angiosuite.com)
   a) Software is downloaded to an iphone or an ipad with a camera. Two dimensional angiogram images of the aneurysm are captured with the camera and then used to estimate aneurysm volume. Dropdown menus listing all commercially available coils are used to estimate packing density; coils can be selected for their effect on packing density during the coiling procedure.
2) AngioCalc (www.angiocalc.com)
   a) All calculations are done on the website. Aneurysm volume estimation is relatively crude compared to AngioSuite; the website allows selection of several different shapes (spherical, elliptical, bilobed, etc.) and the volume is calculated by typing in the dimensions of the aneurysm. Coils are then selected to calculate packing density.

Adjunctive Techniques for the Treatment of Wide-Necked Aneurysms

Wide-necked aneurysms, generally defined as having a dome-to-neck ratio of <2:1, can be difficult to treat with coiling alone. Several strategies exist to coil wide-necked aneurysms using adjunctive techniques.

Balloon-Assisted Coiling

1) "Balloon remodeling" of wide-necked aneurysms is based on the concept that framing coils, placed in the aneurysm with the temporary support of a balloon, can "ovalize" the aneurysm and create a stable structure for coil packing (Fig. 5.8).
2) Systemic heparinization is critical. Consider pretreatment with anti-platelet agents. Guide catheter: Must be large enough to accommodate both a balloon catheter and a microcatheter – use a 6F guide catheter or larger.
3) Attach a two-headed RHV to the guide catheter and attach a continuous heparinized saline infusion to the RHV.
4) Watch out for bubbles in the system.
5) Place a balloon catheter (HyperGlide™ or HyperForm™ ev3, Irvine, CA), deflated, in the parent vessel adjacent to the aneurysm.

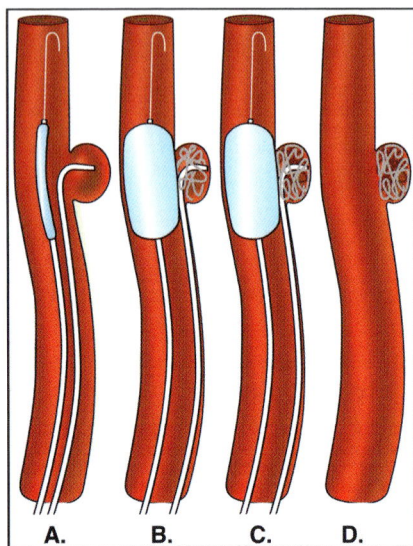

Fig. 5.8 Balloon remodeling technique. Inflating a temporary balloon adjacent to a wide-necked aneurysm (**a**) permits placement of a framing coil, which "ovalizes" the aneurysm dome and allows packing with additional coils (**b**, **c**). The presence of the balloon forces the coils into a shape that they would not normally assume, which further contributes to the stability of the coil mass. (**d**) Final result.

6) Navigate the microcatheter into the aneurysm.
   a) Alternatively, use a balloon with a dual lumen large enough to advance coils. The Ascent™ (Codman Neurovascular, Raynham, MA) can be inflated whilst advancing coils through a central lumen.[30]
7) Insert one loop of coil into the aneurysm so that the tip of the coil points away from the dome. This prevents the catheter tip from getting wedged against the aneurysm dome when the balloon is inflated and limits the risk of aneurysm perforation during coil insertion.
8) Inflate the balloon under roadmap guidance and deploy the first framing coil.
9) Deflate the balloon prior to detachment and assess the stability of the coil. Detach if the first coil appears to be stable.
10) An alternative method is to quickly deploy and detach multiple coils during the first inflation.
    a) This method has been described as *balloon-assisted rapid intermittent sequential coiling* (BRISC) and may be a way to more fully stabilize the coil mass with multiple intertwining coils.[31]
11) Place additional framing coils during temporary inflation of the balloon.
    a) Caution: Coil deployment with the inflated balloon can interfere with the smooth delivery of coils by diminishing the to- and fro- motion of the microcatheter tip.[32] This effect can be compensated for, to some degree, by gentle, slight movement of the catheter forward or backward as the coil is deployed.
12) As further coils are deployed, the balloon should be deflated, at least intermittently, after each coil is placed. This prevents too great a volume of coils and blood to accumulate in the aneurysm and to allow reperfusion of the affected circulation.
13) Often, once a stable framing construct of coils has been created, additional filling and finishing coils can be safely inserted without inflating the balloon.
14) The remove the microcatheter, inflate the balloon a final time to stabilize the coil mass as the microcatheter is withdrawn.

15) Balloon remodeling tips
   a) Balloon inflation times have not been found to be related to ischemic events.[33]
   b) The HyperForm™ balloon is highly compliant, and can adapt to vessel anatomy better than less compliant balloons like the HyperGlide™. This makes the HyperForm™ the most suitable device for treating non-side-wall aneurysms, such as bifurcation aneurysms.[34]
   c) A significant advantage of balloon remodeling is that the balloon can provide temporary occlusion in the event of intraprocedural rupture.

Stent-Assisted Coiling

Presently there are two stents designed specifically for stent-assisted coiling of wide necked intracranial aneurysms available in the US: the Neuroform3™ stent (Stryker Neurovascular, Fremont CA) and the Enterprise™ Vascular Reconstruction Device and Delivery System (Codman Neurovascular, Raynham, MA). Both devices consist of a self-expanding Nitinol stent that is deployed in the parent vessel adjacent to the aneurysm neck; the stent then acts as a scaffold to hold coils in place inside the aneurysm (Fig. 5.9). Incredibly, years after the introduction of both stent systems, and after the world-wide sales of tens of thousands of Neuroform and Enterprise stents, both devices are still under a Humanitarian Device Exemption; they can only be used under a protocol approved by each institution's Investigational Review Board (IRB). Differences in the design between the two devices are discussed below. Although there was some initial hope that the use of stents would improve long-term occlusion rates of aneurysms,[35] a recent study[36] failed to detect a difference in long-term occlusion rates between stenting or other techniques including balloon remodeling and double catheter technique (also see below). The use of these devices requires treatment with a dual antiplatelet regimen, and therefore they are most useful in the treatment of unruptured aneurysms. Stent-assisted coiling should be avoided when possible in patients with subarachnoid haemorrhage; bleeding complications are more frequent in SAH patients after stent-assisted coiling because of dual antiplatelet therapy.[37–39] Stent-assisted coiling should be used SAH patients only when other techniques for treatment of the aneurysm, including partial coiling (see below) are not possible. For completeness' sake it is worth mentioning that flow diverting stents, such as the Pipeline device, can also be used along with coils (see below).

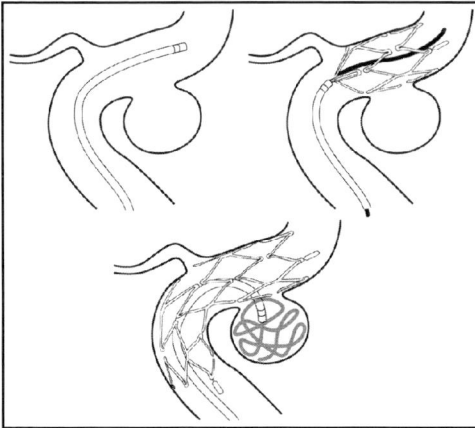

Fig. 5.9 Stent-assisted coiling technique. Advance a microcatheter across the neck of the aneurysm (*upper left*). Deploy the stent across the aneurysm neck (*upper right*), and the coil the aneurysm by placing a microcatheter through the stent and into the aneurysm (*lower*).

Neuroform vs. Enterprise

Each device has advantages and disadvantages.
1. Neuroform
    (a) Advantages:
        • Older, more established device (available in the US since 2002).
        • Easy-to-see marker bands.
        • Open-cell design may allow stent to conform to the vessel wall in sharp curves.
    (b) Disadvantages:
        • Stiffer and harder to track than the Enterprise.
        • Designed to be tracked over an exchange-length microwire.
2. Enterprise
    (a) Advantages:
        • More flexible and easier to navigate and deploy than the Neuroform.
        • Is designed to be deployed primarily, without first placing an exchange-length microwire.
        • May be pulled back into the microcatheter (recaptured) for repositioning during deployment, provided that no more than 80% of the stent has been placed outside of the microcatheter.
        • Flared ends of the stent make it easier to advance a microcatheter into the lumen of the deployed stent (in contrast to the Neuroform, which has a tendency to cause microcatheters to snag on the proximal markers).
    (b) Disadvantages:
        • Closed cell design makes it more vulnerable to "cobra-necking," when it is positioned in arteries with a tight curve, such as the carotid siphon (Fig. 5.10). That is, the closed cell design of the stent makes it act like a metal tube that can kink and flatten out in tight curves, which can make navigation through the stent after deployment difficult.
        • Current size selection is more limited than it is for Neuroform™.
        • Markers are harder to see on fluoroscopy.
        • The distal end of the delivery wire is larger in diameter than the wire immediately proximal to it (i.e., the part that is within the stent prior to deployment). This size step-off causes the delivery wire to snag on the stent after deployment in some cases.
        • May show delayed proximal migration of the stent, especially in the posterior circulation.[40,41]

General Considerations for Stent-Assisted Coiling Procedures

1. Case selection.
    (a) Wide-necked aneurysms are generally defined as those with a neck width ≥4 mm or a dome-to-neck ratio of <2.
2. Antiplatelet therapy:
    (a) Aspirin 325 mg PO QD for ≥3 days prior to the procedure and
    (b) Clopidogrel (Plavix®) 75 mg PO QD for ≥3 days prior to the procedure.
        • Alternatively, a loading dose of Aspirin 325 mg PO and clopidogrel 300 mg PO or NG can be given the day before or at least 5 h before the procedure.
        • If the stent is used on an urgent basis (e.g., as a bail-out maneuver in procedure in which the use of a stent was not anticipated), a GPIIb/IIIa inhibitor infusion can be administered until a loading dose of aspirin and clopidogrel has had time to take effect. The authors of this handbook favour abciximab, because the agent can be reversed, if needed, with platelet transfusion.
            – Abciximab 0.025 mg/kg IV bolus followed by infusion at 10 µg/min IV for 12 h.
                (a) Note: If an NG tube is going to be used for administration of clopidogrel, the tube should be placed prior to giving abciximab, to minimize the risk of nasopharyngeal bleeding.

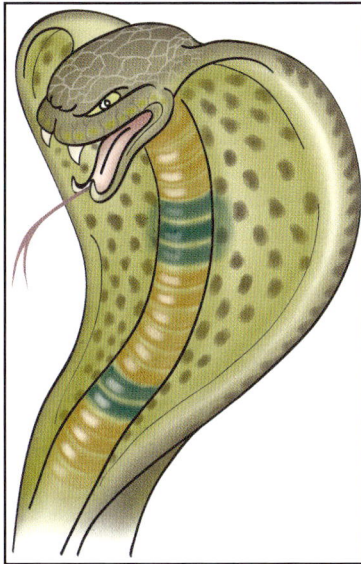

Fig. 5.10 A cobra and its neck. The closed-cell design of stents such as the Enterprise, Pipeline and Silk stents make the devices susceptible to kinking (i.e., cobra-necking) when deployed in a tightly curving artery, such as a closed carotid siphon. The kinked part of the device can impede navigation through the stent.

3. Make measurements of the parent vessel and aneurysm neck width and select a stent.
4. In most cases, the stent can be deployed and the aneurysm coiled during the same case. In situations where the stent placement procedure is difficult or prolonged, staging the procedure by bringing the patient back on another day for coiling can be helpful. After several weeks, the stent is endothelialized and is more stable, making trans-stent coiling somewhat easier.
5. Post-procedure management
    (a) If manual or c-clamp compression is used when the sheath is removed, an extended compression time is needed because of the presence of aspirin and clopidogrel. Usually, 40 min is sufficient, compared to 15–20 min in patients without platelet therapy on board.
    (b) Clopidogrel, 75 mg PO daily, should be continued for 1 month after the stent is deployed. Aspirin, either 325 mg or 81 mg PO daily, should be continued indefinitely.

Neuroform Technique

1) Devices
    a) The Neuroform stent comes from the manufacturer pre-loaded in a 3F microdelivery catheter, and is positioned in the parent vessel adjacent to the aneurysm neck. A "stabilizer" hypotube, which is also pre-loaded in the microdelivery catheter, is then used to stabilize and deploy the stent as the microdelivery catheter is withdrawn. The stent consists of a fine wire mesh that cannot be seen on standard fluoroscopy; platinum marker bands (four at each end) can be seen. The interstices of the fully-expanded stent are large enough to accommodate a microcatheter tip size 2.5F or smaller (realistically, <2.0F) for coiling.

b) The Neuroform3™ is most often used but as of the writing the Neuroform2™ is still available. Neuroform3™ has more interconnects between cells of the stent to limit prolapse of the stent into the neck of the aneurysm, whereas the fewer interconnects between cells on the Neuroform2 makes it easier to perform Y-stent technique with this stent. (see below)

c) The Neuroform EZ® is the latest version of the Neuroform delivery and does not require delivery over an exchange-length wire. This system is similar to the Enterprise™ Vascular Reconstruction Device.

d) Stent sizes:
   i) Diameters (mm): 2.5, 3.0, 3.0, 3.5, 4.0, 4.5
   ii) Lengths (mm): 15, 20, 30

e) Stent selection. The stent must be long enough to extend at least 4 mm proximal and 4 mm distal to the aneurysm neck to avoid stent migration.

f) Microcatheter
   i) Neuroform
      (1) The regular Neuroform comes pre-loaded in a Renegade® HI-FLO™ microcatheter.
   ii) Neuroform EZ
      (1) The best microcatheter to use with the Neuroform EZ is the Marksman™ (ev3, Irvine, CA). The Marksman is braided and is less prone to ovalize in curves than the Renegade® HI-FLO™ microcatheter.

g) Device preparation
   i) Neuroform
      (1) Remove the stent deployment catheter from the package and irrigate it with heparinized saline. Instructions for irrigation are on the plastic package. Avoid irrigating too forcefully, as the stent may be pushed distally within or even ejected from the microdelivery catheter.
   ii) Neuroform EZ
      (1) The stent comes loaded on a microwire inside of a clear plastic introducer sheath. Insert the introducer sheath halfway into the RHV and gently close the RHV around the sheath. Turn on the flush in the RHV until heparinized saline begins dripping out of the proximal end of the sheath. *Do not cinch the RHV too tightly around the introducer sheath, as this may damage the stent and/or microwire inside. The Neuroform EZ introducer sheath is not as resistant to compression as the corresponding device for the Enterprise stent is, and therefore the Neuroform EZ system is more vulnerable to damage in this way.* Once the sheath is irrigated advance the sheath tip into the hub of the RHV and transfer the stent into the delivery catheter by advancing the microwire.

2) Deployment technique
   a) Neuroform
      i) Navigate a microcatheter and microwire (0.010 in. or 0.014 in.) distal to the aneurysm under roadmap guidance.
      ii) Remove the microwire and replace it with an exchange-length 0.014 in. microwire with a soft, J-shaped distal curve. Soft wires such as Transend™ EX 0.014 in. 300 cm Floppy tip (Stryker, Fremont, CA) preferred.
      iii) *Always keep the tip of the exchange wire in sight on fluoroscopy to ensure that it does not enter a small branch or perforate the vessel.*
      iv) Wipe the microwire with a saline-soaked Telfa™ (Covidien, Mansfield, MA), and thread the delivery catheter containing the Neuroform3™ stent onto the exchange-length microwire using the brown plastic peel-away introducer.
      v) Grasp the distal end of the delivery catheter between thumb and index finger and apply gentle pressure to the delivery catheter just proximal to the stent to prevent the stent from sliding back as the catheter is advanced. The peel-away introducer is removed just before the tip of the microdelivery catheter enters the RHV.
      vi) *While the tip of the exchange-length microwire is monitored by fluoroscopy*, the microdelivery catheter is advanced over the wire and into a position across the neck of the aneurysm.
      vii) Hold the stabilizer firmly in place as the delivery catheter is pulled back over the stabilizer and microwire to unsheath the stent. The marker bands spread out as the stent expands.

viii) Maintain position of the proximal stent markers as the stent unfurls. If there is any instability in the system the catheter and stent may migrate – or jump – proximally during deployment.

ix) *Important*: Preserve microwire access during and after deployment of the stent. Maintaining "wire access" will ensure that the coiling microcatheter will pass within the stent and through the interstices, rather than outside the stent and between the stent and the parent vessel wall.

x) The delivery catheter and stabilizer are then removed over the exchange-length wire. A standard-length microcatheter is then advanced over the microwire until it is past the stent. The exchange-length microwire is then removed and replaced with a standard-length microwire for navigation into the aneurysm.

b) Neuroform EZ

   i) First position the delivery catheter, (a Marksman™ or a Renegade®) across the aneurysm neck using a microwire such as a Synchro®-14 0.014 in. (Stryker, Fremont, CA). These catheters are relatively stiff and in some situations it is easier to obtain access with a smaller microcatheter and then exchange that microcateheter for the delivery catheter.

   ii) Advance the Neuroform EZ® over the delivery microwire to the tip of the microcatheter.

   iii) Similar to the deployment technique used for the Enterprise™ Vascular Reconstruction Device and Delivery System (Codman Neurovascular, Raynham, MA) (see below), the stent delivery microwire is advanced so that the radio-opaque markers are well positioned on either side of the aneurysm neck. Stabilize the microwire and deploy the stent by pulling the microcatheter back over the microwire.

3) Neuroform tips:

   a) The stent should be "unstuck" from its original position within the microcatheter, prior to deployment, by gently pushing on the stent with the stabilizer, with the stent in a relatively straight segment. Unsticking the stent will make it easier to deploy.

   b) If the stent is pushed back in the microdelivery catheter during its passage through the parent vessel on the way to the aneurysm, the stent can be re-advanced to the tip of the microdelivery catheter by placing the distal end of the microdelivery catheter in a relatively straight intracranial vessel (e.g., the M1 segment or the basilar artery). Straightening out the distal portion of the microdelivery catheter, will minimize the resistance as the stabilizer is used to push the stent back into optimal position 1–2 mm proximal to the tip of the microdelivery catheter.

   c) The Neuroform stent may be navigated into a position primarily (without exchanging over an exchange-length microwire), if the anatomy is favourable (i.e., non-tortuous) and the guide catheter can be placed in a very distal position. The Neuron™ guide catheter (Penumbra, Inc., San Leandro, CA) is nicely suited for this.

   d) *"Y" configuration*. A single Neuroform stent placed across the neck of a basilar apex aneurysm can decrease the effective size of the neck to facilitate coiling. Some basilar apex aneurysms are so wide-necked that two stents, placed in a "Y" configuration, are required.[42] In this technique, one stent is positioned in the basilar artery, extending into one P1. A second Neuroform stent is guided through the interstices of the first stent, from the basilar artery and extending into the opposite P1 (Fig. 5.11).

   e) *Double barrel Neuroform technique*. Flow diversion was accomplished in a symptomatic fusiform basilar artery aneurysm by laying down, side by side, a total of six Neurform 2 4.5 × 30 mm stents.[43]

   f) *Stent malpositioning*. Inadvertent deployment of a Neuroform stent so that one end of the device is close to the aneurysm neck, or actually extends into the aneurysm, can be managed in one of two ways:

      i) In some situations, if a part of the stent has prolapsed into the aneurysm, coiling can be done successfully. Deploy the coils so that they encircle the stent struts or rest against the stent.

      ii) Deploy a second Neuroform stent can be deployed through the interstices of the first. It is important to maintain microwire access after placement of the first stent for this technique to be used.

   g) Hydrocoils® (MicroVention, Inc., Aliso Viejo, CA). Using Hydrocoils in combination with a Neuroform stent can be tricky. Once the hydrogel has

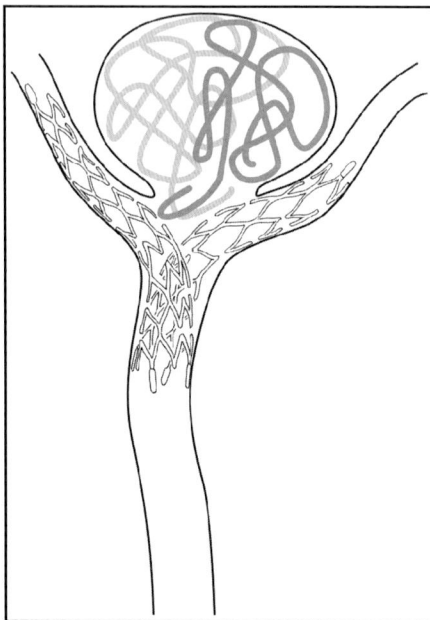

Fig. 5.11 "Y" configuration. A basilar apex aneurysm with a very wide neck is treated by extending one Neuroform stent into one P1, and another Neuroform stent into the opposite P1.

expanded after contact with blood, there is a potential for binding or resistance between the gel and the stent struts, should the Hydrocoil® need to be withdrawn or repositioned through the stent. Hydrocoils should be used with caution with Neuroform stents or avoided altogether.

Enterprise Technique

1) Devices.
   a) The Enterprise™ Vascular Reconstruction Device and Delivery System (Codman Neurovascular, Raynham, MA) comes from the manufacturer within a plastic sheath (the "dispenser loop"). A Prowler® Select® Plus microcatheter (Codman Neurovascular, Raynham, MA) is first positioned across the neck of the aneurysm with an ordinary microwire; the microwire is then withdrawn and replaced with the stent/delivery wire assembly for stent positioning and deployment.
   b) Delivery wire. A delivery wire is preloaded within the stent, and both the stent and delivery wire come from the manufacturer in the dispenser loop. The delivery wire has three radiopaque zones: the proximal wire, the "stent positioning marker," (which indicates where the undeployed stent is loaded, and runs the length of the stent) and the distal tip.
   c) Stent. The stent struts cannot be seen on standard fluoroscopy; each end of the four platinum marker bands can be seen, but are considerably more difficult to see compared to the markers on the Neuroform stent. The

interstices of the fully-expanded Enterprise stent are large enough to accommodate a microcatheter tip with an outer diameter size ≤2.3F for coiling.

    i) Stent sizes

        (1) Enterprise is indicated for use when the parent vessel diameter is 2.5–4.0 mm.

        (2) Diameter: 4.5 mm

    ii) Lengths (mm): 14, 22, 28, 37

d) Stent selection. The stent must be long enough to extend at least 4 mm proximal and 4 mm distal to the aneurysm neck to avoid prolapse of the stent into the aneurysm or stent migration.

e) Device preparation. Do not shape the tip of the delivery wire. The stent comes loaded on a microwire inside of a clear plastic "dispenser loop," or sheath.

2) Deployment technique

a) Navigate a Prowler® Select® Plus microcatheter (Codman Neurovascular, Raynham, MA) and microwire (0.010 in. or 0.014 in.) past the aneurysm using a roadmap. The tip is positioned at least 12 mm distal to the neck of the aneurysm. The Prowler microcatheter is relatively stiff and in some situations it is easier to obtain access with a smaller microcatheter first and then exchange the Prowler into position.

b) Remove the microwire and insert the Enterprise stent into the Prowler® Select® Plus microcatheter by placing the tip of the dispenser loop in the RHV and advancing the delivery wire.

    i) As a final preparation, the distal end of the dispenser loop is placed in the RHV so that, the tip is about halfway in. The RHV is then tightened securely around the dispenser, and the RHV is vigorously flushed to back-irrigate the dispenser loop and purge the system of bubbles.

    ii) Once the dispenser loop is irrigated advance the tip of the dispenser loop into the hub of the RHV and transfer the stent into the delivery catheter by advancing the microwire.

c) Advance the delivery wire without fluoroscopy until the marker on the wire is at the RHV. The marker on the delivery wire is 150 cm from the distal tip.

d) Navigate the delivery wire and stent into position across the neck of the aneurysm under roadmap guidance.

e) Position the stent for deployment by aligning the stent positioning marker on the delivery wire with the target site.

f) Deploy the stent by holding the delivery wire firmly in place while carefully retracting the microcatheter.

g) If the stent position is not satisfactory, the stent may be recaptured by advancing the microcatheter. Do not attempt to recapture it by pulling on the delivery wire. Stent recapture may be done provided that <80% of the stent has been deployed; this is "recapturability limit" is indicated by the proximal end of the stent positioning marker. If the proximal end of the stent positioning marker is still within the microcatheter, it is okay to recapture the stent.

h) The stent should be recaptured only once.[44] If further repositioning is needed, the stent should be removed and a new one is used.

    i) After the Enterprise is deployed, remove Prowler® Select® Plus microcatheter and wire. Advance a new microcatheter and microwire into the aneurysm for coiling.

3) Enterprise tips:

a) If the delivery wire snags on the stent after deployment, readvance the microcatheter into the stent to recapture the wire.

b) The Enterprise stent is less effective when it is deployed in a tight curve. Two problems can occur in a tight curve:

    i) Apposition of the stent to the wall of the vessel can be impaired.[45]

    ii) Cobra-necking (kinking) of the Enterprise stent in a tight curve can make it difficult to re-advance a microcatheter through the stent.

Jailing Technique for Stent-Assisted Coiling

The jailing technique involves placement of the microcatheter in the aneurysm prior to deployment of the stent (Fig. 5.12). The advantages of this technique are that the coiling microcatheter is more stable – being held in place by the stent – and it obviates the need to navigate through the stent after deployment.

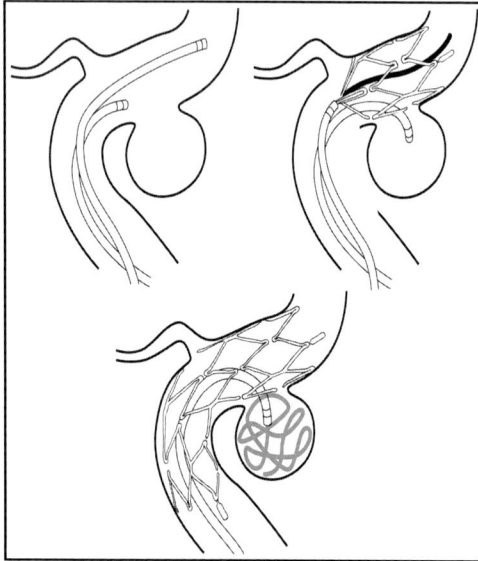

Fig. 5.12 Jailing technique. Park the coiling microcatheter proximal to the aneurysm as the stent microcatheter is advanced into position (*upper left*). Then place the coiling microcatheter inside the aneurysm and deploy the stent (*upper right*). Coil the aneurysm with the stent in place (*lower*). Finally, withdraw the coiling microcatheter carefully under fluoroscopic visualization.

1) Use a guide catheter that is large enough to accommodate both the stent deployment microcatheter and the coiling microcatheter (e.g., Neuron 6F 070 or a 6F Cook Shuttle)
2) Attach a double-headed RHV to the guide catheter.
3) Advance both microcatheters through the guide catheter simultaneously.
4) Position the coiling microcatheter just proximal to the aneurysm, then advance the stent deployment microcatheter across the mouth of the aneurysm.
    a) Optional: deploy a single loop of coil immediately prior to deploying the stent. The loop of coil will serve to stabilize the coiling microcatheter during stent deployment.
5) Deploy the stent while carefully maintaining coiling microcatheter position.
6) When coiling is complete, carefully remove coiling microcatheter.
7) The "semi-jailing" technique involves partially deploying the stent, then coiling the aneurysm, followed by complete deployment of the stent.[46] This variation on the jailing technique allows for manipulation of the coiling microcatheter during the coiling part of the procedure.

Double Catheter Coiling Technique

Some wide-necked aneurysms can be treated by using two microcatheters to simultaneously place coils across the neck of the aneurysm.[47] One of the coils is detached in the aneurysm, and the other coil is left attached to its pusher wire to stabilize the coil construct (Fig. 5.13). The major problem with this technique is that long-term durability of the occlusion of the aneurysm with this technique may not be very good,[48] possibly because tight coil packing of aneurysms is less feasible without the use of a balloon or stent.

1. For guide catheter access use a single large device such as a 6 or 7F Envoy® (Codman Neurovascular, Raynham, MA), a 6F 0.070 in Neuron catheter (Penumbra, Inc., San Leandro, CA), or a 90 cm Cook Shuttle® (Cook Inc., Bloomington, IN).

2. Attach either a two-headed RHV or two single RHVs in series to the guide catheter and attach a continuous heparinized saline infusion.

3. Watch out for bubbles in the system. The more connections on the catheter, the greater the chance of bubbles.

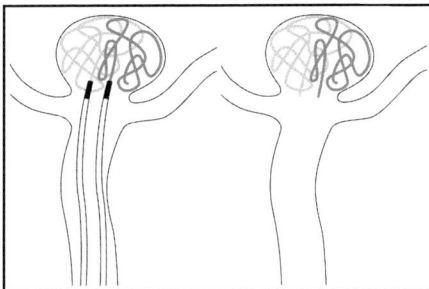

Fig. 5.13 Double microcatheter technique for coiling wide-necked aneurysms. With two microcatheters placed in the aneurysm, one coil is positioned but not detached, to act as a stabilizer as additional coils are deployed from the other microcatheter.

4. Insert two low-profile microcatheters with preloaded microwires into the RHVs. Advance each microcatheter one after the other a few centimeters at a time in a "leap-frog" fashion until they are positioned in the aneurysm.

5. Advance a coil through one microcatheter. Select the coil so that it is as large as possible but not so large that it prolapses into the parent artery.

6. After multiple loops are in the aneurysm, advance a similar sized coil though the other microcatheter.

7. Position both coils in the aneurysm, then do a guide catheter angiogram. If the positioning is adequate, detach the coil with the least number of loops across the neck (this is usually the second coil deployed). When the coil detaches, remove the pusher-wire.

8. Do not detach the other coil yet. The other coil is a stabilizer for the coil mass.

9. Advance another, slightly smaller coil through the microcatheter and detach it once it is properly positioned.

10. As long as the coil construct seems stable, alternate placing and detaching coils between the two microcatheters, to help assure uniform packing of the entire aneurysm.

11. Always be sure to have one coil positioned within the aneurysm, but not yet detached, to stabilize the system as each additional coil is advanced, positioned, and detached.

12. Confusion can arise about which coil is being detached and which is being left in place. It can help to cover the hub of the microcatheter containing the stabilizing coil with a sterile towel, to prevent mistakenly detaching that coil.

13. Note that with bare platinum GDC® (Stryker Neurovascular, Fremont, CA) coils, one may get unintended "sympathetic detachment" of a coil in contact with one which is intended to be detached. This is rare, but can be avoided using coated coils or other coil types, especially coils not using electrical detachment mechanisms.

14. Continue this process until the desired packing density is achieved, until the microcatheter kicks back or the coil begins to prolapse into the parent artery.

Partial Coiling

In subarachnoid haemorrhage, the use of adjunctive techniques to coil wide-necked aneurysms adds complexity and risk to the procedure.[49] In addition, stent-supported coiling requires combination antiplatelet therapy to prevent in-stent thrombosis, which can increase the risk of rehaemorrhage, and is problematic if additional surgical procedures, such as ventriculostomy, are anticipated. An alternative strategy is to partially coil the aneurysm, to protect against rehaemorrhage in the acute phase, and undertake additional treatment, if necessary, in the future. Aneurysmal haemorrhage usually occurs due to a rent in the aneurysm dome, or from a daughter sack, if present. "Capping" of the aneurysm, or coiling of the apex of the dome, can protect against rebleeding in the short term. The patient can be brought back for more definitive treatment at a later date.

Flow Diversion

Flow diversion is the latest rage in neurointervention. Hoards of neurointerventionalists have been running across the steppe to learn and use a handful of recently introduced flow-diverters for the treatment of intracranial aneurysms. See Chap. 13 for an in-depth discussion of the devices and published literature about them. Presently, only the Pipeline™ embolization device (PED) (ev3, Irvine, CA) is both FDA-approved and CE mark-approved. The Silk (Balt Extrusion, Montmorency, France) is CE mark-approved.

Pipeline Technique

The Pipeline Embolization Device is currently FDA-approved for the treatment of large or giant wide-necked intracranial aneurysms of the ICA from the petrous to the superior hypophyseal segments in patients age 22 and older. See Table 5.1 for a glossary of Pipeline terms.
1) Devices
   a) The Pipeline stent is a woven wire mesh tube consisting of 25% platinum and 75% cobalt-nickel alloy. It provides 30–35% surface coverage of the target vessel with a pore size of 0.02–0.05 mm^2 at nominal diameter. It is attached to a stainless steel pusher wire and is compatible with a 3F (0.027 in.) microcatheter. The pusher wire has platinum coil tip that extends 15 mm beyond the distal end of the stent. The device comes from the manufacturer loaded inside of an introducer sheath, similar to how the Enterprise stent is packaged.
   b) Stent sizes
      i) The expanded, unconstrained diameter is 0.25 mm larger than the labeled diameter.
      ii) Diameters (mm): 2.50, 2.75, 3.00, 3.25, 3.50, 3.75, 4.00, 4.25, 4.50, 4.75, 5.00
      iii) Lengths (mm): 10, 12, 14, 16, 18, 20, 25, 30, 35
   c) Stent selection
      i) Choose a stent with a diameter that approximates the diameter of the parent vessel and a length that is at least 6 mm longer than the aneurysm neck.

Table 5.1 Pipeline glossary

Pipeline stenting is tricky. It is much more challenging than using, say, the Neuroform or Enterprise devices. A small vocabulary has evolved to help operators communicate clearly and succinctly during Pipeline cases

Capture coil	Attachment to delivery wire that holds the distal end of the stent in place. Aka "protective coil."
Cigar	Initial shape of the Pipeline device as it is unsheathed with the distal end of the stent still constrained within the capture coil.
Corking	Retrieval of partly deployed stent by pulling on the delivery wire to trap the stent between the capture coil and the tip of the microcatheter.
Fluffing	The gentle process of alternating forward motion of the delivery wire with pulling back on the microcatheter to deploy the stent in an optimal position.
Load (or loading the microcatheter)	To advance the microcatheter during deployment. This is necessary when the partially deployed stent appears to be too elongated or is beginning to twist. Loading the microcatheter has the effect of expanding and shortening the portion of the partially deployed stent adjacent to the microcatheter tip.
Tip coil	The 15 mm long part of the delivery wire that is distal to the capture coil.

ii) When the parent vessel diameter proximal to the aneurysm is different from the parent vessel diameter distal to the aneurysm:
   (1) Either size the stent to the larger diameter, or
   (2) Use two Pipeline devices, with each sized to the proximal or distal parent vessel diameter. Deploy the distal one first.
2) Deployment technique
   a) Guide catheter
      i) Use a large guide catheter, such as a 6F Neuron™ 070 (Penumbra, Inc., San Leandro, CA) or a 6F Cook Shuttle® (Cook, Inc., Bloomington, IN). Larger, more stable guide catheters provide stability during stent deployment and also permit good-quality guide catheter angiograms with the Marksman microcatheter in position.
   b) Working views
      i) Find PA and lateral working views that show optimal views of the proximal and distal landing zones within the parent artery. This is different from aneurysm coiling technique, in which visualization of the aneurysm neck is most important. Obtain a 3-D angiogram once the guide catheter is in place to find the best working views.
   c) Microcatheter access
      i) The Pipeline is designed to be used with the Marksman™ (ev3, Irvine, CA) microcatheter.
      ii) Under roadmap guidance, advance the Marksman™ microcatheter over a microwire and place the microcatheter tip at least 20 mm past the distal edge of the aneurysm neck, preferably in a straight segment (such as the M1).
      iii) Partially withdraw the microwire and gently retract the microcatheter to take slack out of the microcatheter.
      iv) Remove the microwire.
   d) Insertion
      i) Remove the introducer sheath and delivery wire from the packaging. Grasp the introducer sheath and delivery wire together to prevent the stent from being inadvertently deployed (i.e., *deployus prematurus*).
      ii) Insert the introducer sheath about halfway into the RHV and cinch down the rotating valve onto the introducer sheath. The introducer sheath is braided and can withstand a lot of force from the valve. Irrigate via the RHV until heparinized saline is dripping out of the proximal end of the introducer sheath, then advance the introducer sheath until it is snuggly inserted into the RHV.
      iii) Advance the stent into the microcatheter by pushing on the delivery wire. ***Do not torque or pull back on the delivery wire while the stent is being advanced through the microcatheter***.
      iv) Gently advance the 15 mm tip coil beyond the tip of the microcatheter and align the distal end of the stent with the distal tip of the microcatheter.
      v) Carefully and slowly pull the microcatheter back into position to begin deploying the stent. The distal end of the stent should be at least 3 mm past the distal edge of the aneurysm neck.
   e) Deployment (Fig. 5.14)
      i) Unsheath the Pipeline by slowly retracting the microcatheter whilst maintaining the position of the Pipeline by holding the delivery wire steady. A "cigar" will appear, as the stent begins to expand while the distal end of the stent is still held in place by the capture coil. Once the cigar appears, continue the deployment by gently pushing the delivery wire forward. Deployment of the stent is accomplished by alternating briefly pulling on the microcatheter with briefly pushing on the delivery wire. Gently nudge the cigar so that it is in a central position within the parent artery, and not eccentric to one side of the vessel.
      ii) Releasing the distal end of the stent:
         (1) The distal end of the stent is held in place by the "capture coil" (or "protective coil") located at just proximal to the 15 mm distal tip. This capture coil holds the distal end of the stent while the stent is first unsheathed, causing the cigar to appear. In about half of cases, the distal end of the stent will spring open spontaneously after the device is unsheathed for several mm. If this does not happen, then the distal end of the stent can be released by rotating

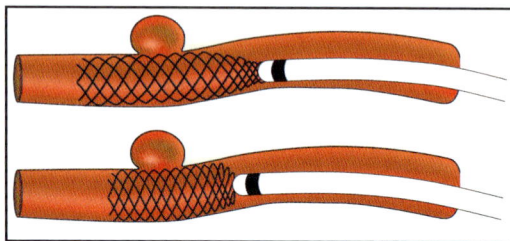

Fig. 5.14 Pipeline deployment technique. The Pipeline stent takes the shape of a funnel as it exits the microcatheter while it is being deployed. This funnel should be broad (*bottom*) and not narrow (*top*). A wide shape of the funnel ensures that the stent is optimally apposed to the walls of the parent vessel and keeps the size of the stent interstices to a minimum (which maximizes surface area coverage).

the delivery wire clockwise for several turns. *Do not rotate the delivery wire for more than 10 turns.* Over-rotation may fracture the delivery wire. If the distal end of the stent does not release with ten turns of the delivery wire, then the stent, delivery wire, and microcatheter should be completely removed as one unit.

iii) Deploy the stent slowly by alternately advancing the delivery wire and pulling gently on the microcatheter. Carefully mold the stent to the parent vessel wall as it is unsheathed. It is critical to obtain very close approximation of the stent to the parent vessel wall; a gap between the stent and the artery wall can lead to thrombosis of the space between the stent and the artery wall and closure of side branches.

iv) Avoid allowing the stent to twist on itself. A twisted Pipeline device can cause occlusion of the parent vessel.

v) After the entire stent has been deployed, carefully advance the microcatheter through the stent to recapture the delivery wire. Once the microcatheter tip is beyond the deployed stent, recapture the delivery wire in a straight segment of the parent vessel. Gently pull the delivery wire while rotating the wire clockwise to ease the capture coil into the microcatheter.

vi) If the capture coil becomes stuck on the deployed stent, rotate the delivery wire clockwise while advancing the delivery wire to release it.

f) Pipeline remodeling

i) After the Pipeline has been fully deployed, carefully inspect the device on fluoroscopy to ensure that it is not twisted and that the stent is fully apposed to the vessel wall. If there is twisting or lack of apposition is present, then the stent should be remodeled. There are two methods for this:

(1) Microwire massage. This will work only for stents with imperfect apposition (not for twisted stents). Form a J-shape with the tip of a microwire such as a Transend® EX 0.014 in. (Stryker Neurovascular, Fremont, CA) and advance the microwire, through a microcatheter, into the stent. Gently move the J-shaped tip back and forth along the region of the stent to expand the stent. It is surprising how easily the Pipeline device will further expand with a gentle microwire massage.

(2) Balloon remodeling. A balloon can be used to either further expand a stent with suboptimal apposition or to expand a slightly twisted stent. Use a compliant balloon, such as a 4 mm diameter HyperGlide™ (ev3, Irvine, CA). Gently advance the balloon catheter into the stent and inflate under fluoroscopy.

g) Using more than one Pipeline stent
  i) Use of multiple stents can be necessary for the following reasons:
    (1) For coverage of very large aneurysms
    (2) When the diameter of the parent vessel is significantly different between the pre-aneurysm and post-aneurysm segments.
    (3) To improve surface coverage across the aneurysm neck.
    (4) When the first stent is in suboptimal – but adequate – position.
  ii) Note: it is more difficult to visualize additional stents placed within an already-deployed stent. Pipeline devices are easier to see on fluoroscopy than on roadmap images.
h) Pipeline removal
  i) Occasionally, a Pipeline stent will be malpositioned during or after deployment, or it will become irreversibly twisted on itself within the parent vessel, which can cause parent vessel occlusion. There are three ways to remove a Pipeline stent:
    (1) Corking. If the stent has not yet been completely deployed, the delivery wire can be pulled back while the microcatheter and stent are held in place. The delivery wire is then used to "cork" (i.e., trap) the stent between the capture coil and the distal tip of the microcatheter. The delivery wire, stent and microcatheter are then removed as one unit.
    (2) Alligator™ Retrieval Device (ev3, Irvine, CA). If the Pipeline stent must be removed after it is deployed, an appropriately sized Alligator device, usually 3 mm can be advanced through the Marksman microcatheter to grasp and remove the stent.
    (3) Snare. Another way to remove a fully deployed stent is to use a 3 mm snare. The snare is advanced through the microcatheter to ensnare and remove the stent. If the stent is partially deployed, the monorail snare technique can be used (Fig. 5.14).
3) Post-procedure management
  a) Long-term dual antiplatelet therapy (aspirin 325 mg QD and clopidogrel 75 mg QD) is necessary (at least 6 months).
  b) Do a follow-up angiogram at 6 months
    i) If the aneurysm has thombosed, discontinue the clopidogrel and continue the aspirin indefinitely.
    ii) If the aneurysm has not yet completely thrombosed, then continue dual antiplatelet therapy for another 6 months and do another follow-up angiogram at that time.
  c) Post-procedure headaches are common after Pipeline treatment, presumably due to thrombosis of the aneurysm. These headaches usually respond to a short course of steroids.
4) Pipeline tips
  a) Choose Pipeline cases appropriately. Avoid using the device in inappropriate anatomy, such as severe pre- or post-aneurysm parent vessel stenosis.
  b) Do not place a Pipeline in vessels that have previously been stented with a different stent system.
  c) Keep in mind that the Pipeline foreshortens considerably (by 50–60%) during deployment.
  d) Rotate the delivery wire in a clockwise direction only.
  e) The stents are easier to see on fluoroscopy than on DSA images. Pipeline are best visualized with an unsubtracted "single shot" angiogram image.
  f) For very large and giant aneurysms, consider partially filling the aneurysm with coils prior to Pipeline insertion. Partial coiling prior to Pipeline stenting will promote thrombosis of the aneurysm and may minimize the risk of delayed rupture of the aneurysm due to thrombotic inflammation and erosion of the aneurysm wall (see Chap. 13 for further discussion of this phenomenon).

Silk Technique

The Silk stent is a flow-diverting self-expanding stent that is CE mark approved and available in most of the world outside the United States. It has generally been used in large or giant aneurysms but also very small side-wall aneurysms that are not easily treated by endovascular coiling.

1) Devices
    a) The original Silk stent had problems with deployment and wall apposition, which has prompted evolution to the current Silk+, which has 15% increased radial force. It is formed of 48 braided nitinol and platinum wires. Eight sinusoidal woven platinum wires increase the radio-opacity of the stent in addition to four markers at the ends. The ends of the unrestrained stent are flared outwards to improve stability of the deployed stent. It provides 35–55% surface coverage when properly matched to vessel size with a pore size of 110–250 μm. The stent is deliverable through a 2.4F 0.021 in. braided microcatheter (Vasco+21, Balt, Montmorency, France) for 2.0 mm to 4.5 mm diameter stents and a 3.0F 0.027 catheter (Vasco+27, Balt, Montmorency, France) for 5.0 mm and 5.5 mm stents. The delivery wire has a soft platinum tip that extends only 9 mm distal to the stent. It is retractable and resheathable until deployed over 90% of its length.
    b) Stent sizes
        i) Silk stents may be sized to vessels up to 0.5 mm smaller, or up to 0.25 mm larger than the nominal diameter of the stent.
        ii) Diameters (mm): 2.0, 2.5, 3.0, 3.5, 4.0, 4.5, 5.0, 5.5
        iii) Lengths (mm): 15, 20, 25, 30, 35, 40
        iv) Note that there is significant shortening of the stent after deployment; the unrestrained length is usually no more than 50% of the length inside of the deployment catheter.
        v) Two 30 mm long tapered stents are available:
            (1) Proximal diameter 4 mm; distal diameter 3 mm
            (2) Proximal diameter 4.5 mm, distal diameter 3.5 mm
    c) Stent selection
        i) A rule of thumb is to choose a stent with nominal diameter as close as possible to or no more than 0.25 mm smaller than the diameter of the parent artery.
        ii) Length should be at least three times the vessel diameter plus the width of the aneurysm neck.[50]
        iii) When there is a significant difference in vessel size proximal and distal to the aneurysm:
            (1) Consider a tapered stent.
            (2) Size it to the larger diameter.
            (3) Place two stents sized to the different diameters, first deploying a smaller distal stent, then overlap with a larger proximal stent.
2) Deployment technique
    a) Guide catheter
        i) It is important to obtain good guide catheter access close to the site of intended stent deployment is key. Position either a Fargo (Balt Extrusion, Montmorency, France) or Neuron™ (Penumbra, Inc., San Leandro, CA) in the intracranial carotid artery or vertebral artery near the aneurysm.
    b) Working views
        i) PA and lateral working views that show optimal views of the proximal and distal landing zones within the parent artery. Obtain a 3-D angiogram once the guide catheter is in place to find the best working views.
    c) Microcatheter access
        i) Silk stents are intended to be used with the Vasco microcatheter (Balt Extrusion, Montmorency, France).
            (1) Vasco+21 is used for stents 2.0 to 4.5 mm diameter and Vasco+27 for stents 5.0 and 5.5 mm diameter.
            (2) Marksman™ (ev3 Neurovascular, Irvine, CA) or Headway® (Microvention/Terumo, Tustin, CA) may be used as alternative microcatheters.
            (3) Under roadmap guidance, advance the Vasco microcatheter over a 0.014 in wire to a position at least 10–20 mm distal to the aneurysm and in a straight segment of the vessel.
            (4) Partially withdraw the wire and remove any slack in the microcatheter.
            (5) Remove the wire.
        ii) Insertion
            (1) Insert the introducer sheath containing the stent into the RHV and allow saline to irrigate the introducer sheath.

(2) Advance the introducer to the hub of the microcatheter and gently tighten up the valve on the RHV to prevent back-bleeding.

(3) Carefully advance the stent by advancing the delivery wire.

(4) Under roadmap guidance, position the stent at the tip of the microcatheter, always watching to ensure that the tip of the delivery wire does not traumatize the vessel.

(5) Slowly, carefully pull the microcatheter back into position to deploy the stent. Ensure that the stent is centered over the aneurysm and keep in mind that shortening of the stent will occur when deployed.

iii) Deployment

(1) Unsheath the self-expanding Silk stent by slowly retracting the microcatheter whilst holding the delivery wire stable. Often there may be friction between the stent and the microcatheter requiring considerable force on the delivery wire to stabilize it.

(2) As the stent unfolds, gently nudge the entire assembly slightly forward from time to time to ensure good wall apposition, especially along curves.

iv) Releasing the stent

(1) As the last portion of the stent begins to exit the microcatheter, ensure that the stent is well positioned across the aneurysm neck, and not kinked or twisted. It may still be possible to resheath and reposition the stent at this point if necessary.

(2) Especially in parent vessels under 3 mm diameter, it is helpful to do a guide catheter angiogram prior to final deployment, since the stent can still be removed if it is occluding the parent artery.[50]

(3) When 90% of the stent has left the microcatheter, the die is cast and the stent must be fully deployed.

(4) After the stent has been deployed, carefully advance the microcatheter through the stent to capture the delivery wire.

v) Silk remodeling

(1) Do a follow-up angiogram and carefully inspect the deployed stent for good wall apposition. Two strategies are available to handle stents that have not been optimally deployed:

(a) Balloon remodeling: Advance a Hyperglide™ balloon (ev3 Neurovascular, Irvine, CA) into the stent and gently inflate it to angioplasty the stent. Do not over-inflate; this may cause the stent to prolapse into the aneurysm.

(b) If the stent is hopelessly twisted and compromising flow, placement of a suitably sized Wingspan™ stent can restore patency.[50]

(2) Use of multiple Silk stents is necessary when:

(i) Increased coverage across aneurysm neck is necessary to slow flow into the aneurysm.

(ii) A large aneurysm neck requires more than one stent.

(iii) There is a large discrepancy between parent vessel sizes proximal and distal to the aneurysm.

3) Post-procedure management

a) Long-term dual antiplatelet therapy (aspirin 325 mg QD and clopidogrel 75 mg QD) for ≥6 months is recommended.

b) A follow-up angiogram should be done at 6 months.

i) If the aneurysm is thrombosed, discontinue clopidogrel but continue aspirin indefinitely.

ii) If there is still flow in the aneurysm, continue dual antiplatelet therapy for another 6 months, and do a repeat angiogram at that time.

iii) If signs of parent artery stenosis are seen on follow-up imaging, continue dual antiplatelet therapy indefinitely.

c) Post-procedure headaches are common and may be treated with a short course of steroids.

4) Silk tips

a) Silk should be used with caution in curved vessels. They can be very difficult to deploy in tortuous anatomy.

b) Always remember that significant (50–60%) shortening that will occur and choose the length of the stent accordingly.

c) Avoid placement of a Silk stent in a vessel previously stented with a different system.

d) Large and giant aneurysms should be coiled prior to stent placement in hopes of preventing the dreaded delayed rupture of flow-diverted aneurysms (see Chap. 13).

Willis Covered Stent

The Willis covered stent (Microport, Shanghai, China)[51] is a cobalt chromium alloy stent with an outer polytetrafluoroethylene (PTFE) expandable membrane that is deployed by balloon inflation, similar to the Jostent™ (Abbott Vascular, Redwood City, CA). As a covered stent, it can be expected to occlude side branches covered by the stent. Consider performing a test occlusion with a balloon at the expected deployment site of the stent to evaluate potential deficits produced by the side branch occlusions.

1) Devices
   a) The Willis stent is a rapid exchange system that does not require an exchange-length wire.
   b) The stent is made with relatively thin 0.06 mm wire in an open cell design. The membrane is also relatively thin, consisting of 30–50 μm thick PTFE. These design properties result in a fairly flexible device for intracranial navigation.[52]
   c) Crossing diameter of the stent mounted on the balloon:
      i) 3.8F (1.27 mm)
   d) Stent sizes:
      i) 2.5 to 5 mm diameter
      ii) 7 to 15 mm length
   e) Stent selection:
      i) In general, choose a diameter that matches or is <1 mm larger than the parent artery diameter.
      ii) If there is a minor mismatch in size between the proximal and distal landing zones, select a stent diameter by averaging the two parent vessel diameters.
      iii) If there is a ≥1 mm mismatch in parent vessel diameter size, deploy a smaller stent distally and second, larger stent proximally.
      iv) The length of the stent should include a ≥3 mm landing zone on each side of the aneurysm neck, i.e., the overall length of the stent should be ≥ the neck length + 6 mm.

2) Deployment technique
   a) Guide catheter
      i) Use a 6F Envoy® catheter (Codman Neurovascular, Raynham, MA) for most cases.
         (1) A 6F 0.070 in Neuron™ (Penumbra, Inc. San Leandro, CA) is useful for distal, more-supportive access in tortuous vessels.
         (2) A 90 cm sheath such as a 6F Shuttle® (Cook, Inc., Bloomington, IN) or Destination® (Terumo Medical, Somerset, NJ) provide great stability and a very large lumen.
   b) Working views.
      i) Select biplane working views to show a pathway to the aneurysm and well beyond it into a straight segment of the middle cerebral artery. This will allow easy advancement of the microwire necessary to position the stent delivery catheter.
      ii) Once the microwire is in place, choose working views to clearly show the landing zones for the stent in the parent artery. At least one projection should include the guide catheter and at least one should provide a clear view of the tip of the microwire.
   c) Microcatheter access
      i) Microwire access into a position well past the aneurysm neck is required for advancement of the stent. A Transend™ EX 0.014 in. Floppy tip (Stryker, Fremont, CA) is preferred.
         (1) For proximal aneurysms with fairly straight vessels, or if using a Neuron® 070 guide catheter (Penumbra, Inc., San Leandro, CA) positioned near the aneurysm, the microwire

may be primarily advanced straight from the guide catheter. A 200 cm microwire is sufficient for this technique.

    (2) In more challenging anatomy, it is easier to position the wire using any appropriate microcatheter that will accommodate a 0.014 in microwire. Use a 300 cm exchange length microwire to maintain microwire position.

    (3) Keep the microwire in constant position until the stent has been satisfactorily deployed.

d) Wipe the microwire with a saline-soaked Telfa™ (Covidien, Mansfield, MA) and load the delivery balloon catheter on which the Willis stent is mounted onto the microwire.

e) Hold the valve of the RHV with the left hand and carefully position the stent delivery catheter on the 0.014 wire with the right hand and advance it up to the RHV.

    i) It takes some finesse to open the RHV valve just enough to get the stent in without having a lot of back-bleeding. Be careful not to damage the stent with the RHV.

    ii) Once the stent is fully in the RHV, the valve can be slightly tightened to prevent back-bleeding, but not too tight to impair advancement of the catheter.

f) Advance the rapid exchange balloon catheter over the wire while holding the wire steady and keeping its tip visualized on fluoroscopy.

g) Position the stent across the neck of the aneurysm.

h) Gently pull back to remove all slack in the balloon catheter and microwire. Watch on fluoroscopy to make sure that the markers are properly positioned across the aneurysm neck.

    i) Slowly inflate the balloon under roadmap guidance. The stent will deploy at the "recommended" inflation pressure, usually five atmospheres.

j) Deflate the balloon and do a follow-up angiogram. Confirm that the stent is properly positioned and the aneurysm does not fill.

k) *Endoleak*

    i) If there is still some filling of the aneurysm, this is termed an "endoleak." Reinflate the balloon to a slightly higher pressure to post-dilate the stent. Avoid inflating the balloon larger than the diameter of the parent artery. If the endoleak persists or worsens, consider placing a second overlapping stent. Carefully evaluate the angiogram pictures and evaluate the site of the endoleak. The second stent should be centered on the site of the leak. Residual small endoleaks, if slow with stasis of contrast in the aneurysm, may be left since these usually resolve on follow-up.[52]

3) Post-procedure management

    a) The developers of the Willis stent keep their patients heparinized for 48 h after the procedure.[52] The benefit of post-procedure heparin is uncertain.

    b) Long-term dual antiplatelet therapy (aspirin 325 mg QD and clopidogrel 75 mg QD) (at least 6 months) is recommended.

    c) Do a follow-up angiogram at 6 months

        i) If the aneurysm has thombosed, discontinue the clopidogrel and continue the aspirin indefinitely.

        ii) If the aneurysm has not yet completely thrombosed, then continue dual antiplatelet for another 6 months and do another follow-up angiogram at that time.

4) Willis stent tips

    a) Carefully select cases for the use of the Willis stent. Since it is balloon-expandable, the stent should not be deployed in very tortuous vessels and since it is a stent-graft, expect to occlude any side branches in the stented vessel.

    b) Stable guide catheter position close to the target lesion greatly facilitates easy stent placement.

    c) Always maintain microwire access across the neck of the aneurysm until it is absolutely certain that the aneurysm is satisfactorily occluded. The microwire comes in handy when additional balloon inflations or overlapping stents are needed to manage an endoleak.

    d) Dual antiplatelets agents before and long term after the procedure are absolutely necessary and patients should be warned that noncompliance may result in thrombosis of the stent.

5.3.   Complications: Avoidance and Management

Overview of Complications and Complication Rates with Coiling

1. Recent large series report overall complication rates ranging from 8.4% to 18.9%[49,53–55]
2. Risk factors for complications:
    (a) Subarachnoid haemorrhage
    (b) Adjunctive techniques (i.e., balloon-assisted and stent-assisted coiling)
    (c) Small and large aneurysms
3. Experience counts: The odds of occurrence of a complication decreased with increasing operator experience.[56]
   For every five cases, the odds ratio declined by 0.69, P = 0.03.

Aneurysm or Vessel Perforation

1. Mechanisms: Extrusion of the microwire, microcatheter, or a coil is most common; perforation can also occur during guide catheter angiograms.[57]
2. Frequency
    (a) A meta-analysis of 17 reports found a significant difference in the frequency of perforations between ruptured and unruptured aneurysms.[58]
        • Ruptured: 4.1%
        • Unruptured: 0.5% (p < 0.001)
    (b) Risk factors
        • Small aneurysm size is an established risk factor for aneurysm perforation.[59–61]
        • *Vessel perforation*. Procedures involving tracking of devices with relatively high resistance (e.g., balloons and stents).
3. Avoidance
    (a) Exercise extra caution when treating smaller aneurysms.
    (b) Take measures to minimize anterograde force on the microcatheter and microwire
    (c) Tighten the RHV around the microcatheter when doing guide catheter angiograms (to prevent the contrast injection from carrying the microcatheter forward).
    (d) Avoid excessive packing.
    (e) Avoid deploying coils between the framing coil and the dome of the aneurysm.
    (f) *Vessel perforation*:
        • Attempt to keep the microwire in relatively larger, proximal vessels (e.g., M3 branches rather than M4 branches if possible).
        • Minimize motion of the microwire.
4. Management
    (a) Recognition is the first step: An abrupt rise in blood pressure or ICP, or a sudden slowing of the heart rate should prompt an immediate guide catheter angiogram.
    (b) *Resist the impulse to pull back on the perforating device!* The perforating microwire or microcatheter may occlude or partially occlude the perforation, and withdrawal of the device may worsen the perforation.
    (c) Reverse heparin anticoagulation with protamine.
    (d) Continue deployment of coils, if possible. This may seal off the perforation.
        • If the microcatheter has perforated the aneurysm wall, a coil can be partially deployed into the subarachnoid space, then the microcatheter can be pulled back slightly until the microcatheter tip is inside the aneurysm again, and the remaining portion of the coil can be deployed within the aneurysm.

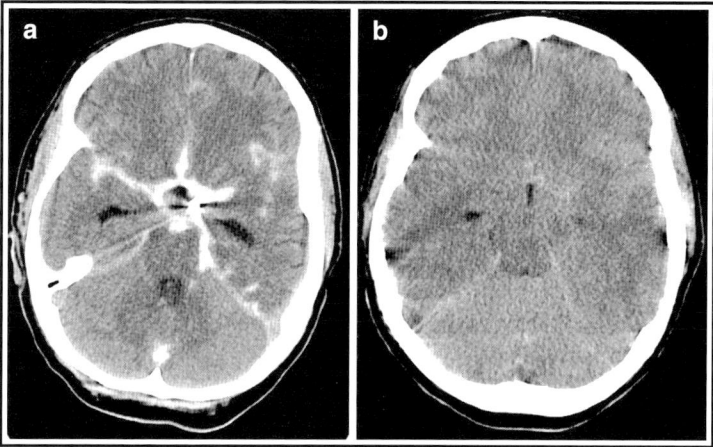

Fig. 5.15 Contrast extravasation on CT. A head CT done immediately after (**a**) and 1 day after (**b**) a re-rupture of a posterior communicating artery aneurysm during coiling. The presence of contrast created the appearance of more blood in the subarachnoid space than there actually was; the contrast in the subarachnoid space typically clears within a day. This particular patient was discharged from the hospital neurologically intact.

    (e) Second microcatheter technique:[62] While the perforating microwire or microcatheter is left in place, a second microcatheter can be navigated into the aneurysm to continue coiling the aneurysm.
    (f) Injection of N-butyl-2-cyanoacrylate (NBCA) has been reported.[63]
    (g) Occasionally, the tear in the aneurysm dome may extend into the parent vessel. In this situation, coil-occlusion of the parent vessel may be the only way to stop the haemorrhage. Obviously, this is a salvage maneuver and the patient's outcome will depend on the presence or absence of collateral circulation.
    (h) Once the aneurysm is secured, a ventriculostomy may be necessary, particularly if the patient remains hypertensive (i.e., if there is ongoing evidence of elevated ICP).
        (i) Once the patient is stabilized, obtain a head CT.
        • Tip: A head CT done immediately after an aneurysm perforation during coiling will always look ferocious, and often much worse than it actually is, due to the presence of contrast material (Fig. 5.15).

Thromboembolism

1. Mechanisms:
    (a) Platelet-rich thrombus formation on devices used during the procedure
        • In an MRI study of thromboembolic events associated with endovascular treatment of basilar apex aneurysms, a majority of diffusion-weighted imaging lesions were found to be in arterial territories proximal to the aneurysm, indicating that most thrombi arose from catheters, wires, and balloons.[64]
    (b) Thrombus formation at the anode (coil) during electrolytic GDC detachment.[65]
    (c) Slowing of flow in the parent vessel caused by vasospasm or occlusion by the guide catheter.

(d) Risk factors:
Wide-necked aneurysms.[66-68]
Balloon-assisted coiling technique.[69]
Loops of coil protruding into the parent vessel.[70]

2. Frequency
(a) Symptomatic thromboembolism: 2–8% of cases[3,66,67,70-72]
- Majority of neurological complications due to thromboembolism are transient[64,67]
(b) "Asymptomatic" thromboembolism (evident on MRI): 28–61%[64,67,73]
(c) Thrombus was identified at the coil-parent artery interface (i.e., at the neck of the aneurysm during coiling) in 4.3% of cases[68]

3. Avoidance
(a) Continuous flushing of all catheters with heparinized saline and meticulous attention to keeping all devices clear of bubbles and clot is essential.
(b) Take steps to prevent stasis of flow around the guide catheter
- Adjust the position of the guide catheter if guide catheter-induced vasospasm is flow-limiting.
(c) Systemic anticoagulation with heparin. Although many operators use routine anticoagulation with IV heparin during aneurysm coiling, data to support its use is lacking.
(d) Prophylactic aspirin. Some operators routinely place patients on aspirin prior to coiling procedures.[74] In a review, Qureshi and colleagues found a lower incidence of thromboembolic events in patients treated concurrently with aspirin (6.4%) compared to patients who did not receive aspirin (8.9%)[3]

4. Management
(a) Recognition is the first step: Guide catheter angiograms should be done frequently to monitor for evidence of thrombosis, such as a filling-defect within the parent vessel adjacent to the aneurysm neck, or vessel drop-out.
(b) Most thrombotic material that appears during coiling, is likely to be platelet-rich; therefore, anti-platelet therapy is the first approach.
- Abciximab[75] 0.25 mg/kg IV rapid bolus followed by 125 µg/kg/min infusion (to a maximum of 10 mg/min) for 12 h.
  - *Caution: Partial dosing of Abciximab should be avoided.* The authors recommend a full loading dose followed by IV infusion for 12 h, unless the threat of hemorrhagic complications is prohibitive. Experimental data and evidence from the interventional cardiology literature have identified a paradoxical drug-induced platelet activation effect with lower levels of platelet inhibition with abciximab, and a corresponding increase in thrombotic complications.[76-78] In fact, the authors have observed two aneurysm coiling cases in which intra-arterial thrombosis seemed to worsen after partial doses of abciximab were given.
- A 2 mm diameter Amplatz Goose Neck microsnare (Microvena, White Bear Lake, MN) can be used to retrieve the thrombus,[79] or break it up, to increase the surface area of the thrombus to be exposed to the anti-platelet agent.
(c) Thrombolytic agents are associated with a risk of significant haemorrhage, particularly during the treatment of ruptured aneurysms,[80] and should be avoided.

Coil Dislodgement or Embolization

1) Mechanism
   a) Unstable or malpositioned coil.
   b) Wide-necked aneurysms carry the greatest risk for this complication.
2) Frequency
   a) Uncommon – 0.5% of cases in one recent series.[55]
3) Avoidance
   a) Meticulous coiling technique and adjunctive techniques for wide-necked aneurysms, such as stent-assisted or balloon-assisted coiling.

4) Management
  a) Several devices can be used to retrieve lost coils:
     i) 2 or 4 mm Amplatz Goose Neck™ microsnare (Microvena, White Bear Lake, MN)
     ii) The Alligator™ Retrieval Device (ev3 Neurovascular, Irvine, CA)[81]
     iii) Micro™ Elite snare (Vascular Solutions, Minneapolis, MN)
     iv) The Merci® Retriever device (Concentric Medical, Mountain View, CA)

Coil Stretching

1. Mechanism
   (a) A distal portion of the coil becomes trapped inside the aneurysm, and attempted withdrawal of the coil results in stretching of the coil. Trapping of a coil can occur when a part of the coil become ensnared in the aneurysm coil mass, jammed between the coil mass and the aneurysm dome, or hooked on a stent. Trapping can also occur if the microcatheter comes out of the aneurysm, and cannot be repositioned inside the aneurysm, after most of the coil has been deployed. Sugiu and colleagues distinguished between "stretching" of the coil, in which the distal part of the coil is trapped and the coil is only slightly elongated, and "unraveling," in which the coil is elongated for some distance and is uncontrollable.[82]
2. Frequency
   (a) Uncommon. Reports from the dawn of the coiling era (i.e., the mid 1990s) described coil unraveling in 2% or less of cases.[83]
3. Avoidance
   (a) During deployment of a coil, do not allow any part of the coil to pass between the existing coil mass and the dome of the aneurysm.
   (b) Do not "force" the coil; if coil resistance increases significantly during deployment, try withdrawing the coil by a small amount and re-deploying, change the position of the microcatheter tip, or try a different coil.
4. Management
   (a) First step: Prompt recognition that the coil is trapped; avoid stretching the coil any further than it has already been stretched. A "stretched" – but not "unraveled" – coil can still be deployed with the following techniques:
     • Stent placement.[84] A Neuroform or Enterprise stent can be used to trap a segment of coil that cannot be advanced into the aneurysm (Fig. 5.16).
     • "Rescue balloon procedure." A non-detachable balloon can be positioned adjacent to the aneurysm neck, and using balloon-assisted coiling technique, the remaining segment of the coil can be advanced into the aneurysm.[82]
   (b) When a coil becomes unraveled to the point that it can no longer be advanced or withdrawn, the unraveled, elongated coil can extend for a long distance (1–2 m or more). Three salvage maneuvers:
     • Monorail snare technique.[85] A microsnare can be used to grasp and withdraw a stretched coil (Fig. 5.17).
     • The elongated portion of coil can be withdrawn from the parent vessel and secured in an extracranial vessel. For example, if aneurysm is in the anterior circulation, the unraveled segment can be placed in the external carotid artery, where antegrade flow will stabilize the coil and prevent it from embolizing into the intracranial circulation. The axillary artery can be used in the same way for posterior circulation aneurysms.
     • The elongated portion of coil can be withdrawn all the way to the femoral artery and secured there.

Vessel Dissection

1. Mechanism: Wire or guide catheter-induced injury to intima.
2. Frequency
   (a) 0.6–3.6% of cases.[54,55,86]
   (b) Vertebral artery dissections seem to be more common than carotid dissections.

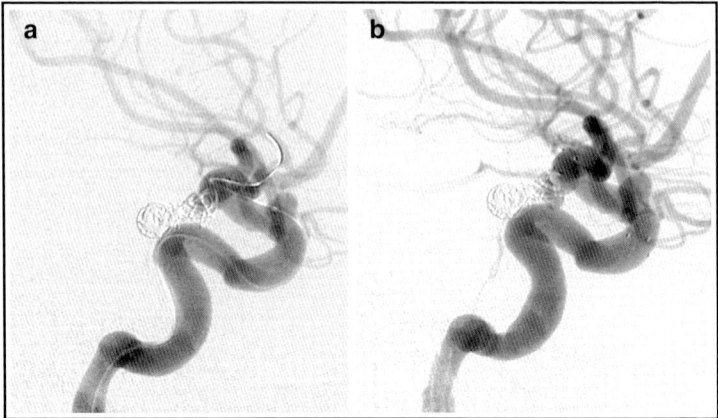

Fig. 5.16 Stent salvage of extruded coil loops. During coiling of a posterior communicating artery aneurysm, loops of coil prolapsed into the adjacent ICA (**a**). A Neuroform stent was deployed across the neck of the aneurysm (**b**); the extruded coil loops were pushed back into the aneurysm by the stent. The stent markers can be seen within the ICA.

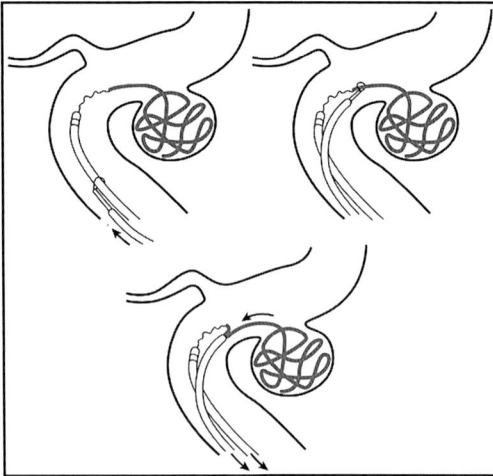

Fig. 5.17 Microsnare technique for retrieval of a stretched coil. Place a 2-mm Amplatz Goose Neck microsnare (Microvena Corp., White Bear Lake, MN) through a second microcatheter. Cut the hub of the indwelling microcatheter away with a scalpel and remove it, leaving the coil pusher wire intact. Then advance the open snare over the outside of the microcatheter containing the pusher wire (*upper left*). Advance the snare and second microcatheter into the guide catheter over the indwelling microcatheter until the snare is in position, past the first microcatheter, to engage the unstretched portion of the coil (*upper right*). Pull the snare back to grasp the coil, and then remove both microcatheters as one unit (*lower*).

     (c) This complication is probably under-reported, as many operators do not do routine surveillance angiograms of the access vessel (i.e., the cervical carotid or vertebral artery) at the completion of the case, and therefore do not identify asymptomatic dissections.

3. Avoidance
     (a) Take steps to minimize intimal trauma (see *Guide catheter placement technique* above).

4. Management
     (a) Always do a guide catheter angiogram of the access vessel at the end of the case.
     (b) Antiplatelet therapy is usually sufficient; aspirin 325 mg suppository during or after the procedure, then PO daily. Add a second antiplatelet agent if possible (e.g., clopidogrel 75 mg PO daily).
     (c) Consider anticoagulation with IV heparin, in addition to antiplatelet therapy, if the dissection is flow-limiting and carries a risk of thrombosis.
     (d) Consider placing a stent across the lesion if it becomes necessary to continue to work in the affected vessel or if the lesion is flow-limiting.
     (e) Follow-up imaging with MRA or CTA should be done in 3–6 months (or at same time as the routine post-coiling angiogram is done. Most dissections treated with antiplatelet therapy will heal within 3–6 months.

Aneurysm Recurrence

1. Aneurysm *recurrence* is defined as recanalization of the aneurysm on follow-up imaging necessitating additional treatment of the aneurysm. Although aneurysm recurrence is generally not a procedural risk, it is a potential complication and should be discussed with the patient during the informed consent process.

2. Mechanism
     (a) Coil mass compaction – thought to be the most common cause of aneurysm recurrence.
     (b) Growth of aneurysm neck or dome.

3. Frequency
     (a) UCLA series: Overall rate of aneurysm recanalization (defined as >10% increase in contrast filling of the aneurysm compared to the immediate post-procedure angiogram), 20.9% over a mean angiographic follow-up period of 11 months.[55]
     (b) Montreal series: "Major recurrence" (defined as a recurrence that is saccular and would permit re-treatment with coils), 20.7% at a mean angiographic follow-up of 16.49 months.[87]
     (c) 15% [86] Twelve (16%) other restudied patients have been found to have significant residual aneurysm or coil compaction/regrowth at the neck.[71]
     (d) Systematic review, posterior circulation: 22.2%[54]

4. Avoidance
     (a) Tight packing of the aneurysm

5. Management
     (a) Repeat coiling procedure.[88] or surgery.

5.4.   Parent Vessel Sacrifice

Indications and Contraindications

General Indications

1. Large or giant aneurysms that cannot be readily treated without sacrificing the adjacent parent vessel
2. Some cavernous segment aneurysms
3. Arteriovenous fistulas (e.g., direct carotid-cavernous fistulas)
4. Vascular neoplasms

5. Carotid blow-out syndrome
6. Traumatic injury

Relative Contraindications

1. Failure of balloon test occlusion (discussed in Chap. 6).
2. Existence of alternative strategies to treat the lesion while preserving the flow in the parent vessel.

Endovascular Technique

The key step in the sacrifice of any large artery, such as the ICA or the vertebral artery, is temporary proximal flow arrest to prevent inadvertent embolization into the cerebral vasculature during the procedure. In general, the artery should be occluded either at or immediately proximal to the lesion. Vessel occlusion can be done with either detachable coils or detachable balloons. Although detachable balloons are not commercially available in the US at the present time, they are available in Europe and Japan.

Patient Preparation and Vascular Access

1) Demonstrate adequate collateral circulation should be demonstrated by balloon test occlusion (Chap. 6). If surgical bypass is planned, then endovascular sacrifice should follow the surgical procedure promptly, to minimize the risk of graft thrombosis due to low flow.
2) Establish guide catheter access in the parent vessel.
3) The 6F 90 cm Shuttle® sheath (Cook Inc., Bloomington, IN) is best for this. It has an inner diameter large enough to accommodate two microcatheters.
   a) Alternatively, two 5F or 6F guide catheters can be used.
      i) Drawback: requires puncturing both femoral arteries.
4) Give a loading dose of IV heparin (5,000 units or 70 units/kg) and 5 min later, draw a 5 mL specimen of blood from the sheath for an activated clotting time (ACT). The ACT should be kept between 250 and 300 s for the duration of the procedure.

Coil Embolization

1) Under roadmap guidance, position the microcatheter to be used for the coils in the artery where occlusion is planned. Place the non-detachable balloon ((HyperForm® balloon (ev3, Irvine, CA) or a Guardwire® balloon (Medtronic AVE, Santa Rosa, CA)) in a proximal segment of the artery.
2) Inflate the balloon and confirm temporary flow arrest by doing a guide catheter angiogram.
3) Deploy the first coil. 18-system 3-D coils with a diameter about twice the diameter of the artery are usually effective. Briefly deflate the balloon prior to detachment to confirm that the first coil is stable. If there is no movement of the first coil with restoration of flow, the balloon is re-inflated and the first coil is detached.
4) Deploy additional coils as necessary to achieve tight packing of the vessel for several cm.
5) Deflate the balloon and obtain final angiogram images.

Detachable Balloon Embolization

The Goldballoon™ balloon (Balt Extrusion, Montmorency, France) is available in most of the world outside of the United States. U.S. operators are advised not to hold their breath waiting for availability in the North American market. Balloons are quicker than coils in achieving complete stasis of flow, but require a little more prepa-ration. Occlusion of an artery with detachable balloons should always be done with two balloons, placed end-to-end, with the proximal balloon functioning as a "safety" bal-loon to minimize the chance of distal migration of the balloons. It is never a good policy to count on just one balloon to occlude a large artery. Valves can fail and balloons deflate and migrate. Silicone balloons can migrate distally, even if fully inflated, although the latex Goldballoon™ (Balt, Montmorency, France) is less likely to do so.

1) Use a large guide catheter and choose a balloon size that is slightly larger than the diameter of the artery to be occluded.

2) Prepare two balloons according to the manufacturer's recommendations. Test the balloon valve with sterile water, as saline or contrast can gum up the valve.

3) Attach the balloons to their recommended delivery catheters. Balt's Magic or Baltacci catheters with extended tips work well. The coaxial catheter system provides stability during detachment. Prime the catheter with 50:50 contrast in saline. Be careful not to damage the balloon or valve as it is placed on the catheter.

4) Attach an RHV to the balloon catheter and a one-way stopcock or FloSwitch™ (BD Medical, Franklin Lakes, NJ) to the RHV. Fill the entire system with 50:50 contrast.

5) Advance the two balloons simultaneously through the guide catheter and into the vessel to limit the risk of premature detachment.

6) Position the balloons in a relatively straight segment if possible. They will be less likely to move forward or backward than if they are placed within a curve or at a branch point. Avoid inflating balloons next to a calcified atherosclerotic plaque. Calcified structures can puncture and deflate the balloon.

7) Inflate the balloons with 50:50 contrast when they are in proper position. If the balloons are properly sized, they will flatten out and elongate as they are inflated. Do not exceed the recommended maximum inflation volume of the balloon.

8) Leave the balloons inflated in place for a while (~5 min), even if a balloon test occlusion has already been done. Observation for several minutes prior to detachment will help ensure that the balloons are stable in that position.

9) Detach the distal balloon first. When the balloon position and stability appears to be satisfactory, detach the distal balloon by slowly, gently and steadily retrac-tion of the balloon catheter. If the balloon doesn't want to detach, gently pull it back against the more proximal balloon to allow it to separate from its catheter.

10) Remove the catheter when the balloon detaches. Watch the balloon for a few minutes to ensure that it stays inflated and in position.

11) Now detach the proximal balloon.

a) If the balloon does easily detach by pulling on its delivery catheter or looks like it is sliding back proximally, gently advance the guide catheter so that it is just proximal to the balloon. This will stabilize the balloon as the deliv-ery catheter is pulled back. Alternatively, position a non-detachable balloon to just below the proximal balloon and inflate it to stabilize the balloon.

b) Another option to facilitate balloon detachment is to have a 4 or 5F cath-eter in a coaxial position over the delivery catheter prior to detachment of the balloon. This extra catheter can greatly facilitate balloon detach-ment, as the balloon can be stabilized with the coaxial catheter. However, this technique makes it nearly impossible to use two catheter systems in one guiding catheter. Therefore, both femoral arteries should be used for this strategy, with two separate guide catheters, to simultaneously place two balloons.

5.5. Appendix: Primer on Imaging of Intracranial Aneurysms

by Joel K. Curé, M.D.

Imaging techniques for intracranial aneurysms include CTA, MRA, catheter angiog-raphy and indocyanine green videoangiography. Evaluation of suspected aneurysmal subarachnoid hemorrhage typically begins with non-contrast computed tomography.

Computed Tomography

Non-contrast computed tomography (CT) is the first-line imaging modality for patients suspected of having an aneurysmal subarachnoid hemorrhage. The most common diagnostic error leading to failure to correctly diagnose SAH is failure to obtain a non-contrast brain CT.[89] Using xanthochromia on lumbar puncture as the gold standard, CT performed on a third generation scanner was 98% sensitive for detecting SAH within 12 h of symptom onset.[90] The sensitivity of CT for SAH decreases with time after the hemorrhage and with small-volume hemorrhages.[91] The most common cause of rebleeding soon after aneurysm surgery is failure to obliterate the offending aneurysm, and this in turn is most commonly due to failure to identify the aneurysm at angiography.[92] The thickness and distribution of the intracranial hemorrhage and aneurysm contour are useful in predicting the site of the offending aneurysm on subsequent angiography.[93,94] The amount of subarachnoid blood on CT (Fisher scale) correlates with the risk of vasospasm.[95] While most aneurysm ruptures produce subarachnoid hemorrhage, aneurysms that have become adherent to the brain surface may produce both subarachnoid and intraparenchymal hemorrhage,[96] entirely intraparenchymal hemorrhage,[97] or more rarely primarily intraventricular hemorrhage.[98] CT in a substantial number of patients with non-aneurysmal SAH demonstrates a characteristic pattern of SAH surrounding the midbrain, the so-called "perimesencephalic subarachnoid hemorrhage" pattern.

Catheter Angiography

Conventional catheter digital subtraction angiography, more recently supplemented with 3D rotational angiography, is still regarded as the gold standard for imaging of intracranial aneurysms.[89] It is considered by many to be the initial study of choice for evaluation of the patient with SAH, particularly in centers with 24/7 availability of a dedicated neurointerventional team.[99,100] DSA provides the highest spatial resolution (0.124 mm pixel size)[91] and is the optimal imaging technique for preoperative assessment of aneurysm anatomy and for evaluating morphological features that have a direct bearing on endovascular or open surgical treatment.[99] The complication rate for catheter angiography by neurointerventionalists in an academic setting has been estimated at 0.3%.[101] No source of hemorrhage is identified in up to 25% of initial catheter angiograms performed for SAH. Repeat catheter angiography discovers an initially unidentified aneurysm in an additional 1–2% of cases.[89]

CT Angiography

CT angiography (CTA) employs a thin-slice high resolution rapidly acquired helical CT scan of the brain during the rapid intravenous infusion ("bolus") of 80–120 cc of iodinated contrast material. Imaging is performed during peak arterial opacification, ideally before significant venous opacification occurs. Sub-millimeter thickness slices can be achieved on modern multi-detector CT scanners with a maximum pixel size of 0.35 mm.[91] Scan time depends on the number of available detectors, but is less than 1 min for a 64 detector scanner with coverage from the foramen magnum to the vertex. Scanners with up to 320 detectors are currently available (Toshiba Aquilion One), the latter enabling whole-brain coverage with a single rotation of the CT gantry. Finally, a CTA evaluation can initiated and completed immediately upon detection of SAH on a non-contrast CT study. This can be accomplished far more quickly than a Neurointerventional team can be mobilized to complete a conventional angiogram under the best of circumstances.

The acquired images are reconstructed and available for multiplanar and 3D viewing at the CT scanner console within approximately 5 min, although network transmission via a PACS system for enterprise-wide review requires a variably longer time interval. The resulting axial source images are reviewed on a PACS viewing station. This is followed by a review of 2D maximum intensity projection (MIP) "sliding slabs" in the coronal, axial, and sagittal planes and of color 3D volume rendered images on an integrated thin client 3D workstation. Review of the source images and 2D reconstructions is particularly helpful for detecting aneurysms that are near or within bone (i.e. in or near the skull base and anterior clinoid processes). 2D reformatted and 3D volume rendered images can be generated to optimally demonstrate the relationship of the aneurysm to adjacent vascular (e.g. parent artery, adjacent perforating vessels) or osseous structures (e.g. the anterior clinoid process), but review of the "source" images is essential.

Several recent studies have supported the use of CTA as the initial imaging modality for suspected intracranial aneurysms. In a recent study of 179 patients (with 239 DSA-documented aneurysms) presenting with SAH to a single institution who underwent CTA and DSA, sensitivity of CTA was 99.6% and specificity was 100% [102] Notably, 19% of the aneurysms in this study were ≤2.9 mm. A recent meta-analysis of 45 studies comparing CTA to DSA for detection of suspected intracranial aneurysms found an overall sensitivity of 97.2% for CTA (95% CI, 95.8–98.2%). CTA specificity was 97.9% (95.7–99.0). Subgroup analysis demonstrated significantly greater sensitivity for 16 and 64 detector CT scanners than for single or 4 detector scanners, especially for smaller (≤4 mm) aneurysms. This was most likely linked to the availability of thinner (sub-millimeter) slices on the 16 and 64 detector CT scanners.[103] Factors affecting the sensitivity and specificity of CTA for aneurysm detection include: aneurysm size and location, vascular tortuosity, radiologist experience, mode of image acquisition and presentation.[89] CTA advantages compared to DSA include ability to demonstrate mural calcification, intraluminal thrombus, orientation of the aneurysm with respect to intraparenchymal hemorrhage, and relationship of the aneurysm to adjacent bony structures. Disadvantages include concealment of aneurysms by bony structures or aneurysm clips and decreased ability to demonstrate small vessels.[89]

MR Angiography

3D time of flight (3D TOF) MR angiography (MRA) is the most commonly used MR angiographic technique for imaging intracranial aneurysms. This technique is based on a T1 weighted 3D Fourier transform spoiled gradient echo MRI sequence (3D-SPGR). Here, the combined use of a short TR and small flip angle produces location-specific signal suppression in stationary tissues due to saturation. Inflowing blood that has not experienced these repeated RF pulses appears "bright" in contrast to the stationary background tissue. The individual imaging "slices" obtained in this fashion are subjected to a maximum intensity projection algorithm that creates a three dimensional angiogram. The data can also be subjected to 3D volume rendering similar to that employed in CT angiographic post-processing.

Advantages of MRA include no requirement for injected contrast (beneficial in patients with renal failure or pregnancy). Use of MR angiography may be limited by patient stability, inability to remain motionless for the study, or by contraindications to MRI, in particular implanted ferromagnetic surgical devices or pacemakers. While modern non-ferromagnetic aneurysm clips and endovascular coils are not contraindications to MRI/MRA, local field distortions and susceptibility effects produced by aneurysm clips compromise vascular analysis in the immediate region of the device as well as downstream from the device. Sensitivity of 3D TOF MRA for cerebral aneurysms ranges from 55–93%. Sensitivity is greatest with larger aneurysms, with a sensitivity of 85–100% reported for aneurysms ≥5 mm.[89] Considering the many logistical barriers to MR scanning of unstable patients in the acute setting and generally higher sensitivity and spatial resolution of CTA and conventional angiography, CTA has become the primary non-invasive modality for aneurysm diagnosis at most centers.

Follow-up of Treated Aneurysms

Follow-up imaging of treated aneurysms is standard for both clipping and coiling. Imaging is necessary to ensure adequate treatment of the aneurysm, and long-term follow-up imaging has the additional advantage of identifying de novo aneurysm formation, which occurs in patients with a history of aneurysmal SAH at a rate of 1–2% per year.[89,104] DSA remains the gold standard for follow-up imaging of both clipped and coiled aneurysms.[105] CTA can provide adequate imaging of some previously clipped aneurysms, but beam-hardening and streak artifacts preclude effective post-coiling evaluation. MRA can provide excellent imaging of coiled aneurysms but is useless with clipped aneurysms because of artifact. The authors of this handbook use DSA for early post-operative assessment of clipped aneurysms and MRA for routine surveillance imaging of coiled aneurysms.

Follow-up of Clipped Aneurysms: CTA

Early post-treatment goals for post-clipping angiography include assessing completeness of aneurysm occlusion, ruling out arterial narrowing or occlusion by the aneurysm clip, and evaluating for possible vasospasm. Late goals of imaging in clipped aneurysms include assessing the stability of the clipped aneurysm and ruling out de novo aneurysms in other intracranial arteries.[105] Susceptibility artifacts generated by aneurysm clips limit the use of MRA for evaluation of clipped aneurysms. Anatomy in the region of the clipped aneurysm and flow within arteries located "downstream" from the clip-related artifact are often impossible to visualize due to these effects. DSA or CTA is therefore required for follow-up of these patients. Recently, CTA has been assuming a larger role in post-clipping evaluation. Reports comparing CTA to DSA for detection of post-clip aneurysm residuals have yielded variable results that may reflect differences in the types of aneurysm clips employed and different MDCT systems and scanning and post-processing techniques. CTA is less useful in patients in whom multiple surgical clips have been used for reconstruction, or in patients with cobalt alloy-containing clips.[106,107] Reported CTA sensitivities for aneurysm remnants have tended to be highest (100%) in studies where only titanium clips were used.[108,109] A recent series of 31 consecutive patients undergoing both DSA and 64-detector CTA after aneurysm clipping with a variety of aneurysm clips (including cobalt-alloy clips) found an overall CTA sensitivity and specificity of only 50% and 100% respectively for aneurysm remnants. When only considering remnants measuring >2 mm on DSA, the sensitivity and specificity of CTA improved to 67% and 100%, respectively. The authors noted: "Conventional DSA remains the most accurate postoperative radiological examination to evaluate the quality of the clipping in every circumstance."[110] The sensitivity of CTA for evaluating vessel patency adjacent to the clipped aneurysm is also lower than that of DSA.[108,110] Post-processed CTA data in which clips have been digitally "removed" with a bone removal software package improves the sensitivity of CTA for detection of postoperative aneurysm residual.[111]

Follow-up of Coiled Aneurysms: MRA

MRA is well-suited to for non-invasive follow up of coiled aneurysms since coil-related artifacts on MR are mild and can be minimized with use short echo time (TE) 3DTOF MRA acquisitions and/or contrast enhanced MRA.[112,113] Contrast enhanced MRA is performed with a very short TE that minimizes susceptibility effects produced by aneurysm coils and signal loss due to turbulent flow (intravoxel phase dispersion). Intravascular contrast also reduces signal loss due to these factors and reduces the loss of signal in slowly flowing blood that occurs due to spin saturation.[114] Finally, use of elliptic centric view-order sampling of κ-space enables data filling of the central portions of K-space responsible for image contrast during early arterial phase of the gadolinium injection, helping to reduce the effects of venous contamination. While some studies have found no added benefit of contrast administration for MRA of coiled aneurysms.[22], others have found contrast enhanced centric phase encoded MRA more sensitive for residual flow in coiled aneurysms.[114], and especially aneurysms treated with stent-assisted coiling.[115] Residual aneurysm filling may be difficult to detect within coiled aneurysms with DSA ("the gold standard") against the opaque coil mass or due to subtraction artifacts. Therefore, it is difficult to compare sensitivity of MRA versus DSA. Some have observed that contrast enhanced MRA.[23] or 3DTOF MRA at 3T may actually demonstrate contrast filling within the coil mass more clearly than DSA.[116] Finally, use of MRA (including contrast enhanced MRA) has been found to be more cost-effective than follow-up with intra-arterial DSA.[24]

MRA Protocol for Imaging of Coiled Aneurysms:[117]

- NVPA Coil
- Axial plane
- Pulse sequence: Vascular TOF SPGR
- Imaging options: Variable bandwidth, Fast, 2ip512, Zip2, Smart Prep
- TE: Minimum
- Flip angle: 45
- Bandwidth: 41.67

- Freq: 320
- Phase: 224
- Nex: 1
- Phase FOV: 0.75
- Scan time: 1:01
- FOV: 22
- Slice thickness: 1.4
- LOCS per slab: 60
- Frequency direction: AP
- User CVs screen
- Maximum monitor period: 30
- Image acquisition delay: 5
- Turbo mode (1) Faster
- Elliptical Centric (1) on

Indocyanine Green Videoangiography

Microscope-integrated indocyanine green (ICG) videoangiography is a useful imaging technique during aneurysm surgery[118,119] and other kinds of neurosurgical procedures. ICG is a near-infrared fluorescent dye that binds tightly to plasma globulins and remains intravascular with normal vascular permeability. It has a half-life of 3–4 min and is eliminated exclusively by the liver. Following an IV injection of ICG, fluorescence is induced with a microscope-integrated light source with a wavelength of 700–850 nm and is imaged with a video camera. It is useful in aneurysm surgery to (1) check for complete exclusion of the aneurysm after clipping and (2) make sure the adjacent parent vessels are still patent. ICG is only visible within exposed vessels in the surgical field; it cannot be visualized through tissue.

1) Additional applications. Aside from aneurysm surgery, ICG has been used in surgery for:
    a) Dural arteriovenous fistulas.[120]
    b) EC-IC bypass.[121]
    c) Decompressive craniectomy for stroke.[122]
    d) Brain tumors.[123,124]
    e) Spinal vascular lesions.[125–127]
2) Devices and drug
    a) The microscope (Zeiss Pentero) must be outfitted with the ICG videoangiography module (FLOW 800, Carl Zeiss, Oberkochen, Germany)
    b) IC-Green™ (Akorn, Inc., Buffalo Grove, IL) comes in 25 mg vials. The drug contains 5% sodium iodine. It should not be given to patients with a history of adverse reactions to iodine or iodinated contrast media.
        i) Dose: 25 mg per dose, one-size-fits-all.
        ii) Alternative dose: 0.2–0.5 mg/kg; daily dose should not exceed 5 mg/kg.[128]
3) Technique
    a) Consent. Informed consent should include the risk of anaphylaxis (1 in 500)[129]
    b) Just prior to completing the surgical exposure, have the anesthesiologist prepare the ICG.
    c) Activate video recording on the microscope.
    d) Inject the ICG.
    e) Continue recording until the bolus of dye passes through the area of interest.
4) Tips:
    a) Repeat doses can be given 20 min or less after the most recent dose without significant residual fluorescence interference from the previous injection.
    b) Oxygen saturation measurements may show falsely low values during the first pass of the drug.[130]

References

1. Qureshi AI, Suri MF, Khan J, et al. Endovascular treatment of intracranial aneurysms by using Guglielmi detachable coils in awake patients: safety and feasibility. J Neurosurg. 2001; 94:880–5.
2. Ogilvy CS, Yang X, Jamil OA, et al. Neurointerventional procedures for unruptured intracranial aneurysms under procedural sedation and local anesthesia: a large-volume, single-center experience. J Neurosurg. 2011;114:120–8.
3. Qureshi AI, Luft AR, Sharma M, Guterman LR, Hopkins LN. Prevention and treatment of thromboembolic and ischemic complications associated with endovascular procedures: part II – clinical aspects and recommendations. Neurosurgery. 2000;46: 1360–75; discussion 75–6.
4. Qureshi AI, Luft AR, Sharma M, Guterman LR, Hopkins LN. Prevention and treatment of thromboembolic and ischemic complications associated with endovascular procedures: part I – pathophysiological and pharmacological features. Neurosurgery. 2000;46:1344–59.
5. Hwang G, Jung C, Park SQ, et al. Thromboembolic complications of elective coil embolization of unruptured aneurysms: the effect of oral antiplatelet preparation on periprocedural thromboembolic complication. Neurosurgery. 2010;67:743–8; discussion 8.
6. Kwon BJ, Im SH, Park JC, et al. Shaping and navigating methods of microcatheters for endovascular treatment of paraclinoid aneurysms. Neurosurgery. 2010;67:34–40; discussion 40.
7. Kiyosue H, Hori Y, Matsumoto S, et al. Shapability, memory, and luminal changes in microcatheters after steam shaping: a comparison of 11 different microcatheters. AJNR Am J Neuroradiol. 2005;26:2610–6.
8. Murayama Y, Tateshima S, Gonzalez NR, Vinuela F. Matrix and bioabsorbable polymeric coils accelerate healing of intracranial aneurysms: long-term experimental study. Stroke. 2003;34:2031–7.
9. Wakhloo AK, Gounis MJ, Sandhu JS, Akkawi N, Schenck AE, Linfante I. Complex-shaped platinum coils for brain aneurysms: higher packing density, improved biomechanical stability, and midterm angiographic outcome. AJNR Am J Neuroradiol. 2007;28:1395–400.
10. Quasar Grunwald I, Molyneux A, Kuhn AL, Watson D, Byrne JV. Influence of coil geometry on intra-aneurysmal packing density: evaluation of a new primary wind technology. Vasc Endovascular Surg. 2010;44:289–93.
11. Kallmes DF, Fujiwara NH. New expandable hydrogel-platinum coil hybrid device for aneurysm embolization. AJNR Am J Neuroradiol. 2002;23:1580–8.
12. Slob MJ, van Rooij WJ, Sluzewski M. Coil thickness and packing of cerebral aneurysms: a comparative study of two types of coils. AJNR Am J Neuroradiol. 2005;26:901–3.
13. Kawanabe Y, Sadato A, Taki W, Hashimoto N. Endovascular occlusion of intracranial aneurysms with Guglielmi detachable coils: correlation between coil packing density and coil compaction. Acta Neurochir (Wien). 2001;143:451–5.
14. Sluzewski M, van Rooij WJ, Slob MJ, Bescos JO, Slump CH, Wijnalda D. Relation between aneurysm volume, packing, and compaction in 145 cerebral aneurysms treated with coils. Radiology. 2004;231:653–8.
15. Slob MJ, Sluzewski M, van Rooij WJ. The relation between packing and reopening in coiled intracranial aneurysms: a prospective study. Neuroradiology. 2005;47:942–5.
16. Morales HG, Kim M, Vivas EE, et al. How do coil configuration and packing density influence intra-aneurysmal hemodynamics? AJNR Am J Neuroradiol. 2011;32(10): 1935–41.
17. D'Agostino SJ, Harrigan MR, Chalela JA, et al. Clinical experience with Matrix2 360 degrees coils in the treatment of 100 intracranial aneurysms. Surg Neurol. 2009;72:41–7.
18. Meyers PM, Lavine SD, Fitzsimmons BF, et al. Chemical meningitis after cerebral aneurysm treatment using two second-generation aneurysm coils: report of two cases. Neurosurgery. 2004;55:1222.
19. Brisman JL, Song JK, Niimi Y, Berenstein A. Treatment options for wide-necked intracranial aneurysms using a self-expandable hydrophilic coil and a self-expandable stent combination. AJNR Am J Neuroradiol. 2005;26:1237–40.
20. Lubicz B, Lefranc F, Levivier M, et al. Endovascular treatment of intracranial aneurysms with a branch arising from the sac. AJNR Am J Neuroradiol. 2006;27:142–7.
21. Kwee TC, Kwee RM. MR angiography in the follow-up of intracranial aneurysms treated with Guglielmi detachable coils: systematic review and meta-analysis. Neuroradiology. 2007;49:703–13.
22. Sprengers ME, Schaafsma JD, van Rooij WJ, et al. Evaluation of the occlusion status of coiled intracranial aneurysms with MR angiography at 3T: is contrast enhancement necessary? AJNR Am J Neuroradiol. 2009;30:1665–71.
23. Agid R, Willinsky RA, Lee SK, Terbrugge KG, Farb RI. Characterization of aneurysm remnants after endovascular treatment: contrast-enhanced MR angiography versus catheter digital subtraction angiography. AJNR Am J Neuroradiol. 2008;29:1570–4.
24. Schaafsma JDMD, Koffijberg HP, Buskens EMDP, Velthuis BKMDP, van der Graaf YMDP, Rinkel GJEMD. Cost-effectiveness of magnetic resonance angiography versus intra-arterial digital subtraction angiography to follow-up patients with coiled intracranial aneurysms. Stroke. 2010;41: 1736–42.
25. Kovacs A, Moehlenbruch M, Hadizadeh DR, Seifert M, Willinek WA, Greschus S, Flacke S, Clusmann H, Urbach H. Non-invasive imaging after stent-assisted coiling of intracranial aneurysms: comparison of 3T-MRI and 64-MDCT. In: European Society of Radiology. Vienna, Austria; 2011.
26. Pierot L, Barbe C, Spelle L, investigators A. Endovascular treatment of very small unruptured aneurysms: rate of procedural complications, clinical outcome, and anatomical results. Stroke. 2010;41:2855–9.
27. Brinjikji WBS, Lanzino GMD, Cloft HJMDP, Rabinstein AMD, Kallmes DFMD. Endovascular treatment of very small (3 mm or smaller) intracranial aneurysms: report of a consecutive series and a meta-analysis. Stroke. 2010;41:116–21.
28. Lum C, Narayanam SB, Silva L, et al. Outcome in small aneurysms (<4 mm) treated by endovascular coiling. J Neurointerv Surg. 2012;4(3):196–8.
29. Goddard JK, Moran CJ, Cross 3rd DT, Derdeyn CP. Absent relationship between the coil-embolization ratio in small aneurysms treated with a single detachable coil and outcomes. AJNR Am J Neuroradiol. 2005;26:1916–20.
30. Kirmani JF, Paolucci U. Ascent: a novel balloon microcatheter device used as the primary coiling microcatheter of a basilar tip aneurysm. J Neuroimaging. 2012;22(2):191–3.
31. Modi J, Eesa M, Menon BK, Wong JH, Goyal M. Balloon-assisted rapid intermittent sequential coiling (BRISC) technique for the treatment of complex wide-necked intracranial aneurysms. Interv Neuroradiol. 2011;17:64–9.
32. Phatouros CC, Halbach VV, Malek AM, Dowd CF, Higashida RT. Simultaneous subarachnoid hemorrhage and carotid cavernous fistula after rupture of a paraclinoid aneurysm during balloon-assisted coil embolization. AJNR Am J Neuroradiol. 1999;20:1100–2.
33. Spiotta AM, Bhalla T, Hussain MS, et al. An analysis of inflation times during balloon-assisted aneurysm coil embolization and ischemic complications. Stroke. 2011;42:1051–5.
34. Cekirge HS, Yavuz K, Geyik S, Saatci I. HyperForm balloon remodeling in the endovascular treatment of anterior cerebral, middle cerebral, and anterior communicating artery aneurysms: clinical and angiographic follow-up results in 800 consecutive patients. J Neurosurg. 2011;114:944–53.
35. Lawson MF, Newman WC, Chi YY, Mocco JD, Hoh BL. Stent-associated flow remodeling causes further occlusion of incompletely coiled aneurysms. Neurosurgery. 2011;69:598–604.
36. Hwang G, Park H, Bang JS, et al. Comparison of 2-year angiographic outcomes of stent- and nonstent-assisted coil embolization in unruptured aneurysms with an unfavorable

INTRACRANIAL ANEURYSM TREATMENT

configuration for coiling. AJNR Am J Neuroradiol. 2011;32(9):1707–10.

37. Tumialán LM, Zhang YJ, Cawley CM, Dion JE, Tong FC, Barrow DL. Intracranial hemorrhage associated with stent-assisted coil embolization of cerebral aneurysms: a cautionary report. J Neurosurg. 2008;108:1122–9.

38. Kim DJ, Suh SH, Kim BM, Kim DI, Huh SK, Lee JW. Hemorrhagic complications related to the stent-remodeled coil embolization of intracranial aneurysms. Neurosurgery. 2010;67:73–9.

39. Kung DK, Policeni BA, Capuano AW, et al. Risk of ventriculostomy-related hemorrhage in patients with acutely ruptured aneurysms treated using stent-assisted coiling. J Neurosurg. 2011;114:1021–7.

40. Lubicz B, Francois O, Levivier M, Brotchi J, Baleriaux D. Preliminary experience with the enterprise stent for endovascular treatment of complex intracranial aneurysms: potential advantages and limiting characteristics. Neurosurgery. 2008;62:1063–9; discussion 9–70.

41. Lavine SD, Meyers PM, Connolly ES, Solomon RS. Spontaneous delayed proximal migration of enterprise stent after staged treatment of wide-necked basilar aneurysm: technical case report. Neurosurgery. 2009;64:E1012; discussion E.

42. Perez-Arjona E, Fessler RD. Basilar artery to bilateral posterior cerebral artery 'Y stenting' for endovascular reconstruction of wide-necked basilar apex aneurysms: report of three cases. Neurol Res. 2004;26:276–81.

43. Bain M, Hussain MS, Spiotta A, Gonugunta V, Moskowitz S, Gupta R. "Double-barrel" stent reconstruction of a symptomatic fusiform basilar artery aneurysm: case report. Neurosurgery. 2011;68:E1491–6.

44. Codman neurovascular. Instructions for use. codman enterprise vascular reconstuction device and delivery system. Codman and Shurtleff, Inc. Raynham, MA 2010.

45. Heller RS, Malek AM. Parent vessel size and curvature strongly influence risk of incomplete stent apposition in enterprise intracranial aneurysm stent coiling. AJNR Am J Neuroradiol. 2011;32(9):1714–20.

46. Hong B, Patel NV, Gounis MJ, et al. Semi-jailing technique for coil embolization of complex, wide-necked intracranial aneurysms. Neurosurgery. 2009;65:1131–9.

47. Baxter BW, Rosso D, Lownie SP. Double microcatheter technique for detachable coil treatment of large, wide-necked intracranial aneurysms. AJNR Am J Neuroradiol. 1998;19:1176–8.

48. Terada T, Tsuura M, Matsumoto N, et al. Endovascular treatment of unruptured cerebral aneurysms. Acta Neurochir Suppl. 2005;94:87–91.

49. Henkes H, Fischer S, Weber W, et al. Endovascular coil occlusion of 1811 intracranial aneurysms: early angiographic and clinical results. Neurosurgery. 2004;54:268–80; discussion 80–5.

50. Lubicz B, Collignon L, Raphaeli G, et al. Flow-diverter stent for the endovascular treatment of intracranial aneurysms: a prospective study in 29 patients with 34 aneurysms. Stroke. 2010;41:2247–53.

51. Tan H-Q, Li M-H, Zhang P-L, et al. Reconstructive endovascular treatment of intracranial aneurysms with the Willis covered stent: medium-term clinical and angiographic follow-up. J Neurosurg. 2011;114:1014–20.

52. Li MH, Li YD, Tan HQ, Luo QY, Cheng YS. Treatment of distal internal carotid artery aneurysm with the willis covered stent: a prospective pilot study. Radiology. 2009;253:470–7.

53. Brilstra EH, Rinkel GJ, van der Graaf Y, van Rooij WJ, Algra A. Treatment of intracranial aneurysms by embolization with coils: a systematic review. Stroke. 1999;30:470–6.

54. Lozier AP, Connolly Jr ES, Lavine SD, Solomon RA. Guglielmi detachable coil embolization of posterior circulation aneurysms: a systematic review of the literature. Stroke. 2002;33:2509–18.

55. Murayama Y, Nien YL, Duckwiler G, et al. Guglielmi detachable coil embolization of cerebral aneurysms: 11 years' experience. J Neurosurg. 2003;98:959–66.

56. Singh V, Gress DR, Higashida RT, Dowd CF, Halbach VV, Johnston SC. The learning curve for coil embolization of unruptured intracranial aneurysms. AJNR Am J Neuroradiol. 2002;23:768–71.

57. McDougall CG, Halbach VV, Dowd CF, Higashida RT, Larsen DW, Hieshima GB. Causes and management of aneu-

rysmal hemorrhage occurring during embolization with Guglielmi detachable coils. J Neurosurg. 1998;89:87–92.

58. Cloft HJ, Kallmes DF. Cerebral aneurysm perforations complicating therapy with guglielmi detachable coils: a meta-analysis. AJNR Am J Neuroradiol. 2002;23:1706–9.

59. Ricolfi F, Le Guerinel C, Blustajn J, et al. Rupture during treatment of recently ruptured aneurysms with Guglielmi electrodetachable coils. AJNR Am J Neuroradiol. 1998;19:1653–8.

60. Doerfler A, Wanke I, Egelhof T, et al. Aneurysmal rupture during embolization with guglielmi detachable coils: causes, management, and outcome. AJNR Am J Neuroradiol. 2001;22:1825–32.

61. Sluzewski M, Bosch JA, van Rooij WJ, Nijssen PC, Wijnalda D. Rupture of intracranial aneurysms during treatment with Guglielmi detachable coils: incidence, outcome, and risk factors. J Neurosurg. 2001;94:238–40.

62. Willinsky R, terBrugge K. Use of a second microcatheter in the management of a perforation during endovascular treatment of a cerebral aneurysm. AJNR Am J Neuroradiol. 2000;21:1537–9.

63. Farhat HI, Elhammady MS, Aziz-Sultan MA. N-butyl-2-cyanoacrylate use in intraoperative ruptured aneurysms as a salvage rescue: case report. Neurosurgery. 2010;67:E216–7.

64. Soeda A, Sakai N, Sakai H, et al. Thromboembolic events associated with guglielmi detachable coil embolization of asymptomatic cerebral aneurysms: evaluation of 66 consecutive cases with use of diffusion-weighted MR imaging. AJNR Am J Neuroradiol. 2003;24:127–32.

65. Guglielmi G, Vinuela F, Sepetka I, Macellari V. Electrothrombosis of saccular aneurysms via endovascular approach. Part 1: electrochemical basis, technique, and experimental results. J Neurosurg. 1991;75:1–7.

66. Vinuela F, Duckwiler G, Mawad M. Guglielmi detachable coil embolization of acute intracranial aneurysm: perioperative anatomical and clinical outcome in 403 patients. J Neurosurg. 1997;86:475–82.

67. Pelz DM, Lownie SP, Fox AJ. Thromboembolic events associated with the treatment of cerebral aneurysms with Guglielmi detachable coils. AJNR Am J Neuroradiol. 1998;19:1541–7.

68. Workman MJ, Cloft HJ, Tong FC, et al. Thrombus formation at the neck of cerebral aneurysms during treatment with guglielmi detachable coils. AJNR Am J Neuroradiol. 2002;23:1568–76.

69. Soeda A, Sakai N, Murao K, et al. Thromboembolic events associated with guglielmi detachable coil embolization with use of diffusion-weighted MR imaging. Part II. Detection of the microemboli proximal to cerebral aneurysm. AJNR Am J Neuroradiol. 2003;24:2035–8.

70. Derdeyn CP, Cross 3rd DT, Moran CJ, et al. Postprocedure ischemic events after treatment of intracranial aneurysms with Guglielmi detachable coils. J Neurosurg. 2002;96:837–43.

71. Ross IB, Dhillon GS. Complications of endovascular treatment of cerebral aneurysms. Surg Neurol. 2005;64:12–8.

72. Kanaan H, Jankowitz B, Aleu A, et al. In-stent thrombosis and stenosis after neck-remodeling device-assisted coil embolization of intracranial aneurysms. Neurosurgery. 2010;67:1523–33.

73. Rordorf G, Bellon RJ, Budzik Jr RF, et al. Silent thromboembolic events associated with the treatment of unruptured cerebral aneurysms by use of guglielmi detachable coils: prospective study applying diffusion-weighted imaging. AJNR Am J Neuroradiol. 2001;22:5–10.

74. Bendok BR, Hanel RA, Hopkins LN. Coil embolization of intracranial aneurysms. Neurosurgery. 2003;52:1125–30; discussion 30.

75. Ng PP, Phatouros CC, Khangure MS. Use of glycoprotein IIb-IIIa inhibitor for a thromboembolic complication during guglielmi detachable coil treatment of an acutely ruptured aneurysm. AJNR Am J Neuroradiol. 2001;22:1761–3.

76. Steinhubl SR, Talley JD, Braden GA, et al. Point-of-care measured platelet inhibition correlates with a reduced risk of an adverse cardiac event after percutaneous coronary intervention: results of the GOLD (AU-Assessing Ultegra) multi-center study. Circulation. 2001;103:2572–8.

77. Quinn MJ, Plow EF, Topol EJ. Platelet glycoprotein IIb/IIIa inhibitors: recognition of a two-edged sword? Circulation. 2002;106:379–85.

78. Kleinman N. Assessing platelet function in clinical trials. In: Quinn M, Fitzgerald D, editors. Platelet function assessment, diagnosis, and treatment. Totowa: Humana Press; 2005. p. 369–84.

79. Fourie P, Duncan IC. Microsnare-assisted mechanical removal of intraprocedural distal middle cerebral arterial thromboembolism. AJNR Am J Neuroradiol. 2003;24:630–2.

80. Cronqvist M, Pierot L, Boulin A, Cognard C, Castaings L, Moret J. Local intraarterial fibrinolysis of thromboemboli occurring during endovascular treatment of intracerebral aneurysm: a comparison of anatomic results and clinical outcome. AJNR Am J Neuroradiol. 1998;19:157–65.

81. Henkes H, Lowens S, Preiss H, Reinartz J, Miloslavski E, Kuhne D. A new device for endovascular coil retrieval from intracranial vessels: alligator retrieval device. AJNR Am J Neuroradiol. 2006;27:327–9.

82. Sugiu K, Martin JB, Jean B, Rufenacht DA. Rescue balloon procedure for an emergency situation during coil embolization for cerebral aneurysms. Technical note. J Neurosurg. 2002;96:373–6.

83. Cognard C, Weill A, Castaings L, Rey A, Moret J. Intracranial berry aneurysms: angiographic and clinical results after endovascular treatment. Radiology. 1998;206:499–510.

84. Fessler RD, Ringer AJ, Qureshi AI, Guterman LR, Hopkins LN. Intracranial stent placement to trap an extruded coil during endovascular aneurysm treatment: technical note. Neurosurgery. 2000;46:248–51; discussion 51–3.

85. Fiorella D, Albuquerque FC, Deshmukh VR, McDougall CG. Monorail snare technique for the recovery of stretched platinum coils: technical case report. Neurosurgery. 2005;57:E210; discussion E.

86. Friedman JA, Nichols DA, Meyer FB, et al. Guglielmi detachable coil treatment of ruptured saccular cerebral aneurysms: retrospective review of a 10-year single-center experience. AJNR Am J Neuroradiol. 2003;24:526–33.

87. Raymond J, Guilbert F, Weill A, et al. Long-term angiographic recurrences after selective endovascular treatment of aneurysms with detachable coils. Stroke. 2003;34:1398–403.

88. Kang HS, Han MH, Kwon BJ, Kwon OK, Kim SH. Repeat endovascular treatment in post-embolization recurrent intracranial aneurysms. Neurosurgery. 2006;58:60–70; discussion 60–70.

89. Bederson JB, Connolly Jr ES, Batjer HH, et al. Guidelines for the management of aneurysmal subarachnoid hemorrhage: a statement for healthcare professionals from a special writing group of the Stroke Council, American Heart Association. Stroke. 2009;40:994–1025.

90. van der Wee N, Rinkel GJ, Hasan D, van Gijn J. Detection of subarachnoid haemorrhage on early CT: is lumbar puncture still needed after a negative scan? J Neurol Neurosurg Psychiatry. 1995;58:357–9.

91. Provenzale JM, Hacein-Bey L. CT evaluation of subarachnoid hemorrhage: a practical review for the radiologist interpreting emergency room studies. Emerg Radiol. 2009;16:441–51.

92. Hino A, Fujimoto M, Iwamoto Y, Yamaki T, Katsumori T. False localization of rupture site in patients with multiple cerebral aneurysms and subarachnoid hemorrhage. Neurosurgery. 2000;46:825–30.

93. Karttunen AI, Jartti PH, Ukkola VA, Sajanti J, Haapea M. Value of the quantity and distribution of subarachnoid haemorrhage on CT in the localization of a ruptured cerebral aneurysm. Acta Neurochir (Wien). 2003;145:655–61; discussion 61.

94. Tryfonidis M, Evans AL, Coley SC, et al. The value of radioanatomical features on non-contrast CT scans in localizing the source in aneurysmal subarachnoid haemorrhage. Clin Anat. 2007;20:618–23.

95. Fisher CM, Kistler JP, Davis JM. Relation of cerebral vasospasm to subarachnoid hemorrhage visualized by computerized tomographic scanning. Neurosurgery. 1980;6:1–9.

96. Pasqualin A, Bazzan A, Cavazzani P, Scienza R, Licata C, Da Pian R. Intracranial hematomas following aneurysmal rupture: experience with 309 cases. Surg Neurol. 1986;25:6–17.

97. Thai QA, Raza SM, Pradilla G, Tamargo RJ. Aneurysmal rupture without subarachnoid hemorrhage: case series and literature review. Neurosurgery. 2005;57:225–9; discussion 225–9.

98. Flint AC, Roebken A, Singh V. Primary intraventricular hemorrhage: yield of diagnostic angiography and clinical outcome. Neurocrit Care. 2008;8:330–6.

99. Kallmes DF, Layton K, Marx WF, Tong F. Death by nondiagnosis: why emergent CT angiography should not be done for patients with subarachnoid hemorrhage. AJNR Am J Neuroradiol. 2007;28:1837–8.

100. Moran CJ. Aneurysmal subarachnoid hemorrhage: DSA versus CT angiography – is the answer available? Radiology. 2011;258:15–7.

101. Fifi JT, Meyers PM, Lavine SD, et al. Complications of modern diagnostic cerebral angiography in an academic medical center. J Vasc Interv Radiol. 2009;20:442–7.

102. Prestigiacomo CJ, Sabit A, He W, Jethwa P, Gandhi C, Russin J. Three dimensional CT angiography versus digital subtraction angiography in the detection of intracranial aneurysms in subarachnoid hemorrhage. J Neurointerv Surg. 2010;2:385–9.

103. Menke J, Larsen J, Kallenberg K. Diagnosing cerebral aneurysms by computed tomographic angiography: meta-analysis. Ann Neurol. 2011;69:646–54.

104. Bruneau M, Rynkowski M, Smida-Rynkowska K, Brotchi J, De Witte O, Lubicz B. Long-term follow-up survey reveals a high yield, up to 30% of patients presenting newly detected aneurysms more than 10 years after ruptured intracranial aneurysms clipping. Neurosurg Rev. 2011;34:485–96.

105. Wallace RC, Karis JP, Partovi S, Fiorella D. Noninvasive imaging of treated cerebral aneurysms, part II: CT angiographic follow-up of surgically clipped aneurysms. AJNR Am J Neuroradiol. 2007;28:1207–12.

106. Sagara Y, Kiyosue H, Hori Y, Sainoo M, Nagatomi H, Mori H. Limitations of three-dimensional reconstructed computerized tomography angiography after clip placement for intracranial aneurysms. J Neurosurg. 2005;103:656–61.

107. van der Schaaf IC, Velthuis BK, Wermer MJ, et al. Multislice computed tomography angiography screening for new aneurysms in patients with previously clip-treated intracranial aneurysms: feasibility, positive predictive value, and inter-observer agreement. J Neurosurg. 2006;105:682–8.

108. Dehdashti AR, Binaghi S, Uske A, Regli L. Comparison of multislice computerized tomography angiography and digital subtraction angiography in the postoperative evaluation of patients with clipped aneurysms. J Neurosurg. 2006;104:395–403.

109. Chen W, Yang Y, Qiu J, Peng Y, Xing W. Sixteen-row multislice computerized tomography angiography in the postoperative evaluation of patients with intracranial aneurysms. Br J Neurosurg. 2008;22:63–70.

110. Thines L, Dehdashti AR, Howard P, et al. Postoperative assessment of clipped aneurysms with 64-slice computerized tomography angiography. Neurosurgery. 2010;67:844–53; discussion 53–4.

111. Tomura N, Sakuma I, Otani T, et al. Evaluation of postoperative status after clipping surgery in patients with cerebral aneurysm on 3-dimensional-CT angiography with elimination of clips. J Neuroimaging. 2011;21:10–5.

112. Wallace RC, Karis JP, Partovi S, Fiorella D. Noninvasive imaging of treated cerebral aneurysms, part I: MR angiographic follow-up of coiled aneurysms. AJNR Am J Neuroradiol. 2007;28:1001–8.

113. Khan R, Wallace RC, Fiorella DJ. Magnetic resonance angiographic imaging follow-up of treated intracranial aneurysms. Top Magn Reson Imaging. 2008;19:231–9.

114. Kaufmann 3rd TJ, Huston J, Cloft HJ, et al. A prospective trial of 3T and 1.5T time-of-flight and contrast-enhanced MR angiography in the follow-up of coiled intracranial aneurysms. AJNR Am J Neuroradiol. 2010;31:912–8.

115. Lubicz B, Levivier M, Sadeghi N, Emonts P, Baleriaux D. Immediate intracranial aneurysm occlusion after embolization with detachable coils: a comparison between MR angiography and intra-arterial digital subtraction angiography. J Neuroradiol. 2007;34:190–7.

116. Ferre JC, Carsin-Nicol B, Morandi X, et al. Time-of-flight MR angiography at 3T versus digital subtraction angiography in the imaging follow-up of 51 intracranial aneurysms treated with coils. Eur J Radiol. 2009;72:365–9.

117. Cure' JK. Brain MRA protocol for coiled aneurysms. Birmingham; 2006.

118. Raabe A, Beck J, Gerlach R, Zimmermann M, Seifert V. Near-infrared indocyanine green video angiography: a new method for intraoperative assessment of vascular flow. Neurosurgery. 2003;52:132–9; discussion 9.

119. Hanggi D, Etminan N, Steiger HJ. The impact of microscope-integrated intraoperative near-infrared indocyanine green videoangiography on surgery of arteriovenous malformations and dural arteriovenous fistulae. Neurosurgery. 2010;67:1094–103; discussion 103–4.

120. Schuette AJ, Cawley CM, Barrow DL. Indocyanine green videoangiography in the management of dural arteriovenous fistulae. Neurosurgery. 2010;67:658–62; discussion 62.

121. Awano T, Sakatani K, Yokose N, et al. Intraoperative EC-IC bypass blood flow assessment with indocyanine green angiography in moyamoya and non-moyamoya ischemic stroke. World Neurosurg. 2010;73:668–74.

122. Woitzik J, Pena-Tapia PG, Schneider UC, Vajkoczy P, Thome C. Cortical perfusion measurement by indocyanine-green videoangiography in patients undergoing hemicraniectomy for malignant stroke. Stroke. 2006;37:1549–51.

123. Ferroli P, Acerbi F, Albanese E, et al. Application of intraoperative indocyanine green angiography for CNS tumors: results on the first 100 cases. Acta Neurochir Suppl. 2011;109:251–7.

124. Kim EH, Cho JM, Chang JH, Kim SH, Lee KS. Application of intraoperative indocyanine green videoangiography to brain tumor surgery. Acta Neurochir (Wien). 2011;153:1487–95; discussion 94–5.

125. Killory BD, Nakaji P, Maughan PH, Wait SD, Spetzler RF. Evaluation of angiographically occult spinal dural arteriovenous fistulae with surgical microscope-integrated intraoperative near-infrared indocyanine green angiography: report of 3 cases. Neurosurgery. 2011;68:781–7; discussion 7.

126. Trinh VT, Duckworth EA. Surgical excision of filum terminale arteriovenous fistulae after lumbar fusion: value of indocyanine green and theory on origins (a technical note and report of two cases). Surg Neurol Int. 2011;2:63.

127. Oh JK, Shin HC, Kim TY, et al. Intraoperative indocyanine green video-angiography: spinal dural arteriovenous fistula. Spine (Phila Pa 1976). 2011;36(24):E1578–80.

128. Chen SF, Kato Y, Oda J, et al. The application of intraoperative near-infrared indocyanine green videoangiography and analysis of fluorescence intensity in cerebrovascular surgery. Surg Neurol Int. 2011;2:42.

129. Hope-Ross M, Yannuzzi LA, Gragoudas ES, et al. Adverse reactions due to indocyanine green. Ophthalmology. 1994;101:529–33.

130. Raabe A, Beck J, Seifert V. Technique and image quality of intraoperative indocyanine green angiography during aneurysm surgery using surgical microscope integrated near-infrared video technology. Zentralbl Neurochir. 2005;66:1–6; discussion 7–8.

6. Provocative Testing

Provocative testing attempts to predict what, if any, clinical deficit would result from the occlusion of some vessel or resection of the territory supplied by that vessel. Provocative testing may be mechanical, in which a vessel is temporarily occluded, usually using a balloon, or pharmacologically, in which an agent is injected to temporarily anesthetize and inactivate a neuroanatomical territory in the brain, spinal cord, or a nerve. When the provocative test is being done, the patient is examined to check for new neurological deficits that may result from either the lack of blood flow to a vascular territory in the case of balloon test occlusion, or an anesthetic infusion into the neural tissue supplied by the vessel being tested pharmacologically. These procedures may be done preoperatively or as part of a therapeutic endovascular procedure to ensure the safety of occluding a vessel by open surgical or endovascular methods. This chapter focuses on arterial procedures. See Chap. 12 for venous provocative testing.

6.1.   Balloon Test Occlusion

Background

Temporary occlusion of a vessel has been shown to be a safe, predictable way to estimate the effect of permanent vascular occlusion. Test occlusion is done to predict whether occlusion of the vessel will have negative haemodynamic consequences, which can result in ischaemic injury to neural tissue and result in a permanent functional deficit. Temporarily occluding a vessel to predict the functional effects was first reported by Rudolph Matas, a New Orleans surgeon, in the early twentieth century, and therefore, the test occlusion procedure is sometimes referred to as the Matas test.[1, 2] The use of an endovascular balloon allows for reversible occlusion of the vessel in a predictable fashion. Balloon test occlusion is generally performed prior to endovascular or surgical occlusion of a major cerebral artery in the management of aneurysms, tumours and other neurosurgical problems.

There are two conditions that must be met to ensure the reliability of the test occlusion results:

1. The vessel being occluded must be at the proper site and level to simulate the anticipated permanent occlusion. It is important to test-occlude beyond any potential collateral vessels that may still provide flow to the brain during the test, yet may be lost after more distal permanent occlusion. In the carotid circulation, more than half the population has angiographically apparent branches of the proximal intracranial carotid that can be a pathway for collateral flow to the brain, during a test occlusion in the cervical carotid.[3] The ophthalmic artery is a significant collateral pathway in many patients and some patients who pass a test occlusion with a balloon proximal to the ophthalmic, may fail when the balloon is placed at the level of the ophthalmic, occluding the collateral flow via that vessel.[4] *A simple rule of thumb is to perform a test occlusion of a vessel with balloon inflation at the same level as the anticipated permanent occlusion.*

2. The test should reliably predict neurological consequences of the vascular occlusion. Temporary occlusion of a vessel could sufficiently lower the blood flow to an eloquent neuroanatomical region, so that a demonstrable neurological deficit occurs. The situation is simple if the test result is abnormal, and the patient exhibits a neurological deficit during the test: it is very likely that the patient would suffer some haemodynamic ischaemic injury due to permanent occlusion of that vessel. When a neurological change occurs during a test occlusion, it may not always be true that a permanent deficit would occur with permanent occlusion of the artery, thanks to the potential for collateral enlargement (*arteriogenesis*) after occlusion. However, it is never wise to ignore a test occlusion that produces a deficit. Somewhat more problematic is the situation in which no

M.R. Harrigan, J.P. Deveikis, *Handbook of Cerebrovascular Disease and Neurointerventional Technique*, DOI 10.1007/978-1-61779-946-4_6,
© Springer Science+Business Media New York 2013

deficit occurs during the test occlusion. Does this imply that the patient will never have an ischaemic problem from permanent occlusion of the vessel, or is there a potential for false negative test occlusions? Neurological examination during arterial test occlusion is usually combined with additional manoeuvers, when possible, to corroborate the clinical findings. These additional manoeuvers include cerebral blood flow imaging, acetazolamide administration, and pharmacological lowering of blood pressure.

Carotid artery test occlusion is done frequently, and experience with the procedure has shown the predictive power of the test. A systematic review of 254 patients in five studies in which an internal carotid was therapeutically sacrificed without a test occlusion found an average stroke rate of 26%, and mortality of 12%.[5] These results are in contrast to a study of 262 patients in eight studies in which the internal carotid was occluded after performing a test occlusion with an average stroke rate of 13% and mortality of 3%. This difference in stroke and death rate reached statistical significance. The significant morbidity associated with carotid artery occlusion, even with prior test occlusion, indicates that test occlusion is an imperfect predictor with a significant false negative rate. Adjunctive evaluation techniques (the additional manoeuvers mentioned above) were added to the neurological assessment to reduce the chances of a false negative test occlusion. The rationale of the additional these tests is that occlusion of the carotid or other vessels may produce a drop in blood flow that puts the patient at risk for stroke, yet not enough of a drop to produce detectable neurological dysfunction during a trial occlusion for a reasonable period of time. These adjunctive tests look for subtle signs of neurological dysfunction or look for the effects of the vessel occlusion on blood flow to the target territory.

Adjunctive Tests of Neurological Function

1. *Hypotensive* challenge.[6–10] Lowering the blood pressure magnifies the haemodynamic effect of vascular occlusion, making it more likely that a neurological deficit will occur in the case of limited collateral flow. When the carotid artery is occluded and no deficit occurs in a normotensive patient, the blood pressure is pharmacologically lowered to a target pressure (e.g. 66% of mean baseline pressure[6]), or until the patient develops a focal neurological deficit or becomes too nauseated and uncomfortable to allow adequate clinical assessment. Agents that can be used for lowering blood pressure should be fast-acting and quickly reversible, such as nitroprusside or esmolol.
   (a) Advantages: Cheap and easy to perform. Does not require moving the patient from the angiography suite.
   (b) Disadvantages: Headaches and nausea are common, for the patient (and the physician). A small series.[10] had 15% false negative rate, which is no better than just a clinical test occlusion.
2. *Neuropsychological testing.*[9, 11, 12] In addition to simple neurological testing during temporary vessel occlusion, a battery of standardized neuropsychological tests are given to test higher cortical functions.
   (a) Advantages: Cheap and easy to perform. Can be performed in the angiography suite. Standardized tests of higher cortical function can detect subtle signs of neurological dysfunction, even if the patient does not have an apparent motor or sensory deficit.[12]
   (b) Disadvantages: Requires skilled personnel to administer testing in an accurate and consistent manner. Most centers have limited experience with this test. Accuracy is unproven.
3. *Electroencephalography (EEG).*[13, 14] Continuous EEG monitoring is done throughout the procedure. Slowing or other deviations from baseline conditions can be secondary signs of developing ischaemia.
   (a) Advantages: Does not require moving the patient with the balloon in place. Can still be done with patients under light general anesthesia. Monitored results can be recorded and examined carefully at a later time, to look for changes corresponding to events during the procedure.
   (b) Disadvantages: Adds cost and complexity to the procedure. Requires preplacement of EEG leads prior to starting the procedure. Requires skilled personnel to monitor the readings. Careful neurological testing will almost always reveal a deficit when EEG changes are present, making the use of this modality redundant when the patient is awake and can be tested neurologically.

4. *Somatosensory evoked potentials (SSEP)* [15, 16] EEG electrodes are attached and electrical stimulation of a peripheral nerve (usually the median nerve) contralateral to the hemisphere being tested, is performed. Cortical responses are recorded and the timing and amplitude of the response indicates cortical function. Testing is done prior to and following balloon inflation.

  (a) Advantages: Does not require moving the patient with the balloon in place. Can still be done with patients under light general anesthesia. Monitoring results can be recorded and examined carefully at a later time to look for changes corresponding to events during the procedure.

  (b) Disadvantages: Adds cost and complexity to the procedure. Requires preplacement of EEG leads and nerve stimulation leads prior to starting the procedure. Stimulation of the nerve can be uncomfortable and distracting to the patient. Results may be difficult to interpret in the setting of underlying spinal or peripheral nerve disease. Requires skilled personnel to monitor the readings. The value of this test is unclear, compared to standard neurological testing.

5. *Cerebral Oximetry.* [17, 18] Commercially available cerebral oximeter, such as INVOS® (Somanetics, Troy, MI) can be applied to the forehead and allows measurement of frontal lobe oxygenation.

  (a) Advantages: Does not require movement of the patient with the balloon in place. Results seem to correlate with neurological deficits and SPECT imaging. [17]

  (b) Disadvantages: Gives only a limited evaluation of frontal lobe oxygenation. Results can be affected by underlying brain pathology. Sensitivity and specificity are unproven.

Adjunctive Tests of Blood Flow

1. *Angiography.* [19, 20] Cerebral angiography before and during balloon test occlusion allows qualitative, semiquantitative assessment of brain blood flow and potential collateral circulation to the occluded vascular territory. A posterior communicating artery diameter <1 mm is a risk factor for subsequent stroke with carotid occlusion. [21] Similarly, the absence of a functional anterior communicating artery is a risk factor for haemodynamic stroke after carotid occlusion. [22] Semi-quantitative assessment consists of looking for synchronous filling of cortical veins with angiography of the contralateral carotid or vertebral during trial occlusion of a carotid, and measuring the difference between hemispheres in the time it takes to achieve venous filling. [19, 20] This provides a rough approximation of differences in mean transit time between the hemispheres.

  (a) Advantages: Easily done. Does not require moving the patient with the balloon in place. Can limit the time the balloon needs to be inflated. Can be done in patients who are under general anesthesia.

  (b) Disadvantages: Requires use of a second catheter to obtain arteriograms of contralateral carotid and vertebral arteries while the balloon is inflated. This then requires bilateral groin punctures or the use of a GuardWire® (Medtronic Vascular, Santa Rosa, CA) balloon wire and diagnostic catheter placed via the same femoral sheath (as discussed below). Results are somewhat subjective. Published data on the accuracy of this, compared to more direct measurements of blood flow, are lacking.

2) *Back-pressure ("stump-pressure") measurement.* [23,24] Blood pressure is measured through the end-hole of the catheter distal to the site of balloon occlusion. The absolute value of the back-pressure or better yet, a ratio of minimum mean back-pressure to mean systemic blood pressure can be recorded. A ratio of 60% or greater is indicates good collateral flow and predicts tolerance to occlusion. [25]

  (a) Advantages: Quick and easy. Does not require moving the patient with the balloon in place.

  (b) Disadvantages: Requires the use of a double lumen balloon catheter, with a central lumen for a guidewire or pressure measurements, and another lumen for inflating and deflating the balloon. Stump pressure fluctuates over time as the balloon is inflated and may not absolutely correlate with Xenon-CT data. [23] Back-pressure readings can be affected if the balloon catheter is in a curve and the end-hole of the catheter kinks or presses against the vessel wall.

3. *Transcranial Doppler (TCD)* [26–28] Sonographic evaluation of the middle cerebral artery is obtained before and after balloon inflation. Mean blood flow velocity and pulsatility index that do not decrease more than 30% are highly predictive of tolerance to carotid occlusion.[27]
   (a) Advantages: Does not require moving patient with the balloon in place. Can be done in patients under general anesthesia.
   (b) Disadvantages: Adds cost and complexity to the procedure. Visualization of the intracranial vessels can be time consuming and can distract from examination of the patient. Test results may be difficult to interpret in the setting of underlying vascular disease. Requires skilled personnel to perform the study, and results can be operator-dependent. Unproven value compared to standard neurological testing.
4. *[133]Xenon imaging*[29] Radioactive Xenon is administered while the carotid is occluded and the patient's brain is imaged with a detector, and blood flow data calculated.
   (a) Advantages: Can provide quantitative blood flow data.
   (b) Disadvantages: Gives only whole-brain images, so only gross side-to-side differences are visible. Use of the radioactive xenon is cumbersome.
5. *Xenon CT*[5, 30] Dynamic CT imaging is done as the patient inhales non-radioactive xenon gas. Scans are obtained prior to balloon inflation to determine baseline flow, and the study is repeated during balloon occlusion to determine the effect of occlusion on blood flow. Can also be done with acetazolamide injection during balloon inflation to evaluate for the presence of vascular reserve.
   (a) Advantages: Provides accurate blood flow data reliably. The hardware used for the xenon delivery is compatible with most commercially available CT scanners. Can do repeated scans to allow scans with and without balloon inflation, and also after acetazolamide.
   (b) Disadvantages: May require moving a patient into the CT scanner with the balloon in place. The scan may be done without transferring the patient if the angiography and balloon placement is done on the CT scanner table using a portable C-arm.[31]) Xenon gas is not FDA approved, and therefore currently requires an Investigational Drug Exemption (IDE) and all the associated paperwork. The hardware for delivering the gas and software for the CT computations require experienced personnel to obtain good studies. Xenon gas can produce euphoria, agitation, and/or nausea in patients, making it difficult to avoid patient motion, which greatly affects accuracy. Produces images of only a limited area of the brain.
6. *CT perfusion*[32] Dynamic CT imaging with a bolus of intravenous contrast, and post-processing can provide blood flow, blood volume and mean-transit time. Scans are obtained without balloon inflation to determine baseline flow, and the study is repeated with balloon inflation to determine the effect of occlusion on blood flow. CT perfusion can also be done with acetazolamide injection during balloon inflation to evaluate cerebrovascular reserve. See the *Primer on Imaging in Stroke* in Chap. 9 for more detail.
   (a) Advantages: Readily available on most CT scanners. Quick and easy. Uses standard iodinated contrast used for any intravenous contrast-enhanced scan. Blood flow data has been validated by Xenon-CT.[33] Can do repeated scans to allow scans with and without balloon inflation and also after acetazolamide.
   (b) Disadvantages: May require moving a patient into the CT scanner with the balloon in place. Requires large-bore intravenous access. Multiple perfusion studies can add to the amount of iodinated contrast given. Produces images of only a limited section of the brain.
7. *Positron emission tomography (PET)*[34] Short acting, radioactive tracers such as.[15]O H$_2$O are administered and PET scanning done. Postprocessing allows blood flow calculation. Scans are obtained without balloon inflation to determine baseline flow, and the study is repeated with balloon inflation to determine the effect of occlusion on blood flow. Can also be done with acetazolamide injection during balloon inflation, to evaluate for the presence of vascular reserve.
   (a) Advantages: Can give accurate quantitative blood flow data. Can image the entire brain, allowing for visualization of secondary signs of impaired cerebral blood flow, such as crossed cerebellar diaschisis.[35] Crossed cerebellar diaschisis is a reflexive drop in blood flow to the contralateral

cerebellar hemisphere, when a substantial drop in blood flow to a cerebral hemisphere occurs. Can do repeated scans to allow scans with and without balloon inflation and also after acetazolamide.

(b) Disadvantages: Requires moving the patient to the PET scanner with the balloon in place. PET scanners are not universally available. Requires immediate access to a cyclotron for making the radiotracer, such as.[15]O H_2O, which has a very, very short half-life. Cyclotrons are even more scarce than PET scanners. To allow for quantitative blood flow measurements, requires an arterial access such as a larger diameter femoral sheath or a separate radial arterial line.

8. *Single-photon emission computed tomography (SPECT)*[36–39] [99m]Technicium-HMPAO is injected intravenously within 5 min after the balloon is inflated, and the radioactive tracer deposits in the brain in quantities proportional to the regional blood flow. After the test occlusion is completed, SPECT scanning shows activity from the tracer, and asymmetry is detected qualitatively by visual inspection of the scan and by measuring the number of radioactive counts in each region of interest.

(a) Advantages: Quick and easy. The imaging can be done after the procedure is completed, so there is no need to transport the patient with a balloon in the vessel. The entire brain can be imaged, allowing for visualization of secondary signs of impaired cerebral blood flow, such as crossed cerebellar diaschisis.[40, 41]

(b) Disadvantages: Does not allow for accurate quantitative measurement of cerebral blood flow. Reliance on asymmetry without absolute values of cerebral blood flow can result in significant false positive and false negative results.[42] Scans obtained with the balloon inflated and deflated cannot be obtained immediately one after the other.

9. *Magnetic resonance (MR) perfusion*[43,44] Diffusion-weighted scans, perfusion imaging with a bolus of intravenous gadolinium contrast, and post-contrast T1 weighted and FLAIR imaging are performed prior to and following the balloon inflation. The diffusion and post-contrast scans are observed for signs of ischaemia with the balloon inflated. Calculation of cerebral blood volume, mean transit time and blood flow can be done on a computer workstation using the MR perfusion data. See the *Primer on Imaging in Stroke* in Chap. 9 for more detail.

(a) Advantages: Does not add to the iodinated contrast given to the patient. Can image the entire brain.

(b) Disadvantages: Requires MR compatible balloon catheters and patient monitoring leads. Unless one has a combined MR and angiographic interventional suite, requires transfer of patient while the balloon is in place. Quantitative blood flow data is of uncertain validity. Significance of any changes on diffusion imaging or postcontrast scans is uncertain.

10. *Computer simulation*[45, 46] Proprietary software allows computer modeling of blood flow in the intracranial circulation using data from MR and digital subtraction angiography imaging.

(a) Advantages: A small series showed computer flow modeling showing greater than 20% drop in flow in the M1 segment and A3 segment during carotid occlusion, accurately predicted the patients who developed clinical symptoms during test occlusion.[46] May theoretically replace invasive balloon-test occlusion.

(b) Disadvantages: Unproven efficacy.

The bottom line on adjunctive tests: Nothing is perfect. Use at least one or two adjunctive tests in addition to neurological assessment. In most cases the two adjunctive tests are angiography plus cerebral blood flow imaging.

Indications for Test Occlusion

To determine the potential safety of occluding an artery, prior to treatment for:
1. Intracranial haemorrhage
2. Aneurysm
3. Arteriovenous malformation
4. Arteriovenous fistula
5. Tumours involving a vascular structure

Complications of Balloon Test Occlusion

Informed consent prior to the procedure should include an estimate of the risk of complications.

Neurological Complications

1. Thromboembolic stroke; a series of 500 carotid test-occlusions reported 1.6% symptomatic neurological complications, of which two (0.4%) were permanent.[30]
2. Dissection of the target vessel.[6] possibly resulting in a dissecting aneurysm. Dissection was found in 1.2% of cases and dissecting aneurysms were reported in 0.2% of cases in the Pittsburg series.[30]
3. Overly aggressive balloon inflation in intracranial vessels can rupture the artery.
4. In the cavernous ICA, carotid cavernous fistula can result from overinflation of the balloon.

Nonneurological Complications

1. Balloon inflation in the carotid bulb or basilar artery can produce a vasovagal reaction and bradycardia, hypotension, and rarely, cardiac arrest.
2. Balloon inflation in the basilar artery can produce unconsciousness and apnea.
3. Anaphylactic reactions to iodinated contrast or any of the medications used can occur as with any endovascular procedure.
4. Similarly, groin hematomas, femoral or iliac dissections.[6], puncture site infections or other access complications can occur.
5. Use of hypotensive challenges may theoretically provoke cardiac ischaemia.

Balloon Test Occlusion: Technique

Preprocedure Preparation

1. Informed consent.
2. IV access.
3. Foley catheter.
4. Rehearse a brief neurological exam with the patient prior to the case.
5. Place a rubber duckie (see Fig. 4.1) in the contralateral hand if the carotid territory is going to be tested.
6. Sedation and analgesia should be minimized if neurological assessment during the test occlusion is planned.

Vascular Access Phase

See Chap. 4 for a general discussion of access techniques.
1. A 6F sheath is placed in the femoral artery.
   (a) If a second catheter is needed for angiography of collateral vessels during the test occlusion, place a 5F sheath in the contralateral femoral artery.
2. Guide catheter selection.
   (a) 6F Guider (Stryker Neurovascular, Fremont, CA) or Envoy® (Codman Neurovascular, San Jose, CA) are stiff enough to provide support when positioned in the common carotid artery, and have an inner diameter to permit good angiograms when the balloon catheter is in position.
   (b) Sheaths (90 cm) (e.g. Shuttle® sheath, Cook Inc., Bloomington, IN) also work very well as alternative guiding catheters for test occlusions. This allows for extra stability if needed.

3. Guide catheter access is obtained in the usual fashion.
4. Antithrombotic medication. A loading dose of IV heparin is given (5,000 units or 70 units/kg is given after sheath placement and at least 5 min before the test occlusion.
5. Pretreat with 0.3–0.5 mg atropine if planning on inflating a balloon in the carotid bulb or basilar artery and the baseline heart rate is low.

Balloons for Test Occlusion

There are four main categories of devices for test occlusion:

1. Double lumen balloon catheter. This has a central lumen for the microwire and for pressure measurements, and another lumen for inflating and deflating the balloon. These devices are similar to most angioplasty balloons, but high-pressure, low-compliance angioplasty balloons are not recommended for test occlusions, as they can traumatize the vessel. Soft balloons such as those on standard occlusion balloons or even Swan-Ganz balloon catheters can be used. The advantage of these balloons is the ability to measure pressures through the distal lumen, and also these balloons are relatively inexpensive. The disadvantage of these balloons is that they do not manoeuver well, are somewhat traumatic to vessels and consequently should not be used in very small vessels or intracranial vessels, although The Ascent™ (Codman Neurovascular, San Jose, CA) is designed to be used in intracranial vessels.

2. Over-the-wire microballoon. The prototypical balloon in this category is the Hyperform™ (ev3 Neurovascular, Irvine, CA) (see Fig. 11.1). The balloon catheter has single lumen and when the appropriately sized wire is advanced beyond the catheter tip, an O-ring type valve in the balloon catheter seals the tip of the catheter around the wire and allows inflation and deflation of the balloon. These balloons have the advantage that they are soft, atraumatic, and very manoeuverable to almost any destination. The downside is that they have single lumen to inflate the balloon and no way to measure backpressure when the vessel is occluded. These small balloons are advanced through a guide catheter placed in the proximal carotid or vertebral artery, depending on the vessel being tested. Measurement of pressure through the guide catheter will show dampening of the pressure waveform, if the balloon is inflated in the vessel a short distance beyond the guidecatheter tip. The microwire must be advanced through the balloon catheter for at least a short segment distal to the balloon. Thus, it requires a straight segment to place the distal wire and care should be taken to keep the wire tip out of small side-branches or acute bifurcations, to prevent perforations or dissections. The risk of injury caused by the microwire can be minimized by creating a tight J-shaped curve on the guidewire tip. One advantage of the microwire in these single lumen balloons is that, if necessary, the balloon can be rapidly deflated by withdrawing the wire. Other balloon types do not have this option for rapid deflation. These microballoons are the most common balloons currently used for cerebrovascular test occlusions.

3. Inflatable balloon wire. This is typified by the GuardWire® (Medtronic Vascular, Santa Rosa, CA). This system works well especially for carotid test occlusions. This occlusion balloon is mounted on a 0.014-in hypotube (a small diameter wire with an inner lumen) and has a 0.028-in profile for the 2.5–5-cm balloon, or 0.036 in for the 3–6 mm balloon. The larger balloon can easily be advanced through 6F guide catheter. It is inflated with an inflation device, which can be removed from the wire, leaving the balloon inflated. This allows removal of the guide catheter and permits placement of a diagnostic catheter via the same femoral arterial sheath for performance of control angiography of potential collateral vessels, while the balloon occludes the target vessel. Another advantage of this balloon wire is that, it has such a low profile that it allows safe moving of the patient with the balloon in place, for cerebral blood flow imaging with CT perfusion. The disadvantages of the balloon wire is that the distal stump pressure cannot be measured and the wire tip extends for several centimeters distal to the balloon. The GuardWire® has other disadvantages, including the fact that it is stiffer than the microballoons, so, as a general rule, should not be used in intracranial vessels or other small vessels. The need for the inflation device also means that there is a bit of a learning curve to be able to use this device efficiently. The most annoying problem with this device is the length of time required for balloon deflation. The balloon should be inflated with a dilute contrast solution (e.g. 30% contrast in saline) to minimize viscosity and decrease the problems associated with inflating and deflating the balloon.

4. Detachable coils. In extremely small, tortuous distal vessels, it may not be possible to safely advance even the smallest microballoons. However, these vessels may still be accessible using low-profile, ten-system microcatheters. With the microcatheter in the vessel to be tested, a detachable coil can be advanced into the vessel to temporarily occlude it. This method will only work in vessels <3 mm in diameter. Use a 2 or 3 mm diameter coil that is stretch resistant so that it can be easily removed. The coil should also be ultra-soft, to fill the lumen of the vessel without traumatizing the intima. Advance as few loops of coil as necessary to occlude flow. Obviously, the patient must be fully heparized, so that the thrombus does not form in the vessel, and occlusion times must be kept to a minimum. *Given the possibilities of thrombus formation and the remote possibility of coil stretching or inadvertent detachment, this method should not be routinely used for test occlusion unless everything else fails.*

Balloons must be sized to match the vessel being occluded. Measure the target vessel using a previous angiographic study, or obtain an angiogram as part of the procedure to get a measurement of the vessel.

1. The ICA requires balloons at least 5 mm in diameter in most cases.
2. The extracranial ICA can be occluded with Swan-Ganz double-lumen balloon (Edwards Lifesciences, Irvine, CA), 10 mm occlusion balloon catheter (Cook Medical, Bloomington, IN), 7 × 7 mm Hyperform™ microballoon (ev3 Neurovascular, Irvine, CA), or 6 mm GuardWire®(Medtronic Vascular, Santa Rosa, CA).
3. The intracranial ICA is best occluded with a Hyperform™ microballoon (ev3 Neurovascular, Irvine, CA) or the Ascent™ (Codman Neurovascular, San Jose, MA).
4. The vertebral arteries can usually be occluded with 5 mm diameter or larger balloons.
5. The straight segment of the cervical vertebral can be occluded with a 10 mm occlusion balloon or a 7 × 7 mm microballoon listed above.
6. Above the C2 segment of the vertebral artery, where the artery curves laterally, only flexible microballoons such as the Hyperform™ should be used.
7. Intracranial vessels such as ICA and vertebral arteries may be as large as 4–5-mm in diameter. The supraclinoid ICA is usually 3.5 mm and basilar artery is usually 3.2 mm in diameter. More distal branches are generally <3 mm in diameter.
8. Vessels >4 mm can be occluded with the 7 × 7 mm Hyperform™ microballoon, or 6 × 9 mm Ascent™ (Codman Neurovascular, Raynham, MA).
9. Vessels ≤4 mm may be occluded with the 4 × 7 mm Hyperform™ (ev3, Irvine, CA), a 4 × 10 mm Hyperglide™ microballoon (ev3, Irvine, CA) or 4 × 10 mm Ascent™ (Codman Neurovascular, San Jose, CA).

Guidewires

- Steerable hydrophilic wires such as 0.035 or 0.038-in. angled Glidewire® (Terumo Medical, Somerset, NJ) can be used to advance a diagnostic catheter or guiding catheter into the carotid or vertebral artery.
- A 0.025 or 0.035-in. Glidewire® (Terumo Medical, Somerset, NJ) can be used for standard occlusion balloons.
- The Transend™ 10 (Stryker Neurovascular, Fremont, CA), X-pedion™ 10 (ev3, Irvine, CA), or other 0.010-in. microwire is used to advance an over-the-wire microballoon catheter to the target vessel.
- The GuardWire® (Medtronic Vascular, Santa Rosa, CA) balloon is integrated as part of a 0.014-in. wire, and can be used as a wire for relatively soft catheters.

Catheter and Balloon Manipulation

1. Attach all the catheters to RHVs and attach a continuous infusion of saline containing 10,000 units heparin per liter.
2. Through the femoral (or brachial) sheath, advance the guide catheter into the ICA or vertebral artery.
3. Do angiograms to determine the best position for the balloon, and to size the artery for proper balloon selection.

4. Avoid positioning the balloon in any area containing atherosclerotic plaque.
5. Obtain a roadmap mask to allow balloon positioning and inflation under roadmap guidance.
6. Warn patients that the catheter manipulation and balloon inflation may cause a feeling of pressure.
7. Use *extreme* caution when advancing or inflating a balloon in intracranial vessels.
8. Always keep track of where the tip of the guidewire is to avoid vascular perforation or dissection.
9. When the balloon reaches the desired location, pull back on the catheter to remove any slack. This will prevent the balloon from advancing forward as it is inflated.
10. Inflate the balloon only just enough to stop the flow. ***Do not overinflate***.
11. Measure the volume required to inflate the balloon and occlude the vessel. When doing adjunctive blood flow imaging, requiring patient transfer with the balloon in place, this allows for deflation and inflation of the balloon without fluoroscopic control.

Double-Lumen Balloon Catheter Technique

1. Prepare the balloon by attaching a 10 mL syringe partially filled with contrast to the inflation port of the balloon, aspirate any air, and release suction to allow contrast to enter the inflation port.
2. Attach a one-way stopcock to the inflation port, and inflate the balloon with 50:50 contrast:saline mixture, then deflate. Angle the balloon to allow aspiration of any residual air as the balloon is deflated.
3. For those ambitious (or foolish) enough to use a Swan–Ganz (Edwards Lifesciences, Irvine, CA) for test occlusion, expect to struggle getting into the vessel of interest, as these balloons are not designed for arterial catheterization. A 0.010 in. microwire can be used to direct the catheter and to do partial inflations for flow direction, but it is not a pleasant experience in tortuous vessels.
4. For all other balloons, such as the 10 mm occlusion balloon catheter (Cook Medical, Bloomington, IN), it is usually necessary to use an exchange wire, unless the patient is young or has straight cervical arteries that are easily accessible with a straight catheter.
5. Using a diagnostic angiographic catheter of desired size and shape, such as a 5F Angled Glidecath® (Terumo Medical, Somerset, NJ), catheterize the target carotid or vertebral artery that is to be tested.
6. Using a 300 cm, 0.035 in. diameter exchange wire, exchange the diagnostic catheter for the balloon catheter.
7. Advance the balloon catheter so that it is just proximal to the site of intended occlusion, and inject the contrast through the central lumen to obtain a roadmap of the vessel.
8. Advance the balloon to the target site.
9. Prepare to measure pressures through the end-hole of the balloon catheter, either by attaching a pressure line to the stopcock (or manifold) attached to the central lumen of the balloon catheter, or by using a pressure-sensing guidewire.
10. Measure a baseline pressure through the central lumen of the balloon catheter.
11. Gently inflate the balloon just enough to occlude the vessel.
12. Inject contrast through the end-hole of the balloon catheter; pooling of contrast in the artery will confirm complete occlusion.
13. Measure the pressures through the central lumen of the balloon catheter again. When the vessel is occluded, there will be dampening of the pressure waveform. A drop in mean pressure by 50% after balloon inflation is suggestive of insufficient collateral flow to the distal territory.
14. Examine the patient for any neurological deficits and pay particular attention to functions performed by areas of the central nervous system supplied by the vessel being occluded.
15. At some point during the test occlusion, do a cerebral angiogram using an arterial catheter in a contralateral sheath, and check for collateral flow from other arterial pathways.

16. If the patient tolerates the balloon inflation clinically and the back pressure in the balloon catheter does not drop <50% post-inflation, keep the vessel occluded for an extended period (~30 min) to confirm tolerance to occlusion.
17. Consider using a supplementary test to look for other signs of haemodynamic insufficiency, when the balloon is inflated (see below).
18. Signs of test occlusion failure:
    (a) Neurological changes
    (b) Drop in back-pressure
    (c) Evidence of poor collateral flow by angiography
    (d) Adjunctive test evidence of poor collateral flow
19. The procedure is complete when the patient fails the test occlusion, or if they pass for at least 30 min. The balloon should be deflated.
20. Prior to removing the balloon, ensure that the patient's symptoms have resolved. If not, a dissection or a thromboembolic complication may have occurred, and leaving the balloon catheter in place provides access for diagnostic angiography and corrective intervention.
21. Remove the balloon catheter when all testing is complete.

Microballoon Catheter Technique

1. Prepare the Hyperform™ or Hyperglide™ (ev3 Neurovascular, Irvine, CA) by thoroughly flushing the sterile holder housing the balloon to activate the hydrophilic coating.
2. Attach a one-way stopcock, or Flo-switch (BD Medical, Franklin Lakes, NJ) to a rotating haemostatic valve, and attach this to the balloon catheter.
3. Fill the balloon catheter with 50% contrast diluted with saline.
4. Insert the X-pedion™ (ev3 Neurovascular, Irvine, CA) or other 0.010-in. wire through the rotating haemostatic valve and into the balloon catheter.
5. Make a j-tip curve on the shapeable platinum tip of the wire, to limit the risk of the microwire traumatizing or perforating a vessel.
6. Place the guide catheter in the carotid or vertebral artery.
7. Make a roadmap.
8. Advance the balloon to the target site.
9. Gently inflate the balloon just enough to occlude the vessel.
10. Confirm occlusion of the vessel by injecting the contrast through the guide catheter. There will be stasis of the contrast in the vessel proximal to the balloon.
11. Examine the patient for neurological deficits and pay particular attention to functions performed by areas of the central nervous system supplied by the artery being occluded.
12. At some point during the test occlusion, do a cerebral angiogram using an arterial catheter in a contralateral sheath. Check for collateral flow from other arterial pathways.
13. If the patient tolerates the balloon inflation clinically, keep the vessel occluded for an extended period (~30 min) to confirm tolerance to occlusion.
14. Use adjunctive tests to assess for haemodynamic insufficiency when the balloon is inflated (see below).
15. Signs of test occlusion failure:
    (a) Neurological changes
    (b) Drop in back-pressure
    (c) Evidence of poor collateral flow by angiography
    (d) Adjunctive test evidence of poor collateral flow
16. When the patient fails the test occlusion, or if they pass for at least 30 min, the procedure is complete. Then deflate the balloon.
17. Prior to removing the balloon, ensure that the patient's symptoms have resolved. If not, there may be a dissection or a thromboembolic complication, and an angiogram via the guide catheter can determine if any corrective intervention is needed.
18. The balloon catheter and guide catheter can be removed after testing is completed.

Technique: Balloon Wire

1. Prepare the balloon on the GuardWire® (Medtronic Vascular, Santa Rosa, CA) by following the manufacturer's directions.

2. Thoroughly flush the sterile holder housing the wire.
3. Fill the inflator syringe that comes in the package with 30–50% contrast.
4. Attach the tubing from the syringe to the clam-shell shaped inflation device that also comes in the package.
5. Examine the microwire and find the gold marker that indicates where to insert the microwire into the inflation device, and carefully place it in the inflation device.
6. Close the clam-shell device and lock it.
7. Turn the dial on the device to the open position.
8. Aspirate back on the syringe and lock it in the position of maximal suction, in order to purge the balloon of air.
9. After a few seconds of maximum suction, turn and release the plunger on the syringe to release the suction and allow contrast to enter the balloon.
10. Repeat steps eight and nine until it looks like no more air can be aspirated from the system.
11. Turn the dial to inflate the balloon and check that it inflates and deflates properly.
12. Once the balloon is prepared, turn the dial to deflate it, and pull the plunger back on the syringe until the balloon is completely deflated.
13. Make a j-tip curve on the shapeable platinum tip of the wire, to limit the risk of the wire traumatizing or perforating a vessel.
14. Place a 6F guide catheter in the carotid or vertebral artery.
15. Make a roadmap.
16. Advance the balloon to the target site.
17. Gently inflate the balloon by turning the dial on the inflation device just enough to occlude the vessel.
18. Confirm occlusion of the vessel by injecting contrast through the lumen of the guide catheter. There will be stasis of contrast in the vessel proximal to the balloon.
19. Clinically test the patient for any neurological deficits and pay particular attention to functions performed by areas supplied by the vessel being occluded.
20. At some point during the test occlusion, do an angiogram to check for collateral flow from other arterial pathways. This can be done either by puncturing the other femoral artery and placing a second sheath, or by using the guide catheter:
    (a) This is done by opening and removing the clamshell of the inflation device, leaving the Guardwire® balloon inflated, and carefully backing out the guide catheter while gently feeding in the 0.014-in. wire, making sure to not pull back on the Guardwire® or displace it.
    (b) When the guide catheter is completely removed from the sheath, a 4F Glidecath® (Terumo Medical, Somerset, NJ) can be carefully advanced through the sheath alongside the 0.014-in. Guardwire® as long as the sheath is at least 5F, and preferably 6F size, to avoid disturbing the wire as the 4-French catheter is manipulated.
    (c) This catheter can then be used to perform selective arteriography of whatever vessels needed to assess collateral flow, while the balloon is still inflated.
21. If the patient tolerates the balloon inflation clinically, keep the vessel occluded for an extended period (~30) to confirm tolerance to occlusion.
22. Use adjunctive tests to look for other signs of haemodynamic insufficiency when the balloon is inflated.
23. If the patient develops symptoms, or if angiography suggests poor collateral flow, the patient has "failed" the test occlusion.
24. When the patient fails the test occlusion, or if they pass for at least 30 min, the procedure is complete. Insert the gold marker on the Guardwire® into the proper position in the clamshell of the inflation device, then turn the dial to zero, and aspirate on the syringe to deflate the balloon.
25. Prior to removing the balloon, ensure that the patient's examination has returned to or remains at their baseline. If not, a dissection of a thromboembolic complication may have occurred and a guide catheter angiogram should be done to determine if any corrective intervention is needed.
26. Remove the balloon catheter and guide catheter after testing is complete.

Guardwire® Tip

The authors use this balloon frequently for cervical carotid or vertebral test occlusions, and, out of approximately 25 cases, have had only one case in which balloon deflation was a problem, even though dilute contrast was used for inflation. This case involved a somewhat tortuous carotid and possibly the angulation caused the inflation/deflation port in the balloon to be pressed against the balloon material by the vessel wall. This required gently pulling back on the inflated balloon, to straighten the vessel and allow the inflation/deflation port to allow for unimpeded deflation of the balloon.

Postprocedure Care

1) Once the procedure is completed, removed the catheters and sheaths and obtain haemostasis.
2) The patient is kept at bed rest with the leg extended for 2 h if a haemostatic patch is used.

Venous Test Occlusion

See Chap. 12, Venous Procedures, for information.

6.2.   Pharmacologic Provocative Testing

Wada Test: Intracarotid Amobarbital Procedure

A Brief History of the Wada Test

The technique of pharmacologically anesthetizing certain parts of the human brain was first reported in the 1940s. W. James Gardner reported injecting procaine through burr-holes in the head to localize speech centers.[47] Juhn Wada, a Canadian neurologist, began using intracarotid injections of Amytal (amobarbital) initially for treating patients with status epilepticus and also those with schizophrenia undergoing electroconvulsive therapy, and later used it for localizing speech and memory, particularly in patients who were candidates for epilepsy surgery.[48, 49] This procedure was refined at the Montreal Neurological institute and by the early 1960s, became an important part of the preoperative work-up for epilepsy surgery.[50–52] Patients undergoing temporal lobe resection to for treatment of epilepsy are at risk for significant neurological and neuropsychological impairment as a complication from surgery. The carotid amobarbital injections can be used to predict which patients are at risk for developing language deficits[52], and also which patients are at risk for developing memory loss.[53] Although initially, the amobarbital was injected into the carotid artery using direct needle puncture, the appearance of transfemoral catheterization for angiography in the 1960s and 1970s resulted in the adoption of transfemoral catheter technique for Wada tests as well. The availability of microcatheters in the 1980s and 1990s led to superselective Wada tests.[54–56] The supply of amobarbital was interrupted in the early part of the new millennium, when the United States FDA required recertification of the manufacturing facilities after a different corporation acquired the rights to make the drug.[57] This led to the use of anesthetic agents such as methohexital[58], etomidate[59], and propofol.[60, 61] However, amobarbital is now readily available and the intracarotid injection procedure remains a key component in the preoperative workup before epilepsy surgery, and the technique remains little changed from the procedure developed by Dr. Wada in the middle of the twentieth century.

6.2.1.2   Strange, But True

The very same Dr. Wada that invented the Wada test also published on the behavioral and EEG changes produced by intracisternal and intraventricular injection of *extracts from the urine of schizophrenic patients.*[62] The authors of this handbook do not recommend the routine use of this particular technique.

Memory Testing in the Wada Test

Neuropsychological testing during the Wada test is primarily designed to predict disabling memory loss after epilepsy surgery. Verbal and visual/spatial memory is tested during temporary anesthesia of a hemisphere with amobarbital. Items are presented to the patient during the period of anesthetization. The number and types of stimuli that can later be recalled indicate how robust the memory functions are in the contralateral hemisphere. Functions lost during injection of the side of the seizure focus are at the risk of injury during surgery, and, conversely, functions remaining intact during injection of the contralateral side are at risk. Verbal memory is frequently on the left and visual/spatial memory is on the right, but the existence of lesions in the epileptogenic side may displace function, and bilateral lesions can make for unpredictable localization.

The protocol of memory testing done during Wada tests should be rigorously standardized, since the items presented and the manner in which they are presented can affect the results of the testing, and can allow for comparison of results done at different times or at different centers.[63] There are two fairly standardized protocols for memory testing during the Wada test: the Montreal and Seattle tests.[64]

1. Montreal test: a series of word cards and objects are presented to the patient, while the hemisphere is under the influence of amobarbital. The patient is then tested for recall when the effect of the drug has worn off. Items spontaneously recalled are scored higher than those picked in a multiple choice test. The number and type of stimuli (verbal or spatial) recalled indicates the functions localized to the hemisphere contralateral to the injection.

2. Seattle test: repeatedly displaying cards showing line drawings and sentences, which the patient is instructed to name and remember. These are interspersed with a card stating "Recall", at which point, the patient names previously shown items. This process begins prior to amobarbital injection and is continued repeatedly during the period of anesthesia, until the effects have dissipated. If, during this test, the patient fails to recall items just presented, then that memory function is localized to that hemisphere.

The Montreal test has a 46% predictive value and the Seattle test a 76% predictive value for memory deficits after epilepsy surgery.[64]

Temporal lobectomy is used to treat medically refractory seizures, and this may involve wide resections of the temporal lobe[65] or more focal resections of the medial temporal lobe (amygdalohippocampectomy).[66] The hippocampal regions are usually supplied by the anterior choroidal artery anteriorly, and posterior cerebral arteries posteriorly. Single photon emission computed tomography (SPECT) studies of brain inactivated by the amobarbital have shown that the Wada test inactivates the hippocampus less than 40% of the time.[67] This issue of the arterial supply to the hippocampus prompted the development of superselective injections in the anterior choroidal and posterior cerebral arteries.[54, 56] However, superselective tests require specialized equipment and expertise, may not localize speech function, and may have a higher risk of complications.[55] Despite the lack of direct perfusion of the hippocampus on carotid injection, there still seems to be a functional effect on the hippocampus when amobarbital is injected into the ICA.[68] The importance of the frontal lobe in forming memories may explain why carotid injections can still localize memory dominance.[69] Moreover, patients who underwent temporal lobectomy in spite of a Wada test localizing memory to the surgical side, had more postoperative deficits than those whose memory was located contralateral to the surgical side on Wada testing.[70] Therefore, the standard internal carotid artery Wada test remains the mainstay for pre-operative evaluation in epilepsy patients.

Confounding Factors That Can Affect the Results of the Wada Test

- Time allowed to elapse between amobarbital injections: To prevent lingering effects of an initial amobarbital injection from confounding the results of the contralateral injection, some advocate performing the right and left injections on separate days.[71] Electroencephalographic studies have shown that less than a 40-min delay between injections can interfere with the results on the second injection.[72]

- The order of which side is injected first: Most centers inject the side of the epileptogenic focus first, so that useful data may still be obtained even if the patient decompensates, becomes too sleepy, or the angiographic equipment fails. However, there is evidence that cerebral hemispheres containing an epileptogenic focus may take longer to recover from the effects of amobarbital than a normal hemisphere.[73] This is another reason to wait for at least 40 min between amobarbital injections.

- Bizarre behavior: The focal anesthesia produced by selective amobarbital can occasionally result in disinhibited behavior (in the patient, that is) which can be disruptive and prevent successful completion of the procedure.[74, 75] Unfortunately, disruptive behavioral outbursts are unpredictable, but fortunately, they are rare.[76]
- Epilepsy without a unilateral medial temporal lobe onset: The results of Wada memory testing may not be as accurate in predicting post-operative memory deficits if portions of the hemisphere other than the temporal lobe are resected.[77]
- Multilingual patients: Multilingual patients may have variable localization of language centers for the different languages[78] and Wada testing may not necessarily accurately predict post-operative language deficits.[79]
- Carbonic anhydrase inhibiting drugs: Patients receiving medications such as topiramate, zonisamide, hydrochlorothiazide, or furosemide may display very rapid recovery from amobarbital or even no effect at all.[80, 81] The patient should be taken off of these medications at least 8 weeks prior to the Wada test.

Indications for the Wada Test

Patients being considered for surgery for:
1. Medically refractory seizures
2. Arteriovenous malformations
3. Tumours

Complications of the Wada Test

Informed consent prior to the procedure should include an estimate of the risk of complications.

NEUROLOGICAL COMPLICATIONS
1. There is a risk of thrombosis of the structures catheterized, with resultant stroke.
2. Dissection of the target vessel may occur, possibly with resultant occlusion or pseudoaneurysm formation.
3. Amytal in the basilar artery (e.g. in cases with a persistent trigeminal artery) can produce unconsciousness and apnea.
4. Seizures.
5. Cerebral edema may occur if the drug is mixed incorrectly.

NONNEUROLOGICAL COMPLICATIONS
1. Anaphylactic reactions to iodinated contrast or any of the medications used can occur as with any endovascular procedure.
2. Similarly, groin hematomas, femoral or iliac dissections, puncture site infections or other access complications can occur.

More Strange, But True

One reported complication of Wada testing in a patient scheduled for epilepsy surgery is that the seizures resolved and the surgery was no longer necessary. A patient had an embolic stroke during the procedure that caused an infarction of the epileptic focus and a cure of the seizures.[82] The authors of this handbook do not recommend routinely creating embolic strokes in hopes of achieving a similar result.

Wada Test: Technique

PREPROCEDURE PREPARATION
1. Brief neurological exam should be done to establish a baseline.
2. Pertinent historical findings:

(a) Has the patient has received medications with a carbonic anhydrase inhibitory effect such as topomirate, zonisamide or various diuretics? If there has been treatment with these agents in the last 8 weeks, it can make the amobarbital ineffective.

(b) When is the last time he or she had a seizure? This is to make sure that the patient is not in a post-ictal state, which can confuse the results of the Wada testing.

(c) Recent sleep history. If they are not well rested, it can make it difficult for the patient to pay attention during the Wada test

3. Evaluate the patient's prior imaging and EEG studies to determine the expected side containing the seizure focus. That side is generally tested first.
4. Informed consent.
5. EEG leads are placed prior to procedure, if used.
6. One IV.
7. A Foley catheter is not necessary.
8. Sedation should be avoided.

PERSONNEL REQUIREMENTS
- Scrubbed angiographic operator
- Scrubbed assistant(s)
- Circulating nurse(s)
- Radiographic technologist(s)
- EEG technologist
- Neuropsychologist or neurologist to do the neuropsychogical testing
- Assistant(s) to record the results of that testing

Suggested Catheters and Guidewires for the Wada Test

- Diagnostic angiography catheters (4 or 5F) are useful for angiographic studies and for injecting the amobarbital. The authors use a 4F Angled Glidecath® catheter (Terumo Medical, Somerset, NJ).
- Hydrophic, steerable wires such as 0.035 or 0.038-in. Glidewire® (Terumo Medical, Somerset, NJ) allow for safe, accurate catheter placement. Ensure that the wire size is matched to the recommended wire size of the catheter.

Procedures

VASCULAR ACCESS

See Chap. 4 for a general discussion of access techniques.
1. A 5F sheath is placed in the femoral artery.
2. Once arterial access is obtained, obtain a baseline ACT and fully heparinize the patient to at least double the baseline ACT (normally 80–150 s). Heparin (50–100 unit per kilogram bolus) will usually get the ACT around 250–300.

AMOBARBITAL PREPARATION
1. Obtain 500-mg vial of amobarbital (Amytal® Lilly, Indianapolis, IN) and sterile water
2. Under sterile conditions, mix 500 mg with 20-mL sterile water
3. Ensure all the powder is dissolved
4. Draw it up in a 20-mL syringe
5. Transfer the solution (25-mg amobarbital per milliliter) to sterile, labeled syringes using a filter needle

AMOBARBITAL DOSAGE

Most practitioners inject 125 mg of amobarbital per hemisphere, and this dosage is used in the procedural descriptions below. Some use 2 mg per kg body weight. Still others inject 25 mg/s, until the patient becomes hemiplegic in the contralateral arm. These variable dosages can make it difficult to compare the results of tests performed at different times or at different institutions.

6.2. Pharmacologic Provocative Testing

CATHETER PREPARATION
1. Choose a catheter for the procedure, usually a 4 or 5F diagnostic cerebral catheter.
2. As soon as it is removed from its sterile package, connect it to the stopcock system to be used during the procedure.
3. Connect a syringe of heparinized saline to the stopcock, and carefully inject saline until a drop is seen from the distal tip of the catheter, measuring the volume of the dead-space of the catheter/stopcock assembly. For a 4F catheter attached to a three-way stopcock, the dead-space of the catheter is approximately 1.2 mL, and slightly more for a larger catheter system.
4. Record the dead space measured, and then flush the system thoroughly as per usual angiographic technique.

CATHETER MANIPULATION
1. Attach all catheters to rotating haemostatic valves and attach a three-way stopcock and continuous infusion of saline containing 10,000 units heparin per liter.
2. Advance the catheter into the desired internal carotid. First do the side of the seizure focus, then later the side opposite to the seizure focus.
3. Do an angiogram first to estimate the expected distribution of the barbiturate, to ensure that there are no anomalous connections to the basilar artery (which could constitute a contra-indication for intracarotid amobarbital injection) and also to rule out incidental cerebral vascular disease.

TECHNIQUE: AMOBARBITAL TEST
1. Using a wet-to-wet connection, connect the labeled amobarbital syringe to the stopcock attached to the catheter. At least 5 mL of amobarbital 25 mg/mL, plus the dead-space of the catheter, should be in the syringe, or 6.2 mL for a 4-French catheter. This allows injection of single bolus of 125 mg into the patient.
2. Hold the syringe vertical so that bubbles in the syringe will rise away from the catheter.
3. Place a sterile half-sheet over the sterile field over the patient's thorax, to prevent contamination of the field during testing.
4. The patient then raises his or her arms and squeezes the examiner's fingers.
5. The patient begins counting backwards from 20.
6. When the patient counts back to 15, begin to inject the 6.2 mL (or slightly more for larger catheters) over 5 s into the ICA.
7. Immediately disconnect the labeled amobarbital syringe, attach a 10-mL syringe and aspirate several milliliters of blood to remove any amobarbital left in the catheter.
8. Double flush the catheter with heparinized saline.
9. If the patient shows the expected hemiparesis contralateral to the site of amobarbital injection, the catheter is pulled back into the descending aorta or removed altogether.
10. In the meantime, after the barbiturate is injected, neuropsychological testing is done as the patient is shown objects and cards to test speech and memory.
11. The patient is asked a standard battery of questions to distract from the previously shown objects, and to determine when the effect of amobarbital has worn off. The EEG is checked to ensure that the tracings are returned to baseline.
12. The patient is allowed to rest for 5–10 min, and the patient is then tested to determine if he or she remembers the items shown. Items spontaneously recalled are scored higher than those picked from multiple choice questions.
13. By the time the neuropsychological testing is completed, it is now approximately 20 min after the initial amobarbital injection.
14. Wait an additional time for a total of at least 40 min between amobarbital injections.
15. The process is then repeated for the contralateral internal carotid.

POSTPROCEDURE CARE
1. Once the procedure is completed, removed the catheters and sheaths and obtain haemostasis.
2. The patient is kept at bed rest with the leg extended for 2 h if a haemostatic patch is used.

Other Pharmacological Agents for Wada Testing

- Sodium methohexital (Brevital® JHP Pharmaceuticals, Parsippany, NJ):[58] This is a very short acting agent with less associated drowsiness even after successive injections. The drug is reconstituted to a concentration of 1 mg/mL. Three milligrams are injected first and the patient is tested for speech function, then, when hemiparesis resolves, a second injection of 2 mg is given and memory testing can be done. If the drug effect wears off before the items are presented for memory testing, another 2 mg injection can be given.
- Etiomidate:[59] A bolus of 0.03–0.04 mg/kg, followed by drip infusion of 0.003–0.004 mg/kg/min, which continues until all items are presented for memory testing. The drug wears off within 4 min of stopping the infusion. In a small series of cases, no complications occurred, but some confusing EEG responses occurred.[59]
- Propofol:[60] Mixed as 10 mg in 10-mL saline, an initial bolus of 10 mg is injected, followed by an additional 3 mg as needed to produce contralateral hemiplegia. In a series of 58 patients, one third experienced some involuntary movements or increased muscle tone that was sometimes disruptive to the neuropsychological testing.[61]

Superselective Wada Test

Indications for Superselective Wada Testing

Indications for superselective Wada testing are the same as for standard Wada testing, but with these added conditions:
- When standard Wada testing is contraindicated due to anomalous connections from carotid to basilar (e.g. persistent trigeminal artery).
- When standard Wada testing results in confusing or unreliable due to excessive sleepiness or inattention after amobarbital injection.
- When standard Wada testing results are suspect due to lack of clinical effect of intracarotid amobarbital, in cases of severe hemispheric injury, or with an arteriovenous malformation.
- For memory testing, superselective posterior cerebral[54,55] or (less commonly) anterior choroidal catheterization is done.[56]
- Middle cerebral catheterization is done for language or motor function localization.[83]

Complications of the Superselective Wada Test

Complications are similar to those of the standard Wada test, but with the added risks of superselective catheterization. There is a higher risk of thromboembolic complications, and local vascular injury in the intracranial circulation. In a series of 45 cases of attempted posterior cerebral arter superselective Wada tests, one case was complicated by post-procedure hemiplegia.[54]

Technique for Superselective Wada Testing

Similar to standard Wada testing with the following exceptions and caveats:
1. A 5 or 6F sheath is used.
2. A 5 or 6F guide catheter is placed in the carotid or vertebral artery.
3. A microcatheter is used for catheterization of the intracranial vessel of choice. For patient comfort, use a soft, flow-directed catheter such as Magic® (Balt/Advanced Interventional Technology, Miami,FL), or Ultraflow® (ev3, Irvine, CA).

4. Select a microwire that is suitable for the particular microcatheter. For the Ultraflow, use a 0.008-in. Mirage® (ev3, Irvine, CA).
5. Systemic heparinization during the procedure is mandatory.
6. RHVs, three-way stopcocks, and continuous heparinized saline infusions are attached to the all catheter lumens.
7. The microcatheter is carefully advanced using roadmap guidance to the target vessel.
8. For posterior cerebral artery testing, place the catheter tip in the P2 segment. In the middle cerebral artery, position it in the distal M1 or M2 segment.
9. Pull back on the microcatheter to relieve any slack.
10. Perform a gentle contrast injection with a 3-mL syringe for a superselective arteriogram to ensure that the desired brain parenchyma is being perfused.
11. To limit the dead-space of the microcatheter, remove the RHV and attach a three-way stopcock to the microcatheter
12. Attach a 3 mL syringe containing amobarbital to the microcatheter stopcock.
13. When ready for neuropsychological testing, inject 30–50 mg of amobarbital into the target vessel, at a rate of 10 mg/s.
14. For posterior cerebral artery testing, adequate anesthesia is confirmed by development of a contralateral hemianopia. For middle cerebral artery testing, check for a contralateral hemiplegia.
15. Once it appears that adequate anesthesia for Wada testing is obtained, slowly withdraw the guide catheter and microcatheter from the patient, leaving the sheath in place.
16. If indicated, perform either a standard Wada test of the contralateral carotid, or a superselective test, as necessary.

Alternatives to Wada Testing

Language Testing

Functional magnetic resonance imaging (fMRI) allows noninvasive localization of brain function by detecting the areas of increased oxygen utilization in the brain, while the patient performs tasks related to that brain function. This technique can be used to localize language dominance, and fMRI gave concordant results compared to Wada testing in 91% of 100 patients who underwent both procedures.[84] The incidence of false lateralization was highest when there was an epileptogenic focus outside the temporal lobe. Language mapping has also been done with noninvasive stimulation by magnetoencephalography (MEG) which correlated with results of Wada testing in 87% of 100 cases.[85] Studies using augmentation of middle cerebral blood flow velocity during a language task to locate speech lateralization have shown a high correlation with Wada test results.[86–88]

Memory Testing

Lateralization of memory dominance can be done noninvasively using.[18]F fluorodeoxyglucose PET imaging, and the medial temporal lobe with hypometabolism tends to be the side that does not support memory function on Wada testing.[89, 90] More recently, fMRI imaging has been used to lateralize verbal memory in epilepsy patients.[91, 92]

The Bottom Line

The Wada test is not yet dead. It remains the gold standard for preoperative evaluation of epilepsy surgery candidates. Other tests are less proven and may require hardware, software, or technical expertise that may not be as widely available in medical centers as the Wada test is. However, as fMRI becomes increasingly available as a clinical diagnostic modality, and accuracy improves, it may in many cases supplant the catheter-based Wada test just as MR angiography has replaced catheter angiography for many applications.

Pre-embolization Provocative Testing

Provocative testing can be done during embolization procedures, to confirm that it is safe to occlude the intended target of the embolization. Before embolizing a lesion, the artery is injected with an anesthetic agent, and if no neurological deficit occurs, it is assumed that it is safe to occlude the vessel. The usual agent for this is amobarbital[93, 94], although methohexital[95] or thiopental[96] can be used as a substitute. Arteries that may supply a peripheral nerve can be tested with lidocaine injection.[97] Lidocaine injections into arteries feeding the brain can cause seizures.[98] Therefore a strategy of first testing with amobarbital, then, if no deficit occurs, testing with lidocaine can greatly reduce the chances for adverse reactions to lidocaine, yet significantly increase the sensitivity of detecting deficits over the use of amobarbital alone.[99] Patients are tested clinically to determine if new neurological deficits are referable to the vascular territory at risk. Greater sensitivity of this test can be obtained by using a battery of cognitive neuropsychological tests during the amobarbital infusion.[100] Larger studies using EEG as well as clinical testing for superselective amobarbital showed greater sensitivity using the EEG data.[101, 102] Amobarbital testing prior to AVM embolization in 109 tests showed 23 abnormal tests by EEG criteria, but only 12 of them were abnormal by clinical testing, yet three showed false negative tests by EEG compared to clinical testing.[101] Amobarbital and lidocaine testing was shown to be helpful in 52 spinal arteriovenous malformations using neurophysiological monitoring with somatosensory and motor evoked potentials, and only one neurological complication that occurred even when the procedure was done under general anesthesia.[103]

The problem with provocative testing during embolization procedures is that there is little evidence concerning the true impact of this testing on patient outcome. Provocative testing should be done whenever possible in awake, cooperative patients, in whom the results would be expected to be most reliable. In embolization procedures that require general anesthesia, the provocative testing should be reserved for high-risk cases in eloquent locations and as long as good neurophysiological monitoring is available.

Procedures

Drug Preparation

1. Amobarbital
   (a) Obtain 500-mg vial of amobarbital (Amytal® Lilly, Indianapolis, IN) and sterile water
   (b) Under sterile conditions, mix 500 mg with 20 mL sterile water
   (c) Ensure all the powder is dissolved
   (d) Draw it up in a 20-mL syringe
   (e) Transfer the solution (25 mg amobarbital per mL) to sterile, labeled syringes using a filter needle.
2. Alternatively: Brevital® may be used
   (a) Obtain 500-mg vial of sodium methohexital (Brevital® JHP Pharmaceuticals, Parsippany, NJ) and sterile water
   (b) Under sterile conditions, mix 500 mg with 50 mL sterile water
   (c) Ensure all the powder is dissolved
   (d) Draw up 1 mL in a 10-mL syringe, and dilute again with sterile water up to 10 mL.
   (e) Transfer the solution (1 mg Brevital per mL) to sterile, labeled syringes using a filter needle.
3. Lidocaine
   (a) Transfer the contents of a syringe of 2% *cardiac* lidocaine to a sterile, labeled syringe.
   (b) Optional: add 1 mL of 4.2% pediatric bicarbonate to the lidocaine to buffer the acidity and reduce the discomfort on injection.

Adjunctive Testing

For brain embolization procedures, consider using neuropsychological testing, EEG monitoring, or evoked potentials during the provocative testing, and for spinal procedures consider using somotosensory and motor evoked potentials. Any of these adjunctive tests require additional time and skilled personnel to do the testing. With neuropsychological testing, a baseline examination should be performed prior to the procedure. Similarly, when neurophysiological monitoring is done, the leads need to be applied and readings are taken to determine the original status, so that alterations can be more readily detected. These adjunctive tests are generally not required for routine external carotid artery territory provocative testing.

Vascular Access Phase

See Chap. 4 for a general discussion of access techniques.
1. Place a 6F sheath in the femoral artery.
2. Obtain guide catheter access in the usual fashion.
3. Position the microcatheter in the target vessel under roadmap guidance.
4. Perform a superselective arteriogram.
5. Study the superselective arteriogram for filling of the brain or spinal cord either directly, or indirectly via dangerous anastamoses.
6. If there is visible supply to normal neurological territory, there are three options:
   (a) Do not embolize the vessel, and try a different vessel.
   (b) If possible, reposition the microcatheter beyond any connection to normal territory, then repeat the superselective arteriogram.
   (c) If it is not possible to place the microcatheter tip beyond connections to normal territory, consider blocking the dangerous anastamosis with a detachable coil to prevent emboli from reaching the normal territory. This is *only* an option if it is certain that other vessels provide adequate flow to the normal territory.
7. Once a safe catheter position is confirmed by superselective arteriography, perform provocative testing.

Technique: Superselective Provocative Testing

1. Remove the RHV and connect a three-way stopcock to the microcatheter.
2. Using a wet-to-wet connection, connect a labeled 3 mL amobarbital syringe to the stopcock attached to the microcatheter.
3. Hold the syringe vertical, such that any bubbles rise away from the catheter.
4. Place a sterile half-sheet over the sterile field over the patient's thorax, to prevent contamination of the field during testing.
5. Inject the amobarbital (usually 30–50 mg) over approximately 5 s into the artery. If using Brevital inject 1–3 mg over 5 s.
6. Immediately disconnect the labeled amobarbital syringe, attach a 3-mL syringe and flush with several milliliters of heparinized saline, to remove any amobarbital left in the catheter.
7. Ask the patient if he or she feels anything abnormal, then do a brief neurological examination, paying particular attention to functions at risk from the vascular territory being tested.
8. If the patient shows a new deficit, the testing is considered abnormal, and the vessel should not be embolized from that catheter position.
9. In the meantime, when the barbiturate is injected, adjunctive testing such as neuropsychological testing or EEG monitoring can be done.
10. If adjunctive testing changes from baseline status, then the testing is also considered abnormal, and the vessel should not be embolized from that catheter position.
11. If there is no change on neurological testing and adjunctive testing, the testing is normal. Proceed to lidocaine testing.
12. Connect a labeled 3-mL lidocaine syringe to the stopcock on the microcatheter.

13. Inject the lidocaine (usually 20–50 mg) over approximately 5 s into the vessel via the microcatheter.
14. Repeat the neurological and adjunctive testing.
15. If no neurological change occurs, and if the patient denies any burning sensation, deficit, and if, the testing is normal and it is safe to embolize.
16. If brain, retina or spinal cord deficit occurs, the testing is abnormal and the vessel should not be embolized from that catheter position. *If the patient reports a burning sensation (i.e., burning dysethesias) then the lidocaine may have reached the spinal cord, and this may also be a sign that embolization into that particular artery should not be done.*
17. If cranial nerve or peripheral nerve deficit occurs after lidocaine, it may still be possible to embolize using larger polyvinyl alcohol particles (> 350 μm size) or detachable coils.
18. During embolization of a vessel, after negative amobarbital and lidocaine testing, a change in flow pattern or visualization of different vessels may be seen after partial occlusion of the artery. Consider repeating the provocative testing again before completing embolization of the feeder.[104]
19. Repeat provocative testing as necessary whenever the microcatheter is placed in a new position. However, remember that the patient can become sleepy after repeated amobarbital injections in a short period of time.

6.2.11 Syringe Safety

Many of the procedures discussed in this book require the use of multiple agents in syringes on the procedure table. For example, embolization procedures with provocative testing require syringes containing local anesthetic, saline flush, contrast, amobarbital, lidocaine, embolic material, etc. It is imperative that these syringes containing different agents, are clearly differentiated, one from another. Confusing syringes with anesthetic agents or embolic materials for contrast or saline flush can lead to disastrous results. The authors of this handbook use customized, labeled, colored syringes (Merit Medical, South Jordan, UT) of various sizes and designs for the various materials. Using the same type of syringe for a certain agent at all times and educating new team members to the routine will minimize confusion and avoid mistakes.

References

1. Matas R. Some of the problems related to the surgery of the vascular system: testing the efficiency of the collateral circulation as a preliminary to the occlusion of the great surgical arteries. Presidential address. Trans Am Surg Assoc. 1910;28:4–54.
2. Wang H, Lanzino G, Kraus RR, Fraser KW. Provocative test occlusion or the Matas test: who was Rudolph Matas? J Neurosurg. 2003;98:926–8.
3. Allen JW, Alastra AJ, Nelson PK. Proximal intracranial internal carotid artery branches: prevalence and importance for balloon occlusion test. J Neurosurg. 2005;102:45–52.
4. Lesley WS, Bieneman BK, Dalsania HJ. Selective use of the paraophthalmic balloon test occlusion (BTO) to identify a false-negative subset of the cervical carotid BTO. Minim Invasive Neurosurg. 2006;49:34–6.
5. Linskey ME, Jungreis CA, Yonas H, et al. Stroke risk after abrupt internal carotid artery sacrifice: accuracy of preoperative assessment with balloon test occlusion and stable xenon-enhanced CT. AJNR Am J Neuroradiol. 1994;15:829–43.
6. Standard SC, Ahuja A, Guterman LR, et al. Balloon test occlusion of the internal carotid artery with hypotensive challenge. AJNR Am J Neuroradiol. 1995;16:1453–8.
7. McIvor NP, Willinsky RA, TerBrugge KG, Rutka JA, Freeman JL. Validity of test occlusion studies prior to internal carotid artery sacrifice. Head Neck. 1994;16:11–6.
8. Dare AO, Gibbons KJ, Gillihan MD, Guterman LR, Loree TR, Hicks Jr WL. Hypotensive endovascular test occlusion of the carotid artery in head and neck cancer. Neurosurg Focus. 2003;14:e5.
9. Marshall RS, Lazar RM, Pile-Spellman J, et al. Recovery of brain function during induced cerebral hypoperfusion. Brain. 2001;124:1208–17.
10. Dare AO, Chaloupka JC, Putman CM, Fayad PB, Awad IA. Failure of the hypotensive provocative test during temporary balloon test occlusion of the internal carotid artery to predict delayed hemodynamic ischemia after therapeutic carotid occlusion. Surg Neurol. 1998;50:147–55; discussion 155–6.
11. Lazar RM, Marshall RS, Pile-Spellman J, et al. Continuous time estimation as a behavioural index of human cerebral ischaemia during temporary occlusion of the internal carotid artery. J Neurol Neurosurg Psychiatry. 1996;60:559–63.
12. Marshall RS, Lazar RM, Mohr JP, et al. Higher cerebral function and hemispheric blood flow during awake carotid artery balloon test occlusions. J Neurol Neurosurg Psychiatry. 1999;66:734–8.
13. Morioka T, Matsushima T, Fujii K, Fukui M, Hasuo K, Hisashi K. Balloon test occlusion of the internal carotid artery with monitoring of compressed spectral arrays (CSAs) of electroencephalogram. Acta Neurochir (Wien). 1989;101:29–34.
14. Cloughesy TF, Nuwer MR, Hoch D, Vinuela F, Duckwiler G, Martin N. Monitoring carotid test occlusions with continuous EEG and clinical examination. J Clin Neurophysiol. 1993;10:363–9.
15. Schellhammer F, Heindel W, Haupt WF, Landwehr P, Lackner K. Somatosensory evoked potentials: a simple neurophysiological monitoring technique in supra-aortal balloon test occlusions. Eur Radiol. 1998;8:1586–9.
16. Su CC, Watanabe T, Yoshimoto T, Ogawa A, Ichige A. Proximal clipping of dissecting intracranial vertebral aneurysm–effect of balloon Matas test with neurophysiological monitoring. Case report. Acta Neurochir (Wien). 1990;104:59–63.
17. Kaminogo M, Ochi M, Onizuka M, Takahata H, Shibata S. An additional monitoring of regional cerebral oxygen saturation to HMPAO SPECT study during balloon test occlusion. Stroke. 1999;30:407–13.
18. Takeda N, Fujita K, Katayama S, Tamaki N. Cerebral oximetry for the detection of cerebral ischemia during temporary carotid artery occlusion. Neurol Med Chir (Tokyo). 2000;40:557–62; discussion 562–3.
19. Abud DG, Spelle L, Piotin M, Mounayer C, Vanzin JR, Moret J. Venous phase timing during balloon test occlusion as a criterion for permanent internal carotid artery sacrifice. AJNR Am J Neuroradiol. 2005;26:2602–9.
20. van Rooij WJ, Sluzewski M, Slob MJ, Rinkel GJ. Predictive value of angiographic testing for tolerance to therapeutic occlusion of the carotid artery. AJNR Am J Neuroradiol. 2005;26:175–8.
21. Schomer DF, Marks MP, Steinberg GK, et al. The anatomy of the posterior communicating artery as a risk factor for ischemic cerebral infarction. N Engl J Med. 1994;330:1565–70.
22. Miralles M, Dolz JL, Cotillas J, et al. The role of the circle of Willis in carotid occlusion: assessment with phase contrast MR angiography and transcranial duplex. Eur J Vasc Endovasc Surg. 1995;10:424–30.
23. Barker DW, Jungreis CA, Horton JA, Pentheny S, Lemley T. Balloon test occlusion of the internal carotid artery: change in stump pressure over 15 minutes and its correlation with xenon CT cerebral blood flow. AJNR Am J Neuroradiol. 1993;14:587–90.
24. Kurata A, Miyasaka Y, Tanaka C, Ohmomo T, Yada K, Kan S. Stump pressure as a guide to the safety of permanent occlusion of the internal carotid artery. Acta Neurochir (Wien). 1996;138:549–54.
25. Morishima H, Kurata A, Miyasaka Y, Fujii K, Kan S. Efficacy of the stump pressure ratio as a guide to the safety of permanent occlusion of the internal carotid artery. Neurol Res. 1998;20:732–6.
26. Giller CA, Mathews D, Walker B, Purdy P, Roseland AM. Prediction of tolerance to carotid artery occlusion using transcranial Doppler ultrasound. J Neurosurg. 1994;81:15–9.
27. Eckert B, Thie A, Carvajal M, Groden C, Zeumer H. Predicting hemodynamic ischemia by transcranial Doppler monitoring during therapeutic balloon occlusion of the internal carotid artery. AJNR Am J Neuroradiol. 1998;19:577–82.
28. Bhattacharjee AK, Tamaki N, Wada T, Hara Y, Ehara K. Transcranial Doppler findings during balloon test occlusion of the internal carotid artery. J Neuroimaging. 1999;9:155–9.
29. Marshall RS, Lazar RM, Young WL, et al. Clinical utility of quantitative cerebral blood flow measurements during internal carotid artery test occlusions. Neurosurgery. 2002;50:996–1004; discussion1004–5.
30. Mathis JM, Barr JD, Jungreis CA, et al. Temporary balloon test occlusion of the internal carotid artery: experience in 500 cases. AJNR Am J Neuroradiol. 1995;16:749–54.
31. Barr JD, Lemley TJ, McCann RM. Carotid artery balloon test occlusion: combined clinical evaluation and xenon-enhanced computed tomographic cerebral blood flow evaluation without patient transfer or balloon reinflation: technical note. Neurosurgery. 1998;43:634–7; discussion 637–8.
32. Jain R, Hoeffner EG, Deveikis JP, Harrigan MR, Thompson BG, Mukherji SK. Carotid perfusion CT with balloon occlusion and acetazolamide challenge test: feasibility. Radiology. 2004;231:906–13.
33. Wintermark M, Thiran JP, Maeder P, Schnyder P, Meuli R. Simultaneous measurement of regional cerebral blood flow by perfusion CT and stable xenon CT: a validation study. AJNR Am J Neuroradiol. 2001;22:905–14.
34. Brunberg JA, Frey KA, Horton JA, Deveikis JP, Ross DA, Koeppe RA. [15]O2O positron emission tomography determination of cerebral blood flow during balloon test occlusion of the internal carotid artery. AJNR Am J Neuroradiol. 1994;15:725–32.
35. Brunberg JA, Frey KA, Horton JA, Kuhl DE. Crossed cerebellar diaschisis: occurrence and resolution demonstrated with PET during carotid temporary balloon occlusion. AJNR Am J Neuroradiol. 1992;13:58–61.
36. Moody EB, Dawson 3rd RC, Sandler MP. 99mTc-HMPAO SPECT imaging in interventional neuroradiology: validation of balloon test occlusion. AJNR Am J Neuroradiol. 1991;12:1043–4.
37. Peterman SB, Taylor Jr A, Hoffman Jr JC. Improved detection of cerebral hypoperfusion with internal carotid balloon test occlusion and 99mTc-HMPAO cerebral perfusion SPECT imaging. AJNR Am J Neuroradiol. 1991;12:1035–41.

38. Monsein LH, Jeffery PJ, van Heerden BB, et al. Assessing adequacy of collateral circulation during balloon test occlusion of the internal carotid artery with 99mTc-HMPAO SPECT. AJNR Am J Neuroradiol. 1991;12:1045–51.

39. Tomura N, Omachi K, Takahashi S, et al. Comparison of technetium Tc 99m hexamethylpropyleneamine oxime single-photon emission tomograph with stump pressure during the balloon occlusion test of the internal carotid artery. AJNR Am J Neuroradiol. 2005;26:1937–42.

40. Eckard DA, Purdy PD, Bonte F. Crossed cerebellar diaschisis and loss of consciousness during temporary balloon occlusion of the internal carotid artery. AJNR Am J Neuroradiol. 1992;13:55–7.

41. Nathan MA, Bushnell DL, Kahn D, Simonson TM, Kirchner PT. Crossed cerebellar diaschisis associated with balloon test occlusion of the carotid artery. Nucl Med Commun. 1994;15:448–54.

42. Yonas H, Linskey M, Johnson DW, et al. Internal carotid balloon test occlusion does require quantitative CBF. AJNR Am J Neuroradiol. 1992;13:1147–52.

43. Michel E, Liu H, Remley KB, et al. Perfusion MR neuroimaging in patients undergoing balloon test occlusion of the internal carotid artery. AJNR Am J Neuroradiol. 2001;22:1590–6.

44. Ma J, Mehrkens JH, Holtmannspoetter M, et al. Perfusion MRI before and after acetazolamide administration for assessment of cerebrovascular reserve capacity in patients with symptomatic internal carotid artery (ICA) occlusion: comparison with (99m)Tc-ECD SPECT. Neuroradiology. 2007;49(4):317–26.

45. Kailasnath P, Dickey PS, Gahbauer H, Nunes J, Beckman C, Chaloupka JC. Intracarotid pressure measurements in the evaluation of a computer model of the cerebral circulation. Surg Neurol. 1998;50:257–63.

46. Charbel FT, Zhao M, Amin-Hanjani S, Hoffman W, Du X, Clark ME. A patient-specific computer model to predict outcomes of the balloon occlusion test. J Neurosurg. 2004;101:977–88.

47. Gardner W. Injection of procaine into the brain to locate speech area in left-handed persons. Arch Neurol Psychiatry. 1941;46:1035–8.

48. Wada J. Clinical experimental observations of carotid artery injections of sodium amytal. Igaku To Seibutsugaku. 1949;14:221–2.

49. Wada JA. Clinical experimental observations of carotid artery injections of sodium amytal. Brain Cogn. 1997;33:11–3.

50. Rovit R, Gloor P, Rasmussen T. Effect of intracarotid injection of sodium amytal on epileptiform EEG discharges: a clinical study. Trans Am Neurol Assoc. 1960;85:161–5.

51. Rovit RL, Gloor P, Rasmussen T. Intracarotid amobarbital in epileptic patients. A new diagnostic tool in clinical electroencephalography. Arch Neurol. 1961;5:606–26.

52. Branch C, Milner B, Rasmussen T. Intracarotid sodium amytal for the lateralization of cerebral speech dominance: observations in 123 patients. J Neurosurg. 1964;21:399–405.

53. Milner B, Branch C, Rasmussen T. Study of short-term memory after intracarotid injection of sodium amytal. Trans Am Neurol Assoc. 1962;87:224–6.

54. Jack Jr CR, Nichols DA, Sharbrough FW, Marsh WR, Petersen RC. Selective posterior cerebral artery Amytal test for evaluating memory function before surgery for temporal lobe seizure. Radiology. 1988;168:787–93.

55. Jack Jr CR, Nichols DA, Sharbrough FW, et al. Selective posterior cerebral artery injection of Amytal: new method of preoperative memory testing. Mayo Clin Proc. 1989;64:965–75.

56. Wieser HG, Muller S, Schiess R, et al. The anterior and posterior selective temporal lobe amobarbital tests: angiographic, clinical, electroencephalographic, PET, SPECT findings, and memory performance. Brain Cogn. 1997;33:71–97.

57. Grote CL, Meador K. Has amobarbital expired? Considering the future of the Wada. Neurology. 2005;65:1692–3.

58. Buchtel HA, Passaro EA, Selwa LM, Deveikis J, Gomez-Hassan D. Sodium methohexital (brevital) as an anesthetic in the Wada test. Epilepsia. 2002;43:1056–61.

59. Jones-Gotman M, Sziklas V, Djordjevic J, et al. Etomidate speech and memory test (eSAM): a new drug and improved intracarotid procedure. Neurology. 2005;65:1723–9.

60. Takayama M, Miyamoto S, Ikeda A, et al. Intracarotid propofol test for speech and memory dominance in man. Neurology. 2004;63:510–5.

61. Mikuni N, Takayama M, Satow T, et al. Evaluation of adverse effects in intracarotid propofol injection for Wada test. Neurology. 2005;65:1813–6.

62. Wada J, Gibson WC. Behavioral and EEG changes induced by injection of schizophrenic urine extract. AMA Arch Neurol Psychiatry. 1959;81:747–64.

63. Mader MJ, Romano BW, De Paola L, Silvado CE. The Wada test: contributions to standardization of the stimulus for language and memory assessment. Arq Neuropsiquiatr. 2004;62:582–7.

64. Dodrill CB, Ojemann GA. An exploratory comparison of three methods of memory assessment with the intracarotid amobarbital procedure. Brain Cogn. 1997;33:210–23.

65. Serafetinides EA, Falconer MA. The effects of temporal lobectomy in epileptic patients with psychosis. J Ment Sci. 1962;108:584–93.

66. Wieser HG, Yasargil MG. Selective amygdalohippocampectomy as a surgical treatment of mesiobasal limbic epilepsy. Surg Neurol. 1982;17:445–57.

67. Setoain X, Arroyo S, Lomena F, et al. Can the Wada test evaluate mesial temporal function? A SPECT study. Neurology. 2004;62:2241–6.

68. Urbach H, Kurthen M, Klemm E, et al. Amobarbital effects on the posterior hippocampus during the intracarotid amobarbital test. Neurology. 1999;52:1596–602.

69. Ojemann JG, Kelley WM. The frontal lobe role in memory: a review of convergent evidence and implications for the Wada memory test. Epilepsy Behav. 2002;3:309–15.

70. Lacruz ME, Alarcon G, Akanuma N, et al. Neuropsychological effects associated with temporal lobectomy and amygdalohippocampectomy depending on Wada test failure. J Neurol Neurosurg Psychiatry. 2004;75:600–7.

71. Grote CL, Wierenga C, Smith MC, et al. Wada difference a day makes: interpretive cautions regarding same-day injections. Neurology. 1999;52:1577–82.

72. Selwa LM, Buchtel HA, Henry TR. Electrocerebral recovery during the intracarotid amobarbital procedure: influence of interval between injections. Epilepsia. 1997;38:1294–9.

73. Bengner T, Haettig H, Merschhemke M, Dehnicke C, Meencke HJ. Memory assessment during the intracarotid amobarbital procedure: influence of injection order. Neurology. 2003;61:1582–7.

74. Terzian H. Behavioural and EEG effects of intracarotid sodium amytal injection. Acta Neurochir (Wien). 1964;12:230–9.

75. Masia SL, Perrine K, Westbrook L, Alper K, Devinsky O. Emotional outbursts and post-traumatic stress disorder during intracarotid amobarbital procedure. Neurology. 2000;54:1691–3.

76. de Paola L, Mader MJ, Germiniani FM, et al. Bizarre behavior during intracarotid sodium amytal testing (Wada test): are they predictable? Arq Neuropsiquiatr. 2004;62:444–8.

77. Kanemoto K, Kawasaki J, Takenouchi K, et al. Lateralized memory deficits on the Wada test correlate with the side of lobectomy only for patients with unilateral medial temporal lobe epilepsy. Seizure. 1999;8:471–5.

78. Rapport RL, Tan CT, Whitaker HA. Language function and dysfunction among Chinese- and English-speaking polyglots: cortical stimulation, Wada testing, and clinical studies. Brain Lang. 1983;18:342–66.

79. Gomez-Tortosa E, Martin EM, Gaviria M, Charbel F, Ausman JI. Selective deficit of one language in a bilingual patient following surgery in the left perisylvian area. Brain Lang. 1995;48:320–5.

80. Kipervasser S, Andelman F, Kramer U, Nagar S, Fried I, Neufeld MY. Effects of topiramate on memory performance on the intracarotid amobarbital (Wada) test. Epilepsy Behav. 2004;5:197–203.

81. Bookheimer S, Schrader LM, Rausch R, Sankar R, Engel Jr J. Reduced anesthetization during the intracarotid amobarbital (Wada) test in patients taking carbonic anhydrase-inhibiting medications. Epilepsia. 2005;46:236–43.

82. Ammerman JM, Caputy AJ, Potolicchio SJ. Endovascular ablation of a temporal lobe epileptogenic focus – a complication of Wada testing. Acta Neurol Scand. 2005;112:189–91.

---

83. Urbach H, Von Oertzen J, Klemm E, et al. Selective middle cerebral artery Wada tests as a part of presurgical evaluation in patients with drug-resistant epilepsies. Epilepsia. 2002;43:1217–23.

84. Woermann FG, Jokeit H, Luerding R, et al. Language lateralization by Wada test and fMRI in 100 patients with epilepsy. Neurology. 2003;61:699–701.

85. Papanicolaou AC, Simos PG, Castillo EM, et al. Magnetocephalography: a noninvasive alternative to the Wada procedure. J Neurosurg. 2004;100:867–76.

86. Knecht S, Deppe M, Ringelstein EB, et al. Reproducibility of functional transcranial Doppler sonography in determining hemispheric language lateralization. Stroke. 1998;29:1155–9.

87. Rihs F, Sturzenegger M, Gutbrod K, Schroth G, Mattle HP. Determination of language dominance: Wada test confirms functional transcranial Doppler sonography. Neurology. 1999;52:1591–6.

88. Knake S, Haag A, Hamer HM, et al. Language lateralization in patients with temporal lobe epilepsy: a comparison of functional transcranial Doppler sonography and the Wada test. Neuroimage. 2003;19:1228–32.

89. Salanova V, Morris 3rd HH, Rehm P, et al. Comparison of the intracarotid amobarbital procedure and interictal cerebral 18-fluorodeoxyglucose positron emission tomography scans in refractory temporal lobe epilepsy. Epilepsia. 1992;33:635–8.

90. Hong SB, Roh SY, Kim SE, Seo DW. Correlation of temporal lobe glucose metabolism with the Wada memory test. Epilepsia. 2000;41:1554–9.

91. Rabin ML, Narayan VM, Kimberg DY, et al. Functional MRI predicts post-surgical memory following temporal lobectomy. Brain. 2004;127:2286–98.

92. Richardson MP, Strange BA, Thompson PJ, Baxendale SA, Duncan JS, Dolan RJ. Pre-operative verbal memory fMRI predicts post-operative memory decline after left temporal lobe resection. Brain. 2004;127:2419–26.

93. Vinuela F, Fox AJ, Debrun G, Pelz D. Preembolization superselective angiography: role in the treatment of brain arteriovenous malformations with isobutyl-2 cyanoacrylate. AJNR Am J Neuroradiol. 1984;5:765–9.

94. Pelz DM, Fox AJ, Vinuela F, Drake CC, Ferguson GG. Preoperative embolization of brain AVMs with isobutyl-2 cyanoacrylate. AJNR Am J Neuroradiol. 1988;9:757–64.

95. Peters KR, Quisling RG, Gilmore R, Mickle P, Kuperus JH. Intraarterial use of sodium methohexital for provocative testing during brain embolotherapy. AJNR Am J Neuroradiol. 1993;14:171–4.

96. Han MH, Chang KH, Han DH, Yeon KM, Han MC. Preembolization functional evaluation in supratentorial cerebral arteriovenous malformations with superselective intraarterial injection of thiopental sodium solution. Acta Radiol. 1994;35:212–6.

97. Horton JA, Kerber CW. Lidocaine injection into external carotid branches: provocative test to preserve cranial nerve function in therapeutic embolization. AJNR Am J Neuroradiol. 1986;7:105–8.

98. Usubiaga JE, Wikinski J, Ferrero R, Usubiaga LE, Wikinski R. Local anesthetic-induced convulsions in man–an electroencephalographic study. Anesth Analg. 1966;45:611–20.

99. Deveikis JP. Sequential injections of amobarbital sodium and lidocaine for provocative neurologic testing in the external carotid circulation. AJNR Am J Neuroradiol. 1996;17:1143–7.

100. Moo LR, Murphy KJ, Gailloud P, Tesoro M, Hart J. Tailored cognitive testing with provocative amobarbital injection preceding AVM embolization. AJNR Am J Neuroradiol. 2002;23:416–21.

101. Rauch RA, Vinuela F, Dion J, et al. Preembolization functional evaluation in brain arteriovenous malformations: the superselective Amytal test. AJNR Am J Neuroradiol. 1992;13:303–8.

102. Paiva T, Campos J, Baeta E, Gomes LB, Martins IP, Parreira E. EEG monitoring during endovascular embolization of cerebral arteriovenous malformations. Electroencephalogr Clin Neurophysiol. 1995;95:3–13.

103. Niimi Y, Sala F, Deletis V, Setton A, de Camargo AB, Berenstein A. Neurophysiologic monitoring and pharmacologic provocative testing for embolization of spinal cord arteriovenous malformations. AJNR Am J Neuroradiol. 2004;25:1131–8.

104. Rauch RA, Vinuela F, Dion J, et al. Preembolization functional evaluation in brain arteriovenous malformations: the ability of superselective Amytal test to predict neurologic dysfunction before embolization. AJNR Am J Neuroradiol. 1992;13:309–14.

7. Intracranial Embolization Procedures

Intracranial embolization procedures are therapeutic endovascular occlusions of vessels involved in vascular lesions of the cerebral circulation. One can imagine more catchy phrases to describe the procedure such as "intentional cerebral embolism" (ICE), but common parlance uses the less colourful and more awkward "intracranial embolization procedure." This chapter covers transarterial embolization in the intracranial circulation aside from intracranial aneurysm treatment, and is divided into four parts:
1. Indications and contraindications
2. General devices and techniques for intracranial vascular access and embolization
3. Techniques specific to particular disease processes
4. Complication avoidance and management
Basic access concepts are discussed in Chap. 4, specific embolization procedures on intracranial aneurysms in Chap. 5, and transvenous embolization procedures in Chap. 12.

7.1.   Intracranial Embolization: Indications and Contraindications

Common Indications

1. Intracranial aneurysms (covered in Chap. 5)
2. Intracranial arteriovenous malformation (AVM)
   (a) Pre-operative embolization
   (b) Pre-radiosurgery
   (c) Curative embolization (reported in from 4% to 27% of patients treated[1–5])
   (d) Palliative embolization for inoperable AVMs (controversial)
      • Attempt to reduce neurological deficits from arterial steal and/or venous hypertension
      • Palliation of intractable headaches
      • Targeted embolization of higher risk AVM components (e.g. associated aneurysms[6–8])
3. Intracranial arteriovenous fistulas (AVFs)
   (a) Carotid cavernous fistula
   (b) Dural AVFs
   (c) Pial AVFs
   (d) Vein of Galen malformations
   (e) Post-traumatic fistulas
   (f) Post-surgical fistulas
4. Bleeding intracranial vessels
   (a) Usually when it occurs as a complication of an endovascular procedure
   (b) Rarely, for post-operative or post-traumatic bleeding
5. Intracranial vascular tumors
   (a) Pre-operative embolization
   (b) Palliative treatment for inoperable tumors

M.R. Harrigan, J.P. Deveikis, *Handbook of Cerebrovascular Disease and Neurointerventional Technique*, DOI 10.1007/978-1-61779-946-4_7, © Springer Science+Business Media New York 2013

Relative Contraindications

1. Vascular anatomy that is prohibitive (e.g., *en passage* feeding arteries that also supply eloquent brain or exaggerated vessel tortuosity).
2. Significant atherosclerotic disease or high-flow vasculopathy affecting the parent vessel (e.g., occlusion or stenosis of the access vessel).
3. Iodinated contrast allergy.
4. Coagulation disorders or heparin hypersensitivity.
5. Active bacterial infection (i.e. bacteremia at time of endovascular treatment).

7.2. Intracranial Vascular Access and Embolization: Techniques and Devices

Evaluation

1. History and physical
2. Neurological exam
3. Blood work (CBC, BUN, Creatinine, PT, PTT)
4. Imaging
   (a) Head CT or MRI
   (b) CTA or MRA
   (c) Preferably a catheter angiogram.
   (d) Imaging considerations:
      - Lesion location, potential brain territories at risk from the procedure, size and configuration.
      - Flow patterns (e.g., high flow vs. low flow arteriovenous shunt).
      - Parent vessel anatomy.
      - Angiographic architecture of lesion (e.g. nidal AVM vs. high-flow AVF vs. mixed lesion)
      - Presence of associated vascular lesion (e.g. aneurysm associated with AVM).
      - Planned site of intended deposition of embolic material.
      - Access vessel anatomy (e.g., dominant versus hypoplastic vertebral artery or ACA, degree of tortuosity).
      - Presence or absence of atherosclerosis or fibromuscular dysplasia in the access vessel.
      - Presence of recent or remote hemorrhage.
      - Associated brain oedema or encephalomalacia.

Treatment Strategy

Prior to the case, preferably the previous day or earlier, the patient should be assessed and all available imaging reviewed in preparation for the case. Decisions about the overall treatment strategy and the role of embolization in that strategy should be made well ahead of time. Plans should include:

1. Choice of access vessel
2. Guide catheter selection
3. Microcatheter and microwire selection
4. Embolic agent to be used
5. Target vessels to be treated
   (a) For most AVMs: Select feeding arteries that allow microcatheter access as close to the nidus as possible.
   (b) In situations in which arterial access is not feasible, successful transvenous embolization has been reported.[9] (see Chap. 12)

6. Staged multiple procedure vs. single embolization
7. Prepare for methods to ensure preservation of neurological function (e.g., provocative testing, neuophysiological monitoring)

Preprocedure Preparation

1. Place two peripheral IVs.
2. NPO for 6 h, except for medications.
3. Patients on insulin for hyperglycemia should get half their normal dose prior to the procedure.
4. Place Foley catheter.
5. Place thigh-high sequential compression device (SCD) sleeves on both legs for deep vein thrombosis prophylaxis.
6. Make sure that all devices that may be needed are available in the angio suite prior to the procedure.
7. If stent-assisted coiling is planned, as in stent-assisted coiling of a carotid-cavernous fistula, pre-treatment with antiplatelet therapy may be indicated:
    (a) Aspirin 325-mg PO QD for ≥3 days prior to the procedure *and*
    (b) Clopidogrel (Plavix®, Sanofi-Aventis, Bridgewater, NJ) 75-mg PO QD for ≥3 days prior to the procedure (or 300-mg PO 5 h prior to the procedure).
8. Some operators recommend pretreatment with dexamethasone, 2 mg PO/IV Q6 hours for 2–3 days before any intracranial embolization procedure to attempt to reduce the risk of swelling. This is based on a positive effect of steroids in the setting of various brain tumors and experimental evidence of success in maintaining intact blood brain barrier using dexamethasone.[10] Some animal data suggests that the dexamethasone reduces the effects of ischemia.[11], which can be a complication of embolization. On the other hand, many studies have found that in acute ischemia, steroids either do not help[12], or may worsen the amount of ischemic damage.[13, 14] Dexamethasone may not aggravate ischemia if it is not given for an extended period before the procedure[15] but given the limited evidence of efficacy and questions about aggravation of ischemia, the authors of this handbook do not use steroids routinely for embolization procedures, except in tumor cases.
9. Patients with recent intracranial hemorrhage
    (a) Arterial line and central venous access are established prior to the procedure
    (b) If a ventriculostomy is present, the catheter must be attached to a monitor, to permit continuous ICP monitoring during the case.
        • ICP is an "early warning system" for AVM rupture or re-rupture during embolization.
        • The ventriculostomy should be "on monitor" (and not "to drain") if possible during the entire procedure, to permit continuous monitoring. Open the drain only intermittently if CSF drainage during the procedure is necessary.

7.3.　Endovascular Technique

The technique of intracranial embolization treatment varies considerably from case to case. The following is a general outline of the procedures and devices used by the authors for most patients. The case is divided into a vascular *access* phase, a microcatheter *access* phase, and an *embolization* phase. Each phase requires choosing a system of devices and techniques to achieve the therapeutic goals.

Awake or Asleep?

Some operators prefer to use general anesthesia for embolization cases whereas others prefer to do them with the patient awake. Each approach has advantages. Embolization with the patient awake permits continuous neurological monitoring, eliminates the risks of general anesthesia, can shorten the length of the case, and is done in many centers. Embolizing with the patient awake is less practical in patients with reduced mental status and in those with small or very distal lesions in which a small amount of patient motion can lead to vessel perforation or inadvertent occlusion of normal vessels. Very distal catheterization, and even more proximal catheterization with larger microcatheter systems can cause considerable pain due to the sensitivity of the proximal intradural vessels, and that pain makes it difficult for even sedated patients to remain motionless. General anesthesia can eliminate this discomfort and patient mobility, allows the operator to focus on the procedure rather than on coaching and assessing the patient, can be much more palatable for anxious patients, and permits tight blood pressure and intracranial pressure control. The lower systemic pressure attainable under general anesthesia also allows some flow control in high flow AVMs or AVFs perhaps providing a lower risk of migration of embolic agents from their intended destination. Intra-operative embolization also definitely requires general anesthesia. Neurophysiological monitoring can still be accomplished under anesthesia using EEG and/or evoked potentials. The authors of this handbook prefer to use general anesthesia in nearly all cases of intracranial embolization, except for rare cases in which medical issues place the patient at elevated risk with anesthesia (e.g., severe heart disease).

Vascular Access Phase

See Chap. 4 for a general discussion of access techniques.

1. A 6F sheath is placed in the femoral artery.
   (a) A 7 or (rarely, 8F) sheath should be used if arterial monitoring through the sheath is planned, or if adjunctive techniques, such as balloon-assisted coil embolization or detachable balloon embolization, are anticipated.
2. (a) Examination of the carotid or vertebral artery is necessary for guide catheter selection, and to check for the presence of atherosclerosis and fibromuscular dysplasia.
   (b) Intracranial images at the beginning of the case are necessary for comparison later, to assess for arterial thromboembolic complications or venous occlusions.
3. Guide catheter selection and positioning
   (a) Depends on intracranial target
      i. Large-lumen guide catheters (Guider and Envoy) are spacious and stable but distal positioning is usually not feasible
         (1) Straight or angled?
            (a) Straight guide catheter
               (i) Useful in relatively straight vessels, or in situations where the guide catheter will be gently navigated through a convoluted vessel over a wire or co-axially over a microcatheter.
               (ii) Preferred for the vertebral artery
               (iii) Preferred for glue embolization since an angle can cause the tip of the guide catheter to indent the microcatheter, and can squeeze ("milk") glue out of the microcatheter if it is pulled back though the guide catheter.
            (b) Angled guide catheter
               (i) Useful when the guide catheter is advanced primarily (without exchanging)
               (ii) Useful when the final position of the catheter tip is in a vessel curve
      ii. The 6F 0.53 in. Neuron guide catheter is good for distal positioning, especially in tortuous vessels, but has a smaller lumen.

4. Anticoagulation.
   (a) The use of prophylactic systemic anticoagulation during intracranial embolization is quite variable. One group advocates systemic heparin in embolization of small AVMs, but not in those larger than 3 cm in diameter.[16] Some never use heparin and others always use it. The authors of this handbook favour heparinization.
      i) Dosing for heparin: Loading dose of IV heparin (5,000 units or 70 units/kg).
   (b) Protamine on stand-by – *Critical*
      i) A syringe containing protamine, enough to reverse the total amount of heparin the patient has received, should be constantly available in the endovascular suite for easy access to the operator, should haemorrhage occur during the case.

Microcatheter Phase

Once a stable guide catheter position is achieved, a microcatheter is coaxially advanced to a position from which the embolic material can be delivered to the target lesion.
1. Roadmap guidance:
   (a) Absolutely critical for safe and effective intracranial catheterization
   (b) Contrast is injected and a mask image of the vascular tree is saved, and superimposed digitally on the live fluoroscopic image.
   (c) Roadmapping ensures safe and expeditious navigation through the complicated and tortuous intracranial vascular anatomy.
   (d) Biplane roadmapping is best.
   (e) 3D roadmapping is available on newer angiographic suites.
   (f) If the patient moves or if a different projection is required to negotiate a turn, another roadmap mask can be obtained.
2. Microcatheter selection
   (a) There are many microcatheters to choose from (Tables 7.1 and 7.2), and the optimal one depends on how large or how distal the target vessel is, what embolic agent will be used, and the training and experience of the operator.
   (b) Microcatheters for AVM embolization come in three varieties:
      i. Over-the-wire microcatheters. By far the most common kind of microcatheter. A curved microwire is manipulated toward the target position and the microcatheter is passively advanced over the wire until it reaches the proper position. Current versions of this type of catheter tend to have more gradual gradations from one degree of stiffness to another and have braiding or stiffeners in the wall to improve forward transmission of pushing power and to prevent kinking of the catheter as it takes sharp turns. Hydrophilic coating reduces friction between the microcatheter and guiding catheter, and with the vessels. It also may reduce the risk of clot accumulation on the catheter.[17]
         1. Advantages:
            (a) Versatile.
            (b) Stable positioning is possible.
            (c) Relatively large lumen accepts various microwires and various types of embolic agents.
            (d) Most are somewhat flexible.
            (e) The distal tip can be steam shaped and some have available pre-shaped curves.
         2. Disadvantages:
            (a) Somewhat stiff.
            (b) May traumatize very small, very tortuous vessels.
            (c) The microwire can traumatize or puncture small vessels when it is advanced beyond the tip.

Table 7.1 Common microcatheters for intracranial embolization

Catheter	Manufacturer	Length (cm)	Outer diameter (French size)	Inner diameter (in.)	Comments
Echelon™ 10	ev3	150	2.1–1.7 distally	0.017	DMSO compatible. Two pre-shaped curves available
Echelon™ 14	ev3	150	2.4–1.9 distally	0.017	DMSO compatible. Two pre-shaped curves available
Excelsior® SL-10	Stryker Neurovascular	150	2.4–1.7 distally	0.0165	Five pre-shaped curves available
Excelsior® 1018®	Stryker Neurovascular	150	2.6–2.0 distally	0.019	Five pre-shaped curves available
Prowler® 10	Codman	70 or 150 or 170	2.3–1.7 distally	0.015	Five pre-shaped curves available.
Prowler® 14	Codman	70 or 150 or 170	2.3–1.9 distally	0.0165	Three pre-shaped curves available.
Prowler® Plus	Codman	150 or 170	3.0–2.3 distally	0.021	Three pre-shaped curves available.
Headway® 17	Microvention/ Terumo	150	2.4–1.7 distally	0.017	Regular, extra-support and advanced for increasing distal support
Nautica™ 14 XL	ev3	150	2.8–2.2 distally	0.018	10 and 18 coil compatible
Rebar® 18	ev3	110 or 153	2.8–2.3 distally	0.021	DMSO compatible
Rebar® 027	ev3	110 or 145	2.8	0.027	DMSO compatible
Renegade® 18	Stryker Neurovascular	150	3.0–2.5 distally	0.021	

Table 7.2 Common flow-directed microcatheters

Catheter	Manufacturer	Length (cm)	Outer diameter (French size)	Inner (distal) diameter (in.)	Comment
Magic®	AIT-Balt	155 or 165	2.7–1.8 distally	0.013	Various distal floppy segments and also "olive-shaped tip" available
Magic® 1.5	AIT-Balt	155 or 165	2.7–1.5 distally	0.010	Various distal floppy segments and also "olive-shaped tip" available
Magic® 1.2	AIT-Balt	165	2.7–1.2 distally	0.008	Various distal floppy segments and also "olive-shaped tip" available
Marathon™	ev3	165	2.7–1.3 distally	0.013	DMSO compatible. High burst pres-sure. Not very flow-directable
Ultraflow™	ev3	165	3.0–1.5 distally	0.012 or 0.013	DMSO compatible. More flow-directed than Marathon, but not as burst-resistant

ii. Flow-directed microcatheters. There are only a small number of flow-directed microcatheters, and some are more flow-directed than others. The only true flow-directed system is the Magic® microcatheter (AIT-Balt, Miami, FL). These microcatheters are so flexible distally that the tip is pulled along by blood flow, making this a good choice for high flow lesions such as AVMs.

    (1) Advantages:

        (a) Very flexible and atraumatic to the vessel.

        (b) Can be advanced very distally in tortuous vessels.

        (c) The ideal microcatheter for vessels less than 2 mm in diameter.

        (d) Distal tip can be steam shaped.

        (e) Flow direction limits need to use a wire beyond the tip of the catheter, reducing the risk of vessel trauma or perforation by the wire.

    (2) Disadvantages:

        (a) Small lumen limits the size of usable micro-guide-wires and also limits the type of embolic agent.

        (b) Catheter position may be less stable compared to over-the-wire types.

iii. Steerable microcatheters. These are the least common kind of microcatheter and are basically over-the-wire catheters that have the added benefit of a steerable tip of the microcatheter.

    (1) Advantages:

        (a) Steerable tip may allow access to difficult angulated branches.

        (b) Distal tip is steam shapeable.

        (c) Tend to be very stable once positioned.

    (2) Disadvantages:

        (a) The stiffest of all microcatheters.

        (b) Not suitable for very small or very distal vessels.

        (c) The microwire can traumatize small vessels.

(c) The smaller "10-size" microcatheters are fairly flexible, although not as flexible as flow-directed microcatheters. Larger "14-size" are stiffer, and the "18-size" systems are extremely stiff, but have a much larger lumen. The over-the-wire microcatheter is most appropriate for relatively proximal intracranial catheterizations and where large particles or microcoils are the embolic agent of choice. If Onyx® (ev3, Irvine, CA) is used, a DMSO-compatible microcatheter must be used.

3. Steam shaping technique:

    (a) Shape the wire mandrel into the desired shape, with an exaggerated degree of curvature (as the microcatheter will recoil to some degree after steam-shaping).

    (b) Hold over steam for 10 s.

    (c) Cool in sterile water and remove mandrel.

    (d) Non-braided (e.g., Magic®) and fiber-braided (e.g., Excelsior®) microcatheters are more likely to retain their shape after steam shaping than metal coil-braided (e.g., Prowler and Echelon™) microcatheters.[18]

4. Microwire selection

    (a) A wide variety of microwires are available, with differing properties such as size, softness, visibility on fluoroscopy, shapeability, and steerability, trackability, and torque control.

    (b) All microwires suitable for neuroendovascular procedures are hydro-phillically coated to reduce friction.

    (c) Wires can have a shapeable distal tip or may come pre-shaped from the manufacturer.

    (d) Shapeable tips are usually made of platinum, which makes them visible on fluoroscopy

(e) Sizes of microwires range from 0.008 in. for the tiny Mirage™ (ev3, Irvine, CA) to a variety of 0.10 in. and even more 0.014-in. wires up to the robust 0.016-in. Headliner™ (Microvention/Terumo, Tustin, CA). Larger diameter wires are available, but are generally a tight fit in commonly used microcatheters and are too stiff for safe intracranial navigation.

(f) In general, 0.010 in. or smaller wires are used in flow-directed catheters, 0.014-in. wires are used in most other microcatheters. Any of the wires larger than 0.014 in. are only used rarely when a large lumen microcatheter is used and added torque or support is needed.

(g) Microwires can be broadly classified according to the design and composition of the core wire that forms the backbone of the microwire:
    i. Stainless steel core wires like Mirage™ or Silverspeed® (ev3, Irvine, CA) or Agility® (Codman Neurovascular, Raynham, MA).
        (1) Superior torque control, compared with many other microwires.
        (2) Heightened radio-opacity makes the platinum tip easy to see on fluoroscopy.
        (3) Shapeable tip.
        (4) Easily kinked.
    ii. Nitinol core wires like the Headliner™ (Terumo Medical Corporation, Somerset, NJ)
        (1) Tip shape supplied by manufacturer.
        (2) J-tip is quite atraumatic to the vessel walls.
        (3) Best suited for uncomplicated vessel anatomy (tends to follow the straightest vessel).
        (4) Very kink-resistant.
    iii. Composite alloy flat-cores like Transend™ EX (Stryker Neurovascular, Fremont, CA)
        (1) Superior torque control than most other wires.
        (2) Kink resistance tends to be more than that of stainless steel core, but less than that of nitinol core wires.
        (3) The tip is shapeable. Note: The tip should be shaped in the direction of the natural curve of the wire to take advantage of the torque characteristics of the flat core.
    iv. Synchro®-14 0.014 in. (Stryker Neurovascular, Fremont, CA)
        (1) Very soft, flexible distal tip, good for navigation into small vessels or through difficult anatomy.
    v. Neuroscout®-14 0.014 in. (Codman Neurovascular, Raynham, MA)
        (1) Similar to Synchro®

5. Microcatheter irrigation

    (a) Continuous irrigation of the microcatheter as well as the guide catheter with heparinized saline (5,000-U heparin per 500-mL saline) is important.

    (b) A three-way stopcock connects the heparinized saline flush-line to an RHV to allow continuous infusion of saline.

    (c) Heparinized saline infusion ensures hydration of the hydrophilic coating on the microwire and minimizes friction.

    (d) Meticulous attention to the microcatheter (and guide catheter) RHV throughout the case is necessary to identify thrombus or bubbles, should they appear.

    (e) The heparinized saline drip should be periodically monitored to ensure that it is dripping slowly, but continuously, and there is still sufficient fluid in the saline bag to last for the case.

6. Microcatheter/microwire preparation

    (a) Flush the plastic hoop housing the microcatheter with heparinized saline to hydrate the hydrophilic coating.

    (b) If necessary, steam-shape the tip of the microcatheter.

    (c) The hub of the microcatheter is attached to an RHV and the lumen of the RHV and microcatheter are flushed with heparinized saline to purge all air from the system.

    (d) Before shaping the microwire, insert it into the RHV and advance the tip of the microwire beyond the tip of the microcatheter.

(e) Shape the tip of the microwire with a microintroducer. A 90° curve or a slightly J-shaped curve is best for most cases.

(f) Attach a torque device to the microwire, pull the microwire tip into the microcatheter, and insert into the RHV of the guide catheter.

7. Microcatheter technique:

(a) The microcatheter is advanced with the left hand and the torque device is controlled with the right hand.

(b) Under roadmap guidance, carefully advance the microwire into the vascular system, and follow with the microcatheter.

(c) In straight segments of the vessel, the catheter tip can be advanced beyond the wire, which limits the risk of vessel damage or perforation.

(d) Around sharp turns or where the vessel branches, the microwire is carefully guided around the curve by rotating the wire.

(e) To reduce the friction between microcatheter and microwire, the wire can be gently pulled back and/or rotated.

(f) The guide catheter position should be monitored periodically during microcatheter positioning, since any resistance to forward motion of the microcatheter will inevitably create back-pressure on the guide catheter.

(g) Gently pull back on the microcatheter periodically to remove redundancy.

(h) Also, periodically check that the heparinized saline flush lines attached to the guide catheter and microcatheter are dripping and bubble-free.

(i) When the microcatheter reaches the target, remove the microwire while observing the tip of the microcatheter on fluoro, since moving the microwire can often release stored energy in the microcatheter, causing it to move (usually forward).

(j) Inject a small amount of contrast through the microcatheter to confirm catheter positioning, and also to confirm patency of the microcatheter. Too much resistance during injection can indicate kinking of the microcatheter. This kinking can be resolved by pulling back on the microcatheter before proceeding further. Injection of contrast or embolic material in a kinked catheter can result in catheter rupture, which is a *disaster*.

(k) When all slack is removed, do a high-magnification microcatheter angiogram.

(l) Evaluate the superselective arteriogram to determine:
   i. the desired position has been reached.
   ii. there are no normal brain vessels filling.
   iii. the flow-rate in order to choose an embolic agent and the injection rate needed.
   iv. there is no sign of contrast exiting the microcatheter proximal to the distal tip. *This would indicate that the microcatheter has been irreparably damaged or even ruptured and must not be used for embolization.*

(m) Once the microcatheter is in position provocative testing may be performed if necessary (see below). Otherwise, the embolization phase begins (also see below).

8. Flow-directed microcatheter technique:

(a) Flow-directed microcatheters are often used for liquid embolic delivery. The high flow state in AVMs and dAVFs greatly makes for rapid and accurate placement of the microcatheter to the desired position. A DMSO-compatible microcatheter must be used if Onyx® (ev3, Irvine, CA) is to be used.

(b) Most flow-directed microcatheters are packaged with a long mandrel that can be used to stiffen the catheter and allow insertion through the RHV into the guide catheter. *Never* advance the mandrel beyond the tip of the microcatheter or use it like a guidewire in the vascular system. The mandrel is not soft enough for intravascular use.

(c) Flush the plastic hoop in which the microcatheter is packaged to hydrate the hydrophilic coating.

(d) Remove the catheter from the hoop and immerse the catheter in a large bowl of sterile, heparinized saline.

(e) If packaged with a mandrel, remove the mandrel from the microcatheter. Having the microcatheter immersed in saline prevents aspirating air into the catheter as the mandrel is withdrawn.

(f) Attach an RHV and flush the system to purge all air.

(g) Insert a microwire (0.010 in. or smaller) through the RHV and into the microcatheter to the distal tip. The authors use the 0.008-in. Mirage™ (ev3, Irvine, CA).

(h) Insert the microcatheter into the RHV of the guide catheter and advance it to the distal tip of the guide catheter. Both the Marathon™ and Ultraflow™ (ev3, Irvine, CA) have a marker on the shaft of the catheter that indicates that the tip is approaching the end of a 90-cm guide catheter, to limit fluoro time.

(i) Under roadmap guidance, advance the flow-directed microcatheter into the vascular system. Note that the tips of most flow-directed microcatheters are quite small and tend to move very quickly, so good fluoroscopic imaging equipment and a watchful eye are needed to keep the tip in view.

(j) Let the blood flow carry the tip forward, and advance the catheter forward at a rate fast enough to keep the catheter moving, but not so fast that redundant loops form in the neck. It is helpful to have one plane of a biplane roadmap system include the tip of the guide catheter to ensure that the microcatheter does not loop in the neck or displace the guide catheter.

(k) Keep the microwire within the microcatheter most of the time and do not advance it beyond the tip. Arteries can be damaged or perforated with a microwire more easily than with a soft catheter.

(l) A curved microwire can be rotated within the microcatheter to direct the tip of the catheter.

(m) If the tip of the microcatheter does not advance as the microcatheter shaft is advanced at the groin, sometimes pulling the microwire back gently will cause the tip to advance.

(n) Only in rare situations when a very sharp angle must be negotiated, the microwire may need to be *cautiously* advanced beyond the tip of a flow-directed microcatheter and torqued into a sharp curve or sharply angulated side-branch.

(o) Note: there can be considerable friction between the soft microcatheter and the microwire, especially with Magic® microcatheters (AIT-Balt, Miami, FL). This can cause the microwire to jump forward if advanced too vigorously or cause the catheter to "accordion" and crumple on itself as the wire is pulled back. These problems can be minimized by gently rotating the wire or moving it in and out slightly to break the friction.

    i. Also note: the microwire cannot be safely advanced beyond the tip of the Magic® 1.2 microcatheter (AIT-Balt, Miami, FL), since the distal lumen is only 0.008 in.

(p) Another technique that can be used to facilitate catheter advancement is to remove the microwire and gently puff saline or contrast through the microcatheter. This will cause the tip of the microcatheter to move proximally a millimeter or two and allow flow to carry the tip in a different direction.

(q) Steam-shaping a 45° curve on the microcatheter can also help keep the tip of the microcatheter in the center of the vessel when making a turn.

(r) Another solution to the problem of insufficient flow-direction is to switch to a different microcatheter. The Ultraflow™ (ev3, Irvine, CA) is more flow directed than the Marathon™ (ev3, Irvine, CA) and the Magic® Standard microcatheter (AIT-Balt, Miami, FL) is far more flow directed than either ev3 catheter. In the line-up of Magic® microcatheters, the "Olive" version has a widened tip and is carried more by the flow. The very floppy Magic® 1.2 microcatheter is extremely flow directed, and can even be obtained in an "Olive" version as well.

(s) If one cannot negotiate a sharp turn into a branch from a larger vessel, position a balloon catheter such as the Hyperglide™ (ev3, Irvine, CA) in the main vessel beyond the branch. Use the balloon to temporarily occlude flow distal to the side-branch. This will allow flow to carry the microcatheter into the branch. This technique adds to the complexity of the case and the presence of another intravascular catheter can add friction and impair the flow-directional capabilities of the microcatheter. Therefore this method is not recommended except in very unusual circumstances where no other options are available.

(t) Gently pull back on the microcatheter periodically to remove redundancy.

(u) Inject a small amount of contrast through the microcatheter to confirm catheter positioning, and also to confirm patency of the microcatheter. When all slack is removed, perform a high-resolution superselective arteriogram.

(v) Do a microcatheter angiogram to determine:
   i. the desired position has been reached.
   ii. there are no normal brain vessels filling.
   iii. the flow-rate in order to choose an embolic agent and the injection rate needed.
   iv. there is no sign of contrast exiting the microcatheter proximal to the distal tip. *This would indicate that the microcatheter has been irreparably damaged or even ruptured and must not be used for embolization.*

(w) Once the microcatheter is in position, provocative testing may be performed if necessary or the embolization phase may begin.

9. Provocative testing (see Chap. 6) is done in an effort to confirm that the vessel being embolized does not supply eloquent neurological territory. Drugs such as amobarbital are injected in the vessel prior to embolization and the patient is tested for new signs of neurological dysfunction. Although usually used on awake patients, it can be done under general anesthesia using electroencephalography (EEG), somatosensory evoked potentials (SSEP), brainstem evoked responses (BAER) and/or motor evoked potentials (MEP). It is controversial whether these tests add safety to the procedure, but provocative testing using EEG has been shown to predict some neurological complications in AVM embolization.[19] SSEPs have been reported to aid in intracranial aneurysm embolization.[20] Monitoring is not free from false negatives, and one should avoid a false sense of security even when testing suggests it is safe to embolize. This is particularly true in high-flow lesions such as AVMs and dAVFs. Careful attention to the microcatheter angiogram may be just as sensitive as provocative testing to rule out normal territories at risk. The technique for provocative testing is as follows:

(a) Position the microcatheter in the desired artery.

(b) Remove the RHV on the microcatheter and connect a three-way stopcock to the microcatheter.

(c) Using a wet-to-wet connection, connect a labeled 3 mL amobarbital (25 mg/mL) syringe to the stopcock attached to the microcatheter.

(d) Hold the syringe in a vertical position to make bubbles rise away from the catheter.

(e) With awake patients, place a sterile half-sheet over the sterile field over the patient's thorax, to prevent contamination of the field during testing.

(f) Inject the amobarbital (usually 30–50 mg, depending on the vessel size and flow-rate) over approximately 5 s into the vessel.

(g) Immediately disconnect the amobarbital syringe and flush the microcatheter with a 3 mL syringe containing heparinized saline to remove any amobarbital left in the catheter.

(h) Ask the patient if he or she feels anything abnormal, then do a brief neurological examination, paying particular attention to functions at risk from the vascular territory being tested. If the patient shows a new deficit, the testing is considered abnormal, and the vessel should not be embolized from that catheter position.

i. In patients under anesthesia, when the barbiturate is injected, adjunctive testing with EEG, SSEP, BAER, and/or MEP can be done. If adjunctive testing changes from baseline status, then the testing is also considered abnormal, and the vessel should not be embolized from that catheter position.

(j) If no change occurs with neurological testing and adjunctive testing, the testing is normal and suggests that it may be safe to embolize, or at least it is safe to proceed to test with lidocaine. Lidocaine may be more sensitive to nerve and white-matter tract supply than is amobarbital. *Do not inject lidocaine if the barbiturate testing is abnormal.*
    i.   Connect a labeled 3-mL syringe of 2% cardiac lidocaine to the stopcock on the microcatheter.
    ii. Inject the lidocaine (usually 20–50 mg) over approximately 5 s into the vessel.
    iii. Repeat the appropriate neurological and/or adjunctive neurophysiological testing. If no change occurs, the testing is normal and it is safe to embolize. If a neurological or neurophysiological deficit occurs, the testing is abnormal and the vessel should not be embolized from that catheter position.

(k) During embolization of an artery after negative amobarbital and lidocaine testing, a change in flow pattern or visualization or different vessels may be seen after a partial occlusion of the vessel. Additional provocative testing may be necessary when additional arteries are targeted.[21]

Syringe Safety

Many of the procedures discussed in this handbook require the use of multiple agents in syringes on the procedure table. For example, an embolization procedure that may involve provocative testing requires syringes containing local anesthetic, saline flush, contrast, amobarbital, lidocaine, embolic material, etc. It is imperative that these syringes containing different agents are clearly differentiated from one another. Confusing syringes with anesthetic agents or embolic materials for contrast or saline flush can lead to disastrous results. Use customized, labeled, coloured syringes (Merit Medical, South Jordan, UT) of various sizes and designs for the various materials. Using the same type of syringe for a certain agent at all times and educating new team members to the routine will minimize confusion and avoid mistakes.

Embolization Phase

With the microcatheter in optimal position, the time is has come for occluding the vessel with an appropriate embolic agent. The microcatheter angiogram with the microcatheter is in its final position will confirm that the originally chosen embolic agent is still appropriate for the flow rate and distance to the lesion. A variety of embolic materials are available and some are more effective than others. The single most important principle of the selection process is for the operator to use the system with which he or she is most experienced and comfortable.

Embolization Strategy

Several fundamental truths have emerged over several decades of global experience with brain AVM embolization:
1. A complete plan for AVM obliteration must formulated prior the beginning of treatment.
    (a) For instance, piecemeal, random embolizations of larger AVMs should be avoided.
2. Medium and large-sized brain AVMs should not be completely embolized in a single session. Complete occlusion of these lesions carries a higher risk of haemorrhage.[22]

3. Priority should be given to embolizing high-flow fistulas within the AVM[23], or intranidal aneurysms, or regions of venous stenosis, rather than randomly embolizing parts of the nidus.
4. Embolization of brain Avms decreases the effectiveness of radiosurgery.[24–26]
    (a) Nevertheless, embolization followed by radiosurgery may be reasonable in some cases.

Liquid Embolics

These agents are supplied in a liquid state and are easily injected through small microcatheters. They are the most commonly used embolic agents used in intracranial embolization procedure.
1. Cyanoacrylates (aka "glue")
    (a) These are acrylic agents that polymerize when they contact hydroxyl ions in blood. Historically, they have been the dominant embolic agents used for intracranial embolization[27], although a precipitated polymer (Onyx) has become more popular in recent years. Although recanalization may occur[28], glue is generally considered to produce an effectively permanent occlusion.[29] The most common acrylic agent used in the United States is n-butyl cyanocrylate n-BCA Trufill® (Codman Neurovascular, Raynham, MA). Polymerization time can be modified by the addition of oil-based contrast agents such as ethiodized oil (Ethiodol,® Savage Laboratories, Melville, NY) (whose hydrophobic medium "hides" the acrylic monomer from hydroxyl ions) or glacial acetic acid (the acid binds with the hydroxyl ions).[28, 30] Longer chain monomers can slow the polymerization and alter adhesive properties.[31] Neuracryl M 2-hexyl cyanoacrylate (Prohold Technologies, El Cajon, CA) is a promising agent, but is not yet approved by the FDA.[32]
        i. Advantages: n-BCA is nearly always permanently occlusive.[29] Speed of polymerization is adjustable using by using Ethiodol® and/or glacial acetic acid. Very visible on fluoro when Ethiodol® or tantalum powder added. With proper technique, it can be used in low or high flow states. In some cases n-BCA can be "pushed" to the target lesion with dextrose solution even if microcatheter is some distance from the lesion. Can be delivered via flow-directed microcatheter.
        ii. Disadvantages: Polymerization time is dependent on numerous factors, including temperature, formulation of glue and Ethiodol®, rate of blood flow, rate of injection, etc. Liquid agent can enter dangerous anastamoses easily. Requires considerable training and experience to avoid problems. Its adhesive property makes it possible to glue the catheter in the vessel. Polymerized glue is firmer than other agents, which can increase the difficulty of the surgical excision of a lesion post-embolization.
2. Precipitated polymers (aka non-adhesive liquid embolic agents)
    (a) These agents are polymers which are insoluble in blood or water and are delivered while dissolved in a non-aqueous solvent. When injected into the vascular system, the solvent disperses and the polymer precipitates to form a solid occlusive agent. Onyx® (ev3, Irvine, CA) is the dominant example of the precipitated polymer and is FDA approved for use in Avms. It consists of ethylene-vinyl copolymer (aka EVAL or EVOH) dissolved in dimethyl sulfoxide (DMSO) with added tantalum powder to make it radio-opaque. It comes in several versions for Avms: Onyx® 18 consists of 6% EVOH and is used for deeper penetration of the nidus; the thicker Onyx® 34 is 8% EVOH and is used for high-flow AVF feeders. When the mixture is injected into the vascular system, the DMSO diffuses away and the EVOH precipitates into a non-adhesive, soft, spongy material. Another embolic agent that forms a stable gel when injected is calcium alginate. It has shown promise in experimental AVM models, but it requires a double lumen microcatheter to simultaneously inject the alginate and the calcium chloride reactant.[33]
        i. Advantages: Onyx® creates a soft, spongy solid precipitate easier to handle than glue during surgical excision of embolized lesions.[34] There is less of an inflammatory response compared to that of glue.[35] Non-adhesive, so that very long, and thorough injections can be made with less fear of gluing the microcatheter in place.

Less stressful to use than adhesive agents. Very visible on imaging. With proper technique, Onyx can be used both low-flow and high flow lesions.

ii. Disadvantages: Onyx® requires DMSO-compatible microcatheters, which are less flexible than non-compatible catheters such as the Magic.® DMSO can be toxic to endothelium and painful for awake patients when injected quickly. *Onyx stinks*: The DMSO diffuses out of the precipitated Onyx and causes the patient to smell of DMSO metabolites (rather unpleasant) for several days. The microcatheter must be positioned very close to the lesion. The ability to slowly inject the Onyx® with less fear of gluing the catheter in place can make one over-confident and occlude more than may be safe.

3. Sclerosing agents
   (a) Sclerosing agents are liquid materials that cause both thrombosis and necrosis of the intima. These agents are readily available and are toxic in high concentrations, but relatively benign in low concentrations. This dependence on concentration is why sclerosing agents work best in slow flow situations like tumors and worst in high flow conditions like AVFs. Absolute ethanol is medical-grade ethanol that is dehydrated sufficiently to be close to 100% pure ethanol. Absolute ethanol is very thrombogenic and very toxic at this concentration. Ethanol is the most frequently used sclerosing agent for intracranial embolization.[36] Even 30% ethanol, mixed with particulate emboli, will induce thrombosis; although this is not as permanent as pure ethanol, it is sufficient for pre-operative embolization.[37–39] Other intracranial sclerosing agents include 50% dextrose solution for low-flow fistulas[40] and a solution of phenytoin in saline, 25 mg/mL[41] for meningiomas.
      i. Advantages: Inexpensive and readily available. Low viscosity allows easy injection through a small microcatheter. Since the toxic effect is diminished when the agent is diluted, small amounts of reflux into a large vessel may be well tolerated. High-concentration ethanol can produce permanent occlusion.[36]
      ii. Disadvantages: Can cause extreme pain in awake patients if the vessels injected are near a meningeal surface. The sclerosing agent is not radio-opaque. Occlusion occurs in a delayed fashion, so it can be difficult to determine when to stop. These agents may require excessive volumes to occlude higher flow lesions. May not work in very high flow fistulas. The risk of systemic toxicity with larger doses of ethanol risk is low, but cardiovascular collapse has been reported.[42] Ethanol permeates beyond the vascular system and increases the permeability of the vessels, which can allow for extravascular contrast extravasation.[43] This permeability effect may contribute to a 47% rate of neurological complications and a 11% mortality rate in studies of brain AVMs embolized with ethanol.[36] The authors of this handbook do not approve of routine use of ethanol or other sclerosing agents for intracranial embolization.

Particles

These are agents that are supplied in a solid state but are individually small enough to be easily injected through small microcatheters, when mixed with diluted contrast material. There are too many available particulate agents to discuss in detail, but all are similar. All particulate agents work best in lesions with a capillary bed, such as tumors. All have a tendency to clog the microcatheter if the particles are too large or injected in too large a quantity. All require a similar technique for their use.

1. Polyvinyl alcohol foam (aka "PVA")
   (a) These are irregularly shaped particles of PVA Examples: Contour® emboli (Boston Scientific, Natick, MA) or PVA Foam Embolization Particles (Cook Medical, Bloomington, IN). The particles are mixed with diluted contrast and are injected through the microcatheter.[44]
      i. Advantages: Inexpensive. Easy to use. If sized appropriately, can be carried by the flow to the lesion even if the microcatheter tip is very proximal to lesion. Occlusion of target vessels occurs very rapidly because the particles are irregular and fit together like jigsaw puzzle pieces.

ii. Disadvantages: Although they can be mixed with contrast, the PVA particles are not radio-opaque, so it is difficult to tell where they are ending up on fluoroscopy. Vessel occlusion is partly related to the thrombus forming around the particles. The vessel may re-open over time as the thrombus breaks down. Clumping of irregular particles can occlude the microcatheter, especially with smaller sized catheters. Particles may fragment as being injected and these fragments may produce a more distal occlusion than anticipated. Not effective for high-flow fistulas. When used for AVMs, may be associated with higher risk or hemorrhagic complications than nBCA glue.[45, 46]

2. Spherical emboli
   (a) These particles are manufactured to have a smooth, spherical shape. Examples: Spherical Contour SE™ (Boston Scientific, Natick, MA), Bead Block™ (Terumo Medical, Somerset, NJ) and Embospheres® (Biosphere Medical, Rockland, MA). All the three are similar in behavior, although a comparative in vitro study showed that Bead Block™ stayed suspended in contrast better than the other products and was somewhat easier to deliver through the microcatheter.[47]
       i. Advantages: Less likely than traditional PVA to clump and clog microcatheter or produce occlusion more proximal than desired.
       ii. Disadvantages: Smoother particles may pass through anastamoses or go more distally than intended. May still clog the microcatheter if particles are too large or in too concentrated a mixture. Vessels occluded may still recanalize over time. Not effective for high-flow fistulas. Embolization procedures take longer with spheres than with PVA.

3. Silk suture
   (a) Small segments of thrombogenic silk suture can be propelled into the vessel through the microcatheter by injecting contrast or saline. Other types of suture material can be used in this fashion, but are less thrombogenic.
       i. Advantages: Inexpensive and universally available. Small segments of 3-O or 5-O suture can be injected through the tiny lumen of a flow-directed microcatheter. More thrombogenic than other particulate agents.
       ii. Disadvantages: Very tedious and time consuming to cut and load individual suture fragments into the microcatheter. Can clog the microcatheter. May require high pressures to flush suture through microcatheter. Not effective for high-flow fistulas. Intense inflammatory response to foreign proteins in silk can often produce fevers, chill, and pain after embolization.

4. Detachable balloons
   (a) These devices are small balloons attached to a microcatheter that are designed to be navigated to the desired site of occlusion, inflated to produce occlusion of the vessel, then detached from the catheter and permanently implanted. The balloons stay inflated thanks to a valve that seals once the balloon detaches. They are typically inflated with contrast to make it visible on fluoroscopy, and the integrity of the balloon and its valve are all that keeps it from deflating. However, nearly all balloons eventually leak and deflate. Polymers such as the hydrophilic 2-hydroxy-ethyl methacrylate (HEMA) can be used to inflate the balloon and ensure long-term stability of the occlusion.[48] At the time of this writing, the Balt Goldballoons (Balt, Monorency, France) have CE mark approval and are available in most of the world outside of the United States. No detachable balloon currently has FDA approval for the U.S. market.
       i. Advantages: Quick, predictable occlusion of large vessels. Can be flow-directed to high-flow fistulas.
       ii. Disadvantages: Require large guide catheters for delivery. During manipulation, balloons may prematurely detach and embolize. Smooth, deformable balloons may migrate distally to an undesired location after detachment. Balloons may rupture if over inflated or inflated against an irregular surface. Virtually all detachable balloons eventually leak and deflate. Valves are easily damaged during preparation, causing balloons to prematurely deflate.

5. Pushable coils
   (a) Small, usually platinum coils that can be delivered through a microcatheter. A wide variety of coils is available from many different companies, including Cook, Boston Scientific and Codman.

6. Detachable platinum coils.
   (a) These include the GDC® (Stryker Neurovascular, Fremont, CA), but similar systems include Trufill® DCS (Codman Neurovascular, Raynham, MA) ACT™ Spherical or Helipaq™ (Micrus/Codman, San Jose, CA) or Microplex™ (Microvention/Terumo Medical, Tustin, CA), or Axium™ (ev3, Irvine, CA). These are bare platinum coils that remain attached to its delivery wire until the operator detaches it. These must be deployed via 150 cm, two tip-marker over-the-wire microcatheters. Detachable coils are discussed further in Chap. 5.
      i. Advantages: Can be positioned and repositioned easily. Platinum is very visible on imaging. Many variably sized and shaped coils are available.
      ii. Disadvantages: Expensive. Unless the coil is well anchored in place, it may pass through fistulas or go more distally than intended in high flow states. It can take many, many coils to occlude high-flow fistulas. Vessels occluded with coils may recanalize over time. Not effective for very distal vessel occlusion. Not suitable for use in flow-directed catheters.
7. Fibered detachable coils
   (a) These are a hybrid of the pushable fibered coil and detachable coil. Examples include the Sapphire NXT™ fibered coils (ev3, Irvine, CA) or Fibered GDC® (Styker Neurovascular, Fremont, CA), although the availability of these may be limited.
      i. Advantages: Very thrombogenic, yet with all the control of a detachable coil.
      ii. Disadvantages: Very stiff. May displace microcatheter from its desired position and may not deploy in tortuous vessels. Requires larger lumen microcatheters. Much more expensive than pushable coils.
8. Augmented detachable coils
   (a) Platinum coils augmented with additional materials were developed to promote healing and decrease the recanalization of aneurysms treated with these coils. These include, among others, the Matrix™ (Styker Neurovascular, Fremont, CA) and Hydrocoil® (Microvention/Terumo Medical, Aliso Viejo, CA). They are discussed further in Chap. 5.
      i. Advantages: Can be used wherever bare platinum coils can be used.
      ii. Disadvantages: Expensive. May be somewhat more difficult to deploy than bare platinum coils. They have no proven benefit over other detachable coils in other intracranial embolization procedures.

Global Gem

Many devices for endovascular therapy in the head, neck and spine are available worldwide, although not in the United States. There are niche products that were previously sold by U.S. companies, presumably because low sales volumes were not felt to justify the cost of manufacture and FDA requirements. These niche items include small platinum injectable coils (the former Berenstein liquid coils) detachable balloons (the former silicone DSB) and steerable microcatheters (the former Pivot). Balt Extrusion (Montmorency, France) makes the soft platinum Flowcoils and detachable latex Goldballoons, and Scientia Vascular (Reno, NV) makes the Plato™ steerable microcatheter which are CE mark approved and sold across the globe. The use of flow diversion for aneurysm treatment is much more prevalent outside the U.S. and many of the devices such are the Silk stent (Balt Extrusion, Montmorency, France), Willis covered stent (Micro-Port, Shanghai, China) and Surpass (Surpass Medical, Tel-Aviv, Israel) are not available for use in the U.S. Companies based in the United States tend to roll out innovative products first in Europe. Some of these include the Luna™ (Nfocus, Palo Alto, CA) multilayer nitinol aneurysm plug, and the Trevo™ (Stryker Neurovascular, Fremont, CA) stent-retriever for stroke.

The effort and expense required to get products approved by the FDA may mean that practitioners in the U.S. may not have access to the latest products or be the first to report their use in the literature. On the other hand, it can save patients and practitioners the embarrassment and risk of using some of the devices that are later found to be problematic. For example, the tungsten MDS coils (Balt, Montmorency, France) used for endovascular therapy were in many ways quicker and easier to use than the other available coils at that time, but had a habit of corroding and dissolving over time.[49–51] The mid-term follow-up of patients treated with these coils led to the eventual discontinuance of their usage.[52] Those in the United States were never involved in this controversy.

N-BCA Embolization Technique

1. Place the microcatheter in the target vessel.
2. Create a blank roadmap mask so that the glue injection can be well visualized under digital subtraction.
3. Set up a second sterile back table that is physically separate from the other sterile areas, so that sodium chloride ions cannot come into contact with the glue before it is injected.
   (a) All people near the sterile field should wear glasses or other eye protection. If a connection comes loose during injection, the glue can spray and stick to whatever it touches.
4. Glue preparation:
   (a) Set out:
      i. Sterile 5% dextrose solution
      ii. 10–15 3-mL syringes
      iii. 2 18-gauge needles
      iv. A pack of blue towels
   (b) Glue concentration:
      i. Examine the microcatheter angiogram to see how long the contrast takes to reach the lesion.
      ii. As a rule of thumb, if the transit time is <1 s, at least a 70% glue mixture (three parts n-BCA to one part Ethiodol®) is required. Transit time >2 s requires a 50% (one n-BCA to one Ethiodol) or more dilute mixture.
      iii. Draw up the Trufill® n-BCA (Codman Neurovascular, Raynham, MA) from its tube using a labeled, glue-compatible 3-mL syringe (avoid polycarbonate plastic...it softens).
   (c) Draw up the Ethiodol® in a labeled syringe, and add the proper volume to the glue syringe to achieve the desired concentration.
   (d) Tantalum powder greatly increases the radio-opacity of glue, but is not absolutely necessary unless the glue mixture is greater than 70% n-BCA. Tantalum is messy and can clump, so most practitioners rarely use it.
5. Fill several 3 mL syringes 5% dextrose solution.
6. Attach a glue-compatible stopcock directly to the microcatheter. Cook Medical (Bloomington, IN) makes a high-pressure, white nylon plastic one-way, and three-way stopcocks with Luer lock fittings that hold up well during glue injections. One-way stopcocks are sufficient, but three-way are preferred since they allow a flush syringe of dextrose to remain attached even when the glue syringe is attached. This works well for doing the push technique (see below).
7. Thoroughly flush the microcatheter with several 3 mL syringes of 5% dextrose solution.
8. Injection techniques: There are four methods for injecting n-BCA (Fig. 7.1)

Fig. 7.1 Four techniques for AVM glue embolization. *Full column technique*: The microcatheter tip (*MC*) is positioned close to the target and beyond all normal arteries. Glue (*shaded*) is steadily injected as a continuous column, filling the vessel lumen. If the glue polymerization time and injection rate are properly controlled, the glue will reach the nidus before polymerizing. The injection is stopped if the glue reaches the vein or begins to reflux back to the microcatheter tip. Arrows indicate blood flow. *Wedge technique*: A microcatheter is gently flow-directed into a vascular channel in the nidus no bigger than the catheter tip, effectively blocking the blood flow beyond the tip. A dilute glue mixture (*shaded*) is then slowly injected, filling the nidus. The slowly polymerizing mixture does not get washed into the veins by the flowing blood because the wedged catheter controls the flow. *Push technique*: The microcatheter tip is some distance to the lesion, and a small bolus (0.1 mL) of glue (*shaded*) is propelled into the vessel with a bolus of 5% dextrose solution. Blood flow (*arrows*) plus momentum from the dextrose bolus (*hatched arrows*) carries the glue toward the lesion until it polymerizes. This technique is the safest way to inject high concentration (ultra-fast polymerizing) glue mixtures without gluing the microcatheter in place. *Dribble technique*: This can be used with the microcatheter tip somewhat proximal to a relatively low-flow lesion that has a capillary bed or nidus with small channels. A full column of relatively dilute glue (*shaded*) is very, very slowly injected so that the blood flow fragments the glue as it exits the microcatheter. The small drops of glue are then carried by the blood flow (*arrows*) into the nidus, where they wedge into the small spaces. This technique is usually used for preoperative tumor or small AVM embolization.

(a) *Continuous column injection technique*:
    i. The "continuous column technique" is the most common n-BCA injection method.
    ii. At the time of injection, fill the Luer-lock connection fully with dextrose and attach a 3-mL syringe loaded with the prepared glue mixture.
    iii. The glue injection is quick but controlled. Polymerization usually occurs within a few seconds.

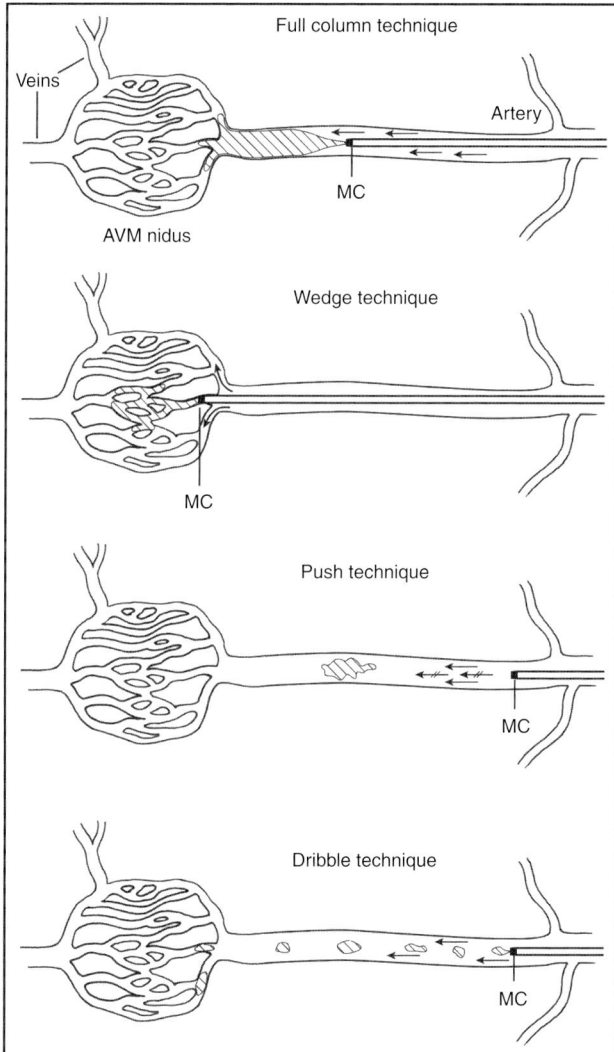

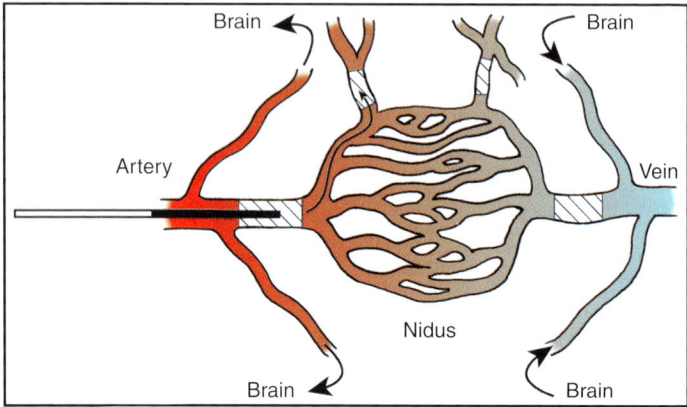

Fig. 7.2 Safety zones for AVM embolization. The artery feeding the AVM may be occluded distal to all normal vessels feeding the brain. *Hatch marks* indicate the safe zones in the artery and the vein. Occlusion proximal to the safe zone can cause an ischemic stroke. The nidus is safe to occlude because it supplies no normal structures. The vein beyond the nidus may be occluded before any inputs from normal brain veins or even veins supplying other segments of the AVM. Occlusion downstream from the safe zone in the vein carries a risk of haemorrhage from remaining nidus or venous infarction of brain.

    iv. Steadily inject the glue under direct visualization using roadmap image. Make sure that the glue column is continuously moving forward during the injection.

    v. Fill the arterial feeder and as much of the nidus as possible.

    vi. Be alert for any signs of reflux of glue back along the catheter, passage of glue into the vein, or reflux of glue from the nidus into other arterial branches feeding the lesion.

    vii. If any of these conditions is occurring and one is using dilute glue, briefly pause the injection, then resume cautiously. Sometimes the glue will find another pathway through the nidus.

    viii. The embolic agent should be deposited in the "safety zone" consisting of AVM nidus and only the artery beyond all normal branches, and vein before other venous inputs beyond the occluded nidus. (Fig. 7.2)

    ix. When the injection is complete or if there is any question that the glue is refluxing or going somewhere it shouldn't, stop injecting, aspirate the syringe to create negative pressure in the microcatheter, and quickly, smoothly withdraw the microcatheter completely from the patient and discard it.

    x. Examine the rotating hemostatic valve of the guide catheter for any retained droplets of glue, then aspirate and double flush the stopcock, RHV, and guide catheter.

    xi. Do a follow-up guide catheter angiogram.

(b) *Wedge injection technique*

    i. The wedge technique is similar to the full-column technique, except that the microcatheter tip is wedged in the nidus or small vessel and much more dilute glue can be used.

    ii. In wedged position, very slow, prolonged injections with dilute glue (less than 30% glue) can be done over several minutes (which seems like hours).

    iii. When glue begins to enter the vein, or to reflux along the microcatheter, one should stop injecting, wait for polymerization, aspirate back from the glue syringe, then pull the catheter out.

(c) *Push technique*

    i. The microcatheter is generally some distance proximal to the lesion, but still beyond normal brain vessels.

ii. When ready to embolize, the microcatheter is flushed with dextrose solution.
iii. A three way stopcock is attached to the hub of the microcatheter, and a syringe of 5% dextrose flush is attached to one connection, and the appropriately mixed glue to another.
iv. Depending on the size of the vessel being embolized, 0.1–0.2 mL of glue mixture is injected into the microcatheter, the stopcock is turned and, under roadmap visualization, the glue is flushed into the vessel using the dextrose flush syringe.
v. Generally, the microcatheter should be removed at this point. The exception would be when the glue bolus travels quite distal to the tip of the microcatheter, and if contrast injections via the guide catheter confirm persistent patency of the feeding vessel being embolized. A second glue bolus may be injected and pushed with dextrose as long as the microcatheter remains patent.

(d) *Dribble injection technique*
i. The dribble technique is similar to the full column technique, except that the glue is injected very, very slowly, to allow the blood flow to fragment the glue and form small particles. These tend to travel along with the blood flow until they impact on a small nidus or capillary bed.

9. *Special situation*: *High concentration (aka "pure glue") n-BCA embolization*:
(a) Occasionally required for very high flow fistulas.
(b) Pure glue embolization is akin to holding a burning object in one's bare hands: It is possible to get burned.
(c) Everything must be done quickly and there is a real risk of refluxing glue into proximal vessels and/or gluing the microcatheter in place.
(d) If the mixture is less than 30% Ethiodol then tantalum powder must be added to the n-BCA to make it visible fluoroscopically.
(e) In extreme high flow states, when using little or no Ethiodol, the pure glue may instantly polymerize in the microcatheter.
(f) Consider putting the glue on ice or in a freezer until immediately before use or gently flushing the microcatheter with 50% dextrose to slow the polymerization just enough to prevent clogging the microcatheter.
(g) Only a 0.1- to 0.3-mL bolus of glue is loaded into the dextrose-flushed microcatheter and pushed into the vessel with a quick injection of dextrose. *Do not hesitate*.
(h) *Immediately pull the microcatheter*. It is best to have at least two people involved: one to inject and the other to pull the guide-catheter/microcatheter assembly as a unit. *No hesitation*.
(i) Now is the time to change one's underwear and prepare to do a control angiogram to see what was accomplished.

10. *Methods to slow down glue polymerization*
(a) Most common method: Add Ethiodol.
(b) Adding tiny amounts of glacial acetic acid.[30] Twenty microliters affect polymerization more profoundly than several mL of Ethiodol[53] and do not increase the viscosity of the mixture like the oily Ethiodol does.[54]
(c) Cooling the glue also slows polymerization, but glue can warm rapidly under ambient room temperature
(d) Injecting 5% dextrose solution via the guide catheter can flood the local circulation with inhibitory dextrose during the n-BCA injection.[55]

Onyx® Embolization Technique

1. Have several vials of Onyx® (ev3, Irvine, CA) agitating on an automatic shaker for at least 30 min while performing other parts of the procedure. The Onyx® technique is similar to the N-BCA except that dimethyl sulfoxide (DMSO)-compatible catheters such as the Rebar® (ev3, Irvine, CA) or more flexible Marathon™ (ev3, Irvine, CA) must be used. Provocative testing can give a false sense of security since Onyx® can easily find its way into places that may not be predicted by superselective angiography or barbiturate injections.
2. Place the microcatheter in position. Select angiogram projections that show the microcatheter tip and its relationship to any curves in the arterial feeder distal

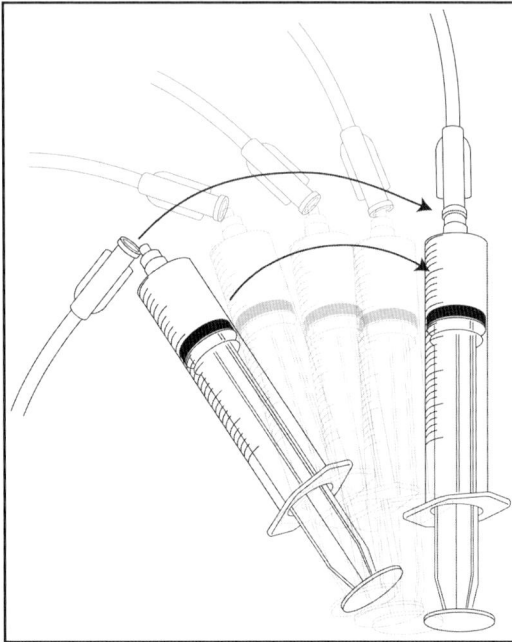

Fig. 7.3 Syringe loading technique for Onyx. (1) Draw up the Onyx® into the syringe specified by the manufacturer. Agitate it back and forth if it will not be injected for more than a few minutes to keep the tantalum suspended. (2) Attach the DMSO syringe directly to the hub of the microcatheter and fill the dead-space of the microcatheter (usually 0.2–0.3 mL) with DMSO over 1–2 min. (3) Remove the DMSO syringe from the microcatheter, and, keeping the hub upright, fill the hub with DMSO. (4) Holding both the catheter hub and Onyx® syringe at 45° to one another, quickly connect the syringe to the hub, and then keep the syringe vertical, plunger down. This keeps a sharp demarcation between the heavier Onyx® in the syringe, and lighter DMSO in the hub of the catheter. It is easier to see the Onyx® fluoroscopically if it is not allowed by be diluted by DMSO.

to the catheter tip, any normal branches proximal to it, and whether the tip is wedged. Study the microcatheter angiograms to determine the arteriovenous transit time, the morphology of the target arterial feeder and venous structures where you will deposit the Onyx®.

3. Select the Onyx® depending on the size of the feeder and degree of arteriovenous shunting. Big feeders with fast flow need Onyx® 34 and Onyx® 18 should be used for small feeders and slower shunting fistulas.

4. Using the proper syringe supplied by ev3, draw up 1 mL of DMSO. The technique for handling the Onyx syringes is illustrated in Fig. 7.3.

5. Using a blank roadmap mask, slowly inject the Onyx® under roadmap visualization at a rate of approximately 0.16 mL/min. Rates of injection over 0.3 mL/min risk vascular injury due to DMSO toxicity.

6. Continue injecting Onyx® as long as it is flowing forward into desired areas of the abnormal vessels.

7. If it refluxes along the catheter, passes into the proximal part of the vein, or refluxes into other arterial feeders, pause the injection for 15 s, then resume injecting. If the Onyx® continues to flow in the wrong direction, pause again for 15–30 s, then try again. If the Onyx® finds another, more desirable pathway, continue the slow injection.

8. Obtain a new mask for roadmap periodically. This makes the newly injected material easier to see. Guide catheter angiograms during the Onyx® injection are helpful too.
9. The Onyx® injection should be done patiently and may take many minutes.
10. Some reflux back along the catheter tip is not a problem, due to the non-adhesive nature of the product. *Avoid more than 1 cm of reflux, however, since even Onyx® may glue a microcatheter into the vessel.*
11. Do not pause the injection for more than 2 min, for the Onyx® may solidify and clog the microcatheter.
12. *Never try to inject against resistance. A clogged microcatheter may burst if the injection is forced.*
13. When adequate filling of the target is achieved, or if the Onyx® repeatedly flows in the wrong direction, stop injecting, aspirate back on the syringe, and slowly and steadily pull back on the microcatheter, disengage it from the deposited Onyx® and remove it. The heavy-duty catheters used for Onyx® can usually be pulled back on their own, without pulling the guide catheter as well.
14. After the microcatheter is withdrawn from the guide catheter, examine the RHV of the guide catheter for any retained droplets of Onyx®, then aspirate and double flush the guide catheter.
15. Once the guide catheter is thoroughly inspected and flushed, do a follow-up guide catheter angiogram.

Ethanol Embolization Technique

Although ethanol is not recommended routinely for intracranial embolization, there may be rare situations in which nothing else is available. When ethanol is added to mixtures of particles, the technique is essentially the same as standard particulate embolization (see below). When used without particles, the technique is more like the technique for glue. Some recommend prophylactic placement of a Swan-Ganz catheter for AVM embolizations with ethanol to monitor for pulmonary hypertension.

1. Be sure to use syringes, stopcocks and microcatheter hubs will not degrade when exposed to ethanol. Usually anything that can be used with glue or DMSO can be used with ethanol, but it is wise to test it first. Since ethanol embolization is not an FDA-approved procedure, manufacturers often state that their products are not approved for use with ethanol.
2. Position the microcatheter. When ready to embolize, perform test injections of contrast through the microcatheter to estimate the rate and volume required to opacify the territory that is to be occluded.
3. If the flow is very rapid, consider placing a coil or two to slow the flow.
4. Flush the microcatheter with saline, since ethanol can cause contrast to precipitate.
5. Inject the absolute ethanol at a rate similar to that which opacified the vessel, but use only approximately 50% of the volume of contrast used.
6. Wait a few minutes and then repeat the contrast injection. If the vessel remains patent, inject another small bolus of ethanol, and wait again.
7. If spasm is seen on repeat test injections, wait until it resolves and decrease the volume of ethanol boluses.
8. After a few boluses have been given, wait at least 5–10 min between ethanol injections before checking for patency of the vessel.
9. If there is no change after 20 mL of ethanol, consider placement of additional coils to slow the flow and help the ethanol work, or try a better embolic agent.
10. Remember that ethanol can work on the endothelium for some time and can also spread through the vessel wall into the tissues, so it is best to keep the ethanol volumes to a minimum. *One mL per kg body weight is the absolute maximum dose.*

Particle Embolization Technique

1. Most particles are similar in how they are handled for intracranial embolization.
2. To avoid clogging the microcatheter, use one of the larger lumen over-the-wire types of microcatheters.

3. The microcatheter tip must be close to the lesion being embolized and in a stable position distal to normal branches.
4. Confirm safe positioning with a microcatheter angiogram and provocative testing, when possible.
5. Choose a particle size depending on the size of the vessels in the target lesion. In general, tumors with a capillary bed are treated with particles <300 μm in diameter, and AVMs require particles over 300 μm.
6. Mix the particles with 50:50 contrast and draw up the emboli in a 10 mL syringe. The syringe acts as a reservoir for emboli.
7. The particles should be fairly dilute to limit the risk of clogging the microcatheter.
8. Attach the syringe to one female connection on a high-pressure three-way stopcock and attach a 3 mL luer-lock syringe to the other female connection. This syringe is used to inject the embolic mixture through the microcatheter.
9. The stopcock is then attached to the hub of the microcatheter.
10. The stopcock is then turned to connect the 10 and 3 mL syringes, and the contrast/emboli mixture is flushed into the 3 mL syringe and then back into the 10-mL syringe, back and forth several times, to ensure uniform suspension of particles.
11. The 3 mL syringe is then filled with 1–2 mL of the emboli suspension.
12. Make a blank roadmap and under fluoroscopic guidance slowly inject the emboli in small (0.2 mL) increments and ensure that the contrast freely flows from the microcatheter tip.
13. Increase or decrease the rate of injection depending on the speed of runoff away from the microcatheter.
14. After every injection of 3–5 mL of embolic suspension, or sooner if emboli are seen to collect in the hub of the microcatheter, disconnect the 3-mL syringe and reconnect another labeled 3-mL syringe filled with dilute 50:50 contrast.
15. Gently flush the microcatheter with the contrast under fluoroscopy, remembering that the microcatheter is still full of emboli.
16. As long as a good runoff of contrast is seen, reconnect the 3-mL emboli syringe, refill it with embolic mixture, and continue to inject emboli.
17. When the 10-mL syringe is empty, consider obtaining a control superselective angiogram via the microcatheter to see whether the flow pattern is changing.
18. If an entire vial of emboli is injected with no change in the flow pattern, consider modifying the flow with a coil or two, or switching to a different embolic agent.
19. Avoid creating reflux of the embolic mixture back along the microcatheter when injecting. Slow or stop the injections if reflux is seen.
20. If resistance is encountered during the injection, stop, disconnect the 3-mL embolic syringe and check the hub of the microcatheter. If emboli are bunched up in the hub, it may be possible to rinse them out with a needle or guidewire introducer and then attempt to flush with contrast. If resistance persists, *do not attempt to force the emboli through by a forceful injection, and do not use a 1 mL syringe to achieve higher pressures*. Attempting to inject through a microcatheter clogged with particles can cause the microcatheter to rupture and even break into pieces.
21. When the flow in the feeder is significantly slowed, the injection of emboli is stopped.
22. If more definitive closure of the vessel is desired after particle embolization, a coil may be deposited to finish the job. Be sure to flush the microcatheter with contrast or saline before inserting a coil. Retained particles in the microcatheter can cause the coil to bind in the microcatheter.
23. Even if the microcatheter seems free of particles, it is best to withdraw and discard the used microcatheter prior to attempting catheterization of another feeder with a new microcatheter.

Silk Suture Embolization Technique

1. Selection of the microcatheter depends on the size of the silk suture being used. An Excelsior® SL-10 (Boston Scientific, Natick, MA) works well with 4–0 silk suture.
2. Obtain several microwire introducers to use as introducers for the silk sutures. An 18-gauge plastic intravenous catheter can also be used for this purpose.
3. Open a sterile package of 4-O silk suture.
4. Insert a 5–10-mm segment of silk into the blunt, distal end of the introducer.

5. Attach a 3 mL syringe of sterile saline to the luer-connector hub of the intro-ducer and flush to expel air. Be careful not to flush the silk out of the introducer.
6. When the microcatheter is properly positioned, check that all slack is removed and there are no kinks. These can impede the injection of silk.
7. Also ensure that the RHV of the guide catheter is just tight enough to prevent back-bleeding, but not too tight to pinch the microcatheter.
8. There should be an RHV with continuous infusion of heparinized saline already attached to the microcatheter hub as well.
9. Insert the introducer containing the silk suture fragment through the RHV of the microcatheter and seat it with its blunt tip in the hub of the microcatheter.
10. Inject the silk into the microcatheter with a small bolus of heparinized saline.
11. Remove the introducer from the RHV and tighten the valve of the RHV.
12. Flush the microcatheter with heparinized saline using a 3 mL or larger syringe to flush the silk into the vessel. There will be a build up of pressure, then a release as the silk is expelled from the microcatheter.
13. The position of the microcatheter should be checked fluoroscopically since the force of these injections can cause the tip to move.
14. Periodic contrast injections are done via the microcatheter to check or changes in the flow.
15. It may take several silk fragments to produce an effect on flow in the target vessel.
16. Consider using particles and/or coils in conjunction with silk to facilitate occlusion.
17. Avoid using a 1 mL syringe for flushes or test injections because this syringe generates sufficient pressure to rupture most microcatheters.
18. If the microcatheter does not flush easily, it may be clogged by the silk.
19. In some cases, a clogged microcatheter may be unclogged by passing a coil pusher through it, but in most cases it must be removed and another microcath-eter used to re-access the vessel to be embolized.
20. The end-point for embolization may be difficult to assess, since silk induces a slow thrombosis that may unpredictably occlude the vessel, so frequent test injections of contrast should be done to prevent reflux of emboli proximally from the occluded vessel.

Detachable Balloon Technique

1. *Preparation*
   (a) Choose a balloon diameter that is slightly larger than the space intended for occlusion.
   (b) Bench-test the balloon by inflating it with sterile water using a blunt-tip 25-gauge needle attached to a 3 mL syringe.
   (c) Insert the needle very carefully into the valve of the balloon and inflate 0.1–0.3 mL, but to no more than the rated volume of the balloon.
   (d) Withdraw the needle and confirm that the balloon remains inflated. If the balloon does not stay inflated, discard it and obtain another balloon.
   (e) Re-insert the blunt needle and deflate it, making sure to tilt the balloon to remove any air bubbles as the water is aspirated.
   (f) Inflate the balloon with an approximately 50:50 contrast solution.
   (g) Attach an RHV with a one-way stopcock to an appropriate balloon deliv-ery microcatheter. In general, the outer diameter of the tip should be less than 2F.
   (h) Flush the RHV and microcatheter with 50:50 contrast.
   (i) Preload a microwire, stiff end first, into the microcatheter and advance it just to the catheter tip. The wire should be small enough such that con-trast can be injected through the microcatheter around the wire.
   (j) Carefully load the prepared balloon onto the microcatheter. It may deflate somewhat as the microcatheter enters the balloon valve.
   (k) Keeping a contrast syringe attached to the open stopcock on the RHV, slowly withdraw the wire, injecting contrast to fill the dead-space of the microcatheter.
   (l) Re-insert the wire, soft end first, back into the microcatheter after form-ing the desired curve on its tip. Advance it to the tip of the microcatheter, but do not advance it into the balloon. Attach a torque device to the microwire.

(m) A very large-lumen guide catheter (or 90-cm sheath) large enough to accept the balloon and another balloon catheter should be in the brachio-cephlic artery supplying the lesion to be embolized.

(n) Attach a two-headed RHV (or 2 RHVs in tandem) to the guide catheter.

2. *Navigation*

(a) Carefully insert the balloon-tipped microcatheter into one RHV, and a second, non-detachable balloon catheter, such as a Hyperform™ (ev3, Irvine, CA), into the other RHV. Alternatively, each balloon can be inserted in a separate, smaller guide catheter inserted via a separate groin puncture.

(b) Advance the two balloons into the vessel.

(c) If possible, advance the detachable balloon catheter without inflation of the balloon to the desired site.

(d) It may be possible to turn the tip of the microcatheter by rotating the wire inside it.

(e) Avoid entering the balloon with the wire, since it may damage or prema-turely detach it.

(f) In some cases it may be necessary to inflate the balloon slightly to let the flow carry it forward.

(g) Never pull back on a partly or fully inflated balloon: It may detach inadvertently.

(h) The second balloon can sometimes be used to facilitate proper positioning of the detachable balloon. It can be inflated next to the detachable balloon to nudge it into a turn, or can be inflated distal to a fistula, to direct all the flow, and the detachable balloon directly to the fistula.

(i) When the balloon is at the target, the second balloon should be positioned proximal to the detachable balloon and slightly inflated to control the flow.

3. *Inflation and detachment*

(a) Fully inflate the detachable balloon. Remember that flow tends to carry balloons forward as they are inflated. The balloon should therefore be slightly proximal to the desired position before inflation, or proximal flow should be stopped by fully inflating the proximal nondetachable balloon.

(b) Do guide catheter angiograms to confirm that the desired position and occlusion have been achieved. If not, the balloon should be deflated, moved to the desired position, and then re-inflated.

(c) When the desired position is confirmed, one could do a test occlusion, if necessary (see Chap. 6).

(d) Inflate the non-detachable balloon fully just proximal to the detachable balloon. This can help stabilize it.[56]

(e) Slowly, steadily, pull back on the microcatheter, continuously watching the inflated balloon. Silicone balloons may slide back in the vessel as trac-tion is put on the microcatheter if insufficiently sized for the vessel or if no proximal support balloon is used.

(f) The valve side of the balloon can often be seen to stretch as the microcath-eter is pulled back, then relax suddenly as the valve slides off the micro-catheter and the balloon detaches.

(g) Place a second balloon or some microcoils adjacent to the first balloon to ensure a stable occlusion if the valve leaks.

Pushable Coil Technique

1. Use a large-lumen microcatheter. Most 18-system fibered coils require at least a 0.021-in. diameter lumen.
2. When the microcatheter is properly positioned, check that all slack is removed and there are no kinks. These can impede the placement of the coil.
3. Also ensure that the RHV of the guide catheter is just tight enough to prevent back-bleeding, but not too tight to pinch the microcatheter.
4. There should be an RHV with continuous infusion of heparinized saline already attached to the microcatheter hub as well.
5. Select an appropriately sized coil to fit in the vessel tightly.
6. For very high-flow states, or when precise coil positioning is required, consider using a detachable coil first.

7. Use the introducer to push the coil into the microcatheter with the plunger supplied by the manufacturer. Alternatively, most coils can be injected into the microcatheter using a small bolus of heparinized saline.
8. Remove the introducer from the RHV, and tighten the valve of the RHV.
9. To flow-inject smaller (up to 10 mm long) microcoils, inject the microcatheter with heparinized saline using a 3 mL or larger syringe to flush the coil into the vessel. This can be monitored fluoroscopically.
10. To deposit the coil in a more controlled fashion use a coil pusher.
11. Do not use a microwire to push pushable coils because microwires can over-ride the coil and wedge it in the microcatheter.
12. The authors of this handbook favour the TruPush® (Codman Neurovascular, Raynham, MA) for 18-system coils and the Pusher 10 (Boston Scientific, Natick, MA) when a smaller, ten-system coil is used in a ten-system microcatheter.
13. Do not push the tip of the coil pusher beyond the tip of the microcatheter. The relatively stiff pusher can traumatize the vessel.
14. Place additional pushable coils as needed.
15. If a coil does not pass easily through the microcatheter, there may be a sharp turn or kink in the microcatheter. Gently pulling it back slightly, or occasionally pushing it forward may relieve the obstruction.
16. The position of the microcatheter should be checked fluoroscopically since the placement of the coils and any catheter manipulation can displace the tip of the microcatheter.
17. Do periodic microcatheter angiograms.
18. It may take several coils to produce an effect on the flow.
19. In high-flow fistulas, consider using a liquid embolic agent (glue or Onyx™) to fill spaces between coils and produce a secure occlusion

Detachable Coil Technique

1. Use of detachable coils is discussed in excruciating detail in the Chap. 5.
2. These coils require the use of 150 cm, two tip marker microcatheters.
3. As a rule, deposit coils in a distal-to-proximal direction.
4. Another rule: begin with the biggest and longest coil. Start with a coil that is oversized to the diameter of the vessel being occluded. If the coil does not appear stable when it's in position, *do not detach it*. Remove it and try a larger diameter coil or a 3D configuration coil.
5. Occasionally coils can be stabilized by placing a loop or two in a side branch or sharp curve in the vessel.
6. Once one coil adequately frames the vessel and is stable, detach it and then place additional detachable coils to further frame and fill the space. The softest possible coils work best to maximize the packing density.
7. If the microcatheter is large enough, use it to intersperse some fibered coils to induce thrombosis. Be careful not to displace the microcatheter with the stiffer coils or jam the coils in the microcatheter, and use detachable fibered coils instead of pushable coils to improve the precision and controllability of the occlusion.
8. For a large vessel or high-flow fistula, it will take many, many coils to block the flow. Consider using a liquid embolic agent to complete the occlusion.
9. Do periodic guide catheter angiograms to assess flow in the vessel and determine when to stop coiling.

Technique for Stent-Assisted Treatment of AV Fistulas

Stent-assisted coiling can be useful for treatment of some fistulas, particularly direct carotid-cavernous fistulas. Stent-assisted coiling is discussed in excruciating detail in Chap. 5.

1. Dual antiplatelet therapy is necessary prior to any stent procedure (see Chap. 4).
2. The Neuroform™ and Jostent® devices require the use of 300 cm 0.014 wire. The Enterprise™ does not.

3. Size the stent appropriately for the parent artery (usually a little wider than the parent artery) and for the lesion being stented (usually at least 4 mm on each side of the lesion).
4. As a rule, place the wire comfortably distal to the lesion by first advancing a standard microcatheter, then, after placement of the 300 cm wire (with a J-shaped tip) the microcatheter is carefully removed, leaving the wire in place.
5. Always keep the wire tip in view and ensure that it stays in a larger vessel and does not injure the vessel wall.
6. It is important to have distal wire access to provide support, particularly with high-flow fistulas.
7. Advance the stent delivery catheter (for Neuroform™ or Jostent®) over the wire, gently pulling back on the wire to make sure the tip remains in a stable position.
8. Once the stent is in position, remove any slack in the wire and stent delivery catheter. *This is critical for obtaining easy and accurate deployment.*
9. If the stent is not in proper positioning, change the position and repeat the arteriogram.
10. Deploy the stent when it is in good position.
11. Do a follow-up guide catheter angiogram to confirm adequate positioning of the stent.
12. The stent delivery catheter can then be removed, and a microcatheter navigated through the stent into the fistula. Coiling of the fistula can then proceed.
13. *Special situations*:
    (a) Consider placing a nondetachable balloon in the stent for inflation as the coils are inserted. This prevents loops of coils from finding their way through the stent and into the parent artery. This is particularly important for cases in which many coils are deployed into the venous side of the fistula, totally obscuring the parent artery on fluoroscopy. It is also important if liquid embolic agents are used on the venous side to keep them from embolizing the artery.
    (b) Jostent® technique:
        i. The Jostent® GraftMaster covered stent (Abbott Vascular, Santa Clara, CA) is a fairly rigid balloon-mounted stent. It is available under a Humanitarian Device Exemption for the treatment of arterial perforations in coronary vessels ≥2.75 mm in diameter. It can be used in the carotid siphon to treat defects in the ICA, although navigation of the device can be challenging in this territory. The stent is deployed by slowly inflating the balloon under roadmap guidance to match the size of the parent artery. Do not exceed the maximum recommended pressure
        ii. When it appears that the stent is opened up to the proper size, deflate the balloon and carefully disengage it from the open stent. It may be stuck to the stent and require another inflation/deflation cycle to free it up. Be careful not to move the stent when trying to pull back on the balloon.
        iii. Once the balloon is deflated and disengaged, perform a follow-up arteriogram via the guide catheter.
        iv. If the stent is not fully apposed to the vessel wall, re-insert the balloon into the stent and attempt to dilate further. Do not exceed maximum pressure for the balloon. If necessary, the balloon could be exchanged for a new low-compliance coronary angioplasty balloon sized to the vessel diameter and no longer than the stent.
        v. Remember that the outer diameter of the stent is more than that of the inner lumen, so the vessel will be dilated around the stent to a greater degree than expected for the size of the balloon used.
        vi. Assuming that the stent was properly sized and positioned in the first place, it should nicely fit the vessel and occlude the fistula when fully deployed. If not, consider navigating a microcatheter from the venous side and place some coils to occlude the shunt.
    (c) Enterprise™ technique:
        i. A 0.021-in. lumen microcatheter like the Prowler Plus™ is navigated over a suitable microwire into the vessel of interest and positioned with its tip approximately 1.5 cm distal to the lesion being covered. Always use roadmap guidance.
        ii. The microwire is removed, and slack removed from the microcatheter.

iii. The stent is mounted on a delivery wire and this is advanced into the microcatheter to the tip of the microcatheter.

iv. The microcatheter can be moved forward or backward until the stent markers are lined up at the desire position for the stent.

v. If there is any question as to the proper positioning, a follow-up arteriogram via the guide catheter prior to stent deployment will confirm whether the markers are appropriately positioned.

vi. The stent is deployed by slowly pulling back on the microcatheter as the delivery wire is stabilized to unsheath the stent.

vii. If it appears to be too proximal or distal, it can be resheathed, repositioned, and redeployed if not already deployed more than 70%. Do not resheath and redeploy it more than a couple of times.

viii. Once it is properly positioned and deployed, the stent delivery catheter can then be removed, and a microcatheter navigated through the stent into the fistula. Coiling of the fistula can then proceed.

Postprocedure Management

1. Do a neurological exam immediately after the procedure or immediately after the patient awakens from general anesthesia.
2. Admit to the NICU or to a step-down unit with vital signs, neuro exams and groin checks Q 1 h.
   (a) It is common after intracranial embolization procedures for patients to have a headache. A head CT should be obtained to exclude haemorrhage when the headache is severe. Most post-embolization headaches are presumably due to irritation and inflammation produced by thrombosis of the lesion.
3. Patients with a stent should receive antiplatelet therapy.
4. Strict blood pressure control will minimize the risk of post-procedure haemorrhage and also help with management of headaches.[57]
5. Most patients undergoing uncomplicated procedures can be discharged to home on post-procedure day 1. Occasionally, patients having pre-surgical embolization should be kept in the hospital for observation until the surgery is done. For patients having multiple staged embolizations, it is usually best to wait at least 7 days between stages.

Tips on Specific Disease Processes

1. Intracranial aneurysms – see Chap. 5.
2. Intracranial arteriovenous malformation (AVM)
   (a) There is no evidence that incomplete embolization improves risk of haemorrhage.[58]
   (b) Most AVM embolizations are done prior to surgery.
   (c) The use of any invasive treatment of unruptured AVMs is controversial and serious questions arise as to whether the benefits of treatment are justified by the risks.[59, 60]
   (d) AVMs that have bled should be treated to complete cure when possible.
   (e) Some low Spetzler-Martin grade AVMs can usually undergo successful surgery without embolization.
   (f) For ruptured AVMs, embolization should be done at least a week after haemorrhage to prevent swelling from the haemorrhage adding to swelling caused by embolization.
   (g) Pre-operative embolization should target feeders difficult to access surgically. Depending on the planned surgical approach, this may include feeders from the posterior or anterior cerebral, large perforators, high flow fistulas, or associated aneurysms.
   (h) Targeted pre-op embolization is less risky than being too aggressive and attempting to cure the AVM. Decide on the goal of embolization ahead of time and stick to the plan.

(i) When doing embolization prior to radiosurgery, use a permanently occlusive liquid embolic, target high risk features like intranidal aneurysms, and attempt to occlude large, contiguous segments of the nidus (not just feeders) to avoid creating separate islands of residual nidus.

(j) For inoperable AVMs, staged embolization with a goal of curative embolization may be attempted, but AVMs that can be completely obliterated with embolization alone are uncommon.

(k) For curative embolization the technique is similar to that for pre-radiosurgery embolization: Occlude contiguous segments of nidus with liquid embolic and avoid creating isolated islands of nidus.

(l) Onyx embolization may be more effective than n-BCA for the treatment of brain AVMs[2, 3], although a multicenter randomized trial of Onyx versus n-BCA did not find a difference between the agents in terms of rates of AVM volume reduction, surgical resection time, or blood loss.[61]

(m) Intranidal injections of dilute glue can be curative.[4, 16] The addition of large amounts of Ethiodol does not appear to affect the biological response or long-term occlusiveness of the n-BCA.[62]

3. Direct carotid cavernous fistulas

(a) Direct, high flow fistulas should be treated urgently if impending vision loss, high intraocular or intracranial pressure, or if clinical signs of venous hypertension or angiographic signs of venous reflux into cerebral cortical or brainstem veins.[63]

(b) CCFs can be treated with transarterial, transvenous, or combined approaches.

(c) Coil embolization of direct CCFs can be effective, especially those with a small-hole.[64, 65]

(d) Stent assisted coiling is often effective, but for high flow fistula may also require liquid embolic injection within the coil mass to occlude shunt.[66–68]

(e) Balloons should be placed to temporarily occlude the artery at the site of the fistula during liquid embolic injection to prevent reflux into the artery.[68]

(f) Adding fibered coils or Hydrocoils to the coil mass can speed the occlusion.[69]

(g) Transvenous occlusion is a helpful option in many cases with difficult or unsafe arterial access, especially in patients with collagen vascular syndromes.[70, 71] See Chap. 12.

(h) Covered stent occlusion of the fistula is a very quick, elegant solution.[72], but the available stents are stiff and difficult to navigate intracranially and long term patency of covered stents is uncertain.

(i) Parent artery occlusion may be the only option in cases with severe disruption of the ICA, such as in some post-traumatic CCFs. Be sure that there is sufficient collateral flow to the occluded hemisphere. This is often obvious angiographically. A balloon test occlusion can be done if there is a question, but, if possible, should be done with the balloon distal to the fistula, since a false positive test occlusion may occur due to a steal through the fistula. On rare occasion, a high-flow fistula may divert flow away from the cerebral circulation, and over a long period of time, collateral circulation to the affected brain territory may progress. In this situation, the patient may fail an ICA test occlusion but then pass at a later date as collateral flow improves.

(j) When doing parent artery occlusion of a fistula, it is best to first coil distal to the fistula, then pack the fistula itself, and occlude the vessel proximal to the occlusion as the last step. Proximal occlusion alone will ensure that the fistula remains via back-flow via the ICA distal to the fistula. This was why carotid ligation resulted in frequent recurrences of the symptoms in the era before endovascular treatment was developed.

(k) Most symptoms of diplopia and proptosis improve within a week after successful occlusion of CCFs, although it is not unusual for symptoms to persist for some months since it can take time for edema and mass effect to subside.[73]

(l) Some patients can transiently worsen post procedure when the cavernous sinus thromboses.

(m) If symptoms worsen or do not recover quickly, and there is evidence of a bruit or the patient hears pulsatile tinnitus, do an angiogram to check for a persistent or recurrent fistula.

4. Intracranial dural arteriovenous fistulas (dAVFs)

(a) Most dural fistulas are accessed through external carotid artery feeders.
(b) Rare intracranial feeders may supply dural fistulas, including pial collaterals from very distal anterior, middle, or posterior cerebral feeders.
(c) If there are relatively few feeders, they may be accessed and embolized via a transarterial route using glue embolization delivered via a flow-directed microcatheter. Complete cure was seen in 34 out of 53 dAVF patients treated with glue.[74]
(d) Curative Onyx embolization of dAVFs with cortical venous drainage was reported in eight consecutive cases.[75]
(e) More commonly, when there are pial contributors to dural fistulas, they are multiple and not easily accessible via an endovascular route. A more sensible alternative is transvenous embolization (Chap. 12) or open surgical disconnection.
(f) The presence of pial arterial collaterals per se are not a risk factor for haemorrhage or neurological decline; *the presence or absence of pial venous drainage is a more important indication of how aggressively to treat these lesions*.

5. Pial arteriovenous fistulas
   (a) True pial AVFs (not associated with AVM or dural AVF) are rare, with less than 100 cases published in the literature.[76]
   (b) They may be associated with hereditary hemorrhagic telangiectasion (Rendu-Osler-Weber) syndrome, and may be multiple.
   (c) Some are extremely high flow lesions, presenting with high-output cardiac failure.
   (d) High-flow AVFs are a challenge for endovascular treatment, given the likelihood that any deposited embolic device might be sucked into the giant veins usually associated with these lesions.
   (e) Detachable balloons can be used to treat these fistulas, but often require two balloons simultaneously navigated to the fistula, and simultaneously inflated, to prevent the high flow from pulling a partially inflated balloon off its delivery microcatheter and out into the veins. Balloon detachment in these large, distal fistulas can be difficult, because the balloons may slide back in the large feeding arteries as the microcatheter is pulled back.
   (f) Because detachable balloons are not currently available in the United States, high concentration glue, with, or without microcoil placement is the mainstay of endovascular therapy for pial AVFs.[76–78]
   (g) When successfully occluded, these patients should be closely monitored for signs of brain edema (normal perfusion breakthrough).
   (h) Keeping the patient slightly hypotensive for a day or two may help.
   (i) Another cause of post-procedure headache and neurological decline is thrombosis of large venous varices draining the fistula.[79] Treatment with steroids and heparin may help those symptoms.

6. Vein of Galen malformations (see also Chap. 14, Appendix: Vein of Galen Malformations)
   (a) May require urgent treatment in very young patients with high-output cardiac failure.
   (b) The primary goal of treatment is to maintain cardiac and brain function and allow for normal development by interruption of arterial inputs to the fistula. Complete angiographic cure is much less important.[80]
   (c) Rarely, spontaneous occlusion of the fistula may occur.[81–83] This is often associated with angiographic signs of slow AV shunting and venous outlet stenosis.[81] Patients with spontaneous cures tend to have excellent clinical outcomes.[83]
   (d) Vein of Galen malformations may occasionally present with haemorrhage, but this does not necessarily imply a poor prognosis.[84]
   (e) Transarterial glue embolization in the primary mode of treatment.[80]
   (f) Transvenous embolization may be technically easier[85], but outcomes are worse. Normal brain veins may drain into the anomalous venous pouch that is the usual target of transvenous coil embolization.[86] As a rule, transvenous embolization should be done only to facilitate transarterial embolization either by loosely placing a coil or two to prevent the migration of transarterial embolic agents through the fistula into the veins, or by retrograde catheterization and occlusion of arterial feeders through the vein.
   (g) In newborns, the procedures are limited by fluid and contrast load. Keep the flush and contrast injections to a minimum.

(h) Anesthetic and critical care management of infants with heart failure can be challenging. Pulmonary hypertension can be treated with inhaled nitric oxide.[87]

(i) Use noninvasive imaging (ultrasound and MRA) to get an idea of vascular anatomy to minimize the angiographic studies needed for diagnosis and treatment planning.

(j) Using a 4F pediatric catheter as a guide catheter, flow directed microcatheters can be used for intracranial navigation. In some cases, an over-the-wire microcatheter can be navigated directly from the groin (or umbilical access) all the way intracranially, but that means that only one glue injection can be done without having to re-access the arterial system.

(k) The highest-flow feeders should be embolized first, and each session should seek to occlude as many feeders as are safely possible, given the limitations on time under anesthesia and contrast load for the child.

(l) As in any intracranial embolization, occlude the feeders distal to any normal brain branches.

(m) High-concentration glue or coils may be necessary to slow the flow in the high flow feeders.

(n) Stage the embolization as necessary, following the child's neurocognitive development, growth, and check periodic MRIs to rule out development of hydrocephalus or leukomalacia and atrophy. If the child does well, further embolization can wait longer than if there is evidence that the venous hypertension is impairing brain development.

(o) Morbidity from invasive procedures is higher in children less than 12 months, so it is best to wait until after the child's first birthday for more extensive embolizations if possible.

(p) It may not be necessary to do shunt surgery for treatment of the hydrocephalus, since transarterial embolization may reduce the venous hypertension and mass effect from the vein and improve CSF dynamics. Some children with vein of Galen malformation may also decline neurologically after shunting.

7. Post-traumatic or post surgical fistulas

(a) Other than carotid cavernous fistulas, intracranial fistulas after closed or penetrating trauma or iatrogenic trauma are rare.

(b) The most important step is to first understand the vascular anatomy and how it affects brain blood flow. Fistulas draining into meningeal veins or dural sinuses may be watched expectantly, since some may spontaneously thrombose. Those draining into cerebral veins require treatment.

(c) Coils and/or liquid embolic agents are the endovascular treatment of choice.

8. Bleeding intracranial vessels

(a) Usually, endovascular treatment of bleeding intracranial vessels is done as management of a complication of an endovascular procedure. It is done occasionally for post-operative or post-traumatic bleeding.

(b) Angiographically apparent active bleeding is a much more ominous sign than a pseudoaneurysm that is not bleeding.

(c) This is an acute emergency since uncontrolled intracranial bleeding can be fatal if not quickly controlled.

(d) Ventriculostomy can decompress the intracranial hypertension and be life-saving.

(e) Placement of a balloon guide catheter or nondetachable balloon catheter proximal to the bleeding site can slow the bleeding while a microcatheter is navigated to the bleeding site.

(f) Parent artery occlusion with coils and/or glue is often the only option. Keep the length of vascular occlusion to a minimum to maximize potential collateral flow and minimize the size of ischemic damage.

(g) Avoid doing a proximal occlusion only; parent vessel occlusion must be done both proximal-to and distal-to the opening in the artery. Proximal occlusion only will not stop bleeding from collateral sources and burns bridges since direct access to the lesion is then blocked.

(h) Disruptions of very proximal intracranial vessels (e.g. carotid or vertebral) may be treated by deployment of a covered Jostent® GraftMaster covered stent (Abbott Vascular, Santa Clara, CA) (see above).

9. Intracranial tumors

(a) Pre-operative embolization indications:[88]

 i. Control surgically inaccessible arterial feeders

 ii. Decrease surgical morbidity by reducing blood loss

 iii. Shorten operative time

 iv. Increase the chance of complete resection

 v. Decrease risk of damage to adjacent normal tissue

        vi. Decrease chance of tumor recurrence
        vii. Allow better visualization of the surgical field
    (b) Most commonly embolized intracranial tumors include meningiomas, paragangliomas, and hemangioblastomas.
    (c) Feeding vessels to the tumor are often external carotid branches that are easily and safely embolized. (See Chap. 8)
    (d) Intracranial feeders from the carotid and vertebral or more distal intracranial branches may supply tumors.
    (e) For tumor embolization, particles are used most commonly, although liquid embolic agents can be useful as well.
    (f) For each feeder, a risk/benefit ratio should be determined. Is the feeder easily and safely catheterized? Would occlusion provide sufficient reduction in the risk of surgery to justify the risk of embolization?
    (g) Treat with dexamethasone before and after tumor embolizations to limit tumor swelling and brain edema.
    (h) Choice of embolic agent
        i. The authors of this handbook favour particle embolization for tumors. PVA, Beadblock (Terumo Medical Corporation, Somerset, NJ), Embospheres (Biosphere Medical, Rockland, MA) and gelfoam powder may all yield adequate results. Recanalization after embolization is not a threat when surgery is planned relatively soon after embolization.
        ii. Beadblock and Embosphere particles may be preferable to PVA foam particles because they are spherical in shape and penetrate the tumor vasculature better. PVA particles are irregularly shaped and form agglomerates that occlude more proximally.[89]
        iii. Particle size selection. Smaller particles (<150 μm) are able to penetrate more deeply into the tumor and result in more complete devascularization.[67] Other data suggest a higher risk of haemorrhage with smaller particles.[17]
    (i) Smaller-to-intermediate size particles (100–300 μm) are appropriate for most tumors.
    (j) Timing of surgery after embolization
        i. Controversial: Some authors recommend surgery soon after embolization[90–92], while some recommend waiting 1–2 weeks, to permit necrosis and softening of the tumor.[92]
        ii. In a review of 45 patients with surgery for meningiomas after embolization, resectability was greatest when surgery was done 7–9 days after embolization.[93]
            (1) However, some patients develop delayed tumor edema and/or haemorrhage after embolization, necessitating urgent surgery.[17, 94]
            (2) Another argument against delayed surgery after embolization is that embolized tumors, such as meningiomas, may be erroneously over-graded on histological examination because of embolization-induced necrosis and reactive changes.[95, 96]
        iii. The authors of this handbook prefer to time surgery immediately after embolization or on the morning after. Occasionally, patients awaiting surgery develop post-embolization edema or intratumoral haemorrhage, necessitating prompt surgery; minimizing this risk by doing early surgery provides a greater benefit than any possible optimization of tumor resectability.
    (k) Steroids before and after treatment are important.
    (l) Dexamethasone, 10 mg IV prior to embolization and then 4-mg PO/IV Q6 hours for 24–48 h after embolization.

7.4. Intracranial Embolization: Complication Avoidance and Management

Informed consent prior to the procedure should include a thorough discussion of the risk of complications.

Neurological Complications

1. Access-related complications include perforation or rupture of intracranial vascular structures[97], causing subarachnoid, intra-parenchymal or rarely subdural bleeding.
2. Thromboembolic complications can occur from clot formation or errant embolic material.
3. There is a risk of AVM rupture and associated intraparenchymal haemorrhage if one occludes draining intracranial venous structures.[98] Haemorrhages can occur acutely or in a delayed fashion.
4. Malignant brain edema may occur after occlusion of a high-flow fistula or AVM.[99]
5. Microcatheters may be glued in place and/or the catheter may break and embolize to an intracranial artery.
6. Brain abscess has been reported after intracranial embolization.[100]
7. Seizures may occur after any intracranial procedure.
8. Tumors may swell and even bleed after embolization, producing a precipitous decline in neurological condition of the patient.

Non-neurological Complications

1. Coils, glue[101], particles[102] or other embolic agents might embolize to the pulmonary circulation.
2. Anaphylactic reactions to iodinated contrast or any of the medications used can occur as with any endovascular procedure.
3. Similarly, groin hematomas or other groin arterial injury can occur, as in any endovascular procedure.
4. Deep venous thrombosis and pulmonary embolism can occur.
5. Anesthesia-related complications can occur.
6. Patients with vascular fragility syndromes like Ehlers Danlos can experience a wide variety of complications related to their connective tissue fragility, including retroperitoneal hematoma and bowel perforation.[71, 103]

Complications of Brain AVM Embolization: The Big Picture

A systematic review of 1,246 patients up to 1995 found temporary morbidity in 10%, permanent morbidity in 8% and mortality in 1% after AVM embolization.[1] More recent studies report 14% neurological complications with 2% persistent disabling deficit and 1% death.[104] Another study found permanent nondisabling stroke in 2.6% and permanent disabling stroke or death in 1.6%.[105] The risk of complications has been reported to correlate with patient age, the number of embolization procedures performed[104], basal ganglia location[105], number of branches embolized[106], deep venous drainage, Spetzler-Martin Grade III to V, and the presence of a peri-procedural bleed.[107]

Another important question: How does embolization affect the annual risk of bleeding? Unfortunately, there have not yet been randomized, prospective studies looking for the effect of embolization on risk of bleeding. Embolization targeted at certain parts of AVMs that are associated with haemorrhage, such as intranidal aneurysms and venous stenosis, is a controversial strategy that some operators believe lowers the risk of AVM haemorrhage. Targeted embolization resulted in approximately 3.6% annual hemorrhage rate.[108] A less specific treatment regimen had patients with a 5.4% annual risk of bleeding and 1% risk of dying after embolization.[58] A lesser degree of occlusion and whether the patient had bled prior to the procedure were the main determinants of whether the patient haemorrhaged in the follow-up.

Complications of Intracranial Tumor Embolization

1. Most common reported complications of tumor embolization are fever and localized pain.[88]
2. The Accreditation Council on Graduate Medical Education set a threshold total complication rate of 5% for head, neck and brain tumor embolization (the term "threshold" meant that a review should be prompted if any individual center's complication rate exceeds that level).[88]
3. Meningiomas. Most commonly embolized intracranial tumor.
   (a) Overall neurological complication rate: 2.5%.[109]
   (b) Other potential complications include intratumoral haemorrhage[17], scalp necrosis[110], and retinal embolization.
4. Hemangioblastomas.
   (a) Total complication rates with hemangioblastoma embolization from 5.6% to 12.5%.[94, 111, 112]
   (b) Tumor haemorrhage or swelling are the most common complications.
   (c) A recent review of reported cases found an overall complication rate of 43% with particle embolization of cerebellar hemangioblastomas.[113]

Management of Selected Complications

Vessel Perforation

1. Mechanism: Microwire perforation is the most common cause. Less commonly the microcatheter tip or a forceful contrast injection may perforate a vessel.[114]
2. Frequency
   (a) One microwire perforation out of over 150 vessels treated by an experienced team using flow-directed microcatheters.[16]
   (b) A large series showed a 1.9% rate of perforations in glue embolization cases and 5.8% in PVA embolization cases.[46] The lower rate of perforation with glue may be due to the greater use of flow-directed microcatheters.
3. Risk factors
   (a) Use of over-the-wire microcatheters.
   (b) Procedures involving tracking of devices with relatively high resistance (e.g., balloons, stiff catheters, and stents).
4. Avoidance
   (a) Always be cautious.
   (b) Always use roadmap guidance for intracranial catheter navigation.
   (c) Always have the wire tip in view fluoroscopically.
   (d) Minimize anterograde force on the microcatheter and microwire. If there is bucking of the wire, it is meeting resistance; any further pushing can cause problems. Better to pull back slightly then rotate the wire to get around the obstacle.
   (e) Use a tight J-tip curve on the wire whenever possible. Keep the microwire in the largest diameter artery possible. Avoid entering small branches (e.g. lenticulostriates, basilar perforators) unnecessarily.
   (f) Tighten the RHV around the microcatheter when doing guide catheter angiograms (to prevent the contrast injection from carrying the microcatheter forward).
5. Management
   (a) Recognition is the first step: An abrupt rise in blood pressure or ICP, or a sudden slowing of the heart rate should prompt an immediate guide catheter angiogram.
   (b) *Resist the impulse to pull back on the perforating device!* The device may occlude or partially occlude the perforation, and withdrawal of the device may worsen the perforation.
   (c) Reverse heparin anticoagulation with protamine.

(d) Sealing of the perforation must be done quickly, and occlusion of normal vascular territories should be minimized.

(e) If possible, quickly puncture the contralateral groin and advance a second guide catheter into the vessel feeding the perforation. An appropriate nondetachable balloon (e.g. Hyperform™) can then be placed proximal to the perforation to provide proximal control and slow the bleeding. This buys time for the operator to think, consider the options and get the perforation sealed in a controlled fashion.

(f) Occasionally, the tear in abnormal vessel may extend into the normal vessel. In this situation, coil-occlusion of the parent vessel may be the only way to stop the haemorrhage. Obviously, this is a salvage maneuver and the patient's outcome will depend on the presence or absence of collateral circulation.

(g) If the patient is not already under anesthesia, he or she may need to be intubated to protect their airway. This scenario is one reason why it is helpful to have all intracranial embolization procedures done under general anesthesia.

(h) Once the perforation is secured, a ventriculostomy will probably be necessary, particularly if the patient remains hypertensive (i.e., if there is ongoing evidence of elevated ICP).

(i) Once the patient is stabilized, obtain a head CT.

(j) If there is a parenchymal haemorrhage with significant mass effect, emergent craniotomy with evacuation should be considered.

Thromboembolism

1. Mechanisms:
   (a) Platelet-rich thrombus formation on devices used during the procedure.
   (b) Thrombus formation in the guide catheter or microcatheter due to inadequate flushing technique.
   (c) Slowing of flow in the parent vessel caused by vasospasm or occlusion by the guide catheter or microcatheter.
   (d) Air emboli.
   (e) Inadvertent embolization of normal territories with embolic agent or device due to:
      i. Reflux of liquid or particulate emboli due to overly forceful injections.
      ii. Displacement of guide catheter or microcatheter during embolization due to catheter instability or redundancy.
      iii. Breaking, stretching, or premature detachment of detachable coils or balloons during manipulation.
      iv. Rupture of microcatheter during injection of liquid or particulate embolic agent.
      v. Fracture and separation of catheter or wire segments during manipulation.
      vi. Retained microcatheter after inadvertently gluing it in a vessel, especially if it breaks at the level of the aortic arch and the proximal end of the retained catheter can be pushed cephalad by the flow.

2. Frequency:
   (a) Symptomatic thromboembolism: Approximately 9–10%.[115]
   (b) A study comparing n-BCA to PVA for embolization found a 3.8% risk of stroke and a 1.9% risk of thromboembolism for glue AVM embolization and a risk of 5.8% stroke and 1.9% risk of thromboembolism in PVA embolization.[46]

3. Avoidance
   (a) Continuous flushing of all catheters with heparinized saline and meticulous attention to keeping all devices clear of bubbles and clot.
   (b) Measures to prevent stasis of flow around the guide catheter
      i. Adjust catheter position if guide catheter-induced vasospasm around the catheter is flow-limiting.
   (c) Systemic anticoagulation with heparin. Although most operators undertake routine anticoagulation with IV heparin during embolization, prospective data to support its use are lacking.

(d) Prophylactic antiplatelet agents. Some operators recommend routine antiplatelet therapy for neurointerventional procedures such as aneurysm coiling.[116, 117]

(e) Remove slack in guide catheter and microcatheter prior to embolization.

(f) Remove any wire or catheter or embolic device immediately if there is a suspicion that it is damaged.

(g) Neurophysiological monitoring (i.e. SSEPs) may detect early signs of a problem.

4. Management

(a) Recognition is the first step: Guide catheter angiograms should be done frequently to monitor for evidence of thrombosis, such as a filling-defect within the parent vessel adjacent to the aneurysm neck, or vessel dropout.

(b) Ensure that the patient is well hydrated and consider pharmacologically augmenting blood pressure to maximize the collateral flow to the impaired territory.

(c) Most thrombotic material that appears during embolization is likely to be platelet-rich; therefore, anti-platelet therapy is the first approach.

   i. Abciximab 0.25 mg/kg IV rapid bolus followed by 125 mcg/kg/min infusion (to a maximum of 10 mg/min) for 12 h. See Chap. 4 for more detail.

(d) A 2-mm diameter Amplatz Goose Neck microsnare (Microvena, White Bear Lake, MN), Merci Retriever® (Concentric Medical, Mountain View, CA), or Alligator™ Retrieval Device (Chestnut Medical Technologies, Menlo Park, CA) can be used to remove clot, fractured wires or catheters or embolic devices.

(e) Occasionally a balloon or stent can be used to restore flow in a vessel.

(f) At each step, evaluate the potential risks and benefits and be prepared to accept a small stroke to avoid potentially worse consequences from unrestrained attempts to open a vessel at all costs.

(g) Craniotomy and surgical removal of the embolic material is an option when there is an experienced cerebrovascular neurosurgeon available.

(h) Thrombolytic agents are associated with a risk of significant haemorrhage, particularly when used on patients with recent haemorrhage. Thrombolytics should be used sparingly, if at all.

AVM Rupture

1. Mechanisms

(a) A generally accepted cause of AVM bleeding after AVM embolization is reduction or obstruction of venous outflow from the AVM without sufficient reduction of inflow.[98]

(b) Another possibility is that partial embolization of the AVM redirects flow into areas unaccustomed to higher flow.

(c) Associated aneurysms may rupture after the change in flow.

2. Frequency

(a) The rate of haemorrhage with AVM embolization ranges from 1.6%[105] to 10.6%.[22]

(b) Rates of death or disability after embolization run from 3% to 11%.[104–107]

3. Avoidance

(a) Avoid embolic material to get into the draining veins. Use a faster-polymerizing glue, or place a proximal coil when necessary to reduce flow.

(b) Treat associated aneurysms whenever possible.

(c) Avoid treating too much of the AVM in one sitting. Medium- and large-sized AVMs should be embolized in stages. Occlusion of >60% of the AVM nidus is associated with an 18 times higher risk of bleeding.[22]

4. Management

(a) First step: Prompt recognition is essential, as always. Look for a sudden headache, sudden increase in blood pressure or ICP, and worsening neurological status.

(b) If not intubated already, consider intubation to protect airway and allow for mechanical hyperventilation.

(c) Emergent CT.

(d) Ventriculostomy if necessary.

(e) If intracranial pressure high from a parenchymal haematoma, lower it with hyperventilation and pharmacological means (e.g. mannitol, hypertonic saline, propofol, etc.) but also be prepared for urgent surgical evacuation of haematoma.[118]

(f) Craniotomy and evacuation of the clot, if necessary.

Postembolization Edema or Hemorrhage (aka Normal Perfusion Breakthrough Syndrome)

Oedema and haemorrhage can occur after abrupt closure of a high flow AV shunt during treatment of an AVM or high flow AVF.

1. Mechanism
   (a) Sudden occlusion of a long-standing AV shunt, exposing vessels with disturbed autoregulation to increased flow.[99]
   (b) Venous thrombosis or occlusion may play a role as well
   (c) Residual AVM nidus may also explain some cases.

2. Frequency
   (a) Uncommon
   (b) AVF series: 5 out of 185 cases of carotid and vertebral fistulas treated, tended to be patients with longstanding fistula that had progressive symptoms of arterial steal from the fistula prior to treatment.[119]
   (c) Three cases were reported in a series of 66 AVM patients treated surgically.[120]

3. Avoidance
   (a) Consider doing cerebral blood flow imaging in patients with AVM-related steal symptoms to assess autoregulation.
   (b) Do staged embolizations to give the brain a chance to recover between sessions.[121, 122]
   (c) Monitor and manage blood pressure closely during and after treatment.[57]
   (d) Avoid causing venous occlusion with residual arteriovenous shunting

4. Management
   (a) Use strict blood pressure control during and after the procedure.
   (b) Monitor intracranial pressure when a ventriculostomy is in place and treat intracranial hypertension aggressively.
   (c) Indomethacin is an option.[123] Indomethacin causes cerebral vasoconstriction.
   (d) Consider surgical decompression if the patient does not respond to medical management.

Arterial Dissection

1. Mechanism: Wire or guide catheter-induced injury to vessel.

2. Frequency
   (a) 1.9% of cases.[46]
   (b) Vertebral artery dissections seem to be more common than carotid dissections.
   (c) This complication is probably under-reported, as many operators do not do routine surveillance angiograms of the access vessel (i.e., the cervical carotid or vertebral artery) at the completion of the case, and therefore do not identify asymptomatic dissections.

3. Avoidance
   (a) Take steps to minimize intimal trauma during the access phase (see Chap. 4).

4. Management
   (a) Always do a guide catheter angiogram of the access vessel at the end of the case.
   (b) Antiplatelet therapy is usually sufficient; aspirin 325 mg suppository during or after the procedure, then PO daily. Add a second antiplatelet agent if possible (e.g., clopidogrel 75-mg PO daily).
   (c) Consider anticoagulation with IV heparin, in addition to antiplatelet therapy, if the dissection is flow-limiting and carries a risk of thrombosis.

(d) Consider placing a stent across the lesion if it becomes necessary to continue to work in the affected vessel, or if further access through that vessel is anticipated.

(e) Follow-up imaging should be done in 3–6 months. Most dissections treated with antiplatelet therapy will heal within 3–6 months.

Retained Microcatheter (aka Glued-in Microcatheter)

Any liquid embolic material that comes into contact with the microcatheter can trap the microcatheter. This is a well-known complication of n-BCA embolization but it can also occur with Onyx. Pulling back on the microcatheter will sometimes cause it to break free, but if it is solidly glued in, then pulling the microcatheter just pulls on the intracranial arteries, so in some cases it is best to leave the microcatheter in place and permanently implant it by cutting off the microcatheter where it enters the femoral artery.[124] Microcatheters left in place in this manner tend to be stable; blood flow down the aorta keeps the microcatheter taut against the side of the artery and allows it to become endothelialized over time.[125] If the microcatheter breaks above the level of the aortic arch during attempted removal, blood flow may carry the smaller fragments up into the intracranial vessels and cause problems.[126] There have been case reports of delayed local complications in the lower extremity after this maneuver.[124, 127]

1. Mechanism
    (a) Usually related to technique – the glue mixture is too concentrated, injected too quickly, reflux of agent around catheter tip not recognized, not pulled quickly enough.
    (b) Similarly, Onyx injected too quickly and allowed to reflux too much for too long may result in a stuck microcatheter.
2. Frequency
    (a) 7.4% of 54 patients treated with glue in the n-BCA vs. PVA trial.[46] None of the microcatheters used for PVA got stuck.
    (b) 8.5% of 47 cases treated with Onyx had retained microcatheters.[128]
3. Avoidance
    (a) Minimize reflux around the microcatheter.
    (b) Have good working views showing microcatheter tip during injection of the liquid embolic.
    (c) Remove slack in the system before injection.
    (d) Remove the microcatheter quickly as soon as the embolic material begins to approach catheter tip.
    (e) Avoid allowing Onyx to reflux more than 1.0 cm along the microcatheter or to stay in contact the microcatheter for more than a few minutes.
    (f) When withdrawing the microcatheter, also pull the guide catheter.
4. Management
    (a) Try continuous gentle traction on the microcatheter for at least 5–10 min; occasionally the microcatheter will pop out safely.
    (b) The monorail snare technique can be used to grasp catheters trapped in Onyx.[129]
    (c) An intermediate catheter can help. If one can be advanced up over the stuck microcatheter to the site of occluding embolic material, counter pressure can be applied if the microcatheter is pulled back as the DAC is advanced. This can facilitate microcatheter extraction.[130]
    (d) If all else fails, the microcatheter is put under tension and the cut at the groin to permanently implant it.
    (e) Consider surgical extraction if blood flow to the brain is impaired.
    (f) Surgical removal after a day or so is problematic because the catheter gets stuck along the vessel by fibrin, and later can become endothelialized.
    (g) A microcatheter that breaks at or above the level of the aortic arch has risk of becoming an embolus to the intracranial circulation. This microcatheter fragment could be grasped with a microsnare, and pulled taut and the end pulled up into an external carotid branch and secured in place with a balloon, coil, or glue with a second microcatheter (obviously, be careful not to glue the snare or second microcatheter in place.) An easier alternative is to secure the microcatheter along the periphery of the vessel by deploying a self-expanding stent in the parent artery. This requires dual antiplatelet therapy after the procedure.

(h) Keep patients on aspirin indefinitely after a retained microcatheter is left in place.
  i. Delayed complications from the implanted catheter, such as vessel thrombosis or pseudoaneurysm, may require surgical repair.

A Poetic Interlude

Sticky

It's old friends that stay and stay and stay and drink up all your beer,
And the song that never ends but always stays inside your ear.
It's the evidence the Lady can't just go and wash away,
And your research fellows that won't write until it's Judgement Day.
It's a ketchup spot that found its way onto your fav' rite tie,
And the slimy, gooey stuff you find all over Baby's eye.
It's the bubble gum that's always found beneath your fav' rite shoe.
And the catheter you left inside because of too much glue.
It's decisions made you hate to have, and hate to say you made 'em,
And the first path that was chosen has to be the one that's taken.
It's the words that play again within the mind when you're alone,
And the patient you should never treat who calls you on the phone.

Guide Catheter-Induced Vasospasm

1. An ounce of prevention is worth a pound of cure: *Be gentle*.
2. Withdraw the catheter into a lower segment of the vessel when significant catheter-induced vasospasm appears.
3. Keep the catheter tip away from kinks and bends in the vessel if possible.
4. A curvaceous carotid or proximal vertebral artery can sometimes be straightened by tilting the patient's head toward the opposite shoulder.
5. Use a smaller guide catheter.
6. Use a soft-tipped guide catheter (e.g., Guider Softip™ XF guide catheter (Stryker Neurovascular, Fremont, CA)).
7. Use Visipaque™ (GE Healthcare, Princeton, NJ) contrast instead of Omnipaque; according to the manufacturer, this contrast material is less spasmogenic than Omnipaque®.
8. Use a guide catheter with an inner obturator (e.g., Northstar® Lumax® Flex Catheter (Cook Inc., Bloomington, IN))
9. Selective injection of IA nitroglycerin (30 mcg/injection).
10. This can help distinguish vasospasm from vessel dissection, if a dissection is suspected.
11. Nitroglycerin paste on the patient's neck ipsilateral to the access vessel
    (a) Dose: 1–5 in.
    (b) Efficacy is unclear
    (c) Drawback: Can cause hypotension and a headache in awake patients. In patients under general anesthesia, the dose (i.e., the number of inches) of paste is adjusted to maintain the blood pressure within normal limits.

References

1. Frizzel RT, Fisher 3rd WS. Cure, morbidity, and mortality associated with embolization of brain arteriovenous malformations: a review of 1246 patients in 32 series over a 35-year period. Neurosurgery. 1995;37:1031–9; discussion 9–40.

2. van Rooij WJ, Sluzewski M, Beute GN. Brain AVM embolization with onyx. AJNR Am J Neuroradiol. 2007;28:172–7; discussion 8.

3. Weber W, Kis B, Siekmann R, Kuehne D. Endovascular treatment of intracranial arteriovenous malformations with onyx: technical aspects. AJNR Am J Neuroradiol. 2007;28:371–7.

4. Yu SC, Chan MS, Lam JM, Tam PH, Poon WS. Complete obliteration of intracranial arteriovenous malformation with endovascular cyanoacrylate embolization: initial success and rate of permanent cure. AJNR Am J Neuroradiol. 2004;25:1139–43.

5. Mounayer C, Hammami N, Piotin M, et al. Nidal embolization of brain arteriovenous malformations using onyx in 94 patients. AJNR Am J Neuroradiol. 2007;28:518–23.

6. Marks MP, Lane B, Steinberg GK, Snipes GJ. Intranidal aneurysms in cerebral arteriovenous malformations: evaluation and endovascular treatment. Radiology. 1992;183:355–60.

7. Meisel HJ, Mansmann U, Alvarez H, Rodesch G, Brock M, Lasjaunias P. Cerebral arteriovenous malformations and associated aneurysms: analysis of 305 cases from a series of 662 patients. Neurosurgery. 2000;46:793–800; discussion 2.

8. Piotin M, Ross IB, Weill A, Kothimbakam R, Moret J. Intracranial arterial aneurysms associated with arteriovenous malformations: endovascular treatment. Radiology. 2001;220:506–13.

9. Kessler I, Riva R, Ruggiero M, Manisor M, Al-Khawaldeh M, Mounayer C. Successful transvenous embolization of brain arteriovenous malformations using onyx in five consecutive patients. Neurosurgery. 2011;69:184–93.

10. Forster C, Kahles T, Kietz S, Drenckhahn D. Dexamethasone induces the expression of metalloproteinase inhibitor TIMP-1 in the murine cerebral vascular endothelial cell line cEND. J Physiol. 2007;580:937–49.

11. Tuor UI, Simone CS, Barks JD, Post M. Dexamethasone prevents cerebral infarction without affecting cerebral blood flow in neonatal rats. Stroke. 1993;24:452–7.

12. Zausinger S, Westermaier T, Plesnila N, Steiger HJ, Schmid-Elsaesser R. Neuroprotection in transient focal cerebral ischemia by combination drug therapy and mild hypothermia: comparison with customary therapeutic regimen. Stroke. 2003;34:1526–32.

13. Adachi N, Chen J, Liu K, Tsuboto S, Arai T. Dexamethasone aggravates ischemia-induced neuronal damage by facilitating the onset of anoxic depolarization and the increase in the intracellular Ca2+ concentration in gerbil hippocampus. J Cereb Blood Flow Metab. 1998;18:274–80.

14. Tsuboto S, Adachi N, Chen J, Yorozuya T, Nagaro T, Arai T. Dexamethasone changes brain monoamine metabolism and aggravates ischemic neuronal damage in rats. Anesthesiology. 1999;90:515–23.

15. Koide T, Wieloch TW, Siesjo BK. Chronic dexamethasone pretreatment aggravates ischemic neuronal necrosis. J Cereb Blood Flow Metab. 1986;6:395–404.

16. Aletich VA, Debrun GM, Koenigsberg R, Ausman JI, Charbel F, Dujovny M. Arteriovenous malformation nidus catheterization with hydrophilic wire and flow-directed catheter. AJNR Am J Neuroradiol. 1997;18:929–35.

17. Kallmes DF, McGraw JK, Evans AJ, et al. Thrombogenicity of hydrophilic and nonhydrophilic microcatheters and guiding catheters. AJNR Am J Neuroradiol. 1997;18:1243–51.

18. Kiyosue H, Hori Y, Matsumoto S, et al. Shapability, memory, and luminal changes in microcatheters after steam shaping: a comparison of 11 different microcatheters. AJNR Am J Neuroradiol. 2005;26:2610–6.

19. Paiva T, Campos J, Baeta E, Gomes LB, Martins IP, Parreira E. EEG monitoring during endovascular embolization of cerebral arteriovenous malformations. Electroencephalogr Clin Neurophysiol. 1995;95:3–13.

20. Liu AY, Lopez JR, Do HM, Steinberg GK, Cockroft K, Marks MP. Neurophysiological monitoring in the endovascular therapy of aneurysms. AJNR Am J Neuroradiol. 2003;24:1520–7.

21. Rauch RA, Vinuela F, Dion J, et al. Preembolization functional evaluation in brain arteriovenous malformations: the ability of superselective Amytal test to predict neurologic dysfunction before embolization. AJNR Am J Neuroradiol. 1992;13:309–14.

22. Heidenreich JO, Hartlieb S, Stendel R, et al. Bleeding complications after endovascular therapy of cerebral arteriovenous malformations. AJNR Am J Neuroradiol. 2006;27:313–6.

23. Yuki I, Kim RH, Duckwiler G, et al. Treatment of brain arteriovenous malformations with high-flow arteriovenous fistulas: risk and complications associated with endovascular embolization in multimodality treatment. Clinical article. J Neurosurg. 2010;113:715–22.

24. Sure U, Surucu O, Engenhart-Cabillic R. Embolization before radiosurgery reduces the obliteration rate of arteriovenous malformations. Neurosurgery. 2008;63:E376; author reply E.

25. Back AG, Vollmer D, Zeck O, Shkedy C, Shedden PM. Retrospective analysis of unstaged and staged Gamma Knife surgery with and without preceding embolization for the treatment of arteriovenous malformations. J Neurosurg. 2008;109(Suppl):57–64.

26. Andrade-Souza YM, Ramani M, Scora D, Tsao MN, terBrugge K, Schwartz ML. Embolization before radiosurgery reduces the obliteration rate of arteriovenous malformations. Neurosurgery. 2007;60:443–52. 10.1227/01.NEU.0000255347.25959.D0.

27. Kerber CW, Wong W. Liquid acrylic adhesive agents in interventional neuroradiology. Neurosurg Clin N Am. 2000;11:85–99, viii–ix.

28. Brothers MF, Kaufmann JC, Fox AJ, Deveikis JP. n-Butyl 2-cyanoacrylate–substitute for IBCA in interventional neuroradiology: histopathologic and polymerization time studies. AJNR Am J Neuroradiol. 1989;10:777–86.

29. Wikholm G. Occlusion of cerebral arteriovenous malformations with N-butyl cyano-acrylate is permanent. AJNR Am J Neuroradiol. 1995;16:479–82.

30. Spiegel SM, Vinuela F, Goldwasser JM, Fox AJ, Pelz DM. Adjusting the polymerization time of isobutyl-2 cyanoacrylate. AJNR Am J Neuroradiol. 1986;7:109–12.

31. Barr JD, Hoffman EJ, Davis BR, Edgar KA, Jacobs CR. Microcatheter adhesion of cyanoacrylates: comparison of normal butyl cyanoacrylate to 2-hexyl cyanoacrylate. J Vasc Interv Radiol. 1999;10:165–8.

32. Komotar RJ, Ransom ER, Wilson DA, Connolly Jr ES, Lavine SD, Meyers PM. 2-Hexyl cyanoacrylate (neuracryl M) embolization of cerebral arteriovenous malformations. Neurosurgery. 2000;59:ONS464–9; discussion ONS9.

33. Becker TA, Preul MC, Bichard WD, Kipke DR, McDougall CG. Calcium alginate gel as a biocompatible material for endovascular arteriovenous malformation embolization: six-month results in an animal model. Neurosurgery. 2005;56:793–801; discussion 793–801.

34. Akin ED, Perkins E, Ross IB. Surgical handling characteristics of an ethylene vinyl alcohol copolymer compared with N-butyl cyanoacrylate used for embolization of vessels in an arteriovenous malformation resection model in swine. J Neurosurg. 2003;98:366–70.

35. Duffner F, Ritz R, Bornemann A, Freudenstein D, Wiendl H, Siekmann R. Combined therapy of cerebral arteriovenous malformations: histological differences between a non-adhesive liquid embolic agent and n-butyl 2-cyanoacrylate (NBCA). Clin Neuropathol. 2002;21:13–7.

36. Yakes WF, Krauth L, Ecklund J, et al. Ethanol endovascular management of brain arteriovenous malformations: initial results. Neurosurgery. 1997;40:1145–52; discussion 52–4.

37. Pelz DM, Fox AJ, Vinuela F, Drake CC, Ferguson GG. Preoperative embolization of brain AVMs with isobutyl-2 cyanoacrylate. AJNR Am J Neuroradiol. 1988;9:757–64.

38. Fox AJ, Pelz DM, Lee DH. Arteriovenous malformations of the brain: recent results of endovascular therapy. Radiology. 1990;177:51–7.
39. Lylyk P, Vinuela F, Vinters HV, et al. Use of a new mixture for embolization of intracranial vascular malformations. Preliminary experimental experience. Neuroradiology. 1990;32:304–10.
40. Phatouros CC, Higashida RT, Malek AM, Smith WS, Dowd CF, Halbach VV. Embolization of the meningohypophyseal trunk as a cause of diabetes insipidus. AJNR Am J Neuroradiol. 1999;20:1115–8.
41. Kasuya H, Shimizu T, Sasahara A, Takakura K. Phenytoin as a liquid material for embolisation of tumours. Neuroradiology. 1999;41:320–3.
42. Wong GA, Armstrong DC, Robertson JM. Cardiovascular collapse during ethanol sclerotherapy in a pediatric patient. Paediatr Anaesth. 2006;16:343–6.
43. Phatouros CC, Halbach VV, Malek AM, Meyers PM, Dowd CF, Higashida RT. Intraventricular contrast medium leakage during ethanol embolization of an arteriovenous malformation. AJNR Am J Neuroradiol. 1999;20:1329–32.
44. Tadavarthy SM, Moller JH, Amplatz K. Polyvinyl alcohol (Ivalon)–a new embolic material. Am J Roentgenol Radium Ther Nucl Med. 1975;125:609–16.
45. Wallace RC, Flom RA, Khayata MH, et al. The safety and effectiveness of brain arteriovenous malformation embolization using acrylic and particles: the experiences of a single institution. Neurosurgery. 1995;37:606–15; discussion 15–8.
46. The n-BCA Trial Investigators. N-butyl cyanoacrylate embolization of cerebral arteriovenous malformations: results of a prospective, randomized, multi-center trial. AJNR Am J Neuroradiol. 2002;23:748–55.
47. Lewis AL, Adams C, Busby W, et al. Comparative in vitro evaluation of microspherical embolisation agents. J Mater Sci Mater Med. 2006;17:1193–204.
48. Taki W, Handa H, Yamagata S, Ishikawa M, Iwata H, Ikada Y. Radiopaque solidifying liquids for releasable balloon technique: a technical note. Surg Neurol. 1980;13:140–2.
49. Weill A, Ducros V, Cognard C, Piotin M, Moret J. Letter. "Corrosion" of tungsten spirals. A disturbing finding. Interv Neuroradiol. 1998;4:337–40.
50. Reul J. Editorial comment. "Corrosion of tungsten spirals" by Weill et al. Interv Neuroradiol. 1998;4:341–2.
51. Peuster M, Kaese V, Wuensch G, et al. Dissolution of tungsten coils leads to device failure after transcatheter embolisation of pathologic vessels. Heart. 2001;85:703–4.
52. Pelz D. Potential hazards in the use of tungsten mechanical detachable coils. Radiology. 2000;214:602–3.
53. Gounis MJ, Lieber BB, Wakhloo AK, Siekmann R, Hopkins LN. Effect of glacial acetic acid and ethiodized oil concentration on embolization with N-butyl 2-cyanoacrylate: an in vivo investigation. AJNR Am J Neuroradiol. 2002;23:938–44.
54. Lieber BB, Wakhloo AK, Siekmann R, Gounis MJ. Acute and chronic swine rete arteriovenous malformation models: effect of ethiodol and glacial acetic acid on penetration, dispersion, and injection force of N-butyl 2-cyanoacrylate. AJNR Am J Neuroradiol. 2005;26:1707–14.
55. Moore C, Murphy K, Gailloud P. Improved distal distribution of n-butyl cyanoacrylate glue by simultaneous injection of dextrose 5% through the guiding catheter: technical note. Neuroradiology. 2006;48:327–32.
56. Masaryk TJ, Perl 2nd J, Wallace RC, Magdinec M, Chyatte D. Detachable balloon embolization: concomitant use of a second safety balloon. AJNR Am J Neuroradiol. 1999;20:1103–6.
57. Massoud TF, Hademenos GJ, Young WL, Gao E, Pile-Spellman J. Can induction of systemic hypotension help prevent nidus rupture complicating arteriovenous malformation embolization?: analysis of underlying mechanism achieved using a theoretical model. AJNR Am J Neuroradiol. 2000;21:1255–67.
58. Raupp EF, Fernandes J. Does treatment with N-butyl cyanoacrylate embolization protect against hemorrhage in cerebral arteriovenous malformations? Arq Neuropsiquiatr. 2005;63:34–9.
59. Deruty R, Pelissou-Guyotat I, Amat D, et al. Complications after multidisciplinary treatment of cerebral arteriovenous malformations. Acta Neurochir (Wien). 1996;138:119–31.

60. Hartmann A, Mast H, Mohr JP, et al. Determinants of staged endovascular and surgical treatment outcome of brain arteriovenous malformations. Stroke. 2005;36:2431–5.
61. Loh Y, Duckwiler GR. A prospective, multicenter, randomized trial of the onyx liquid embolic system and N-butyl cyanoacrylate embolization of cerebral arteriovenous malformations. J Neurosurg. 2010;113:733–41.
62. Sadato A, Wakhloo AK, Hopkins LN. Effects of a mixture of a low concentration of n-butylcyanoacrylate and ethiodol on tissue reactions and the permanence of arterial occlusion after embolization. Neurosurgery. 2000;47:1197–203; discussion 204–5.
63. Halbach VV, Hieshima GB, Higashida RT, Reicher M. Carotid cavernous fistulae: indications for urgent treatment. AJR Am J Roentgenol. 1987;149:587–93.
64. Guglielmi G, Vinuela F, Duckwiler G, Dion J, Stocker A. High-flow, small-hole arteriovenous fistulas: treatment with electro-detachable coils. AJNR Am J Neuroradiol. 1995;16:325–8.
65. Siniluoto T, Seppanen S, Kuurne T, Wikholm G, Leinonen S, Svendsen P. Transarterial embolization of a direct carotid cavernous fistula with guglielmi detachable coils. AJNR Am J Neuroradiol. 1997;18:519–23.
66. Suzuki S, Lee DW, Jahan R, Duckwiler GR, Vinuela F. Transvenous treatment of spontaneous dural carotid-cavernous fistulas using a combination of detachable coils and onyx. AJNR Am J Neuroradiol. 2006;27:1346–9.
67. Wakhloo AK, Perlow A, Linfante I, et al. Transvenous n-butyl-cyanoacrylate infusion for complex dural carotid cavernous fistulas: technical considerations and clinical outcome. AJNR Am J Neuroradiol. 2005;26:1888–97.
68. Luo CB, Teng MM, Chang FC, Chang CY. Transarterial balloon-assisted n-butyl-2-cyanoacrylate embolization of direct carotid cavernous fistulas. AJNR Am J Neuroradiol. 2006;27:1535–40.
69. Marden FA, Sinha Roy S, Malisch TW. A novel approach to direct carotid cavernous fistula repair: HydroCoil-assisted revision after balloon reconstruction. Surg Neurol. 2005;64:140–3; discussion 3.
70. Russell EJ, Reddy V, Rovin R. Combined arterial and venous approaches for cure of carotid-cavernous sinus fistula in a patient with fibromuscular dysplasia. Skull Base Surg. 1994;4:103–9.
71. Chuman H, Trobe JD, Petty EM, et al. Spontaneous direct carotid-cavernous fistula in Ehlers-Danlos syndrome type IV: two case reports and a review of the literature. J Neuroophthalmol. 2002;22:75–81.
72. Gomez F, Escobar W, Gomez AM, Gomez JF, Anaya CA. Treatment of carotid cavernous fistulas using covered stents: midterm results in seven patients. AJNR Am J Neuroradiol. 2007;28:1762–8.
73. Yang ZJ, Li HW, Wu LG, et al. Prognostic analysis and complications of traumatic carotid cavernous fistulas after treatment with detachable balloon and/or coil embolization. Chin J Traumatol. 2004;7:286–8.
74. Guedin P, Gaillard S, Boulin A, et al. Therapeutic management of intracranial dural arteriovenous shunts with leptomeningeal venous drainage: report of 53 consecutive patients with emphasis on transarterial embolization with acrylic glue. J Neurosurg. 2010;112:603–10.
75. van Rooij WJ, Sluzewski M. Curative embolization with onyx of dural arteriovenous fistulas with cortical venous drainage. AJNR Am J Neuroradiol. 2010;31:1516–20.
76. Wang YC, Wong HF, Yeh YS. Intracranial pial arteriovenous fistulas with single-vein drainage. Report of three cases and review of the literature. J Neurosurg. 2004;100:201–5.
77. Itami H, Sugiu K, Tokunaga K, Ono S, Onoda K, Date I. Endovascular treatment of adult pial arteriovenous fistula. No Shinkei Geka. 2007;35:599–605.
78. Limaye US, Siddhartha W, Shrivastav M, Anand S, Ghatge S. Endovascular management of intracranial pial arterio-venous fistulas. Neurol India. 2004;52:87–90.
79. Vinuela F, Drake CG, Fox AJ, Pelz DM. Giant intracranial varices secondary to high-flow arteriovenous fistulae. J Neurosurg. 1987;66:198–203.
80. Lasjaunias PL, Chng SM, Sachet M, Alvarez H, Rodesch G, Garcia-Monaco R. The management of vein of Galen aneurysmal malformations. Neurosurgery. 2006;59: S184–94; discussion S3–13.

81. Hurst RW, Kagetsu NJ, Berenstein A. Angiographic findings in two cases of aneurysmal malformation of vein of Galen prior to spontaneous thrombosis: therapeutic implications. AJNR Am J Neuroradiol. 1992;13:1446–50.

82. Kuroki K, Uozumi T, Arita K, Takechi A, Matsuura R, Fujidaka M. Spontaneous disappearance of an aneurysmal malformation of the vein of Galen. Neuroradiology. 1995;37:244–6.

83. Nikas DC, Proctor MR, Scott RM. Spontaneous thrombosis of vein of Galen aneurysmal malformation. Pediatr Neurosurg. 1999;31:33–9.

84. Meyers PM, Halbach VV, Phatouros CP, et al. Hemorrhagic complications in vein of Galen malformations. Ann Neurol. 2000;47:748–55.

85. Mickle JP, Quisling RG. The transtorcular embolization of vein of Galen aneurysms. J Neurosurg. 1986;64:731–5.

86. Gailloud P, O'Riordan DP, Lehmann CU. Confirmation of communication between deep venous drainage and the vein of galen after treatment of a vein of Galen aneurysmal malformation in an infant presenting with severe pulmonary hypertension. AJNR Am J Neuroradiol. 2006;27:317–20.

87. Ashida Y, Miyahara H, Sawada H, Mitani Y, Maruyama K. Anesthetic management of a neonate with vein of Galen aneurysmal malformation and severe pulmonary hypertension. Paediatr Anaesth. 2005;15:525–8.

88. American Society of Interventional and Therapeutic Neuroradiology, Head, neck, and brain tumor embolization. AJNR Am J Neuroradiol. 2001;22:S14–5.

89. Laurent A, Wassef M, Chapot R, Houdart E, Merland JJ. Location of vessel occlusion of calibrated tris-acryl gelatin microspheres for tumor and arteriovenous malformation embolization. J Vasc Interv Radiol. 2004;15:491–6.

90. Rodesch G, Lasjaunias P. Embolization of meningiomas. In: Al-Mefty O, editor. Meningiomas. New York: Raven; 1991. p. 285–97.

91. Nelson PK, Setton A, Choi IS, Ransohoff J, Berenstein A. Current status of interventional neuroradiology in the management of meningiomas. Neurosurg Clin N Am. 1994;5:235–59.

92. Ahuja A, Gibbons KJ. Endovascular therapy of central nervous system tumors. Neurosurg Clin N Am. 1994;5:541–54.

93. Kai Y, Hamada J, Morioka M, Yano S, Todaka T, Ushio Y. Appropriate interval between embolization and surgery in patients with meningioma. AJNR Am J Neuroradiol. 2002;23:139–42.

94. Eskridge JM, McAuliffe W, Harris B, Kim DK, Scott J, Winn HR. Preoperative endovascular embolization of craniospinal hemangioblastomas. AJNR Am J Neuroradiol. 1996;17:525–31.

95. Ng HK, Poon WS, Goh K, Chan MS. Histopathology of post-embolized meningiomas. Am J Surg Pathol. 1996;20:1224–30.

96. Perry A, Chicoine MR, Filiput E, Miller JP, Cross DT. Clinicopathologic assessment and grading of embolized meningiomas: a correlative study of 64 patients. Cancer. 2001;92:701–11.

97. Halbach VV, Higashida RT, Dowd CF, Barnwell SL, Hieshima GB. Management of vascular perforations that occur during neurointerventional procedures. AJNR Am J Neuroradiol. 1991;12:319–27.

98. Hademenos GJ, Massoud TF. Risk of intracranial arteriovenous malformation rupture due to venous drainage impairment. A theoretical analysis. Stroke. 996;27:1072–83.

99. Spetzler RF, Wilson CB, Weinstein P, Mehdorn M, Townsend J, Telles D. Normal perfusion pressure breakthrough theory. Clin Neurosurg. 1978;25:651–72.

100. Pendarkar H, Krishnamoorthy T, Purkayastha S, Gupta AK. Pyogenic cerebral abscess with discharging sinus complicating an embolized arteriovenous malformation. J Neuroradiol. 2006;33:133–8.

101. Pelz DM, Lownie SP, Fox AJ, Hutton LC. Symptomatic pulmonary complications from liquid acrylate embolization of brain arteriovenous malformations. AJNR Am J Neuroradiol. 1995;16:19–26.

102. Kline JN, Ryals TJ, Galvin JR, Loftus CM, Hunter JH. Pulmonary embolization and infarction. An iatrogenic complication of transcatheter embolization of a cerebral arteriovenous malformation with polyvinyl alcohol sponge. Chest. 1993;103:1293–5.

103. Horowitz MB, Purdy PD, Valentine RJ, Morrill K. Remote vascular catastrophes after neurovascular interventional therapy for type 4 Ehlers-Danlos syndrome. AJNR Am J Neuroradiol. 2000;21:974–6.

104. Hartmann A, Pile-Spellman J, Stapf C, et al. Risk of endovascular treatment of brain arteriovenous malformations. Stroke. 2002;33:1816–20.

105. Jayaraman MV, Marcellus ML, Hamilton S, et al. Neurologic complications of arteriovenous malformation embolization using liquid embolic agents. AJNR Am J Neuroradiol. 2008;29:242–6. Epub 2007 Nov 1.

106. Kim LJ, Albuquerque FC, Spetzler RF, McDougall CG. Postembolization neurological deficits in cerebral arteriovenous malformations: stratification by arteriovenous malformation grade. Neurosurgery. 2006;59:53–9; discussion 9.

107. Ledezma CJ, Hoh BL, Carter BS, Pryor JC, Putman CM, Ogilvy CS. Complications of cerebral arteriovenous malformation embolization: multivariate analysis of predictive factors. Neurosurgery. 2006;58:602–11; discussion 11.

108. Meisel HJ, Mansmann U, Alvarez H, Rodesch G, Brock M, Lasjaunias P. Effect of partial targeted N-butyl-cyanoacrylate embolization in brain AVM. Acta Neurochir (Wien). 2002;144:879–87; discussion 88.

109. Probst EN, Grzyska U, Westphal M, Zeumer H. Preoperative embolization of intracranial meningiomas with a fibrin glue preparation. AJNR Am J Neuroradiol. 1999;20:1695–702.

110. Chan RC, Thompson GB. Ischemic necrosis of the scalp after preoperative embolization of meningeal tumors. Neurosurgery. 1984;15:76–81.

111. Friedrich H, Hansel-Friedrich G, Zeumer H. Intramedullary vascular lesions in the cervical region: transoral and dorsal surgical approach. Two case reports. Neurosurg Rev. 1990;13:65–71.

112. Takeuchi S, Tanaka R, Fujii Y, Abe H, Ito Y. Surgical treatment of hemangioblastomas with presurgical endovascular embolization. Neurol Med Chir (Tokyo). 2001;41:246–51; discussion 51–2.

113. Cornelius JF, Saint-Maurice JP, Bresson D, George B, Houdart E. Hemorrhage after particle embolization of hemangioblastomas: comparison of outcomes in spinal and cerebellar lesions. J Neurosurg. 2007;106:994–8.

114. Hong JW, Baik SK, Shin MJ, Choi HY, Kim BG. Successful management with glue injection of arterial rupture seen during embolization of an arteriovenous malformation using a flow-directed catheter: a case report. Korean J Radiol. 2000;1:208–11.

115. Qureshi AI, Luft AR, Sharma M, Guterman LR, Hopkins LN. Prevention and treatment of thromboembolic and ischemic complications associated with endovascular procedures: part II–clinical aspects and recommendations. Neurosurgery. 2000;46:1360–75; discussion 75–6.

116. Kang HS, Han MH, Kwon BJ, et al. Is clopidogrel premedication useful to reduce thromboembolic events during coil embolization for unruptured intracranial aneurysms? Neurosurgery. 2010;67:1371–6; discussion 6.

117. Hwang G, Jung C, Park SQ, et al. Thromboembolic complications of elective coil embolization of unruptured aneurysms: the effect of oral antiplatelet preparation on periprocedural thromboembolic complication. Neurosurgery. 2010;67:743–8; discussion 8.

118. Carvi y Nievas M, Haas E, Hollerhage HG. Severe intracranial bleedings during endovascular procedures: outcome of surgically treated patients. Neurol Res. 2007;29:81–90.

119. Halbach VV, Higashida RT, Hieshima GB, Norman D. Normal perfusion pressure breakthrough occurring during treatment of carotid and vertebral fistulas. AJNR Am J Neuroradiol. 1987;8:751–6.

120. Luessenhop AJ, Ferraz FM, Rosa L. Estimate of the incidence and importance of circulatory breakthrough in the surgery of cerebral arteriovenous malformations. Neurol Res. 1982;4:177–90.

121. Spetzler RF, Martin NA, Carter LP, Flom RA, Raudzens PA, Wilkinson E. Surgical management of large AVM's by staged embolization and operative excision. J Neurosurg. 1987;67:17–28.

122. Andrews BT, Wilson CB. Staged treatment of arteriovenous malformations of the brain. Neurosurgery. 1987;21:314–23.
123. Hansen PA, Knudsen F, Jacobsen M, Haase J, Bartholdy N. Indomethacin in controlling "normal perfusion pressure breakthrough" in a case of large cerebral arteriovenous malformation. J Neurosurg Anesthesiol. 1995;7:117–20.
124. Bingol H, Sirin G, Akay HT, Iyem H, Demirkilic U, Tatar H. Management of a retained catheter in an arteriovenous malformation. Case report. J Neurosurg. 2007;106:481–3.
125. Zoarski GH, Lilly MP, Sperling JS, Mathis JM. Surgically confirmed incorporation of a chronically retained neurointerventional microcatheter in the carotid artery. AJNR Am J Neuroradiol. 1999;20:177–8.
126. Mizoue T, Arita K, Nakahara T, Kawamoto H, Kurisu K. A case of cerebral arteriovenous malformation with accidental migration of a microcatheter during endovascular procedure. No Shinkei Geka. 1997;25:443–6.
127. Ruckert RI, Bender A, Rogalla P. Popliteal artery occlusion as a late complication of liquid acrylate embolization for cerebral vascular malformation. J Vasc Surg. 1999;29:561–5.
128. Weber W, Kis B, Siekmann R, Jans P, Laumer R, Kuhne D. Preoperative embolization of intracranial arteriovenous malformations with onyx. Neurosurgery. 2007;61:244–52; discussion 52–4.
129. Kelly ME, Turner RT, Gonugunta V, Rasmussen PA, Woo HH, Fiorella D. Monorail snare technique for the retrieval of an adherent microcatheter from an onyx cast: technical case report. Neurosurgery. 2008;63:ONSE89; discussion ONSE.
130. Binning MJ, Yashar P, Orion D, et al. Use of the outreach distal access catheter for microcatheter stabilization during Intracranial arteriovenous malformation embolization. AJNR Am J Neuroradiol. 2011 Jul 14 [Epub ahead of print]

8. Extracranial Embolization

Extracranial embolization procedures are therapeutic endovascular occlusions of vessels outside the cranial cavity. This chapter covers:
1. Head and neck transarterial embolization procedures
2. Percutaneous procedures
3. Spinal embolization

8.1.   Head and Neck Transarterial Embolization

Indications

1) Bleeding
   a) Idiopathic epistaxis (exceedingly common)
   b) Post-traumatic (common)
   c) Post surgical (occasionally)
   d) Bleeding tumours (occasionally)
   e) Post-radiation changes (occasionally)
2) Carotid blow-out syndrome (a particularly problematic combination of (c)–(e), above)
3) Extracranial vascular tumours, pre-operative embolization (common) or palliative embolization (rare)
   a) Juvenile nasopharyngeal angiofibroma
   b) Paraganglioma (aka chemodectoma, glomus tumour)
   c) A wide variety of other primary and metastatic vascular tumours.
4) Extracranial arteriovenous malformations (AVM) (uncommon)
   a) Superficial AVMs
   b) Intraosseous AVMs
   c) Diffuse AVMs
   d) Intraorbital AVMs
5) Extracranial arteriovenous fistulas (AVF)
   a) Congenital fistulas (Very rare)
   b) Dural AVFs (Covered in Chaps. 7 and 12)
   c) Post-traumatic fistulas (occasionally)
   d) Post-surgical fistulas (occasionally)

Relative Contraindications

1. Feeding vessels feed eloquent structures (e.g., brain, eye, or spinal cord)
2. Vascular anatomy that is difficult for endovascular access (e.g., exaggerated vessel tortuosity, vascular anomalies).
3. Significant atherosclerotic disease or high-flow vasculopathy affecting the parent vessel (e.g., occlusion or stenosis of the access vessel).
4. Life-threatening contrast allergy.
5. Coagulation disorders or heparin hypersensitivity.
6. Active bacterial infection (i.e., bacteremia at time of endovascular treatment).

M.R. Harrigan, J.P. Deveikis, *Handbook of Cerebrovascular Disease and Neurointerventional Technique*, DOI 10.1007/978-1-61779-946-4_8,
© Springer Science+Business Media New York 2013

8.2. Techniques and Devices

Evaluation

1) History and physical.
2) Neurological exam.
3) Blood work (CBC, BUN, Creatinine, PT, PTT)
4) Imaging
   a) CT or MRI of the lesion
   b) CTA or MRA
   c) If possible, a catheter angiogram.
   d) Imaging considerations
      i) Lesion location, potential territories at risk from the procedure, size and configuration.
      ii) Whether there is involvement of the skull or spine.
      iii) Flow patterns (e.g., high flow vs. low flow arteriovenous shunt).
      iv) Parent vessel anatomy.
      v) Angiographic architecture of lesion (e.g., nidal AVM vs. high-flow AVF vs. mixed lesion vs. tumour)
      vi) Presence of associated vascular lesion (e.g., aneurysms, multiple AVMs or AVFs).
      vii) Plan site of intended deposition of embolic material.
      viii) Access vessel anatomy.
      ix) Presence or absence of stenosis in the access vessel.

Treatment Strategy

Assess the patient and available imaging prior to the case, and preferably prior to the day of the procedure. Decisions about the overall treatment strategy and the role of embolization in that strategy should be made well ahead of time. Plans should include:

1) Choice of access vessel
2) Guide catheter selection
3) Microcatheter and microwire selection
4) Embolic agent to be used
5) Target vessels to be treated
6) Single procedure versus staged multiple procedures
7) Preparation for methods to ensure preservation of neurological function (e.g., provocative testing, neuophysiological monitoring)

Preprocedure Preparation

1) One or two peripheral IVs.
2) NPO for 6 h, except for medications.
3) Patients on insulin for hyperglycemia should get half their normal dose prior to the procedure.
4) Place Foley catheter.
5) Make sure that all devices that may be needed are available in the angio suite prior to the procedure.
6) Many practitioners routinely pre-treat patients with dexamethasone, 2 mg PO/IV Q 6 h for 2–3 days before any tumour embolization procedure to attempt to reduce the risk of swelling.
7) *Patients with a recent hemorrhage*:
   a) Arterial line and large-caliber venous access are established prior to the procedure.
   b) If the airway is threatened, the patient should be intubated and ventilated.

Awake or Asleep?

1) As a rule, extracranial embolization procedures should be done awake.
2) Exceptions: Children, patients with unstable airways (e.g., some epistaxis patients) and cases that are anticipated to be very long in duration.

Vascular Access Phase

See Chap. 4 for a general discussion of access techniques.
1) A 6F sheath is placed in the femoral artery.
   a) A 7F sheath is necessary if arterial monitoring is going to be done with the sheath, or if a need for a proximal balloon catheter is anticipated. An even larger sheath may be needed if stent-grafting is going to be done.
2) Systemic anticoagulation.
   a) Thromboembolic complications can occur during any vascular catheterization. The senior author of this handbook favours universal use of systemic heparin for all embolization procedures whereas the junior author almost never uses heparin.
      i) Who is right, and who is wrong? Systemic anticoagulation with IV heparin appears to carry relatively little risk in patients without active bleeding, and judicious use of heparin appears to be of relatively low-risk particularly since the drug can be rapidly reversed with protamine.
      ii) IV heparin dose: 5,000 units or 70 units/kg, followed by 1,000 units per additional hour.
3) Guide catheter selection
   a) Large-bore, stiff guide catheters are best for external carotid artery positioning and embolization. The large ID permits the use of large microcatheters and allows for good-quality angiograms with injection of contrast into the guide catheter while the microcatheter is in position.
      i) Envoy® (Codman Neurovascular, Raynham, MA)
      ii) Guider Softip™ XF guide catheter (Stryker Neurovascular, Fremont, CA)
      iii) Cook Shuttle® (Cook Medical, Bloomington, IN)
      iv) 4F Berenstein II (Cordis Endovascular, Miami Lakes, FL)
         (1) This guide catheter is particularly useful for external carotid territory embolizations because it can easily be placed in the distal external carotid or even superselectively in individual branches with little trauma to the vessels. It acts like a mini-Envoy®.
4) Guide catheter positioning
   a) Carotid system.
      i) Using a roadmap, advance the guide catheter over a hydrophilic wire into the ECA and into a straight segment proximal to the origin of the branch feeding the lesion. A "high position" of the guide catheter maximizes the stability of the guide catheter and improves control over the microcatheter and microwire. When the target involves proximal branches of the ECA, like the ascending pharyngeal artery or the superior thyroid artery, it may be necessary to position the tip of the guide catheter in the distal segment of the common carotid. In a very curved ECA, the guide catheter can be should be positioned immediately proximal to the curve. Moderate curves in the vessel usually cannot be straightened out by guiding a relatively stiff catheter around them, and the guide catheter can cause spasm or even a dissection. Therefore, it is better to settle for a relatively proximal guide catheter position. If added stability is necessary, a relatively stiff 0.014 in. wire can be advanced through the guide catheter as a "buddy wire," and if the catheter has a large enough lumen, a microcatheter can be advanced alongside it. The buddy wire will help keep the guide catheter in place.
   b) Subclavian artery.
      i) Using a roadmap, position the guide catheter adjacent to the target branch. The thyrocervical and costocervical trunks may sometimes be directly catheterized with a guide catheter, but more often, the guide catheter must be placed in the proximal subclavian artery.
      ii) A buddy wire is often needed during embolizations with the guide catheter in the proximal subclavian artery.

c) Do a guide catheter angiogram once it is in position to assess the configuration of the vessel around the tip and to check for the presence of vasospasm or vessel dissection around the tip. If catheter tip-induced vasospasm is present and flow limiting, withdrawal of the catheter tip by several millimeters is often sufficient to restore flow.

d) Attached an RHV with continuous saline infusion to the hub of the catheter.

Microcatheter Access Phase

Once a stable guide catheter position has been obtained, advance a microcatheter is advanced into a position from which embolic material can be delivered to the target.

1) Working views
    a) Obtain high magnification PA and lateral working views and make sure that the guide catheter is visible on at least one view.
    b) Use biplane roadmaps during navigation.

2) Microcatheter selection
    a) There are many microcatheters, and the optimal choice depends on how large or how distal the target vessel is, what embolic agent will be used, and the training and experience of the operator. See Chap. 7 for more detail about microcatheters.
    b) Microcatheters for extracranial embolization:
        i) Over the wire microcatheters. These are by far the most common and are quite sufficient for nearly all procedures.
        (1) Examples: Excelsior® 10–18 (Stryker Neurovascular, Fremont, CA) Prowler® (Codman Neurovascular, Raynham, MA), Echelon™ (ev3 Neurovascular, Irvine, CA)
    c) Flow-directed microcatheters. These are *so* flexible distally that they are ideal for catheterizing very small vessels in an atraumatic fashion. However, they are quite flimsy and unstable and are rarely used for extracranial embolization, except in some AVM cases.
        i) Examples: Magic® (AIT-Balt, Miami, FL) Marathon™ or Ultraflow™ (ev3 Neurovascular, Irvine, CA)
    d) Steerable microcatheters. These are the least common and are basically over-the-wire catheters that have the added benefit of a steerable tip of the microcatheter.
        i) Example: Plato™ Microcath (Scientia, Reno, NV).
    e) Two-marker, over-the-wire microcatheters, rather than single-marker catheters, are necessary for the use of detachable coils. The two markers in microcatheters used in detachable coils are always 3 cm apart to determine that the coil is properly deployed. This feature can also be used for calibration and measurements. These two markers may make the distal 3 cm minimally stiffer than one marker catheters, but do not preclude the use of embolic agents other than detachable coils.

3) Microwire selection
    a) A wide variety of microwires is available, with differing properties such as size, softness, visibility on fluoroscopy, shapeability, and steerability, trackability, and torque control. All microwires suitable for neuro-endovascular procedures are hydrophillically coated to reduce friction.
    b) Wires can have a shapeable distal tip or may come pre-shaped from the manufacturer. Shapeable tips are usually made of platinum, which makes them visible on fluoroscopy.
    c) Sizes of microwires range from 0.008 in. for the tiny Mirage™ (ev3 Neurovascular, Irvine, CA) to a variety of 0.010 in. and even more 0.014-in. wires up to the robust 0.016-in. Headliner™ (Microvention/Terumo, Tustin, CA). Larger diameter wires are available, but are generally a tight fit in commonly used microcatheters and are too stiff for navigation in small vessels.
    d) In general, 0.014-in. wires are used for extracranial embolizations, since they are torquable and will be compatible with most over-the-wire microcatheters.
    e) The Synchro® or Transend® EX (Stryker Neurovascular, Fremont, CA) are very flexible, manoeuvrable wires that work efficiently in most instances.
    f) The authors of this handbook often use the slippery and atraumatic J-tip Headliner™ (Microvention/Terumo, Tustin, CA) in tortuous external carotid branches.

4) Microcatheter irrigation
   a) Continuous irrigation of the microcatheter as well as the guide catheter with heparinized saline (5,000 U heparin per 500 mL saline) is important. Heparinized saline infusion ensures hydration of the hydrophilic coating on the microwire and minimizes friction.
   b) Meticulous attention to the microcatheter (and guide catheter) RHV throughout the case is necessary to identify thrombus or bubbles, should they appear.
   c) The heparinized saline drip should be periodically monitored to ensure that it is dripping slowly, but continuously, and there is still sufficient fluid in the saline bag to last for the case.
5) Microcatheter/microwire preparation
   a) Remove the microcatheter from the package and flush the plastic hoop to hydrate the hydrophilic coating.
   b) If necessary, the tip of the microcatheter can be steam shaped over the small mandrel that usually comes packaged with the catheter.
   c) Insert the microwire into the microcatheter, extend the tip of the microwire beyond the tip of the microcatheter, and shape the tip of the microwire with an introducer. Attach the torque device to the microwire.
   d) Tighten the RHV on the microcatheter just enough to prevent leakage of flush and to allow easy use of the microwire.
6) Microcatheter navigation
   a) Carefully insert the microcatheter into the RHV of the guide catheter and advance it to the distal tip of the guide catheter. Both the Echelon™ and Rebar® (ev3 Neurovascular, Irvine, CA) have a marker on the shaft of the catheter that indicates that the tip is approaching the tip of a 90 cm guide catheter, to limit the need for fluoroscopy up to that point.
   b) Carefully advance the microwire and follow with the microcatheter under roadmap guidance. It is acceptable to advance the tip of the microcatheter without the microwire in straight segments of the vessel.
   c) Carefully guide the microwire around sharp curves and beyond branches by rotating the microwire.
   d) Fixing the microwire in space, the microcatheter can be advanced over the wire and around turns.
   e) To break the friction between microcatheter and microwire, the wire can be gently pulled back and/or rotated.
   f) Monitor the guide catheter position at all times because any resistance to forward motion of the microcatheter will inevitably create backpressure on the guide catheter.
   g) Gently pull back slightly on the microcatheter periodically to remove redundancy.
   h) Also periodically check that the heparinized saline flush lines attached to the guide catheter and microcatheter are dripping and bubble-free.
   i) When the microcatheter reaches the target, remove the microwire and observe the tip of the microcatheter fluoroscopically, since moving the wire can often release stored energy in the microcatheter, causing it to move (usually forward).
   j) Do a microcatheter angiogram to confirm microcatheter positioning and to confirm patency of the microcatheter. Too much resistance during injection can indicate kinking of the microcatheter. Kinking can be resolved by pulling back on the catheter before proceeding further. Forced injection of contrast or embolic material into a kinked catheter can result in catheter rupture, which can be a disaster.
   k) The microcatheter arteriogram shows:
      i) Whether the desired position has been reached
      ii) Whether there are dangerous anastamoses filling
      iii) The flow-rate in order to choose an embolic agent and the injection rate needed
      iv) That there is no sign of contrast exiting the microcatheter proximal to the distal tip. When this happens it is a sign that the microcatheter has been irreparably damaged and must not be used for embolization
   l) Once the microcatheter is in position and a microcatheter angiogram is done, provocative testing may be performed if necessary (see below).
   m) The embolization phase may now begin (also see below).

7) Flow-directed microcatheter navigation:
   a) Flow-directed microcatheters are commonly used for liquid embolic delivery, usually for treatment of AVMs or AVFs. The high flow state in these conditions greatly facilitates rapid and accurate navigation of the microcatheter to the target. However, in the extracranial circulation, flow rates are less than those in the intracranial circulation, even in hypervascular lesions. Therefore, the flow-directed characteristics of these microcatheters do not assist navigation in the extracranial circulation to any great extent. These catheters can still be used, but technique is virtually the same as that for over-the-wire microcatheters, except that 0.010 or smaller microwires must be used. Again, if Onyx® (ev3, Irvine, CA) is to be used as an embolic agent in the case, a DMSO-compatible microcatheter must be used.
8) Steerable microcatheter navigation:
   a) Steerable microcatheters are seldom needed for extracranial embolization. They are most appropriate for coil embolization. Their positioning technique is very similar to over-the-wire technique, with a number of idiosyncrasies, given the special steerable characteristics of the catheter. The Plato™ Microcath (Scientia, Reno, NV) is a radically different microcatheter, although it is approved only in Europe at the time of this writing. It is virtually the only true steerable microcatheter available, even it is not readily available at the time of this writing. Further discussions on the use of this microcatheter are in Chaps. 5 and 7.
9) Provocative testing (see Chap. 6) is done to confirm that the vessel being embolized does not supply dangerous anastamoses to the central nervous system or cranial nerves. Pharmacologic agents such as amobarbital and lidocaine are injected in the vessel prior to embolization and the patient is tested for new signs of neurological dysfunction. Amobarbital injections test for nerve cell body supply in the central nervous system and lidocaine injections test for nerve axons such as cranial nerves.[1] Most provocative testing is done on awake patients, although it can be done while the patient is under general anesthesia using neurophysiological monitoring with electroencephalography (EEG), somatosensory evoked potentials (SSEP), brainstem evoked responses (BAER) and/or motor evoked potentials (MEP).[2–4] Monitoring is not free from false negatives,[2] and the practitioner should never be lulled into a false sense of security even when testing suggests it is safe to embolize, since the pharmacological agents can go preferentially by flow to the abnormal territory. This is especially true in high flow lesions such as AVM or AVF. Careful attention to microcatheter angiograms may be just as sensitive as provocative testing to rule out normal territories at risk. After embolization of a vessel after negative amobarbital and lidocaine testing, a change in flow pattern or visualization or different vessels may be seen after partial occlusion of the vessel. Consider repeating the provocative testing again, and only proceed with further embolization if the provocative testing remained negative.[5]

Syringe Safety

Many of the procedures discussed in this book require the use of multiple agents in syringes on the procedure table. For example, an embolization procedure that involves provocative testing requires syringes containing local anesthetic, saline flush, contrast, amobarbital, lidocaine, embolic material, etc. It is imperative that these syringes containing different agents are clearly differentiated, one from another. Confusing syringes with anesthetic agents or embolic materials for contrast or saline flush can lead to disastrous results. Use customized, labeled, coloured syringes (Merit Medical, South Jordan, UT) of various sizes and designs for the various materials. Using the same type of syringe for a certain agent at all times and educating new team members to the routine will minimize confusion and avoid mistakes.

Embolization Phase

A variety of embolic agents are available and some are more effective than others. The single most important principle of the selection process is that the operator uses the system with which he or she is most experienced and comfortable.

1) Embolic material selection
   a) Liquid embolics. The most commonly used intracranial embolic agents.
      i) Cyanoacrylates. (aka glue)
         (1) These are acrylic agents that are in a liquid state and polymerize when they contact hydroxyl ions in blood and are mainly used for intracranial embolization. The most common acrylic agent used in the United States is n-butyl cyanocrylate (n-BCA) Trufill® (Codman Neurovascular, Raynham, MA). Polymerization time can be modified by the addition of oil-based contrast agents such as Ethiodol® (Savage Laboratories, Melville, NY) or glacial acetic acid. Glue tends to cause considerable pain on injection of extracranial vessels, so it is used mainly for spinal embolization, for rare high-flow fistulas in the head and neck for actively bleeding vessels or for direct percutaneous embolization of vascular tumors via needle puncture.
      ii) Precipitated polymer. (aka non-adhesive liquid embolic agent)
         (1) These agents are polymers that are insoluble in blood or water and come dissolved in a non-aqueous solvent. When injected into the vascular system, the solvent disperses and the polymer precipitates to form a solid occlusive agent. Onyx® (ev3, Irvine, CA) is the dominant example of the precipitated polymer and is FDA-approved for use in AVMs. The agent is slowly infused through the microcatheter so is not a particularly useful agent for most applications in the extracranial circulation. The DMSO solvent in the Onyx is locally toxic and causes pain on injection. Another issue with Onyx® is the dark tantalum used to make it radio-opaque which may be visible through the skin if injected in superficial vessels. Consequently it, like the acrylic glue, is also uncommonly used in extracranial procedures.
   b) Sclerosing agents
      i) Sclerosing agents are liquid agents that promote thrombosis and necrosis of the intima to prevent recanalization. Absolute ethanol is medical-grade ethanol that is dehydrated sufficiently to be close to 100% pure ethanol. Absolute ethanol is very thrombogenic and toxic at this concentration. Alcohol should be avoided or only used with utmost caution when treating lesions anywhere near the central nervous system because of this toxicity. It is also extremely painful when injected in vessels in awake patients, and can cause skin necrosis if used in superficial vessels. Consequently, absolute ethanol is usually reserved for attempted palliative embolization for tumours and direct percutaneous sclerotherapy for vascular malformations or tumours in the head and neck. Absolute alcohol should not be confused with Absolut Vodka (Pernod Ricard, Paris, France), which is a trendy alcoholic beverage.
   c) Particles
      i) Particles are the most common agents used in the extracranial head and neck circulation. All particulate agents work best in lesions with a capillary bed, such as tumours. All have a tendency to clog the microcatheter if the particles are too large or injected in too large a quantity. All require a similar technique for their use, and are mixed with contrast and injected via a microcatheter.
         (1) Polyvinyl alcohol foam. (aka "PVA")
            (a) These are irregularly shaped particles of PVA Examples: Contour® emboli (Boston Scientific, Natick, MA) or PVA Foam Embolization Particles (Cook Medical, Bloomington, IN).
         (2) Spherical emboli
            (a) These particles are manufactured to have a smooth, spherical shape. Examples Spherical Contour SE™ (Boston Scientific, Natick, MA) or Bead Block™ (Terumo Medical, Somerset, NJ) or Embospheres® (Biosphere Medical, Rockland, MA).
   d) Silk suture
      i) Small segments of silk suture can be loaded into a microcatheter and then propelled into the vessel by injecting contrast or saline. Other types of suture material can be used in this fashion, but are less thrombogenic.

e) Detachable balloons
   i) Detachable balloons are attached to a microcatheter, navigated to the desired site of occlusion, inflated to produce occlusion of the vessel, then detached from the catheter and permanently implanted. They are used on rare occasion in the extracranial circulation for high-flow fistulas or for large vessel occlusion. At the time of this writing, the Goldballoon™ balloon (Balt Extrusion, Montmorency, France), is available in most of the world outside of the United States, but no detachable balloons are currently approved for the North American market.
f) Pushable coils.
   i) These are platinum coils with thrombogenic fibers that are pushed through the microcatheter with a wire pusher. Examples include Trufill® pushable coils (Codman Neurovascular, Raynham, MA), Hilal and Tornado® Microcoils (Cook Medical, Bloomfield, IN), Fibered Platinum, and Vortx® coils (Boston Scientific, Natick, MA). Small coils such as 2 mm or 5 mm straight coils or 2 mm × 20 mm helical coils can also be propelled through the microcatheter and into the vessel using rapid injections of saline or contrast. Since these are effective in producing vascular occlusion and are inexpensive, they are the most common coils used for extracranial embolization. Still, it is rare that medium sized vessels need occlusion with coils in the extracranial circulation. These coils are best used in the extracranial territories mainly to block anastamotic vessels and prevent particles or liquid emboli from entering the dangerous territory.
g) Detachable platinum coils.
   i) Detachable coils are rarely used in extracranial embolizations. They are more expensive and not as effective in inducing thrombosis as fibered pushable coils, and are also much slower to deploy. The added precision and security they provide are not usually needed outside the cerebral circulation. They are discussed further in Chap. 5.
h) Detachable fibered coils
   i) These are a hybrid of the pushable fibered coil and detachable coil. Examples include the Sapphire NXT™ fibered coils (ev3, Irvine, CA). They provide the same features as pushable fibered coils but with added precision. This precision is usually unnecessary in the extracranial circulation.
i) Stents
   i) Stents are rarely used for embolization in the extracranial circulation such as for the occasional dissecting aneurysm or arteriovenous fistulas that may require stent-assisted coil embolization. The Neuroform™ (Stryker Neurovascular, Fremont, CA) and Enterprise™ (Codman Neurovascular, Raynham, MA) stents may be used in smaller vessels (up to 4.5-mm diameter), but would be used off-label if used in the extracranial circulation. When dealing with AV fistula or pseudoaneurysm arising from larger vessels, the larger self-expanding carotid stents including NexStent® (Boston Scientific, Natick, MA) or Acculink™ (Abbott Laboratories, Abbott Park, IL) can be used for preservation of flow in large or medium sized vessels in extracranial embolization procedures. Coils can be placed in the pseudoaneurysm or on the venous side of the AV fistula, while the stent in the artery prevents herniation of coils into the parent artery. The authors of this handbook have done stent-assisted coiling in cases of wide necked post-traumatic extracranial carotid pseudoaneurysms, or large post-traumatic AVF in the carotid or vertebral artery. It may also be helpful to temporarily inflate a non-detachable balloon, like the Hyperform™ (ev3, Irvine, CA) within the stent during placement of coils or liquid embolic agents in the aneurysm or fistula to provide added assurance that the coils, or other agents do not find their way through the openings of the stent into the parent artery.
      (1) Standard low surface coverage-area intracranial stents like the Neuroform™ or Enterprise™ can sometimes channel flow away from a side-wall aneurysm to induce thrombosis without

placing coils. This spontaneous thrombosis after stent placement would not be expected in the case of an AV fistula due to the higher flow conditions. An alternative to this are covered stents, such as the Jostent® (Abbott, Abbot Park, IL). This over-the-wire balloon inflatable covered stent allows rapid occlusion of a fistula without necessarily using coils. The stent is FDA-HDE approved for repair of ruptured coronary vessels 3–5 mm in diameter, and therefore use elsewhere in the body is off-label. Larger vessels (4–7.5 mm) require the Wallgraft™ (Boston Scientific, Natick, MA). This is a self-expanding stainless steel stent-graft is less traumatic than balloon inflatable stents, but requires a large (>8F) sheath. The Viabahn® (W. L. Gore, Flagstaff, AZ) is a heparin coated self-expanding nitinol stent graft that has the added benefit of being MRI compatible. These latter stent-grafts require 7F sheaths for the smaller stents (5 or 6 mm) or 8F for the larger stents (7 or 8 mm). None of these covered stents is FDA-approved for use in the brachiocephalic vessels, but can be life-saving in some cases of active bleeding of a major vessel.[6]

2) n-BCA embolization technique. See Chap. 7 for an in-depth discussion of glue injection technique.

    a) Place a flow-directed or over-the-wire microcatheter close to the target and beyond any potential connections to the brain, eye, cranial nerves or spinal cord. Also, avoid getting glue in muscular or cutaneous branches since it may cause considerable pain. Do provocative testing if necessary.

    b) Glue preparation

        i) Set up a separate sterile back table for n-BCA preparation. All personnel working at this table should be free of any contact with saline and should wear eye protection. If a connection comes loose during injection, the glue can spray and stick to whatever it touches.

        ii) Examine the microcatheter angiogram to determine how long the contrast takes to reach the lesion. Rule of thumb: if that time is <1 s, use at least 70% glue mixture (three parts n-BCA to one part Ethiodol®) is required. Contrast transit time >2 s requires a 50% (one n-BCA to one Ethiodol) or more dilute mixture.

        iii) Tantalum powder greatly increases the radio-opacity of glue, but is not absolutely necessary unless the glue mixture is >70% n-BCA. Tantalum is messy and can clump, and also the pigment may be visible through the skin in superficial vessels, so most practitioners almost never use it in the extracranial circulation.

        iv) Draw up the Trufill® n-BCA (Codman Neurovascular, Raynham, MA) from its tube using a labeled, glue-compatible 3-ml syringe (avoid polycarbonate plastic…it softens).

        v) Draw up the Ethiodol® in a labeled syringe, and add the proper volume to the glue syringe to achieve the desired concentration.

        vi) Have 10–15 labeled 3-ml syringes filled with 5% dextrose solution ready.

    c) Injection technique

        i) Pull back slightly on the microcatheter to remove any slack, and slightly loosen the rotating hemostatic valve so that it just barely prevents back-flow of blood in the guide catheter, without binding the microcatheter too tightly.

        ii) Attach a glue-compatible stopcock directly to the microcatheter. Cook Medical (Bloomington, IN) makes a high-pressure, white nylon plastic one, and three-way stopcocks with Luer lock fittings that hold up well during glue injections.

        iii) Three-way are preferred because they allow a flush syringe of dextrose to remain attached even when the glue syringe is attached. This works well for doing the push technique (see below).

        iv) Thoroughly flush the microcatheter with 5% dextrose solution. Generally, approximately 5–10 ml is sufficient to clear all saline and/or blood from the microcatheter lumen.

        v) As the last dextrose is being injected, close the stopcock to prevent blood backflow into the microcatheter.

        vi) Holding the stopcock upright, fill the Luer-lock connection fully with dextrose.

vii) Create a blank roadmap to help visualize the glue injection and attach a 3-ml syringe loaded with the prepared glue mixture.

viii) Swiftly and steadily inject the glue using while watching the roadmap image. Fill the arterial feeder and as much of the nidus as possible.

ix) Be alert for any signs of reflux of glue back along the catheter, passage of glue into the vein, or reflux of glue from the nidus into other arterial branches feeding the lesion. If any of these conditions is occurring and one is using dilute glue, one might be able to briefly pause the injection, then resume cautiously. Sometimes the glue will find another pathway through the nidus.

x) The glue injection is quick but controlled. Polymerization occurs within a few seconds. The embolic agent should be deposited in the "safety zone" consisting of AVM nidus and only the artery beyond all normal branches, and vein before other venous inputs beyond the occluded nidus (see Fig. 7.2). If there is any question that the glue is refluxing or going somewhere it shouldn't, or if finished filling the desired space with glue, stop injecting, aspirate the syringe to create negative pressure in the microcatheter, and quickly, smoothly withdraw the microcatheter completely from the patient and discard it.

xi) Examine the rotating hemostatic valve of the guiding catheter for any retained droplets of glue, then aspirate and double flush the stopcock, rotating hemostatic valve, and guide-catheter.

xii) Once the guide catheter is thoroughly inspected and flushed, re-insert it to the arterial territory of interest, and perform a follow-up arteriogram to ensure that the desired result is obtained.

3) Onyx® embolization technique

a) Preparation

i) Have several vials of Onyx® (18 and/or 34) agitating in an automatic mixer for 30 min while performing other parts of the procedure. The Onyx technique is similar to the technique using n-BCA glue except that a dimethyl sulfoxide (DMSO)-compatible microcatheter must be used, such as the Rebar® (ev3, Irvine, CA) or more flexible Marathon™ (ev3, Irvine, CA).

ii) Note that provocative testing can give a false sense of security since Onyx® can easily find its way into places that may not be predicted by microcatheter angiography or barbiturate injections.

iii) Confirm proper catheter positioning with a microcatheter angiogram. Select a projection that shows the microcatheter tip and its relationship to any curves in the arterial feeder distal to the catheter tip, any normal branches proximal to it, and whether the tip is wedged.

iv) Study the microcatheter angiogram to determine the arteriovenous transit time and to visualize the morphology of the target vessels.

v) Select a pre-mixed viscosity of the agent depending on the size of the feeder and degree of arteriovenous shunting. Big feeders with fast flow need Onyx® 34 and small feeders or slower shunting should be treated with Onyx® 18.

vi) Draw up 1 ml of DMSO and the Onyx® using the syringes provided in the kit. Agitate the Onyx back and forth if it will not be injected for more than a few minutes to keep the tantalum from precipitating

vii) Attach the DMSO syringe directly to the hub of the microcatheter and fill the dead-space of the microcatheter (usually 0.2–0.3 ml) with DMSO over 1–2 min.

viii) Remove the DMSO syringe from the microcatheter, and, keeping the hub upright, fill the hub with DMSO.

ix) Holding both the catheter hub and Onyx® syringe at 45° to one another, quickly connect the syringe to the hub, and then keep the syringe vertical with the plunger down (see Fig. 7.3). This method keeps a sharp demarcation between the heavier Onyx® in the syringe and lighter DMSO in the hub of the catheter and makes it easier to see radiographically than if the DMSO and Onyx® are allowed to mix together.

b) Onyx injection technique
   i) Using a blank roadmap, slowly inject the Onyx® at a rate of approximately 0.16 ml/min. Rates of injection >0.3 ml/min risk vascular injury due to DMSO toxicity.
   ii) Continue injecting Onyx® as long as it is flowing forward into desired areas of the abnormal vessels. If it refluxes along the catheter, passes into the proximal part of the vein, or refluxes into other arterial feeders, pause the injection for 15 s, then resume injecting. If the Onyx® continues to flow in the wrong direction, pause again for 15–30 s, then try again. If the Onyx® finds another, more desirable pathway, continue the slow injection.
   iii) Make a new roadmap mask periodically. New roadmaps subtract out the already deposited embolic agent and makes the newly injected material easier to see. Guide catheter angiograms can be done during the Onyx injection to determine if there are still portions of the feeding artery or nidus that could be occluded from this microcatheter position.
   iv) The Onyx® injection requires patience and usually takes at least several minutes.
       (1) Some reflux back along the catheter tip is not a problem, due to the non-adhesive nature of the product. Avoid more than 1 cm of reflux, however, since even Onyx® may glue a microcatheter into the vessel.
       (2) Do not pause the injection for >2 min at a time because the Onyx® may solidify and clog the microcatheter.
       (3) Never try to inject against resistance. A clogged microcatheter may burst if the injection is forced.
   v) When adequate filling of the desired vascular spaces is achieved, or if the Onyx® repeatedly flows in the wrong direction, stop injecting, aspirate back on the syringe, and steadily pull back on the microcatheter, disengage it from the deposited Onyx® and remove it.
   vi) After the microcatheter is withdrawn from the guide catheter, examine the RHV of the guide catheter for any retained droplets of Onyx®, then aspirate and double flush the stopcock, RHV, and guide catheter.
   vii) Do a guide catheter angiogram once the guide catheter is thoroughly inspected and flushed to see what has been accomplished.
4) Ethanol embolization technique
   a) Ethanol embolization is seldom done for extracranial embolization. It is useful for occasional situations in which the microcatheter tip is very close to the lesion, and for direct puncture of superficial tumours or vascular malformations (see below).
   b) Some operators use Swan-Ganz catheter monitoring for AVM embolization with ethanol, to watch for signs of pulmonary hypertension due to the pulmonary effects of ethanol.
   c) When added to particles, the technique is essentially the same as standard particulate embolization (see below). When used without particles, the technique is more like that for glue.
   d) Be sure to use syringes, stopcocks and microcatheter hubs will not degrade when exposed to ethanol. Often, those that can be used with glue or DMSO will withstand ethanol, but it is wise to test it first. Since ethanol is not an FDA-approved embolic material, manufacturers state that their products are not approved for use with ethanol.
   e) Position the microcatheter and do provocative testing as needed.
   f) Prior to embolizing, do test injections of contrast through the microcatheter to estimate the rate and volume required to fill the vessels that will be treated. If the flow is very rapid, consider placing a coil or two to slow the flow.
   g) Flush the microcatheter with saline because ethanol can cause contrast to precipitate.
   h) Inject the absolute ethanol at a rate similar to the rate that was used for the microcatheter angiogram but use only approximately 50% of the volume of contrast that was used for the microcatheter angiogram.
   i) Wait a few minutes, then repeat the contrast injection. If the target vessels remain patent, inject another small bolus of ethanol, and wait again.

j) If spasm is seen on repeat test injections, wait until it resolves and decrease the volume of the ethanol bolus.

k) After a few boluses of ethanol have been given, wait at least 5–10 min between ethanol injections before checking for patency of the vessel.

l) If there is no change after 20 mL of ethanol, consider placement of additional coils to slow the flow and help the ethanol work, or try a better embolic agent.

m) Remember that ethanol can work on the endothelium for some time and can also spread through the vessel wall into the adjacent tissues, so it is best to keep the total ethanol volume to a minimum.

5) Particle embolization technique

a) Most particles are used in a similar fashion for extracranial embolization.

b) To avoid major problems with particles clogging the microcatheter, use a larger lumen microcatheter, such as a RapidTransit® (Codman Neurovascular, Raynham, MA).

c) The microcatheter tip must be close to the lesion being embolized and in a stable position distal to normal branches.

d) Choose a particle size depending on the size of the vessels in the target lesion. In general, use particles <300 µm in diameter for tumors and particles >300 µm for AVMs.

e) If there are potential connections to cranial nerves use particles >300 µm.

f) Mix the particles with 50:50 contrast in saline and draw up the emboli in a labeled 10-ml syringe. This acts as a reservoir for emboli.

g) The particles should be fairly dilute to limit the risk of clogging the microcatheter.

h) Attach the syringe to one female connection on a 3-way stopcock and attach a labeled 3-ml Luer-lock syringe to the other female connection. This syringe is used to inject the embolic mixture through the microcatheter.

i) The stopcock is then attached to the hub of the microcatheter.

j) The stopcock is turned to connect the 10 and 3 mL syringes, and the contrast/emboli mixture is flushed into the 3-ml syringe and then back into the 10-ml syringe, back and forth several times, to ensure uniform suspension of particles.

k) The 3-ml syringe is then filled with 1–2 mL of the emboli suspension.

l) Using a blank roadmap, slowly inject the emboli in small (0.2 mL) increments and ensure that the contrast freely flows from the microcatheter tip.

m) Increase or decrease the rate of injection, depending on the speed of run-off away from the microcatheter.

n) Every 3–5 mL of embolic suspension, or sooner if emboli are seen to collect in the hub of the microcatheter, disconnect the 3 mL syringe and reconnect another labeled 3 mL syringe filled with dilute 50:50 contrast.

o) Gently flush the microcatheter with the contrast under fluoroscopy, remembering that the microcatheter is still full of emboli.

p) As long as a good runoff of contrast is seen, reconnect the 3-ml embolic syringe, refill it with embolic mixture, and continue to inject emboli.

q) When the 10 mL syringe is empty, consider obtaining a control superselective angiogram via the microcatheter to see whether the flow pattern is changing.

r) Especially with AVMs it may require some time and a considerable amount of emboli to occlude a feeder.

s) If an entire vial of emboli is injected with no change in the flow pattern, consider modifying the flow with a coil or two, or switching to a different embolic agent.

t) Avoid creating reflux of the embolic mixture back along the microcatheter when injecting. Slow or stop the injections if reflux is seen.

u) If resistance is encountered during the injections, stop, disconnect the 3 mL embolic syringe and check the hub of the microcatheter. If emboli are bunched up in the hub, it may be possible to rinse them out with a needle or guidewire introducer, then attempt to gently flush with contrast.

v) If resistance continues, do not attempt to force the emboli through by a forceful injection, and do not use a 1 mL syringe to achieve higher pressures. Forcibly injecting through a microcatheter clogged with particles can cause the microcatheter to rupture and even break into pieces.

w) When the flow in the feeder is significantly slowed, injections of emboli are stopped.

x) If more definitive closure of the vessel is needed after particle embolization, a coil or a tiny pledget of Gelfoam may be deposited to finish the job.

y) Be certain to flush out the microcatheter with contrast or saline before inserting a coil. Particles in the microcatheter can cause the coil to bind in the microcatheter.

z) Even if the microcatheter seems free of particles, it is best to withdraw and discard the used microcatheter prior to attempting catheterization of another feeder with a new microcatheter.

6) Silk suture embolization technique.
   a) See Chap. 7.

7) Detachable balloon technique.
   a) See Chap. 7.

8) Pushable coil technique
   a) See Chap. 7.

9) Detachable coil technique
   a) Use of detachable coils is discussed in excruciating detail in the Intracranial Aneurysms Procedure Chap. 5. Use of detachable coils for fistulas is covered in Chap. 7.

10) Stent placement for AVF technique
    a) The use of stents for aneurysm coiling is discussed in Chap. 15 and for AV fistulas in Chap. 7.

11) Stent-graft placement for active bleeding
    a) Begin by obtaining large guide catheter access (a 6F Cook Shuttle is best). Consider placing a second sheath in the opposite femoral artery; this will allow a temporary balloon catheter to be placed in the target vessel to buy time to prepare for stenting. During the access phase, external packing may control the bleeding while the endovascular procedure is underway. In a dire situation, someone may need to manually compress the bleeding site until it is controlled, but their hands will be exposed in the X-ray field and potentially make fluoroscopic imaging difficult.

    b) In the setting of a massive bleeding from trauma or a carotid blow-out or, pretreatment with antiplatelet agents is not advisable. Loading the patient with clopidogril (usually 300–600 mg) only after the stent placement and only after the bleeding has stopped seems to be the most prudent way to handle antiplatelet therapy in this setting.

    c) Size the stent-graft appropriately for the parent artery (usually a little wider than the parent artery) and for the lesion being stented (usually at least 4 mm coverage on either side of the lesion).

    d) Obtain a good roadmap that shows the bleeding site to be treated and also the vessel proximally and distally as much as possible. Consider placing an external radio-opaque marker over the bleeding site to ensure coverage by the stent-graft even if the patient moves.

    e) Advance a microcatheter with a 0.014 in., 300 cm exchange as distal as possible to the lesion being stented. Then remove the microcatheter and leave the exchange-length microwire in place. Take care not to traumatize the bleeding vessel during this process. Always keep the wire tip in view and ensure that it stays in a larger vessel and does not injure the vessel wall.

    f) Advance the stent delivery catheter over the wire, gently pulling back on the wire to make sure the tip remains in a stable position.

    g) Once the stent is in position, remove any slack in the wire and stent delivery catheter. This is critical for obtaining easy and accurate deployment.

    h) Do a guide-catheter angiogram. If the stent is not in proper position, change the position and repeat the angiogram.

    i) When a good position is achieved across the neck of the lesion, the stent is ready for deployment.

    j) Self-expanding stent technique
       i) The use of self expanding stent-grafts for bleeding vessels is similar to the placement of self expanding carotid stents, as is covered in Chap. 10.
       ii) The Wallgraft™ and Viabahn® stents require a large sheath. A 6F Cook Shuttle™ is suitable.

iii) Once the guide catheter or sheath is in place, advance a 300-cm microwire distal to the lesion.

iv) Advance the stent delivery catheter over the microwire while gently pulling back on the wire to make sure the tip remains in a stable position.

v) As with other self-expanding stents, the stent-graft is deployed by stabilizing the inner part of the delivery system as the outer part of the delivery catheter is pulled back, exposing the stent, and allowing it to expand.

vi) Remove the stent delivery catheter and do a guide catheter angiogram to determine whether the stent-graft has sealed the bleeding site.

vii) If the stent is not fully apposed to the vessel wall, do a post-stent angioplasty. Use the minimum pressure required to slightly dilate the stent. Do not allow the balloon to inflate outside of the stent.

viii) If a continued leak is present, consider using a second self-expanding stent or stent-graft.

k) Balloon-expandable stent technique

i) For a Jostent®, the stent is deployed by inflating the balloon under roadmap guidance to match the size of the parent artery. Do not exceed the maximum recommended pressure, and be careful not to disrupt the site of bleeding.

ii) When it appears that the stent is opened up to the proper size, deflate the balloon and carefully disengage it from the open stent. It may be stuck to the stent and may require another inflation/deflation cycle to free it up. Be careful not to move the stent when trying to pull back on the balloon.

iii) Once the balloon is deflated and disengaged, do a guide catheter angiogram.

iv) If the stent is not fully apposed to the vessel wall, re-insert the balloon into the stent and attempt to dilate further. Do not exceed maximum pressure for the balloon. If necessary, the balloon could be exchanged for a new low-compliance coronary angioplasty balloon sized to the vessel diameter and no longer than the stent.

v) Remember that the outer diameter of the stent is more than that of the inner lumen, so the vessel will be dilated around the stent to a greater degree than expected for the size of the balloon used.

vi) Assuming that the stent was properly sized and positioned in the first place, it should nicely fit the vessel and occlude the lesion when fully deployed. If not, consider a second stent-graft.

Post-procedure Management

1. Complete the neurological exam.
2. Admit to the ICU with vital signs, neuro exams and groin checks Q 1 h.
   a) It is not uncommon for patients undergoing embolization procedures to have some pain in the area treated the evening after the procedure.
3. IV fluids (normal saline) at 100 mL/h until the patient is taking oral fluids well.
4. Stented patients require dual antiplatelet therapy (clopidogril 75 mg and aspirin 325 mg daily). Other post-embolization patients are not routinely treated with antithrombotic agents.
5. Pay close attention to blood pressure after embolization of a high flow AVF or an actively bleeding artery.
6. Patients who do not have planned surgery after extracranial embolization procedures can be discharged to home on post-procedure day 1.
7. Patients undergoing embolization of tumours should be observed for a few days to watch for signs of swelling and/or venous congestion.
8. Depending on the lesion treated, there may or may not be a need for routine radiographic follow-up. Most patients are followed clinically and with cross-sectional imaging.

8.3.   Tips on Specific Disease Processes

Head and Neck Embolization

1) Extracranial arteriovenous malformation (AVM)
    a) Indications: pre-operative flow reduction or palliation for bleeding, cosmetic deformity, pain or tinnitus.
    b) Since these are infiltrative lesions that intimately involve normal structures, complete cure is rare, even with radical embolization plus surgery.
    c) Particle embolization is effective for preoperative embolization, but is not useful for palliative treatment since the occlusion will be temporary and the clinical benefits transient.
    d) Embolization with n-BCA glue will be permanent the glue is placed within the nidus. The microcatheter tip must be placed as close to the nidus as possible.
    e) An alternative to transarterial embolization is direct puncture and embolization with glue[7] or sclerotherapy with ethanol[8] (see below). In patients whose external carotid arteries have been previously ligated in a desperate attempt to treat the lesion, embolization may still be possible by a direct needle puncture of the feeding vessels and embolization with glue distal to the ligation.[9]
    f) Flow control with either transarterial embolization or percutaneous needle injection can be achieved by direct external compression of external draining veins during the glue or ethanol injection.
    g) A more complicated solution is to surgically reconstruct the ligated vessel, which can be a reasonable option if ischemic symptoms are present in the territory distal to the ligation.[10]
    h) Take extreme care to not allow the occlusive agent to enter dangerous anastamoses to the brain, spinal cord, or eye (see Chap. 1 for a listing of anastamoses).
    i) Keep the glue, ethanol, or even small (less than 300 μm) particles out of the vessels supplying cranial nerves, by doing provocative testing, if possible, or at least keeping the embolic agent strictly within the nidus.
    j) Also, keep liquid embolics or small particles out of cutaneous branches of the superficial temporal or facial arteries. Embolization of these arteries will cause pain, blistering, and necrosis of the skin.
    k) The bottom line: Less is more. Do not be too aggressive and the risk of complications will be reduced.
2) Extracranial arteriovenous fistula (AVF)
    a) Congenital head and neck AVFs are rare, but often present with a pulsatile mass, tinnitus, or high-output cardiac failure. They have a predilection for arising from the internal maxillary artery.[11,12]
    b) These congenital AVFs were previously treated with detachable balloons, but more recently, transarterial embolization using GDC coils and glue has been successful.[13]
    c) The goal is to occlude the fistula directly because proximal occlusion is destined to fail thanks to the presence of generous facial collaterals.
    d) In high-flow AVFs, care must be taken to size the coils (or balloon) large enough to prevent passage through the fistula into the veins and eventually into the lungs.
    e) Post-traumatic and post-surgical AVFs in the head and neck can occur in a wide variety of locations and the treatment depends on the symptoms and vascular anatomy.
    f) In an expendable vessel, such as an external carotid branch, coil and/or glue occlusion of both the fistula and parent artery may be an option. When possible the fistula and proximal vein should be occluded to prevent collateral vessels from maintaining patency of the fistula.
    g) If there is adequate collateral flow to the brain, occlusion of the carotid or vertebral artery can be done to treat some fistulas. Prior test occlusion is mandatory (Chap. 6).

h) Case reports of stent-grafts to treat carotid or vertebral AVFs have shown the devices are effective in occluding the fistula and maintaining the flow in the parent artery, at least in the acute phase.[14–16] However, the long-term patency of these devices is unknown.

i) Vertebrovenous AVFs are usually post-traumatic, but may be spontaneous,[17,18] especially in children, or those with an underlying collagen vascular such as Ehlers Danlos or neurofibromatosis. These fistulas can often be treated with balloons or coils on the venous side of the fistula preserving flow.[19,20]

3) Idiopathic epistaxis

a) Endovascular treatment for nosebleeds consists of selective catheterization and particle embolization of the nasal vessels, usually the sphenopalatine arteries.

b) Coil embolization *should not be done* for idiopathic epistaxis: Coils only block access for later re-embolization should bleeding recur.

c) A study of 70 patients treated with embolization for epistaxis found that 86% had effective relief of bleeding, and only one (1.4%) had a serious neurological complication.[20a]

d) Two other reports of over 100 patients each found acute complication rates of up to 17% and a 1–2% rate of long-term neurological deficits.[21,22]

e) Complications can be minimized by careful attention to angiographic anatomy and awareness of dangerous anastamoses. Provocative testing with amobarbital and lidocaine prior to embolization is an added safety factor.[1]

f) Always check the contralateral sphenopalatine artery angiographically, even if the bleeding is obviously unilateral, because there can be side-to-side collaterals.[23] The authors of this handbook nearly always embolize the sphenopalatine arteries bilaterally.

g) Smaller particles may be used on the side of active bleeding, but always use large particles (≥500 µm) on the contralateral side to minimize the risk of nasal mucosal necrosis. Remember: large particles call for large microcatheters.

h) Ethmoidal branches from the ophthalmic artery may be the cause of treatment failure after embolization of the internal maxillary artery. There has been a case report of embolization of the ophthalmic artery for epistaxis[24] but this is not recommended due to the risk of vision loss and the availability of a fairly easy and safe surgical procedure to ligate these vessels.

i) Accessory meningeal arteries may also rarely be a source of bleeding in epistaxis and can be embolized.[25]

j) A review of embolization compared to internal maxillary ligation suggested that ligation was more effective and, although the complications were more frequent than for embolization, the major complications of embolization (stroke) were more serious.[26]

k) In some centers, endoscopic ligation of the sphenopalatine artery is becoming a minimally invasive, safe, and effective first choice for the treatment of epistaxis.[27]

l) Embolization may become a second line choice after a failed endoscopic ligation, or where the expertise for endoscopic ligation is unavailable.

4) Post-traumatic and post-surgical bleeding

a) Treatment of post-traumatic or post-surgical bleeding is very similar to treatment of post-traumatic and post-surgical AVF (above). The main difference is the urgency of the situation.

b) A general rule: Damaged, bleeding vessels must be occluded definitively, except in cases when an obvious major neurological deficit will result.

c) For quick and definitive closure of the bleeding vessels, the main endovascular tools are detachable coils (for larger vessels), n-BCA (for smaller vessels) and detachable balloons (if available).

d) Consider the use of a proximal balloon catheter in the parent artery to control bleeding while catheterization and embolization of the damaged is going on.

e) Coiling of bleeding pseudoaneurysms extending into sinuses should always be avoided. The walls of pseudoaneurysms are too fragile to contain a coil mass beyond the acute phase, and the coils will inevitably erode through the walls of the pseudoaneurysm. The authors of this handbook have managed a patient with a previously coiled ICA pseudoaneurysm that extended into the sphenoid sinus; 1 year after treatment, the patient presented with coil strands coming out of his nose and down his throat.[28]

f) If occlusion of the carotid does not appear to be an option, based on limited collateral flow to the brain or a positive test occlusion, stent-graft placement may be the only endovascular option.

g) Prior to any major vascular occlusion, consider surgical options such as vascular repair or bypass, if the anatomic location is favorable.

5) Bleeding tumours

a) Embolization of tumours is usually done with particles, since they tend to lodge in the small vessels of the tumour bed and produce sufficient devascularization for surgical excision.

b) Particles may also be used for actively bleeding tumours, but, if possible, it may be quicker and more definitive to stop the bleeding with n-BCA, as long the microcatheter is positioned close to the lesion and no dangerous anastamoses are present.

c) If endovascular microcatheter access to the bleeding vessel is not possible, direct needle puncture and glue injection may be feasible.

6) Carotid blow-out syndrome

a) Carotid blow-out syndrome is catastrophic, sudden bleeding from the carotid in patients after surgical treatment for head and neck malignancy.[29] In popular jargon the term often refers to any sudden, spontaneous bleeding from the carotid.

b) Carotid blow-outs occur in ≤5% cases of advanced cancer patients after surgery and does not seem to be necessarily related to preoperative radiation therapy[30] although anecdotally, it may be seen soon after radiation therapy.[31] In any case, carotid blow-outs tend to occur in patients whose carotid may be minimally covered by healthy connective tissue.

c) Carotid blow-out is one of the most urgent situations imaginable, since patients can bleed to death, often drowning in their own blood, in minutes.

d) The airway should be secured by intubation, if not already done.

e) The bleeding site is packed to control bleeding and emergent angiography is helpful if there is time, since often the exact site of bleeding may be uncertain.

f) A large caliber sheath should be placed to maximize options for devices.

g) In patients that are not actively bleeding at the time of the arteriogram, a pseudoaneurysm is the usual angiographic sign of the bleeding site.[32]

h) Parent artery occlusion is the usual treatment, unless the collateral flow is limited by angiographic criteria. Test occlusion could be performed if the patient is clinically stable.

i) Delayed ischemic complications occur in 15–20% of cases with carotid occlusion, so stent-graft placement seems to be an attractive option, when feasible.[6] Reported results with self-expanding stent-grafts have been promising, but long-term patency rates are unknown. In a series of three patients treated for carotid blow-out with stent-grafts two went on to be thrombosed and/or exposed.[33]

j) Carotid blow-out syndrome can be a long-term problem in some patients; multiple episodes of massive bleeding were reported in 26% of patients with carotid blow-out syndrome.[34]

7) Tips for large vessel occlusion (see also Chaps. 5 and 7)

a) Indications

  i) Post-traumatic bleeding

  ii) Carotid blow-out syndrome

  iii) Pre-operative occlusion of large vessel involved with a tumor

  iv) Treatment of certain difficult aneurysms, pseudoaneurysms, AVFs, AVMs

b) Whenever possible, perform a test occlusion first.

  i) In emergency situations, tolerance of a large vessel occlusion may be estimated by angiographic evaluation of collaterals.

c) Whenever possible, use proximal flow control such as with a Merci balloon guide

8) Extracranial vascular tumours

a) Juvenile nasopharyngeal angiofibroma

  i) Hypervasular tumour in young boys that usually presents with nasal bleeding and nasal obstruction. In females, haemangiopericytoma can have a similar clinical presentation.

  ii) Angiographically, these lesions show an intense tumour blush supplied mainly by the distal internal maxillary artery branches with variable contributions from the accessory meningeal and ascending pharyngeal arteries. Larger tumours may be supplied from the petrous and cavernous carotid branches, the middle meningeal artery, and even the transverse facial artery.

iii) Preoperative particle embolization of the feeding arteries is effective in reducing blood loss, especially in larger tumours.[35]

iv) Vision loss from central retinal artery embolization[36] and facial nerve palsy[37] have been reported as a complication of angiofibroma embolization. These complications underscore the need for careful attention to technique, vigilance for dangerous anastamoses, and the use of provocative testing.

v) Direct tumour needle puncture and embolization with glue is an option for these tumors.[38] Tumours may have feeders from the carotid, potentially allowing retrograde flow of glue to the carotid, so constant vigilance for visualization of dangerous collaterals during the glue injection is mandatory.

b) Paragangioma (aka chemodectoma, glomus tumour)

i) These tumors include glomus jugulare, glomus tympanicum, carotid body tumours, glomus vagale, or rare paragangliomas of the larynx, orbit, paranasal sinuses, or elsewhere in the head and neck.

ii) The jugulare, tympanicum, carotid body, and vagale tumours all tend to have dominant vascular supply from one or more branches of the ascending pharyngeal artery. On angiography, these lesions have an intense tumour blush, often with some arteriovenous shunting.

iii) When these tumors become very large, it is sometimes difficult to determine from which location they have arisen. Larger tumors may have intracranial, even intradural extension, usually in the posterior fossa, with blood supply from the anterior inferior cerebellar artery or other intracranial branches in the posterior fossa.

iv) The primary indication for endovascular treatment is preoperative embolization. Rarely, palliative embolization may be done for inoperable lesions to slow progression of the tumour.

v) Embolization is usually done with particles from a transarterial route.[39] Provocative testing should be done because of the tendency of feeding vessels to also supply cranial nerves (Chap. 6). If a neurological deficit occurs with provocative lidocaine injection, embolization with larger particles (>300 µm) can still be done, because these particles are too large to get into branches going to cranial nerves.

vi) Onyx® embolization of both the arteries and veins may provide good hemostasis for the surgeon removing large paragangliomas.[40]

vii) Vascular tumours may also be directly punctured with a needle and injected with n-BCA.[41–44] Direct puncture with glue embolization still carries a risk of stroke through reflux of glue into carotid branches.[45]

c) Other vascular tumours

i) Preoperative or palliative embolization can be helpful for vascular metastases and other rare tumours in the head and neck.

ii) Transarterial particle embolization is most commonly done for any lesion with a capillary bed to trap small particles.

iii) Rarely, direct puncture with glue injection may be done when arterial access is difficult.[41,43]

d) Special situation: Kasabach Merritt syndrome

i) Kasabach Merritt syndrome is a consumptive coagulopathy with platelet and fibrinogen consumption associated with a large vascular lesion, often in the head and neck.

(1) Classically, the tumours were called involuting infantile haemangiomas, but more recently these have been diagnosed as Kaposiform haemangioendotheliomas (KHE).[46]

(2) Medical therapy with aspirin, steroids, vincristine and alpha interferon has been helpful controlling the coagulopathy.[47–49]

(3) Transarterial embolization of the primary feeding vessels with particles appears safe and effective and does not prevent re-embolization if needed.[47,48,50]

(4) A single case report touts Onyx as a good agent for KHE.[51] However, the dark tantalum in the agent can stain very superficial lesions and the occlusion of feeding arteries can prevent access for later embolization.

8.4. Complications of Head and Neck Embolization

Informed consent prior to any interventional procedure must include a discussion of the risk of complications. Published reports of series of embolization procedures should not be relied on to indicate the true risk of complications. It is human nature to rush to publicize good results and gloss over the bad. Especially in the case of extracranial embolization, the procedures are widely varied in the techniques and agents used and territories involved, so results and complications of, for example, epistaxis embolization with particles cannot be used to predict results from facial AVMs with n-BCA. The operator's personal experience and complication rates should also be disclosed if known.

Neurological Complications

1) Head and neck embolization carries a 1–2% risk of stroke due to thromboembolism. Stroke, blindness, or spinal cord infarct may occur from reflux of embolic material or passage through dangerous anastamoses.
2) Cranial nerve defect can occur with embolic material entering the blood supply to the nerve.
3) In spinal AVMs and AVFs passage of emboli into the veins, or even thrombosis induced by the embolization, may worsen venous congestion of the cord and cause worsening symptoms.[52,53]
4) AVFs with large draining veins may swell and compress neural structures after embolization.
5) Access complications can occur with dissection of access vessels, specifically the common carotid or subclavian.
6) Microcatheters or wires may fracture and embolize.
7) Use of liquid embolics can cause the microcatheter to be glued in place.

Non-neurological Complications

1) Embolization of superficial vessels in the head and neck can result in ischemia and necrosis of skin, mucosa, and other tissue.
2) In AV fistulas, embolic material may travel to the pulmonary circulation.[54,55]
3) Anaphylactic reactions to iodinated contrast or any of the medications used can occur as with any endovascular procedure.
4) Similarly, groin haematomas or other groin arterial injury can occur, as in any endovascular procedure.
5) Deep venous thrombosis and pulmonary embolism can occur.
6) Anesthesia-related complications can occur if using general anesthesia.
7) Use of Onyx in the external carotid circulation can cause bradycardia and asystole, presumably by induction of the trigeminocardiac reflex by toxic effects of the DMSO.[56] Reflexive bradyarrhythmia occurred in 7.5% of dural AVFs treated with Onyx.[57]

How to Avoid Extracranial Embolization Complications in Ten Easy Steps

1) Carefully study the angiograms and cross sectional imaging of the lesion and surrounding structures to have a clear understanding of the anatomy and pathology in the case.
2) Do microcatheter angiograms prior to embolization to look for reflux into normal territories or filling of dangerous anastamoses.

3) Familiarize yourself with the devices that will be used during the case, particularly if it is a device not commonly used (like a stent-graft or detachable balloons).
4) Focus on basic techniques such as flushing and microcatheter navigation.
5) In awake patients do provocative testing with amobarbital and lidocaine.
6) Use neurophysiological monitoring and provocative testing even when using general anesthesia in spinal embolization cases.
7) When embolizing with any agent, inject no faster than was done for the contrast injection during the microcatheter angiogram.
8) Immediately stop injecting when reflux occurs or if different vessels (potentially dangerous anastamoses) appear.
9) Do periodic guide catheter and microcatheter angiograms to monitor progress and to decide when to stop.
10) Pay constant attention to the patient: vital signs, neurological status, neurophysiological monitoring, and comfort level. It is all too easy to expend all of one's attention on the procedural aspects and forget the person underneath the sterile drape.

8.5. Percutaneous Procedures

Indications

1) Superficial venous and lymphatic malformation
   a) These lesions are usually cosmetic problems that were present at birth and can usually be accurately diagnosed on MRI imaging.
   b) These lesions can be differentiated from AVMs by the absence of a bruit and thrill.
   c) Unlike AVMs, there is no role for transarterial embolization of any kind. Sadly, the authors of this handbook have seen too many patients who have been misdiagnosed and even previously treated by transarterial embolization with absolutely no benefit.
   d) Percutaneous sclerotherapy and/or laser treatments and/or surgical excision are the effective treatments.[8]
2) Superficial arteriovenous malformations
   a) These lesions are percutaneously accessible vascular tumours. Embolization is done pre-operatively (common) or for palliation (rare).
3) Juvenile nasopharyngeal angiofibroma
4) Paraganglioma (aka chemodectoma, glomus tumour)
5) A wide variety of other primary and metastatic vascular tumours.

Percutaneous Sclerotherapy: Technique

This technique is used for the treatment of superficial arteriovenous malformations as well as venous and lymphatic malformations.[8] It has also been used for preoperative or definitive treatment of haemangiomas.[58] When using the sclerotherapy technique for arteriovenous malformations, an arterial catheter is used to angiographically localize the target lesion and monitor progress. Angiographic catheters are not used when treating venous or lymphatic malformations.
1) Sclerosing agents
   a) Ethanol
      i) Advantage: Readily available. Cheap. Very effective sclerosant.
      ii) Disadvantage: Requires high concentration. *Painful.*[59] Higher risk of local complications.[59] Can have systemic complications in high doses.
   b) Bleomycin
      i) Advantages: Much fewer local and systemic complications than ethanol make it the preferred choice for venous and lymphatic malformations.[59] Less painful.

ii) Disadvantages: Must be treated with the same precautions as any chemotherapy drug. Usually must be specially mixed by hospital pharmacy. Requires more sessions of sclerotherapy to achieve the same clinical result

2) Anesthesia
   a) Percutaneous ethanol sclerotherapy is almost always performed under general anesthesia because the ethanol injection is very painful.
   b) Bleomycin is less painful, although many practitioners still use anesthesia

3) Access
   a) The area of the lesion is localized by palpation or ultrasonic localization, or in the case of AVM, by contrast injection in the feeding artery for road-map guidance.
   b) For an AVM, the lesion can accessed by puncturing the artery close to the nidus, the nidus itself, or the proximal vein close to the nidus. For venous and lymphatic malformations, the ideal puncture site is the larger cavernous spaces within the lesion. The skin overlying the lesion is prepared and draped and local anesthetic injected intradermally at the site of the expected needle puncture.
   c) Insert a 22 gauge spinal needle for deep lesions or butterfly for superficial lesions. Place the tip at the expected depth of the lesion. Check for return of blood or lymphatic fluid. Reposition the needle if good return is not obtained. Bright red pulsatile blood indicates that AVM has been punctured; dark blue blood indicates puncture of venous malformation, and straw-colored or slightly bloody fluid is seen with puncture of lymphatic malformations. Once good return from the needle is seen, do a digital subtraction angiogram with injection of contrast through the needle.
   d) For venous and lymphatic malformations, a second needle may be used to puncture another part of the now contrast-filled malformation. The second needle allows drainage of fluid from the lesion as the ethanol is injected to remove the diluting blood or fluid and reduce the risk of over-pressurizing the lesion with ethanol and creating leakage back along the needle.[60]

4) Injection
   a) Study the angiogram images to ensure that the needle is in a vascular space, and that it fills the lesion. Estimate the rate and volume required to opacify the territory that is to be occluded.
   b) If the flow is extremely rapid, consider placing a coil or two through the needle to slow the flow. Ten-system fibered coils will pass through a 22-gauge needle; 18-system coils will pass through thin-wall 19 gauge or any 18 gauge needle. Most cases will not require coils, especially if the flow can be manually slowed by manual compression of the draining veins, or by placement over the area of a compressive O-ring affixed to the skin over the lesion. Do a repeat percutaneous angiogram when the venous outlets are compressed, to assess the change in flow and to check the rate and volume required to opacify the lesion.
   c) Flush the needle with saline because ethanol can cause contrast to precipitate. It is usually easiest to attach a short extension tubing to the needle with a one-way stopcock at the end of the tubing to control back-bleeding through the needle.
   d) Inject absolute ethanol at a rate similar to that which opacified the vessel, but use only approximately 50% of the volume of contrast used. If a second needle is positioned in the lesion, remove the stylet and let it back-bleed during the ethanol injection to relieve the pressure within it.
   e) After the first injection, let at least 5 min elapse and then release the pressure on the veins and check for back-bleeding from the injected needle. If rapid return is obtained, inject another dose of ethanol equal to 50% of the volume of contrast needed to opacify the lesion. After waiting another 5 min, again check for return from the needle. If the return is still brisk, repeat the contrast injection. If the vessel remains patent, inject another small bolus (1 or 2 ml) of ethanol, and wait again.
   f) If vasospasm is seen on repeat test injections, wait until it resolves and decrease the volume of ethanol boluses.
   g) Stop the ethanol injection when there is no longer blood return or if blanching or discoloration of the skin is seen to prevent damage to the soft tissues and skin.
   h) If there is no change after 20 mL of ethanol, consider placement of additional coils to slow the flow and help the ethanol work, or try n-BCA as the embolic agent.

i) Remember that ethanol can work on the endothelium for some time and can also spread through the vessel wall into the adjacent tissues, so it is best to keep the ethanol volumes to a minimum.

j) To minimize local tissue damage, it is best to stage the procedure rather than attempting to cure the lesion with a single session. The maximum recommended ethanol dose per session is 1 mL per kg body weight.[60,61]

k) When the puncture cavity appears to be thrombosed, wait another 5 min and then remove the needle and hold manual pressure for approximately 5–10 min or when hemostasis is obtained.

l) If only a few ml of ethanol have been injected, a second needle puncture (use a new needle) and additional ethanol injections may be done.

m) It is time to stop when swelling or discoloration at the puncture site is seen or if the ethanol dose gets over 20–30 ml, and absolutely if 1 ml/kg is reached.[61]

n) When using bleomycin, inject a volume approximately 1 mL at a time and plan on injecting approximately the total volume of contrast required to fill the space.

o) Wait 5 min between injections and be certain to check that blood or fluid can be aspirated between injections. Note that thrombosis of the space is not as common with bleomycin.

p) Keep the total dose of bleomycin each day to less than 0.5 units /kg body weight.

Percutaneous n-BCA Injection: Technique

This technique involves direct puncture and glue embolization of feeding vessels that may have been ligated[9] or direct puncture and embolization of AVMs[62] or vascular tumours in the head and neck[41–43] or spine.[63]

1) Access

a) Park an arterial catheter in the feeding artery to the vascular lesion to allow for roadmap imaging and control angiography.

b) Prep and drape the skin overlying the target and inject local anesthetic (2% lidocaine).

c) Using a roadmap, plan a trajectory to allow direct needle access to the target without hitting any vital structures. Biplane or 3D roadmapping is particularly useful.

d) For very superficial lesions plan an oblique trajectory to allow the skin and tissues to stabilize the needle once it is positioned in the lesion.

e) Insert a 22 gauge spinal needle with a metal hub under roadmap guidance to the desired position. Remove the stylet when the needle seems deep enough to look for blood return. If no return is obtained the needle should be advanced or withdrawn until good blood flow is obtained.

f) In the scalp and face the tumour or vessels may be mobile and it may take some manipulation to puncture the lesion and not glance off it.

g) Once good blood return is obtained, do an angiogram with injection of contrast through the needle to:
   i) Confirm proper positioning
   ii) Look for any filling of normal vessels or dangerous anastomoses
   iii) Time the volume required to fill the lesion
   iv) Determine the arteriovenous transit time

2) n-BCA preparation

a) Prepare the n-BCA on a second sterile back table that is saline-free. As always when using glue, all persons near the sterile field should wear glasses or other eye protection. If a connection comes loose during injection, the glue can spray and stick to whatever it touches.

b) Rule of thumb: For high-flow fistulas use a concentrated mixture such as a 70% glue (three parts n-BCA to one part Ethiodol®). Most tumours require a dilute mixture, such as 20% (one part n-BCA to four parts Ethiodol).

c) Tantalum powder greatly increases the radio-opacity of glue, but is not absolutely necessary unless the glue mixture is greater than 70% n-BCA. Tantalum is messy and can clump, and also the pigment may be visible through the skin in superficial vessels, so most operators usually avoid it in the extracranial circulation.

d) Draw up the Trufill® n-BCA (Codman Neurovascular, Raynham, MA) using a labeled, glue-compatible 3 mL syringe (avoid polycarbonate plastic...it softens).

e) Draw up the Ethiodol® in a labeled syringe, and add the proper volume to the glue syringe.

f) Have several labeled 3 mL syringes filled with 5% dextrose solution ready.

3) Injection

a) Re-confirm proper needle positioning with a small contrast injection.

b) Select a projection that shows the needle tip and its relationship to any curves in the arterial feeder distal to the needle, any visible normal branches, and the lesion.

c) Attach a glue-compatible stopcock directly to the needle. One-way stopcocks are sufficient, but three-way are preferred since it allows a flush syringe of dextrose to remain attached even when the glue syringe is attached. Be careful not to move the needle when attaching stopcocks or syringes.

d) Thoroughly flush the needle with 5% dextrose solution. About 2–3 mL is sufficient to clear all saline and/or blood from the needle lumen. As the last mL of dextrose is being injected, close the stopcock to prevent blood backflow into the needle.

e) Make a blank roadmap to make the glue easy to visualize.

f) Attach a 3 mL syringe loaded with the glue mixture and slowly and steadily inject the glue using the blank roadmap. Watch to make sure that the glue column is continuously moving forward during the injection. Fill the arterial feeder and as much of the nidus or tumour bed as possible.

g) Be on the alert for reflux of glue back along arterial feeders, passage of glue into the vein, or reflux of glue through the nidus or tumour bed into other potentially dangerous arterial branches feeding the lesion. If any of these conditions is occurring and one is using dilute glue, one might be able to aspirate to stop forward motion, then after a brief pause, resume cautiously. Sometimes the glue will find another pathway through the nidus.

h) In high flow AVMs, flow can be controlled during the glue injection by manual compression of draining veins or by placement of a compressive dressing or O-ring[7] over the skin overlying superficial lesions.

i) Close the stopcock when the glue injection is complete and wait. Polymerization will be complete within a few minutes. Rotate the needle to break the bond with the injected glue and then remove it.

j) Once the needle is removed and hemostasis obtained at the puncture site, do a follow-up arteriogram to ensure that the desired result is obtained. If other segments of the lesion remain patent, addition needle punctures and glue injections may be done.

Complications of Percutaneous Injection Procedures

Informed consent prior to any interventional procedure must include a discussion of the risk of complications.

Neurological Complications

1. Nerve damage is possible, particularly to the facial nerve, if the sclerosing agent is injected near the nerve.
2. Cranial nerve injury can occur with embolic material entering the blood supply to the nerve.
3. Stroke, blindness, and spinal cord infarction can occur from embolic material reflux or passage through dangerous anastamoses.
4. Large lesions may swell and compress neural structures after treatment.

Non-neurological Complications

1. Sclerotherapy in the head and neck can result in ischemia and necrosis of skin, mucosa, or other tissues.
2. Pulmonary embolization is possible during treatment of AV fistulas and venous malformations.
3. Anaphylactic reactions to iodinated contrast or any of the medications used can occur as with any endovascular procedure.
4. Similarly, groin haematomas and other groin arterial injury can occur, as in any endovascular procedure.
5. Anesthesia-related complications can occur.

8.6.   Spinal Embolization

Indications: Spinal Embolization

1. Type I spinal dural arteriovenous fistula (dAVF) (not common, but not rare)
   (a) Preoperative embolization
   (b) Definitive embolization
2. Type II spinal intramedullary AVM (rare)
   (a) Preoperative embolization
   (b) Palliative embolization for symptom reduction
   (c) Focused embolization of features at risk for bleeding (e.g., intranidal aneurysms)
3. Type III juvenile AVM (very rare)
   (a) Palliative embolization for symptom reduction
4. Type IV perimedullary AVF (very rare)
   (a) Definitive embolization
   (b) Pre-operative embolization
5. Spinal vascular tumours: Pre-operative embolization
   (a) Haemangioblastoma (rare)
   (b) Primary bone lesions (e.g., aneurysmal bone cyst) (uncommon)
   (c) Vascular metastatic tumours (e.g., renal cell cancer, thyroid cancer) (very common)

Awake or Asleep?

Use of glue or ethanol can cause considerable pain due to the toxic nature of these agents, and the pain makes it difficult for even sedated patients to remain motionless. General anesthesia eliminates this discomfort and allows the operator to focus on the procedure rather than on coaching and assessing the patient. It can make the procedure much more palatable for anxious patients. Another advantage of general anesthesia is that it allows for patient immobility including prolonged interruption of respiration while imaging tiny spinal vessels. The limited ability to monitor the neurological status of the patient during general anesthesia may be partially mitigated by the use of neurophysiological monitoring, such as somatosensory and/or motor evoked potentials. Neurophysiological monitoring adds to the cost and complexity of the procedure, and may not be readily available or reliable, depending on the institution. However, the authors of this handbook find monitoring very useful for spinal embolization, and use it for virtually all embolization of intramedullary lesions, even in awake patients. Less complicated bone or paraspinal soft tissue tumour embolization can be easily done under local anesthesia with minimal sedation, and adequate image quality is possible in cooperative patients.

Embolization with the patient awake permits continuous neurological monitoring, eliminates the risks of general anesthesia, can shorten the length of the case, and is done in many centers. The authors of this handbook prefer to do most cases of embolization other than intramedullary spinal embolization awake with conscious sedation, to allow for provocative testing. Vascular navigation in the extracranial circulation is also much less challenging than in intracranial embolization procedures, so it is less critical that the patient remains motionless.

Guide Catheters for Spinal Embolization

Guide catheters for spinal intervention have two special characteristics:
- They have complex curves that allow the catheter to have relatively stable positioning in the transversely-oriented spinal branches.
- They are relatively short (60–80 cm), since that is all that is needed to access these vessels.

1) Standard spinal angiography catheters, like the 5F Mikaelsson and the 5F Simmons I (Merit Medical, South Jordan, UT), are complex-curved catheters that can readily engage side-branches of the aorta.
   a) *Advantages*: Reverse curve provides stability in transverse branches of the aorta. Non-hydrophilic coating makes the catheter more stable in the vessel.
   b) *Disadvantages*: These catheters are soft and may back out and disengage from the vessel as the microcatheter is advanced through it. Microcatheters fit tightly in these catheters, so guide catheter angiograms cannot usually be done while the microcatheter is in place.

2) 4F angled Glidecath® (Terumo Medical, Somerset, NJ)[5] or 4F Berenstein II (Cordis Endovascular, Miami Lakes, FL)[64] can be advanced distally into the intercostal or lumbar arteries. The usual technique for these catheters is use a standard spinal angiography catheter to first engage the spinal artery and then exchange it for the 4F catheter over an exchange-length wire.[64]
   a) *Advantages*: Soft, atraumatic tip. Minimizes risk of vasospasm and dissection in narrow and tortuous vessels. When placed distally in a segmental vessel, these catheters are a fairly stable platform for 10-system microcatheters.
   b) *Disadvantages*: Relatively flimsy and prone to become displaced, especially when the vasculature is tortuous. Requires the use of an exchange wire to access the lumbar or intercostal artery. Larger caliber microcatheters may not easily pass through these catheters. Even small microcatheters are a tight fit and it is not possible to inject contrast around the microcatheter.

3) 6 or 7F coronary guide catheters like the Runway™ (Boston Scientific, Natick, MA) can be obtained with various curves such as the Amplatz left or allRight™ curve that can engage segmental spinal vessels.
   a) *Advantages*: Very stable platforms. Gigantic internal lumen. Will accept various devices and microcatheters with room to spare for contrast injections.
   b) *Disadvantages*: These are big, stiff catheters can be traumatic to the vessel and not easily used in tortuous vessels. May not engage vessels that arise at a sharp angle from the aorta. Often require the use of an exchange wire to access the vessel of interest.

4) Standard 5 or 6F guide catheters such as the Envoy® (Codman Neurovascular, Raynham, MA) or Guider Softip™ XF (Stryker Neurovascular, Fremont, CA) work well if spinal vessels in the cervical or upper thoracic region are accessed through subclavian artery branches.

Guide Catheter Technique: Segmental Spinal Arteries

1) *Direct navigation method*. Useful in young patients with non-tortuous, non-atherosclerotic vessels, and when using a catheter with a complex, reverse curve shape.
   a) Flush the catheter with heparinized saline and attach it to an RHV with continuous flush.
   b) Advance the hydrophilic wire to the tip of the guide catheter to stiffen it and allow passage through the valve in the hub of the sheath. Use the peel-away introducer to insert the tip of the catheter into the sheath, but

do not peel it off. Just slide it back to the hub of the catheter to keep it out of the way and available to use again if needed.

   c) Advance the catheter over the hydrophilic wire into the abdominal aorta. Reconstitute the shaped catheter by one of two methods:
       i) If the hydrophilic wire can easily be advanced into the contralateral iliac artery or a renal artery, the curve of the complex curve catheter (e.g. Mikaelsson or Simmons) may be formed by advancing the catheter just enough to engage the renal or iliac artery. Then, withdraw the hydrophilic wire into the catheter and gently push and rotate the catheter to form the curve.
      ii) Alternatively, advance the catheter into the aortic arch. When the hydrophilic wire is pulled back, the catheter usually reconstitutes as the catheter is rotated.

   d) Withdraw the wire completely and double flush the catheter with heparinized saline.

   e) Position the tip of the catheter at the target spinal level. With small puffs of contrast, gently rotate and manipulate the catheter tip into the origin of the segmental artery. Gently pull the catheter back to advance it into the segmental artery for 1–2 cm to obtain a stable position.
       i) If the catheter does not advance into the vessel when it is pulled back, park it at the origin of the artery and place a microcatheter into the artery over a microwire. The guide catheter can then be pulled back, advanced forward, or rotated *very gently* into a more stable position. Movement that is too vigorous will push the guide catheter back into the aorta.

   f) Occasionally, in younger patients with large segmental spinal arteries, a simple curved guide catheter can be manipulated into a segmental artery using a steerable hydrophilic wire such as a 0.035 in. or 0.038 in. Glidewire® (Terumo Medical, Somerset, NJ).

2) *Exchange method.* Useful when using a 4F guide catheter and also often when using larger coronary-type guide catheters.
   a) Place a 5F diagnostic spinal catheter in the segmental spinal artery over an exchange length (270–300 cm) wire, usually a hydrophilic wire like Glidewire® (Terumo Medical, Somerset, NJ).
   b) Advance the tip of the wire into a distal branch of the artery using a roadmap.
   c) Exchange the diagnostic catheter for the guide catheter under fluoroscopy.

3) *Optimizing guide catheter position in spinal cases*
   a) Guide catheter stability can be a huge problem in spinal embolization cases given the continual movement of the vessels with respiration and the fairly proximal guide catheter position that is necessary in many cases. In a lumbar or intercostal artery with a significant proximal curve, the guide catheter may easily advance beyond the origin of the vessel. Moderate curves in the vessel usually cannot be straightened out by guiding a relatively stiff catheter around them, and may cause spasm or even dissection. If added guide catheter stability is needed, a relatively stiff 0.014 in. wire can be advanced through the guide catheter as a buddy wire, and if the catheter has a large enough lumen, a microcatheter can be advanced alongside it. The buddy wire will help keep the guide catheter in place. Buddy wires cannot be used when 5F or smaller catheters are used as guide catheters.
   b) Many times only very tenuous catheter positioning is possible, and one must keep an eye on the guide catheter position *constantly* during the case and gently adjust its position as necessary.

4) *Guide catheter irrigation*
   a) Continuous irrigation of the guide with heparinized saline (5,000 U heparin per 500 mL saline) is important.

5) *Contrast injections*
   a) Frequent puffing of contrast can be used to help manipulate the guide catheter into spinal segmental arteries. A 20 mL syringe containing contrast can be left attached to the catheter for these injections, and then used immediately for hand injections of contrast for angiographic runs. As is done in the cerebral arteries, the syringe is held vertically with care not to allow bubbles to enter the catheter. Spinal arteries are best imaged with hand injections of contrast, to allow for modulation of

the injection rate and volume, depending on the size of the vessel and stability of the catheter.

6) *Maintaining guide catheter position*
   a) Monitor the position of the guide catheter constantly during the microcatheter access and embolization phases of the procedure.
   b) The guide catheter may become displaced during microcatheter navigation, which can result in kinking of the microcatheter and can cause sudden, undesired displacement of the microcatheter.
   c) Any displacement of the guide catheter tip should be corrected. If the guide catheter becomes too unstable, consider replacing it with a more stable guide catheter.

Techniques and Tips on Spinal Embolization for Specific Lesions

Type I Spinal Dural Arteriovenous Fistula (dAVF)

1) Particle embolization of dAVFs has been shown to be a temporary solution, and recurrence is by far the rule, not the exception.[65,66] Embolization with n-BCA is more effective, with 55% improvement in gait and a 15% recurrence rate.[67] Embolization with Onyx has also been reported.[68]
2) A contraindication to embolization is a spinal cord feeder arising from the same radicular artery supplying the fistula, which is present in approximately 6% of cases.[69]
3) Endovascular treatment consists of full-column n-BCA injection in the radicular artery feeding the fistula with glue dilute enough to be pushed through the fistula into the intradural vein.
4) The authors of this handbook frequently place a microcoil in the lumbar or intercostal feeder beyond the radicular branch, to prevent the glue from entering muscular branches. *Embolization of muscular branches can cause severe pain.*[70]
5) A post-embolization CT, confirming intradural venous location of the glue column, is a good way to predict who will have a long-term cure.[52]
6) Both surgery and endovascular treatment can lead to improvement in gait but not bladder dysfunction if the symptom duration prior to treatment is >1 year.[71]
7) Several groups advocate an attempt at endovascular treatment first, reserving surgical treatment for unsuccessful embolization.[72,73]
8) Close clinical and imaging follow-up is needed in all spinal fistula patients. Recurrence of symptoms after successful treatment should prompt a full angiographic workup, since collaterals may enlarge to supply the fistula and even remote new fistulas may develop.[69]

Type II Spinal Intramedullary AVM

1) Carefully study the spinal angiogram to determine all arterial feeders, draining veins, and the relationship of the AVM with normal spinal cord vessels. Look for associated feeding artery and intranidal aneurysms. *Do not treat the lesion until the anatomy is thoroughly understood and a plan of action has been formulated.*
2) Slow PVA particle embolization has been advocated for intramedullary AVMs.[74,75] The endpoint of particle embolization can be objectively determined by serial provocative testing (stop when the provocative testing shows neurological changes) and/or serial pressure measurements from the microcatheter (stop when the microcatheter pressure rises to 90% of systemic pressure).[5] However, AVMs treated with particle embolization frequently recanalize.[65,76]
3) Embolization with n-BCA may be more effective and safer than particle embolization in experienced hands.[2,77]
4) Monitoring with SSEPs and MEPs, as well as provocative testing prior to embolization, may reduce the risk of complications.[2–4,78]

5) Catheterization of the nidus with a flow-directed microcatheter is the goal, with a careful full column glue injection after a negative provocative testing.
6) Aneurysms associated with the AVM should be specifically targeted for embolization to reduce the risk of AVM bleeding.[79]
7) A study 17 patients with intramedullary AVMs treated with Onyx® embolization reported a 37% acute cure rate; 82% had a good clinical result with no permanent neurological procedural complications.[80,81]
8) A study of functional and emotional quality of life in spinal cord AVM patients after embolization showed significantly worse scores compared to patients with post-traumatic spinal cord problems.[82] This suggests that further improvements in treatment of these patients are necessary.

Type III Juvenile AVM

1) These diffuse AVMs with cord and segmental spinal and paraspinal nidus are difficult to treat, or at least to cure, but are extremely rare.
2) Palliative embolization with glue or Onyx® for symptom reduction has been reported.[83,84]
3) Successful surgical resection following embolization has been reported.[85–88] Combined arterial and venous embolization followed by surgical resection of a large AVM associated with Cobb syndrome has also been reported.[89]

Type IV Perimedullary AVF

1) These lesions are rare perimedullary fistulas without an intervening nidus. They can present with hemorrhage or progressive myelopathy. They can have multiple arterial feeders and prominent congestion of the perimedullary veins that can make the angiogram challenging to figure out.
2) As with all spinal vascular malformations, a high quality spinal angiogram and a though visualization and understanding of the vascular anatomy and pathology are mandatory before considering treatment.
3) Preoperative embolization via a transarterial route has been successful and reported in several small series.[90–93]
4) Surgical treatment reserved for accessible fistulas and for those in which embolization failed to occlude the fistula.[94,95]
5) Conus and filum terminale AVFs are usually best treated surgically.[77,95]
6) Some large fistulas (so-called Type IV-c lesions) can be treated with transvenous coiling either via a standard transfemoral venous approach[94] or though surgical access to the dilated veins.[96]
7) Primary endovascular treatment for giant fistulas with detachable balloons in 10 patients reported six good clinical results and one complication caused by migration of the balloon into the draining vein.[53]
8) A French study of glue transarterial n-BCA embolization reported a 67% rate of angiographic cure; 22% had transient neurological deficits, but all had improvement in all at follow-up.[97] Clinical improvement was stable in cases in which complete angiographic cure was not obtained.[98]
9) Use highly concentrated n-BCA preparations (≥70%) for high flow fistulas.
10) Careful and complete angiographic follow-up is needed in these patients, since they can develop co-existing separate Type I dural fistulas, which likely develop because of venous hypertension.[99]

Epidural and Paraspinal AVF

1) These are rare congenital or acquired fistulas often presenting with radiculopathy, but occasionally with myelopathy if venous drainage backs up into the spinal cord veins.[100,101]
2) Treatment may be transarterial embolization, or surgical interruption of the radicular veins that provide the conduit for arterialized blood to the intradural veins.

Spinal Vascular Tumours: Pre-operative Embolization

1) Preoperative embolization of spinal cord haemangioblastomas has been reported.[102,103] One of four patients undergoing preoperative embolization for thoracolumbar haemangioblastomas had transient worsening myelopathy.[104]

2) Vascular tumours in the spinal region, most commonly metastatic renal cell cancer or less commonly thyroid cancer, seem to benefit greatly from preoperative particle embolization.[105–107]

3) Primary bone lesions (e.g., aneurysmal bone cyst) can benefit from preoperative particle embolization.

4) Do a *vigilant* angiographic search for collateral connections to normal spinal cord arteries. Serial provocative testing with clinical and/or SSEP and MEP monitoring can reduce the risk of inadvertent passage of emboli to the spinal cord circulation.[106]

5) Symptomatic spinal osseous haemangiomas may benefit from transarterial preoperative embolization[108] or percutaneous vertebroplasty.[109] These lesions may also be treated with direct needle puncture and ethanol injection, but the total ethanol volume should be kept <15 mL to prevent complications.[110]

References

1. Deveikis JP. Sequential injections of amobarbital sodium and lidocaine for provocative neurologic testing in the external carotid circulation. AJNR Am J Neuroradiol. 1996;17: 1143–7.
2. Niimi Y, Sala F, Deletis V, Setton A, de Camargo AB, Berenstein A. Neurophysiologic monitoring and pharmacologic provocative testing for embolization of spinal cord arteriovenous malformations. AJNR Am J Neuroradiol. 2004;25: 1131–8.
3. Katayama Y, Tsubokawa T, Hirayama T, Himi K, Koyama S, Yamamoto T. Embolization of intramedullary spinal arteriovenous malformation fed by the anterior spinal artery with monitoring of the corticospinal motor evoked potential–case report. Neurol Med Chir (Tokyo). 1991;31:401–5.
4. Sala F, Niimi Y, Krzan MJ, Berenstein A, Deletis V. Embolization of a spinal arteriovenous malformation: correlation between motor evoked potentials and angiographic findings: technical case report. Neurosurgery. 1999;45:932–7; discussion 937–8.
5. Touho H, Karasawa J, Ohnishi H, Yamada K, Ito M, Kinoshita A. Intravascular treatment of spinal arteriovenous malformations using a microcatheter – with special reference to serial xylocaine tests and intravascular pressure monitoring. Surg Neurol. 1994;42:148–56.
6. Lesley WS, Chaloupka JC, Weigele JB, Mangla S, Dogar MA. Preliminary experience with endovascular reconstruction for the management of carotid blowout syndrome. AJNR Am J Neuroradiol. 2003;24:975–81.
7. Ryu CW, Whang SM, Suh DC, et al. Percutaneous direct puncture glue embolization of high-flow craniofacial arteriovenous lesions: a new circular ring compression device with a beveled edge. AJNR Am J Neuroradiol. 2007;28:528–30.
8. Deveikis JP. Percutaneous ethanol sclerotherapy for vascular malformations in the head and neck. Arch Facial Plast Surg. 2005;7:322–5.
9. Gobin YP, Pasco A, Merland JJ, Aymard AA, Casasco A, Houdart E. Percutaneous puncture of the external carotid artery or its branches after surgical ligation. AJNR Am J Neuroradiol. 1994;15:79–82.
10. Riles TS, Berenstein A, Fisher FS, Persky MS, Madrid M. Reconstruction of the ligated external carotid artery for embolization of cervicofacial arteriovenous malformations. J Vasc Surg. 1993;17:491–8.
11. Halbach VV, Higashida RT, Hieshima GB, Hardin CW. Arteriovenous fistula of the internal maxillary artery: treatment with transarterial embolization. Radiology. 1988;168: 443–5.
12. Gabrielsen TO, Deveikis JP, Introcaso JH, Coran AG. Congenital arteriovenous fistulas supplied by a single branch of the maxillary artery. AJNR Am J Neuroradiol. 1994;15: 653–7.
13. Kim BS, Lee SK, terBrugge KG. Endovascular treatment of congenital arteriovenous fistulae of the internal maxillary artery. Neuroradiology. 2003;45:445–50.
14. Redekop G, Marotta T, Weill A. Treatment of traumatic aneurysms and arteriovenous fistulas of the skull base by using endovascular stents. J Neurosurg. 2001;95:412–9.
15. du Toit DF, Leith JG, Strauss DC, Blaszczyk M, Odendaal JV, Warren BL. Endovascular management of traumatic cervicothoracic arteriovenous fistula. Br J Surg. 2003;90:1516–21.
16. Schonholz CJ, Uflacker R, De Gregorio MA, Parodi JC. Stent-graft treatment of trauma to the supra-aortic arteries. A review. J Cardiovasc Surg (Torino). 2007;48:537–49.
17. Yoshida S, Nakazawa K, Oda Y. Spontaneous vertebral arteriovenous fistula–case report. Neurol Med Chir (Tokyo). 2000;40:211–5.
18. Passos Filho PE, Mattana PR, Pontalti JL, Silva FM. Endovascular treatment of spontaneous vertebral arteriovenous fistula in children: case report. Arq Neuropsiquiatr. 2002;60:502–4.
19. Merland JJ, Reizine D, Riche MC, et al. Endovascular treatment of vertebral arteriovenous fistulas in twenty-two patients. Ann Vasc Surg. 1986;1:73–8.
20. Halbach VV, Higashida RT, Hieshima GB. Treatment of vertebral arteriovenous fistulas. AJR Am J Roentgenol. 1988; 150:405–12.
20a. Christensen NP, Smith DS, Barnwell SL, Wax MK. Arterial embolization in the management of posterior epistaxis. Otolaryngol Head Neck Surg. 2005;133:748–53.
21. Tseng EY, Narducci CA, Willing SJ, Sillers MJ. Angiographic embolization for epistaxis: a review of 114 cases. Laryngoscope. 1998;108:615–9.
22. Elden L, Montanera W, Terbrugge K, Willinsky R, Lasjaunias P, Charles D. Angiographic embolization for the treatment of epistaxis: a review of 108 cases. Otolaryngol Head Neck Surg. 1994;111:44–50.
23. Shaw SM, Kamani T, Ali A, Manjaly G, Jeffree M. Sphenopalatine-sphenopalatine anastomosis: a unique cause of intractable epistaxis, safely treated with microcatheter embolization: a case report. J Med Case Reports. 2007;1: 125.
24. Moser FG, Rosenblatt M, De La Cruz F, Silver C, Burde RM. Embolization of the ophthalmic artery for control of epistaxis: report of two cases. Head Neck. 1992;14:308–11.
25. Duncan IC, Dos Santos C. Accessory meningeal arterial supply to the posterior nasal cavity: another reason for failed endovascular treatment of epistaxis. Cardiovasc Intervent Radiol. 2003;26:488–91.
26. Cullen MM, Tami TA. Comparison of internal maxillary artery ligation versus embolization for refractory posterior epistaxis. Otolaryngol Head Neck Surg. 1998;118:636–42.
27. Snyderman CH, Goldman SA, Carrau RL, Ferguson BJ, Grandis JR. Endoscopic sphenopalatine artery ligation is an effective method of treatment for posterior epistaxis. Am J Rhinol. 1999;13:137–40.
28. Zhuang Q, Buckman CR, Harrigan MR. Coil extrusion after endovascular treatment. Case illustration. J Neurosurg. 2007;106:512.
29. Borsanyi SJ. Rupture of the carotids following radical neck surgery in radiated patients. Eye Ear Nose Throat Mon. 1962;41:531–3.
30. Marcial VA, Gelber R, Kramer S, Snow JB, Davis LW, Vallecillo LA. Does preoperative irradiation increase the rate of surgical complications in carcinoma of the head and neck? A Radiation Therapy Oncology Group Report. Cancer. 1982;49:1297–301.
31. Gupta S. Radiation induced carotid artery blow out: a case report. Acta Chir Belg. 1994;94:299–300.
32. Chaloupka JC, Putman CM, Citardi MJ, Ross DA, Sasaki CT. Endovascular therapy for the carotid blowout syndrome in head and neck surgical patients: diagnostic and managerial considerations. AJNR Am J Neuroradiol. 1996;17:843–52.
33. Warren FM, Cohen JI, Nesbit GM, Barnwell SL, Wax MK, Andersen PE. Management of carotid 'blowout' with endovascular stent grafts. Laryngoscope. 2002;112:428–33.
34. Chaloupka JC, Roth TC, Putman CM, et al. Recurrent carotid blowout syndrome: diagnostic and therapeutic challenges in a newly recognized subgroup of patients. AJNR Am J Neuroradiol. 1999;20:1069–77.
35. Moulin G, Chagnaud C, Gras R, et al. Juvenile nasopharyngeal angiofibroma: comparison of blood loss during removal in embolized group versus nonembolized group. Cardiovasc Intervent Radiol. 1995;18:158–61.
36. Onerci M, Gumus K, Cil B, Eldem B. A rare complication of embolization in juvenile nasopharyngeal angiofibroma. Int J Pediatr Otorhinolaryngol. 2005;69:423–8.
37. Ikram M, Khan K, Murad M, Haq TU. Facial nerve palsy: unusual complication of percutaneous angiography and embolization for juvenile angiofibroma. J Pak Med Assoc. 1999;49:201–2.
38. Tranbahuy P, Borsik M, Herman P, Wassef M, Casasco A. Direct intratumoral embolization of juvenile angiofibroma. Am J Otolaryngol. 1994;15:429–35.
39. Valavanis A. Preoperative embolization of the head and neck: indications, patient selection, goals, and precautions. AJNR Am J Neuroradiol. 1986;7:943–52.

40. Rimbot A, Mounayer C, Loureiro C, et al. Preoperative mixed embolization of a paraganglioma using Onyx. J Neuroradiol. 2007;34:334–9.

41. Casasco A, Herbreteau D, Houdart E, et al. Devascularization of craniofacial tumors by percutaneous tumor puncture. AJNR Am J Neuroradiol. 1994;15:1233–9.

42. Abud DG, Mounayer C, Benndorf G, Piotin M, Spelle L, Moret J. Intratumoral injection of cyanoacrylate glue in head and neck paragangliomas. AJNR Am J Neuroradiol. 2004;25:1457–62.

43. Chaloupka JC, Mangla S, Huddle DC, et al. Evolving experience with direct puncture therapeutic embolization for adjunctive and palliative management of head and neck hypervascular neoplasms. Laryngoscope. 1999;109: 1864–72.

44. Harman M, Etlik O, Unal O. Direct percutaneous embolization of a carotid body tumor with n-butyl cyanoacrylate: an alternative method to endovascular embolization. Acta Radiol. 2004;45:646–8.

45. Krishnamoorthy T, Gupta AK, Rajan JE, Thomas B. Stroke from delayed embolization of polymerized glue following percutaneous direct injection of a carotid body tumor. Korean J Radiol. 2007;8:249–53.

46. Mukerji SS, Osborn AJ, Roberts J, Valdez TA. Kaposiform hemangioendothelioma (with Kasabach Merritt syndrome) of the head and neck: case report and review of the literature. Int J Pediatr Otorhinolaryngol. 2009;73:1474–6.

47. Komiyama M, Nakajima H, Kitano S, Sakamoto H, Kurimasa H, Ozaki H. Endovascular treatment of huge cervicofacial hemangioma complicated by Kasabach-Merritt syndrome. Pediatr Neurosurg. 2000;33:26–30.

48. Bornet G, Claudet I, Fries F, et al. Cervicofacial angioma and the Kasabach-Merritt syndrome. Neuroradiology. 2000;42:703–6.

49. Drucker AM, Pope E, Mahant S, Weinstein M. Vincristine and corticosteroids as first-line treatment of Kasabach-Merritt syndrome in kaposiform hemangioendothelioma. J Cutan Med Surg. 2009;13:155–9.

50. Stanley P, Gomperts E, Woolley MM. Kasabach-Merritt syndrome treated by therapeutic embolization with polyvinyl alcohol. Am J Pediatr Hematol Oncol. 1986;8:308–11.

51. Wolfe SQ, Farhat H, Elhammady MS, Moftakhar R, Aziz-Sultan MA. Transarterial embolization of a scalp hemangioma presenting with Kasabach-Merritt syndrome. J Neurosurg Pediatr. 2009;4:453–7.

52. Cognard C, Miaux Y, Pierot L, Weill A, Martin N, Chiras J. The role of CT in evaluation of the effectiveness of embolisation of spinal dural arteriovenous fistulae with N-butyl cyanoacrylate. Neuroradiology. 1996;38:603–8.

53. Ricolfi F, Gobin PY, Aymard A, Brunelle F, Gaston A, Merland JJ. Giant perimedullary arteriovenous fistulas of the spine: clinical and radiologic features and endovascular treatment. AJNR Am J Neuroradiol. 1997;18:677–87.

54. Pelz DM, Lownie SP, Fox AJ, Hutton LC. Symptomatic pulmonary complications from liquid acrylate embolization of brain arteriovenous malformations. AJNR Am J Neuroradiol. 1995;16:19–26.

55. Pukenas BA, Satti SR, Bailey R, Weigele JB, Hurst RW, Stiefel MF. Onyx pulmonary artery embolization after treatment of a low-flow dural arteriovenous fistula: case report. Neurosurgery. 2011;68:E1497–500; discussion E500.

56. Puri AS, Thiex R, Zarzour H, Rahbar R, Orbach DB. Trigeminocardiac reflex in a child during pre-Onyx DMSO injection for juvenile nasopharyngeal angiofibroma embolization. A case report. Interv Neuroradiol. 2011;17:13–6.

57. Lv X, Jiang C, Zhang J, Li Y, Wu Z. Complications related to percutaneous transarterial embolization of intracranial dural arteriovenous fistulas in 40 patients. AJNR Am J Neuroradiol. 2009;30:462–8.

58. Weiss I, TM O, Lipari BA, Meyer L, Berenstein A, Waner M. Current treatment of parotid hemangiomas. Laryngoscope. 2011;121:1642–50.

59. Spence J, Krings T, TerBrugge KG, Agid R. Percutaneous treatment of facial venous malformations: a matched comparison of alcohol and bleomycin sclerotherapy. Head Neck. 2011;33:125–30.

60. Puig S, Aref H, Brunelle F. Double-needle sclerotherapy of lymphangiomas and venous angiomas in children: a simple technique to prevent complications. AJR Am J Roentgenol. 2003;180:1399–401.

61. Mason KP, Michna E, Zurakowski D, Koka BV, Burrows PE. Serum ethanol levels in children and adults after ethanol embolization or sclerotherapy for vascular anomalies. Radiology. 2000;217:127–32.

62. Han MH, Seong SO, Kim HD, Chang KH, Yeon KM, Han MC. Craniofacial arteriovenous malformation: preoperative embolization with direct puncture and injection of n-butyl cyanoacrylate. Radiology. 1999;211:661–6.

63. Schirmer CM, Malek AM, Kwan ES, Hoit DA, Weller SJ. Preoperative embolization of hypervascular spinal metastases using percutaneous direct injection with n-butyl cyanoacrylate: technical case report. Neurosurgery. 2006;59:E431–2; author reply E431–2.

64. Fanning NF, Pedroza A, Willinsky RA, terBrugge KG. Segmental artery exchange technique for stable 4F guiding-catheter positioning in embolization of spinal vascular malformations. AJNR Am J Neuroradiol. 2007;28:875–6.

65. Hall WA, Oldfield EH, Doppman JL. Recanalization of spinal arteriovenous malformations following embolization. J Neurosurg. 1989;70:714–20.

66. Nichols DA, Rufenacht DA, Jack Jr CR, Forbes GS. Embolization of spinal dural arteriovenous fistula with poly-vinyl alcohol particles: experience in 14 patients. AJNR Am J Neuroradiol. 1992;13:933–40.

67. Song JK, Gobin YP, Duckwiler GR, et al. N-butyl 2-cyano-acrylate embolization of spinal dural arteriovenous fistulae. AJNR Am J Neuroradiol. 2001;22:40–7.

68. Nogueira RG, Dabus G, Rabinov JD, Ogilvy CS, Hirsch JA, Pryor JC. Onyx embolization for the treatment of spinal dural arteriovenous fistulae: initial experience with long-term follow-up. Technical case report. Neurosurgery. 2009;64:E197–8; discussion E198.

69. Niimi Y, Berenstein A, Setton A, Neophytides A. Embolization of spinal dural arteriovenous fistulae: results and follow-up. Neurosurgery. 1997;40:675–82; discussion 682–3.

70. Doppman JL, Di Chiro G. Paraspinal muscle infarction. A painful complication of lumbar artery embolization associated with pathognomonic radiographic and laboratory findings. Radiology. 1976;119:609–13.

71. Song JK, Vinuela F, Gobin YP, et al. Surgical and endovascular treatment of spinal dural arteriovenous fistulas: long-term disability assessment and prognostic factors. J Neurosurg. 2001;94:199–204.

72. Westphal M, Koch C. Management of spinal dural arteriovenous fistulae using an interdisciplinary neuroradiological/neurosurgical approach: experience with 47 cases. Neurosurgery. 1999;45:451–7; discussion 457–8.

73. Van Dijk JM, TerBrugge KG, Willinsky RA, Farb RI, Wallace MC. Multidisciplinary management of spinal dural arteriovenous fistulas: clinical presentation and long-term follow-up in 49 patients. Stroke. 2002;33:1578–83.

74. Horton JA, Latchaw RE, Gold LH, Pang D. Embolization of intramedullary arteriovenous malformations of the spinal cord. AJNR Am J Neuroradiol. 1986;7:113–8.

75. Theron J, Cosgrove R, Melanson D, Ethier R. Spinal arteriovenous malformations: advances in therapeutic embolization. Radiology. 1986;158:163–9.

76. Biondi A, Merland JJ, Reizine D, et al. Embolization with particles in thoracic intramedullary arteriovenous malformations: long-term angiographic and clinical results. Radiology. 1990;177:651–8.

77. Meisel HJ, Lasjaunias P, Brock M. Modern management of spinal and spinal cord vascular lesions. Minim Invasive Neurosurg. 1995;38:138–45.

78. Sala F, Beltramello A, Gerosa M. Neuroprotective role of neurophysiological monitoring during endovascular procedures in the brain and spinal cord. Neurophysiol Clin. 2007;37:415–21.

79. Konan AV, Raymond J, Roy D. Transarterial embolization of aneurysms associated with spinal cord arteriovenous malformations. Report of four cases. J Neurosurg. 1999;90:148–54.

80. Molyneux AJ, Coley SC. Embolization of spinal cord arteriovenous malformations with an ethylene vinyl alcohol copolymer dissolved in dimethyl sulfoxide (Onyx liquid embolic system). Report of two cases. J Neurosurg. 2000;93:304–8.

81. Corkill RA, Mitsos AP, Molyneux AJ. Embolization of spinal intramedullary arteriovenous malformations using the liquid embolic agent, Onyx: a single-center experience in a series of 17 patients. J Neurosurg Spine. 2007;7:478–85.

82. Lundqvist C, Andersen O, Blomstrand C, Svendsen P, Sullivan M. Spinal arteriovenous malformations. Health-related quality of life after embolization. Acta Neurol Scand. 1994;90:337–44.

83. Miyatake S, Kikuchi H, Koide T, et al. Cobb's syndrome and its treatment with embolization. Case report. J Neurosurg. 1990;72:497–9.

84. Soeda A, Sakai N, Iihara K, Nagata I. Cobb syndrome in an infant: treatment with endovascular embolization and corticosteroid therapy: case report. Neurosurgery. 2003;52:711–5; discussion 714–5.

85. Touho H, Karasawa J, Shishido H, Yamada K, Shibamoto K. Successful excision of a juvenile-type spinal arteriovenous malformation following intraoperative embolization. Case report. J Neurosurg. 1991;75:647–51.

86. Menku A, Akdemir H, Durak AC, Oktem IS. Successful surgical excision of juvenile-type spinal arteriovenous malformation in two stages following partial embolization. Minim Invasive Neurosurg. 2005;48:57–62.

87. Kalhorn SP, Frempong-Boadu AK, Mikolaenko I, Becske T, Harter DH. Metameric thoracic lesion: report of a rare case and a guide to management. J Neurosurg Spine. 2010;12:497–502.

88. Fairhall JM, Reddy R, Sears W, Wenderoth JD, Stoodley MA. Successful endovascular and surgical treatment of spinal extradural metameric arteriovenous malformation. Case report. J Neurosurg Spine. 2010;13:784–8.

89. Spiotta AM, Hussain MS, Masaryk TJ, Krishnaney AA. Combined endovascular and surgical resection of a giant lumbosacral arteriovenous malformation in a patient with Cobb syndrome. J Neurointerv Surg. 2011;3:293–6.

90. Barrow DL, Colohan AR, Dawson R. Intradural perimedullary arteriovenous fistulas (type IV spinal cord arteriovenous malformations). J Neurosurg. 1994;81:221–9.

91. Hida K, Iwasaki Y, Goto K, Miyasaka K, Abe H. Results of the surgical treatment of perimedullary arteriovenous fistulas with special reference to embolization. J Neurosurg. 1999;90:198–205.

92. Sure U, Wakat JP, Gatscher S, Becker R, Bien S, Bertalanffy H. Spinal type IV arteriovenous malformations (perimedullary fistulas) in children. Childs Nerv Syst. 2000;16:508–15.

93. Mourier KL, Gobin YP, George B, Lot G, Merland JJ. Intradural perimedullary arteriovenous fistulae: results of surgical and endovascular treatment in a series of 35 cases. Neurosurgery. 1993;32:885–91; discussion 891.

94. Halbach VV, Higashida RT, Dowd CF, Fraser KW, Edwards MS, Barnwell SL. Treatment of giant intradural (perimedullary) arteriovenous fistulas. Neurosurgery. 1993;33:972–9; discussion 979–80.

95. Cho KT, Lee DY, Chung CK, Han MH, Kim HJ. Treatment of spinal cord perimedullary arteriovenous fistula: embolization versus surgery. Neurosurgery. 2005;56:232–41; discussion 232–41.

96. Touho H, Monobe T, Ohnishi H, Karasawa J. Treatment of type II perimedullary arteriovenous fistulas by intraoperative transvenous embolization: case report. Surg Neurol. 1995;43:491–6.

97. Rodesch G, Hurth M, Alvarez H, Tadie M, Lasjaunias P. Spinal cord intradural arteriovenous fistulae: anatomic, clinical, and therapeutic considerations in a series of 32 consecutive patients seen between 1981 and 2000 with emphasis on endovascular therapy. Neurosurgery. 2005;57:973–83; discussion 973–83.

98. Rodesch G, Hurth M, Alvarez H, David P, Tadie M, Lasjaunias P. Embolization of spinal cord arteriovenous shunts: morphological and clinical follow-up and results–review of 69 consecutive cases. Neurosurgery. 2003;53:40–9; discussion 49–50.

99. Krings T, Coenen VA, Weinzierl M, et al. Spinal dural arteriovenous fistula associated with a spinal perimedullary fistula: case report. J Neurosurg Spine. 2006;4:241–5.

100. Cognard C, Semaan H, Bakchine S, et al. Paraspinal arteriovenous fistula with perimedullary venous drainage. AJNR Am J Neuroradiol. 1995;16:2044–8.

101. Silva Jr N, Januel AC, Tall P, Cognard C. Spinal epidural arteriovenous fistulas associated with progressive myelopathy. Report of four cases. J Neurosurg Spine. 2007;6:552–8.

102. Tampieri D, Leblanc R, TerBrugge K. Preoperative embolization of brain and spinal hemangioblastomas. Neurosurgery. 1993;33:502–5; discussion 505.

103. Eskridge JM, McAuliffe W, Harris B, Kim DK, Scott J, Winn HR. Preoperative endovascular embolization of craniospinal hemangioblastomas. AJNR Am J Neuroradiol. 1996;17:525–31.

104. Biondi A, Ricciardi GK, Faillot T, Capelle L, Van Effenterre R, Chiras J. Hemangioblastomas of the lower spinal region: report of four cases with preoperative embolization and review of the literature. AJNR Am J Neuroradiol. 2005; 26:936–45.

105. Breslau J, Eskridge JM. Preoperative embolization of spinal tumors. J Vasc Interv Radiol. 1995;6:871–5.

106. Guzman R, Dubach-Schwizer S, Heini P, et al. Preoperative transarterial embolization of vertebral metastases. Eur Spine J. 2005;14:263–8.

107. Olerud C, Jonsson Jr H, Lofberg AM, Lorelius LE, Sjostrom L. Embolization of spinal metastases reduces peroperative blood loss. 21 patients operated on for renal cell carcinoma. Acta Orthop Scand. 1993;64:9–12.

108. Smith TP, Koci T, Mehringer CM, et al. Transarterial embolization of vertebral hemangioma. J Vasc Interv Radiol. 1993;4:681–5.

109. Acosta Jr FL, Dowd CF, Chin C, Tihan T, Ames CP, Weinstein PR. Current treatment strategies and outcomes in the management of symptomatic vertebral hemangiomas. Neurosurgery. 2006;58:287–95; discussion 287–95.

110. Doppman JL, Oldfield EH, Heiss JD. Symptomatic vertebral hemangiomas: treatment by means of direct intralesional injection of ethanol. Radiology. 2000;214:341–8.

9. Treatment of Acute Ischaemic Stroke

9.1. Endovascular Treatment for Acute Stroke: General Considerations

The elements of successful treatment for acute stroke are:
1. Rapid evaluation and decision making
2. Careful patient selection
3. Rapid and effective pharmacologic or mechanical thrombolysis

Speed is critical. Approach any potential candidate for endovascular therapy with an eye towards first administering IV t-PA, or getting the patient on the angio suite table as soon as possible. The overall strategy consists of the following steps:
1. Make a correct diagnosis of acute ischaemic stroke and determine the time of onset.
2. Focus on the patient examination, *essential tests*, and imaging.
3. For IA cases:
   a. Alert the angio suite technicians and nurses as soon as possible, to permit room and device preparation.
   b. Obtain vascular access for the endovascular procedure as soon as possible.
      - If the patient is unable to undergo the procedure awake, he or she should be transferred to the angio suite, placed on the table, and have a femoral artery sheath placed while the anesthesia service is called. Do a quick diagnostic angiogram prior to the induction of anesthesia; if necessary, withdraw the catheter into the aortic arch while the patient is intubated.
   c. Obtain and prepare the devices and thrombolytic medications as soon as possible.
      - Place catheters, wires, thrombolytic drugs, and other anticipated devices on the sterile table and prepare them while the patient is being brought to the angio suite, or while the vascular access is being obtained.
   d. Make a decision about the thrombolysis technique (i.e., drug vs. mechanical thrombolysis) as soon as the first angiographic images of the craniocervical circulation are obtained.
   e. IA thrombolysis often requires a combination of techniques (e.g., thrombolytic drug infusion plus angioplasty and stenting). As each maneuver is done, the next step should be anticipated and planned.

The Need for Speed

Numerous thrombolysis trials have demonstrated that the earlier the treatment, the better the chance of a favourable outcome. Treatment within 90 min is superior to treatment within 3 h,[1,2] and treatment within 3 h is superior to treatment within 6 h,[3,4] and so on. Therefore, evaluate and treat every ischaemic stroke patient as swiftly and efficiently as possible. The importance of speed was underscored by the scientific statement published by the American Heart Association in 2006 entitled "Reducing Delay in Seeking Treatment by Patients with Acute Coronary Syndrome and Stroke":[5]
1. Defer non-essential tests, and prepare the treatment methods (i.e., the angio suite or t-PA) rapidly.
   - Do not allow non-essential tests, such as a CXR in most cases, to interfere with the work-up. A CXR is not necessary during the initial work-up for most patients with acute stroke.[6]
2. According the 2003 *Guidelines for the Early Management of Patients With Ischaemic Stroke*, patients who are candidates for pharmacologic thrombolysis should complete the CT examination within 25 min of arrival at the emergency

department, and the study should be interpreted within an additional 20 min (door to interpretation time of 45 min).[7]

3. Importantly, *do not delay CT perfusion examination and/or transportation of the patient to the angio suite while awaiting the blood test results.*

    a. Serum creatinine measurement is typically required prior to the procedures using iodinated contrast. However, the 2010 *American College of Radiology Manual on Contrast Media* recommends checking of creatinine only for patients who have established risk factors for contrast-induced nephropathy.[8] The authors of this handbook proceed with CT perfusion and with angiography in patients with acute ischaemic stroke prior to the blood test results, if necessary, on the grounds that checking of creatinine is really not necessary in many patients, and that the benefit of rapid diagnosis and treatment justifies the relatively low risk of nephropathy.[9,10]

    b. Likewise, do not delay transportation of the patient to the angio suite pending platelet count and coagulation studies, if IA thrombolysis is anticipated. The endovascular procedure can be started and the vascular access can be accomplished while awaiting the laboratory results.

4. Implement effective triage; bump or reschedule elective cases and other clinic activities to accommodate the patient suffering from acute stroke.

Thrombolytic Agents

Several thrombolytic agents are available (Table 9.1). Most work by converting plasminogen to plasmin. Plasmin then cleaves the fibrin meshwork of the thrombus, leading to lysis. Urokinase and streptokinase are the first-generation agents and are not fibrin- (i.e., clot) specific. Urokinase, a naturally occurring serine protease with low antigenicity, was withdrawn from the market in the United States for several years due to manufacturing issues, but has recently been reintroduced. Streptokinase, an activator of plasminogen but not an enzyme, despite the name, has limited usefulness because many patients have pre-formed anti-streptococcal antibodies and have the potential for an anaphylactic reaction to this agent. Second-generation agents are fibrin-specific and include prourokinase (aka pro-UK, or saruplase) and alteplase. They have the drawback of lowering the levels of fibrinogen and plasminogen, leading to an increased risk of haemorrhagic complications. Prourokinase is a precursor of urokinase and is converted on the surface of the thrombus to urokinase by fibrin-bound plasmin, resulting in superior fibrin specificity and lytic efficacy, compared to urokinase. Prourokinase has the distinction of being the agent used in the Prolyse in Acute Cerebral Thromboembolism (PROACT) trials,[11,12] but is not currently available for clinical use in the US. Presently, t-PA is the only agent approved by the FDA specifically for IV thrombolysis for ischaemic stroke. Third-generation agents include reteplase and tenecteplase and offer the theoretical advantages of longer half-lives and greater penetration into the thrombus matrix when compared to the second-generation agents. Reteplase is a deletion mutant in which the finger, epidermal growth factor, and kringle-1 domains have been deleted from the wild-type t-PA molecule. Tenecteplase is also a t-PA mutant.

Three main thrombolytic agents are currently available in the United States: alteplase (Activase, Genentech, San Francisco, CA); urokinase (Abbokinase, Abbott

Table 9.1 Intra-arterial thrombolytic agents

		Half-life (min)	Intra-arterial dose	Description
First generation	Urokinase	14–20	500,000–1,000,000 units	Serine protease
Second generation	Prourokinase (NA)	20	6–9 mg	Proenzyme precursor of urokinase
	Alteplase (t-PA)	3–5	5–40 mg	Serine protease
Third generation	Reteplase	15–18	4–8 units	Deletion mutant of t-PA

NA not available, *t-PA* recombinant tissue plasminogen activator

Laboratories, Abbott Park, IL); and reteplase (Retavase, Centocor, Malvern, PA). Five milligrams of alteplase are equivalent to 1 unit (U) of reteplase. Although each agent has its own theoretical advantages, a direct comparison of the effectiveness of these agents in acute stroke is not available. In a retrospective comparison of t-PA to urokinase for IA thrombolysis, no differences in recanalization rates were found with respect to the thrombolytic agent or dosage.[13] Reversal of all thrombolytics can be done by administering fresh frozen plasma in the event of haemorrhagic complication.

Other novel fibrinolytic agents are tenecteplase and desmetoplase. Tenecteplase is a genetically modified form of t-PA, that has 14-fold greater fibrin specificity, a longer half-life, and 80-fold greater resistance to inhibition by plasminogen activator inhibitor type-1.[14] Treatment with tenecteplase has been found to avoid the systemic plasminogen activation and plasmin generation commonly seen after t-PA therapy. In addition, the absence of a procoagulant effect that can occur with thrombolytics may reduce the risk of early re-occlusion.[15] In a pilot dose-escalation study, 75 stroke patients were treated with IV tenecteplase for <3 h after symptom onset.[16] The patients were treated with one of the three doses of tenecteplase: 0.1, 0.2, and 0.4 mg/kg. No case of symptomatic intracranial haemorrhage was observed during the first 72 h after treatment. A larger phase IIB/III trial of IV tenecteplase for stroke was stopped prematurely because of slow enrollment.[17]

Desmetoplase is one of the four proteases found in the saliva of the blood-feeding vampire bat *Desmodus rotundus*, collectively referred to as *D rotundus* salivary plasminogen activators (DSPAs). Desmetoplase is the α1 variant among the DSPAs and has >72% of amino acid sequence identity with human t-PA. DSPAα-1 induces faster and more sustained recanalization than t-PA, and produces less anti-plasmin consumption and fibrinogenolysis. Furthermore, unlike t-PA, DSPAα-1 does not enhance *N*-methyl-D-aspartate–mediated neurodegeneration.[18] Desmetoplase has shown promise in two phase 2 ischaemic stroke trials.[19,20]

Ancrod is a protease derived from Malaysian pit viper venom. In contrast to thrombolytic agents which act on plasminogen, ancrod produces a rapid decrease in serum fibrinogen by accelerating cleavage of the fibrinogen A-α chain.[21] Reduction in serum fibrinogen levels produces anticoagulation by depleting the substrate needed for thrombus formation. Depletion of fibrinogen also reduces blood viscosity.[22]

Patient Preparation

Evaluation
1. History, physical, and neurological exam.
2. Make an accurate diagnosis and pinpoint the time of onset of the stroke symptoms.
   a. For patients with stroke symptoms, upon awakening, the time of onset is assumed to be the time the patient was last known to be symptom-free.
3. Localize the stroke symptoms and assess the severity of the stroke (see below: Appendix 2: NIH Stroke Scale).
   a. Several conditions can mimic stroke:[7,23,24]
      i. Conversion disorder ⎤
      ii. Complicated migraine ⎬ three most common stroke mimics.[23]
      iii. Seizures ⎦
      iv. Confusional state
      v. Syncope
      vi. Toxic or metabolic syndromes
      vii. Hypoglycemia
      viii. Subdural hematoma
      ix. Brain tumor
4. Blood test (CBC, Cr, PT, PTT).
5. EKG
6. Imaging
7. Essential: Noncontrast head CT.
   a. The primary role of CT is to check for an intracranial haemorrhage, which is present in some 15% of the patients presenting with acute stroke. Other potential findings on CT, such indications of cerebral ischaemia, are secondary (see below: Appendix 1: Primer on Imaging in Stroke).
   b. In some cases, a rapid CT can be done in the angio suite immediately prior to the IA procedure (e.g., XperCT or DynaCT).

8. Optional but helpful: CT perfusion/CT angiography
   a. The 2009 American Heart Association Scientific Statement recommended that a vascular imaging study *should not* delay the start of IV thrombolysis in patients presenting within 3 h of onset of ischaemic stroke.[25]
   b. Vascular imaging (e.g., CT perfusion) can help with patient selection for IA treatment. Routinely combining a CT perfusion and CT angiography study with the screening CT scan for all patients with ischaemic stroke eliminates the need for two separate trips to the CT scanner and streamlines the decision making process.

Pre-procedure Preparation
1. IV thrombolysis cases: Obtain t-PA.
2. IA cases: Call the angio suite and make sure that all the nurses, technicians, devices that may be needed are available in the angio suite prior to the procedure.
3. Place two peripheral IVs.
   • Glucose-containing solutions should be avoided.[7]
4. Place Foley
5. NPO except for medications

9.2. Patient Selection for Thrombolysis

The following applies mostly to patients with anterior circulation stroke; patient selection for basilar artery thrombolysis is discussed separately below.

Indications

1. Acute ischaemic stroke with an onset of symptoms within 3–8 h prior to anticipated treatment
2. Significant neurological symptoms (NIHSS >4 except for patients with isolated aphasia or hemianopia)
3. Exclude other causes of acute neurological symptoms (e.g., intracranial haemorrhage, seizures, confusional states, toxic or metabolic states, and brain tumors).

Absolute Contraindications

1. Acute intracranial haemorrhage
2. Large hypoattenuating region or mass effect on CT

Relative Contraindications

1. Improving neurological symptoms
2. Lacunar stroke
3. Coma
4. Seizure
5. Major stroke (NIHSS >30)
6. Recent history of surgery or intracranial haemorrhage
7. Recent myocardial infarction.[26]
8. History of anaphylaxis to thrombolytic drugs or iodinated contrast media

Decision-making: IV or IA Thrombolysis?

Although IV thrombolysis is FDA-approved for the treatment of selected patients with acute ischaemic stroke, IA thrombolysis has emerged as a valid alternative for

Table 9.2 Patient selection for intravenous or intra-arterial thrombolysis

IV thrombolysis	
Relative indications	**Relative contraindications**
Symptom onset <3 h prior to treatment	Major stroke (NIHSS >22)
Mild to moderate symptoms (NIHSS <20)	Minor symptoms, such as isolated sensory loss, dysarthria, or ataxia
Small, distal vessel occlusion	Improving neurological symptoms
Significant territory (>20% of affected volume) of salvageable tissue on per-fusion imaging	Hypertension: SBP >185 mmHg; DBP >110 mmHg
Intolerance to iodinated contrast	Head trauma, prior stroke, or myocardial infarction within 3 months
High risk for anesthesia complications (if use of general anesthesia is needed for IA thrombolysis)	Gastrointestinal or urinary tract haemorrhage within 21 days
Age <75	Major surgery within 14 days
	Arterial puncture at a noncompressible site within 7 days
	History of previous intracranial haemorrhage
	Evidence of active bleeding or acute trauma
	Blood glucose concentration <50 mg/dL (2.7 mmol/L)
	Age > 75
	Early signs of ischaemia on CT (>30% of hemisphere)
	INR >1.5 or platelet count <100,000/mm³
	Recent history (within 21 days) of head injury or other trauma, major operation, myocardial infarction, or bleeding
	Age > 75
	On antiplatelet agents at time of onset[27]
	Length of M1 thrombus >8 mm by CT[28]
IA thrombolysis	
Relative indications	**Relative contraindications**
Symptom onset due to ICA or MCA occlusion <6–8 h prior to treatment	Elongated aortic arch or otherwise difficult vascular access
Symptom onset due to vertebrobasilar occlusion <12–24 h prior to treatment	High risk for anesthesia complications (if use of general anesthesia is anticipated)
Significant territory (>20% of affected volume) of salvageable tissue on per-fusion imaging	Anticipated delay in beginning interventional procedure
Angio suite and staff is promptly available	Intolerance to iodinated contrast
Contraindications to IV thrombolysis (e.g., recent surgery or head injury)	Major stroke (NIHSS >22)
Accessible vascular anatomy	INR >1.5
Concomitant arterial stenosis or dissection	Recent history (within 14 days) of larger ischaemic stroke
Hyperdense MCA sign	Age >80[29]
Suspected "hard embolus" (i.e., calcified debris or some other occlusive material that may respond better to mechanical embolectomy than IV thrombolysis)	
Failure to improve after systemic thrombolysis	
On antiplatelet agents at time of onset[27]	

Source: References[7,19,20,30–33]

some patients, depending on the clinical setting. Selection between the two treatments requires consideration of a number of factors (Table 9.2). In brief, the most suitable candidates for IV thrombolysis are patients with relatively small regions of affected cerebral territory who can be treated within 4.5 h of symptom onset. The most suitable candidates for IA thrombolysis are those with larger vessel occlusions, who can be treated within 6–8 h of symptom onset. A detailed discussion of the factors that favour each particular approach follows the table.

Patient Selection for IV Thrombolysis

Subgroup analysis of the IV t-PA trials have identified a number of factors that predict a favourable result with IV thrombolysis: NIHSS <10[34] or NIHSS <20,[1,35] a normal baseline CT scan, a normal pretreatment blood glucose level, normal pretreatment blood pressure,[34] and age <75[1,35]

Size Is Important
A recent study showed that the length of a middle cerebral artery thrombus was predictive of the outcome from intravenous thrombolysis.[28] A thrombus measuring 8 mm in length or longer measured by noncontrast CT was associated with a lack of recanalization and a poor outcome on follow-up. Could this be a strong indication for endovascular intervention?

Patient Selection for IA Thrombolysis

The clinical criteria for enrollment in the PROACT studies may be considered during patient evaluation for IA therapy of acute stroke. The PROACT selection criteria should not be regarded as rigid criteria for day-to-day decision-making, as they were formulated in the setting of a randomized trial, and patients with complicated issues, such as coexisting arterial dissection, may have confounded the results of the trial and were necessarily excluded. The leading factor in patient selection in the PROACT studies was the time from symptom onset, generally within 6 h for anterior circulation occlusions. In PROACT II, the typical interval, from initiation of IA infusion of thrombolytic drug to completion of recanalization, was 90–120 min; therefore, the 6-h treatment window may be viewed as an 8-h recanalization window.[12] Thus, for situations in which recanalization can be accomplished more rapidly than in the PROACT trials, such as with mechanical thrombolysis, the time window for recanalization may be extended to 8 h. For patients with basilar artery occlusions, IA thrombolysis can be undertaken up to 24 h after symptom onset.[30,31] Additional clinical inclusion criteria for PROACT II were a minimum NIHSS score of 4, except for isolated aphasia or hemianopia, and ages 18–85 years.

Angiographic findings were graded according to the TIMI scale (Table 9.3). Only patients with angiographic evidence of complete occlusion (TIMI grade 0) or contrast penetration with minimal perfusion (TIMI grade 1) were included. Exclusion criteria for PROACT II are listed in Table 9.4.

The TIMI scale is limited by not considering occlusion location or collateral circulation; Qureshi and colleagues introduced an alternative classification scheme for acute ischaemic stroke that incorporates these angiographic findings (Table 9.5).[38]

Table 9.3 Thrombolysis in myocardial infarction (TIMI) scale

Grade	Definition
0	No flow
1	Some penetration past the site of occlusion but no flow distal to occlusion
2	Distal perfusion but delayed filling in distal vessels
3	Distal perfusion with adequate perfusion of distal vessels

Adapted from Chesebro et al[36]

Table 9.4 Exclusion criteria for PROACT II

NIHSS
Coma
Rapidly improving neurologic signs
Stroke within the previous 6 weeks
Seizures at onset of presenting stroke
Clinical presentation suggestive of subarachnoid haemorrhage
Previous intracranial haemorrhage, neoplasm, or subarachnoid haemorrhage
Septic embolism
Suspected lacunar stroke
Surgery, biopsy of a parenchymal organ, trauma with internal injuries or lumbar puncture within 30 days
Head trauma within 90 days
Active or recent haemorrhage within 30 days
Known haemorrhagic diathesis, baseline international normalized ratio >1.7, activated partial thromboplastin time >1.5 times normal, or baseline platelet count <100 × 10⁹/L
Known sensitivity to contrast agents
Uncontrolled hypertension defined by a blood pressure ≥180 mmHg systolic or ≥100 mmHg diastolic on three separate occasions at least 10 min apart or requiring IV therapy
CT evidence of haemorrhage, intracranial tumors except for small meningiomas, significant mass effect from the infarction, and acute hypodense parenchymal lesion or effacement of cerebral sulci in more than one-third of the MCA territory
Angiographic evidence of arterial dissection, arterial stenosis precluding safe passage of a microcatheter into the MCA, nonatherosclerotic arteriopathy, no visible occlusion, or occlusion of an artery other than the M1 or M2 segments of the MCA

From Furlan et al [12], with permission

Table 9.5 Qureshi grading system for acute ischaemic stroke[a]

Grade 0	No occlusion		
Grade 1	MCA occlusion (M3 segment)	ACA occlusion (A2 or distal segments)	1 BA/VA branch occlusion
Grade 2	MCA occlusion (M2 segment)	ACA occlusion (A1 and A2 segments)	≥2 BA/VA branch occlusions
Grade 3	MCA occlusion (M1 segment)		
3A	Lenticulostriate arteries spared and/or leptomeningeal collaterals visualized		
3B	No sparing of lenticulostriate arteries nor leptomeningeal collaterals visualized		
Grade 4	ICA occlusion (collaterals present)	BA occlusion (partial filling direct or via collaterals)	
4A	Collaterals fill MCA	Anterograde filling[a]	
4B	Collaterals fill ACA	Retrograde filling[a]	
Grade 5	ICA occlusion (no collaterals)	BA occlusion (complete)	

From Qureshi.[37], with permission
ACA anterior cerebral artery, *BA* basilar artery, *ICA* internal carotid artery, *MCA* middle cerebral artery, *VA* vertebral artery
[a]The predominant pattern of filling

9.3. Intravenous Thrombolysis for Acute Ischaemic Stroke

Intravenous t-PA is currently the only FDA-approved treatment for acute ischaemic stroke in selected patients.

IV t-PA Protocol[7]

1. Infuse 0.9 mg/kg (maximum of 90 mg) over 60 min with 10% of the dose given as a bolus over 1 min.
   - Mnemonic for remembering the dose: 0–9–9–0 (0.9 mg/kg for max 90 mg)
2. Admit the patient to the ICU or a stroke unit.
3. Neurological exam Q 15 min during the infusion and Q 30 min for next 6 h, then Q 1 h for a total of 24 h after treatment.
4. Vital signs Q 15 min for first 2 h, Q 30 min for 6 h, and Q 1 h for a total of 24 h after treatment. Maintain SBP <180 mmHg and SBP <105 mmHg.
   - Antihypertensive medication regimen:
     i. Labetalol 10 mg IV over 1–2 min; may repeat every 10–20 min as needed to a maximum dose of 300 mg. Alternatively, start with a labetalol bolus and use an infusion of 2–8 mg/min.
     ii. If blood pressure is not controlled, start an infusion of sodium nitroprusside at 0.5 mg/kg/min.
5. Discontinue the infusion (if the drug is still being given) and obtain a head CT if the patient develops severe headaches, acute hypertension, nausea.
6. Avoid placement of NG tubes, Foley catheters, or intra-arterial catheters.

Ultrasound Augmentation of IV Thrombolysis

Transcranial Doppler (TCD) can augment IV thrombolysis. Ultrasound can induce reversible changes in the thrombus fibrin mesh, creating microstreams of plasma through the thrombus and accelerating the transport and penetration of t-PA into the clot, resulting in more complete and faster clot lysis.[39] Three techniques for ultrasound-enhanced thrombolysis have been studied:

1. Low frequency ultrasound (300 kHz). A randomized trial comparing IV tPA + low frequency ultrasound to IV tPA alone was terminated after a significantly higher rate of haemorrhage was observed in the ultrasound group.[40]
2. High frequency TCD (2 MHz) with or without addition of gaseous microbubbles.[37,41,42]
   a. A randomized trial of 2 MHz TCD in patients receiving IV t-PA for MCA occlusion showed a significantly higher rate of recanalization in the TCD group without a difference in the rate of symptomatic haemorrhage.[37,43,44]
   b. A randomized phase 2 trial of 2 MHz TCD coupled with increasing doses of perflutren-lipid microspheres in patients receiving IV tPA for proximal intracranial arterial occlusions showed that perflutren microspheres can be safely combined with systemic tPA and ultrasound at a dose of 1.4 mL. However, safety concerns due to increased rates of symptomatic ICH in the second dose tier (2.8 mL) resulted in the premature termination of the trial.[44]
3. High frequency colour-coded duplex.[45–47]

A systematic review found a higher rate of complete recanalization in patients receiving a combination of high frequency ultrasound + IV tPA compared to patients getting IV tPA alone, without an increased risk of symptomatic intracranial haemorrhage.[48]

Patient Management After Thrombolysis

1. Admit to a Neurological ICU.
2. Monitor blood pressure closely. An increase in post-thrombolysis BP is a sign of intracranial haemorrhage.[49]
3. No anticoagulation or antiplatelet therapy for 24 h.
4. Surveillance head CT on post-procedure day 1 to monitor for haemorrhage.

Complications (*management* of complications is discussed below)

   A pooled analysis of data on 2,639 patients in 15 studies of IV t-PA for acute stroke, found a rate of symptomatic intracerebral haemorrhage of 5.2%.[50] The rate of all haemorrhage (symptomatic and asymptomatic) was 11.5%. The mean total death rate was 13.4%, and the proportion of patients achieving a very favourable outcome was 37.1%. Other reported risks associated with IV thrombolysis include:

1. Hemi-orolingual angioedema occurs in 1.3–5.1% of patients.[51–53]
2. Myocardial rupture may occur in patients who were given IV thrombolytic, within a few days of myocardial infarction (MI).[26] In a series of patients receiving IV thrombolysis for MI, 1.7% had a myocardial rupture. Most occurred in patients receiving thrombolytic within 48 h of the MI, and all were fatal.

9.4. Intra-arterial Thrombolysis for Acute Ischaemic Stroke

Endovascular Technique

Thrombolysis cases can be divided into an access phase and a thrombolysis phase. Access consists of femoral artery puncture, brief diagnostic angiography, and placement of a guide catheter in the carotid or vertebral artery. The thrombolysis phase concerns reopening of the occluded cervical or intracranial vessel.

Awake or Asleep?

General anesthesia is associated with worse outcomes with IA treatment of stroke.[54] Although it is not clear that anesthesia *causes* worse outcomes in this setting,[55] general anesthesia can lengthen the time of the procedure and add anesthesia-associated risks, so it makes sense to avoid general anesthesia when possible. Patients with non-dominant hemisphere strokes can often tolerate emergent angiography and thrombolysis, with adequate coaching. Good results have been obtained even in aphasic patients with dominant hemisphere ischaemic strokes, in whom the vascular anatomy was favourable, and the procedure could be accomplished swiftly. Intubation and sedation should be used in patients with posterior circulation strokes and others who simply cannot cooperate adequately. To save time, patients requiring general anesthesia should be intubated in the emergency room or in the angio suite while vascular access is underway. A key point is that a vascular access and a diagnostic angiogram can be accomplished prior to the induction of anesthesia, if necessary.

Access Phase

See Chap. 4 for a general discussion of access techniques.

1. Prep and drape the right or left groin, and infiltrate the skin with local anesthesia.
2. Place a sheath in the femoral artery.
    a. Use as large a sheath as possible (6, 7, or 8F).
    b. Use a micropuncture set: It may reduce the risk of potential bleeding at the puncture site.[56]

3. Obtain a focused diagnostic angiogram using a diagnostic catheter. The objectives are to confirm the diagnosis of a major arterial occlusion and to map out the pertinent anatomy.
4. Cervical PA and lateral views of the involved carotid or vertebral artery, and intracranial PA and lateral views of the affected arterial system are usually all that is necessary.
5. Image additional vessels only if they can be catheterized rapidly. A complete four-vessel angiogram, only if time permits, could provide information about collateral circulation and filling of vessels distal to the acute occlusion, but is usually not needed, especially if CTA is available.
6. An aortic arch angiogram could be helpful in elderly patients who have a tortuous aortic arch.
7. If the occluded intracranial artery is difficult to discern, then look at a "stroke-o-gram" (Fig. 9.1). Manipulation of the contrast and brightness of the digital subtraction image of the intracranial capillary phase of the arteriogram can make the affected brain territory more apparent.
8. Exchange the diagnostic catheter for a 6F guide catheter, and place it as high as possible in the cervical carotid or vertebral artery.
9. Guide catheter options:
   a. *Best Option*: A 6F 90 cm sheath (e.g. Shuttle® sheath, Cook Inc., Bloomington, IN)
      i. This catheter is large enough to allow use of the largest Penumbra reperfusion catheter, and is also necessary if extracranial angioplasty and stenting are anticipated.
   b. Envoy® (Cordis Neurovascular, Miami Lakes, FL)
      i. Advantages: Relatively rigid, provides a good platform in tortuous vessels, large internal lumen. Good choice in many stroke patients, as they tend to be elderly and have ectatic vessels.
      ii. Disadvantages: Stiff, sharp-edged tip.

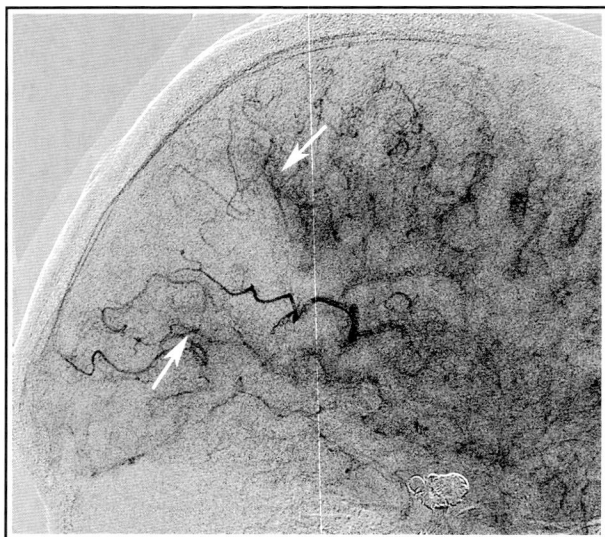

Fig. 9.1 Stroke-o-gram. Capillary phase of ICA angiogram showing a filling defect in the parietal region, corresponding to an occluded distal MCA branch in a patient with an acute ischemic stroke. The contrast has been dialed up and the brightness turned down of this DSA image to accent the region of filling defect (*arrows*).

c. Guider Softip™ XF guide catheter (Stryker Neurovascular, Fremont, CA).
  i. Advantages: Soft, atraumatic tip. Minimizes risk of vasospasm and dissection in narrow, tortuous vessels.
  ii. Disadvantages: Relatively flimsy, prone to fall into the arch when the vasculature is tortuous.
d. Merci balloon guide catheter – if the Merci device is going to be used.
e. Alternatively, to save time, a guide catheter can be advanced into the carotid or vertebral system primarily, and be used for the initial diagnostic angiogram. This strategy is usually the most successful in younger patients with straightforward anatomy.
f. A 6F Simmons 2 Envoy® (Codman Neurovascular, Raynham, MA) catheter can be advanced primarily into the common carotid artery in many patients with tortuous anatomy.
  i. Disadvantage: Less stable than other guide catheters which can be placed in the upper cervical internal carotid artery.

Heparin or No Heparin?

Some operators use full systemic heparinization for all intracranial interventions. In the setting of thrombolysis for acute stroke, systemic heparin may exacerbate potential bleeding related to thrombolytic enzyme infusion. The authors of this handbook prefer to reserve systemic heparin for selected cases, usually in which there is stasis of flow caused by the guide catheter. If IV heparin is given, a 5,000 unit bolus and a 500 unit per hour infusion is commonly used, and a syringe containing protamine is kept on the back table for emergent use, should haemorrhage occur during the case.

Thrombolysis Phase

Obtain a good working view once the guide catheter is in position. The working view should be under high magnification and should demonstrate the occluded vessel, as well as a clear intravascular path to the occlusion. It is also important to keep the guide catheter in view on at least one projection (PA or lateral) during the whole procedure, to permit correction of the guide catheter, should the catheter be pushed down (which is not uncommon) or become unstable during passage of the microcatheter. Real-time TCD monitoring during the procedure is relatively easy to do and can detect reocclusion, hyperperfusion, thromboembolism and air embolism.[57]

Device Selection
1. Microcatheter
   The choice of microcatheter depends on two factors: How difficult microcatheter access is likely to be, and whether thrombolytic drug infusion alone is planned, or if mechanical thrombolysis in combination with drug infusion is anticipated.
   a. Penumbra Reperfusion catheters come in four sizes and can be used to do suction thrombectomy and/or infusion of thrombolytics (see below).
   b. The UltraFlow™ microcatheter (ev3, Irvine, CA) is relatively easy to maneuver in tortuous anatomy and into distal vessels. It requires a small microwire and cannot be used with a snare.
   c. If the use of a snare is anticipated, requiring an ID ≥0.018 in., then the following microcatheters will work:
     i. Rapid Transit™ microcatheter (Codman Neurovascular, Raynham, MA)
     ii. Prowler™ Plus microcatheter (Codman Neurovascular, Raynham, MA)
     iii. Excelsior™ 1018 microcatheter (Stryker Neurovascular, Fremont, CA)
2. Microwire
   A relatively soft-tipped microcatheter should be used, to minimize the chance of vessel perforation. Stiffer microwires should be avoided. Preferred microwires for most stroke cases:
   a. Mirage™ 0.008 in. (ev3, Irvine, CA). Good for use with the UltraFlow™ microcatheter.
   b. J-tipped Headliner® 0.012 in. (Microvention/Terumo, Tustin, CA)
   c. Synchro®-14 0.014 in. (Stryker Neurovascular, Fremont, CA)
   d. Transend™ EX 0.014 in. Soft Tip (Stryker Neurovascular, Fremont, CA)

Pharmacological Thrombolysis

1. Microcatheter technique and infusion of thrombolytic.
   a. Form a J-shape at the tip of the microwire.
   b. Using a road map, gently navigate the microwire into the occluded vessel and into the region of occlusion. Avoid jabbing small perforating vessels with the microwire.
   c. Once the microwire tip is in or slightly beyond the region of occlusion, pin the microwire and carefully advance the microcatheter tip into the region of occlusion.
   d. Advance the microcatheter tip for a distance likely to be distal to the embolus or thrombus. This point is typically at the next branch point of the occluded vessel (e.g., in M1 occlusion, the embolus is often lodged in the vessel at the MCA bifurcation).
   e. Withdraw the microwire and do a gentle microcatheter angiogram to clarify the extent and position of the occlusion.
   f. Next, draw the microcatheter back into the occluded portion of the vessel and inject the thrombolytic agent. Inject slowly, over several minutes. Move the microcatheter tip through the clot as the thrombolytic agent is injected, to distribute the thrombolytic throughout the clot.
   g. Do a guide catheter angiogram after each dose to track the progress of thrombolysis, and to monitor for vessel perforation by looking for contrast extravasation. Periodic microcatheter angiograms can be helpful too.
      Caveat: Microcatheter injections of contrast may be associated with a higher incidence of intracranial haemorrhage.[58]
   h. Mechanical thrombolysis maneuvers can be done to supplement drug infusion (see below)
2. Choice of thrombolytic drug
   The authors of this handbook prefer to use whichever thrombolytic agent can be obtained and prepared quickly. Although each has advantages and disadvantages, no particular agent has been found to be superior to the others in direct comparison. Each agent is listed in Table 9.1.
3. When to stop
   The procedure is complete once recanalization of the vessel has been obtained or when the maximum dose of the thrombolytic agent has been administered and all other maneuvers, such as mechanical thrombolysis, have been done. Another signal to stop is any sign of possible haemorrhage, such as severe headache or nausea, or an abrupt change in blood pressure or heart rate (although patients can expect a bad headache after any intracranial thrombolysis procedure).
   a. *Migrating clot.* In some cases the large vessel thrombus may break up and migrate into distal branches. The temptation in this situation is to chase the clot into the distal branches and continue to infuse thrombolytic. However, occluded distal branches will often recanalize spontaneously after successful reopening of the proximal vessel, due to increased flow in the vessels and after the distal branches have incubated for a period of time with the thrombolytic agent that is already present. Also, it is generally not worth the added risk to continue to infuse additional thrombolytic drug, after the larger vessels have been reopened.
   b. *Reocclusion.* Reocclusion of a vessel, such as an M1 segment, is not uncommon after thrombolysis. This may be due to vasospasm, a platelet-rich thrombus, pre-existing atherosclerosis, or an iatrogenic dissection. There can even be a paradoxical procoagulant effect of tPA.[15] Options include:
      i. IA infusion of nitroglycerin, 30–60 µg, into the affected area. The vessel will usually reopen quickly, if vasospasm is present. This can be effective as a diagnostic maneuver as well as a therapeutic one.
      ii. Addition of an antiplatelet agent, such as a GP IIB/IIIA inhibitor. Pharmacological and mechanical thrombolysis can disrupt the endothelium and cause the formation of a platelet-rich thrombus. Angiographic evidence of this may be present, such as a fluffy filling defect in the region of reocclusion. IA or IV infusion of an antiplatelet agent may dissolve the clot, however, this will increase the chance of haemorrhagic complications. The wisdom of adding an antiplatelet agent should be weighed against the cost of continued reocclusion of the vessel.
      iii. Atherosclerotic stenosis or a dissection can be treated with intracranial angioplasty and stenting. Again, these manoeuvres increase the risk of bleeding and should be used only when the weight of the evidence indicates that the reocclusion will be long-lasting and clinically significant. See Sect. 9.5.4.

Postprocedure Care

1. The femoral artery sheath may be left in place while the thrombolytic drug wears off, and removed later.
2. Get a head CT to check for haemorrhage.
3. Admit to the intensive care unit for observation and blood pressure control.

Mechanical Embolectomy
An array of mechanical thrombolysis techniques exist, which may be employed as an alternative to or in combination with pharmacological thrombolysis:
1. Merci® Retriever: Discussed separately below.
2. Snares. Microsnares can be used to retrieve foreign bodies, such as detached coils or catheter fragments, or to treat acute ischaemic stroke. Although snare-retrieval of intracranial arterial thrombi can be done,[59–62] the authors of this handbook prefer to use snares in combination with a fibrinolytic drug, to break up the thrombus and increase the surface area available for lysis. Other authors have found the device to be most useful in the treatment of basilar artery occlusion.[63]
   a. *Devices.*
      i. Amplatz Goose Neck® microsnare (ev3, Irvine, CA). Available sizes: 2, 4 and 7 mm.
      ii. Microcatheter. Any microcatheter with an ID ≥0.018 in. is large enough. The following microcatheters will work:
         A. Rapid Transit™ microcatheter (Codman Neurovascular, Raynham, MA)
         B. Prowler™ Plus microcatheter (Codman Neurovascular, Raynham, MA)
         C. Excelsior™ 1018 microcatheter (Stryker Neurovascular, Fremont, CA)
   b. *Technique.*
      i. *Clot retrieval.*[62] Position the microcatheter so that the tip is just proximal to the occlusion. Advance a snare with a diameter slightly larger than the occluded vessel out of the microcatheter so that the loop of the snare is opened fully. Push the microcatheter together with the snare into the clot. Pull the snare back into the microcatheter, so that only a small portion of the snare can be seen outside of the microcatheter tip on fluoroscopy. Withdraw the microcatheter and snare several centimeters into a relatively straight segment. Do a guide catheter angiogram with gentle injection of contrast, to avoid disengaging of the thrombus. If the clot is caught in the snare, withdraw the microcatheter and snare as a unit into the guide catheter while applying suction to the proximal end of the guide catheter with a 60 mL syringe.
      ii. *Clot maceration.* Position the microcatheter in the occluded vessel and infuse the thrombolytic drug. If guide catheter angiograms show persistent occlusion, advance the microcatheter is past the occlusion and deploy a 4 mm snare. Gently withdraw the microcatheter and snare so that the snare is within the thrombus. Move the microcatheter and snare back and forth to macerate the clot and increase the surface area available for pharmacologic thrombolysis.
         A soft, J-tip guidewire can also be used for clot maceration. Use a guidewire smaller than the inner diameter of the microcatheter (e.g. J-Tip Headliner® 0.012 in. (Microvention/Terumo, Tustin, CA)) to allow constant, gentle clot maceration during the thrombolytic infusion.
3. Alligator™ Retriever device. This is a claw-like micro-forceps deliverable though a microcatheter. It works well to grasp and retrieve misplaced coils and other intravascular foreign bodies. It can also be used to retrieve thrombus.[64]
   a. *Devices.*
      i. Alligator™ Retriever device (ev3 Neurovascular, Irvine, CA). Available sizes: 2, 3, 4 and 5 mm. For best results, the nominal size should match the size of the vessel containing the obstructive object.
      ii. Guide catheter: If possible use a large-diameter Merci® balloon guide catheter to permit temporary occlusion and aspiration during removal of the clot.

iii. Microcatheter. Any microcatheter with an ID ≥0.021 in. is large enough. The following microcatheters will work:
- Merci® 18 L™ microcatheter (Stryker Neurovascular, Fremont, CA)
- Prowler™ Plus microcatheter (Codman Neurovascular, Raynham, MA)
- Renegade® microcatheter (Stryker Neurovascular, Fremont, CA)

b. *Techniques*

i. Clot retrieval. Position the microcatheter so that the tip is just proximal to the occlusion. Insert the Alligator into the microcatheter using the supplied introducer. Advance the Alligator to the tip of the microcatheter, but not yet into the vessel. Do not rotate the device. Then pull the microcatheter back and stabilize the Alligator wire to unsheathe the jaws of the Alligator. Very carefully advance the Alligator forward into the clot. Then advance the microcatheter over the stabilized Alligator wire so that the jaws begin to close. Keep tension on the Alligator wire but do not pull it completely into the microcatheter, as that will release whatever is grasped in the jaws. Withdraw the microcatheter and Alligator as a unit. Apply suction to the proximal end of the guide catheter with a 60 mL syringe to remove the Alligator and microcatheter without disengaging the clot. Completely withdraw the microcatheter from the guide catheter and thoroughly aspirate any clot from the guide catheter. If blood does not freely aspirate, a large thrombus may be present and the guide catheter must be removed from the patient and flushed.

ii. Foreign body retrieval. The steps are the same as clot retrieval, but it is much easier to determine if a radio-opaque coil or other foreign body is effectively grasped by the Alligator by fluoroscopic imaging.

4. Suction thrombectomy. Proximal large vessel occlusions can be treated with suction thrombectomy.[65–67]

a. *Technique*. Navigate a 6 or 7F guide catheter over a hydrophilic wire and placed the tip in the proximal third of the thrombus. Aspirate the thrombus with a 60 mL syringe while moving the guide catheter in and out of the thrombus several times. Continue aspirating for about 10 s each time.

b. Distal suction thrombectomy is done with the Penumbra Retrieval system (see below).

5. Intracranial angioplasty. Balloon angioplasty can augment thrombolysis in occlusions with underlying stenosis caused by atherosclerosis or a dissection. Angioplasty is most useful in the treatment of M1 segment thrombosis, which can be the result of thrombosis superimposed on atherosclerotic lesions, in contrast to distal basilar occlusions, which are more commonly embolic.[68] Angioplasty in this setting can reduce the risk of rethrombosis.[69] Several authors have reported favourable results with *rescue angioplasty*, in which angioplasty is used to obtain recanalization in vessel occlusions that are resistant to thrombolytic agents alone. Two retrospective series have reported recanalization using angioplasty in a total of 10 of 16 occluded arteries that were resistant to pharmacologic thrombolysis.[70,71] Caveat: Rescue angioplasty after failed thrombectomy was found to be associated with an increased risk of SAH.[72]

a. *Technique*. Do thrombolytic drug infusion and mechanical embolectomy first. Once these attempts at recanalization of the vessel are unsuccessful, measure the diameter of the proximal segment of the occluded artery on angiography to determine the appropriate size of the angioplasty balloon. Always undersize the balloon compared to vessel size. Advance a microwire past the occlusion into a distal vessel; place the microwire tip in the most distal position that is safely possible to maximize microwire purchase. Then advance the angioplasty balloon to the point of stenosis under roadmap guidance and inflate to nominal pressure. Oscillate the balloon 1–2 atmospheres above nominal pressure for 10–30 s before deflation. Withdraw the balloon into a larger proximal artery to permit follow-up angiography.

b. *Devices*. Small, noncompliant coronary angioplasty balloons useful in this setting, such as a 2×9 mm Maverick2™ Monorail™ Balloon Catheter (Boston Scientific, Natick, MA).

1. Intracranial stenting. An underlying atherosclerotic plaque may be the source of the occluding thrombus, and stenting may help prevent re-thrombosis after successful recanalization. Even when there is not an underlying atherosclerotic stenosis, placement of a stent can trap thrombus against the wall of the vessel and provide

immediate restoration of flow. Reports of rescue stenting of intracranial thrombosis after failure of other modalities have shown successful recanalization.[73,74]

    a. *Technique.* Attempt thrombolytic drug infusion and/or mechanical embolectomy first. Once these attempts at recanalization of the vessel are unsuccessful, measure the diameter of the proximal segment of the occluded artery on angiography to determine the appropriate size of the stent. Self-expanding stents may be sized to no more than the measured vessel size. *Always undersize balloon-expandable stents.* The stent should cover the entire length of thrombus, if possible. Advance an exchange-length microwire distal to the occlusion into a distal vessel; place the microwire tip in the most distal position that is safely possible to maximize microwire purchase. Then advance the balloon mounted stent to the point of occlusion under roadmap guidance and very slowly inflate to nominal pressure. If using a self-expanding stent, position it with the distal end just beyond the occlusion and slowly deploy it. When the stent is fully deployed, withdraw the delivery catheter into a larger proximal artery to permit follow-up angiography.

    b. *Devices.* Balloon expandable coronary stents are available in the various sizes but may be difficult to navigate in tortuous vessels and may rupture vessels due pressures required to deploy them. Self-expanding stents made for the intracranial circulation are much less traumatic to the vessels. Neuroform™ (Stryker Neurovascular, Fremont, CA) and especially Enterprise™ (Codman Neurovascular, San Jose, CA) are easier to deploy, but their HDE status makes off-protocol use in stroke problematic outside of an FDA-approved trial. Wingspan™ stents (Stryker Neurovascular, Fremont, CA) can be used for a symptomatic atherosclerotic stenosis but it is also an HDE product and its use for thrombotic occlusions without an underlying stenosis also requires careful consideration of these regulatory issues. Use of HDE products on an emergency basis outside of their approved protocol requires prompt notification of the hospital IRB, the device manufacturer, and the FDA. Solitaire™ (ev3 Neurovascular, Irvine, CA) is self-expanding and also has the option of being retrievable (see below). This allows the stent to be recaptured in a large guide catheter so it can be used as a retriever, with a reported high success rate recanalizing vessels.[75] This device was recently approved by the FDA.

Merci Retriever

    The Merci® Retrieval system (Stryker, Fremont, CA) was the first FDA-approved treatment for acute stroke aside from IV t-PA. The Merci Retriever is based on a flexible nitinol wire that assumes a helical shape once it emerges from the tip of the microcatheter. The microcatheter, containing the wire, is passed distal to the thrombus, the catheter is withdrawn, and the helical configuration taken by the wire ensnares the clot for removal from the vasculature. Arteries amenable to embolectomy with the Merci devices include the ICA, M1 and M2 segments, vertebral artery, basilar artery, and PCA. The Merci Retriever (Models X5 and X6) first received FDA 510(k) clearance for sale in the US in August 2004, based on data from the MERCI trial.[76] The Centers for Medicare and Medicaid Services established an ICD-9 procedure code (39.74) for Merci retrievers in October 2006. FDA 510(k) clearance for the L5 model was granted in February 2007, based on data from the Multi-Merci trial.[77] In 2011 the developer Concentric Medical was acquired by Stryker.

    1. Devices (Fig. 9.2)

        a. *Merci® Balloon Guide catheter.* The balloon guide catheter is designed to allow temporary occlusion of the carotid or vertebral artery during clot retrieval. It is available in 7, 8 and 9F sizes; in general the 7F is recommended for a small vertebral artery and the 9F is for a large carotid artery. It is packaged with an obturator for smooth vessel introduction and may be inserted through a femoral artery sheath, or exchanged directly into the femoral artery without a sheath. Usage without a sheath is usually not recommended, as the guide catheter may frequently get clogged as clots are extracted, and this may require removal of the guide catheter. The proximal end of the guide catheter includes a straight hub for device insertion and an angled hub for distal balloon inflation. Always connect an RHV with a three-way stop clock to the hub, to allow continuous flushing with heparinized saline. The compliant silicone balloon at the distal end of the guide catheter inflates to a 10 mm diameter with the maximum inflation volume of 0.8 mL is used. Use a 3 mL syringe, prepared with 50% contrast in saline, for balloon inflation.

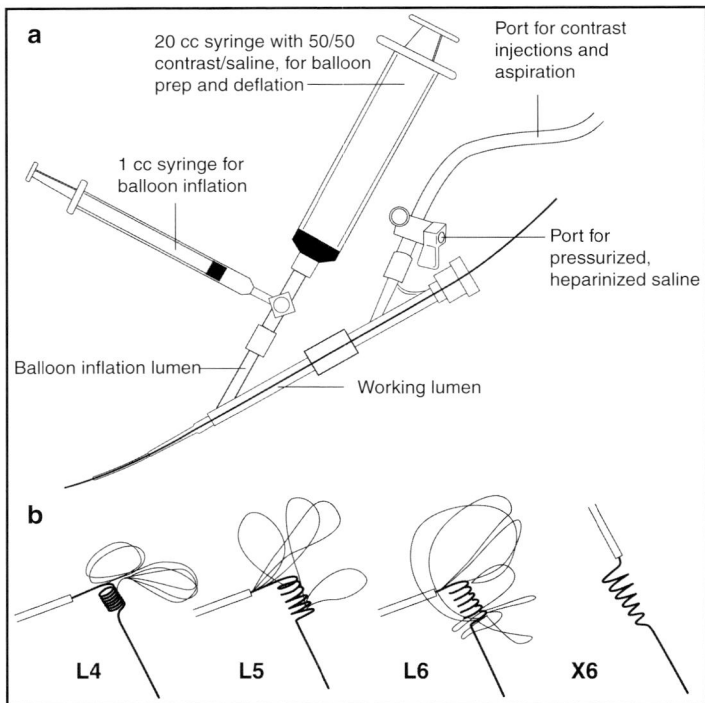

Fig. 9.2 The Merci® Balloon guide catheter set up (**a**), the Merci® Retrievers (**b**).

    b. *Microwire*. Use a microwire to advance the Merci microcatheter into the target vessel. The 0.012 in. J-tip Headliner™ (Microvention/Terumo, Tustin, CA) is preferred.

    c. *Merci® Microcatheters*. These microcatheters have a single radio opaque marker at the tip.

        i. *14X microcatheter*. Used only for X-6 retrievers, it has a 0.017 in. inner lumen.

        ii. 18 L *microcatheter*. Used for L and V-series retrievers and has a 0.021 in. lumen.

    d. *Merci® Retrievers* The retrievers are mounted on nitinol pusher wires, and each retriever is packaged with an introducer and a torque device.

        i. X-series retrievers. The X6 retriever has six tapered helical loops from 3 mm down to 1.5 mm and looks like a corkscrew. The X5 retriever has been discontinued.

        ii. V-series retrievers. These are a hybrid of both the X and L series retrievers.

        iii. L-series retrievers. The L4, L5 and L6 retrievers have four, five and six non-tapering helical loops, respectively. These are arranged at a 90° angle to the pusher wire. These are the "hairy retrievers" with suture threads bound to the nitinol wire to augment thrombus engagement. Loop diameter of the helix is 2.0 mm on the L4, 2.5 mm on the L5 and 2.7 mm on the L6. The L6 having a stiffer coil design, is more stretch resistant than the L5, and is most suitable for use in the larger and more proximal vessels (i.e. M1, ICA).

e. Distal Access Catheter (DAC). The DAC is an intermediate-sized catheter designed to be used in a triaxial system to provide additional support to the microcatheter (see Chap. 4). The DAC comes in numerous sizes and lengths:
   i. DAC 038. OD 3.9F, ID 0.038 in. Comes in two lengths: 125 and 136 cm.
   ii. DAC 044. OD 4.3F, ID 0.044 in. Comes in three lengths: 115, 130, and 136 cm.
   iii. DAC 057. OD 5.2F, ID 0.057 in. Comes in two lengths: 115 and 125 cm.
   iv. DAC 070. OD 6.3F, ID 0.070 in. Comes in two lengths: 105 and 120 cm.
f. *3 and 60 mL syringes*. Use a 3 mL syringe to inflate the guide catheter balloon and the 60 mL syringe for aspiration through the guide catheter during clot retrieval.

2. Technique
   a. Obtain femoral artery access and place a diagnostic catheter in the target carotid, subclavian, or vertebral artery.
   b. Give IV heparin (5,000 unit bolus and a 500 unit per hour infusion). A syringe containing protamine (50 mg) should be on the back table in case a haemorrhage occurs.
   c. Prepare the balloon guide catheter.
   d. Purge the balloon of air with the 3 mL syringe containing 50% contrast in saline.
   e. Flush the catheter with heparinized saline.
   f. Exchange the diagnostic catheter over a hydrophilic wire for the balloon guide catheter. Alternatively, the balloon guide catheter may be navigated directly into the carotid or vertebral artery over the hydrophilic wire. The balloon guide catheter should be positioned as distally as possible in the ICA or vertebral artery. *Note: the Merci balloon guide catheter is flimsier than most other guide catheters, and distal positioning will help stabilize it.*
   g. Consider using a DAC as an intermediary catheter to stabilize the microcatheter (see below).
   h. Advance the Merci microcatheter over a microwire with a J-tip curve into the target vessel. Navigate the microwire delicately past the clot, then stabilize the microwire and navigate the microcatheter into the artery distal to the clot. Remove the microwire and do a microcatheter angiogram (using a gentle injection with a 3 mL syringe containing 100% contrast) to confirm that the microcatheter tip is distal to the clot and that a vessel perforation has not occurred.
   i. Advance the Merci Retriever through the microcatheter until up to four loops of the helix are visible past the tip of the microcatheter. Withdraw the microcatheter and the retriever as a unit into the clot. Tighten the retriever loops by rotating the retriever wire counterclockwise by two revolutions. Advance the remaining loops by stabilizing the retriever and withdrawing the microcatheter. Allow the loops to deploy into the thrombus and turn the retriever wire counter-clockwise as many as five times to further engage the clot. Do not overdo the rotations, as over-aggressive rotation can kink or fracture the retriever.
      i. Anticipate that withdrawal of the retriever will be very painful for the patient, so now would be a good time to give conscious patients a dose of intravenous analgesics.
   j. Inflate the balloon on the guide catheter to stop antegrade flow in the ICA or vertebral artery. The balloon is adequately inflated when "ovalization" of the balloon is seen on fluoroscopy, indicating that the compliant balloon has conformed to the walls of the surrounding vessel.
   k. *Very, very slowly*, pull the engaged clot-retriever-microcatheter assembly back as a unit into the guide catheter and then out of the patient while applying forceful suction with the 60 mL syringe to the angled port of the RHV.
   l. Thoroughly aspirate all debris before flushing the guide catheter with heparinized saline.
   m. Deflate the balloon and do a guide catheter angiogram.
   n. Several passes with the retrieval device may be required.
   o. When a retriever is re-used for another pass, inspect it to be certain that it is undamaged and free of clot fragments. Manually straighten it out as it is back-loaded into the introducer.

p. The L4, 5, and 6 retrievers are usually not re-used because they often get twisted and the fibers get tangled after a single pass.

q. Do not attempt more than three passes of the retriever to minimize the chance of vessel injury.

r. Femoral artery access site closure. The sizable hole in the femoral artery created by the 8 or 9F Merci Balloon catheter can still be closed effectively with a Perclose ProGlide device (Abbott Laboratories, Abbott Park, IL).[78]

3. Merci Technique Tips

a. The balloon guide catheter may be positioned in the subclavian artery – rather than the vertebral artery – for posterior circulation cases, if access to the vertebral artery itself is difficult.

b. Distal Access Catheter (DAC) provides support for the microcatheter and can improve traction on the retriever (Fig. 9.3).

i. Advance a coaxial assembly of microwire, in the 18 L microcatheter, in the DAC through the balloon guide catheter as a unit and to the target vessel.

ii. The 057 DAC can get to the M1 segment without too much difficulty. Smaller DACs are used for smaller vessels and the 070 for large clots in the proximal carotid.

iii. Choose the shortest length of a DAC that will get near the target.

iv. If the DAC will not advance distally to the desired location, position the microcatheter beyond the clot, deploy the MERCI retriever, and gently pull back on the microcatheter/retriever assembly as the DAC is advanced. Almost always the DAC will easily advance quite distally using the counter-traction from the retriever.

v. Pulling on the microcatheter/retriever assembly while stabilizing the DAC provides a direct vector of force on the retriever with less straightening and distortion of vessels.

vi. For even greater traction, position the DAC up to the face of the clot and "sandwich" the clot between the Merci retriever and the tip of the DAC. Pulling on the entire assembly can often capture large thrombi.

vii. Aspirate through the DAC as well as through the balloon guide catheter during clot extraction to aid removal of all clot fragments. One can aspirate only through the DAC if not using the balloon guide catheter.

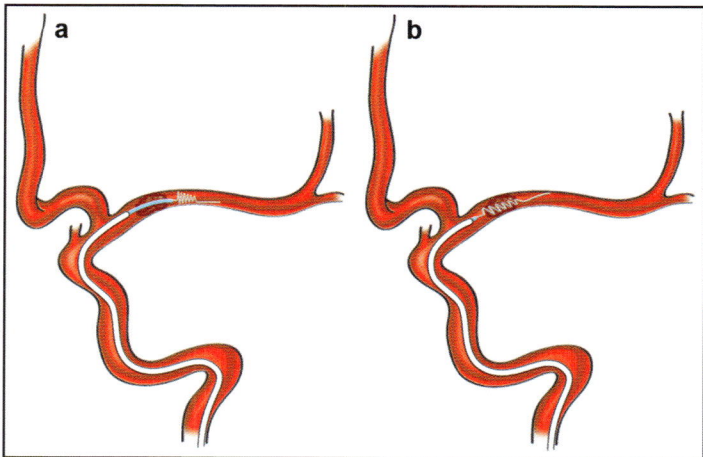

Fig. 9.3 Distal Access Catheter (DAC) technique. The microcatheter is advanced within the DAC to the edge of the clot. The DAC provides support during deployment and retrieval of the Merci® Retriever.

viii. Use of the DAC does not appear to add significant risk to the procedure. A series of over 100 procedures including a DAC had no complications related to its use.[79]

c. The Merci system may be used in patients who have been treated with IV t-PA. In the Multi-Merci trial, the use of IV t-PA before conventional angiography and attempted thrombectomy with the device did not increase the incidence of intracranial haemorrhage compared to patients not treated with IV t-PA.[77]

d. The Merci system may be augmented with IA fibrinolytic infusion. In the Multi-Merci trial, use of up to 24 mg t-PA was allowed in cases of treatment failure with the device, or to treat distal emboli that were not accessible with the device after successful proximal embolectomy.[77] Recanalization was achieved in 72% of patients in whom adjunctive IA t-PA was used, compared to 64% of patients treated with the device only; rates of haemorrhage were similar between the groups.

e. Caveat: A more recent study of the National Inpatient Sample showed the intracranial haemorrhage rate in patients undergoing endovascular therapy was significantly higher (20% vs. 15.5%) with associated use of thrombolytics.[29]

Penumbra System™

The Penumbra System™ (Penumbra, Inc., San Leandro, CA) was the second FDA-approved mechanical treatment for acute stroke. It does clot aspiration using a microcatheter attached to an electrical aspiration pump capable of producing 25 mmHg of suction. The Separator™ is a soft wire with a tear-drop-shaped enlargement of 6 mm proximal to its tip and is inserted via the microcatheter to physically break up the clot and keep the microcatheter tip from clogging. A major advantage over the Merci system is the fact that the Penumbra System works at the proximal face of the clot, eliminating the need to blindly position the microcatheter distal to the occlusion.

1. Devices
   a. *Guide catheter.*
      i. Use the largest guide catheter possible.
         A. The Penumbra reperfusion system works best with large guide catheters: 6F Cook Shuttle or Neuron 088 MAXX. This allows use of the 054 Reperfusion catheter.
         B. The Neuron 053 6F guide catheter can only accommodate the 026 Reperfusion catheter.
         C. The Neuron 070 6F guide catheter can also accommodate the 032 Reperfusion catheter.
   b. *Microwire.* Any soft microwire can be used to advance the Reperfusion microcatheter into the target vessel, but be aware that using microwires much smaller than the lumen of the catheter may create an overhanging shelf at the catheter tip, which can cause the catheter to hang up on branch points. To solve this problem:
      i. Use a larger diameter wire (0.016 or 0.018 in.) in the 026 and 032 catheters.
      ii. Use coaxial placement of an Excelsior® SL-10 (Stryker Neurovascular, Fremont, CA) microcatheter within the 041 Reperfusion catheter, all over a 0.014 in. microwire.
      iii. For the 054 Reperfusion catheter try a coaxial assembly using a 032 Reperfusion catheter.
   c. *Reperfusion microcatheters.* These microcatheters consist of a proximal stainless steel hypotube for pushability and stability, and stainless steel wire reinforcement distally for more flexibility. Stainless steel is not as kink resistant as other materials, so caution must be exercised in tortuous vessels to avoid kinking the catheter. These microcatheters have a single radio opaque marker at the tip.
      i. 026 microcatheter: 150 cm length, 3.9F tapering to 2.8F distally with a 0.026 in. lumen. Used for clot retrieval in small, distal vessels.
      ii. 032 microcatheter. 150 cm length, 4.1F tapering to 3.4F distally with a 0.032 in. lumen. Used for middle sized arteries.
      iii. 041 microcatheter. 137 cm length, but a generous 4.1F both proximal and distal and a 0.041 in. lumen. Used for larger vessel, proximal clots.
      iv. 054 microcatheter. 0.064 in. proximal lumen tapering to 0.054 distally with ability to rapidly aspirate large amounts of thrombus. Can be used in carotid or even proximal M1 segment, but usually

requires coaxial advancement over the 0.032 microcatheter to keep from hanging up on curves or branch points, such as the ophthalmic origin.

d. *The Separator™*. These wires are used to break up clot and keep the distal Reperfusion catheter clear of obstruction. A tear-drop bulbous swelling on the wire, of about 6 mm from its tip is indicated by a radioopaque gold marker. Each Separator is sized and matched to the corresponding Reperfusion catheter. All are 200 cm long and have a soft tip. The Separator™ has stainless steel core and can get mangled after a short period of use. The Separator™ FLEX has a nitinol core and is fairly indestructible.

    i. 026. Sized for the PSC026 catheter. Proximal wire is 0.018 in. with a 30 cm distal 0.010 in. segment.

    ii. 032. Sized for the PSC032 catheter. Proximal wire is 0.018 in. with a 20 cm distal 0.010 in. segment.

    iii. 041. Only works in the big PSC041 catheter. Proximal 0.020 wire with distal 43 cm 0.014 in. segment.

    iv. 054. Only for the PSC054 catheter. Wire size is 0.014 with a 0.045 distal bulb.

e. Aspiration Pump and connecting tubing. The necessary sterile connecting tubing for the aspiration pump, comes packaged with the Penumbra System devices.

2. Technique

a. Obtain femoral artery access and place a diagnostic catheter in the target carotid, subclavian, or vertebral artery.

b. Determine the size of the vessel occluded and choose appropriately sized reperfusion and guide catheters.

c. Give IV heparin (5,000 unit bolus and a 500 unit per hour infusion). A syringe containing protamine (50 mg) should be on the back table in case a haemorrhage occurs.

d. Prepare the guide catheter. Generally, a 6F or larger guide catheter is needed.

    i. Note: the Penumbra 6F 053 Neuron guide catheter can only be used for the 026 Penumbra Reperfusion catheters. The Penumbra 6F 070 guide catheter can be used with the 032 Reperfusion catheter. In other cases, a 6F Shuttle is necessary.

e. Exchange the diagnostic catheter over a hydrophilic wire (0.035 or 0.038 in.) for the guide catheter. Alternatively, the guide catheter may be navigated directly into the carotid or the vertebral artery over the hydrophilic wire. Position the guide catheter as distally as possible.

f. Advance the Reperfusion catheter over a microwire with a J-tip curve into the target artery. It is only necessary to navigate the just proximal to the clot. Do a guide catheter angiogram to confirm that the microcatheter tip is at the proximal face of the clot and that a vessel perforation has not occurred.

g. Tips for reperfusion catheter access

    i. Larger catheters (041 or 054) are more easily advanced in a coaxial fashion over a smaller microcatheter.

    ii. To position the 054 Reperfusion catheter above a tricky ophthalmic segment in the setting of an M1 clot, pull the catheter forward using the "grappling hook technique":[80] Coaxially advance an 18 L microcatheter (Stryker, Fremont, CA) through a 054 catheter and position it distal to the M1 clot. Deploy a Merci Retriever in the M1 clot and *very gentle* traction on the Retriever can create enough alteration in the angle and tension on the reperfusion catheter to pull it forward into the M1 segment.

h. Advance the Separator through the microcatheter until the gold radioopaque marker is visible just past the opaque tip of the microcatheter. There can be significant resistance in tortuous arteries.

i. Connect the microcatheter to the Aspiration Pump using the supplied sterile tubing. Flush the tubing with heparinized saline and tighten the connections.

j. Turn on the Aspiration Pump and gently move the Separator in and out of the microcatheter to fragment clot and keep the tip of the catheter free of obstructing clot.

k. Be gentle with the Separator and keep in mind that the tip extends beyond the tip of the catheter and can injure the vessel, especially if it is advanced into a small branch or at a sharp curve.

l. Only aspirate for short periods at a time and do frequent guide catheter angiograms to assess progress.
m. A large flow of blood through the catheter may indicate that the Reperfusion catheter tip is too proximal.
n. If the follow-up guide catheter angiogram shows incomplete arterial recanalization, consider adding an intra-arterial thrombolytic agent and/or additional passes with the Penumbra system. Several passes (2–3) with the device are often required.
o. Firm occlusions that do not respond to aspiration may require a pass with a Merci retriever, an Alligator, or a larger Penumbra Reperfusion catheter.

Solitaire™ Neurovascular Remodeling Device

The Solitaire™ device (ev3, Neurovascular, Irvine, CA) is a self-expanding closed-cell design stent that can be fully deployed and then completely retrieved if not detached. The stent can be used as an embolectomy device for patients with acute ischaemic stroke.[75,81,82] It is currently CE mark-approved in Europe and FDA-approved in the U.S. The Solitaire™ AB is detachable and the Solitaire™ FR device is non-detachable. The Solitaire™ FR With the Intention For Thrombectomy (SWIFT) study compared the Solitare device to MERCI for treatment of acute stroke; the study is currently closed to enrollment but the results have not yet been released.[83]

1. Devices
   a. Stents. The Solitaire™ stent is open-ended (unlike the Trevo™ device, which is close-ended) and has a closed-cell design. It is mounted on a 0.016 in wire.
      i. 4 mm by 15 mm; 4 mm by 20 mm
         (1) Recommended vessel diameter: 3.0–4.0 mm
      ii. 6 mm by 20 mm; 6 mm by 30 mm
         (1) Recommended vessel diameter: 5.0–6.0 mm
   b. Microcatheter
      i. Manufacturer recommends the Rebar™ Microcatheter (ev3, Irvine, CA)
         (1) 4 mm diameter Solitaire: Rebar 18
         (2) 6 mm diameter Solitaire: Rebar 27
2. Technique
   a. Use a 6F or larger guide catheter.
      i. A balloon guide catheter such as the Merci® Balloon Guide Catheter (Stryker, Fremont, CA) is recommended.
   b. Advance the Rebar microcatheter over a 0.014 in. microwire into the target vessel and through the clot. Position the tip of the microcatheter just distal to the clot.
   c. Exchange the microwire for the Solitaire stent.
   d. Deploy the stent in the clot by slowly withdrawing the microcatheter until the stent is fully deployed.
   e. Allow the stent to be deployed for 1–2 min, and then retrieve it by gently pulling it into the microcatheter.
   f. Withdraw the microcatheter and retrieved stent into the guide catheter whilst aspirating through both the microcatheter and the guide catheter continuously; if a balloon guide catheter is being used, inflate the balloon for this maneuver.
   g. Remove the microcatheter and stent together to irrigate and clear the Solitaire of clot.
   h. 1–3 passes may be necessary. The Solitaire should not be deployed and retrieved more than three times.

Trevo™ Stentriever™

The Trevo™ device (Stryker, Fremont, CA) is a self-expanding closed-cell design stent that can be fully deployed and then completely retrieved if not detached. The design is similar to the Solitaire™ device (see above).

3. Devices
   a. Stent. The Trevo™ stent is close-ended (unlike the Solitaire™ stent, which is open-ended) and has a closed-cell design.
      i. 4 mm by 20 mm
         (1) Recommended vessel diameter: 3.0–4.0 mm
   b. Microcatheter
      i. Manufacturer recommends the Trevo™ 18 Microcatheter (Stryker, Fremont, CA)
      ii. The Rebar™ Microcatheter (ev3, Irvine, CA) will also work.

4. Technique
   a. Use a 6F or larger guide catheter.
      i. A balloon guide catheter such as the Merci® Balloon Guide Catheter (Stryker, Fremont, CA) is recommended.
   b. Advance the microcatheter over a 0.014 in. microwire into the target vessel and through the clot. Position the tip of the microcatheter just distal to the clot.
   c. Exchange the microwire for the Trevo stent.
   d. Deploy the stent by slowly withdrawing the microcatheter until the stent is fully deployed.
   e. Allow the stent to be deployed for 1–2 min, and then retrieve it by gently pulling it into the microcatheter.
   f. Withdraw the microcatheter and retrieved stent into the guide catheter whilst aspirating through both the microcatheter and the guide catheter continuously; if a balloon guide catheter is being used, inflate the balloon for this maneuver.
   g. Remove the microcatheter and stent together, then irrigate and clear the Trevo of clot.
   h. Up to six passes may be necessary. An individual Trevo device should not be deployed and retrieved more than three times.

EKOS® Neurowave™ Micro-Infusion System

The EKOS system (EKOS Corporation, Bothell, WA) uses ultrasound energy and infusion of tPA to breakup clot in patients with ischaemic stroke. Ultrasonic energy causes the fibrin strands to relax and allow deeper penetration of the tPA. This device is currently approved by the U.S. FDA for infusion of contrast into the neurovasculature; use of the device with tPA and for the treatment of ischaemic stroke is considered off-label. Preliminary trial results with this device for the treatment of stroke have been positive.[84,85] The device is currently being used in the Interventional Management of Stroke III (IMS-III) trial.

1. Devices
   a. Micro-infusion catheter
      This 150 cm disposable microcatheter tapers from 3.0F (1 mm) at the proximal end to 2.8F at the distal end. It has a single central lumen that accommodates a 0.014 in microwire. The central lumen permits navigation over a microwire; the microwire is then removed to allow infusion of contrast and tPA. There is a piezoelectric ultrasound element (the "tip treatment zone") at the distal end of the microcatheter. The tip treatment zone is 2 mm long and 1 mm in diameter, and emits ultrasound energy at a frequency of 1.4–1.9 MHz in a 360° radial pattern perpendicular to the long axis of the catheter. An electrical connector at the proximal end of the catheter connects to the catheter interface cable that plugs into the control unit.
   b. Control unit
      The control unit connects to the micro-infusion catheter via the catheter interface cable and delivers electrical power to the tip treatment zone. The control unit also monitors the delivered electrical power, load impedance phase, catheter tip temperature, and radiofrequency leakage during operation. Both the control unit and the catheter interface cable are nonsterile and reusable.

2. Technique
   a. Use a guide catheter that is ≥6F.
      Use a large-enough guide catheter (e.g., a Neuron 070 6F) to permit frequent guide catheter angiograms while the micro-infusion catheter is in position.
   b. Give loading dose of IV heparin.
   c. Attach the micro-infusion catheter to an RHV with heparinized saline flush and advance it over a 0.014 in microwire into the target artery under roadmap guidance. The micro-infusion catheter is somewhat stiff, and primary navigation of the catheter into the target may be difficult. An alternative is to obtain microcatheter access with another microcatheter first and then exchange the microcatheter over an exchange-length microwire (e.g., 300 cm Synchro-2) for the micro-infusion catheter.
   d. Advance the tip of the micro-infusion catheter past the thrombus and do a microcatheter angiogram to confirm that the tip is beyond the thrombus. Then, pull the micro-infusion catheter back so that the tip is within the thrombus.
   e. Prepare tPA: 0.5 mg/mL saline.

f. Gently hand-inject a total of 2.0 mg (4 mL) tPA over 4 min. Activate the ultrasound at the beginning of the infusion.

g. Continue the infusion at a rate of 10 mg/h (for up to 120 min and maximum 22 mg tPA) as needed to recanalize the artery. Do a guide catheter angiogram every 15 min or so to monitor progress.

3. EKOS tips

a. Use of EKOS should be limited to accessible, relatively large intracranial arteries that are accessible such as the ICA, MCA (M1 or M2 segments), vertebral artery or basilar artery.[85] EKOS should not be used in the ACA, PCA, SCA or PICA, AICA. EKOS should also be avoided in situations in which safe navigation of a 0.014 in microwire is questionable, such as arterial dissections, chronic atherosclerosis, vasculitis, vasospasm, moyamoya, arteriopathy, and fibromuscular dysplasia.

b. Keep an eye on the control unit monitor throughout the procedure. Numerous alarm icons are used by the control unit to indicate various problems.

c. The micro-infusion catheter tip temperature is monitored by the control unit continuously; the control unit is programmed to stop power deliver if the temperature is <32°C or >43°C.

d. Never transmit electrical energy to the micro-infusion catheter when the tip is in the air. Electrical energy should only be transmitted when the catheter is in the patient and infusion fluid is flowing through the central lumen.

Additional Devices for Mechanical Thrombectomy

A number of devices are presently available for foreign body retrieval or are in evaluation in clinical trials for use in acute ischaemic stroke:

1. *En Snare® (Merit Medical, South Jordan, UT).* The En Snare device is FDA-approved for foreign body retrieval. The En Snare has a tulip-shaped three-loop design requiring a catheter with a 0.027-in. lumen. It opens distally, which may not allow sufficient capture of emboli.[63]

2. *Angiojet® (Possis Medical, Inc., Minneapolis, MN).* The Angiojet is a two-lumen device that combines local suction with mechanical disruption, an approach that has been termed *rheolytic thrombectomy*. Multiple retrograde high pressure saline jets are directed into the primary evacuation lumen of the catheter to create a vortex that draws in, traps, and fragments thrombus. The debris is simultaneously removed by suction via the recovery lumen. The Angiojet was originally developed for coronary and peripheral artery revascularization; neurovascular uses have been essentially limited to the carotid artery or intracranial venous sinuses.[63,86,87] The 5F AngioJet can be advanced through a 6F guide catheter and guided over a 0.014 in. microwire.

    The Neurojet (Possis Medical) was a smaller, single-lumen device that can be advanced through a 3F catheter. It was designed for the intracranial circulation, but development of this device was halted after vessel dissection was noted in an initial feasibility and safety trial.[88]

3. *The Phenox® Clot Retriever (Phenox, GmbH., Bochum, Germany)* has a dense network of firm polyamid fibers attached to a wire core, and can be passed via a >0.021 in. inner lumen microcatheter to extract occlusive intracranial thrombi.[89] It has advantages over other mechanical retrievers, in that it is less likely to fragment the clot.[90] This device is currently not available in the United States.

4. *The Catch (Balt Extrusion, Montmorency, France)* is a wind-sock basket retriever deployed distal to the clot and pulled back to remove the thrombus. Catch has a 4 × 19 mm diameter basket and is deployed with the Vasco+21 microcatheter. Catch9 has a 9 × 37 mm basket and is used with the Vasco+35. In a head-to-head comparison with the Merci® system, the Merci® system had a higher success in restoring flow (90%) compared to the Catch (70%) and caused less fragmentation of clot.[91] The Catch is not available in the United States.

Perfusion Augmentation: The NeuroFlo™ System

This system is radically different from other devices to improve blood flow to the brain. It involves placement of a large diameter double balloon NeuroFlo™ catheter (CoAxia, Maple Grove, MN) in the abdominal aorta and the balloons are temporarily inflated to partially obstruct flow in the abdominal aorta and divert blood flow to the brain. This system appears to provide some benefit both by cerebral blood flow parameters and by clinical outcome in the setting of symptomatic vasospasm after subarachnoid haemorrhage,[92,93] and the device was given a Humanitarian Device Exemption (HDE) by the FDA in March 2005 for this application. The SENTIS (Safety and Efficacy of Neuroflo Technology in Ischaemic Stroke) trial compared the use of NeuroFlo plus standard medical therapy to standard medical therapy alone in 515 stroke patients.[94] This trial did not find a significant difference in outcomes between the groups, but it did meet the primary safety endpoint, and post hoc analysis suggested that NeuroFlo is associated with better outcomes in patients presenting within 5 h of stroke onset and in those older than age 70. The system is simple to use and is relatively low risk, and may become a useful option for stroke treatment in centers without expertise in intracranial thrombolysis or thrombectomy techniques.

Patient Management After IA Stroke Treatment

1. Admit the patient to the ICA or a stroke unit.
2. Neurological exam Q 15 min during the infusion and Q 30 min for next 6 h, then Q 1 h for a total of 24 h after treatment.
3. Vital signs Q 15 min for first 2 h, Q 30 min for 6 h, and Q 1 h for a total of 24 h after treatment. Maintain SBP <180 mmHg and SBP <105 mmHg.
   a. Antihypertensive medication regimen
      i. Nicardipine infusion 5 mg/h IV to start; titrate as needed to a maximum of 15 mg/h.
      ii. Labetalol 10 mg IV over 1–2 min; may repeat every 10–20 min as needed to a maximum dose of 300 mg. Alternatively, start with a labetalol bolus and use an infusion of 2–8 mg/min.
      iii. If blood pressure is not adequately controlled, start an infusion of sodium nitroprusside at 0.5 mg/kg/min.
4. Obtain a head CT if the patient develops severe headaches, acute hypertension, nausea.
   In PROACT II, symptomatic ICH occurred in IA thrombolysis patients on an average of 10.2 h after the start of treatment; mortality was 83% in these patients.[95]
5. For patients treated with thrombolytics, avoid placement of NG tubes, Foley catheters, or intra-arterial catheters until the day after treatment if possible.
6. As with IV t-PA use, avoid antithrombotic agents (e.g. heparin, aspirin) for 24 h.
7. Surveillance head CT on post-procedure day 1 to monitor for haemorrhage.
   a. Antithrombotics can then be started if the CT shows no bleed.

Complications (management of complications is discussed below)
   A pooled analysis of data on 852 patients in 27 studies of IA thrombolysis found a rate of symptomatic intracerebral haemorrhage of 9.5%.[96] The death rate was 27.2% and the proportion of patients achieving a favourable outcome was 41.5%. In PROACT II, procedural complications included systemic haemorrhage (primarily hemorrhages at the puncture site) in 7% of patients, worsening of neurologic symptoms (1%) and anaphylaxis (1%).[12]

Combined IV + IA Strategies

Treatment with early administration of IV thrombolytics followed by IA thrombolysis (aka *bridging*) has been investigated in several studies. The ongoing Interventional Management of Stroke III (IMS III) trial is evaluating IV p-PA treatment in combination with mechanical thrombectomy.[97] Preliminary trials of IV GP IIB/IIIA inhibitor combined with IA thrombolysis have also been done or are in progress.
1. IV + IA t-PA.
   a. In the Emergency Management of Stroke Bridging Trial, 35 patients were randomized to receive either IV t-PA (0.6 mg/kg, 60 mg maximum over 30 min) or placebo, followed by IA injection of t-PA (average dose 11 mg).[98] There were no difference in the outcomes between the groups, but the TIMI 3 recanalization rate was better in the IV/IA group compared to the placebo/IA group (55% vs. 10%, $P = 0.03$). There was only one symptomatic ICH, in an IV/IA patient.

b. In the NIH Interventional Management of Stroke (IMS) trial, 80 patients with an NIHSS ≥10 received IV t-PA (0.6 mg/kg, 60 mg maximum over 30 min) within 3 h of symptom onset. Additional t-PA was then administered via microcatheter at the site of the thrombus up to a total dose of 22 mg over 2 h.[99] Compared to historical controls treated with conventional IV t-PA, rates of mortality and haemorrhage were not significantly different. The combined IV/IA patients showed a modest trend to improved outcome at 3 months (odds ratios ≥2).

c. The Recanalization using Combined intravenous Alteplase and Neuro-interventional Algorithm for acute Ischaemic StrokE (RECANALISE) trial was a nonrandomized prospective cohort study of 160 patients comparing treatment with IV alteplase only (n = 107) to treatment with both IV alteplase and IA treatment (n = 53).[100] Only patients who presented within 3 h after onset were included.
   i. Recanalization
      1. IV only: 52%
      2. IV + IA: 87% (p = 0.0002)
   ii. Symptomatic intracranial haemorrhage
      1. IV only: 11%
      2. IV + IA: 9% (p = 0.73)
   iii. Favourable outcome (mRSS 0–2 at 90 days)
      1. IV only: 44%
      2. IV + IA: 57% (p = 0.35)

d. A case–control study from Spain compared IV to IV + IA in stroke patients who did not respond to IV.[101] A total of 42 patients who received IA therapy after IV tPA treatment failed (defined as a lack of clinical improvement or recanalization 1 h after tPA bolus) were compared to 84 matched IV-only patients.
   i. Recanalization at 24 h
      1. IV only: 25.3%
      2. IV + IA: 46.3% (p = 0.016)
   ii. Symptomatic intracranial haemorrhage
      1. IV only: 6%
      2. IV + IA: 11.9% (p = 0.205)
   iii. Favourable outcome (mRSS 0–2 at 3 months)
      1. IV only: 14.9%
      2. IV + IA: 40% (p = 0.012)

e. The Interventional Management of Stroke III (IMS-III) is an ongoing multicenter NIH-sponsored randomized trial comparing IV only to IV plus IA treatment within 3 h of onset.[97] Enrollment of 900 patients is planned; as of this writing 656 subjects were enrolled. Enrollment was stopped on May 2, 2012.

2. IV GP IIB/IIIA + IA
   a. In the Combined Local Fibrinolysis and Intravenous Abciximab in Acute Vertebrobasilar Stroke Treatment study, 47 patients were treated with an IV bolus of abciximab (0.25 mg/kg) followed by a 12-h infusion (0.125 µg kg/min) and low-dose IA t-PA (median dosage: 20 mg).[102] Additional angioplasty and/or stenting was done in 14 patients. Compared to historical controls treated IA t-PA only (median dosage: 40 mg), symptomatic ICH was not significantly different, but the rates of TIMI 3 recanalization and favourable outcome were significantly higher in the combined treatment group.

   b. A German study of 75 patients with basilar artery occlusion compared IA thrombolysis alone with IV abciximab + IA thrombolysis.[103] Patients receiving the combined treatment had a better recanalization rate (83.7% vs. 62.5%, respectively P = 0.03) and a higher survival rate (58.1% vs. 25%, P = 0.02). Rates of symptomatic intracerebral haemorrhage were comparable in both groups (14% vs. 18.8%, P = 0.41).

Thrombolysis Complications: Management

1. Intracranial Haemorrhage
   a. Obtain a head CT to check for haemorrhage:
      i. IV thrombolysis: Obtain a head CT for any patient complaining of a severe headache or exhibiting a neurologic change. A surveillance post-thrombolysis head CT hospital day 2 is standard in some centers.

ii. IA thrombolysis: Obtain a CT immediately after the endovascular procedure to establish a baseline. It is common to see minor extravasation of contrast in the affected region of the brain ("*contrastoma*"), particularly in the basal ganglia; this is often *not* a sign of haemorrhage. Obviously, a head CT should be obtained in any patient with a severe headache or neurologic change. A CT on hospital day 2 is also commonly done.

   b. Asymptomatic and small haemorrhages (<30 mL) are managed conservatively.
      i. Reverse blood thinning agents.
         A. Reverse heparin if patient is heparinized (protamine IV, 10 mg per 1,000 units of heparin).
         B. Consider fresh frozen plasma and platelet transfusion.
      ii. Tight blood pressure control (maintain SBP ≤160 mmHg).
      iii. Frequent neuro exams, keep patient in ICU.
   c. Symptomatic, significant haemorrhage (>30 mL).
      i. Reverse blood thinning agents.
         A. Reverse heparin if patient is heparinized (protamine IV, 10 mg per 1,000 units of heparin).
         B. Consider fresh frozen plasma and platelet transfusion.
      ii. Intubate, if needed to control airway.
      iii. Mannitol 50 g IV.
      iv. Consider ventriculostomy if symptomatic hydrocephalus is present.
      v. Consider craniotomy for evacuation of clot.

2. Femoral artery haemorrhage
   a. Most common site of extracranial haemorrhage with IA thrombolysis.
   b. Signs of groin haemorrhage:
      i. Obvious bleeding at site or an enlarging subcutaneous haematoma.
      ii. *Ripping*, severe pain at the puncture site (a sign of a dissection).
      iii. Hypotension and bradycardia.
   c. Management:
      i. Manual compression.
      ii. Pelvic and abdominal CT scan to check for haemorrhage.
      iii. If the sheath is still in place, upsize to a larger-gauge sheath.
      iv. Volume expansion with IV fluids and transfusions if needed. Consider Vascular Surgery consultation for surgical repair of vessel.
      v. Consider reversal of anticoagulation and antiplatelet agents (i.e., platelet transfusion) if the haemorrhage is life-threatening.

3. Angioedema
   a. Defined as localized swelling of the tongue, lips or oropharynx within 6 h after the start of IV thrombolytic infusion.[104]
   b. Symptoms are typically mild, transient, and contralateral to the ischaemic hemisphere; in some cases, however, progression can be rapid and life-threatening due to airway obstruction.
   c. Patients on angiotensin-converting-enzyme inhibitors appear to be at increased risk of this complication.[53] Evidence of frontal and insular ischaemia on CT is also an associated risk factor.[51]
   d. Management:
      i. Prepare for intubation or cricothyroidotomy, if needed for airway control.
      ii. Obtain a CT of the face and head to rule out tongue haemorrhage.
      iii. Consider a brief course of high-dose steroids (e.g., Decadron 10 mg IV, then 6 mg IV Q 6 × 24 h).

9.5.   Special Situations

Basilar Artery Occlusion

The incidence of acute basilar artery occlusion is about 25% that of acute MCA occlusion.[105] Vertebrobasilar artery occlusion syndromes are discussed in detail in Chap. 17.

Radiographic Evaluation

Imaging in patients with posterior circulation acute stroke is somewhat different from that in patients with anterior circulation stroke. Of course, all patients must be evaluated for the presence of intracranial haemorrhage; noncontrast CT is adequate for this purpose. Because of bone artifact and the difficulty with imaging the brainstem and cerebellum, CT perfusion is less useful in this setting, although PCA territory ischaemia may be well characterized. CT angiography (CTA) can be very helpful in patients with basilar artery occlusion,[106] particularly in defining the extent of the occlusion and in assessing collateral circulation. A CTA can be obtained at the same time as the initial screening CTA, and some centers routinely combine CTA with CT perfusion for the evaluation of all patients with acute ischaemic stroke. MRI, combined with MR angiography (MRA) can also be helpful.

Patient Selection for Thrombolysis

Patient selection criteria for thrombolysis for basilar artery occlusion are controversial,[107,108] largely because the condition is uncommon, two modalities exist (IA and IV thrombolysis), and because all of the existing published data comes from small, nonrandomized series, except for one randomized trial, which was terminated because of poor enrollment.[109] The Basilar Artery International Cooperation Study (BASICS) was an international prospective nonrandomized observational study of 592 patients with acute basilar artery occlusion.[110] Outcomes were assessed at 1 month. The overall rate of a poor outcome (mRSS of 4, 5 or death) was 68%. Treatment with anticoagulation only was compared to treatment with IV thrombolytics or IA therapy. Although some subgroups within the treatment arms did better than others, the authors concluded that the study results did "not support unequivocal superiority of IA treatment over IV thrombolytics, and the efficacy of IA treatment versus IV thrombolytics needs to be assessed in a randomized controlled trial."

Inclusion Criteria

1. Acute or progressive onset of significant brainstem, cerebellar, or PCA territory symptoms within 12–24 h of treatment.[111]
   In the Australian Urokinase Stroke Trial, a 24 h window was not associated with an increased rate of adverse outcomes.[109]
2. Basilar artery occlusion, as shown by CTA, angiography, or MRA.
3. Relative inclusion criteria (i.e., factors that predict a favourable response to thrombolysis)
   a. Embolic origin of occlusion.[30]
   b. Distal basilar artery occlusion, or short segment occlusion.[30,112]
   c. Evidence of good collateral circulation.
   d. Younger patient.

Exclusion Criteria

1. Acute intracranial haemorrhage.
2. Examination compatible with brain death, or near-brain death.
3. Widespread, severe ischaemic injury on imaging (e.g., hypoattenuation and brain edema throughout the brainstem and cerebellum on CT).
4. Relative exclusion criteria:
   a. Atherosclerotic occlusion.[30]
   b. Proximal basilar artery occlusion, or longer segment occlusion.[30,112]
   c. Older patient.

Techniques

1. IA therapy
   a. Obtain femoral artery access and place a diagnostic catheter in the subclavian artery proximal to the origin of the vertebral artery.

b. Select the vertebral artery that is largest in caliber and patent. Angiograms of both vertebral arteries may be necessary if pre-procedure CTA or MRA was not done. Be sure to image the origin of the vertebral artery prior to placing the diagnostic catheter in the vessel to check for atherosclerosis at the origin of the artery. Bilateral ICA angiograms are also helpful in some cases to assess collateral circulation via the P-comms.

c. If both vertebral arteries are occluded, angiograms of the thyrocervical costocervical trunks and ICAs should be done. IA thrombolysis by injection of t-PA into the ascending cervical branch of the thyrocervical trunk has been reported.[113]

d. Give IV heparin (5,000 unit bolus and a 500 unit per hour infusion). A syringe containing protamine (50 mg) should be on the back table in case a haemorrhage occurs.

e. The diagnostic catheter is then exchanged for a guide catheter, which is positioned as distal as possible within the vertebral artery.

f. Do thrombectomy or thrombolysis as described above in Sect. 9.4.1.

2. IV thrombolysis
a. IV thrombolytic treatment can be effective for basilar artery occlusion. A systematic review concluded that recanalization rates are better for patients treated with IA thrombolysis, but the clinical outcome is similar for either modality.[114]

b. Regimen for IV t-PA: 0.9 mg/kg (maximum of 90 mg) over 60 min with 10% of the dose given as a bolus over 1 min.

Outcomes and Complications

The following data are from a systematic review of series consisting of 420 patients treated with IA (344 patients) or IV thrombolysis (76 patients) for basilar artery occlusion.[114]

1. Frequency of recanalization
   a. IA: 65%
   b. IV: 53% ($p = 0.05$)
2. Death or dependency
   a. IA: 76%
   b. IV: 78% ($p = 0.82$)
3. Survival rates
   a. IA: 45%
   b. IV: 50% ($p = 0.48$)
4. Good outcome rates
   a. IA: 24%
   b. IV: 22% ($p = 0.82$)
   c. Without recanalization: 2%

Associated Carotid Stenosis + Stroke

Acute ischaemic stroke in the presence of atherosclerotic carotid stenosis can be effectively treated with IA thrombolysis and carotid angioplasty and stenting (CAS) during the same procedure. CAS procedures are discussed in detail in Chap. 10. The key issues for combined thrombolysis and CAS are:

1. If thrombus is present in the cervical ICA, thrombolysis or thrombectomy in this vessel should be done prior to CAS.
2. Antiplatelet therapy is mandatory to avoid acute stent thrombosis due to platelet activation. Parenteral GP IIB/IIIA inhibitors are the fastest-acting antiplatelet agents available; the authors of this handbook prefer abciximab, because it is reversible with platelet transfusion if necessary.
   (a) Note: Use of antiplatelet agents, in addition to thrombolytics, increases the risk of haemorrhage. Therefore, the use of thrombolytic drugs should be minimized as much as possible if a stent is to be used.

Technique

1. Obtain femoral artery access and place a diagnostic catheter in the CCA.
2. If the angiogram shows significant stenosis of the cervical ICA (>50%), prepare for CAS:
   a. Give antiplatelet agents.
   b. Select and prepare CAS devices.
3. Place an exchange-length hydrophilic wire in the ECA (or use an Amplatz Extra Stiff Guidewire 0.035″ (Cook Inc., Bloomington, IN) if the ECA is not accessible). Exchange the diagnostic catheter over the wire for a 6F 90 cm sheath (e.g. Shuttle® sheath, Cook Inc., Bloomington, IN) or an 8F guide catheter.
4. Give heparin IV (2,000 unit bolus and a 500 unit per hour infusion). Have protamine on stand-by.
5. Navigate a microwire and microcatheter into the ICA past the region of stenosis. Do a microcatheter angiogram to clarify the anatomy distal to the stenosis. There are two possible locations for the symptomatic occlusion, and each calls for a different strategy:
   a. *Cervical ICA*. A relatively small amount of thrombus in the cervical ICA may respond to selective injection of a lytic agent through the microcatheter. Larger, occlusive thrombosis can be handled in several ways:
      i. *Microcatheter navigation into the intracranial vessels*. Gently navigate a microwire (with a "J" shape at the tip) and a microcatheter through the occlusion.[115]
      ii. *Suction thrombectomy*. A large clot in the ICA may be treated with suction thrombectomy by aspiration through the guide catheter. However, use caution when positioning the guide catheter adjacent to the origin of the ICA, as a friable atherosclerotic plaque may be disrupted or a dissection may occur. Alternatively, a 4 or 5F diagnostic catheter may be used for suction.
   b. *Intracranial vessel*. If the anatomy permits, guide a microwire and microcatheter through the stenotic ICA and into the occluded intracranial vessel. Recanalization of the vessel via selective administration of a thrombolytic drug or thrombectomy is then followed by CAS.
      i. Note: once the cervical carotid is revascularized and antegrade flow is improved, intracranial occluded and stenotic regions may then significantly improve. In elective CAS, it is axiomatic that distal tandem stenoses will often improve after treatment of the proximal lesion.
      ii. If a 054 Penumbra reperfusion catheter can be advanced across the stenosis and used to aspirate symptomatic clot in the middle cerebral artery, it can then be used to deploy an EPD to do the CAS.[116]
6. Thrombolytic agent. Options include:
   a. *GP IIB/IIIA inhibitor*. Intra-arterial injection of a GP IIB/IIIA inhibitor accomplishes two things:
      i. Acute thrombi, even predominantly fibrin-rich ones (i.e., "red clot") will dissolve with direct administration of a GP IIB/IIIA inhibitor;
      ii. The drug will provide anti-platelet protection after deployment of the stent.
      iii. *Abciximab dose*: Use the systemic loading dose: 0.25 mg/kg in a concentration of 2 mg/mL saline. Infuse the drug over several minutes. Follow the IA dose with a 12 h IV infusion at a rate of 10 μg/min.
      iv. Note: Avoid partial loading doses of abciximab, as there is data in the cardiology literature to indicate that partial loading doses of abciximab have a paradoxical pro-thrombotic effect.[117–119]
   b. *Fibrinolytic*. If a fibrinolytic drug is used, such as t-PA, minimize the amount of drug used to reduce the risk of haemorrhage (e.g., tight blood pressure control), as simultaneous administration of both fibrinolytic and antiplatelet drugs elevates the risk of haemorrhage.
7. Once the distal lesion has been treated, standard CAS procedure is used to treat the stenotic lesion.

8. After the procedure, if not already done, give the patient a loading dose of aspirin and clopidogrel (aspirin 325 mg PO/NG/PR and clopidogrel 300 mg PO/NG), followed by aspirin (325 mg PO QD) and clopidogrel (75 mg PO QD) for 1 month. Continue aspirin indefinitely.

Extracranial Carotid or Vertebral Dissection + Stroke

Spontaneous or traumatic dissection of the cervical vessels can cause stroke one or both of two mechanisms:
1. Thromboembolism (most common)
2. Haemodynamic impairment (less common)

Angiographic findings that indicate a dissection, rather than atherosclerotic stenosis, include a tapering stenosis, string sign, double lumen, and scalloping.[120] Extracranial dissection syndromes are discussed in Chap. 18.

In most arterial dissection cases, thrombolysis without stenting is sufficient. Non-flow limiting dissections frequently cause some degree of thrombosis at the dissection site, which is usually platelet-rich (i.e., "white clot") and will respond to treatment with antiplatelet agents. A common scenario is a non-occlusive dissection with associated thrombus and embolization with occlusion of intracranial vessels. In these situations, the authors of this handbook have obtained good results with IA or IV injection of a GP IIB/IIIA inhibitor, followed by long-term treatment (3 months) with a combination antiplatelet regimen (e.g., aspirin and clopidogrel).

Stenting is usually only necessary when:
1. The dissection is flow-limiting and the patient is symptomatic because of haemodynamic failure.
2. Treatment of the dissection is necessary to provide access to a distal lesion.

Technique

1. Obtain femoral artery access and place a diagnostic catheter in the target vessel proximal to the lesion.
2. Do an angiogram. If stenting is necessary, then:
3. Exchange the diagnostic catheter for a guide catheter.
   a. 6F 90 cm sheath (e.g. Shuttle® sheath, Cook Inc., Bloomington, IN) or an 8F guide catheter.
   b. In rare cases, the dissection originates in the aortic arch or subclavian artery. In these situations, the access catheter should be positioned in the aorta or subclavian proximal to the dissection; stabilization of the guide catheter can be obtained by passage of a "buddy wire" into the subclavian or innominate artery.
4. Give IV heparin (5,000 unit bolus and a 500 unit per hour infusion). Have protamine on stand-by.
5. *Gently* navigate a microwire with a J-shaped tip and microcatheter into and past the region of dissection. Do a microcatheter angiogram to determine if the microcatheter is in the true lumen rather than the false lumen. It is critical to obtain access to the true lumen distal to the dissection. Inadvertent stenting of the false lumen will cause a complete occlusion.
6. If thrombus is present in the dissection site, then IA infusion of a GP IIB/IIIA inhibitor or a thrombolytic agent may dissolve the thrombus and permit stenting of the lesion without the risk of embolization.
   a. Note: Use of antiplatelet agents, in addition to thrombolytics, increases the risk of haemorrhage. Therefore, minimize the use of thrombolytic drugs as much as possible if a stent is used.
   b. The authors of this handbook prefer to use abciximab in these cases. Abciximab is reversible with platelet transfusions should bleeding complications arise, and it will provide the necessary protection against platelet activation once the stent is deployed.
      i. Abciximab dose: Use the systemic loading dose: 0.25 mg/kg in a concentration of 2 mg/mL saline. Infuse the drug over several minutes. Follow the IA dose with a 12 h IV infusion at a rate of 10 μg/min.

Note: Avoid partial loading doses of abciximab, as there is data in the cardiology literature to indicate that partial loading doses of abciximab have a paradoxical pro-thrombotic effect.[117–119]

7. Advance an embolic protection device across the lesion and deploy it in the true lumen of the vessel distal to the dissection.
Always use an embolic protection device in this setting when feasible. Even in cases where there is no apparent thrombus or atherosclerosis associated with the stenosis, non-angiographically apparent debris may be released when the stent is deployed.

8. Advance and deploy a self-expanding stent. Size and position the stent to extend from the normal vessel proximal to the dissection and cover as much of the dissection as possible. For long dissections, particularly spiral dissections that extend from the CCA into the ICA, coverage of the proximal portion of the dissection may be sufficient, to plaster the dissection flap against the wall of the vessel and re-establish antegrade flow.

9. After the procedure, if not already done, give the patient a loading dose of aspirin and clopidogrel (aspirin 325 mg PO/NG/PR and clopidogrel 300 mg PO/NG), followed by aspirin (325 mg PO QD) and clopidogrel (75 mg PO QD) for 1 month. Continue aspirin indefinitely.

Associated Intracranial Stenosis + Stroke

Atherosclerotic stenosis may underlie an acute occlusion. This combination of disorders – acute thrombosis on top of a stenotic lesion – may be apparent immediately on imaging, or only after thrombolysis fails to reopen a narrowed segment. Indications of concomitant stenosis on imaging in acute stroke include:

1. Calcification in the wall of the affected vessel on CT or CTA.
2. Long segment occlusion.
3. Clinical risk factors for atherosclerosis.

Treatment options include angioplasty or angioplasty with stent placement. The optimal strategy depends largely on the size and accessibility of the lesion. Angioplasty alone has the advantages of (1) not requiring antiplatelet therapy, (2) being easier and safer than stenting, particularly in tortuous anatomy. Stenting is more likely to maintain patency of the vessel, at least for the short term, and is the best option for treatment of occlusive dissections.

Technique

Intracranial angioplasty technique is discussed in detail in Chap. 11.

1. Establish an accurate diagnosis of significant intracranial stenosis. This often comes after an attempt at primary thrombectomy or thrombolysis.
2. Once guide catheter is established, advance a microwire and microcatheter past the area of stenosis. Remove the microwire and do a microcatheter angiogram to assess the distal vessels and further characterize the region of stenosis.
3. Preparation:
   a. Make measurements to determine the size of the angioplasty balloon and/or stent that is needed.
   b. For atherosclerotic stenosis, use a non-compliant coronary angioplasty balloon such as the Maverick2™ Monorail™ balloon catheter (Boston Scientific, Natick, MA).
   c. If a dissection is the cause of the stenosis, stenting without angioplasty may be sufficient.
   d. *Device size*: Select a balloon with a diameter slightly smaller than the normal diameter of the artery. The length of the balloon should be relatively short to maximize the ease of navigation of the balloon into the target vessel.
   e. Prepare the balloon and indeflator (balloon inflation/deflation device). Load the indeflator with 50/50 contrast in heparinized saline.
4. Advance an exchange-length microwire through the microcatheter and then exchange the microcatheter for the balloon catheter.
5. Gently guide the angioplasty balloon into the proximal region of stenosis or occlusion and inflate it to nominal pressure. Keep the balloon inflated for 40–50 s and then deflate.

6. Do a guide catheter angiogram after each inflation to reassess the lesion and check for contrast extravasation. Several balloon inflations are often necessary to reopen an occluded, atherosclerotic intracranial artery.
7. Addition of a stent is indicated for some atherosclerotic vessels that will not stay open despite angioplasty and for dissections.
8. If stent deployment is planned, then antiplatelet therapy is important.
   a. An IV GP IIB/IIIA inhibitor will provide immediate antiplatelet protection once the stent is deployed. Later, the patient may be given aspirin and a loading dose of clopidogrel for long-term antiplatelet therapy.
   b. Note: Addition of antiplatelet agents significantly increases the risk of haemorrhagic complications.
9. Choice of stent:
   a. A self-expanding stent, such as the Wingspan™ Stent System (Stryker Neurovascular, Fremont, CA), is first-line in most situations. This device was developed specifically for the treatment of intracranial stenosis and is highly trackable and flexible. Wingspan technique is discussed in detail in Chap. 11. Neuroform stent-assisted revascularization for acute stroke has been reported.[121]
   b. Humanitarian Device Exemption products such as Wingspan, Enterprise, and Neuroform stents must have an IRB protocol and whenever used for stroke or other uses outside their approved protocol there must be prompt reporting and justification of a protocol violation to the IRB, the manufacturer, and the FDA.
   c. Coronary balloon-expandable stents are rigid and difficult to maneuver safely through the carotid siphon or distal vertebral artery. Use of these stents to treat intracranial stenosis is associated with complication rates in the neighbourhood of 20–25%.[122,123] Balloon-expandable stents are acceptable in carefully selected cases in which stent-assisted recanalization is critical and an appropriate self-expanding stent is not available.
   d. *Sizing of stent*: The stent diameter should be about 0.5 mm less than the normal diameter of the vessel.
10. *Post-procedure antiplatelet therapy*: Dual antiplatelet therapy is standard in any stent procedure: Clopidogrel 75 mg PO/NG QD for 1 month and aspirin 325 PO/NG QD indefinitely.

Central Retinal Artery Occlusion

Central retinal artery occlusion is rare, occurring in 1.3 per 100,000 people per year.[124] The retina is irrigated primarily by the central retinal artery. Experimental occlusion of the central retinal artery up to 97 min in rhesus monkeys causes no detectable damage.[125] Ischaemic injury occurs beyond 98 min and correlates with the length of occlusion, and occlusion for 240 min results in massive, irreversible retinal damage.

A number of small, retrospective studies have reported that IA thrombolysis for acute central retinal artery occlusion benefits a minority of patients, ranging from 15% to 30% of cases.[126–133] The success rate with IA thrombolysis declines with time since onset of symptoms, with the best results occurring in patients treated within 6 h of onset.[127,130,134] Although good results have been obtained in some 9% of patients treated >14 h after symptom onset,[130] this may not be significantly different from the natural history, in which 8% of patients report significant recovery without therapy.[134,135] A prospective, randomized, multicenter trial of IA thrombolysis by the European Assessment Group for Lysis in the Eye (EAGLE) did not show a benefit with IA treatment, however, the time-to-treatment was long (12.78 h, see below).[136] The most important predictors of a good response to IA thrombolysis includes a short time since symptom onset and younger age.[129] Risk factors for complications with IA thrombolysis are advanced age and high grade ipsilateral ICA atherosclerotic stenosis.[128]

Diagnosis

1. Central retinal artery occlusion manifests as sudden, painless, unilateral visual loss.
   a. In contrast, occlusion of the ophthalmic artery can cause orbital and eye pain and conjunctival injection, in addition to visual loss.

b. *Branch retinal artery occlusion* most commonly affects the temporal retinal vessels, and the resulting visual deficit is characteristically incomplete.[137]
c. Central retinal *vein* occlusion can be identified by the presence of retinal vein dilatation in all four quadrants and retinal haemorrhages. Central retinal vein occlusion may occur along with central retinal artery occlusion.
    i. IA thrombolysis for central retinal vein occlusion led to improvement in visual acuity in 23% of the patients in one series.[138]
2. Although sudden, painless loss of vision in one eye is almost always due to central retinal artery occlusion, an ophthomological examination is necessary to confirm the diagnosis. Funduscopic examination findings include ischaemic macular edema, a cherry red spot, and reduced or no retinal blood flow.
3. Brain MRI may show restricted diffusion in the distal part of the affected optic nerve.[139]

European Assessment Group for Lysis in the Eye (EAGLE)

Multicenter, randomized trial in Germany and Austria comparing IA thrombolysis (44 patients) to conservative therapy (40 patients) for central retinal artery occlusion.[136] The IA group received tPA infusion into the ophthalmic artery (maximum, 50 mg).

1. Mean interval between symptom onset was 12.78 h for the IA group and 10.99 h for the conservative therapy group.
2. Vision improved significantly in both groups, and did not differ between the groups.
3. Two patients in the conservative group and 13 patients in the IA group had adverse reactions.
4. A noteworthy finding of this study was that the conservative management group did better than patients in previous reports of conservative management, suggesting that the medical management used in this study (see below) is efficacious.
5. *The biggest limitation of this study was the relatively long time to treatment for the IA group.*

Technique: IA Treatment of Central Retinal Artery Occlusion

Despite the findings of the EAGLE trial, IA treatment of central retinal artery occlusion remains a reasonable option in younger patients who present within a relatively short period of time, such as within 3–8 h (the standard time period for consideration of IA treatment of ischaemic stroke).

1. Do a diagnostic cerebral angiogram. Isolated occlusion of the central retinal artery is usually not apparent on a diagnostic angiogram, but concomitant abnormalities in the carotid or ophthalmic arteries, such as intraluminal thrombus or atherosclerosis, should be checked for. Also, a baseline intracranial angiogram is important, to check for the presence of other vessel occlusions and to establish a baseline, should an intracranial thromboembolic event occur later in the case or afterwards.
2. Give IV heparin (5,000 unit bolus). Have protamine on stand-by.
3. Obtain guide catheter access. The higher in the ICA, the better.
4. Place a microcatheter in the ophthalmic artery under roadmap guidance. The tip of the microcatheter does not have to be in a very distal position for the access to the central retinal artery.
    a. Any small microcatheter and microwire will do. The authors of this handbook prefer to use an UltraFlow™ microcatheter (ev3, Irvine, CA) or Magic® (AIT-Balt, Miami, FL) and Mirage™ 0.008 in. microwire (ev3, Irvine, CA).
    b. If the ICA or ophthalmic artery is occluded, or if the ophthalmic artery cannot be accessed, then the selective injection of thrombolytic into the distal internal maxillary artery can be done.

5. Do a microcatheter angiogram.
6. *Note*: The choroidal blush on angiography should not be confused with the retina. The choroidal blush results from contrast filling of the ciliary arteries; the presence or absence of the choroidal blush has no bearing on the outcome of IA thrombolysis.[127]
7. Infuse the thrombolytic agent into the ophthalmic artery over approximately 1 h.
   a. Favourable results have been reported with both t-PA and urokinase.
      i. t-PA: 15–50 mg.[128,140,141]
      ii. Urokinase: 100,000–1,000,000 units.[127–130]
8. Ophthomological examinations may be done during the infusion of the thrombolytic drug; funduscopic evidence of retinal artery recanalization sometimes occurs during the procedure.
9. Stop the procedure when vision is significantly improved or when the maximum dose of thrombolytic agent (40–50 mg t-PA or 900,000–1,000,000 units urokinase) has been given.
10. Do final post-procedure intracranial angiograms.

Non-endovascular Treatment

Contrary to popular belief, spontaneous improvement in both visual acuity and visual fields does occur, mainly during the first 7 days.[142] A variety of non-interventional management options exist, and the efficacy of the various techniques is controversial.[143]
1. The following protocol was used for the patients in the conservative therapy arm of the EAGLE trial:[136]
   a. Isovolemic haemodilution to keep hematocrit ≤40%
   b. *Ocular massage*. Repeated increased pressure is applied to the globe for 10–15 s, followed by a sudden release with an in-and-out movement using a 3-mirror contact lens for 3–5 min.
   c. A single drop of topical timolol 0.5%.
   d. Acetazolamide, 500 mg IV.
   e. All patients in both arms of the EAGLE trial were treated with twice-daily dose-adjusted heparin for five days and aspirin, 100 mg a day for at least four weeks.
2. Other methods:
   a. Anterior chamber paracentesis. Intraocular pressure can be reduced by direct aspiration of aqueous fluid.
   b. IV tPA. A randomized trial of IV tPA, using the same dosing scheme as for IV tPA treatment of ischaemic stroke, was terminated early because of a lack of efficacy and because a patient treated with tPA had an intracranial haemorrhage.[144]

Venous Occlusion

Treatment of intracranial venous occlusion is discussed in Chap. 12.

9.6. Appendix 1: Primer on Imaging in Stroke
by Joel K. Curé, M.D.

Imaging goals in ischemic stroke:
1. Confirming a diagnosis of ischemic stroke and exclusion of non-vascular (e.g. tumor) causes of the clinical ictus
2. Exclusion of hemorrhage and estimation of the risk of hemorrhagic transformation
3. Selection of patients for reperfusion therapy by distinguishing ischemic but viable (i.e., the penumbra) from infarcted tissue and excluding those for whom the therapeutic risk exceeds the anticipated benefit
4. Identifying large-vessel occlusion that may complicate or represent a target for therapy

The 2007 *Guidelines for the Management of Patients with Acute Ischemic Stroke* noted: "Both CT and MRI are options for imaging the brain, but for most cases and at most institutions, CT remains the most practical initial brain imaging test".[145] This may change with increasing availability of MRI. MRI is more sensitive than CT for detection of acute infarction, is able to detect both acute and chronic hemorrhage as effectively as CT, and demonstrates higher interobserver and intraobserver reliability than CT for ischemic stroke diagnosis, even in readers with little experience.[146]

Stroke location and distribution at imaging reflects mechanism.[147] Most strokes are thromboembolic and their imaging appearance reflects the territory of the occluded artery less any portion of that territory that is adequately perfused by collateral blood supply. Solitary or multiple unilateral cortical or cortical/subcortical infarcts may be secondary to either cardiogenic emboli or large arterial occlusion. Cardiogenic emboli typically account for bilateral acute infarcts in both the anterior and posterior circulations, especially in the absence of definable intracranial arterial occlusions on CTA, MRA, or transcranial Doppler. However, multiple synchronous infarcts may be encountered in patients with occlusive vasculopathies (e.g. CNS vasculitis) or coagulopathies. Lacunar infarcts, due to small arterial occlusion, are typically small (< 1.5 cm) and imaging abnormalities correspond to the territory of the occluded perforating artery. These infarcts most commonly occur in the basal ganglia, thalamus, brainstem, or deep cerebellar white matter. Arterial border zone infarcts occur in regions of brain that lie between major arterial territories. These include deep cerebral hemispheric regions such as the centrum semiovale, corona radiata, and cortical zones between the ACA and MCA and the MCA and PCA territories. Arterial border zone infarcts may occur bilaterally in cases of global cerebral hypoperfusion or unilaterally in patients with severe ICA stenosis or MCA stenosis plus A1 segment hypoplasia.

Noncontrast CT Diagnosis of Acute Infarction

In CT scan interpretation the terms, "hypoattenuation" and "hyperattenuation" are preferred to "hypodense" and "hyperdense". Attenuation indicates the degree of x-ray absorption that occurs within tissue. In patients with stroke, hypoattenuating tissue tends to be edematous, and hyperattenuating tissue tends to be hemorrhagic.

Brain edema associated with hemispheric stroke may be detectable within 1–2 h of stroke onset. CT identifies ischemic lesions with a sensitivity of 65% and a specificity of 90% within 6 h of stroke onset.[148] However, the sensitivity of CT for acute ischemic stroke within the first 3 h of symptom onset has been reported to be as low as 7%.[146] CT is insensitive for small acute infarcts, especially in the posterior fossa[1-9] and is less sensitive than diffusion weighted MRI in the acute setting.[150] The peak period for identifying brain ischemia on CT is 3–10 days after the ictus, well beyond the thrombolytic time window. The value of early CT in acute stroke is therefore not chiefly diagnostic, but prognostic. A large hypoattenuation area detected within 6 h of stroke onset is an indication of irreversible tissue injury,[148] portends an increased risk of hemorrhagic transformation in patients treated with rTPA,[151] and is associated with an increased risk of fatal brain edema.[152] ECASS-1 and subsequent analyses of its CT and patient data led to the "one third rule". Patients with CT-identified early ischemic changes (EIC) involving less than one third of the MCA territory had an improved functional outcome after IV thrombolysis compared to patients with EIC in more than one third of the MCA territory or who had no EIC on CT.[153] However, the unreliability of volume estimation with the one third rule and lack of demonstrable evidence of an effect on treatment modification led to development of the ASPECTS scoring system. This scoring system assigns one point each to ten regions within the MCA territory. A point is deducted for each of the ten regions demonstrating EIC. In patients undergoing intravenous thrombolysis at less than 3 h from symptom onset, a baseline ASPECTS score less than or equal to seven predicted patients who were unlikely to achieve independent functional outcome.[154] Sensitivity of CT for acute intracranial hemorrhage approaches 100%.[155]

Early CT Finding That Suggest Infarction

1. Loss of gray–white differentiation may be detected within 6 h of onset of stroke symptoms in 82% of patients with MCA territory ischemia.[156] Cytotoxic edema reduces the attenuation of gray matter into the range of white matter, thereby decreasing gray-white matter contrast.

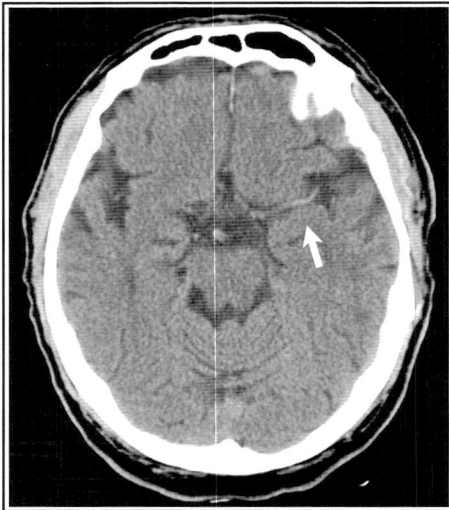

Fig. 9.4 MCA sign. Hyperattenuation of the M1 segment due to thromboembolism (*arrow*).

     (a) *"Insular ribbon sign"*: Loss of gray-white matter differentiation in the insular cortex can be an early sign of MCA ischemia.[157]
     (b) *Obscuration of the lentiform nucleus* reflects cytotoxic edema within the involved basal ganglia, again decreasing gray–white matter contrast.[158]
  2. *Cortical sulcal effacement* due to swelling of edematous gyri.
  3. *"MCA sign."* Hyperattenuation of the M1 segment (or other intracranial arteries, e.g. the posterior cerebral artery) due to thromboembolism.[159–161](Fig. 9.4)
  4. *Sylvian dot sign.* Distal MCA (M2 or M3 branches) occlusion indicated by hyperattenuation in the Sylvian fissure.[162] Sensitivity 38%, specificity 100%, positive predictive value 100%, negative predictive value 68%.[163]

The combined presence of the insular ribbon sign (Fig. 9.5), hemispheric sulcal effacement, and decreased attenuation of the lentiform nucleus is predictive of ICA occlusion.[164]

Since "time is brain", it is held that eligible patients presenting with acute stroke within the 4.5 h time window should receive intravenous tPA prior to performance of additional advanced imaging (including vascular or "penumbral" imaging with CT or MR perfusion techniques).[165] The identification of ischemic penumbra may be useful in three scenarios:
  1) Offering treatment to patients who do not qualify for treatment under current guidelines (e.g. beyond the "time window").
  2) Identifying patients for whom treatment within the current time window is likely to be futile.
  3) Identifying IV-tPA non-responders to whom endovascular therapies might be offered.[166]

CT Perfusion

CT perfusion provides quantitative data about CBF, and is becoming widely available on multidetector CT scanners. CT perfusion involves repeated ("cine") helical CT imaging of the brain during the transit of an injected bolus of iodinated contrast through the intracranial vasculature. Measurements of the change in tissue attenuation during passage of the contrast bolus are used to generate quantitative information about CBF as well as CBV and time-to-peak (TTP) or mean transit time (MTT).

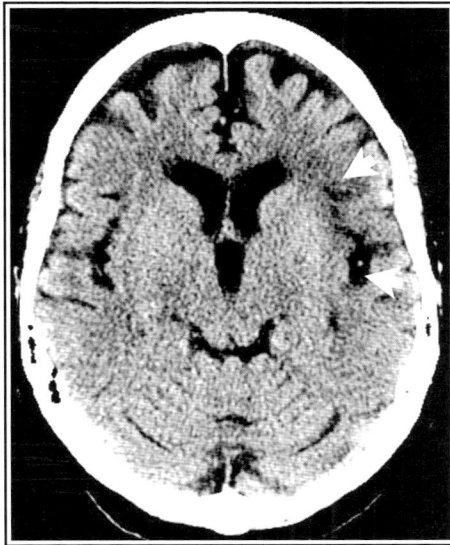

Fig. 9.5 Insular ribbon sign. Loss of gray-white differentiation in the insula (*arrow heads*) can be an early sign of MCA territory ischaemia.

Acquisition and processing of the data are accomplished seconds to minutes. The concept of CT perfusion was introduced more than 20 years ago,[167] but had to await the development of high-speed helical CT scanners, fast computers, and software capable of rapid data analysis to make the technique clinically useful.

Normal Values of CBF and CBV

Cerebral blood flow is normally maintained within a narrow range by autoregulation. Normal CBF is approximately 80 mL per 100 g/min in human gray matter and approximately 20 mL per 100 g/min in white matter. Global CBF, as well as average CBF in the cortical mantle, which is roughly a 50:50 mix of gray matter and white matter, is approximately 50 mL per 100 g/min. Protein synthesis in neurons ceases when CBF falls below 35 mL per 100 g/min.[168] At a CBF ≤20 mL per 100 g/min, however, electrical failure occurs and synaptic transmission between neurons is disturbed, leading to loss of function of still-viable neurons.[169–171] Metabolic failure and cell death occur at CBF ≤12 mL per 100 g/min.[170] CBV is defined as the amount of blood in a given quantity of brain tissue. Normal CBV is approximately 4–5 mL per 100 g.[172,173] CBV can be decreased or increased during cerebral ischemia, depending on the efficacy of cerebral autoregulation and patency of collateral arterial pathways.[173–176]

CT Perfusion Technique

Parameters

CT perfusion produces the following data:

1. Cerebral blood flow (CBF), measured in mL per 100 g of brain tissue per minute (mL/100 g/min) or as mL per 100 mL of brain tissue per minute (mL/100 mL/min).
2. Cerebral blood volume (CBV), measured in mL/100 g or mL/100 mL.

Table 9.6 CT perfusion methods

	First-pass techniques		Whole brain method
	Deconvolution method	**Maximum slope method**	**Whole brain method**
Parameters	CBF, CBV, MTT	CBF, CBV, TTP	PBV
Amount of brain imaged	4–8 slices	4–8 slices	Entire brain
Amount of contrast material	40–50 ml	50 mL	100 mL
Rate of contrast injection	4 mL/s	8 mL/s	3 mL/s
Principle sources of error	Choice of AIF, blood–brain barrier leakage, recirculation of contrast material	Delay in appearance of contrast material in the brain (e.g., due to diminished cardiac output or proximal vessel occlusion)	Diminished cardiac output or proximal vessel occlusion or stenosis

AIF arterial input function, *CBF* cerebral blood flow, *CBV* cerebral blood volume, *MTT* mean transit time, *TTP* time to peak, *PBV* perfused cerebral blood volume

3. Time to peak (TTP) is defined as the time delay (in seconds) between the first arrival of contrast within major arteries included in the section imaged and the peak attenuation of the brain tissue.
4. Mean transit time (MTT) indicates the time (in seconds) required for contrast material to pass from the arterial side to the venous side of the intracranial circulation. Blood and intravascular contrast material pass through vascular pathways of varying length and complexity in the brain's vascular network. The average of all of these possible transit times is MTT.
   (a) TTP and MTT are parameters unique to CBF techniques (e.g., CT perfusion and MRI perfusion) that utilize an intravascular indicator and track the passage of the indicator through the brain over the course of time to determine CBF.

Concepts

There are two commonly applied methods of CT perfusion (Table 9.6). These methods, known as the first pass bolus tracking techniques, are based on the indicator dilution principle and provide information about CBF, CBV, and MTT, and TTP. A known amount of a nondiffusible tracer (e.g., iodinated contrast material) is injected into an antecubital vein, and its concentration is repeatedly measured during its first pass through an intracranial vessel. Contrast transit through the intracranial vasculature produces a transient change in brain tissue attenuation. This change is linearly proportional to the serum concentration of the contrast agent. With helical CT scanning, these changes can be graphed as a time-attenuation curve for every voxel in a CT-imaging slice.

Two different mathematical approaches are commonly used to calculate CT perfusion data from the time-attenuation curve: *deconvolution* and *maximum slope*. With deconvolution methodology, the attenuation values of an artery in the field of view (the arterial input function), such as the anterior cerebral artery, are integrated with time-attenuation information of the brain tissue on a voxel-by-voxel basis in a mathematical operation called deconvolution. In mathematical terms:

$$C_t(t) = CBF \cdot [C_a(t) \otimes R(t)]$$

where $C_t(t)$ is the tissue time-attenuation curve; $C_a(t)$ is the arterial time-attenuation curve; $R(t)$ is the impulse residue function, and $\otimes$ is the convolution operator. The impulse residue function is an idealized tissue time-attenuation curve that would result if the entire bolus (the *impulse*) of contrast material was administered instantaneously into the artery supplying a given area of the brain. The plateau of impulse residue function reflects the length of time during which the contrast material (the *residue*) is passing through the capillary network. Both $C_t(t)$ and $C_a(t)$ can be measured, and the deconvolution process uses the information to calculate CBF and CBV.

MTT is then derived by using the central volume principle, which relates CBF, CBV, and MTT in the following relationship:

$$CBF = CBV/MTT$$

The accuracy of this method depends upon an intact blood–brain barrier, as leakage of the contrast material out of the intravascular space can lead to artifactually high perfusion parameters. Accuracy can also be influenced by the choice of the reference artery[177] and recirculation of contrast material. The venous output function serves as a reference against which the CTP parametric values are normalized and scaled. Since CBV values are affected by the choice of the venous output function, the chosen ROI for the venous output function should include the voxel demonstrating the maximum area under the time/attenuation curve and the least amount of partial volume averaging.[178]

In the *maximum slope method*, the maximum slope of the time-attenuation curve is used to calculate CBF (Fig. 9.6).[179–181] Values for CBV are calculated from the maximum-enhancement ratio, which is the maximum enhancement of the time-attenuation curve in a given voxel compared to that of the superior sagittal sinus.[179,182,183] Software using this method reports TTP rather than MTT. The accuracy of this method depends on a rapid bolus injection of contrast material, because a delay in the appearance of contrast material in the intracranial vasculature will lead to a decrease in the maximum slope of the time-attenuation curve, and CBF will be underestimated.[179,184]

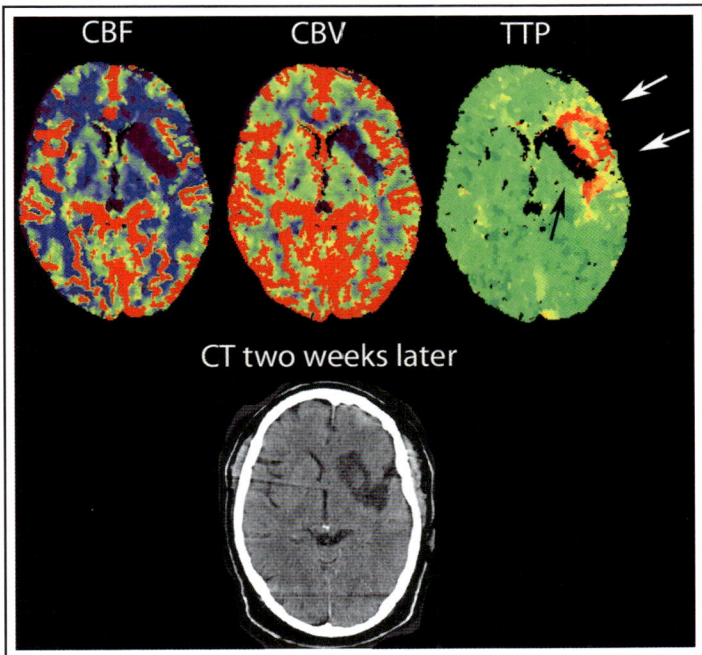

Fig. 9.6 Maximum slope method. In CT perfusion with the maximum slope method (Siemens), regions of completed infarction show up as a "black hole" – dense, black areas on CBF, CBV, and TTP images (*black arrow*). Adjacent areas of abnormality on that are not black (*white arrows*) indicate regions of salvageable tissue. The CT done 2 weeks later shows the black hole region as a completed infarction.

Validation

Quantitative CBF measurement by CT perfusion has been validated by comparison to other techniques for measuring CBF such as microspheres;,[185] xenon CT,[186,187] and PET.[188,189] CT perfusion imaging using the deconvolution technique has been shown to demonstrate little variability within individuals.[188] The use of CT perfusion in the identification of cerebral ischemia has been validated in experimental models.[190–192] Further validation of CT perfusion in human subjects by comparison with other brain imaging techniques in the setting of acute stroke, has been extensive and is discussed below.

Limitations

CT perfusion imaging has several practical limitations. Brain regions close to the skull are difficult to image because of bone artifact. A peripheral IV is required for intravenous administration of the contrast material, which can be a nuisance for some intensive care unit patients. The study requires iodinated contrast, which can be problematic in patients with renal insufficiency or contrast allergy.

An important limitation concerns the use of an intravascular indicator in first-pass CT perfusion methods. As opposed to older techniques like xenon-CT and PET, in which diffusible tracers are used and only capillary perfusion is measured, all intracranial vessels are included in CT perfusion. This difference leads to an over-estimation of CBF in regions that include large vessels, such as around the Sylvian fissure.[193] Moreover, this aspect of CT perfusion makes it difficult to compare CT perfusion results to CBF values obtained by the use of other methods. This situation may be ameliorated by vessel removal using threshold-based segmentation algorithms.[178,189] Finally, variability in quantification between different CT perfusion post-processing software packages limits the ability to generalize parametric thresholds (e.g. CBF threshold representing the infarct core) between platforms.[194]

Interpretation of CT Perfusion Data

Validity has been demonstrated for the commonly used mathematical techniques for CT perfusion by comparison with other CBF measurement techniques. However, each method has inherent limitations and sources of systematic error; hence, the description of CT perfusion as being "semiquantitative" by some authors.[195,196] Assessment of cerebral perfusion based on absolute values for CBF and CBV should be made with caution.[197,198]

In CT perfusion using the deconvolution method, some have found that MTT values >145% the contralateral hemisphere correlate best with tissue at risk for infarction in cases of persistent arterial occlusion, compared to DWI/FLAIR MRI.[199] Using the maximum slope method, a reduction of CBV of 60%, compared to non-ischemic regions of the brain, best identified cerebral ischemia.[196]

Mean transit time is prolonged in regions of cerebral ischemia. In a series of patients with acute ischemic MCA stroke, Eastwood and colleagues found average MTT to be 7.6 s in the affected MCA territories and 3.6 s in the unaffected MCA territories.[200] Areas of reduced perfusion were defined as MTT >6 s because that value represented at least three standard deviations greater than the average MTT values in unaffected MCA territories.

TTP is typically <8 s in normal brain tissue with unimpaired antegrade flow. In ischemic regions, TTP is prolonged, reflecting delayed tracer arrival through alternative pathways such as leptomeningeal vessels. TTP maps are useful for accurate identification of areas of impaired perfusion.[196] A regional TTP >8 s raises the suspicion of cerebral ischemia. However, TTP maps can provide false-positive findings when TTP is prolonged due to carotid stenosis or occlusion and regional CBF is compensated for by collateral vessels.[201]

Both MTT and TTP maps can be used to identify cerebral ischemia. MTT maps offer advantages over CBF and CBV maps. MTT appears to be affected by ischemia at an earlier stage than CBF or CBV, although it is less specific.[202] Color-coded TTP and MTT maps appear to demonstrate regions of cerebral ischemia more readily than CBF and CBV maps. TTP and MTT are usually homogenous in normal areas of brain tissue, permitting easy identification of abnormal hemodynamics.[202] Moreover, CBF and

CBV data are over-estimated when the ROI includes major vessels, such as MCA branches.[189] In comparison, TTP and MTT do not seem to be influenced by the presence of large vessels within ROIs. The absence of regions of extended TTP or MTT is usually a reliable indication that ischemia is not present.

CT Perfusion in Ischemic Stroke

CT perfusion can be done at the same time as the initial screening CT scan in patients with acute ischemic stroke and can distinguish viable tissue from regions of completed infarction.

1. CT perfusion can be used to exclude poor candidates for thrombolysis, such as patients with lacunar strokes and patients with no arterial occlusions, which account for up to 25%[203] and 29%[204] of patients with acute stroke, respectively.
2. CT perfusion imaging can provide prognostic information because patients with profound, widespread ischemia can be expected to have poorer outcomes than those with borderline ischemia.[202,205]

CT perfusion can potentially identify salvageable tissue at risk of infarction.[202,206] Using the deconvolution method, a mismatch between regional MTT, CBF, and CBV maps can indicate the presence of ischemic but potentially salvageable brain (penumbra).[190,195,201,207] Studies attempting to define the parameter that best identifies the infarct core have yielded different results. In a series of patients with acute stroke studied by Wintermark and colleagues, CBV <2.0 mL per 100 g best identified the irreversibly injured infarct core. Regions demonstrating MTT >145% compared to mirror-image voxels in the contralateral hemisphere optimally conformed to the ischemic region (infarct core + penumbra).[199] A more recent study by Campbell, et al found that CBF <31% of the mean contralateral hemispheric CBF best predicted infarct core.[208]

"Prognostic maps" co-demonstrating the ischemic zone (e.g. MTT > 145% contralateral mirror image voxel values = core + penumbra) in green and the infarct core (CBV <2.0 mL per 100 g) in red can be generated to provide an at-a-glance image of these parameters (Fig. 9.6).[209]

Using the maximum slope method, the relative values of CBF and CBV can be used to distinguish infarcted from ischemic tissue. In a series of patients undergoing CT perfusion studies within 6 h of stroke onset, the thresholds for best discrimination between infarcted and non-infarcted tissue were 48% of normal values for CBF, and 60% of normal values for CBV.[196] The lowest relative CBF and CBV values among brain regions not developing infarctions were 29% and 40% of normal values, respectively.

Validation of CT Perfusion in Acute Ischemic Stroke

The deconvolution method has been validated in the diagnosis of acute ischemic stroke by comparison to CT imaging[200] and to MR T2-weighted imaging,[200] diffusion imaging,[202,209] and perfusion imaging (Fig. 9.7).[200] In a series of patients with acute stroke, undergoing both CT perfusion and MRI diffusion studies on admission, infarct size on CBF maps correlated highly with the size of the abnormality on the diffusion-weighted imaging (DWI) map ($r = 0.968$).[209] Similarly, infarct size assessed by CT perfusion studies done on admission in patients with ischemic stroke, correlated highly with infarct size measured by follow-up MRI-DWI maps obtained an average of 3 days after admission ($r = 0.958$).[202] However, a recent study of treated patients who had complete early reperfusion found that CTP prognostic maps were not predictive for irreversibly or reversibly lost neurologic function.[210]

The maximum slope method has been validated in acute stroke by comparison to CT, MRI, and SPECT.[201] In a series of patients with acute stroke, who underwent both CT perfusion and SPECT studies on admission, the areas of ischemia indicated by CT perfusion CBF maps correlated well with those indicated by SPECT imaging ($r = 0.81$).[181] In a series in which ischemic areas on admission of CT perfusion images, were compared to the follow-up CT or MR images showing final infarctions, infarction was found to develop in all patients with >70% CBF reduction and in 50% of patients with 40–70% CBF reduction.[201] Based on a threshold of CBF <60% (compared with CBF in normal vascular territories), CBF maps predicted the extent of infarction with high sensitivity (93%) and specificity (98%). Similarly, TTP >3 s predicted infarction with a sensitivity of 91% and a specificity of 93%. Notably, in the same study, a negative predictive value for TTP >3 s of 99% was found, indicating that the absence of extended TTP is usually accurate in excluding the presence of ischemia. In a series of CT perfusion studies done in patients with acute stroke <6 h after onset, and compared to the follow-up CT or MRI, threshold values of 48% and 60% of normal, for CBF and CBV, respectively, were found to discriminate best between the areas of infarction and the areas of non-infarction.[196]

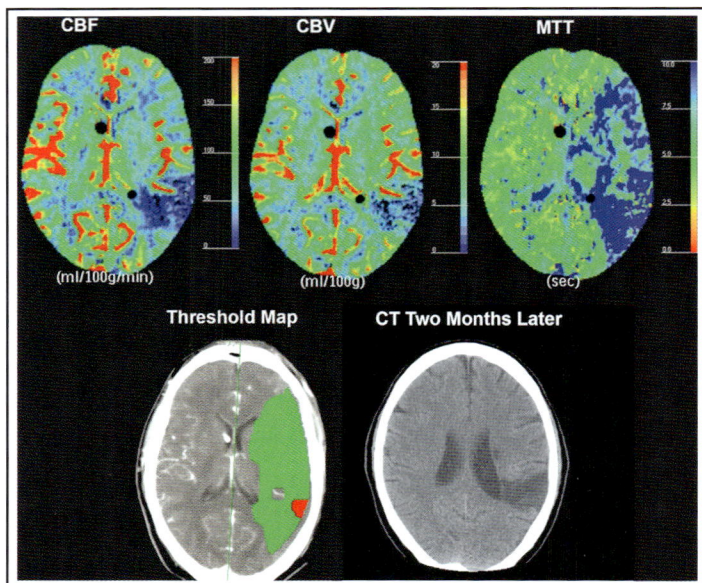

Fig. 9.7 Deconvolution method. In deconvolution CT perfusion (General Electric, Philips), the "black hole" technique is not a reliable way to identify regions of completed infarction. Threshold maps, however, can provide the same information. Here, the ischaemic core (*dark threshold area – red on the colour image*) is defined as absolute CBV <2 mL per 100 g, and the penumbra (*light threshold area – green on the colour image*) is defined as the region of brain with MTT values 1.45 times the MTT values in the corresponding area of the opposite hemisphere.[199] The follow-up CT shows an infarction that corresponds to the ischaemic core region.

CT Angiography

CT angiography (CTA) is useful in identifying large vessel occlusion, and can complement CT perfusion. The time required for acquisition, processing, and analysis of CTA studies of patients with acute ischemic stroke, averages 15 min.[211] Compared to catheter angiography, CTA has sensitivity and specificity for the detection of large vessel occlusion of 98.4 and 98.1%, respectively.[211] CTA may be prone to false-positive results; in two series of CTA in acute stroke, a minority of patients was found to have lesions on CTA that could not be found with catheter angiography.[212,213] CTA can be particularly useful in assessment of vertebrobasilar occlusion,[106] as CT perfusion imaging of the posterior circulation territory is limited because of bone artifact. However, basilar artery lesions can be better assessed with CTA than vertebral artery lesions.[214] CTA combined with CT perfusion shows good agreement with MRI in the assessment of infarct size, cortical involvement, and intracranial cerebral artery occlusion.[215] Finally, some authors have found application of ASPECTS.[154] scoring to CTA source images a robust method (and superior to ASPECT analysis of routine non-contrast brain CT) for early detection of irreversible ischemia and prediction of final infarct volume.[216,217]

Table 9.7 MRI signal characteristics of cerebral infarction

Time since ictus	DWI image	ADC map	FLAIR	T1	T2
Minutes or sooner	Not apparent	Dark	Not apparent	Not apparent	Not apparent
Minutes to hours	Bright	Dark	Not apparent	Not apparent	Not apparent
>6 h	Bright	Dark	Bright	Hazy	Bright
Hours to days	Bright	Dark	Bright	Dark	Very bright
1–2 week	Bright	Not apparent	Bright	Dark	Very bright
>2 weeks	Not apparent or dark	Bright	Bright	Dark	Bright

MRI

Magnetic resonance imaging is based on the interaction between a powerful, uniform magnetic field, radiofrequency (RF) energy, and body tissues. Protons absorb energy from pulsed RF waves (excitation) and are thereby deflected from their alignment with the main magnetic field. As the nuclei return to rest, energy is released and signals are induced in a receiver and converted into diagnostic images. During the process of energy release, spatially encoded voxel-specific relaxation constants can be obtained and, in conjunction with Fourier transform reconstruction, used to construct images that demonstrate specific tissues. A wide array of MRI imaging sequences is available (Table 9.7). Most MRI images accentuate T1 or T2 relaxation; T1 is longitudinal, or spin–lattice relaxation time and T2 is transverse, or spin-spin relaxation time. In T1-weighted images, fat has increased signal (short T1 relaxation) and water appears dark (long T1 relaxation). In T2-weighted images, water has increased signal relative to brain (long T2 relaxation). Brain tissue water content is typically increased in regions of edema, ischemia, and hemorrhage, thus changing the appearance of the tissue on MRI. T2-weighted images usually show only tissue changes caused by severe and prolonged ischemia – apparent only after some 6–24 h following stroke onset – and are therefore not optimal for evaluating acute ischemia.

Diffusion-Weighted Imaging

Diffusion-weighted imaging (DWI) measures the Brownian motion of water protons in tissue. Normal random motion of water protons leads to a loss of signal on diffusion weighted images. Ischemic failure of the ATP-dependent sodium-potassium cellular membrane pumps leads to water migration from the extracellular space to the intracellular space. Random water proton motion in the constricted extracellular space is reduced. Severely ischemic brain tissue appears bright on DWI due to signal preservation in these areas of decreased Brownian motion. These changes occur within minutes after ischemic stroke (Fig. 9.8).[218,219] Areas of ischemia appear bright on DWI in the acute phase and become unapparent or dark after about 2 weeks. DWI images are superior to CT and conventional MRI in the detection of acute ischemia.[149] Sensitivities of 88–100% for acute stroke detection with DWI have been reported, with specificity from 86–100%.[220] Analyzed pooled data from several studies yielded a PPV of 100% and a NPV of 90.6%.[221]

Diffusion-weighted images are influenced by other parameters including spin density and T1 and T2 relaxation effects. Calculation of the apparent diffusion coefficient (ADC) eliminates these influences and provides "pure" diffusion information.[222] Two otherwise identical image sets are obtained, one with a low (but non-zero) b value and one with a b value = 1,000 s/mm^2. The natural logarithm of signal intensity vs. b value for these two values is plotted and the slope of this line is used to determine

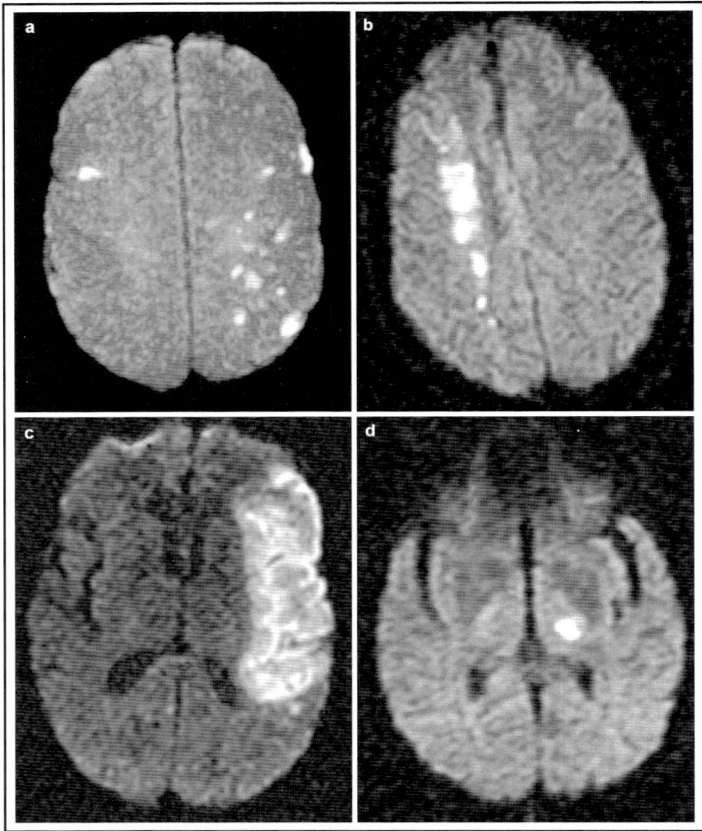

Fig. 9.8 Patterns of acute ischemic stroke on MRI. Diffusion-weighted images of an embolic stroke (**a**); an arterial border zone (aka watershed territory or "rosary" pattern) stroke (**b**); a large artery (MCA) stroke (**c**); and a lacunar stroke (**d**).

ADC for each voxel in the image.[223] The resulting "map" demonstrates the calculated ADC for each pixel in the image, with signal intensity proportional to the magnitude of the ADC. Areas of acute infarction (restrained diffusion) appear bright on diffusion weighted images and have low ADC values (appear dark) on ADC maps. Subacutely, signal on diffusion weighted images within infarcted areas may appear bright due to "T2 shine through", but correlation with the ADC maps will demonstrate that this is a T2 effect, and does not reflect true diffusion restraint. After about 2 weeks, diffusion becomes *facilitated*. Signal in the infarcted area decreases on DWI and increases on ADC maps as a result. Decreased ADC values indicate with good sensitivity (88%) and specificity (90%) that, an infarct is less than 10 days old.[224] Venous infarctions, in contrast, cause an increase in ADC values in the acute phase because of vasogenic edema, although in later stages, the ADC map appearance becomes complex because of the coexistence of cytotoxic and vasogenic edema and the presence of hemorrhage.[225]

Diffusion-weighted imaging can be useful in the workup of patients with TIA.[226] "Dots of hyperintensity" on DWI, indicating microinfarctions that are too small to cause permanent neurological symptoms, are found in some 40–50% of patients with traditionally defined TIA.[227] This has led to a recommendation for a change of the definition of TIA from a clinical to a tissue-based definition, specifically: "A transient episode of neurological dysfunction caused by focal brain, spinal cord, or retinal ischemia, without acute infarction".[228] Patients with clinically transient neurological events in whom asymptomatic diffusion abnormalities are discovered have a high risk of early completed stroke.[229]

Diffusion-weighted imaging and ADC maps are dynamic. Areas of ischemic injury may enlarge by 43% in the first 52 h after onset,[230] although in most patients, lesion size appears to reach a maximum by 24 h.[231] Conversely, all areas demonstrating DWI hyperintensity and ADC map hypointensity may not necessarily be infarcted, as bright regions on DWI can be reversed by reperfusion. In a series of patients with acute stroke, 19.7% demonstrated "normalization" of ADC abnormalities after reperfusion.[232] Tissue with ADC values 75–90% of normal brain are likely to proceed to infarction, whereas tissue with ADC values >90% of normal are more likely to recover.[233] Nevertheless, DWI hyperintensity is a necessary stage on the path to infarction,[226] and the volume of DWI abnormalities do correlate with clinical severity.[230,234]

Perfusion Imaging

MRI perfusion imaging employs a first pass tracking technique and deconvolution method for calculating the brain perfusion parameters. MRI perfusion uses the same deconvolution technique as CT perfusion, which is described in detail above. In MRI perfusion, a bolus of gadolinium is injected rapidly into a peripheral vein, and tissue- and arterial-input curves are used to generate CBF, CBV, TTP and MTT images. The information is not quantitative because, the MR signal change after IV administration of gadolinium is not proportionally related to the plasma concentration of gadolinium. MRI perfusion is subjected to many of the limitations of CT perfusion, such as the dependence of lesion volume on arterial input function selection[235], and controversy about the optimal perfusion parameters for the identification of affected tissue.[236] The value of MRI perfusion imaging lies in the *perfusion–diffusion mismatch* hypothesis. This holds that abnormal regions on perfusion images that appear normal on diffusion weighted imaging, are equal to the penumbra, and represent potentially salvageable tissue. A perfusion–diffusion mismatch pattern is present in some 70% of patients with anterior circulation stroke scanned within 6 h of onset,[237] is strongly associated with proximal MCA occlusion,[237] and resolves on reperfusion.[238,239] A recent study reported low favorable clinical responses and high mortality rates in a small group of patients (N = 8) with *matched* perfusion and diffusion abnormalities who underwent attempted intraarterial thrombolysis, especially those with large infarcts.[240]

The penumbra on perfusion imaging has been defined as regions where DWI is normal and TTP >4 s,[241] although, for practical purposes, any region that is abnormal on perfusion imaging but normal on DWI may represent salvageable tissue.[242] Among MRI perfusion parameters, CBF, MTT and TTP appear to best identify all affected tissue (and thereby distinguish penumbra when compared to DWI),[243,244] and CBV seems to best predict the final infarct volume.[245] Compared to final infarct volumes imaged on MRI, the sensitivities of CBF, CBV, and MTT for detection of perfusion abnormalities were 84%, 74%, and 84%, respectively, and the specificities were 96%, 100%, and 96%, respectively.[245]

Together, perfusion imaging and DWI can identify tissue that is at the risk of infarction but amenable to salvage with revascularization.[246] In a series of patients receiving IV thrombolytics for acute ischemic stroke and imaged both before and after 2 h of treatment, 78% of patients had complete resolution of perfusion lesions and 41% had resolution of DWI lesions.[247] Perfusion–diffusion imaging has been used in clinical trials to select patients for thrombolysis. Intravenous desmoplase was given only to patients with a DWI-PWI mismatch ≥20%, and the drug was found to be potentially effective in improving clinical outcomes.[19,20]

MR Angiography

MRA techniques fall into three categories:
1) Time of flight. Very common MRA technique.
   a) Depends on a strong signal from blood flowing into a plane where stationary tissue signal has been saturated.

i) Advantage: No contrast agent is used.
ii) Disadvantages: Spin dephasing in areas of turbulent flow or magnetic susceptibility (near paramagnetic blood products, ferromagnetic objects, and air/bone interfaces) causes signal loss that may lead to overestimation of stenosis.
2) Phase contrast. Not often used.
   a) Image contrast from the differences in phase accumulated by moving spins in a magnetic field gradient. Stationary spins accumulate no net phase.
      i) Advantages: No contrast agent is used. Less likely to confuse fresh clot for flowing blood as it is strictly flow-dependent.
      ii) Disadvantages: Acquisition times are relatively long.
3) Contrast-enhanced MRA. Common MRA technique.
   a) Based on a combination of rapid 3D imaging and the T1-shortening effect of IV gadolinium.
      i) Advantages: High signal-to-noise ratios, robustness irrespective of blood flow patterns or velocities, and fast image acquisition, allowing for the evaluation of larger anatomic segments (from the aortic arch to the circle of Willis).
      ii) Disadvantage: Requires IV gadolinium, which carries a small risk of complications, particularly in patients with renal insufficiency (see below).

Gadolinium and Nephrogenic Systemic Fibrosis

Gadolinium is a chemical element with an atomic number of 64. It has seven unpaired electrons in its outer shell which hasten T1 relaxation and increase signal in the area of interest. Gadolinium alone is toxic, but not when combined with a chelating agent. Several FDA-approved gadolinium preparations are available. A study of high-dose gadolinium administration in a population with a high prevalence of baseline renal insufficiency, showed no renal failure associated with its administration.[248] The rate of anaphylactic reactions is also very low; in a survey of >700,000 patients receiving gadolinium, the rate of serious allergic reactions was <0.01% and most reactions were limited to mild nausea or urticaria.[249]

Nephrogenic systemic fibrosis (aka nephrogenic fibrosing dermopathy) is strongly associated with gadodiamide (Omniscan™; GE Healthcare, Princeton, NJ).[250,251] Although most patients have a history of exposure to gadoliamide, other gadolinium-based agents have been implicated.[252] It appears to occur only in patients with renal insufficiency, generally in those requiring dialysis,[252] and is dose-dependent.[251] The condition consists of thickening and hardening of the skin of the extremities, due to increased skin deposition of collagen. The condition may develop rapidly and result in wheelchair-dependence within weeks. There may also be involvement of other tissue such as the lungs, skeletal muscle, heart, diaphragm, and esophagus.[253] The mechanism is not understood. An estimate of the incidence of this syndrome comes from an internet-based medical advisory originating in Denmark, which reported that, of about 400 patients with severely impaired renal function, 5% were subsequently diagnosed with nephrogenic systemic fibrosis.[254]

Management consists of correction of renal function (usually dialysis), which may result in a cessation or reversal of symptoms.[255]

Identification of Hemorrhage on MRI

MRI is as sensitive for acute hemorrhage as CT.[146] The appearance of intracranial hemorrhage changes with time as the hemoglobin moiety changes from non-paramagnetic oxyhemoglobin through the paramagnetic forms (deoxyhemoglobin, methemoglobin, and hemosiderin). Subacute blood appearing hyperintense on T1weighted images is in the methemoglobin form. The characteristic T1 shortening here is due to a phenomenon known as "dipole-dipole relaxation enhancement (PEDDRE)." T2 shortening (and the associated signal loss) depend on the presence of an intact cell membrane sequestering paramagnetic hemoglobin moieties from the extracellular space and thereby establishing a local magnetic gradient. Red blood cells usually undergo lysis in the subacute phase (i.e. methemoglobin) of

Table 9.8 MRI signal characteristics of cerebral haemorrhage

Time since ictus (days)	Tissue characteristics	T1-weighted image	T2-weighted image	Susceptibility-weighted image
<1	Oxyhaemoglobin	Isointense to dark	Bright	Isointense to dark
1–3	Deoxyhaemoglobin formation	Isointense to dark	Dark	Dark
3–7	Intracellular methemoglobin	Bright	Isointense to dark	Dark
Weeks	Cell breakdown, extracellular methemoglobin	Bright	Bright	Dark
Long term	Haemosiderin formation	Isointense, may have dark rim	Very dark rim	Dark

parenchymal hemorrhage evolution. Early in the pre-lysis phase, blood appears "bright" on T1 (PEDDRE) and "dark" on T2 weighted images (paramagnetic effect). After RBC lysis, methemoglobin-dominant hematomas still appear bright on T1 (again, PEDDRE), but become "bright" on T2 weighted images due to disruption of the paramagnetic effect by RBC lysis. Deoxyhemoglobin (acute) and hemosiderin (chronic) share similar appearances on T1 (isointense to gray matter) and T2 (hypointense to gray matter) MRI. However, acute hemorrhage is typically associated with vasogenic edema, while chronic hemorrhage is not (the latter may associated with cavitation, gliosis, and focal atrophy). The recurrence of T2 shortening in chronic (hemosiderin) hematomas long after RBC lysis is due to the ingestion of hemosiderin by macrophages.[256]

Acute hemorrhage characteristics on MRI are summarized in Table 9.8. Susceptibility weighted MRI can help identify acute cerebral hemorrhage, "microbleeds," and intravascular clot.[257] Asymptomatic microbleeds are caused by hypertension and amyloid angiopathy, and are found in up to 6% of elderly patients and 26% of patients with prior ischemic stroke.[226] The finding of microbleeds in patients with acute ischemic stroke, may predict an increased risk of hemorrhage transformation after thrombolysis. In a study of patients undergoing IA thrombolysis for acute ischemic stroke, microbleeds were found in 12% of patients prior to treatment.[258] Symptomatic hemorrhages occurred in 20% of patients with an evidence of prior microbleeds, compared to 11% of patients without prior microbleeds. The Bleeding Risk Analysis in Stroke Imaging Before Thrombolysis (BRASIL) study found that the risk of intracranial hemorrhage attributable to microbleeds was small and unlikely to exceed the benefits of thrombolytic therapy. This study could not draw conclusions about the risk of hemorrhage in patients with multiple microbleeds, however.[259]

9.7.   Appendix 2: NIH Stroke Scale

The National Institutes of Health Stroke Scale (NIHSS) is widely used and it provides important prognostic information.[260–263]

A detailed description of the NIHSS can be downloaded at www.ninds.nih.gov/disorders/stroke/strokescales.htm

Higher scores indicate greater stroke severity (Tables 9.9 and 9.10). A score of ≥16 predicts a high probability of death or severe disability whereas a score of ≥6 predicts a good recovery.[263] Some 60–70% of acute ischaemic stroke patients with a baseline NIHSS score <10 will have a favourable outcome after 1 year, compared to only 4–16% of patients with a score >20.[264]

Table 9.9 NIH stroke scale

1(a). Level of consciousness	Alert	0
	Drowsy	1
	Stuperous	2
	Coma	3
1(b). LOC questions	Answers both correctly	0
	Answers one correctly	1
	Incorrect	2
1(c). LOC commands	Obeys both correctly	0
	Obeys one correctly	1
	Incorrect	2
2. Best gaze	Normal	0
	Partial gaze palsy	1
	Forced deviation	2
3.Visual	No visual loss	0
	Partial hemianopia	1
	Complete hemianopia	2
	Bilateral hemianopia	3
4. Facial palsy	Normal	0
	Minor paralysis	1
	Partial paralysis	2
	Complete paralysis	3
5. Motor arm	No drift	0
	Drift	1
	Some effort against gravity	2
	No effort against gravity	3
	No movement	4
	UN = Amputation or join fusion	
6. Motor leg	No drift	0
	Drift	1
	Some effort against gravity	2
	No effort against gravity	3
	No movement	4
	UN = Amputation or join fusion	
7. Limb ataxia	Absent	0
	Present in one limb	1
	Present in two limbs	2
	UN = Amputation or join fusion	
8. Sensory	Normal	0
	Mild-to-moderate sensory loss	1
	Severe to total sensory loss	2
9. Best language	No aphasia	0
	Mild-to-moderate aphasia	1
	Severe aphasia	2
	Mute, global aphasia	3

Table 9.9 (continued)

10. Dysarthria	Normal	0
	Mild-to-moderate dysarthria	1
	Severe dysarthria	2
	UN = Intubated or other physical barrier	
11. Extinction and inattention	No abnormality	0
	Visual, tactile, auditory, spatial, or personal inattention	1
	Profound hemi-inattention or extinction to more than one modality	2

From http://www.ninds.nih.gov/doctors/NIH_Stroke_Scale.pdf
Administer the stroke scale items in the order listed. Record performance in each category after each subscale exam.
Each score should indicate what the patient does, not what the examiner thinks the patient can do

Table 9.10 NIH stroke scale score severity

Group	NIHSS score
Mild	≤6
Moderate	7–10
Moderately severe	11–15
Severe	15–22
Very severe	≤23

From Ezzeddine et al[205], with permission

References

1. The NINDS t-PA Stroke Study Group. Generalized efficacy of t-PA for acute stroke. Subgroup analysis of the NINDS t-PA Stroke Trial. Stroke. 1997;28:2119–25.
2. Marler JR, Tilley BC, Lu M, et al. Early stroke treatment associated with better outcome: the NINDS rt-PA stroke study. Neurology. 2000;55:1649–55.
3. Steiner T, Bluhmki E, Kaste M, et al. The ECASS 3-hour cohort. Secondary analysis of ECASS data by time stratification. ECASS Study Group. European Cooperative Acute Stroke Study. Cerebrovasc Dis. 1998;8:198–203.
4. Hacke W, Donnan G, Fieschi C, et al. Association of outcome with early stroke treatment: pooled analysis of ATLANTIS, ECASS, and NINDS rt-PA stroke trials. Lancet. 2004;363:768–74.
5. Moser DK, Kimble LP, Alberts MJ, et al. Reducing delay in seeking treatment by patients with acute coronary syndrome and stroke: a scientific statement from the American Heart Association Council on Cardiovascular Nursing and Stroke Council. Circulation. 2006;114:168–82.
6. Sagar G, Riley P, Vohrah A. Is admission chest radiography of any clinical value in acute stroke patients? Clin Radiol. 1996;51:499–502.
7. Adams Jr HP, Adams RJ, Brott T, et al. Guidelines for the early management of patients with ischemic stroke: a scientific statement from the Stroke Council of the American Stroke Association. Stroke. 2003;34:1056–83.
8. American College of Radiology. Manual on contrast Media. Version 7. Reston, VA; 2010.
9. Hopyan JJ, Gladstone DJ, Mallia G, et al. Renal safety of CT angiography and perfusion imaging in the emergency evaluation of acute stroke. AJNR Am J Neuroradiol. 2008;29:1826–30.
10. Lima FO, Lev MH, Levy RA, et al. Functional contrast-enhanced CT for evaluation of acute ischemic stroke does not increase the risk of contrast-induced nephropathy. AJNR Am J Neuroradiol. 2010;31:817–21.
11. del Zoppo GJ, Higashida RT, Furlan AJ, Pessin MS, Rowley HA, Gent M. PROACT: a phase II randomized trial of recombinant pro-urokinase by direct arterial delivery in acute middle cerebral artery stroke. PROACT Investigators. Prolyse in Acute Cerebral Thromboembolism. Stroke. 1998;29:4–11.
12. Furlan A, Higashida R, Wechsler L, et al. Intra-arterial prourokinase for acute ischemic stroke. The PROACT II study: a randomized controlled trial. Prolyse in Acute Cerebral Thromboembolism. JAMA. 1999;282:2003–11.
13. Eckert B, Kucinski T, Neumaier-Probst E, Fiehler J, Rother J, Zeumer H. Local intra-arterial fibrinolysis in acute hemispheric stroke: effect of occlusion type and fibrinolytic agent on recanalization success and neurological outcome. Cerebrovasc Dis. 2003;15:258–63.
14. Davydov L, Cheng JW. Tenecteplase: a review. Clin Ther. 2001;23:982–97; discussion 1.
15. Hoffmeister HM, Szabo S, Kastner C, et al. Thrombolytic therapy in acute myocardial infarction: comparison of procoagulant effects of streptokinase and alteplase regimens with focus on the kallikrein system and plasmin. Circulation. 1998;98:2527–33.
16. Haley Jr EC, Lyden PD, Johnston KC, Hemmen TM, the TNKiSI. A pilot dose-escalation safety study of tenecteplase in acute ischemic stroke. Stroke. 2005;36:607–12.
17. Haley EC, Thompson JLP, Grotta JC, et al. Phase IIB/III trial of tenecteplase in acute ischemic stroke. Stroke. 2010;41:707–11.
18. Liberatore GT, Samson A, Bladin C, Schleuning W-D, Medcalf RL. Vampire Bat salivary plasminogen activator (desmoteplase): a unique fibrinolytic enzyme that does not promote neurodegeneration. Stroke. 2003;34:537–43.
19. Hacke W, Albers G, Al-Rawi Y, et al. The Desmoteplase in Acute Ischemic Stroke Trial (DIAS): a phase II MRI-based 9-hour window acute stroke thrombolysis trial with intravenous desmoteplase. Stroke. 2005;36:66–73.
20. Furlan AJ, Eyding D, Albers GW, et al. Dose Escalation of Desmoteplase for Acute Ischemic Stroke (DEDAS): evidence of safety and efficacy 3 to 9 hours after stroke onset. Stroke. 2006;37:1227–31.
21. Ewart MR, Hatton MW, Basford JM, Dodgson KS. The proteolytic action of Arvin on human fibrinogen. Biochem J. 1970;118:603–9.
22. Ehrly AM. Influence of Arwin on the flow properties of blood. Biorheology. 1973;10:453–6.
23. Tsivgoulis G, Alexandrov AV, Chang J, et al. Safety and outcomes of intravenous thrombolysis in stroke mimics: a 6-year, single-care center study and a pooled analysis of reported series. Stroke. 2011;42:1771–4.
24. Winkler DT, Fluri F, Fuhr P, et al. Thrombolysis in stroke mimics: frequency, clinical characteristics, and outcome. Stroke. 2009;40:1522–5.
25. Latchaw RE, Alberts MJ, Lev MH, et al. Recommendations for imaging of acute ischemic stroke: a scientific statement from the American Heart Association. Stroke. 2009;40:3646–78.
26. Becker RC, Hochman JS, Cannon CP, et al. Fatal cardiac rupture among patients treated with thrombolytic agents and adjunctive thrombin antagonists: observations from the Thrombolysis and Thrombin Inhibition in Myocardial Infarction 9 Study. J Am Coll Cardiol. 1999;33:479–87.
27. Diedler JMD, Ahmed NMDP, Sykora MMD, et al. Safety of intravenous thrombolysis for acute ischemic stroke in patients receiving antiplatelet therapy at stroke onset. Stroke. 2010;41:288–94.
28. Riedel CH, Zimmermann P, Jensen-Kondering U, Stingele R, Deuschl G, Jansen O. The importance of size: successful recanalization by intravenous thrombolysis in acute anterior stroke depends on thrombus length. Stroke. 2011;42:1775–7.
29. Brinjikji W, Rabinstein AA, Kallmes DF, Cloft HJ. Patient outcomes with endovascular embolectomy therapy for acute ischemic stroke: a study of the national inpatient sample: 2006 to 2008. Stroke. 2011;42:1648–52.
30. Brandt T, von Kummer R, Muller-Kuppers M, Hacke W. Thrombolytic therapy of acute basilar artery occlusion. Variables affecting recanalization and outcome. Stroke. 1996;27:875–81.
31. Kirton A, Wong JH, Mah J, et al. Successful endovascular therapy for acute basilar thrombosis in an adolescent. Pediatrics. 2003;112:e248–51.
32. Adams HP, del Zoppo GJ, von Kummer R. Management of stroke: a practical guide for the prevention, evaluations and treatment of acute stroke. 2nd ed. Caddo: Professional Communications, Inc.; 2002.
33. Agarwal P, Kumar S, Hariharan S, et al. Hyperdense middle cerebral artery sign: can it be used to select intra-arterial versus intravenous thrombolysis in acute ischemic stroke? Cerebrovasc Dis. 2004;17:182–90.
34. Demchuk AM, Tanne D, Hill MD, et al. Predictors of good outcome after intravenous tPA for acute ischemic stroke. Neurology. 2001;57:474–80.
35. The National Institute of Neurological Disorders and Stroke rt-PA Stroke Study Group. Tissue plasminogen activator for acute ischemic stroke. The National Institute of Neurological Disorders and Stroke rt-PA Stroke Study Group. N Engl J Med. 1995;333:1581–7.
36. Chesebro JH, Knatterud G, Roberts R, et al. Thrombolysis in Myocardial Infarction (TIMI) Trial, phase I: a comparison between intravenous tissue plasminogen activator and intravenous streptokinase. Clinical findings through hospital discharge. Circulation. 1987;76:142–54.
37. Alexandrov AV, Molina CA, Grotta JC, et al. Ultrasound-enhanced systemic thrombolysis for acute ischemic stroke. N Engl J Med. 2004;351:2170–8.
38. Qureshi AI. New grading system for angiographic evaluation of arterial occlusions and recanalization response to intra-arterial thrombolysis in acute ischemic stroke. Neurosurgery. 2002;50:1405–15.
39. Francis CW, Blinc A, Lee S, Cox C. Ultrasound accelerates transport of recombinant tissue plasminogen activator into clots. Ultrasound Med Biol. 1995;21:419–24.
40. Daffertshofer M, Gass A, Ringleb P, et al. Transcranial low-frequency ultrasound-mediated thrombolysis in brain isch-

emia: increased risk of hemorrhage with combined ultrasound and tissue plasminogen activator: results of a phase II clinical trial. Stroke. 2005;36:1441–6.

41. Viguier A, Petit R, Rigal M, Cintas P, Larrue V. Continuous monitoring of middle cerebral artery recanalization with transcranial color-coded sonography and Levovist. J Thromb Thrombolysis. 2005;19:55–9.

42. Molina CA, Ribo M, Rubiera M, et al. Microbubble administration accelerates clot lysis during continuous 2-MHz ultrasound monitoring in stroke patients treated with intravenous tissue plasminogen activator. Stroke. 2006;37:425–9.

43. Alexandrov AV, Mikulik R, Ribo M, et al. A pilot randomized clinical safety study of sonothrombolysis augmentation with ultrasound-activated perflutren-lipid microspheres for acute ischemic stroke. Stroke. 2008;39:1464–9.

44. Molina CA, Barreto AD, Tsivgoulis G, et al. Transcranial ultrasound in clinical sonothrombolysis (TUCSON) trial. Ann Neurol. 2009;66:28–38.

45. Eggers J, Koch B, Meyer K, Konig I, Seidel G. Effect of ultrasound on thrombolysis of middle cerebral artery occlusion. Ann Neurol. 2003;53:797–800.

46. Eggers J, König IR, Koch B, Händler G, Seidel G. Sonothrombolysis with transcranial color-coded sonography and recombinant tissue-type plasminogen activator in acute middle cerebral artery main stem occlusion: results from a randomized study. Stroke. 2008;39:1470–5.

47. Perren F, Loulidi J, Poglia D, Landis T, Sztajzel R. Microbubble potentiated transcranial duplex ultrasound enhances IV thrombolysis in acute stroke. J Thromb Thrombolysis. 2008;25:219–23.

48. Tsivgoulis GMD, Eggers JMD, Ribo MMD, et al. Safety and efficacy of ultrasound-enhanced thrombolysis: a comprehensive review and meta-analysis of randomized and nonrandomized studies. Stroke. 2010;41:280–7.

49. Butcher KMDP, Christensen SP, Parsons MPF, et al. Postthrombolysis blood pressure elevation is associated with hemorrhagic transformation. Stroke. 2010;41:72–7.

50. Graham GD. Tissue plasminogen activator for acute ischemic stroke in clinical practice: a meta-analysis of safety data. Stroke. 2003;34:2847–50.

51. Hill MD, Lye T, Moss H, et al. Hemi-orolingual angioedema and ACE inhibition after alteplase treatment of stroke. Neurology. 2003;60:1525–7.

52. Hill MD, Buchan AM. Thrombolysis for acute ischemic stroke: results of the Canadian Alteplase for Stroke Effectiveness Study. CMAJ. 2005;172:1307–12.

53. Engelter ST, Fluri F, Buitrago-Tellez C, et al. Life-threatening orolingual angioedema during thrombolysis in acute ischemic stroke. J Neurol. 2005;252:1167–70.

54. Abou-Chebl A, Lin R, Hussain MS, et al. Conscious sedation versus general anesthesia during endovascular therapy for acute anterior circulation stroke. Stroke. 2010;41:1175–9.

55. Hemmer LB, Zeeni C, Gupta DK. Generalizations about general anesthesia: the unsubstantiated condemnation of general anesthesia for patients undergoing intra-arterial therapy for anterior circulation stroke. Stroke. 2010;41:e573.

56. Kumpe DA. Thrombolysis of acute stroke syndromes. In: Kandarpa K, Aruny JE, editors. Handbook of interventional radiologic procedures. Philadelphia: Lippincott Williams & Wilkins; 2002. p. 47–62.

57. Rubiera M, Cava L, Tsivgoulis G, et al. Diagnostic criteria and yield of real-time transcranial Doppler monitoring of intra-arterial reperfusion procedures. Stroke. 2010;41:695–9.

58. Khatri P, Broderick JP, Khoury JC, Carrozzella JA, Tomsick TA. Microcatheter contrast injections during intra-arterial thrombolysis may increase intracranial hemorrhage risk. Stroke. 2008;39:3283–7.

59. Chopko BW, Kerber C, Wong W, Georgy B. Transcatheter snare removal of acute middle cerebral artery thromboembolism: technical case report. Neurosurgery. 2000;46:1529–31.

60. Kerber CW, Barr JD, Berger RM, Chopko BW. Snare retrieval of intracranial thrombus in patients with acute stroke. J Vasc Interv Radiol. 2002;13:1269–74.

61. Fourie P, Duncan IC. Microsnare-assisted mechanical removal of intraprocedural distal middle cerebral arterial thromboembolism. AJNR Am J Neuroradiol. 2003;24:630–2.

62. Wikholm G. Transarterial embolectomy in acute stroke. AJNR Am J Neuroradiol. 2003;24:892–4.

63. Nesbit GM, Luh G, Tien R, Barnwell SL. New and future endovascular treatment strategies for acute ischemic stroke. J Vasc Interv Radiol. 2004;15:103S–10.

64. Kerber CW, Wanke I, Bernard Jr J, Woo HH, Liu MW, Nelson PK. Rapid intracranial clot removal with a new device: the alligator retriever. AJNR Am J Neuroradiol. 2007;28:860–3.

65. Lutsep HL, Clark WM, Nesbit GM, Kuether TA, Barnwell SL. Intraarterial suction thrombectomy in acute stroke. AJNR Am J Neuroradiol. 2002;23:783–6.

66. Chapot R, Houdart E, Rogopoulos A, Mounayer C, Saint-Maurice JP, Merland JJ. Thromboaspiration in the basilar artery: report of two cases. AJNR Am J Neuroradiol. 2002;23:282–4.

67. Nedeltchev K, Remonda L, Do DD, et al. Acute stenting and thromboaspiration in basilar artery occlusions due to embolism from the dominating vertebral artery. Neuroradiology. 2004;46:686–91.

68. Cross 3rd DT, Moran CJ, Akins PT, Angtuaco EE, Derdeyn CP, Diringer MN. Collateral circulation and outcome after basilar artery thrombolysis. AJNR Am J Neuroradiol. 1998;19:1557–63.

69. Nakayama T, Tanaka K, Kaneko M, Yokoyama T, Uemura K. Thrombolysis and angioplasty for acute occlusion of intracranial vertebrobasilar arteries. Report of three cases. J Neurosurg. 1998;88:919–22.

70. Mori T, Kazita K, Mima T, Mori K. Balloon angioplasty for embolic total occlusion of the middle cerebral artery and ipsilateral carotid stenting in an acute stroke stage. AJNR Am J Neuroradiol. 1999;20:1462–4.

71. Ringer AJ, Qureshi AI, Fessler RD, Guterman LR, Hopkins LN. Angioplasty of intracranial occlusion resistant to thrombolysis in acute ischemic stroke. Neurosurgery. 2001;48:1282–90.

72. Shi ZS, Liebeskind DS, Loh Y, et al. Predictors of subarachnoid hemorrhage in acute ischemic stroke with endovascular therapy. Stroke. 2010;41:2775–81.

73. Gupta R, Vora NA, Horowitz MB, et al. Multimodal reperfusion therapy for acute ischemic stroke: factors predicting vessel recanalization. Stroke. 2006;37:986–90.

74. Levy EI, Mehta R, Gupta R, et al. Self-expanding stents for recanalization of acute cerebrovascular occlusions. AJNR Am J Neuroradiol. 2007;28:816–22.

75. Castano CMDP, Dorado LMD, Guerrero CMD, et al. Mechanical thrombectomy with the solitaire AB device in large artery occlusions of the anterior circulation: a pilot study. Stroke. 2010;41:1836–40.

76. Smith WS, Sung G, Starkman S, et al. Safety and efficacy of mechanical embolectomy in acute ischemic stroke: results of the MERCI trial. Stroke. 2005;36:1432–8.

77. Smith WS. Safety of mechanical thrombectomy and intravenous tissue plasminogen activator in acute ischemic stroke. Results of the multi Mechanical Embolus Removal in Cerebral Ischemia (MERCI) trial, part I. AJNR Am J Neuroradiol. 2006;27:1177–82.

78. Layton KF, White JB, Cloft HJ, Kallmes DF. Use of the Perclose ProGlide device with the 9 French Merci retrieval system. Neuroradiology. 2006;48:324–6.

79. Spiotta AM, Hussain MS, Sivapatham T, et al. The versatile distal access catheter: the Cleveland Clinic experience. Neurosurgery. 2011;68:1677–86; discussion 86.

80. Hui FK, Hussain MS, Spiotta A, et al. Merci retrievers as access adjuncts for reperfusion catheters: the grappling hook technique. Neurosurgery. 2012;70(2):456–60.

81. Henkes H, Flesser A, Brew S, et al. A novel microcatheter-delivered, highly-flexible and fully-retrievable stent, specifically designed for intracranial use. Technical note. Interv Neuroradiol. 2003;9:391–3.

82. Roth CM, Papanagiotou PM, Behnke SM, et al. Stent-assisted mechanical recanalization for treatment of acute intracerebral artery occlusions. Stroke. 2010;41:2559–67.

83. Solitaire™ FR With the Intention For Thrombectomy (SWIFT) study. 2011. http://clinicaltrials.gov/ct2/show/NCT01054560. Accessed 11 Aug 2011.

84. Mahon BR, Nesbit GM, Barnwell SL, et al. North American clinical experience with the EKOS MicroLysUS infusion catheter for the treatment of embolic stroke. AJNR Am J Neuroradiol. 2003;24:534–8.

85. IMS II Trial Investigators. The Interventional Management of Stroke (IMS) II Study. Stroke. 2007;38:2127–35.

86. Opatowsky MJ, Morris PP, Regan JD, Mewborne JD, Wilson JA. Rapid thrombectomy of superior sagittal sinus and transverse sinus thrombosis with a rheolytic catheter device. AJNR Am J Neuroradiol. 1999;20:414–7.

87. Bellon RJ, Putman CM, Budzik RF, Pergolizzi RS, Reinking GF, Norbash AM. Rheolytic thrombectomy of the occluded internal carotid artery in the setting of acute ischemic stroke. AJNR Am J Neuroradiol. 2001;22:526–30.

88. Molina CA, Saver JL. Extending reperfusion therapy for acute ischemic stroke: emerging pharmacological, mechanical, and imaging strategies. Stroke. 2005;36:2311–20.

89. Henkes H, Reinartz J, Lowens S, et al. A device for fast mechanical clot retrieval from intracranial arteries (Phenox clot retriever). Neurocrit Care. 2006;5:134–40.

90. Liebig T, Reinartz J, Hannes R, Miloslavski E, Henkes H. Comparative in vitro study of five mechanical embolectomy systems: effectiveness of clot removal and risk of distal embolization. Neuroradiology. 2008;50:43–52.

91. Brekenfeld C, Schroth G, El-Koussy M, et al. Mechanical thromboembolectomy for acute ischemic stroke: comparison of the catch thrombectomy device and the Merci Retriever in vivo. Stroke. 2008;39:1213–9.

92. Lylyk P, Vila JF, Miranda C, Ferrario A, Romero R, Cohen JE. Partial aortic obstruction improves cerebral perfusion and clinical symptoms in patients with symptomatic vasospasm. Neurol Res. 2005;27 Suppl 1:S129–35.

93. Alnaami I, Saqqur M, Chow M. A novel treatment of distal cerebral vasospasm. A case report. Interv Neuroradiol. 2009;15:417–20.

94. Shuaib A, Bornstein NM, Diener HC, et al. Partial aortic occlusion for cerebral perfusion augmentation: safety and efficacy of NeuroFlo in Acute Ischemic Stroke trial. Stroke. 2011;42:1680–90.

95. Kase CS, Furlan AJ, Wechsler LR, et al. Cerebral hemorrhage after intra-arterial thrombolysis for ischemic stroke: the PROACT II trial. Neurology. 2001;57:1603–10.

96. Lisboa RC, Jovanovic BD, Alberts MJ. Analysis of the safety and efficacy of intra-arterial thrombolytic therapy in ischemic stroke. Stroke. 2002;33:2866–71.

97. Khatri P, Hill MD, Palesch YY, et al. Methodology of the interventional management of stroke III trial. Int J Stroke. 2008;3:130–7.

98. Lewandowski CA, Frankel M, Tomsick TA, et al. Combined intravenous and intra-arterial r-TPA versus intra-arterial therapy of acute ischemic stroke: Emergency Management of Stroke (EMS) Bridging Trial. Stroke. 1999;30:2598–605.

99. The IMSSI. Combined intravenous and intra-arterial recanalization for acute ischemic stroke: the interventional management of stroke study. Stroke. 2004;35:904–11.

100. Mazighi M, Serfaty JM, Labreuche J, et al. Comparison of intravenous alteplase with a combined intravenous-endovascular approach in patients with stroke and confirmed arterial occlusion (RECANALISE study): a prospective cohort study. Lancet Neurol. 2009;8:802–9.

101. Rubiera M, Ribo M, Pagola J, et al. Bridging intravenous-intra-arterial rescue strategy increases recanalization and the likelihood of a good outcome in nonresponder intravenous tissue plasminogen activator-treated patients: a case–control study. Stroke. 2011;42:993–7.

102. Eckert B, Koch C, Thomalla G, et al. Aggressive therapy with intravenous abciximab and intra-arterial rtPA and additional PTA/stenting improves clinical outcome in acute vertebrobasilar occlusion: combined local fibrinolysis and intravenous abciximab in acute vertebrobasilar stroke treatment (FAST): results of a multicenter study. Stroke. 2005;36:1160–5.

103. Nagel S, Schellinger PD, Hartmann M, et al. Therapy of acute basilar artery occlusion: intraarterial thrombolysis alone vs bridging therapy. Stroke. 2009;40:140–6.

104. Hill MD, Barber PA, Takahashi J, Demchuk AM, Feasby TE, Buchan AM. Anaphylactoid reactions and angioedema during alteplase treatment of acute ischemic stroke. CMAJ. 2000;162:1281–4.

105. Brandt T. Diagnosis and thrombolytic therapy of acute basilar artery occlusion: a review. Clin Exp Hypertens. 2002;24:611–22.

106. Brandt T, Knauth M, Wildermuth S, et al. CT angiography and Doppler sonography for emergency assessment in acute basilar artery ischemia. Stroke. 1999;30:606–12.

107. Schellinger PD, Hacke W. Intra-arterial thrombolysis is the treatment of choice for basilar thrombosis: pro. Stroke. 2006;37:2436–7.

108. Ford GA. Intra-arterial thrombolysis is the treatment of choice for basilar thrombosis: con. Stroke. 2006;37:2438–9.

109. Macleod MR, Davis SM, Mitchell PJ, et al. Results of a multicentre, randomised controlled trial of intra-arterial urokinase in the treatment of acute posterior circulation ischaemic stroke. Cerebrovasc Dis. 2005;20:12–7.

110. Schonewille WJ, Wijman CA, Michel P, et al. Treatment and outcomes of acute basilar artery occlusion in the Basilar Artery International Cooperation Study (BASICS): a prospective registry study. Lancet Neurol. 2009;8:724–30.

111. Davis SM, Donnan GA. Basilar artery thrombosis: recanalization is the key. Stroke. 2006;37:2440.

112. Hacke W, Zeumer H, Ferbert A, Bruckmann H, del Zoppo GJ. Intra-arterial thrombolytic therapy improves outcome in patients with acute vertebrobasilar occlusive disease. Stroke. 1988;19:1216–22.

113. Wang H, Fraser K, Wang D, Alvernia J, Lanzino G. Successful intra-arterial basilar artery thrombolysis in a patient with bilateral vertebral artery occlusion: technical case report. Neurosurgery. 2005;57:E398; discussion E.

114. Lindsberg PJ, Mattle HP. Therapy of basilar artery occlusion: a systematic analysis comparing intra-arterial and intravenous thrombolysis. Stroke. 2006;37:922–8.

115. Nesbit GM, Clark WM, O'Neill OR, Barnwell SL. Intracranial intraarterial thrombolysis facilitated by microcatheter navigation through an occluded cervical internal carotid artery. J Neurosurg. 1996;84:387–92.

116. Hui FK, Hussain MS, Elgabaly MH, Sivapatham T, Katzan IL, Spiotta AM. Embolic protection devices and the Penumbra 054 catheter: utility in tandem occlusions in acute ischemic stroke. J Neurointerv Surg. 2011;3:50–3.

117. Steinhubl SR, Talley JD, Braden GA, et al. Point-of-care measured platelet inhibition correlates with a reduced risk of an adverse cardiac event after percutaneous coronary intervention: results of the GOLD (AU-Assessing Ultegra) multicenter study. Circulation. 2001;103:2572–8.

118. Quinn MJ, Plow EF, Topol EJ. Platelet glycoprotein IIb/IIIa inhibitors: recognition of a two-edged sword? Circulation. 2002;106:379–85.

119. Kleinman N. Assessing platelet function in clinical trials. In: Quinn M, Fitzgerald D, editors. Platelet function assessment, diagnosis, and treatment. Totowa: Humana Press; 2005. p. 369–84.

120. Fisher CM, Ojemann RG, Roberson GH. Spontaneous dissection of cervico-cerebral arteries. Can J Neurol Sci. 1978;5:9–19.

121. Fitzsimmons BFM, Becske T, Nelson PK. Rapid stent-supported revascularization in acute ischemic stroke. AJNR Am J Neuroradiol. 2006;27:1132–4.

122. Kessler IM, Mounayer C, Piotin M, Spelle L, Vanzin JR, Moret J. The use of balloon-expandable stents in the management of intracranial arterial diseases: a 5-year single-center experience. AJNR Am J Neuroradiol. 2005;26:2342–8.

123. Kiyosue H, Okahara M, Yamashita M, Nagatomi H, Nakamura N, Mori H. Endovascular stenting for restenosis of the intracranial vertebrobasilar artery after balloon angioplasty: two case reports and review of the literature. Cardiovasc Intervent Radiol. 2004;27:538–43.

124. Leavitt JA, Larson TA, Hodge DO, Gullerud RE. The incidence of central retinal artery occlusion in Olmsted County, Minnesota. Am J Ophthalmol. 2011;152(5):820–3.

125. Hayreh SS, Zimmerman MB, Kimura A, Sanon A. Central retinal artery occlusion. Retinal survival time. Exp Eye Res. 2004;78:723–36.

126. Beatty S, Au Eong KG. Local intra-arterial fibrinolysis for acute occlusion of the central retinal artery: a meta-analysis of the published data. Br J Ophthalmol. 2000;84:914–6.

127. Weber J, Remonda L, Mattle HP, et al. Selective intra-arterial fibrinolysis of acute central retinal artery occlusion. Stroke. 1998;29:2076–9.

128. Butz B, Strotzer M, Manke C, Roider J, Link J, Lenhart M. Selective intraarterial fibrinolysis of acute central retinal artery occlusion. Acta Radiol. 2003;44:680–4.

129. Arnold M, Koerner U, Remonda L, et al. Comparison of intra-arterial thrombolysis with conventional treatment in patients with acute central retinal artery occlusion. J Neurol Neurosurg Psychiatry. 2005;76:196–9.

130. Schmidt DP, Schulte-Monting J, Schumacher M. Prognosis of central retinal artery occlusion: local intraarterial fibrinolysis versus conservative treatment. AJNR Am J Neuroradiol. 2002;23:1301–7.

131. Aldrich EM, Lee AW, Chen CS, et al. Local intraarterial fibrinolysis administered in aliquots for the treatment of central retinal artery occlusion: the Johns Hopkins Hospital experience. Stroke. 2008;39:1746–50.

132. Mueller AJ, Neubauer AS, Schaller U, Kampik A. Evaluation of minimally invasive therapies and rationale for a prospective randomized trial to evaluate selective intra-arterial lysis for clinically complete central retinal artery occlusion. Arch Ophthalmol. 2003;121:1377–81.

133. Fraser SG, Adams W. Interventions for acute non-arteritic central retinal artery occlusion. Cochrane Database Syst Rev. 2009:CD001989.

134. Schmidt D, Schumacher M, Wakhloo AK. Microcatheter urokinase infusion in central retinal artery occlusion. Am J Ophthalmol. 1992;113:429–34.

135. Atebara NH, Brown GC, Cater J. Efficacy of anterior chamber paracentesis and Carbogen in treating acute nonarteritic central retinal artery occlusion. Ophthalmology. 1995;102:2029–34; discussion 34–5.

136. Schumacher M, Schmidt D, Jurklies B, et al. Central retinal artery occlusion: local intra-arterial fibrinolysis versus conservative treatment, a multicenter randomized trial. Ophthalmology. 2010;117:1367.e1–75.e1.

137. Ros MA, Magargal LE, Uram M. Branch retinal-artery obstruction: a review of 201 eyes. Ann Ophthalmol. 1989;21:103–7.

138. Paques M, Vallee JN, Herbreteau D, et al. Superselective ophthalmic artery fibrinolytic therapy for the treatment of central retinal vein occlusion. Br J Ophthalmol. 2000;84:1387–91.

139. Kilani R, Marshall L, Koch S, Fernandez M, Postel E. DWI findings of optic nerve ischemia in the setting of central retinal artery occlusion. J Neuroimaging. 2011 Jun 23. doi: 10.1111/j.1552-6569.2011.00601.x. [Epub ahead of print]

140. Feltgen N, Neubauer A, Jurklies B, et al. Multicenter study of the European Assessment Group for Lysis in the Eye (EAGLE) for the treatment of central retinal artery occlusion: design issues and implications. EAGLE Study report no. 1: EAGLE Study report no. 1. Graefes Arch Clin Exp Ophthalmol. 2006;244:950–6.

141. Richard G, Lerche RC, Knospe V, Zeumer H. Treatment of retinal arterial occlusion with local fibrinolysis using recombinant tissue plasminogen activator. Ophthalmology. 1999;106:768–73.

142. Hayreh SS. Acute retinal arterial occlusive disorders. Prog Retin Eye Res. 2011;30:359–94.

143. Beatty S, Au Eong KG. Acute occlusion of the retinal arteries: current concepts and recent advances in diagnosis and management. J Accid Emerg Med. 2000;17:324–9.

144. Chen CS, Lee AW, Campbell B, et al. Efficacy of intravenous tissue-type plasminogen activator in central retinal artery occlusion: report from a randomized, controlled trial. Stroke. 2011;42:2229–34.

145. Adams HP Jr, del Zoppo G, Alberts MJ, et al. Guidelines for the early management of adults with ischemic stroke: a guideline from the American Heart Association/American Stroke Association Stroke Council, Clinical Cardiology Council, Cardiovascular Radiology and Intervention Council, and the Atherosclerotic Peripheral Vascular Disease and Quality of Care Outcomes in Research Interdisciplinary Working Groups: the American Academy of Neurology affirms the value of this guideline as an educational tool for neurologists. Stroke. 2007;38:1655–711.

146. Chalela JA, Kidwell CS, Nentwich LM, et al. Magnetic resonance imaging and computed tomography in emergency assessment of patients with suspected acute stroke: a prospective comparison. Lancet. 2007;369:293–8.

147. Wessels T, Wessels C, Ellsiepen A, et al. Contribution of diffusion-weighted imaging in determination of stroke etiology. AJNR Am J Neuroradiol. 2006;27:35–9.

148. von Kummer R, Bourquain H, Bastianello S, et al. Early prediction of irreversible brain damage after ischemic stroke at CT. Radiology. 2001;219:95–100.

149. Mullins ME, Schaefer PW, Sorensen AG, et al. CT and conventional and diffusion-weighted MR imaging in acute stroke: study in 691 patients at presentation to the emergency department. Radiology. 2002;224:353–60.

150. Lansberg MG, Albers GW, Beaulieu C, Marks MP. Comparison of diffusion-weighted MRI and CT in acute stroke. Neurology. 2000;54:1557–61.

151. Larrue V, von Kummer RR, Muller A, Bluhmki E. Risk factors for severe hemorrhagic transformation in ischemic stroke patients treated with recombinant tissue plasminogen activator: a secondary analysis of the European-Australasian Acute Stroke Study (ECASS II). Stroke. 2001;32:438–41.

152. Kasner SE, Demchuk AM, Berrouschot J, et al. Predictors of fatal brain edema in massive hemispheric ischemic stroke. Stroke. 2001;32:2117–23.

153. Menon BK, Puetz V, Kochar P, Demchuk AM. ASPECTS and other neuroimaging scores in the triage and prediction of outcome in acute stroke patients. Neuroimaging Clin N Am. 2011;21:407–23, xii.

154. Barber PA, Demchuk AM, Zhang J, Buchan AM. Validity and reliability of a quantitative computed tomography score in predicting outcome of hyperacute stroke before thrombolytic therapy. ASPECTS Study Group. Alberta Stroke Programme Early CT Score. Lancet. 2000;355:1670–4.

155. Castillo PR, Miller DA, Meschia JF. Choice of neuroimaging in perioperative acute stroke management. Neurol Clin. 2006;24:807–20.

156. von Kummer R, Nolte PN, Schnittger H, Thron A, Ringelstein EB. Detectability of cerebral hemisphere ischaemic infarcts by CT within 6 h of stroke. Neuroradiology. 1996;38:31–3.

157. Truwit CL, Barkovich AJ, Gean-Marton A, Hibri N, Norman D. Loss of the insular ribbon: another early CT sign of acute middle cerebral artery infarction. Radiology. 1990;176:801–6.

158. Tomura N, Uemura K, Inugami A, Fujita H, Higano S. Shishido F. Early CT finding in cerebral infarction: obscuration of the lentiform nucleus. Radiology. 1988;168:463–7.

159. Gacs G, Fox AJ, Barnett HJ, Vinuela F. CT visualization of intracranial arterial thromboembolism. Stroke. 1983;14:756–62.

160. Tomsick TA, Brott TG, Olinger CP, et al. Hyperdense middle cerebral artery: incidence and quantitative significance. Neuroradiology. 1989;31:312–5.

161. Barber PA, Demchuk AM, Hill MD, et al. The probability of middle cerebral artery MRA flow signal abnormality with quantified CT ischaemic change: targets for future therapeutic studies. J Neurol Neurosurg Psychiatry. 2004;75:1426–30.

162. Barber PA, Demchuk AM, Hudon ME, Pexman JH, Hill MD, Buchan AM. Hyperdense sylvian fissure MCA "dot" sign: A CT marker of acute ischemia. Stroke. 2001;32:84–8.

163. Leary MC, Kidwell CS, Villablanca JP, et al. Validation of computed tomographic middle cerebral artery "dot" sign: an angiographic correlation study. Stroke. 2003;34:2636–40.

164. Koga M, Saku Y, Toyoda K, Takaba H, Ibayashi S, Iida M. Reappraisal of early CT signs to predict the arterial occlusion site in acute embolic stroke. J Neurol Neurosurg Psychiatry. 2003;74:649–53.

165. Lyden PD. Advanced brain imaging studies should not be performed in patients with suspected stroke presenting within 4.5 hours of symptom onset. Stroke. 2011;42:2668–9.

166. Selim MH, Molina CA. Conundra of the penumbra and acute stroke imaging. Stroke. 2011;42:2670–1.

167. Axel L. Cerebral blood flow determination by rapid sequence computed tomography. Radiology. 1980;137:679–86.

168. Mies G, Ishimaru S, Xie Y, Seo K, Hossmann KA. Ischemic thresholds of cerebral protein synthesis and energy state following middle cerebral artery occlusion in rat. J Cereb Blood Flow Metab. 1991;11:753–61.

169. Astrup J, Symon L, Branston NM, Lassen NA. Cortical evoked potential and extracellular K+ and H+ at critical levels of brain ischemia. Stroke. 1977;8:51–7.

170. Morawetz RB, Crowell RH, DeGirolami U, Marcoux FW, Jones TH, Halsey JH. Regional cerebral blood flow thresholds during cerebral ischemia. Fed Proc. 1979;38:2493–4.

171. Morawetz RB, DeGirolami U, Ojemann RG, Marcoux FW, Crowell RM. Cerebral blood flow determined by hydrogen clearance during middle cerebral artery occlusion in unanesthetized monkeys. Stroke. 1978;9:143–9.

172. Sakai F, Nakazawa K, Tazaki Y, et al. Regional cerebral blood volume and hematocrit measured in normal human volunteers by single-photon emission computed tomography. J Cereb Blood Flow Metab. 1985;5:207–13.

173. Muizelaar JP, Fatouros PP, Schroder ML. A new method for quantitative regional cerebral blood volume measurements using computed tomography. Stroke. 1997;28:1998–2005.

174. Nabavi DG, Cenic A, Dool J, et al. Quantitative assessment of cerebral hemodynamics using CT: stability, accuracy, and precision studies in dogs. J Comput Assist Tomogr. 1999;23:506–15.

175. Hatazawa J, Shimosegawa E, Toyoshima H, et al. Cerebral blood volume in acute brain infarction: a combined study with dynamic susceptibility contrast MRI and 99mTc-HMPAO-SPECT. Stroke. 1999;30:800–6.

176. Todd NV, Picozzi P, Crockard HA. Quantitative measurement of cerebral blood flow and cerebral blood volume after cerebral ischaemia. J Cereb Blood Flow Metab. 1986;6:338–41.

177. Latchaw RE, Yonas H, Hunter GJ, et al. Guidelines and recommendations for perfusion imaging in cerebral ischemia: a scientific statement for healthcare professionals by the writing group on perfusion imaging, from the Council on Cardiovascular Radiology of the American Heart Association. Stroke. 2003;34:1084–104.

178. Konstas AA, Goldmakher GV, Lee TY, Lev MH. Theoretic basis and technical implementations of CT perfusion in acute ischemic stroke, part 1: theoretic basis. AJNR Am J Neuroradiol. 2009;30:662–8.

179. Klotz E, Konig M. Perfusion measurements of the brain: using dynamic CT for the quantitative assessment of cerebral ischemia in acute stroke. Eur J Radiol. 1999;30:170–84.

180. Miles K. Measurement of tissue perfusion by dynamic computed tomography. Br J Radiol. 1991;64:409–12.

181. Koenig M, Klotz E, Heuser L. Perfusion CT in acute stroke: characterization of cerebral ischemia using parameter images of cerebral blood flow and their therapeutic relevance. Electromedica. 1998;66:61–6.

182. Steiger HJ, Aaslid R, Stooss R. Dynamic computed tomographic imaging of regional cerebral blood flow and blood volume. A clinical pilot study. Stroke. 1993;24:591–7.

183. Hunter GJ, Hamberg LM, Ponzo JA, et al. Assessment of cerebral perfusion and arterial anatomy in hyperacute stroke with three-dimensional functional CT: early clinical results. AJNR Am J Neuroradiol. 1998;19:29–37.

184. Wintermark M, Maeder P, Thiran JP, Schnyder P, Meuli R. Quantitative assessment of regional cerebral blood flows by perfusion CT studies at low injection rates: a critical review of the underlying theoretical models. Eur Radiol. 2001;11:1220–30.

185. Gobbel G, Cann C, Fike J. Measurement of regional cerebral blood flow using ultrafast computed tomography. Theoretical aspects. Stroke. 1991;22:768–71.

186. Gobbel GT, Cann CE, Fike JR. Comparison of xenon-enhanced CT with ultrafast CT for measurement of regional cerebral blood flow. AJNR Am J Neuroradiol. 1993;14:543–50.

187. Wintermark M, Thiran JP, Maeder P, Schnyder P, Meuli R. Simultaneous measurement of regional cerebral blood flow by perfusion CT and stable xenon CT: a validation study. AJNR Am J Neuroradiol. 2001;22:905–14.

188. Gillard JH, Minhas PS, Hayball MP, et al. Assessment of quantitative computed tomographic cerebral perfusion imaging with H2(15)O positron emission tomography. Neurol Res. 2000;22:457–64.

189. Kudo K, Terae S, Katoh C, et al. Quantitative cerebral blood flow measurement with dynamic perfusion CT using the vascular-pixel elimination method: comparison with H2(15)O positron emission tomography. AJNR Am J Neuroradiol. 2003;24:419–26.

190. Nabavi DG, Cenic A, Craen RA, et al. CT assessment of cerebral perfusion: experimental validation and initial clinical experience. Radiology. 1999;213:141–9.

191. Nabavi DG, Cenic A, Henderson S, Gelb AW, Lee TY. Perfusion mapping using computed tomography allows accurate prediction of cerebral infarction in experimental brain ischemia. Stroke. 2001;32:175–83.

192. Hamberg LM, Hunter GJ, Maynard KI, et al. Functional CT perfusion imaging in predicting the extent of cerebral infarction from a 3-hour middle cerebral arterial occlusion in a primate stroke model. AJNR Am J Neuroradiol. 2002;23:1013–21.

193. Roberts H. Neuroimaging techniques in cerebrovascular disease: computed tomography angiography/computed tomography perfusion. Semin Cerebrovasc Dis Stroke. 2001;1:303–16.

194. Kamalian S, Maas MB, Goldmacher GV, et al. CT cerebral blood flow maps optimally correlate with admission diffusion-weighted imaging in acute stroke but thresholds vary by postprocessing platform. Stroke. 2011;42:1923–8.

195. Rother J, Jonetz-Mentzel L, Fiala A, et al. Hemodynamic assessment of acute stroke using dynamic single-slice computed tomographic perfusion imaging. Arch Neurol. 2000;57:1161–6.

196. Koenig M, Kraus M, Theek C, Klotz E, Gehlen W, Heuser L. Quantitative assessment of the ischemic brain by means of perfusion-related parameters derived from perfusion CT. Stroke. 2001;32:431–7.

197. Sorensen AG. What is the meaning of quantitative CBF? AJNR Am J Neuroradiol. 2001;22:235–6.

198. Tomandl BF, Klotz E, Handschu R, et al. Comprehensive imaging of ischemic stroke with multisection CT. Radiographics. 2003;23:565–92.

199. Wintermark M, Flanders AE, Velthuis B, et al. Perfusion-CT assessment of infarct core and penumbra: receiver operating characteristic curve analysis in 130 patients suspected of acute hemispheric stroke. Stroke. 2006;37:979–85.

200. Eastwood JD, Lev MH, Azhari T, et al. CT perfusion scanning with deconvolution analysis: pilot study in patients with acute middle cerebral artery stroke. Radiology. 2002;222:227–36.

201. Mayer TE, Hamann GF, Baranczyk J, et al. Dynamic CT perfusion imaging of acute stroke. AJNR Am J Neuroradiol. 2000;21:1441–9.

202. Wintermark M, Reichhart M, Thiran JP, et al. Prognostic accuracy of cerebral blood flow measurement by perfusion computed tomography, at the time of emergency room admission, in acute stroke patients. Ann Neurol. 2002; 51:417–32.

203. Chamorro A, Sacco RL, Mohr JP, et al. Clinical-computed tomographic correlations of lacunar infarction in the Stroke Data Bank. Stroke. 1991;22:175–81.

204. Derex L, Tomsick TA, Brott TG, et al. Outcome of stroke patients without angiographically revealed arterial occlusion within four hours of symptom onset. AJNR Am J Neuroradiol. 2001;22:685–90.

205. Ezzeddine MA, Lev MH, McDonald CT, et al. CT angiography with whole brain perfused blood volume imaging: added clinical value in the assessment of acute stroke. Stroke. 2002;33:959–66.

206. Koroshetz WJ, Lev MH. Contrast computed tomography scan in acute stroke: "You can't always get what you want but…you get what you need". Ann Neurol. 2002;51:415–6.

207. Cenic A, Nabavi DG, Craen RA, Gelb AW, Lee TY. Dynamic CT measurement of cerebral blood flow: a validation study. AJNR Am J Neuroradiol. 1999;20:63–73.

208. Campbell BC, Christensen S, Levi CR, et al. Cerebral blood flow is the optimal CT perfusion parameter for assessing infarct core. Stroke. 2011;42(12):3435–40.

209. Wintermark M, Reichhart M, Cuisenaire O, et al. Comparison of admission perfusion computed tomography and qualitative diffusion- and perfusion-weighted magnetic resonance imaging in acute stroke patients. Stroke. 2002;33:2025–31.

210. Zhao L, Barlinn K, Bag AK, et al. Computed tomography perfusion prognostic maps do not predict reversible and irreversible neurological dysfunction following reperfusion therapies. Int J Stroke. 2011;6:544–6.

211. Lev MH, Farkas J, Rodriguez VR, et al. CT angiography in the rapid triage of patients with hyperacute stroke to intraar-

terial thrombolysis: accuracy in the detection of large vessel thrombus. J Comput Assist Tomogr. 2001;25:520–8.

212. Verro P, Tanenbaum LN, Borden NM, Sen S, Eshkar N. CT angiography in acute ischemic stroke: preliminary results. Stroke. 2002;33:276–8.

213. Wildermuth S, Knauth M, Brandt T, Winter R, Sartor K, Hacke W. Role of CT angiography in patient selection for thrombolytic therapy in acute hemispheric stroke. Stroke. 1998;29:935–8.

214. Graf J, Skutta B, Kuhn FP, Ferbert A. Computed tomographic angiography findings in 103 patients following vascular events in the posterior circulation: potential and clinical relevance. J Neurol. 2000;247:760–6.

215. Wintermark M, Meuli R, Browaeys P, et al. Comparison of CT perfusion and angiography and MRI in selecting stroke patients for acute treatment. Neurology. 2007;68:694–7.

216. Coutts SB, Lev MH, Eliasziw M, et al. ASPECTS on CTA source images versus unenhanced CT: added value in predicting final infarct extent and clinical outcome. Stroke. 2004;35:2472–6.

217. Camargo EC, Furie KL, Singhal AB, et al. Acute brain infarct: detection and delineation with CT angiographic source images versus nonenhanced CT scans. Radiology. 2007;244:541–8.

218. Li F, Silva MD, Sotak CH, Fisher M. Temporal evolution of ischemic injury evaluated with diffusion-, perfusion-, and T2-weighted MRI. Neurology. 2000;54:689–96.

219. Moseley ME, Cohen Y, Mintorovitch J, et al. Early detection of regional cerebral ischemia in cats: comparison of diffusion- and T2-weighted MRI and spectroscopy. Magn Reson Med. 1990;14:330–46.

220. Kunst MM, Schaefer PW. Ischemic stroke. Radiol Clin North Am. 2011;49:1–26.

221. Davis DP, Robertson T, Imbesi SG. Diffusion-weighted magnetic resonance imaging versus computed tomography in the diagnosis of acute ischemic stroke. J Emerg Med. 2006;31:269–77.

222. Radiological Society of North America. Diffusion imaging: from basic physics to practical imaging. RSNA, 1999. 2007. http://ej.rsna.org/ej3/0095-98.fin/index.htm. Accessed 17 Feb 2007

223. Schaefer PW, Grant PE, Gonzalez RG. Diffusion-weighted MR imaging of the brain. Radiology. 2000;217:331–45.

224. Lansberg MG, Thijs VN, O'Brien MW, et al. Evolution of apparent diffusion coefficient, diffusion-weighted, and T2-weighted signal intensity of acute stroke. AJNR Am J Neuroradiol. 2001;22:637–44.

225. Lovblad KO, Bassetti C, Schneider J, et al. Diffusion-weighted MR in cerebral venous thrombosis. Cerebrovasc Dis. 2001;11:169–76.

226. Sitburana O, Koroshetz WJ. Magnetic resonance imaging: implication in acute ischemic stroke management. Curr Atheroscler Rep. 2005;7:305–12.

227. Gass A, Ay H, Szabo K, Koroshetz WJ. Diffusion-weighted MRI for the "small stuff": the details of acute cerebral ischaemia. Lancet Neurol. 2004;3:39–45.

228. Easton JD, Saver JL, Albers GW, et al. Definition and evaluation of transient ischemic attack: a scientific statement for healthcare professionals from the American Heart Association/American Stroke Association Stroke Council; Council on Cardiovascular Surgery and Anesthesia; Council on Cardiovascular Radiology and Intervention; Council on Cardiovascular Nursing; and the Interdisciplinary Council on Peripheral Vascular Disease. The American Academy of Neurology affirms the value of this statement as an educational tool for neurologists. Stroke. 2009;40:2276–93.

229. Ay H, Koroshetz WJ, Benner T, et al. Transient ischemic attack with infarction: a unique syndrome? Ann Neurol. 2005;57:679–86.

230. Baird AE, Warach S. Magnetic resonance imaging of acute stroke. J Cereb Blood Flow Metab. 1998;18:583–609.

231. Schwamm LH, Koroshetz WJ, Sorensen AG, et al. Time course of lesion development in patients with acute stroke: serial diffusion- and hemodynamic-weighted magnetic resonance imaging. Stroke. 1998;29:2268–76.

232. Fiehler J, Knudsen K, Kucinski T, et al. Predictors of apparent diffusion coefficient normalization in stroke patients. Stroke. 2004;35:514–9.

233. Desmond PM, Lovell AC, Rawlinson AA, et al. The value of apparent diffusion coefficient maps in early cerebral ischemia. AJNR Am J Neuroradiol. 2001;22:1260–7.

234. Kidwell CS, Saver JL, Mattiello J, et al. Thrombolytic reversal of acute human cerebral ischemic injury shown by diffusion/perfusion magnetic resonance imaging. Ann Neurol. 2000;47:462–9.

235. Thijs VN, Somford DM, Bammer R, Robberecht W, Moseley ME, Albers GW. Influence of arterial input function on hypoperfusion volumes measured with perfusion-weighted imaging. Stroke. 2004;35:94–8.

236. Rivers CS, Wardlaw JM, Armitage PA, et al. Do acute diffusion- and perfusion-weighted MRI lesions identify final infarct volume in ischemic stroke? Stroke. 2006;37:98–104.

237. Barber PA, Davis SM, Darby DG, et al. Absent middle cerebral artery flow predicts the presence and evolution of the ischemic penumbra. Neurology. 1999;52:1125–32.

238. Staroselskaya IA, Chaves C, Silver B, et al. Relationship between magnetic resonance arterial patency and perfusion-diffusion mismatch in acute ischemic stroke and its potential clinical use. Arch Neurol. 2001;58:1069–74.

239. Seitz RJ, Meisel S, Moll M, Wittsack HJ, Junghans U, Siebler M. Partial rescue of the perfusion deficit area by thrombolysis. J Magn Reson Imaging. 2005;22:199–205.

240. Sandhu GS, Parikh PT, Hsu DP, Blackham KA, Tarr RW, Sunshine JL. Outcomes of intra-arterial thrombolytic treatment in acute ischemic stroke patients with a matched defect on diffusion and perfusion MR images. J Neurointerv Surg. 2012;4(2):105–9.

241. Sobesky J, Zaro Weber O, Lehnhardt FG, et al. Which time-to-peak threshold best identifies penumbral flow? A comparison of perfusion-weighted magnetic resonance imaging and positron emission tomography in acute ischemic stroke. Stroke. 2004;35:2843–7.

242. Kidwell CS, Alger JR, Saver JL. Beyond mismatch: evolving paradigms in imaging the ischemic penumbra with multimodal magnetic resonance imaging. Stroke. 2003;34:2729–35.

243. Sorensen AG, Copen WA, Ostergaard L, et al. Hyperacute stroke: simultaneous measurement of relative cerebral blood volume, relative cerebral blood flow, and mean tissue transit time. Radiology. 1999;210:519–27.

244. Parsons MW, Yang Q, Barber PA, et al. Perfusion magnetic resonance imaging maps in hyperacute stroke: relative cerebral blood flow most accurately identifies tissue destined to infarct. Stroke. 2002;33:1581–7.

245. Schaefer PW, Hunter GJ, He J, et al. Predicting cerebral ischemic infarct volume with diffusion and perfusion MR imaging. AJNR Am J Neuroradiol. 2002;23:1785–94.

246. Neumann-Haefelin T, Wittsack HJ, Wenserski F, et al. Diffusion- and perfusion-weighted MRI. The DWI/PWI mismatch region in acute stroke. Stroke. 1999;30:1591–7.

247. Chalela JA, Kang DW, Luby M, et al. Early magnetic resonance imaging findings in patients receiving tissue plasminogen activator predict outcome: insights into the pathophysiology of acute stroke in the thrombolysis era. Ann Neurol. 2004;55:105–12.

248. Prince MR, Arnoldus C, Frisoli JK. Nephrotoxicity of high-dose gadolinium compared with iodinated contrast. J Magn Reson Imaging. 1996;6:162–6.

249. Murphy KP, Szopinski KT, Cohan RH, Mermillod B, Ellis JH. Occurrence of adverse reactions to gadolinium-based contrast material and management of patients at increased risk: a survey of the American Society of Neuroradiology Fellowship Directors. Acad Radiol. 1999;6:656–64.

250. Thomsen HS. Nephrogenic systemic fibrosis: a serious late adverse reaction to gadodiamide. Eur Radiol. 2006;16:2619–21.

251. Collidge TA, Thomson PC, Mark PB, et al. Gadolinium-enhanced MR Imaging and nephrogenic systemic fibrosis: Retrospective Study of a Renal Replacement Therapy Cohort. Radiology. 2007;245(1):168–75.

252. Kuo PH, Kanal E, Abu-Alfa AK, Cowper SE. Gadolinium-based MR contrast agents and nephrogenic systemic fibrosis. Radiology. 2007;242:647–9.

253. Cowper SE, Boyer PJ. Nephrogenic systemic fibrosis: an update. Curr Rheumatol Rep. 2006;8:151–7.

254. Stenver DI. Investigation of the safety of MRI contrast medium Omniscan. Danish Medicines Agency. 2006. http://www.dkma.dk/1024/visUKLSArtikel.asp?artikelID=8931. Published 29 May 2006. Accessed 7 Dec 2006.

255. Cowper SE. Nephrogenic systemic fibrosis: the nosological and conceptual evolution of nephrogenic fibrosing dermopathy. Am J Kidney Dis. 2005;46:763–5.

256. Barkovich AJ, Atlas SW. Magnetic resonance imaging of intracranial hemorrhage. Radiol Clin North Am. 1988;26:801–20.

257. Hermier M, Nighoghossian N. Contribution of susceptibility-weighted imaging to acute stroke assessment. Stroke. 2004;35:1989–94.

258. Kidwell CS, Saver JL, Villablanca JP, et al. Magnetic resonance imaging detection of microbleeds before thrombolysis: an emerging application. Stroke. 2002;33:95–8.

259. Fiehler J, Albers GW, Boulanger JM, et al. Bleeding risk analysis in stroke imaging before thromboLysis (BRASIL): pooled analysis of T2*-weighted magnetic resonance imaging data from 570 patients. Stroke. 2007;38:2738–44.

260. Muir KW, Weir CJ, Murray GD, Povey C, Lees KR. Comparison of neurological scales and scoring systems for acute stroke prognosis. Stroke. 1996;27:1817–20.

261. Brott T, Adams Jr HP, Olinger CP, et al. Measurements of acute cerebral infarction: a clinical examination scale. Stroke. 1989;20:864–70.

262. Goldstein LB, Bertels C, Davis JN. Interrater reliability of the NIH stroke scale. Arch Neurol. 1989;46:660–2.

263. Adams Jr HP, Davis PH, Leira EC, et al. Baseline NIH stroke scale score strongly predicts outcome after stroke: a report of the Trial of Org 10172 in Acute Stroke Treatment (TOAST). Neurology. 1999;53:126–31.

264. Kwiatkowski TG, Libman RB, Frankel M, et al. Effects of tissue plasminogen activator for acute ischemic stroke at one year. N Engl J Med. 1999;340:1781–7.

10. Extracranial Angioplasty and Stenting

10.1.   Carotid Bifurcation Lesions

Indications and Contraindications

The indications for carotid angioplasty and stenting (CAS) are in evolution. The original CAS trials and registries examined the use of CAS in patients considered to be at high risk of complications with CEA; therefore, most available clinical data on CAS is in this setting. Guidelines for CAS developed by a collaborative panel of interventional neuroradiolgists (Table 10.1) emphasized that CAS be used in patients at high risk of complications with surgery. On August 30, 2004, the FDA approved the Accunet™ embolic protection device and the Acculink™ stent (Abbott Laboratories, Santa Clara, CA) for the treatment of patients at high risk for adverse events from CEA who require carotid revascularization and meet the following criteria:

1. Patients with neurological symptoms and ≥50% stenosis of the common or internal carotid artery by ultrasound or angiogram OR patients without neurological symptoms and ≥80% stenosis of the common or internal carotid artery by ultrasound or angiogram, and
2. Patients must have a reference vessel diameter within the range of 4.0 and 9.0 mm at the target lesion.

On September 1, 2004, the Centers for Medicare and Medicaid Services (CMS) announced that CAS with EPD is reasonable and necessary and would be covered for the following patients:

1. High risk for CEA, symptomatic, >70% (must use FDA approved device)
2. High risk, symptomatic, >50%, (and enrolled in a post-approval trial)
3. High risk, asymptomatic, >80% (and enrolled in a post-approval trial)

Patients at high risk for CEA were defined as having significant comorbidities or anatomic risk factors (i.e., recurrent stenosis and/or previous radical neck dissection), and would be poor candidates for CEA in the opinion of a surgeon. Significant comorbid conditions included but were not limited to:

1. Congestive heart failure (CHF) class III/IV;
2. Left ventricular ejection fraction (LVEF) <30%;
3. Unstable angina;
4. Contralateral carotid occlusion;
5. Recent myocardial infarction (MI);
6. Previous CEA with recurrent stenosis;
7. Prior radiation treatment to the neck;
8. Other conditions that were used to determine patients at high risk for CEA in the prior carotid artery stenting trials and studies, such as ARCHER, CABERNET, SAPPHIRE, BEACH, and MAVERIC II.

After review of the CREST study results, on May 6, 2011, FDA announced it approved the expanded indication of the use of the Acculink™ stent (Abbott Laboratories, Santa Clara, CA) for the treatment patients having standard risk for adverse events from CEA. The FDA mandated a post-marketing study to follow patients for 3 years. As of the writing of this handbook, there are several other stents FDA approved for CAS but these are still only approved for patients at high risk for CEA. In addition, the CMS has indicated which US facilities are eligible for reimbursement. A list of these centers is available at www.cms.hhs.gov/coverage/carotid-stent-facilities.asp.

M.R. Harrigan, J.P. Deveikis, *Handbook of Cerebrovascular Disease and Neurointerventional Technique*, DOI 10.1007/978-1-61779-946-4_10, © Springer Science+Business Media New York 2013

Table 10.1 Indications and contraindications for carotid angioplasty and stenting

A.	Acceptable indications for CAS	
	1.	Symptomatic, severe stenosis that is surgically difficult to access (e.g., high bifurcation requiring mandibular dislocation)
	2.	Symptomatic, severe stenosis in a patient with a significant medical disease that would make the patient high risk for surgery
	3.	Symptomatic severe stenosis *and* one of the following conditions:
		(a) Significant tandem lesion that may require endovascular therapy
		(b) Radiation-induced stenosis
		(c) Restenosis after CEA
		(d) Refusal to undergo CEA after proper informed consent
		(e) Stenosis secondary to arterial dissection
		(f) Stenosis secondary to fibromuscular dysplasia
		(g) Stenosis secondary to Takayasu arteritis
	4.	Severe stenosis associated with contralateral carotid artery occlusion requiring treatment before undergoing cardiac surgery
	5.	Severe underlying carotid artery stenosis revealed after recanalization of carotid occlusion after thrombolysis for acute stroke (presumed to be the etiology of the treated occlusion) or to enable thrombolysis for acute stroke
	6.	Pseudoaneurysm
	7.	Asymptomatic preocclusive lesion in a patient otherwise meeting criteria 1–3
B.	Relative Contraindications	
	1.	Asymptomatic stenosis of any degree, except in particular circumstances, as described above (A4, A6, A7)
	2.	Symptomatic stenosis associated with an intracranial vascular malformation
	3.	Symptomatic stenosis in a patient with a subacute cerebral infarction
	4.	Symptomatic stenosis in a patient with a significant contraindication to angiography
C.	Absolute Contraindications	
	1.	Carotid stenosis with angiographically visible intraluminal thrombus
	2.	A stenosis that cannot be safely reached or crossed by an endovascular approach

From Barr et al. [14] Reprinted with permission from the American Society of Neuroradiology
Definitions: *Severe stenosis* is 70% or greater diameter stenosis by NASCET measurement criteria. *Preocclusive stenosis* is 90% or greater diameter stenosis by NASCET criteria or NASCET definition of "near occlusion" [5]

Patient Preparation

Evaluation

1. History and physical
2. Neurological exam
3. Blood work (CBC, Cr, PT, PTT)
4. EKG
5. Imaging
   a. Baseline carotid duplex exam
   b. Confirmatory study (e.g. CTA, MRA, or catheter angiogram).

Pre-procedure Preparation

1) Dual antiplatelet therapy
   a) Do platelet function testing if desired (see Chap. 4).
2) Place two peripheral IVs.
3) Place foley catheter.
4) NPO after midnight or 6 h prior to the procedure except for medications.

5) Hold routine antihypertensive medications on the morning of the procedure.
6) Make sure that all devices that may be needed are available in the angio suite prior to the procedure.

Endovascular Technique

The technique of CAS varies slightly from case to case, depending on the clinical situation. The following is a general outline of the procedure used by the authors for most patients. As with any neurointerventional procedure, the case can be divided into an *access* phase, and an *intervention* phase. In CAS, access consists of placing a guide catheter in the common carotid artery; as many patients in this setting have extensive atherosclerotic disease and a tortuous aortic arch and great vessels, a variety of techniques and devices exist to facilitate this procedure. The intervention phase involves negotiating the stenotic lesion, deployment of the embolic protection device, pre-stent angioplasty, stent deployment, post-stent angioplasty, and embolic protection device retrieval. These techniques also call for an assortment of tips and tricks to handle difficult situations.

Access Phase

See Chap. 4 for more detail on access procedures.
1. Position the patient on the angiography table awake.
2. Rehearse an abbreviated neurological exam with the patient prior to draping.
3. Place a 5F sheath in the femoral artery.
4. Give a loading dose of IV heparin (5,000 units or 70 units/kg).
5. Do a three-vessel diagnostic angiogram using a diagnostic catheter. Include PA, lateral, and ipsilateral oblique angiograms of the target vessel and quantitative measurements of the target vessel and stenotic lesion. Do a PA and lateral intracranial angiogram with injection of contrast into the ipsilateral CCA for later comparison to check for the possibility of thromboembolism within the intracranial circulation suspected during or after the procedure.
6. Obtain optimal angiographic views of the carotid bifurcation – usually the lateral view. (Biplane imaging is best.)
7. Calculate diameters of the CCA, the ICA, the region of greatest stenosis, and the length of the lesion (that needs to be covered by the stent).
8. Select devices based on these vessel measurements: Embolic protection device, pre-dilation angioplasty balloon, stent, and post-dilation angioplasty balloon.
9. Place the diagnostic catheter in the target CCA. Advance an exchange-length wire for exchange of the diagnostic catheter for a 6-F 90-cm sheath (e.g. Shuttle® sheath, Cook Inc., Bloomington, IN).
10. If the ECA is widely patent and accessible with the exchange wire without contacting the atherosclerotic plaque, then advance a 0.035 in. stiff 300-cm hydrophilic wire through the diagnostic catheter, and into a distal branch of the ECA, such as the internal maxillary artery or the occipital artery.
11. If the ECA is occluded, or if the atherosclerotic plaque extends into the CCA for a significant degree, advance a stiff J wire (e.g., Amplatz Extra Stiff Guidewire 0.035 in. (Cook Inc., Bloomington, IN) through the diagnostic catheter and positioned in the distal CCA immediately below the lesion.
12. When the stiff guidewire has been positioned, exchange the 5F groin sheath over a tapered obturator, for the 6F 90-cm sheath. Position the distal end of this system approximately 2 cm proximal to the carotid bifurcation (the tip of the Shuttle may undulate up and down with each cardiac cycle; therefore position the tip should at a safe distance from the lesion, yet distal enough in the common carotid to maximize stability of the Shuttle, and to be able to see its tip on the fluoroscopic image). Remove the exchange-length wire and the obturator from the sheath together; 5–10 mL of blood should be aspirated through the RHV into a waste bowl as the wire and obturator are removed. Flush all catheter systems continuously with heparinized saline.
13. 6F 90-cm sheath device options:
    a. Shuttle®–SL Flexor® (Cook Inc., Bloomington, IN).
        i. Robust, stable sheath.
        ii. Tip: Remove the Tuohy-Borst valve that comes with the introducer set and replace it with a standard RHV.

b. Super Arrow-Flex® Percutaneous Sheath (Arrow International, Reading, PA).
  i. Braided sheath, resistant to kinking.
  ii. Disadvantage: It can stretch if pulled back against resistance.
c. Pinnacle® Destination™ Guiding Sheath (Terumo Medical Corp., Somerset, NJ).
    Low profile, slick.

Tips for Difficult Access Cases

1. Femoral artery access is limited (i.e. high grade iliac or femoral artery stenosis or occlusion)
   a. Brachial artery approach.[1]
   b. Angioplasty and possible stenting of the iliac or femoral artery
2. Aortic arch or great vessels are tortuous
   a. Use the ECA to anchor the wire.
      i. During the initial placement of the diagnostic catheter in the CCA, use a 0.035-in. hydrophilic wire to advance the diagnostic catheter into a branch of the ECA.
      ii. Remove the wire and replace it with a stiffer exchange-length wire, such as a 0.038-in. hydrophilic wire or an Amplatz extra-stiff (Cook Medical, Bloomington, IN).
      iii. Exchange the diagnostic catheter for the 90-cm sheath.
          This technique works well in the left CCA using a Simmons 2 catheter as the diagnostic catheter.
   b. "Tower of power" technique to add stability to the 90-cm sheath:
       Advance an 8F guide catheter (e.g., 8F straight Envoy® (Codman Neurovascular, San Jose, CA) inside of an 8F 90-cm sheath.
   c. Larger diameter 90-cm sheath (e.g., 7F or 8F) adds stability.
   d. Buddy wire technique.
       Use a larger diameter 90-cm sheath (e.g., 8F sheath) and a 0.014 or 0.018-in. wire anchored into a branch of the ECA.
   e. Direct percutaneous CAS.[2]
   f. Snare-assisted wire and catheter placement (aka "pull-through technique").[3]
      i. Introduce a wire via micropuncture access to the ipsilateral superficial temporal artery and position it in the aorta.
      ii. Place a snare (e.g. Amplatz Gooseneck® ev3 Endovascular, Plymouth, MN) from a guide catheter via a femoral (or even brachial) access and snare the grab the wire.
      iii. Pull the wire, snare, and guide catheter up as a unit into the carotid.
   g. If access to the carotid is lost during the exchange for the 90-cm sheath, re-access the common carotid artery using a 105 cm 6.5F Slipcath® curved hydrophilic catheter (Cook Inc., Bloomington, IN) placed through the sheath.
      i. Select the origin of the common carotid with the curved catheter, and place a 0.038-in. hydrophillic wire back in the common carotid or external carotid.
      ii. Advance catheter and sheath into position.
3. Tandem stenoses (e.g., atherosclerotic stenosis both at the origin of the CCA and at the bifurcation).
       CAS of the origin lesion (see below), followed by CAS of the bifurcation lesion.
       Note: after CAS of the origin lesion, it is important to maintain wire access through the first stent.
      i. After placement of an ostial stent, with a small amount of the stent extending into the aortic arch (as planned), it is difficult to navigate a wire through the newly placed stent.
      ii. If using an EPD during treatment of the ostial lesion, place the first stent, then recapture the EPD with a retrieval catheter.
      iii. Before withdrawing the retrieval catheter, advance the 90-cm sheath (or guide catheter) over the retrieval catheter and into the CCA through the first stent. Be careful not to get hung up on the end of the stent.

Intervention Phase

Undertake the four-stage procedure for CAS after placing the guide catheter. Obtain high-resolution biplane angiograms after each step and perform neurologic exams to allow for prompt recognition of any changes from the patient's baseline status.

1. Advance EPD.
   a. Make a roadmap
   b. Select a relatively straight segment of the ICA for placement of the distal protection device that will also permit the device to be at least 2–3 cm distal to the lesion.
   c. Guide the EPD through the region of stenosis, slowly and carefully to avoid dislodging plaque.
2. Deploy EPD.
   a. The radio-opaque markers on the EPD should be well visualized and closely apposed to the wall of the vessel.
   b. The tip of the EPD wire should be in view on the fluoroscope (i.e., it should not be allowed to migrate too far into the intracranial ICA).
   c. Do abbreviated neurological exam.
   d. Do angiogram.
3. Pre-dilation angioplasty
   a. Objective: to open the stenotic region only enough to accommodate the stent.
   b. Use a relatively small balloon – typically 2.0 or 2.5-mm diameter angioplasty balloon, and long enough to cover the plaque. Smaller balloons are associated with better results in CAS.[4]
   c. Keep the blood pressure cuff on continuous mode during angioplasty.
   d. A circulating nurse should stand by to administer atropine and dopamine if necessary.
   e. Pre-treat with atropine, 0.75-mg IV, for HR <~60.
      If not pre-treated, administer atropine, 0.75-mg IV if the patient becomes bradycardic during the angioplasty.
   f. Start dopamine infusion at 2–5 μg/kg/min (and increase as needed to a maximum of 50 μg/kg/min) for a significant drop in blood pressure during angioplasty (~SBP $\geq$25% below baseline, or SBP <110 mmHg).
   g. Once the balloon is in position, inflate to nominal pressure *briefly* (for 1–2 s), then deflate.
   h. Brief balloon inflation is usually sufficient to "crack" the plaque while minimizing the chance of bradycardia and hypotension.
   i. Remove the pre-dilation angioplasty balloon.
   j. Do abbreviated neurological exam.
   k. Do angiogram.
4. Stenting
   a. On the angiogram (and roadmap image), decide on the optimal position of the stent, and identify the precise location of the planned distal stent end location (i.e. where the self-expanding stent will begin deployment).
   b. On an *unsubtracted* angiogram image, identify bony landmarks for the stent deployment targets (e.g., middle of the body of C2) that will allow precise deployment of the stent if the patient moves and the roadmap degrades.
   c. Carefully advance the stent into position.
   d. Monitor the EPD position during this manoeuvre.
   e. Do abbreviated neurological exam.
   f. Do angiogram.
   g. Deploy stent.
      Deploy smoothly and swiftly.
   h. It is okay to "jail" the origin of the ECA with the stent.
   i. Do abbreviated neurological exam.
   j. Do angiogram.
5. Post-dilation angioplasty (if needed).
   a. *Do only if really needed*. Remember: Less is more. Post-stenting angioplasty is the riskiest part of CAS.[4–7]
   b. Objectives:

    i. To widen the stenotic region if the degree of stenosis after stent deployment is still significant (>30–40%).

    ii. To seat the stent against the vessel wall if it does not appear to be firmly apposed to the plaque and vessel wall after the initial deployment.

  c. The size of the post-dilation angioplasty balloon is critical

    i. Diameter should be smaller than the diameter of the normal portion of the ICA, to minimize the risk of bradycardia, asystole, and dissection.

    ii. The length of the balloon should be less than the length of the deployed stent; an angioplasty balloon longer than the stent can cause a dissection.

  d. Again, the blood pressure cuff is placed on continuous mode and a circulating nurse should stand by to administer atropine and dopamine if necessary.

  e. Position the balloon entirely within the stent, then inflate to nominal pressure briefly for 1–2 s, then deflate.

  f. Remove the balloon.

  g. Do abbreviated neurological exam.

  h. Do angiogram.

6. Retrieval of EPD.

  a. Advance the retrieval catheter through the stent.

  b. Capture the EPD in a relatively straight segment of the ICA.

  c. Do abbreviated neurological exam.

  d. Do angiogram.

7. Obtain final angiographic images.

    Cervical: PA and lateral, and intracranial: PA and lateral angiograms.

8. Remove the sheath.

  a. Options for management of the femoral artery puncture site:

    i. Exchange the 90-cm sheath over a 150-cm 0.035-in. hydrophilic wire for a closure device.

    ii. Exchange the 90-cm sheath for a short sheath (of equal or greater French size), and remove the short sheath later (when the heparin has worn off) and apply compression to the puncture site.

    iii. Partially withdraw the 90-cm sheath – so that only 10–20 cm remains in the femoral artery – and loop it up and tape it to the patient's groin. Remove it can be removed later, and apply compression.

Post-procedure Management

1. Complete neurological exam.

2. Admit to the NICU or step-down unit with neuro exams and groin checks Q 1 h.

3. Antiplatelet therapy:

  a. Antiplatelet therapy: Aspirin 325-mg PO QD indefinitely *and*

  b. Clopidogrel (Plavix®) 75-mg PO QD for 30 days after the procedure

  Or

  c. Antiplatelet therapy: Aspirin 325-mg PO QD indefinitely *and*

  d. Ticlopidine (Ticlid®) for 30 days after the procedure.

    i. Note: Must monitor for neutropenia (see above)

4. For patients with hypotension, requiring dopamine infusion:

  a. Hypotension after CAS is usually self-limited and resolves within 1–2 days.

  b. Do a cardiac work-up to exclude an MI

    i. EKG

    ii. Cardiac enzymes

5. Routine follow-up carotid duplex exam

  a. After procedure or on post-procedure day 1.

  b. After 1 month.

  c. After 6 months, then annually after that.

  d. Caveat: Closed cell design stents may produce elevated velocities on early follow-up duplex imaging that may suggest a degree of stenosis that may not really be significant.[8]

CAS Tips

1. Operator experience and careful patient selection is critical. Patients with risk factors for complications with CAS (see below) should be managed by experienced operators or not treated by endovascular methods at all. Carotid endarterectomy (CEA) remains the "gold standard" for the treatment of atherosclerotic carotid stenosis.
2. Prepare all of the devices needed for the procedure before the case, immediately prior to the groin stick. Place them in a stack on the back table or at the foot of the patient's table, with each device separated by a sterile towel in the order that they will be used (e.g., put the EPD at the top, followed by the pre-dilation balloon directly underneath, etc.). This will permit rapid and efficient access to each device as it is needed.
3. Use embolic protection whenever possible.
4. Do a hand-injection angiogram after each step, to check for dissections, intraluminal thrombi, positioning of devices, and documentation. If a complication should arise during or after the case, a complete set of angiograms can help sort out and manage the problem.
5. Examine the patient after each step of the procedure (e.g., "Everything's going fine, Mr. Smith. How are you? Wiggle your toes. Squeeze the rubber duck. Show me your teeth. Say, "Today's a sunny day." ").
6. Do not over-dilate during angioplasty. It is better to under-size the angioplasty balloons than to over-size them, to minimize the risk of bradycardia and hypotension and also embolic complications.[9]
7. As long as the stenosis lumen is sufficient to allow passage of a stent delivery catheter and the plaque is not heavily calcified, one study found primary stent placement without any balloon angioplasty could be successful 79% of the time.[10] This is not standard protocol but may reduce the risk of bradycardia, hypotension and also embolic complications.

Other Tips for Handling Difficult CAS Situations

1. The region of stenosis is too narrow to permit navigation of a distal EPD.
   a. Consider careful pre-dilation of the lesion without distal protection, followed by placement of the EPD.
      i. The greatest risk of embolic events appears to occur during stent deployment.[11] Also, emboli can occur during passage of the EPD, even without a high grade stenosis. Therefore, careful pre-dilation with a small-diameter balloon, to permit the use of a distal EPD, can be done in some cases with acceptable risk
   b. Consider using a proximal balloon-occlusion system (e.g., MO.MA. Invatec, Roncadelle, Italy), or a flow reversal device (e.g., Parodi Anti-Emboli System.W.L. Gore & Associates, Newark, DE) if available.
2. The EPD cannot be retrieved (the retrieval catheter cannot be advanced through the stent, or the EPD cannot fold up into the retrieval catheter).
   a. Advance the 90-cm sheath up into and through the stent, if possible
   b. Bring the EPD into the sheath.
   c. Use a curved retrieval catheter.
3. Carotid is too tortuous to deploy EPD
   a. Tilt the patient's head toward the opposite shoulder, to straighten out the vessel
   b. Use a balloon-occlusion device (e.g., Guardwire® Temporary Occlusion and Aspiration System.Medtronic AVE, Santa Rosa, CA)
4. In-stent restenosis
   a. Endovascular retreatment *is only appropriate if the in-stent stenosis is symptomatic.*
      i. CAS changes the physiology of carotid artery disease. Most strokes from carotid atherosclerosis are embolic. CAS stabilizes the plaque, and restenosis after CAS may not have the same natural history as native carotid stenosis.
   b. If retreatment is necessary, consider using a cutting balloon.[12, 13]
      i. Cutting balloon technique:
         A. Pretreat the patient with dual antiplatelet therapy.
         B. Obtain access with a 6F Sheath or 8F guide catheter.

C. Load with IV heparin.
D. Position an embolic protection device distal to the region of stenosis.
E. Select a Flextome® Cutting Balloon® Dilatation Device (Boston Scientific, Natick, MA) to match the desired diameter (≤ diameter of the stent).
F. Inflate to nominal pressure, deflate, and remove devices.

c. Cryotherapy balloons are available (Polarcath™ Boston Scientific, Natick, MA) and may reduce the rate of restenosis caused by intimal hypertophy, but these have not been tested in the carotid system.

Risk Factors for CAS Complications

Patient factors that elevate risk with CAS. Consider strategies to minimize risk in these patients or alternatives such as medical management or CEA.

1. Tortuous anatomy
   a. Can impede access or positioning of the EPD.
   b. Interferes with stability of the devices.
2. Long lesion or multiple lesions
   Plaque debris may overwhelm EPD.
3. Tandem lesions
   a. e.g., CCA origin stenosis and bifurcation disease
   b. Increases complexity of procedure.
4. Ulcerated lesion.
5. Bilateral carotid disease.
6. Intraluminal thrombus
   One of the two published absolute contraindications to CAS.[14]
7. Echolucency on carotid ultrasound (grey-scale median ≤25).[15]
8. Dialysis-dependent renal failure.
   In ARCHeR, patients with dialysis-dependent renal failure had a stroke, death, and myocardial infarction rate of 28.6%.[16]
9. Absence of hypercholesterolemia.[17]

Management of Neurological Complications During or After CAS

1. Prompt recognition of a neurologic change is critical.
2. If a neurological change occurs during the case:
   a. Perform angiograms of the cervical carotid system and the intracranial circulation
   b. Look for intraluminal thrombus, intracranial vessel dropout, or slowing of contrast passage through distal intracranial vessels (indicates a *shower of emboli* into multiple small branches).
   c. Look for signs of dissection caused by the angioplasty balloon or a distal dissection produced by the EPD.
3. Options for thrombolysis if needed:
   a. IV GP IIb/IIIa inhibitor
      i. Advantages: Powerful antiplatelet agents, particularly useful for platelet-rich thrombus, which often is the case in stent deployment.
      ii. Disadvantage: Carries a risk of ICH[18] relatively long half-life.
   b. Abciximab
      Loading dose 0.25 mg/kg, followed by 12 h continuous infusion at 10 μg/min.
   c. Eptifibitide
      Loading dose of 135 μg/kg followed by a 20–24-h infusion of 0.5 μg/kg
   d. The authors of this handbook prefer abciximab, which, unlike eptifibitide, can be reversed with platelet transfusion if necessary.
   e. Intra-arterial thrombolytic (e.g., tPA or urokinase)
      i. Advantage: Short half-life
      ii. Disadvantage: May not be as effective as a GP IIb/IIIa inhibitor if the thrombus is platelet-rich. Also carries a risk of ICH.

4. Suspect ICH:
   a. If angiogram does not show an occlusion to explain neurological change, or shows signs of mass-effect.
   b. Particularly if the patient complains of a headache, and a Cushing's response (i.e., hypertension and bradycardia) occurs.
   c. Obtain a head CT if an ICH is suspected; leave the sheath in place, if possible, for the trip to the scanner
      i. The 90-cm sheath tip can be pulled down into the aorta and secured at the groin by looping and taping the excess sheath to the patient.
      ii. Include a CT perfusion study along with the non-contrast head CT, if there is no evidence of ICH
         May identify ischaemic regions, clarify diagnosis.
      iii. If ICH is identified:
         Reverse heparin with protamine (10 mg IV per 1,000 units of heparin given).
      Maintain vigilant blood pressure control.
5. Hyperperfusion syndrome:
   a. Has been seen to occur in up to 5% of CAS cases;[19] associated with ICH in 0.67%.[16] Also a recognized complication of CEA.
   b. Defined as: ipsilateral headache, nausea, focal seizures, or focal neurologic deficit without radiographic evidence of infarction.
   c. Presumed mechanism: A chronic low blood flow state because of carotid stenosis leads to compensatory cerebral vasodilation in the affected territory, and loss of autoregulatory capacity. With carotid revascularization, an abrupt increase in CBF occurs without autoregulatory control.
   d. Time course: Symptoms can appear 6 h to 4 days after CAS.[20]
   e. Risk factors (derived from CEA literature):[21, 22]
      i. ICA stenosis ≥90%
      ii. Contralateral ICA stenosis or occlusion
      iii. Poor collateral flow
      iv. Hypertension
      v. Recent cerebral ischaemic event
      vi. Younger patient
   f. Management: Close observation, vigilant blood pressure control.
6. Neurological change + unremarkable angiogram: Consider *transient contrast encephalopathy*.[23]
   a. Head CT: cortical enhancement and edema.
   b. Syndrome is self-limited; prognosis is good.
7. Post-procedure neurological change
   a. Some 25–30% of cerebral ischaemic events with CAS occur 2–14 days after the procedure.[17, 24]
   b. Work-up:
      i. Head CT
      ii. Carotid duplex exam
   c. Consider return to the angio suite for a diagnostic angiogram and possible intra-arterial thrombolysis
      Angiographic improvement was seen in 80% of patients but clinical improvement in only 40% and 60% died when intracranial occlusions were treated with IA thrombolysis.[24]
8. When angiography or CT imaging does not explain a neurological change, consider MRI with diffusion-weighted imaging, which can identify subtle ischaemic changes.

CAS Pearls

1. Previously, GP IIb/IIIa inhibitors were standard treatment during CAS. However, an increased risk of ICH was observed with these medications.[18] GP IIb/IIIa inhibitors during CAS are now reserved for select cases.

2. Pre-dilation angioplasty may reduce long-term stroke risk.[25]
   Possible mechanism: improved remodeling of the plaque prior to stent placement may stabilize the plaque.[26]
3. The primary advantage of self-expanding stents for CAS, compared to balloon-mounted stents, is that self-expanding stents are less vulnerable to compression.[27]
4. All filter devices have a pore size of 100 μm or larger; this may explain why the Guardwire® balloon system has been found to capture significantly more particles than filter devices.[28, 29]
5. Intraluminal thrombi are more easily seen on high speed unsubtracted angiograms (7.5 or 15 fps) than on subtracted angiograms.[7]
6. It is not unheard of to see some spasm in the vessel distal to the stent. This will resolve spontaneously. It should be differentiated from residual stenosis not covered by the stent, or a dissection, which may require placement of a second stent to treat the residual stenosis.

Embolic Protection Devices

Cerebral embolization of plaque debris and thombotic material during CAS is a major source of morbidity during CAS. Embolic protection devices have evolved to limit embolization during CAS. The first report of an embolic protection technique described a triple coaxial catheter with a latex balloon mounted at the distal end.[30] The ICA was occluded during stent placement, and debris was flushed and aspirated after stent deployment. Since then, ICA filters and flow-reversal techniques[31] have also been introduced. The use of embolic protection devices has been widespread since about 2000; filter devices are currently most commonly used.

Filter Devices

The primary advantage of filter devices is the preservation of the flow through the ICA. Several devices are available.
1. Accunet™ (Abbott Laboratories, Santa Clara, CA)
   a. Device sizes (target vessel diameter)(mm): 4.5 (3.25–4.0); 5.5 (4.0–5.0); 6.5 (5.0–6.0); 7.5 (6.0–7.0)
   b. Trials: ARCHeR, CREST, CAPTURE
   c. Comments: Polyurethane filter, 150-μm pore size. FDA-approved for CAS in high-risk or standard-risk patients.
2. FilterWire EZ™ (Boston Scientific Corp, Natick, MA)
   a. Size: One size fits all, for vessel diameter 3.5–5.5 mm
   b. Trials: BEACH, CABERNET
   c. Comments: Polyurethane filter, 110-μm pore size. Cleared for marketing in U.S. for saphenous vein grafts.
3. Angioguard™ (Cordis Corp., Miami Lakes, FL)
   a. Device sizes (vessel diameter) (mm): 5 (3.5–4.5); 6 (4.5–5.5); 7 (5.5–6.5); 8 (6.5–7.5)
   b. Trials: SAPPHIRE, CASES
   c. Comments: Polyurethane filter, 100-μm pore size.
4. Emboshield™ (Abbott Laboratories, Abbott Park, Il)
   a. Device sizes (target vessel diameter) (mm): 5.0 (2.5-4.8), 7.2 (4.0-7.0).
   b. Trials: SECuRITY, EXACT
   c. Comments: Nylon filter, 140-μm pore size. Three different degrees of wire stiffness available.
5. SpiderFX™ (ev3, Plymouth, MN)
   a. Sizes (mm): 3.0, 4.0, 5.0, 6.0, 7.0.
   b. Trial: CREATE II
   c. Comments: Wire mesh filter. Design permits advancement of a 0.014-in. microwire alone across stenotic region first, then placement of EPD over the microwire. Crossing profile: 2.9F.
6. Interceptor® PLUS (Medtronic, Inc., Santa Rosa, CA)
   a. Offered in sizes to fit vessel diameters from 4.25mm to 6.25 mm.
   b. Trial: MAVErIC III
   c. Comments: Nitinol wire mesh filter. Crossing profile: 2.7F. Has been commercially released to European markets.

7. Rubicon® (Rubicon Medical, Salt Lake City, UT)

   Crossing profiles: 2.1, 2.4, 2.7 F. 100-μm pore size. Compatible with 6F guide catheters.

Balloon-Occlusion Devices

Balloon occlusion techniques involve inflation of a balloon and interruption of flow in the ICA distal to the stenosis for the duration of the stenting procedure. After CAS, aspiration of the proximal carotid system is done prior to balloon deflation remove embolic material.

1. Guardwire® Temporary Occlusion and Aspiration System (Medtronic AVE, Santa Rosa, CA)
   a. Sizes (mm): 2.5–5.0 and 3.0–6.0.
   b. Trials: MAVErIC I and II.
   c. Crossing profile: 2.9F.
   d. Comments: Formally known as PercuSurge. Approved in the U.S. for saphenous vein grafts. Export® Catheter (Medtronic AVE, Santa Rosa, CA) is designed to be used with the Guardwire® for aspiration of debris.
   e. Transient neurological changes have been seen in up to 5% of patient undergoing CAS with distal balloon occlusion.[32, 33]
2. MO.MA (Invatec, Roncadelle, Italy)
   a. "Endovascular clamping device," emulates surgical clamping by simultaneous endovascular occlusion of the CCA (up to 13 mm in diameter) and the ECA (up to 6 mm in diameter). Blood is aspirated during or after the CAS procedure.
   b. Trials: MO.MA, PRIAMUS.[34]
   c. Comment: FDA approval October, 2006.
3. Medicorp occlusive balloon (Medicorp, Nancy, France).[35]
   Comment: Not available in the U.S.

Flow-Reversal Device

The flow-reversal technique involves placement of balloons in the ECA and CCA to interrupt flow in these vessels and cause retrograde flow in the ICA to prevent embolization into the intracranial circulation.[31]

1. Parodi Anti-Emboli System (W.L. Gore & Associates, Flagstaff, AZ)
   a. Temporarily reverses flow in the ICA during CAS. Balloons are inflated in the CCA and the ECA, and an outside connector with a filter creates an "external arteriovenous fistula" during CAS.
   b. Comments: Requires a gigantic 11F sheath.
   c. The use of flow-reversal devices assumes that considerable collateral flow is present and theoretically has the greatest chance of significantly reducing the cerebral blood flow during CAS. This has not been systematically tested.

Stents

Stents currently in use for CAS are self-expanding stents, and are available in tapered or straight designs. *Open cell* stents have struts that can extend into the lumen and can potentially interfere with passage of the EPD retrieval catheter, whereas *closed cell* stents do not have exposed struts, but may not have good wall apposition in a curved vessel. Selection of the stent is determined by lesion length and the normal diameter of the artery. The stent should be oversized by 1–2 mm more than the normal arterial caliber and should completely cover the lesion. At diameters less than that of full expansion, self-expanding stents exert a chronic outward radial force that serves to maintain apposition of the stent to the vessel wall after deployment. If the stent will extend from the CCA into the ICA the stent should be sized according to the larger caliber of the CCA. Tapered stents are also available to accommodate the tapering of the vessel. In the United States, there are several FDA approved stents and each has approval to be used with a specific EPD. With all the merger and acquisition activity in the medical device industry, companies that market each stent may change from time to time.

1. Acculink™ (Abbott Laboratories, Santa Clara, CA)
   a. Tapered stent diameters (proximal/distal)(mm): 10/7, 8/6.
   b. Tapered stent lengths (mm): 30, 40.
   c. Straight stent diameters (mm): 5, 6, 7, 8, 9, 10.
   d. Straight stent lengths (mm): 20, 30, 40.
   e. Material: Nitinol
   f. Trials: CREST, CREATE II, ARCHeR
   g. Comments: Open cell design. FDA approved *both* for patients high risk *and* standard risk for CEA.
   h. Approved EPD: Accunet™
2. Xact™ (Abbott Laboratories, Abbott Park, IL).
   a. Tapered stent diameters (proximal/distal)(mm): 10/8, 9/7, 8/6.
   b. Tapered stent lengths (mm): 30, 40.
   c. Straight stent diameters (mm): 7, 8, 9, 10.
   d. Straight stent lengths (mm): 20, 30.
   e. Material: Nitinol.
   f. Trials: ACT I, SECuRITY, EXACT.
   g. Comments: Closed cell design. FDA approved for patients high risk for CEA.
   h. Approved EPD: Emboshield NAV.
3. Precise® (Cordis Endovascular, Miami Lakes, FL).
   a. Straight stent diameters (mm): 5, 6, 7, 8, 9, 10.
   b. Straight stent lengths (mm): 20, 30, 40.
   c. Material: Nitinol.
   d. Trials: CASES, CREATE.
   e. Comments: Segmented (open) cell design. FDA approved for patients high-risk for CEA.
   f. Approved EPD: Angioguard®.
4. Wallstent® (Boston Scientific, Natick, MA)
   a. Straight stent diameters (mm): 6, 8, 10.
   b. Straight stent lengths (mm): 20, 30, 40.
   c. Material: Elgiloy® cobalt-chromium-iron-nickel-molybdenum alloy.
   d. Trial: BEACH.
   e. Comments: Closed cell design. Produces extensive artifact on MRI imaging. FDA approved for patients high risk for CEA. Only stent approved for bilateral placement.
   f. Approved EPD: FilterWire EZ™.
5. NexStent (Boston Scientific, Natick, MA)
   a. Tapered stent diameters: self-tapering, all diameters 4–9 mm.
   b. Tapered stent lengths (mm): 30.
   c. Trial: CABERNET, SONOMA
   d. Comments: Open cell design. FDA approved for high risk patients.
   e. Approved EPD: FilterWire EZ™
6. Protege® (ev3, Plymouth, MN)
   a. Tapered stent diameters (proximal/distal)(mm): 10/7, 8/6.
   b. Tapered stent lengths (mm): 30, 40.
   c. Straight stent diameters (mm): 6, 7, 8, 9, 10.
   d. Straight stent lengths (mm): 20, 30, 40, 60.
   e. Material: nitinol.
   f. Trial: CREATE.
   g. Comments: Open cell design. FDA approved for patients high risk for CEA.
   h. Approved EPD: SpiderFX®.

Carotid Stenting for Dissection or Pseudoaneurysm

1. Indication: *Symptomatic, hemodynamically significant* carotid dissection or pseudoaneurysm despite therapy with antiplatelet agents or anticoagulation.
2. Pre-medication with antiplatelet agents is critical. In an emergency, treatment with an IV GP IIb/IIIa inhibitor can be given as a "bridge to therapy," until an appropriate loading dose of ASA and clopidogrel has been given and allowed time to take effect (2–5 h after oral administration).

3. Use an EPD if possible.

   Thromboembolic material may be present in the area of dissection even if not visible on angiography.
4. Cover entire area of dissection with the stent, if possible; if not possible, then cover the proximal part of the dissection.
5. The technique is generally the same as for CAS of atherosclerotic carotid bifurcation disease, although angioplasty is not usually needed for dissections.
6. Be sure the guidewire and EPD are within the true lumen and not subintimal, otherwise stenting can make the dissection worse. If there is any question, advance a catheter distal to the dissection, do a gentle contrast injection for an arteriogram, and check that the catheter is in the true lumen and appropriate branches can be seen.

10.2.   Vertebral Artery Stenosis

This section focuses on the treatment of symptomatic vertebral artery origin stenosis, as symptomatic disease attributable to extracranial vertebral artery stenosis distal to the origin is less common.

Indications

1. Symptoms of VBI (must include at least two of the following symptoms)[36]:
   a. Motor or sensory symptoms
   b. Dysarthria
   c. Imbalance
   d. Dizziness or vertigo
   e. Tinnitus
   f. Alternating paresthesias
   g. Homonymous hemianopia
   h. Diplopia
   i. Other cranial nerve palsies
   j. Dysphagia
2. Although traditionally vertigo or dizziness in the absence of other symptoms has not been regarded as indicative of VBI, recent evidence suggests that the opposite is true.[37]
3. MRI evidence of ischaemic injury to the posterior circulation.
4. ≥50% stenosis of the vertebral artery by CTA, angiography, or MRA.
5. Hypoplasia or stenosis affecting the contralateral vertebral artery.

Contraindication

Intraluminal thrombus.

a. Usually one can treat the patient with anticoagulation, then stent the vertebral after resolution of thrombus.
b. Safe and successful treatment in one case of a vertebral stenosis associated with thrombus has been reported using flow reversal and an EPD.[38]

Patient Preparation

Same as for carotid bifurcation lesions (see previous discussion).

Endovascular Technique (Vertebral Artery Origin Lesions)

The technique for treating vertebral artery origin stenoses is similar to the technique for treating carotid bifurcation lesions, however, the important difference is that balloon-expandable stents are preferred, as these stents allow more precise deployment than self-expanding stents, and are less likely to "watermelon-seed" (i.e. squeezed out of position from the stenosis).

1. Position patient on the angiography table awake.
2. Rehearse an abbreviated neurological exam with the patient prior to draping. Include posterior circulation elements (e.g., visual fields, extraocular movements, facial symmetry).
3. Access the femoral artery; however, an ipsilateral upper extremity approach (i.e., radial artery or brachial artery) may be more favourable, depending on the patient's anatomy.
   (a) 6F or 7F sheath. 5F might be sufficient if a low-profile coronary stent is being used.
4. Do a diagnostic angiogram, including the ipsilateral subclavian artery and vertebral artery. Angiography of the contralateral vertebral artery can help clarify distal vertebrobasilar anatomy.
5. Give a loading dose of IV heparin (5,000 units or 70 units/kg).
6. Place a 6F guide catheter in the subclavian artery adjacent to the vertebral artery.
   a. Stabilize the guide catheter if necessary by placing a supportive 0.014 in. or larger buddy wire into the ipsilateral axillary artery.
   b. Requires a larger guide catheter.
7. Advance and deploy embolic protection device (EPD) if possible.
   a. Use an EPD if:[39]
      i. Vertebral artery diameter is >3.5 mm.
      ii. Ulcerated target lesion.
   b. Deploy EPD in a straight segment of the cervical vertebral artery ≥2 cm distal to lesion.
   c. Do abbreviated neurological exam.
   d. Do angiogram.
8. Pre-dilation angioplasty
   a. Only necessary if the region of stenosis is too small to allow passage of the balloon-mounted stent.
   b. Use a relatively small balloon should be used – typically 2.0 or 2.5-mm angioplasty balloon, long enough to cover the plaque. Position the balloon, inflate to nominal pressure, then deflate.
      Inflation of the balloon for a minute or more is necessary to "crack" the plaque.
   c. Remove the pre-dilation angioplasty balloon.
   d. Do abbreviated neurological exam.
   e. Do angiogram.
9. Advance balloon-mounted stent across the lesion.
   a. Consider off-label use of a coronary drug-eluting stent.
      In a multistudy review, drug-eluting stents had lower rates of restenosis (11%) compared with bare metal stents (30%) in the vertebral artery at a mean follow-up of 24 months.[40]
   b. Measure the diameter of the normal-appearing vertebral artery distal to the lesion and select a stent slightly larger than that diameter (by 0.3–1 mm[41]), and long enough to both cross the region of stenosis and extend distal to the lesion by 3–5 mm.
   c. On the angiogram (and roadmap image), decide on the optimal position of the stent, and identify the precise location of the planned distal stent edge.
      The traditional technique is to position the stent so that it extends just barely into the subclavian artery. This practice has been carried over from literature about treatment of coronary and renal artery ostial lesions[42–46], and has been thought to minimize the chance of "watermelon-seeding" the stent and to decrease the risk of recurrent stenosis. The downside is that it can make it difficult to catheterize distal to the stent if necessary. However, in a recent series of 117 cases, the authors obtained good results with positioning of the stent exactly at the vertebral artery origin.[41] This has the advantage of permitting access to the vertebral artery after stent placement.

d. On an *unsubtracted* angiogram image, identify bony landmarks for the stent deployment targets (e.g., transverse process of T2) that will allow precise deployment of the stent if the patient should move and the road-map become degraded.
e. Carefully advance the stent into position, and then pull back slightly to remove any slack in the system.
    Monitor the EPD position carefully during this manoeuvre.
f. Do abbreviated neurological exam.
g. Do angiogram.
10. Deploy stent.
a. Inflate the balloon to nominal pressure and allow it to stay inflated for 10–15 s if possible, to seat the stent.
b. Deflate the balloon.
c. Do abbreviated neurological exam.
d. Do angiogram.
11. Post-dilation angioplasty (if needed).
    Objective:
    i. To widen the stenotic region if the degree of stenosis after stent deployment is still significant.
    ii. To seat the stent against the vessel wall if it does not appear to be firmly apposed to the plaque after the initial deployment.
12. Retrieve the EPD.
a. Carefully advance the retrieval catheter through the stent.
b. Retrieve the EPD in a relatively straight segment of the vertebral artery.
c. Do abbreviated neurological exam.
d. Do angiogram.
13. Final angiographic images are obtained.
    Cervical PA intracranial PA and lateral angiograms.
14. Note: Obtaining access to the distal vertebral artery can be difficult once the stent is placed (because the stent extends into the subclavian artery). If access to the distal vertebral artery is needed (e.g., for treatment of a tandem stenosis), preserve wire-access to the vertebral artery until all procedures are completed.
    Technique:
    i.   Retrieve the EPD with the EPD retrieval catheter, but keep the EPD retrieval catheter in the vertebral artery, distal to the stent.
    ii. Use the EPD retrieval catheter like a guidewire to navigate the guide catheter into position directly adjacent to the mouth of the stent.
    iii. Advance a guidewire through the stent and into the distal verte-bral artery.
    iv. Remove the EPD retrieval catheter.

Extracranial Vertebral Artery Stenosis Distal to the Origin

Tips

1. Obtain a CTA prior to angioplasty, to exclude the presence of extrinsic compression factors (e.g., osteophytes).[47]
2. Study the vertebral angiograms carefully to determine if spinal cord vessels arise near the stenotic lesion to be treated. Take care to preserve these vessels and protect them from occlusion by emboli or shifting plaque. Consider a balloon test occlusion prior to angioplasty and stent placement if concerned that spinal cord vessels could be at risk of occlusion.
3. Suspect vertebral artery injury if there is a history of cervical spine manipulations and VBI symptoms.[48]
4. Caveat: Balloon expandable stents in very mobile segments of the vertebral (e.g. at the C2 level) may be crushed and kinked with head rotation or neck movement. Self-expanding stents are less prone to kinking when compressed.

5. If VBI symptoms occur with rotation of the head to one side, think *Bow Hunter's Stroke Syndrome* (aka rotational VBI; see Chap. 18):
   a. Characterized by occlusion or stenosis of the vertebral artery at C1–C2 with head rotation
   b. Usually caused by extrinsic compression of the vertebral artery, such as by osteophytes. a fibrous band[49], or a cervical disk herniation.[50]
   c. Associated with a hypoplastic vertebral artery ending in PICA.[51]
   d. Consider surgical decompression.[52–54]

10.3.   Carotid Artery Origin Lesions

Indications

1. Symptomatic stenosis ≥50% by CTA, angiography, or MRA.
2. Significant CCA origin stenosis in tandem with a distal carotid artery lesion for which endovascular treatment is planned.

Contraindication

Intraluminal thrombus.

Patient Preparation

Same as for carotid bifurcation lesions (see above).

Endovascular Technique

The technique for treating CCA origin stenoses is similar to the technique for treating vertebral artery origin lesions, just on a larger scale. Balloon-expandable stents are preferred, as these stents allow more precise deployment than self-expanding stents, and are less prone to watermelon-seed. Begin by the following steps:
1. Place a 90-cm 6F sheath in the aortic arch or innominate artery adjacent to the CCA (for technique see above section under Carotid Bifurcation Lesions, *Access Phase*).
   Stabilize the 90-cm sheath if necessary by passage of a buddy wire into the right axillary artery.
      i.   Wire: 0.035 in. or larger
      ii. Requires a larger 90-cm sheath.
2. Advance and deploy EPD.
   a. Deploy EPD in a straight segment of the CCA ≥2 cm distal to lesion, but only if the vessel is appropriate for the rated size of the EPD. If the CCA diameter is too large, deploy the EPD in the internal carotid.
   b. Do abbreviated neurological exam.
   c. Do angiogram.
3. Pre-dilation angioplasty
   a. Objective:
      To open the stenotic region only enough to accommodate the stent.
   b. Use a relatively small balloon – typically 2.0 or 2.5 mm angioplasty balloon, and long enough to cover the plaque. Position the balloon, inflate to nominal pressure *briefly* (for 1–2 s), then deflate.
      Brief balloon inflation "cracks" the plaque while minimizing the chance of bradycardia and hypotension.
   c. Remove the pre-dilation angioplasty balloon.
   d. Do abbreviated neurological exam.
   e. Do angiogram.

4. Advance balloon-mounted stent across lesion.
   a. Measure the diameter of the normal-appearing CCA distal to the lesion and select a stent matched to that diameter, and long enough to both cover the region of stenosis and extend into the common carotid by 1–2 mm.
   b. On the angiogram (and roadmap image), decide on the optimal position of the stent, and identify the precise location of the planned distal stent end location. The stent should also extend 1–2 mm into the innominate artery or aortic arch.
   c. Carefully advance the stent into position, and remove any slack in the system. Monitor the EPD position during this manoeuvre.
   d. Do abbreviated neurological exam.
   e. Do angiogram.
5. Deploy stent.
   a. Inflate the balloon to nominal pressure and allow it to stay inflated for 10–15 s if possible, to deploy and seat the stent.
   b. Deflate the balloon.
   c. Do abbreviated neurological exam.
   d. Do angiogram.
6. Post-dilation angioplasty (if needed).
   Objective:
   i. To widen the stenotic region if the degree of stenosis after stent deployment is still significant.
   ii. To seat the stent against the vessel wall if it does not appear to be firmly apposed to the plaque after the initial deployment.
   iii. To flare the proximal part of the stent extending into the aorta or innominate.
7. Retrieval of EPD.
   a. Advance the retrieval catheter carefully through the stent.
   b. Retrieve the EPD in a relatively straight segment of the vessel.
   c. Do abbreviated neurological exam.
   d. Do angiogram.
8. Obtain final angiographic images.
   Cervical PA and oblique and intracranial PA and lateral angiograms.
9. Note: Access to the distal carotid artery can be difficult once the stent is placed (because the stent extends into the aortic arch or innominate artery). If this access is needed, preserve wire-access to the CCA until all procedures are completed.
   Technique:
   i. Retrieve the EPD with the EPD retrieval catheter, but keep the EPD retrieval catheter in the CCA, distal to the stent.
   ii. Use the EPD retrieval catheter like a guidewire to navigate the guide catheter into a position directly adjacent to the mouth of the stent.
   iii. Advance a guidewire via the retrieval catheter through the stent and into the distal CCA or ECA.
   iv. Remove the EPD retrieval catheter.

10.4.   Subclavian Artery Origin Lesions

Indications

1. Symptomatic stenosis ≥50% by CTA, angiography, or MRA.
   a. Stenosis or occlusion proximal to the vertebral origin can present with *subclavian steal* symptoms: Transient posterior circulation symptoms often associated with elevation or prolonged exercise of the ipsilateral arm.
   b. In addition to observed asymmetry in arm blood pressure, arm symptoms include arm claudication, emboli to fingers, arm and hand rest pain, numbness and muscle atrophy.
   c. Patients with internal mammary to coronary bypass may have angina.
2. Symptomatic subclavian occlusions.
   82% of chronic total occlusions may still be successfully opened.[55]
3. Significant subclavian origin stenosis in tandem with a vertebral artery lesion for which endovascular treatment is planned.

Contraindication

Lesions that cannot be crossed by a guidewire.

Patient Preparation

Same as for carotid bifurcation lesions (see above).

Endovascular Technique: Femoral Artery Approach

The technique for treating subclavian origin stenoses is similar to the technique for treating common carotid artery origin lesions. Balloon-expandable stents are preferred for an antegrade approach from the groin, as with proximal common carotid stents. An approach from the arm can also allow self-expanding stent deployment (see below).

1. For groin access: place a 90-cm 6F sheath in the aortic arch or innominate artery adjacent to the subclavian artery.
2. EPDs are usually used to protect the vertebral in treating proximal subclavian stenosis.
   a. Dual EPDs may be used to protect the vertebral and internal mammary if an internal mammary to coronary bypass is present.[56]
      To prevent trapping EPDs between stent and vessel wall, consider placing at least one EPD from an arm approach or remove one after pre-dilation angioplasty.
   b. Deploy EPD in a straight segment of the vertebral artery distal to its origin, but only if the vessel is appropriate for the rated size of the EPD.
      If using dual EPDs, place the other in a straight segment of the desired vessel.
   c. Do abbreviated neurological exam.
   d. Do angiogram.
3. Pre-dilation angioplasty.
   a. Objective: To open the stenotic region only enough to accommodate the stent.
   b. Use a relatively small balloon should be used – typically 2.0 or 2.5 mm angioplasty balloon, and long enough to cover the plaque. Position the balloon, inflate to nominal pressure *briefly* (for 1–2 s), then deflate.
      A brief balloon inflation "cracks" the plaque while minimizing the chance of bradycardia and hypotension.
   c. Remove the pre-dilation angioplasty balloon.
   d. Do abbreviated neurological exam.
   e. Do angiogram.
4. Advance stent across lesion.
   a. Measure the diameter of the normal-appearing subclavian distal to the lesion and select a stent matched to that diameter, and long enough to both cross the region of stenosis and extend into the aorta by 1–2 mm.
   b. On the angiogram (and roadmap image), decide on the optimal position of the stent, and identify the precise location of the planned distal stent end location. The stent should extend 1–2 mm into the innominate artery or aortic arch.
   c. Carefully advance the stent into position.
      Monitor EPD position during this manoeuvre.
   d. Do abbreviated neurological exam.
   e. Do angiogram.
5. Deploy stent.
   a. Inflate the balloon to nominal pressure and allow it to stay inflated for 10–15 s if possible, to deploy and seat the stent.
   b. Deflate the balloon.
   c. Do abbreviated neurological exam.
   d. Do angiogram.
6. Post-dilation angioplasty (if needed).
   Objective:
      i. To widen the stenotic region if the degree of stenosis after stent deployment is still significant.
      ii. To seat the stent against the vessel wall if it does not appear to be firmly apposed to the plaque after the initial deployment.
      iii. To flare the part of the stent that hangs into aorta or innominate.

7. Retrieval of EPD.
    a. Advance the retrieval catheter carefully through the stent.
    b. Retrieve the EPD in a relatively straight segment of the vessel.
    c. Do abbreviated neurological exam.
    d. Do angiogram.
8. Obtain final angiographic image.
    Cervical PA and oblique and intracranial PA and lateral angiograms.
9. Note: Access to the distal subclavian or vertebral artery can be difficult once the stent is placed (because the stent extends into the aortic arch or innominate artery). If access distally is needed, preserve wire-access until all procedures are completed.
    Technique:
        i. Retrieve the EPD with the EPD retrieval catheter, but keep the EPD retrieval catheter in the subclavian, distal to the stent.
        ii. Use the EPD retrieval catheter like a guidewire to navigate the guide catheter into a position directly adjacent to the mouth of the stent.
        iii. Advance a guidewire via the retriever catheter through the stent and into the distal subclavian or vertebral.
        iv. Remove the EPD retrieval catheter.

Endovascular Technique: Brachial Approach

This technique may be easier for treating subclavian origin stenoses compared to using femoral arterial access, especially in the presence of difficult, tortuous anatomy. Self-expanding stents can often be used effectively from the arm approach, since they may be more precisely positioned at the origin of the vessel from the aorta or innominate artery. Self-expanding stents may have a lower restenosis rate.[57]

1. Using a micro-puncture access system, access the ipsilateral brachial artery (see Chap. 4).
    Use a Doppler guided needle (Smart-needle®, Vascular Solutions, Minneapolis, MN) (20 gauge or smaller) to allow puncture of a non-palpable vessel.
2. Insert a sheath large enough to deliver the balloons and stent (usually 6 or 7F).
3. Also consider groin access with at least a 5F sheath. Place a guide catheter in the aortic arch or innominate artery adjacent to the subclavian for contrast injections.
4. If possible, use and EPD to protect the vertebral when treating proximal subclavian stenosis.
    a. Use dual EPDs to protect the vertebral and internal mammary if an internal mammary to coronary bypass is present.[56]
    b. When stenting from an arm approach, the angioplasty balloons and stent obviously must be advanced over a separate guidewire.
    c. Deploy EPD in a straight segment of the vertebral artery distal to its origin, but only if the vessel is appropriate for the rated size of the EPD.
5. Pre-dilation angioplasty
    a. Objective:
    To open the stenotic region enough to accommodate the stent.
    b. Advance an appropriately sized wire (usually 0.014) carefully across the stenosis and well into the descending aorta for stability.
    c. A non-compliant angioplasty balloon sized to approximately 80% of the normal diameter distal to the lesion should be used – typically 6.0–8.0 mm, and long enough to cover the plaque. Once the balloon is in position, slowly inflate to nominal pressure, watching fluoroscopically and continually asking the patient how they are doing, then deflate.
        Some pain may be expected at high inflation pressures but severe pain may herald dissection or rupture of the vessel.
    d. Remove the pre-dilation angioplasty balloon.
    e. Do abbreviated neurological exam.
    f. Do angiogram.
    g. If the stenosis has been resolved and there is no dissection, consider deferring stent placement
6. Advance stent across lesion.
    a. Measure the diameter of the normal-appearing subclavian distal to the lesion and select a stent 1–2 mm larger than that diameter, and long enough to both cross the region of stenosis and extend distally by 1–2 mm.
    b. If at all possible, avoid having the stent cover ("jail") the ostium of the vertebral artery.

    c. On the angiogram (and roadmap image), decide on the optimal position of the stent, and identify the precise location of the planned distal stent end location. The stent should extend 1–2 mm into the innominate artery or aortic arch to prevent "watermelon seeding."

    d. Carefully advance the stent across the stenosis with the tip extending into the aorta (or innominate).
       Monitor the EPD and the guidewire tip positions.

    e. Do abbreviated neurological exam.

    f. Do an angiogram, preferably both from the brachial sheath retrograde and the catheter positioned in the aorta.

7. Deploy stent.

    a. Using a self-expanding stent, begin to deploy the stent in the aorta (or innominate), and after it begins to open up, gently pull back so that only a millimeter or two is in the aorta (or innominate).

    b. Then slowly deploy the remainder of the stent.

    c. If using a balloon expandable stent, deploy it by inflating the balloon to nominal pressure and keep inflated for 10–15 s to seat the stent.

    d. Then deflate the balloon.

    e. Do abbreviated neurological exam.

    f. Do angiogram.

8. Post-dilation angioplasty (if needed).
    Objective:
      i. To widen the stenotic region if the degree of stenosis after stent deployment is still significant.
      ii. To seat the stent against the vessel wall if it does not appear to be firmly apposed to the plaque after the initial deployment.
      iii. To flare the portion of stent hanging into the aorta or innominate.

9. Retrieval of EPD.

    a. The retrieval catheter should be advanced carefully over the EPD.

    b. The EPD should be retrieved in a relatively straight segment of the vessel.

    c. Do abbreviated neurological exam.

    d. Do angiogram.

10. Final angiographic images are obtained.
    Cervical PA and oblique and intracranial PA and lateral angiograms.

Tips

1. There is so far insufficient evidence to determine whether stenting has any benefit over angioplasty alone in subclavian stenosis.[58]

2. If the subclavian is totally occluded:

    a. Obtain a roadmap of the proximal and distal extent of the plaque, usually using one catheter in the aorta and another accessed from the arm via a brachial approach

    b. If using only a femoral approach, access both groins and have one catheter in the aorta and one in the contralateral vertebral and opacify the occluded subclavian via the collateral flow in subclavian steal syndrome.

    c. Usually the occluded segment is relatively short, and may be crossed with a stiff guidewire.

    d. Use care to probe the central portion of the plaque, to avoid getting subintimal.

    e. If the wire penetrates the plaque, carefully advance it well distally to provide good support.

    f. EPDs usually cannot be used before the first angioplasty unless a brachial artery access is obtained.

    g. Do a primary angioplasty with a very small (2–3 mm) diameter and gradually dilatate with a slightly larger balloon before any EPD or stent can be placed.

    h. When a channel is made through the occlusion, protect at least the vertebral and possibly also the distal arm with an EPD.

    i. Once a channel is open in the subclavian, consider using a cutting balloon to size it up to 5–6 mm.

    j. Deploy a stent to stabilize the plaque. It will look terrible on angiography after flow is restored.

    k. If any difficulty is encountered, consider surgical carotid-subclavian bypass.[59]

References

1. Al-Mubarak N, Roubin GS, Iyer SS, Gomez CR, Liu MW, Vitek JJ. Carotid stenting for severe radiation-induced extracranial carotid artery occlusive disease. J Endovasc Ther. 2000;7:36–40.

2. Perez-Arjona EA, DelProsto Z, Fessler RD. Direct percutaneous carotid artery stenting with distal protection: technical case report. Neurol Res. 2004;26:338–41.

3. Mitsuhashi Y, Nishio A, Kawakami T, et al. New pull-through technique using the superficial temporal artery for transbrachial carotid artery stenting. Neurol Med Chir (Tokyo). 2009;49:320–4.

4. Jin S-CMD, Kwon OKMD, Oh CWMD, et al. A Technical strategy for carotid artery stenting: suboptimal prestent balloon angioplasty without poststenting balloon dilatation. Neurosurgery. 2010;67:1438–43.

5. North American Symptomatic Carotid Endarterectomy Trial Collaborators. Beneficial effect of carotid endarterectomy in symptomatic patients with high-grade carotid stenosis. N Engl J Med. 1991;325:445–53.

6. Martin JB, Pache JC, Treggiari-Venzi M, et al. Role of the distal balloon protection technique in the prevention of cerebral embolic events during carotid stent placement. Stroke. 2001;32:479–84.

7. Vitek JJ, Roubin GS, Al-Mubarek N, New G, Iyer SS. Carotid artery stenting: technical considerations. AJNR Am J Neuroradiol. 2000;21:1736–43.

8. Pierce DS, Rosero EB, Modrall JG, et al. Open-cell versus closed-cell stent design differences in blood flow velocities after carotid stenting. J Vasc Surg. 2009;49:602–6; discussion 606.

9. Sadato A, Satow T, Ishii A, Ohta T, Hashimoto N. Use of a large angioplasty balloon for predilation is a risk factor for embolic complications in protected carotid stenting. Neurol Med Chir (Tokyo). 2004;44:337–42; discussion 343.

10. Bussiere M, Pelz DM, Kalapos P, et al. Results using a self-expanding stent alone in the treatment of severe symptomatic carotid bifurcation stenosis. J Neurosurg. 2008;109:454–60.

11. Al-Mubarak N, Roubin GS, Vitek JJ, Iyer SS, New G, Leon MB. Effect of the distal-balloon protection system on microembolization during carotid stenting. Circulation. 2001;104:1999–2002.

12. Tamberella MR, Yadav JS, Bajzer CT, Bhatt DL, Abou-Chebl A. Cutting balloon angioplasty to treat carotid in-stent restenosis. J Invasive Cardiol. 2004;16:133–5.

13. Heck D. Results of cutting balloon angioplasty for carotid artery in-stent restenosis in six patients: description of the technique, long-term outcomes, and review of the literature. J NeuroIntervent Surg. 2009;1:48–50.

14. Barr JD, Connors III JJ, Sacks D, et al. Quality improvement guidelines for the performance of cervical carotid angioplasty and stent placement: developed by a Collaborative Panel of the American Society of Interventional and Therapeutic Neuroradiology, the American Society of Neuroradiology, and the Society of Interventional Radiology. AJNR Am J Neuroradiol. 2003;24:2020–34.

15. Biasi GM, Froio A, Diethrich EB, et al. Carotid plaque echolucency increases the risk of stroke in carotid stenting: the Imaging in Carotid Angioplasty and Risk of Stroke (ICAROS) Study. Circulation. 2004;110:756–62.

16. Wholey M. ARCHeR trial: prospective clinical trial for carotid stenting in high surgical risk patients-preliminary 30-day results. In: Paper presented at the American College of Cardiology annual meeting, March 30 2003; Chicago, IL; 2003.

17. Qureshi AI, Luft AR, Janardhan V, et al. Identification of patients at risk for periprocedural neurological deficits associated with carotid angioplasty and stenting. Stroke. 2000;31:376–82.

18. Qureshi AI, Saad M, Zaidat OO, et al. Intracerebral hemorrhages associated with neurointerventional procedures using a combination of antithrombotic agents including abciximab. Stroke. 2002;33:1916–9.

19. Meyers PM, Higashida RT, Phatouros CC, et al. Cerebral hyperperfusion syndrome after percutaneous transluminal stenting of the craniocervical arteries. Neurosurgery. 2000; 47:335–45.

20. Abou-Chebl A, Yadav JS, Reginelli JP, Bajzer C, Bhatt D, Krieger DW. Intracranial hemorrhage and hyperperfusion syndrome following carotid artery stenting: risk factors, prevention, and treatment. J Am Coll Cardiol. 2004;43: 1596–601.

21. Ouriel K, Shortell CK, Illig KA, Greenberg RK, Green RM. Intracerebral hemorrhage after carotid endarterectomy: incidence, contribution to neurologic morbidity, and predictive factors. J Vasc Surg. 1999;29:82–7; discussion 87–9.

22. Sbarigia E, Speziale F, Giannoni MF, Colonna M, Panico MA, Fiorani P. Post-carotid endarterectomy hyperperfusion syndrome: preliminary observations for identifying at risk patients by transcranial Doppler sonography and the acetazolamide test. Eur J Vasc Surg. 1993;7:252–6.

23. Dangas G, Monsein LH, Laureno R, et al. Transient contrast encephalopathy after carotid artery stenting. J Endovasc Ther. 2001;8:111–3.

24. Wholey MH, Wholey MH, Tan WA, et al. Management of neurological complications of carotid artery stenting. J Endovasc Ther. 2001;8:341–53.

25. Bosiers M, Peeters P, Deloose K, et al. Does carotid artery stenting work on the long run: 5-year results in high-volume centers (ELOCAS Registry). J Cardiovasc Surg (Torino). 2005;46:241–7.

26. Wholey MH. What's new in carotid artery stenting. J Cardiovasc Surg (Torino). 2005;46:189–92.

27. Wholey MH, Wholey MH, Tan WA, Eles G, Jarmolowski C, Cho S. A comparison of balloon-mounted and self-expanding stents in the carotid arteries: immediate and long-term results of more than 500 patients. J Endovasc Ther. 2003;10: 171–81.

28. Reimers B, Corvaja N, Moshiri S, et al. Cerebral protection with filter devices during carotid artery stenting. Circulation. 2001;104:12–5.

29. Macdonald S, Venables GS, Cleveland TJ, Gaines PA. Protected carotid stenting: safety and efficacy of the MedNova NeuroShield filter. J Vasc Surg. 2002;35:966–72.

30. Theron J, Courtheoux P, Alachkar F, Bouvard G, Maiza D. New triple coaxial catheter system for carotid angioplasty with cerebral protection. AJNR Am J Neuroradiol. 1990;11: 869–77.

31. Parodi JC, Schonholz C, Ferreira LM, Mendaro E, Ohki T. "Seat belt and air bag" technique for cerebral protection during carotid stenting. J Endovasc Ther. 2002;9:20–4.

32. Whitlow PL, Lylyk P, Londero H, et al. Carotid artery stenting protected with an emboli containment system. Stroke. 2002;33:1308–14.

33. Henry M, Henry I, Klonaris C, et al. Benefits of cerebral protection during carotid stenting with the PercuSurge GuardWire system: midterm results. J Endovasc Ther. 2002;9:1–13.

34. Coppi G, Moratto R, Silingardi R, et al. PRIAMUS - proximal flow blockage cerebral protectIon during carotid stenting: results from a Multicenter Italian registry. J Cardiovasc Surg (Torino). 2005;46:219–27.

35. Henry M, Amor M, Klonaris C, et al. Angioplasty and stenting of the extracranial carotid arteries. Tex Heart Inst J. 2000;27:150–8.

36. Charbel F, Guppy K, Carney A, Ausman J. Extracranial vertebral artery disease. In: Winn H, editor. Youmans neurological surgery. 5th ed. Philadelphia: Saunders; 2004. p. 1691–714.

37. Kumar A, Mafee M, Dobben G, Whipple M, Pieri A. Diagnosis of vertebrobasilar insufficiency: time to rethink established dogma? Ear Nose Throat J. 1998;77(966–9):72–4.

38. Amole AO, Akdol MS, Wood CE, Keyrouz SG, Erdem E. Endovascular management of symptomatic vertebral artery origin stenosis in the presence of an acute thrombus. J NeuroIntervent Surg. 2011 Jun 23. [Epub ahead of print]

39. Wehman JC, Hanel RA, Guidot CA, Guterman LR, Hopkins LN. Atherosclerotic occlusive extracranial vertebral artery disease: indications for intervention, endovascular techniques, short-term and long-term results. J Interv Cardiol. 2004;17:219–32.

40. Stayman AN, Nogueira RG, Gupta R. A systematic review of stenting and angioplasty of symptomatic extracranial vertebral artery stenosis. Stroke. 2011;42:2212–6.

41. Hatano TMDP, Tsukahara TMDP, Miyakoshi AMD, Arai DMD, Yamaguchi SMD, Murakami MMDP. Stent placement for atherosclerotic stenosis of the vertebral artery ostium: angiographic and clinical outcomes in 117 consecutive patients. Neurosurgery. 2011;68:108–16.

42. Rees CR, Palmaz JC, Becker GJ, et al. Palmaz stent in atherosclerotic stenoses involving the ostia of the renal arteries: preliminary report of a multicenter study. Radiology. 1991; 181:507–14.

43. Tuttle KR, Chouinard RF, Webber JT, et al. Treatment of atherosclerotic ostial renal artery stenosis with the intravascular stent. Am J Kidney Dis. 1998;32:611–22.

44. Henry M, Amor M, Henry I, et al. Stents in the treatment of renal artery stenosis: long-term follow-up. J Endovasc Surg. 1999;6:42–51.

45. Fischell TA, Saltiel FS, Foster MT, Wong SC, Dishman DA, Moses J. Initial clinical experience using an ostial stent positioning system (Ostial Pro) for the accurate placement of stents in the treatment of coronary aorto-ostial lesions. J Invasive Cardiol. 2009;21:53–9.

46. Salazar M, Kern MJ, Patel PM. Exact deployment of stents in ostial renal artery stenosis using the stent tail wire or Szabo technique. Catheter Cardiovasc Interv. 2009;74:946–50.

47. Cagnie B, Barbaix E, Vinck E, D'Herde K, Cambier D. Extrinsic risk factors for compromised blood flow in the vertebral artery: anatomical observations of the transverse foramina from C3 to C7. Surg Radiol Anat. 2005;27:312–6.

48. Cagnie B, Jacobs F, Barbaix E, Vinck E, Dierckx R, Cambier D. Changes in cerebellar blood flow after manipulation of the cervical spine using Technetium 99 m-ethyl cysteinate dimer. J Manipulative Physiol Ther. 2005;28:103–7.

49. Mapstone T, Spetzler RF. Vertebrobasilar insufficiency secondary to vertebral artery occlusion from a fibrous band. Case report. J Neurosurg. 1982;56:581–3.

50. Vates GE, Wang KC, Bonovich D, Dowd CF, Lawton MT. Bow hunter stroke caused by cervical disc herniation. Case report. J Neurosurg. 2002;96:90–3.

51. Frisoni GB, Anzola GP. Vertebrobasilar ischemia after neck motion. Stroke. 1991;22:1452–60.

52. Hanakita J, Miyake H, Nagayasu S, Nishi S, Suzuki T. Angiographic examination and surgical treatment of bow hunter's stroke. Neurosurgery. 1988;23:228–32.

53. Shimizu T, Waga S, Kojima T, Niwa S. Decompression of the vertebral artery for bow-hunter's stroke. Case report. J Neurosurg. 1988;69:127–31.

54. Matsuyama T, Morimoto T, Sakaki T. Comparison of C1-2 posterior fusion and decompression of the vertebral artery in the treatment of bow hunter's stroke. J Neurosurg. 1997;86:619–23.

55. Babic S, Sagic D, Radak D, et al. Initial and long-term results of endovascular therapy for chronic total occlusion of the subclavian artery. Cardiovasc Intervent Radiol. 2012; 35:255–62.

56. Omeish AF, Ghanma IM, Alamlih RI. Successful stenting of total left subclavian artery occlusion post-coronary artery bypass graft surgery using dual left vertebral artery and left internal mammary artery protection. J Invasive Cardiol. 2011;23:E132–6.

57. Miyakoshi A, Hatano T, Tsukahara T, Murakami M, Arai D, Yamaguchi S. Percutaneous transluminal angioplasty for atherosclerotic stenosis of the subclavian or innominate artery: angiographic and clinical outcomes in 36 patients. Neurosurg Rev. 2012;35:121–5.

58. Burihan E, Soma F, Iared W. Angioplasty versus stenting for subclavian artery stenosis. Cochrane Database Syst Rev 2011:CD008461.

59. Law MM, Colburn MD, Moore WS, Quinones-Baldrich WJ, Machleder HI, Gelabert HA. Carotid-subclavian bypass for brachiocephalic occlusive disease. Choice of conduit and long-term follow-up. Stroke. 1995;26:1565–71.

11. Endovascular Treatment of Intracranial Stenosis and Vasospasm

This chapter discusses techniques for intracranial angioplasty and stenting for atherosclerotic arterial stenosis, and angioplasty and intra-arterial drug infusion for cerebral vasospasm after aneurysmal SAH.

11.1.　Intracranial Atherosclerotic Stenosis

Indications for Intracranial Angioplasty and Stenting

Position Statement on Intracranial Angioplasty and Stenting for Cerebral Atherosclerosis by the ASITN, SIR, and ASNR[1][:1]

1. For symptomatic patients with >50% intracranial stenosis who have failed medical therapy, balloon angioplasty with or without stenting should be considered.
2. Patients who have an asymptomatic intracranial arterial stenosis should first be counseled regarding optimizing medical therapy. There is insufficient evidence to make definite recommendations regarding endovascular therapy in asymptomatic patients with severe intracranial atherosclerosis. They should be counseled regarding the nature and extent of their disease, monitored for new neurological symptoms, and have periodic noninvasive imaging at regular intervals of 6–12 months (MRA or CTA) initially, and later with cerebral angiography if warranted. Optimal prophylactic medical therapy should be instituted, which might include antiplatelet and/or statin therapy.
3. Continued evaluation and improvements in both pharmacological and catheter-based therapies are needed to reduce the possibility of stroke from intracranial atherosclerosis.

Contraindications

1. Patient inability to have antiplatelet therapy and/or anticoagulation.
2. Highly calcified lesions or anatomy that prevents endovascular access.

Preprocedure Preparation

1) Informed consent.
2) Dual antiplatelet therapy.
   a) Do platelet function testing if desired (see Chap. 4).

---

[1] ASITN, American Society of Interventional and Therapeutic Neuroradiology; SIR, Society of Interventional Radiology; and ASNR, American Society of Neuroradiology.

M.R. Harrigan, J.P. Deveikis, *Handbook of Cerebrovascular Disease and Neurointerventional Technique*, DOI 10.1007/978-1-61779-946-4_11, © Springer Science+Business Media New York 2013

3) Two peripheral IVs.
4) Foley catheter.
5) NPO after midnight or 6 h prior to the procedure except for medications.
6) Ensure all devices required are available in the angio suite prior to the procedure.

Endovascular Technique

The access phase involves placing a guide catheter in the internal carotid or vertebral artery. The intervention phase includes advancing a microwire across the stenotic lesion, followed by angioplasty with or without stent deployment.

Awake or Asleep?

Intracranial angioplasty can be uncomfortable, as stretching and pulling on intracranial vessels are painful. The authors of this handbook use general anesthesia in most cases and the SAMMPRIS protocol required the used of general anesthesia. However, good results have been obtained without anesthesia. Avoiding anesthesia permits continuous neurological surveillance and eliminates anesthesia-associated risks:

1. Patients who are awake should rehearse the neurological exam on the angio suite table prior to draping. A squeeze toy should be placed in the patient's hand contralateral to the side being treated.
2. In a report of 37 intracranial angioplasty and stenting cases without general anesthesia, technical success was achieved in all patients.[2] About 61% experienced intraprocedural symptoms that led to some alteration of the interventional technique. Headache was the most common symptom, and, when persistent, signaled the occurrence of intracranial haemorrhage.

Access Phase

Patients with intracranial atherosclerosis are also prone to extracranial disease. The reader is referred to Chap. 10, *Extracranial Angioplasty and Stenting* for a detailed discussion of access techniques and tips for difficult situations. Compared to other intracranial procedures, angioplasty procedures require extra-rigid guide catheter support.

1. Guide catheter access is obtained in the usual manner (see Chap. 4).
2. Systemic anticoagulation. Thromboembolic complications can occur during angioplasty, when there is slowing of flow in the parent vessel caused by the guide catheter, or in the target vessel by the microwire or angioplasty balloon.
3. A loading dose of IV heparin is given (5,000 units or 70 units/Kg. Additional doses of heparin are necessary only for cases lasting several hours.
4. Protamine on standby – *Critical*:
   a. A syringe containing enough protamine to reverse the total amount of heparin the patient has received should be kept on the back table for easy access to the operator, should haemorrhage occur:
      – Dose of protamine required to reverse heparin: 10 mg protamine/1,000 U heparin.
5. Guide catheter selection and positioning:
   a. The guide catheter should be 90 cm long (and not longer) for use with the Wingspan stent system
   b. Guide catheter support is more important for intracranial angioplasty procedures than most other intracranial interventions. Angioplasty balloons and stents are relatively rigid and difficult to navigate; forward motion of these devices can cause unexpected high amounts of downward-directed force on the guide catheter. Therefore, due caution should be used in guide catheter selection and positioning.
   c. Stiffer guide catheters and positioning of the guide catheter as high as possible helps to maximize support for the intervention.
   d. The catheter tip may slide up and down and rub against the vessel wall with each heart beat; this is to be taken into account when positioning the catheter.

Intervention Phase

Once the guide catheter is in position, a good "working view" must be obtained. The working view should be under high magnification and demonstrate the target lesion and distal vessels, and guide the catheter clearly. In most situations, a microcatheter is advanced through the stenotic intracranial vessel over an exchange-length microwire. The purpose of the microcatheter is to facilitate atraumatic and smooth passage of the microwire into a distal vessel; the microcatheter is then removed and the balloon is guided over the microwire into position within the region of stenosis. If stenting is planned, the "pre-dil" balloon is removed and a self-expanding stent (e.g., Wingspan,™ Stryker, Fremont, CA) is deployed. Alternatively, a balloon-mounted stent (e.g., PHAROS™ Vitesse,™ Codman Neurovascular, San Jose, CA) is navigated into position and the stent is deployed.

Device Selection

Essential devices for intracranial angioplasty include an exchange-length microwire, a microcatheter, and a balloon. The Wingspan™ Stent System with Gateway™ PTA Balloon Catheter (Stryker, Fremont, CA) was specifically designed for intracranial angioplasty and stenting. It is available on a Humanitarian Device Exemption basis; the use of the Wingspan system currently requires IRB approval. The Wingspan devices and technique are discussed in detail in a separate section below. The PHAROS™ Vitesse™ (Codman Neurovascular, San Jose, CA) balloon-expandable stent is an alternative to the Wingspan stent and is also covered in a separate section below.

1) Microwires:
    a) "Beefiness," trackability and torque control are microwire properties that are most important for intracranial angioplasty. A relatively soft distal tip is helpful as well, to minimize the chances of distal vessel vasospasm and perforation.
    b) The authors preferred microwires for most cases:
        i) Transend™ 0.014 in. 300 cm Floppy Tip (Stryker):
            (1) Superior torque control, compared to other microwires.
            (2) Heightened radiopacity makes the tip easy to see on fluoroscopy.
        ii) X-Celerator™ 0.014 in. 300 cm (ev3, Irvine, CA):
            (1) Soft tip, relatively supportive body, very lubricious.
2) Microcatheters:
    a) A low profile, straight microcatheter, usually of any kind, is sufficient.
    b) The 1.7F Echelon-10 microcatheter (ev3, Irvine, CA) can be pushed through tortuous and stenotic vessels better than other microcatheters.
3) Angioplasty balloons:
    a) Noncompliant coronary angioplasty balloons are designed to create sufficient radial force to dilate vessels thickened by atherosclerotic plaque. NC: noncompliant:
        i) Selected balloons:
            (1) Gateway™ PTA Balloon Catheter (to be used with the Wingspan stent – see below).
            (2) Maverick2™ Monorail™ balloon Catheter (Boston Scientific, Natick, MA).
            (3) NC Raptor™ balloon catheter (Cordis, Miami, FL).
            (4) Size:
                (a) The diameter of the balloon should correspond to or be smaller than the normal diameter of the vessel; 2.0–2.5 mm diameter balloons are usually appropriate.
                (b) The length of the balloon should be kept to a minimum, to optimize trackability.
4) Stents:
    a) Wingspan (see below).
    b) Balloon-mounted coronary stents are problematic in intracranial circulation, as they are fairly rigid and difficult to track in tortuous vessels. More importantly, the intracranial arteries, which float freely in CSF, are not surrounded by fibrous connective tissue like coronary arteries and they are more vulnerable to dissection and perforation during deployment

of balloon-mounted stents. Relatively high complication rates have been reported with balloon-mounted coronary stents.[2–4]

  i) If a balloon-mounted coronary stent must be used, cobalt–chromium coronary stents are the easiest to deliver compared to other balloon-mounted stents.[2]
  ii) The recently-introduced PHAROS™ Vitesse™ (Codman Neurovascular, San Jose, CA) is a balloon-mounted stent specifically designed for the intracranial circulation.

Angioplasty Without Stent Deployment

Angioplasty alone is less morbid than angioplasty and stenting with balloon-expandable stent. By itself, angioplasty is a reasonable option for patients with symptomatic intracranial stenosis, particularly because intracranial stenting has not yet been shown to reduce the risk of stroke, and the use of a stent (even the Wingspan system) adds complexity and expense to the procedure. The balloon should be sized to cover the length of the lesion, and the diameter should be ≤ the normal diameter of the vessel. Refer to Wingspan Gateway angioplasty procedure, described below, for a discussion of technique.

Wingspan Procedure

The manufacturer of the Wingspan™ Stent System with Gateway™ PTA Balloon Catheter has obtained a Humanitarian Device Exemption from the United States FDA. The system is authorized for use in improving cerebral artery lumen diameter in patients with intracranial atherosclerotic disease, refractory to medical therapy, in intracranial vessels with ≥50% stenosis that are accessible to the system. An IRB approval is currently necessary to use the system.

1. Devices:
    (a) Guide catheter should be 6F and 90 cm long.
    (b) Microwire. Synchro²™ or Transend™ 0.014 in. Floppy Tip (Stryker, Fremont, CA) is the recommended microwire. Use an exchange-length microwire (300 cm) to maintain microwire access after stent placement in case additional stent placement or post-stent angioplasty is needed.
    (c) Gateway™ PTA balloon catheter:
        • The Gateway is a modified version of the Maverick2™ balloon catheter, with silicone coating on the balloon and hydrophilic coating on the catheter to facilitate access. Radio-opaque markers on the balloon permit visualization of the proximal and distal ends of the balloon on fluoroscopy.
        • Available sizes:
            – Balloon diameters (mm): 1.5, 2.0, 2.25, 2.75, 3.0, 3.25, 3.5, 3.75, 4.0.
            – Balloon lengths (mm): 9, 15, 20.
            – Nominal inflation pressure: 6 atm. Rated burst pressure: 12 atm. (14 atm. for 2.25–3.25 mm diameters only).
        • Size selection:
            – Plan angioplasty to achieve approximately 80% of normal vessel diameter. For example, for a vessel with a 3.0 mm normal diameter, angioplasty to produce a diameter of about 2.4 mm would be appropriate.
            – If the target vessel has different diameters proximal and distal to the lesion, size the balloon to the smaller of the two.
        • Preparation:
            – Use 50/50 mixture of contrast in heparinized saline.
            – Prepare the insufflater and attach it with a three-way stopcock and an empty 20 mL syringe to the balloon catheter.
            – Apply suction to the balloon but do not pre-inflate it.
            – Continuously flush through the lumen of the balloon catheter with heparinized saline via a stopcock and an RHV.
    (d) Wingspan™ Stent:
        • The Wingspan is a 3.5F nitinol over-the-wire (OTW) self-expanding stent. The design is very similar to the Neuroform2™ stent (Boston

Scientific, Natick, MA); it has four platinum markers at each end for visualization, and is deployed from the delivery microcatheter (called the "outer body") with the "inner body"; the inner body is analogous to the "stabilizer" device which is used to deploy Neuroform stents.

- Available sizes:
  - Stent diameters (mm): 2.5, 3.0, 3.5, 4.0, 4.5.
  - Stent lengths (mm): 9, 15, 20.
- Size selection:
  - Select a stent length which extends a minimum of 3 mm on both sides of the lesion.
  - If the target vessel has different diameters proximal and distal to the lesion, size the stent to the larger of the two.
  - After deployment, the stent may shorten up to 2.4% in 2.5 mm stents and up to 7.1% in 4.5 mm stents.[5]
- Preparation
  - The Wingspan system should be flushed with heparinized saline, as indicated in the diagram on the package.
  - The more flushes, the better. Continuous flushes with heparinized saline should be connected via stopcocks and RHVs to both the Wingspan deployment catheter (the "outer body") and the inner body.
  - The tapered tip of the inner body should be loosened slightly, with about 1 mm of space between the spearhead-shaped tip of the inner body and the distal end of the outer body, to allow adequate flushing and prevent "corking," or binding of the inner body tip to the outer body catheter. During flushing, heparinized saline should be seen dripping from the inner lumen and from between the inner and outer bodies.

2. Technique:
   (a) Angioplasty:
   - The Gateway balloon may be taken up primarily, over a nonexchange-length microwire, if the anatomy is favorable. Alternatively, an exchange-length microwire can be advanced into a distal intracranial vessel within a microcatheter, which can be exchanged for the Gateway balloon.
   - After flushing, advance the balloon catheter over the microwire into the guide catheter. When positioned at the RHV, a marker on the balloon catheter shaft indicates the guide catheter tip. This feature saves fluoro time.
   - With roadmap guidance, advance the balloon until the balloon markers are across the lesion. Perform a guide catheter angiogram with the balloon in position, to confirm proper positioning.
   - Inflate the balloon slowly to nominal pressure, at a rate of ~1 atm./10 s, under fluoroscopy. When the balloon is fully inflated, leave it up for another 10–20 s and then deflate. Do a guide catheter angiogram prior to removing the balloon.
   - In most cases a single inflation will be sufficient. Occasionally, a second inflation, at a slightly higher pressure (e.g., 8 atm.) is helpful.
   (b) Stent deployment:
   - Tighten the RHV on the inner body to prevent its migration – and advance the outer body of the Wingspan system over the exchange-length microwire:
     - The delivery system should be advanced only by grasping the outer body, to avoid inadvertently advancing the inner body and prematurely deploying the stent.
   - Advance the outer body slightly past the region of stenosis.
   - Using the marker bands to identify the position of the stent, advance the inner body just proximal to the stent.
   - Pull back on the outer body, to bring the outer body tip into position just past the region of stenosis; this should be the final maneuver prior to stent deployment.
   - Deploy the stent by holding the inner body in a stable position with the right hand, while, with the left hand, slowly withdraw the outer body.
     - Do not attempt to change the position of the stent during deployment.

- Once the stent is deployed, bring the deployment system into the proximal part of the vessel, or into the guide catheter, while leaving the microwire in position. Do a guide catheter angiogram.
3. Gateway and Wingspan tips.[5]:
    (a) Do not over tighten the RHV around the balloon catheter shaft.
    (b) If the balloon is difficult to inflate, remove it and use another device.
    (c) If the balloon watermelon-seeds (i.e., slips forward or backward during inflation)
        - Apply gentle traction to the balloon catheter during inflation, to stabilize the balloon and prevent it from migrating distally during inflation, or
        - Select a longer balloon.
    (d) If the stent system binds with the microwire during navigation through tortuous vessels:
        - Affirm that adequate flush is being applied to both the inner and outer body catheters.
        - Try a softer microwire (e.g., Synchro2®-14, Stryker Neurovascular, Fremont, CA).
    (e) Keep in mind that the tapered tip of the inner body extends for 10–12 mm past the distal tip of the outer body, and is radiolucent (in contrast to the Neuroform system, which does not have anything that extends out of the deployment catheter). Care should be taken to avoid jamming the distal end of the system into a curving vessel.
    (f) Once the stent catheter is advancing over the microwire, advantage may be taken of the forward momentum and tracking continued to a site distal to the lesion. It is easier to move the system from distal to proximal than vice versa.
    (g) If the stent is malpositioned deployment, consider placing a second stent.

Pharos Technique

The Pharos™ Vitesse™ (Micrus, San Jose, CA) is a cobalt chromium open cell silicon carbide-coated balloon-expandable stent. The silicon carbide coating is purported to reduce thrombus formation[6, 7], suppress platelet activation[8, 9], stimulate endothelialization[10], and prevent corrosion.[11] The authors of this handbook wonder if silicon carbide also cures cancer and is effective as a treatment for erectile dysfunction. It is CE mark-approved in Europe but it is currently an investigational device in the U.S. It is presently being evaluated in the industry-sponsored Phase III Study of Pharos™ Vitesse™ Neurovascular Stent System Compared to Best Medical Therapy for the Treatment of Ischaemic Disease (VISSIT). The VISSIT trial protocol is similar to the SAMMPRIS protocol.
1) Devices
    a) Guide catheter should be ≥5F with a length of 90 or 100 cm.
    b) Microwire. Use a 0.014 in. microwire.
    c) Stent
        i) Rapid-exchange system
        ii) Sizes:
            (1) Diameters (mm): 2.0, 2.25, 2.5, 2.75, 3.0, 3.5, 4.0, 4.5, 5.0.
            (2) Lengths (mm): 8, 10, 13, 15, 18, 20, 22, 26, 30, 35.
2) Technique
    a) Obtain guide catheter access.
    b) Angioplasty prior to Pharos stent placement is only necessary for tight stenoses that cannot be directly traversed by the stent system.
    c) Do a guide catheter angiogram and select an appropriate stent. The stent diameter should closely match the diameter of the target artery proximal and distal to the region of stenosis. Match the length of the stent with the length of the stenosis.
    d) Remove the stent from the protective ring and flush it with heparinized saline. Avoid contact with the balloon-mounted stent.
    e) Back-load the proximal end of the microwire into the stent catheter. Shape the tip of the microwire.
    f) Open the RHV widely and carefully insert the stent catheter into the guide catheter.

g) Navigate the stent into position across the target lesion.

h) Attach a 3-way stopcock and an indeflator containing 50:50 contrast in saline. Purge air from the system by applying negative pressure for about 15 s until no bubbles appear in the contrast material.

i) Deploy the stent by slowing inflating the balloon to nominal pressure. Deflate the balloon and apply negative pressure for at least 50 s. Check carefully on fluoroscopy to ensure that the stent has been fully expanded. Remove the balloon catheter.

j) The manufacturer recommends waiting for at least 30 min before removing the guide catheter to ensure that a dissection or thrombosis has not occurred.

3) Pharos tips

a) If a vacuum cannot be held during purging of air from the system prior to deployment, remove the stent and stent catheter. Slowly pull the stent catheter under fluoroscopic visualization to a position just distal to the tip of the guide catheter. Do not attempt to pull an unexpanded stent back through the guide catheter. The stent catheter and guide catheter must be removed as a single unit. During removal of the stent catheter and guide catheter, advance the microwire into a distal position. Tighten the RHV around the stent catheter and remove them together slowly.

b) Do not expand the stent more than 0.5 mm above the nominal diameter.

c) If resistance is met during removal of the delivery system, then the guide catheter and stent catheter should be removed as a single unit.

Postprocedure Management

1. Complete neurological exam.
2. Admit to the NICU or step-down unit with neuro exams and groin checks Q 1 h.
3. Antiplatelet therapy:
   (a) Antiplatelet therapy: Aspirin 325 mg PO QD indefinitely *and*
   (b) Clopidogrel (Plavix®) 75 mg PO QD for ≥30 days after the procedure:
     • Note: Some operators maintain patients on dual antiplatelet therapy for 3–6 months, longer than is usually done for cervical carotid or Neuroform stent cases. Cardiologists are recently moving toward longer periods of dual antiplatelet treatment (3, 6, or 12 months) after coronary angioplasty and stenting.[12] It can be argued that atherosclerotic intracranial arteries are similar in size and pathology to similarly-diseased coronary arteries.
       Or
   (c) Antiplatelet therapy: Aspirin 325 mg PO QD indefinitely *and*
   (d) Ticlopidine (Ticlid®) for 30 days after the procedure:
     • Note: Monitor for neutropenia.
4. Most patients can be discharged from the hospital on postprocedure day 1 or 2.

Intracranial Angioplasty Tips

1. Operator experience and careful patient selection is critical. No Class I data exists yet to show that intracranial angioplasty and stenting is beneficial to patients; therefore, the odds must be stacked in the patient's favor. Patients undergoing intracranial angioplasty should be managed by experienced operators or not treated by endovascular methods at all.
2. All devices needed for the procedure are to be prepared before the case, immediately prior to the groin stick and placed in a stack on the back table or at the foot of the patient's table, with each device separated by a sterile towel in the order that they will be used. This will permit rapid and efficient access to each device as required.
3. A hand-injection angiogram has to be done after each step, to check for contrast extravasation, dissection, intraluminal thrombi, positioning of devices, and

documentation. If a complication should arise during or after the case, a complete set of angiograms can help sort out and manage the problem.
4. If the patient is awake, a brief neurological exam after each step of the procedure has to be completed.
5. Overdilation during angioplasty should be avoided. It is better to undersize the angioplasty balloons than to oversize them.
6. In-stent restenosis:
    (a) Consider endovascular treatment *only if* the in-stent stenosis is symptomatic.
    (b) If treatment is necessary, consider doing a redo angioplasty with or without another stent.

Management of Intracranial Complications During or After Intracranial Angioplasty

1. Prompt recognition of a change is critical.
2. If an abrupt change in blood pressure or heart rate occurs, or if a neurological change occurs in an awake case:
    (a) Obtain AP and lateral intracranial angiograms.
    (b) Look for contrast extravasation and other signs of vessel perforation (such as a wire tip in the wrong location) intraluminal thrombus, intracranial vessel dropout, or slowing of contrast passage through distal intracranial vessels (indicates a shower of emboli into multiple small branches).
    (c) Look for signs of dissection caused by devices.
3. Options for thrombolysis if needed:
    (a) IV GP IIb/IIIa inhibitor (e.g., eptifibitide or abciximab):
        • Advantages: Powerful antiplatelet agent, particularly useful for platelet-rich thrombosis, which can occur with stent deployment.
        • Disadvantages: Carries a risk of ICH[13], relatively long half-life.
        • The authors prefer abciximab, which, unlike eptifibitide, can be reversed with platelet transfusion if necessary:
            – Abciximab:
              Loading dose of 0.25 mg/kg, followed by a 12-h intravenous infusion at a rate of 10 mg/min.
            – Eptifibitide:
              Loading dose of 135 µg/kg followed by a 20–24 h infusion of 0.5 µg/kg/min.
    (b) Intra-arterial thrombolytic (e.g., tPA or urokinase):
        • Advantage: Short half-life.
        • Disadvantage: May not be as effective as a GP IIb/IIIa inhibitor if the thrombus is platelet-rich. Also carries a risk of ICH.
4. Intracranial haemorrhage:
    (a) Suspect a haemorrhage if sudden hypertension or bradycardia occurs, or if the patient complains of a headache.
    (b) Do an angiogram – look for contrast extravasation.
    (c) If ICH is identified:
        • Reverse heparin with protamine (10 mg IV per 1,000 units of heparin given).
        • Maintain tight blood pressure control.
        • Platelet transfusion (to reverse antiplatelet medications).
    (d) Obtain a head CT; leave the sheath in place for the trip to the scanner.
5. Postprocedure neurological change:
    (a) Obtain head CT.
    (b) Consider return to the angio suite for a diagnostic angiogram and possible intra-arterial thrombolysis.
6. When angiography or CT imaging does not explain a neurological change, consider MRI with diffusion-weighted imaging, which can identify subtle ischemic changes.

11.2.   Endovascular Treatment of Cerebral Vasospasm

Indications for Endovascular Treatment of Cerebral Vasospasm

1. New onset of a neurologic change not due to other causes.
2. Radiographic evidence of ischemia due to vasospasm in a brain territory that corresponds to the neurologic deficit, with or without prior treatment with hyperdynamic therapy:
   (a) Some operators advocate a trial of hyperdynamic therapy for vasospasm prior to performing angioplasty[14, 15], while others prefer to do angioplasty on an emergent basis.[16]
   (b) In contrast to treatment of acute ischemic stroke, evidence of infarction on CT is *not necessarily* a contraindication to treatment:
      • In a series of 17 cases in which angioplasty was done despite a CT scan showing a new hypodensity, there was no haemorrhages or worsening of symptoms.[17] There was resolution of the CT hypodensities in 5 of the 17 patients and a majority of the patients improved clinically.
3. *Balloon angioplasty* is an option for symptomatic vasospasm affecting intracranial arteries >1.5 mm in diameter[18], such as the intracranial ICA, the M1, A1, and the vertebral and basilar arteries and P1 segments.
4. *Intra-arterial injection of pharmacologic agents* is an option for vessels that are not accessible or safely treatable with a balloon, such as distal ACA or MCA branches, or the A1 segment (which can be difficult to reach with a balloon).

Awake or Asleep?

Symptomatic vasospasm typically manifests as confusion and a decline in the level of consciousness, making it difficult for patients to cooperate with an endovascular procedure. General anesthesia makes the procedure easier and safer. A practical alternative to general anesthesia is to intubate the patient prior to the procedure (usually in the Neuro ICU) and place him or her on a mechanical ventilator with chemical paralysis and continuous analgesia and sedation.

Techniques

Access Phase

The procedure for carotid or vertebral artery access for vasospasm is nearly identical to that used for angioplasty for atherosclerotic intracranial stenosis as seen above. Several issues pertinent to treatment of vasospasm are:

1. Speed. Endovascular treatment of vasospasm is a variant of endovascular treatment of acute ischemic stroke – see Chap. 9, *Thrombolysis for Acute Ischemic Stroke* – therefore treatment should proceed as swiftly as possible. For example, if general anesthesia is planned but not quickly available, the patient can be brought to the angio suite, prepped, and groin access obtained while anesthesia is arranged.
2. Guide catheter positioning depends on whether balloon angioplasty is planned, or if IA drug infusion only is anticipated. Balloon angioplasty requires the guide catheter be placed as high as possible, for maximal support, whereas drug infusion through a microcatheter can be accomplished with the guide catheter in a relatively low position.

3. Use of systemic heparin:
   (a) Systemic heparinization can be used in selected patients, but is associated with theoretical increased risk of haemorrhage in postcraniotomy patients:
       • Procedural anticoagulation with systemic heparinization can be done safely in SAH patients with a ventriculostomy.[19, 20]
       • Systemic heparinization in patients with a recent craniotomy carries a 1. 8% risk of major haemorrhage.[21]
   (b) Systemic heparin should be reserved for cases in which there is guide catheter-induced interruption of antegrade flow in the access vessel, or a relatively long period of interruption of flow in an intracranial vessel due to the microcatheter or angioplasty balloon:
       • A loading dose of IV heparin is given (70 U/kg) and 5 min later, a 5 mL specimen of blood for an activated clotting time (ACT) is drawn from the sheath. The ACT should be kept between 250 and 300 s for the duration of the procedure.

Balloon Angioplasty

1. Device selection:
   (a) There are two views about the kind of balloon to use to treat vasospasm, i.e., compliant or noncompliant balloons. The arguments for and against each kind of device are summarized in Table 11.1. Good results have been obtained with either device[22]; the authors of this handbook are evenly divided in their preference:
       • Compliant balloons:
           – HyperGlide™ (ev3, Irvine, CA):
             Available sizes: 4×10 mm; 4×15 mm; 4×20 mm; 4×30 mm.
           – HyperForm™ (ev3, Irvine, CA):
             Available sizes: 4×7 mm; 7×7 mm.
           – For most cases the HyperGlide™ 4×10 mm balloon is most suitable.
       • Microwires:
           – X-pedion™ 0.010 in. microwire (ev3, Irvine, CA). This wire comes with the HyperGlide balloon and is useful in most cases.
           – Synchro2®-10 (Boston Scientific, Natick, MA). This wire is more steerable than the X-pedion and has an added advantage of being slightly smaller, so that slow contrast leakage will occur from the balloon when it is inflated, which helps prevent overinflation of the balloon.
       • Noncompliant balloons:
           – Maverick2™ Monorail™ Balloon Catheter (Boston Scientific, Natick, MA).
               (a) A wide range of sizes are available; the 1.5×9 mm and the 2.0×9 mm sizes are most suitable.
           – NC Ranger™ Balloon Catheter (Boston Scientific, Natick, MA).
           – NC Raptor™ (Cordis, Miami, FL).
2. Compliant balloon technique with the HyperGlide system:
   (a) Preparation:
       • Attach the HyperGlide balloon catheter to an RHV and flush using a 10 mL syringe containing 50/50 contrast in heparinized saline.
           – Compliant balloon catheter assembly
       • Fill a 3 mL syringe with 50/50 contrast in heparinized saline and attach it to the side port of the RHV (Fig. 11.1).
       • Insert the X-pedion microwire through the RHV until the distal tip emerges from the distal tip of the balloon catheter, and shape the tip.
       • Note: The microwire should not be allowed to extend more than 10 cm beyond the tip of the balloon catheter; if it extends any further than 10 cm the balloon will not function correctly. To prevent this, advance the microwire until the tip of the microwire is 4–5 cm and then tighten the torque device onto the microwire at the mouth of the RHV.
       • Test inflation. Place the distal end of the balloon catheter in a bowl of sterile saline and use the 3 mL syringe to fully inflate the balloon under direct visualization (the maximum rated volume for the

Table 11.1 Balloon selection for angioplasty for vasospasm

Advantages	Disadvantages
Compliant balloons	
More easily placed in small, tortuous vessels	The diameter of the balloon varies greatly with the amount of inflation. Overdilation and rupture of the vessel is a greater threat than with noncompliant balloons
Balloon and catheter are softer and less traumatic to vessels	
Smaller, softer microwires are less likely to traumatize or perforate the vessel	
Balloon can be inflated and deflated repeatedly, since it deflates completely. (Noncompliant balloons get "krinkly" after one inflation)	Lower inflation pressure may require multiple inflations to adequately dilate the target vessel. Occasionally, the low pressure balloon will not adequately open the affected vessel
With slow, careful, low pressure inflation, the balloon gently teases open the vessel	
Single-lumen balloons, such as the Hyperglide and Hyperform, can be deflated quickly and easily by withdrawing the wire (Note: the balloon cannot be reinflated after it is deflated by pulling back on the wire)	
Noncompliant balloons	
If appropriately sized for the target vessel, they will be less likelihood of overdilation and/or rupture of the vessel, since they reach the nominal size and then stop inflating	Heavier, bulkier, and more rigid than compliant balloons
They are used with a 0.014 in. microwire, which provides more torquability and support than smaller wires	They require a heavier microwire for support, which may carry a greater risk of vessel injury or perforation
Because they are difficult to navigate into small distal vessels, angioplasty is usually limited to larger proximal vessels, where one is less likely to face problems	Noncompliant balloons get "krinkly" after one inflation, increasing possibility of vessel injury when maneuvering a balloon that has already been inflated and deflated

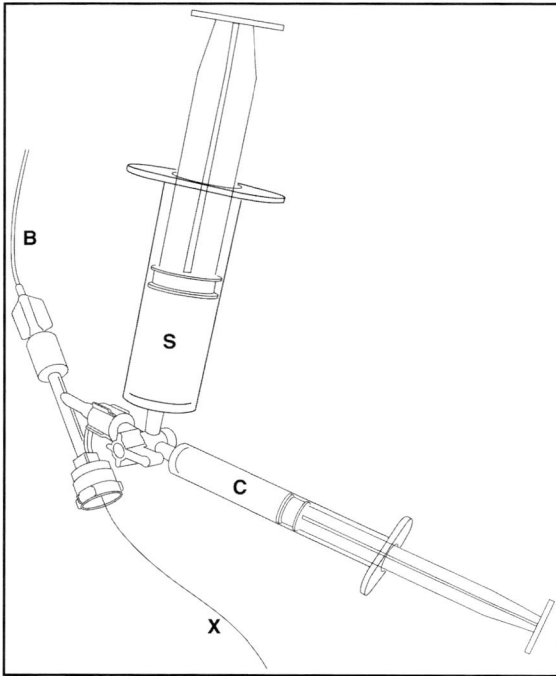

Figure 11.1 Set-up for using the HyperGlide™ and Hyperform™ systems. Three mL syringe (*C*), 10 mL syringe containing 50/50 contrast in heparinized saline (*S*), X-pedion microwire (*X*), and balloon catheter (*B*).

4 × 10 mm HyperGlide balloon in 0.16 mL). During the first inflation, the balloon typically inflates in an eccentric manner, which is why a test inflation is required. Subsequent balloon inflations should be symmetric.

(b) Angioplasty technique:
- Advance the microwire and balloon into the target vessel under roadmap fluoroscopy.
- *Carefully and gently* inflate the balloon under fluoroscopic visualization:
  - For the 4 × 10 mm HyperGlide balloon, see Table 11.2 for infusion volumes required to obtain each balloon diameter.
- Deflate the balloon with the Cadence syringe:
  - Note: Do not withdraw the microwire into the tip of the balloon catheter unless rapid deflation of the balloon is needed, as this will introduce blood into the balloon catheter; the manufacturer recommends the balloon not be inflated once this happens.
- Reposition the balloon for additional angioplasties as needed.

3. Noncompliant balloon technique with the Maverick angioplasty balloon:
  (a) Preparation:
  - Use 50/50 mixture of contrast in heparinized saline.
  - Prepare the insufflater and attach it with a three-way stopcock and an empty 20 mL syringe to the balloon catheter.

Table 11.2 HyperGlide balloon inflation volumes

Infusion volume (mL)	Balloon size (mm)
0.02	2.0
0.04	2.6
0.06	3.0
0.08	3.3
0.10	3.5
0.12	3.7
0.14	3.9
0.16	4.1

Infusion volume required for the 4 × 10 mm HyperGlide balloon. From.[25]

- Apply suction to the balloon but do not pre-inflate it.
- Continuously flush through the lumen of the balloon catheter with heparinized saline via a stopcock and a rotating hemostatic valve.

(b) Angioplasty technique:
- The balloon can be advanced into position primarily, without exchanging over an exchange-length microwire, when the target vessel is fairly proximal, like the ICA or the vertebral artery, and sometimes the basilar artery. For treatment of the M1 and A1 segments, and frequently the basilar artery, exchange-length microwire should be advanced within a microcatheter first. With the microwire tip positioned in a distal vessel, the microcatheter is then exchanged for the balloon catheter.
- The balloon is advanced into position under roadmap guidance and inflated to the appropriate pressure briefly, for 1–2 s. It has to be ensured that the balloon is completely deflated before it is repositioned.
  - Eskridge and Song[23] recommend a four-step angioplasty technique, in which the balloon is sequentially inflated and deflated at progressively larger diameters and advanced a slight distance after each inflation (25 % inflation, deflation, 50 % inflation, deflation, 75 % inflation, deflation, and then 100 % inflation).
- Reposition the balloon for additional angioplasties as needed.

4. Angioplasty tips:
(a) In general, the smaller and shorter the balloon, the better.
(b) Work in a proximal-to-distal direction. Improvement in the caliber of proximal vessels will sometimes lead to the same in distal vessel calibers.
(c) In cases of severe vasospasm, when the target vessel is too constricted to accept the balloon, pretreatment by intra-arterial injection of nitroglycerin, 20 mcg, can help. A microcatheter is positioned in the proximal part of the vessel and the drug is slowly infused. A very limited amount of papaverine is usually safe and effective for this maneuver; other drug options include nitroglycerine, nicardipine and verapamil. Nitroglycerin works faster than other agents used for vasospasm, such as nicardipine and verapamil:
- Some operators recommend that pharmacologic dilation prior to angioplasty should be avoided, on the basis that predilation makes angioplasty less likely to work. Theoretically, angioplasty is effective because it stretches the vessel wall, and dilation of the vessel before angioplasty may make this less likely to occur.
(d) When both the A1 and M1 segments require treatment, angioplasty of the A1 segment should be attempted first.[24] If infusion of a vasodilating agent into the A1 segment after successful treatment of the M1 segment, the drug may be diverted away from the A1 segment and into the M1 segment:
- Alternatively, temporary balloon occlusion of the M1 segment can help divert the drug into the ACA.[23]

Infusion of Pharmacologic Agents

Intra-arterial administration of the calcium channel blockers nicardipine, nimodipine, and verapamil has been reported. No single agent has been shown to be more efficacious than the others. Parenteral nimodipine is not currently available in the United States. IA infusion of these agents can be used to treat vessels that cannot be dealt with, or are difficult to treat with balloon angioplasty, such as distal branches and the A1 segment. IA papaverine administration is no longer recommended. See Chap. 13, *Intracranial Aneurysms and Subarachnoid Haemorrhage*, for a discussion of the published data.

1. Nicardipine.
   (a) Regimen: Nicardipine (Cardene IV; ESP Pharma, Inc., Edison, NJ) is diluted in 0.9% NaCl to a concentration of 0.1 mg/mL. Inject 1 mL aliquots through the microcatheter to a maximal dose of 5 mg per vessel.[25]
2. Verapamil:
   (a) Regimen: Verapamil HCl Injection. Dilute a 5 mg vial with 0.9% NaCl to a concentration of 1 mg/mL. Inject 10–20 mg per vessel for a maximum of 20 mg per carotid. Watch vital signs for transient hypotension and bradycardia.

Treatment-Related Complications

A review of published reports indicate major complications with endovascular treatment was seen at 5%, for vasospasm with an incidence of 1.1% vessel rupture[26]:

1. Reported complications include thromboembolism, arterial dissection, reperfusion haemorrhage, branch occlusion, bleeding from untreated aneurysms, retroperitoneal haemorrhage, groin hematoma, and vessel rupture.[27]

References

1. Higashida RT, Meyers PM, Connors III JJ, Sacks D, Strother CM, Barr JD, Wojak JC, Duckwiler GR. Intracranial angioplasty and stenting for cerebral atherosclerosis: a position statement of the American Society of Interventional and Therapeutic Neuroradiology, Society of Interventional Radiology, and the American Society of Neuroradiology. AJNR Am J Neuroradiol. 2005;26:2323–7.

2. Abou-Chebl A, Krieger DW, Bajzer CT, Yadav JS. Intracranial angioplasty and stenting in the awake patient. J Neuroimaging. 2006;16:216–23.

3. Kiyosue H, Okahara M, Yamashita M, Nagatomi H, Nakamura N, Mori H. Endovascular stenting for restenosis of the intracranial vertebrobasilar artery after balloon angioplasty: two case reports and review of the literature. Cardiovasc Intervent Radiol. 2004;27:538–43.

4. Kessler IM, Mounayer C, Piotin M, Spelle L, Vanzin JR, Moret J. The use of balloon-expandable stents in the management of intracranial arterial diseases: a 5-year single-center experience. AJNR Am J Neuroradiol. 2005;26:2342–8.

5. Stryker Neurovasular. Wingspan Stent System with Gateway PTA Balloon Product Prescriptive Information. Instructions for Use. Fremont, CA 2012.

6. Hansi C, Arab A, Rzany A, Ahrens I, Bode C, Hehrlein C. Differences of platelet adhesion and thrombus activation on amorphous silicon carbide, magnesium alloy, stainless steel, and cobalt chromium stent surfaces. Catheter Cardiovasc Interv. 2009;73:488–96.

7. Schmehl JM, Harder C, Wendel HP, Claussen CD, Tepe G. Silicon carbide coating of nitinol stents to increase antithrombogenic properties and reduce nickel release. Cardiovasc Revasc Med. 2008;9:255–62.

8. Bickel C, Rupprecht HJ, Darius H, et al. Substantial reduction of platelet adhesion by heparin-coated stents. J Interv Cardiol. 2001;14:407–13.

9. Monnink SH, van Boven AJ, Peels HO, et al. Silicon-carbide coated coronary stents have low platelet and leukocyte adhesion during platelet activation. J Investig Med. 1999;47:304–10.

10. Dahm JB, Willems T, Wolpers HG, Nordbeck H, Becker J, Ruppert J. Clinical investigation into the observation that silicon carbide coating on cobalt chromium stents leads to early differentiating functional endothelial layer, increased safety and DES-like recurrent stenosis rates: results of the PRO-Heal Registry (PRO-Kinetic enhancing rapid in-stent endothelialisation). EuroIntervention. 2009;4:502–8.

11. Bolz A, Brem B, Schaldach M. Corrosion behavior of antithrombogenic coating of silicon carbide. Biomed Tech (Berl). 1990;35 Suppl 2:227–9.

12. Coolong A, Mauri L. Clopidogrel treatment surrounding percutaneous coronary intervention: when should it be started and stopped? Curr Cardiol Rep. 2006;8:267–71.

13. Qureshi AI, Saad M, Zaidat OO, et al. Intracerebral hemorrhages associated with neurointerventional procedures using a combination of antithrombotic agents including abciximab. Stroke. 2002;33:1916–9.

14. Macdonald RL. Management of cerebral vasospasm. Neurosurgical Review 2006;29:179–93.

15. Harrigan MR. Hypertension may be the most important component of hyperdynamic therapy in cerebral vasospasm. Crit Care. 2010;14:151.

16. Rosenwasser RH, Armonda RA, Thomas JE, Benitez RP, Gannon PM, Harrop J. Therapeutic modalities for the management of cerebral vasospasm: timing of endovascular options. Neurosurgery. 1999;44:975–9; discussion 979–80.

17. Jabbour P, Veznedaroglu E, Liebman K, Rosenwasser RH. Is radiographic ischemia a contraindication for angioplasty in subarachnoid hemorrhage? In: AANS annual meeting. San Francisco: American Association of Neurological Surgeons; 2006.

18. American Society of Interventional and Therapeutic Neuroradiology. Mechanical and pharmocologic treatment of vasospasm. AJNR Am J Neuroradiol. 2001;22:26S–7S.

19. Bernardini GL, Mayer SA, Kossoff SB, Hacein-Bey L, Solomon RA, Pile-Spellman J. Anticoagulation and induced hypertension after endovascular treatment for ruptured intracranial aneurysms. Crit Care Med. 2001;29:641–4.

20. Hoh BL, Nogueira RG, Ledezma CJ, Pryor JC, Ogilvy CS. Safety of heparinization for cerebral aneurysm coiling soon after external ventriculostomy drain placement. Neurosurgery. 2005;57:845–9; discussion 845–9.

21. Raabe A, Gerlach R, Zimmermann M, Seifert V. The risk of haemorrhage associated with early postoperative heparin administration after intracranial surgery. Acta Neurochir (Wien). 2001;143:1–7.

22. Terry A, Zipfel G, Milner E, et al. Safety and technical efficacy of over-the-wire balloons for the treatment of subarachnoid hemorrhage-induced cerebral vasospasm. Neurosurg Focus. 2006;21:E14.

23. Eskridge JM, Song JK. A practical approach to the treatment of vasospasm. AJNR Am J Neuroradiol. 1997;18:1653–60.

24. Murayama Y, Song JK, Uda K, et al. Combined endovascular treatment for both intracranial aneurysm and symptomatic vasospasm. AJNR Am J Neuroradiol. 2003;24:133–9.

25. ev3 Neurovascular/Covidien. Hyperform Balloon. Instructions for Use. Irvine, CA 2012.

26. Hoh BL, Ogilvy CS. Endovascular treatment of cerebral vasospasm: transluminal balloon angioplasty, intra-arterial papaverine, and intra-arterial nicardipine. Neurosurg Clin N Am. 2005;16:501–16; vi.

27. Sayama CM, Liu JK, Couldwell WT. Update on endovascular therapies for cerebral vasospasm induced by aneurysmal subarachnoid hemorrhage. Neurosurg Focus. 2006;21:E12.

12. Venous Procedures

Venous neuroendovascular procedures include venography, venous test occlusion, venous sampling, transvenous embolization, venous thrombolysis and thrombectomy, and venous stenting. The reader is invited to consult related chapters in the book, which provide additional information on similar topics from an arterial approach.

12.1.   Venous Access: Basic Concepts

Pre-procedure Evaluation

1) Brief neurological exam should be done to establish a baseline, should a neurologic change occur during or after the procedure.
2) The patient should be asked if they have a history of iodinated contrast reactions.
3) The groins should be examined. The femoral arterial pulse provides a landmark for femoral venous access.
4) Ask the patient about any history of deep venous thrombosis that may require using special sites for venous access.
5) Blood work, including a serum creatinine level, serum glucose if diabetic and coagulation parameters, should be reviewed.

Pre-procedure Orders

1) NPO except medications for 6 h prior to the procedure.
2) Patients on insulin for hyperglycemia should get half their normal dose prior to the procedure.
3) Place a peripheral IV.
4) Place Foley catheter if a long, involved procedure is anticipated.

Contrast Agents

Non-ionic contrast agents are well tolerated and are usually used for these procedures. Iohexol (Omnipaque®, GE Healthcare, Princeton, NJ), a low osmolality, non-ionic contrast agent, is relatively inexpensive and is the most commonly used agent in venographic procedures. In patients with a history with severe anaphylactic reactions to iodinated contrast, small quantities of gadolinium-based MR contrast agents may be used instead.

Sedation/Anesthesia

Diagnostic venography and intracranial venous pressure measurements cause minimal discomfort. Intracranial venous interventions, such as venous sinus stenting, can be uncomfortable and may require general anesthesia.

Venous Access

1) Femoral vein access
   a) The most commonly used access.
   b) Technique:

i) Inject local anesthetic
ii) Advance a 22-gauge needle with a syringe half-full of heparinized saline just medial to a palpable femoral arterial pulse.
iii) As the needle is advanced, the continuous suction is applied to the syringe by pulling back on the plunger.
iv) If the arterial pulse is not palpable, the fluoroscopic landmark is that the vein lies over the most medial aspect of the femoral head. In many cases it is medial to the femoral head.
v) In difficult cases, needle puncture of the femoral vein can be facilitated by using Doppler-assisted needle (*Smart*Needle™ Vascular Solutions, Minneapolis, MI).
(1) Venous flow sounds like wind whistling through trees, while arterial flow has that familiar, strongly pulsatile sound on Doppler.
vi) When the vein is punctured, there may not be good spontaneous blood return from the needle. If blood can still be freely aspirated, the needle is in the vein.
vii) Using a micropuncture access kit, a 0.018 in. wire can then be inserted into the needle, the needle is removed, and a coaxial dilator is placed in the vein. The inner dilator is removed.
viii) A J-tip 0.038 in. wire is then carefully advanced under fluoroscopic visualization, and intravenous positioning is confirmed by visualization of the wire to the right of the spine.
ix) The sheath is then advanced into the vein.
(1) A 6F, 25 cm long Pinnacle® (Terumo Medical, Somerset, NJ) sheath is useful for most cases.
(2) Larger sheaths are usually well tolerated.
2) Alternative routes
a) Internal jugular vein. The jugular vein can be used for access to the ipsilateral dural venous sinuses.
i) Retrograde jugular punctures are done using a small vessel access system.
ii) The carotid pulse is palpated and the 22-gauge needle is inserted just lateral to the pulse, angling cephalad. A syringe attached to the needle is gently aspirated as the needle is advanced until dark venous blood freely aspirates. (If the blood is bright red and pulsatile, that is the carotid artery. Pull out and hold pressure for 5–10 min, then try more laterally).
iii) When the needle is in the vein, the 0.018 in. platinum-tip wire of the access kit is advanced carefully up the jugular vein, the needle is removed and the coaxial dilator is inserted.
iv) Microcatheters may be advanced directly through the outer 4F coaxial dilator Always attach a rotating hemostatic valve with a continuous saline flush to the hub of the dilator.
v) If larger catheters are used, the dilator may be exchanged over a 0.035–0.038 in. J-tip wire for a 10 cm long sheath of appropriate size. Since there is less soft tissue support and only a short length of the guidewire can usually be advanced up the jugular, it can be challenging to get the sheath into the vessel without buckling the wire and potentially losing access. Use progressively larger dilators to dilate the tract. Rotating the dilators and sheath as they are advanced over the wire helps.
b) Arm or subclavian veins can also be used to access the venous system. However, angulation at the entry of the jugular veins to the brachiocephalic veins and valves in these locations can make it difficult to access the jugular or more cephalad veins from the arm.

Catheter Navigation

1) Catheters should be advanced over a steerable hydrophilic wire.
2) When the tip of the wire enters the junction of the inferior vena cava and right atrium, keep the curved tip of the wire pointing laterally to facilitate passage into the superior vena cava.
3) Keep an eye on the electrocardiographic (ECG) monitor, since arrhythmias can be induced if the wire irritates the wall of the atrium or if it enters the right ventricle.

4) Once the catheter is advanced into the superior vena cava, it can either be advanced straight up the right internal jugular, or angled sharply to the left to enter the left brachiocephalic vein. It must then be advanced in a cephalad direction if catheterization of the left internal jugular is desired.
5) Valves in the proximal internal jugular veins sometimes can impede advancement of the guidewire up the internal jugular veins. The valves can be gently probed with an angled Glidewire® (Terumo Medical, Somerset, NJ) as the patient breathes deeply. Another useful wire for navigating through venous valves is the 0.016 in. Gold-tip Glidewire® (Terumo Medical, Somerset, NJ). Once the wire is past the valve, the catheter can then be advanced into the more cephalad jugular vein.
6) Catheterization of more cephalad venous structures requires use of a co-axial microcatheter/microwire assembly, usually placed through a 5 or 6F guide catheter.
7) When advancing a microcatheter through any guide catheter, always remember that movement of the microcatheter forward creates retrograde force on the guide catheter.
8) Attempts at advancing the microcatheter very distally can make the guide catheter buckle in the right atrium, causing arrhythmias.
   a) Arrhythmias will resolve when the slack is taken out of the guide catheter.
   b) Buckling of the guiding catheter may be avoided by using a stiffer catheter, such as a 6 or 7F Northstar® Lumax® (Cook Medical, Inc., Bloomington, IN), or a *Tower of Power* arrangement with a 90 cm sheath combined with a 100 cm guide catheter to create a stiffer platform.

Tips for Catheter Navigation in Difficult Situations

- Veins are more mobile than arteries, and are therefore less supportive to the catheter. One generally needs somewhat stiff guide catheters for support.
- Veins are generally tortuous, requiring a steerable soft-tip wire to get to the target vessel.
- Veins are more variable in their anatomy than arteries. Moreover, many pathological venous conditions are associated with venous occlusions.
- When in doubt about where the catheter tip is, periodically inject contrast through the catheter under fluoroscopy or make a roadmap.
- Veins carry blood toward the heart. It can be difficult to navigate against the flow of blood. Stiff, steerable wires, and steerable catheters are helpful in the venous system.
- Direct access to a target in the venous system may be difficult. Sometimes, it is helpful to use a more circuitous route to obtain access in the intracranial venous system. A multiple catheter, snare assisted technique may help in accessing the target in this situation (Fig. 12.1).

Road Mapping

Road mapping is less effective for venous procedures compared to arterial procedures. It is difficult to opacify the venous structures for more than a few centimeters beyond the tip of the catheter, since the contrast is injected against the flow of blood. Excellent roadmap images of the target venous structures can be obtained by injecting contrast in the arterial feeding vessels via a separate angiographic catheter in the arterial side when performing venous catheterization for transvenous embolization of arteriovenous fistulas. A diagnostic catheter can be parked in the internal carotid artery during intracranial venous procedures specifically for making venous-phase roadmaps.

Double Flushing

Double flushing is discussed in Chap. 2. Although small clot emboli are less likely to create clinically evident problems on the venous side, one should utilize good angiographic techniques including double flushing at all times to limit the risk of complications.

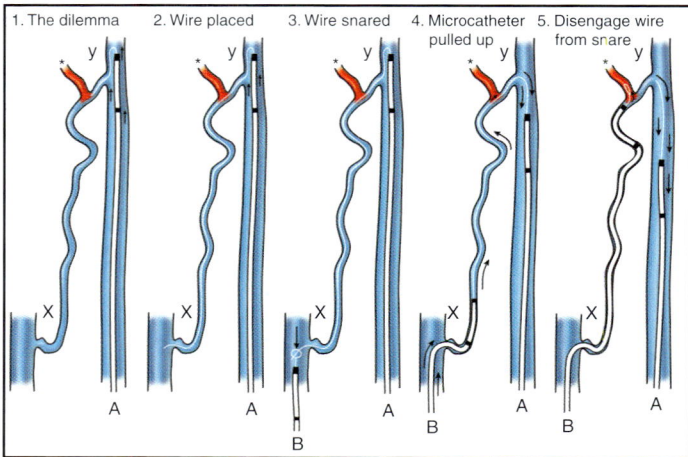

Fig. 12.1 Snare-assisted catheterization. *1. The dilemma.* In an attempt to obtain transvenous access to the site of an arteriovenous fistula (*), difficult angles make it impossible to advance a microcatheter (*A*) directly. Neither the microcatheter nor the microwire can be navigated directly via the small venous channel (*X*). A wire may be advanced into an indirect pathway (*Y*), but the microcatheter cannot make the sharp turn and displaces the wire and pushes beyond the turn. *2. Place the microwire.* Carefully navigate a soft microwire into the small venous channel (*X*), and into the larger vessel below. This microwire does not provide sufficient support to allow the microcatheter to follow around the turn. *3. Snare the microwire.* Position a second microcatheter (*B*) with its tip near the end of the microwire. Advance a snare through this microcatheter and maneuver it around the end of the microwire. Then pull the snare back into the microcatheter to grasp the wire. *4. Pull the microcatheter up.* Gently pull the microwire (now snared) back into the first microcatheter (*A*) and pushe the second microcatheter (*B*) to slowly advance it up the small arterial pedicle (*X*). *5. Disengage the microwire from the snare.* The snare is then pushed out slightly from the second microcatheter (*B*) tip to disengage the wire. The wire and first microcatheter (*A*) can then be withdrawn. The second microcatheter is then advanced to the desired target over either the snare itself, or, preferably, the snare can be removed and a microwire is used to guide the microcatheter into position.

Continuous Saline Infusion

Three-way stopcocks or manifolds must be used to provide a heparinized saline drip through the catheter. One should always use a rotating hemostatic valve on the catheter, so that the catheter hub is never left open to the air. When the catheter is in the venous system, low venous pressure may pull air into the catheter. Careful double flushing is also required if a wire is inserted and removed or if any blood is present in the lumen. The use of multiple hemostatic valves and continuous infusions is mandatory for any coaxial catheterization.

Anticoagulation

Heparinization limits thrombus formation in the catheter system, which can impair normal functioning of these systems. Moreover, thrombus in or around the catheter can cause venous thrombosis, potentially resulting in deep venous thrombosis, pulmonary emboli, and/or local thrombotic occlusion of the cerebral venous structures being catheterized. However, published data on whether systemic heparin is effective in preventing complications of venous procedures is lacking.

Hand Injection

A 10 mL syringe containing contrast should attached to the stopcock on the catheter, and the syringe should be snapped with the middle finger several times to release bubbles stuck to the inside surface of the syringe. The syringe should be held in a vertical position, with the plunger directed upward, to allow bubbles to rise away from the catheter. Contrast injections through a microcatheter are usually done with 3 or 1 mL syringes.

Mechanical Injection

There is generally no role for power injections during venous procedures.

Puncture Site Care

Manual compression should be applied to the femoral vein puncture site for 5–10 min after removal of the sheath. The patient should be kept at strict bed rest with the legs extended for at least 2 h, depending on the sheath size. A SyvekExcel® hemostatic patch (Marine Polymer Technologies, Danvers, MA) can be helpful. Bleeding from venous punctures is less of a concern compared to arterial punctures, and closure devices are not used.

12.2.   Venography

Background

Venography-the imaging of veins is rarely done in the head and neck using direct catheterization, due to the availability of excellent noninvasive imaging techniques, such as magnetic resonance venography (MRV) to study the venous system.[1] Most commonly, direct catheter angiography of the venous system is only performed as part of another venous procedure.

Indications for Venography

1) To confirm catheter placement and to assess venous drainage patterns in venous sampling procedures.
2) To evaluate for stenosis or occlusion in patients with suspected venous hypertension.
3) To evaluate for stenosis or occlusion in patients with unexplained tinnitus.
4) To assess collateral pathways in anticipation of surgical or endovascular occlusion of dural venous sinuses.
5) To evaluate for potential routes of access for transvenous embolization procedures.
6) In cases of transarterial embolization of arteriovenous shunts, venous catheterization may be done to monitor pressure, and determine the degree of reduction of venous hypertension.

Complications of Venography

Informed consent prior to the procedure should include an estimate of the risk of complications.

Neurological Complications

1) Since venography is usually performed as part of another venous procedure, the patient should be informed of the potential complications of the more involved procedure.
2) Statistics on complications of venography alone are lacking, since it is not a commonly performed procedure.
3) Theoretically, there is always a risk of venous infarction and hemorrhage whenever one deals with intracranial venous structures, but the risk of these complications is unknown and probably very low.

Non-neurological Complications

1) Anaphylactic reactions to iodinated contrast or any of the medications used can occur as with any endovascular procedure.
2) Access-site hematomas can occur, but are less common and less severe compared to arterial punctures.
3) Venous thrombosis can occur, producing symptoms of deep venous thrombosis, or pulmonary emboli.

Venography: Procedural Aspects

Suggested Wires and Catheters for Venography

Hydrophilic Wires
1) The 0.035 angled Glidewire® (Terumo Medical, Somerset, NJ) is soft, flexible, and steerable.
2) The 0.038 in. angled Glidewire® (Terumo Medical, Somerset, NJ) is slightly stiffer than the 0.035 and helpful when added wire support is needed, but is too stiff for routine use in smaller veins or intracranial veins.
3) Softer, yet torquable wires such as the Headliner™ (Microvention, Tustin, CA) or Gold-tip Glidewire® (Terumo Medical, Somerset, NJ) can be helpful for navigating the sometimes difficult valves in the lower internal jugular and for accessing the intracranial sinuses.

Catheters for Venography
There is one principle to keep in mind when doing venography: blood flows back toward the heart. Therefore, contrast injected in head or neck veins through a catheter placed via a femoral approach will flow back toward the heart and opacify the vessel caudal to the tip of the catheter. In the larger dural sinuses, it can be difficult to inject contrast more than a few centimeters beyond the tip of the catheter.
1) Soft-tip, simple angle catheters for catheterizing the caudal IPS or jugular bulb:
   a) 4 or 5F Berenstein curve Soft-Vu® (Angiodynamics, Queensbury, NY)
   b) 4 or 5F Angled Glide-catheter® (Terumo Medical, Somerset, NJ).
2) Guiding catheters used for coaxial approach :
   a) 5 or 6F angle-tip Envoy® (Codman Neurovascular, Raynham, MA).
3) Microcatheters used for the coaxial approach should be braided with a relatively large internal lumen:
   a) RapidTransit® (Codman Neurovascular, Raynham, MA).
4) Catheterization of the superior sagittal sinus in adults requires a 170 cm microcatheter
   a) RapidTransit® (Codman Neurovascular, Raynham, MA) is available in a 170 cm length, and works well for this purpose

    b) Remember to use a 200 cm or longer microwire
        i) 0.012 J-Tip Headliner® (Microvention, Tustin, CA)
        ii) 0.014 Soft-Tip Transend™ (Stryker Neurovascular, Fremont, CA)
5) Excellent opacification of dural sinuses can be obtained using intermediate
   catheter systems.
    a) DAC® (Stryker Neurovascular, Fremont, CA), whose 038 and 044 systems
       come in up to 136 cm., which is sufficient for most cases.

Techniques

Femoral Venous Access

Depending on the size of the catheter being used, a 5 or 6F sheath is placed in the right (or left) femoral vein.

Catheter Manipulation

1) Attach all catheters to rotating hemostatic valves and attach a three-way stop-cock and continuous infusion of saline containing 10,000 units heparin per liter.
2) Through the femoral venous sheath, advance the catheter into the desired internal jugular vein.
3) Once in the internal jugular vein, direct the catheter superomedially to point into the inferior petrosal sinuses, or superolaterally to point to the jugular bulb.
4) If the venous structures being studied are more cephalad than the jugular bulb or IPS, advance a large-lumen microcatheter coaxially through the rotating hemostatic valve of the guiding catheter.
5) Warn awake patients that the catheter manipulation may cause discomfort.
6) Carefully and gently advance the microcatheter over a soft-tip guidewire into the venous sinus cephalad to the area to be studied.
7) Do test injections of 1–2 mL of contrast to ensure proper catheter position and to estimate the amount of contrast required for a selective venogram.
8) Intracranial venograms are performed with hand injections of contrast.
9) Large dural venous sinuses may require injection volumes of 3–5 mL or more, and smaller sinuses, like the IPS may only require 1–3 mL
10) Cortical veins or deep veins like the internal cerebral veins should be cautiously injected with small volumes of contrast.
11) Perform venograms with high quality DSA imaging systems using 2–4 frames per second.

Tips for Evaluating Venogram Images

• Inevitably, when using microcatheters for venography of large dural sinuses, a streaming of contrast and unopacified blood from tributary veins will be seen, creating apparent filling defects in the vein.
• Apparent filling defects from streaming will change in size and configuration from frame-to-frame during the angiographic run, and have vague margins, whereas true filling defects or stenoses are static and more clearly demarcated.
• If it is not clear if a filling defect is real or not, adjusting catheter position and repeating the run may help confirm the presence of a real defect.
• Remember that potentially large Pacchionian granulations are normally expected within the dural sinuses, usually in lateral aspect of the transverse sinuses, and smaller ones can be seen in the superior sagittal sinus.

Venous Pressure Measurements

Stenosis seen on venography may or may not be hemodynamically significant. Therefore, patients with suspected venous hypertension should have venous pressure measurements obtained proximal and distal to any potential stenosis. The simplest method is to connect saline-filled extension tubing from a three-way stopcock or manifold connected between the catheter and a standard pressure transducer. For full evaluation of the intracranial sinuses, it is necessary to take the measurements using a microcatheter that can be advanced into the superior sagittal sinus, ipsilateral and contralateral transverse and sigmoid sinuses and jugular veins, obtaining pressure measurements at each of these sites. Waveforms of pressure measurements obtained via a microcatheter will inevitably be inaccurate, but studies have shown the mean values are accurate.[2] If the pressure waveform is completely flat, it may be necessary to change the display scale on the monitor. If the waveform is flat and the pressure measurements do not seem correct, the microcatheter may be wedged against the wall of the vessel, or it may be kinked, so gentle withdrawal of the catheter may improve the reading. More accurate pressure measurements may be obtained by inserting a 0.014 in. PressureWire ™ Certus (St. Jude Medical Systems, St. Paul, MI) in the microcatheter.

Venous pressure measurements can also be useful during transarterial embolization of arteriovenous malformations or fistulas. Particularly in the palliative embolization of extensive lesions, intracranial venous pressure measurements can provide objective data about the effect of embolization on flow through the lesion. Reduction of pressure to more normal levels suggests the patient will gain a clinical benefit from the procedure. In similar fashion, a Doppler guidewire can document alterations in blood flow by measuring changes in velocity in the veins draining arteriovenous shunts as the arterial feeders are embolized.[3]

12.3. Venous Test Occlusion

Background

Venous test occlusion is done to predict whether occlusion of the vein will have negative hemodynamic consequences. However, there are considerable differences between arterial and venous test occlusion. On the arterial side, occlusion of the vessel can quickly cause a sufficient drop in blood flow to a vascular territory to cause a demonstrable neurological deficit. However, there is less of a linear relationship of blood flow to patency of a venous structure; hence neurological deficits may not occur quick enough to be detected during the test. Moreover, many of the potentially disabling signs and symptoms of venous occlusive disease, such as intractable headaches and visual loss, may develop weeks or months after venous occlusion. There are reports of balloon test occlusions failing to predict disastrous venous hypertension and brain swelling after permanent occlusion of the tested venous sinus.[4] Venous sinuses have reportedly been safely occluded when collateral venous flow appears adequate on angiographic studies and if the pressure proximal to the site of occlusion increased by less than 10 mmHg as measured at the time of surgical occlusion.[5,6] Therefore, endovascular venous test occlusion can help assess tolerance for occlusion with multimodal criteria by measuring pressure changes produced by occlusion, evaluation of angiographic drainage patterns with and without occlusion, and clinical testing of the patient.

Indications for Venous Test Occlusion

1) To determine the potential safety of occluding a venous structure, prior to anticipated occlusion as treatment for tumors, arteriovenous malformations or fistulas involving a venous sinus.
2) To determine the potential safety of occluding a venous structure, prior to anticipated occlusion to permit proper surgical exposure when that venous structure is in the way.
3) To confirm a venous etiology in patients with unexplained tinnitus.

Complications of Venous Test Occlusion

Informed consent prior to the procedure should include an estimate of the risk of complications.

Neurological Complications

1) There is a risk of thrombosis of the venous structures catheterized, with resultant venous infarction.
2) Overly aggressive balloon inflation in intracranial vessels can rupture venous structures and produce epidural, subdural, subarachnoid or intracerebral bleeding.
3) Statistics on complications of venous test occlusion alone are lacking, since it is a rarely performed procedure.

Non-neurological Complications

1) There is a risk of a profound vagal response to balloon inflation in the jugular vein or sigmoid sinus, potentially producing bradycardia, hypotension, and even cardiac arrest.
2) Anaphylactic reactions to iodinated contrast or any of the medications used can occur as with any endovascular procedure.
3) Groin hematomas can occur, but are less common and less severe compared to arterial punctures.
4) Venous thrombosis can occur at the site of balloon inflation or anywhere in the venous system.

Venous Test Occlusion: Procedural Aspects

Anti-coagulation

Administer 50–70 units/kg IV heparin bolus and hourly boluses as needed to keep the activated clotting times at least double the baseline value. Also, consider pretreating any patient undergoing test occlusion with a dose of aspirin to limit any cascade of platelet aggregation instigated by intimal injury produced by the balloon.

Sedation/Anesthesia

Most commonly, venous test occlusion is done with the patient conscious, with minimal sedation in order to detect neurological changes produced by the temporary venous occlusion. In some cases, catheterization above the skull base can produce a great deal of discomfort so it can be argued that the procedure should be done under general anesthesia. Given the importance of pressure measurements and angiographic evaluation during these procedures, the neurological examination is of secondary importance. Therefore, if patient discomfort is considerable, venous test occlusion under general anesthesia may still provide useful information. Another option is to use heavy sedation and analgesia during the catheterization phase of the procedure and let it wear off for the actual balloon inflation.

Suggested Wires and Catheters for Venous Test Occlusion

Access Wires
- Steerable hydrophilic wires such as 0.035 or 0.038 in. angled Glidewire® (Terumo Medical, Somerset, NJ) can be used to advance a guiding catheter into the jugular vein.
- Softer, yet torquable wires such as the Headliner™ or Gold-tip Glidewire® (Microvention, Tustin, CA) can be helpful for navigating through pesky valves in the lower internal jugular vein.
- Soft-tip Transend™ (Stryker, Kalamzoo, MI) or other 0.014 in. wire is used to advance the balloon catheter to the target vessel.

Guiding Catheters and Balloons for Venous Test Occlusion
1) Guide catheters used for coaxial approach include standard 5, 6 or 7F large-lumen gauge guide catheters, such as 6F angle-tip Envoy® (Codman Neurovascular, Raynham, MA) or 6F Northstar® Lumax® (Cook Medical, Inc.,

Bloomington, IN). It has to be ensured the internal lumen will accept the outer diameter of the balloon catheter. The balloon catheter package insert will indicate the recommended guide catheter size.

2) A 6F 90 cm sheath (e.g., Shuttle® sheath, Cook Inc., Bloomington, IN) works very well as a guide catheter for test occlusions. It provides extra stability.

3) Balloons must be sized to match the vessel being occluded. The target vessel must be measured using a previous MR venogram, or a venogram obtained as part of the procedure to get a measurement of the vessel.

4) If the target vessel is 6 mm or smaller, a soft flexible balloon, such as the 7 mm Hyperform™ (ev3 Neurovascular, Irvine, CA) can be used. However, significant disadvantage of the Hyperform balloon is that one cannot use these single-lumen balloons to measure pressures beyond the site of occlusion.

5) The Ascent® balloon (Codman Neurovascular, Raynham, MA) is dual lumen and pressure can be measured through the central lumen when the wire is removed, and is available in 4 and 6 mm diameters.

6) Over-the-wire angioplasty balloons also have an internal lumen through which one can measure distal pressure through the end-hole of the catheter.[7]

7) Alternatively the 0.014 in. PressureWire™ (St. Jude Medical Systems, St. Paul, MN) can be inserted through the balloon catheter.

8) The shaft of the balloon catheter must generally be at least 120 cm and preferably 150 cm to reach the target vessel. The Savvy® balloon (Cordis Endovascular, Miami, FL) is available in various balloon diameters and lengths and has a large enough inner lumen for obtaining pressure measurements.

9) A 4 or 5F diagnostic catheter is useful to have in the arterial system, to obtain cerebral arteriography during the test occlusion. This allows visualization of venous drainage patterns as the balloon is inflated.

Procedures

Femoral Access

1) Femoral venous access is obtained as described above.
2) Depending on the size of the catheter being used, an appropriate sheath is placed in the right (or left) femoral vein.
3) In the contralateral groin, the same process is performed, except that the femoral artery has to be aimed at and the diagnostic 4 or 5F catheter inserted and positioned with its tip in the descending aorta, until it is needed for angiographic studies.

Catheter Manipulation

1) Attach all catheters to rotating hemostatic valves and attach a three-way stop-cock and continuous infusion of saline containing 10,000 units heparin per liter.
2) Through the femoral venous sheath, advance the desired guiding catheter into the desired internal jugular vein. A venous-phase arteriogram may be necessary to determine the best access to the venous structure being tested.
3) Once the guide catheter is in the internal jugular vein, advance an appropriately sized balloon catheter coaxially through the rotating hemostatic valve of the guide catheter.
4) Warn awake patients that the catheter manipulation may cause discomfort.
5) Carefully and gently advance the balloon catheter over a soft-tip microwire into the venous sinus up to the site for test occlusion.
6) Do a test injection of 1–2 mL of contrast through the end-hole of the balloon catheter, to ensure proper position.

Test Occlusion

1) With the balloon catheter positioned at the site to be tested, inject contrast through the central lumen of the catheter, to confirm proper positioning and to obtain a roadmap of the vessel.

2) Prepare to measure venous pressures, either by attaching a pressure line to the stopcock (or manifold) attached to the central lumen of the balloon catheter, or by using a pressure-sensing guidewire.
3) Measure a baseline pressure through the central lumen of the balloon catheter.
4) Gently inflate the balloon just enough to occlude the vessel. Less than one atmosphere is required to occlude the vein with an appropriately sized balloon.[7]
5) Measure pressure through the central lumen of the balloon catheter again. This reading indicates the back pressure in the venous system proximal to the occlusion.
    a) Stable pressure indicates adequate collateral flow.
    b) Rising pressure, especially if it increases by at least 10 mmHg, indicates limited collateral venous circulation and is one element of a "failed" test occlusion.
6) Examine and test the patient for any neurological deficits and check for some of the more subtle signs and symptoms, including headache, vertigo, ringing in the ears, and visual changes.
7) Perform a cerebral arteriography using the arterial catheter during the test occlusion to assess venous drainage patterns and look for angiographic signs of venous congestion. These signs include:
    a) Slowing of the arteriovenous transit time
    b) Congestion and dilatation of cortical veins
    c) Stasis of flow in venous sinuses.
    d) It is helpful to compare the flow patterns before and after balloon inflation in the venous structure.
8) If the patient tolerates the balloon inflation clinically and back pressure in the balloon catheter does not rise, keep the vein occluded for an extended period of about 30 min to confirm tolerance to occlusion.
9) Criteria for a "failed" test (one or more constitute failure):
    a) The patient develops symptoms.
    b) The back pressure rises by at least 10 mmHg.
    c) Angiography suggests venous congestion.
10) When the patient fails the test occlusion, or if they pass for at least 30 min, the procedure is complete. The balloon is then be deflated.
    a) Prior to removing the balloon, ensure that the patient's symptoms have resolved and that venous pressure has returned to baseline. If not, some venous thrombosis may have been caused; leaving the balloon catheter in place provides access for any corrective intervention.
    b) In the vast majority of cases, deflating the balloon relieves any symptoms produced. The balloon catheter can then be removed.

12.4.   Venous Sampling Procedures

Background

Endocrine-secreting tumors can produce significant symptoms, even when the tumor is small. Imaging studies may fail to detect very small lesions. This section will focus on venous sampling in the context of Cushing's disease.

Indications for Inferior Petrosal Sinus Sampling (IPSS)

1) ACTH-dependant Cushing's syndrome.
2) When biochemical testing and MRI imaging of the pituitary do not clearly differentiate between pituitary or an ectopic ACTH source.
3) When MRI imaging does not clearly localize the tumor, even if biochemical tests strongly suggest a pituitary location.
4) Any situation in which greater confidence is required to localize the ACTH-producing tumor, such as recurrent Cushing's syndrome after pituitary surgery.

Complications of Petrosal Sinus Sampling

Informed consent prior to the procedure should include an estimate of the risk of complications.

Neurological Complications

1) Permanent neurological complications at highly experienced centers are rare: one out of 1,200, or 0.083%.[8]
2) Realistically, neurological complications may be higher when less experienced operators are involved, but are still generally under 1%.
3) Reported neurological complications include transient or permanent brainstem ischemia[9,10] brainstem hemorrhage[9] subarachnoid hemorrhage[11] and transient sixth cranial nerve palsy.[12]

Non-neurological Complications

1) Anaphylactic reactions to iodinated contrast or any of the medications used can occur.
2) Groin hematomas can occur, but are less common and less severe compared to arterial punctures.
3) Venous thrombosis can occur. Two out of 34 (5.9%) patients undergoing IPSS had deep venous thrombosis, and one of these died from resulting pulmonary embolism.[13]
4) Theoretically, Cushing's patients may be expected to be at increased risk for infectious complications, but these have not been reported after venous sampling procedures.

Inferior Petrosal Sinus Sampling: Technique

Preprocedure Preparations

1) Some time before the procedure, 5 mL purple-top sample tubes are obtained and labeled with the patient information and numbered.
2) Ensure that a vial of ovine corticotrophin releasing hormone (oCRH) will be available.
3) Just prior to the procedure, a container filled with ice should be obtained to transport the samples to the laboratory.

Contrast Agents

For venous sampling procedures, only small amounts of contrast are required to confirmed proper catheter placement.
1) Nonionic contrast agents are well tolerated and are usually used for these procedures. Iohexol (Omnipaque®, GE Healthcare, Princeton, NJ), a low osmolality, nonionic contrast agent, is relatively inexpensive and probably the most commonly used agent in venous sampling procedures.
2) In patients with a history with severe anaphylactic reactions to iodinated contrast, the authors have used small quantities of Gadolinium-based MR contrast agents with good results.
3) In theory, the sampling could be done using no contrast material, since fluoroscopic landmarks could indicate proper catheter placement.

Personnel Requirements

Venous sampling procedures and IPSS procedures in particular require a number of assistants in the room to help obtain the samples and then assist in placing the samples in the laboratory tubes and then organizing them in a meaningful way.

1) Three people are needed to obtain samples from three locations simultaneously.
2) Two or three additional people are needed to obtain the syringes containing the samples. One of them should be responsible for making sure that each sample is placed in its proper vial and then placed in the iced container for transport to the lab.

Sedation/Analgesia

The use of sedation should be minimized, since many drugs can temporarily affect baseline ACTH production.

Suggested Wires and Catheters for Petrosal Sinus Sampling

Hydrophilic Wires

- The 0.035 in. angled Glidewire® (Terumo Medical, Somerset, NJ) is soft, flexible, and steerable.
- The 0.038 in. angled Glidewire® (Terumo Medical, Somerset, NJ) is slightly stiffer than the 0.035 in. and helpful when added wire support is needed, but is too stiff to routinely use it in the petrosal sinuses.
- Softer, yet torquable wires such as the Gold-tip Glidewire® (Terumo Medical, Somerset, NJ) can be helpful for navigating the sometimes pesky valves in the lower internal jugular and in accessing the inferior petrosal sinuses.

Catheters for Inferior Petrosal Sinus Sampling

1) Traditional approach: 4 or 5F catheters placed in the very caudal aspects of the inferior petrosal sinuses.
2) Coaxial approach: A microcatheter is placed in the IPS through a 5F guide catheter in the jugular vein.
3) Examples:
   a) Soft-tip, simple angle catheters for sampling the caudal IPS: 4 or 5F Berenstein curve Soft-Vu® (Angiodynamics, Queensbury, NY) or 4 or 5F Angled Glide-catheter® (Terumo Medical, Somerset, NJ).
   b) Guide catheters used for coaxial approach include standard 5 or 6F large-lumen gauge guide catheters such as the 5 or 6F multi-purpose curve Envoy® (Codman Neurovascular, Raynham, MA).
   c) Microcatheters used for the coaxial approach should be braided with a relatively large internal lumen, such as RapidTransit® (Codman Neurovascular, Raynham, MA).

Procedures

Femoral Venous Access

1) The femoral vein is accessed as described above.
2) A 5 or 6F sheath is placed in the right femoral vein and another in the left femoral vein. When using 5F catheters, for example, one sheath can be 5F and the other 6F, to permit collection of peripheral venous samples from around the catheter in the larger diameter sheath.

Catheter Manipulation

1) Attach the two 5F catheters to rotating hemostatic valves and attach a three-way stopcock and continuous infusion of saline containing 10,000 units heparin per liter.

2) Through each femoral venous sheath, advance a 5F catheter into the contralateral internal jugular vein. This crossed catheterization method allows for optimal mechanical advantage in catheterizing the more difficult left internal jugular from the closer right femoral sheath.

3) Once the catheters are in the internal jugular veins, direct each catheter medially to point into the inferior petrosal sinuses. If the catheter curve matches the angle of the IPS, the catheter can be gently advanced into inferior part of the sinus.

4) If the catheter does not easily pass into the sinus, a steerable, soft tip 0.035 in. or smaller guidewire can *very, very gently* manipulated antero-supero-medially into the IPS, and the catheter gently advanced over the wire.

5) Warn the patient that the catheter manipulation may cause discomfort.

6) Contrast injected at the jugular bulb may opacify a part of the IPS, and can be used as a roadmap. Once one IPS is successfully catheterized, a roadmap for the contralateral IPS can be made with gentle contrast injection. Contrast will travel into the cavernous sinus and across the circular sinus into the contralateral cavernous sinus and IPS.

7) Aim for the largest venous channel draining from the cavernous sinus, since the IPS may consist of a number of distinct vessels.

8) If the wire and or catheter point *infero*medially, it is in the condylar vein and should be redirected. Note that the condylar vein and IPS may connect together as they join the internal jugular vein.

9) Once the right and left IPS catheters are in position, inject 2–5 mL of contrast for a selective venogram. The catheter is in a good position if contrast refluxes up into the cavernous sinus. The venogram is also studied for venous drainage patterns that may affect the lateralization of tumors with the IPS sampling (e.g. dominant drainage of both cavernous sinuses into one IPS).

10) If microcatheters are used to collect the samples:
    a) Place dual 5 or 6F guide catheters in the internal jugular veins pointing toward the IPSs. Gently advance a large lumen (0.021 in. or larger) microcatheter over a soft-tip micro-wire into the IPS using roadmap guidance. The tip should be in the straight part of the IPS, and preferably not below any large connecting veins between right and left IPS.

Venous Access Tips
- Cushing's patients are often obese, which makes palpating the artery difficult. Moreover, the femoral vein may be surprisingly medial on some patients.
- If one femoral vein can be accessed, but not the other, a reverse-curve catheter like Simmons 1 should be advanced through the sheath and into the contralateral iliac vein. A wire can then be advanced into the common femoral vein to fluoroscopically localize the vein or advance the catheter over the wire into the femoral vein, inject contrast, and obtain a roadmap image to guide needle placement in the vein.
- Patients with deep venous thrombosis may have chronic occlusion of the femoral veins. As long as one femoral vein is patent, the vein is usually big enough to place two sheaths in the patent vein, one slightly more distal than the other.
- It is possible to place two sheaths in one femoral vein. This may be necessary in patients having a superficial infection in one groin, or in patients with venous anomalies such as a left iliac vein that does not connect to the inferior vena cava.
- If there is occlusion of one internal jugular, or the IPS has an anomalous connection to the vertebral venous system rather than the jugular bulb, it may not be possible to obtain IPS samples from that side. However, if the other IPS can be catheterized, it may be possible to advance one microcatheter into the ipsilateral cavernous sinus. Then, using a second catheter placed in the same jugular or through the same guiding catheter if a 6 or 7F catheter is used, a second microcatheter may be advanced into the cavernous sinus, then across the posterior intercavernous sinus and into the contralateral cavernous sinus. Thus, bilateral cavernous sinus sampling can be performed even if one internal jugular vein is not accessible.

Inferior Petrosal Sinus Sampling

1) *Simultaneous* 3 mL venous samples are obtained from the right and left IPS catheters as well as a peripheral venous sample obtained from the larger femoral venous sheath. Therefore, three scrubbed operators are needed to draw the samples.

Table 12.1 Colour codes for specimen tube labels

R = Red	Red = right inferior petrosal sinus (RIPSS)
L = Green	Green = left inferior petrosal sinus (LIPSS)
P = Blue	Blue = peripheral

Table 12.2 Inferior petrosal sinus sampling worksheet

	T: –10 min	T: –5 min	T: 0 min	T: 1 min	T: 3 min	T: 5 min	T: 10 min
R IPS							
L IPS							
Peripheral							

2) Before each sample is obtained, attach a "waste syringe" to the catheter and aspirate the dead-space of the catheter, usually 2 mL for a 5F catheter or 0.3 mL for a microcatheter.
3) One or more sets of samples are obtained to determine baseline ACTH values.
   a) The authors of this handbook prefer to obtain three sets of baseline samples, at 5 min intervals, to ensure a greater likelihood that an ACTH peak would be observed, given the known pulsatile secretion of an ACTH.[14,15]
4) Collect the right IPS, left IPS and peripheral venous samples all simultaneously. Aspirate the samples slowly and steadily for approximately 60 s to prevent collapse of the vein around the catheter and to prevent the dilution of the specimen by blood drawn in a retrograde direction from the jugular or condylar veins by excessive aspiration.
5) The three specimen syringes are handed to circulating assistants who place each blood sample into an appropriately labeled tube, which is then put in an ice-filled container.
6) It must be ensured that the correct sample syringe is used to fill the correct sample tube.
   a) Sterile coloured stickers on the syringes are a good idea (Table 12.1). This colour coordination can be used to make a similar sterile marking on the proper stopcock of the respective catheter. The receiving sample tubes are also pre-labeled with an identifying number. A pre-printed worksheet (Table 12.2) with the tube numbers, the time of sampling, and the site acts as a key, allowing one to later interpret the results obtained from the lab.
7) After each sample is obtained, the catheter and sheath are gently flushed with heparinized saline to clear the blood from the lumen.
8) Care must be taken during all these maneuvers to avoid pushing, pulling or torqueing the catheters.
9) Repeat selective venograms should be obtained via the IPS catheters after the baseline samples are obtained, to confirm that good catheter position is maintained.
10) Via a peripheral venous access, the patient is given 1 µg/kg body weight of CRH up to a maximum of 100 µg.
11) At least two sets of samples are obtained at timed intervals after the CRH is flushed into the venous line. The authors obtain sample sets 1, 3, 5, and 10 min after the CRH administration.

Cavernous Sinus Sampling

1. This procedure is very similar to inferior petrosal sinus sampling using microcatheters.
2. Bilateral femoral venous sheaths are inserted, one side is one F larger than the size of the guide catheter used to allow peripheral venous sampling via the sheath.
3. Two 5, 6, or even 7F angled guide catheters are advanced via the femoral sheaths into the contralateral internal jugular veins, pointing toward the inferior petrosal sinuses.
   a. The authors of this handbook use 5F soft-tip catheters, which can be placed in the inferior aspect of the IPS with little discomfort to the patient. The bigger, stiffer catheter sizes should be kept in the jugular to minimize discomfort.
4. Gentle contrast injections can be used to obtain a roadmap.
5. Through an RHV attached to the guide-catheter, advance a large- lumen microcatheter such as RapidTransit® (Codman Neurovascular, Raynham, MA).

6. Advance the microcatheter over a steerable, soft-tip microwire such as a 0.014 in. Soft-tip Transend™ (Stryker Neurovascular, Fremont, CA) into the IPS.
7. Whenever possible, advance the microcatheter though the straight segment of the sinus with the wire pulled back into the catheter, to minimize the risk of wire perforation.
8. Warn the patient that some discomfort may occur as the catheter is advanced through the IPS.
9. Gently position the tip of the microcatheters in the posterior cavernous sinus bilaterally.
10. Blood samples can then be obtained as described above for IPS sampling.

Jugular Venous Sampling

Sampling from the jugular bulb can be obtained in cases in which the IPS is difficult to catheterize directly, or if the operator is inexperienced with catheterization of the sinus.
1) Catheter navigation is the same as for IPS sampling, up to the point of positioning a 5F catheter at each jugular bulb.
2) Samples are obtained from the 5F catheters along with a peripheral sample from one of the femoral sheaths, as described for IPS sampling.

Puncture Site Management

Once the samples are obtained, the catheters are removed and hemostasis is obtained, as discussed above in the general comments. Because Cushing's patients frequently have received insulin for their hyperglycemia, it may not be advisable to use protamine to reverse heparin, as protamine administration can cause hypotension. Unless the patient has never received NPH insulin, it is best to leave the sheaths in place until the ACT returns to normal. The sheaths can then be removed and hemostasis should be obtained by manual pressure. The patient should be kept at strict bed rest with the legs extended for at least 2 h, depending on the sheath size.

Petrosal Sinus Sampling: Tips for Complication Avoidance
1. Use soft-tip catheters and microwires under roadmap guidance, and be extremely gentle to prevent venous injury or perforation.
2. Use systemic heparin and meticulous flushing technique to prevent thrombosis.
3. Pay attention to the patient: Severe pain, dizziness, nausea, facial/oral numbness or double vision could indicate something bad is happening.
4. Unexplained sudden hypertension can be a sign of impending brainstem ischemia, and could indicate that it is time to pull back the catheters.[8]

Venous Sampling: Interpretation of Results

Petrosal Sinus Sampling

Sampling for Cushing's is done to (1) determine whether abnormal ACTH production is due to a pituitary adenoma ("Cushing's disease") or an ectopic source and (2) for pituitary adenomas, determine which side the tumor is on.
1) Pituitary versus ectopic source.
    a) Calculate the ratio of the ACTH level in the IPS to the ACTH level in the peripheral sample.
        i) A ratio of 2:1, IPS:peripheral before CRH administration or 3:1 after CRH administration is diagnostic of a pituitary source of abnormal ACTH secretion.[16]
            (1) Using the 2:1 ratio as a threshold, basal IPS sampling correctly identified 205 out of 215 surgically confirmed cases of Cushing's disease, for a sensitivity of 95% and no false positives for a specificity of 100%.[16]

(2) After CRH administration, and using a 3:1 ratio as a threshold, IPS sampling identified all the Cushing's disease patients, resulting in 100% sensitivity and 100% specificity with no false positives.[16]

(3) Other studies with smaller numbers of patients with somewhat lower success rates, have still shown sensitivity and specificity over 90%.[17-19]

(4) The Italian Study Group[19]found that the best success with IPS:peripheral ratios of 2.1:1 for basal IPS sampling and 2.15:1 for post-CRH sampling, however other reports[20] confirmed the validity of the 2:1 and 3:1 ratios.

2) Side of pituitary adenoma

a) *In vivo* experiments showed that mixing of blood between the cavernous sinuses is minimal, and therefore sampling of blood from the petrosal sinus gives an accurate sample of what is coming from each cavernous sinus.[21]

b) There was early enthusiasm that petrosal sinus sampling could be used to pinpoint the side of the pituitary in which the causative adenoma was located.[22]

c) The NIH group found that, using a threshold of a difference of at least 1.4 times the contralateral IPS that the ACTH-producing lesion would be correctly located about 68% of the time based on baseline samples and 71 after CRH.[16]

d) One cause of unsuccessful lateralization of the tumor by IPS sampling is a hypoplastic IPS[23] associated with asymmetric drainage of both cavernous sinuses to one IPS.

e) Side-to-side IPS ratios were better at lateralizing the lesion when selective venograms showed symmetric drainage of the cavernous sinuses to their respective IPS.[24]

f) There may be a limit to the ability to lateralize the lesion since there is tendency for one side of the pituitary to be dominant, even in normal individuals.[25]

g) Other causes of false lateralization include multiple adenomas, which were found in 13 out of 660 (2%) patients undoing surgery for Cushing's disease.[26]

h) Even more unusual are ectopic adenomas within the cavernous sinus[27] as a potential cause of false localization.

Petrosal Sinus Sampling: Ratios to Remember
- IPS:peripheral ratio of 2 or more pre-CRH indicates a pituitary adenoma producing ACTH (Cushing's disease).
- IPS:peripheral ratio of 3 or more post-CRH indicates Cushing's disease.
- IPS:IPS ratio of 1.4 or more indicates the side of the lesion.
- If the IPS:IPS ratios pre-and post-CRH each suggest a different side of the lesion, the results cannot be relied upon to lateralize the lesion.[28]

Examples of IPSS Results: Three Real-Life Cases

Sample Patient A

	T: −5 min	T: 0 min	T: 3 min	T: 5 min	T: 10 min
R IPS	561	823	12,823	5,796	3,792
L IPS	26	29	611	319	299
Peripheral	10	9	24	27	19

All values are ACTH levels in ng/L; T, time; min, minutes before and after administration of CRH

Discussion: A classic result. IPS: periperal ratio is >2 for all IPS samples before CRH administration and >3 post-CRH. Therefore the source of the ACTH must be in the pituitary. The right IPS is greater than 1.4 times the left IPS, so the lesion should be on the right. All samples dramatically exceed the threshold ratios.

Diagnosis: A right-sided pituitary adenoma was successfully located and removed at surgery.
Sample Patient B

	T: –10 min	T: –5 min	T: 0 min	T: 1 min	T: 3 min	T: 5 min	T: 10 min
R IPS	59	184	127	26	5,154	1,086	1,159
L IPS	321	236	405	266	4,912	1,757	1,422
Peripheral	28	27	26	322	26	50	74

All values are ACTH levels in ng/L; T, time; min, minutes before and after administration of CRH

Discussion: MRI suggested a right pituitary adenoma. All readings show a 2:1 IPS:periperal ratio pre-CRH and almost all readings show at least 3:1 IPS:peripheral ratio post-CRH, indicating Cushing's disease from a pituitary adenoma. Notice at 1 min post-CRH the RIPS value is the same as the previous peripheral value. This likely indicates the samples were mixed up somehow. Note also that at 3 min post-CRH, there is higher ACTH in the right IPS, even though the remaining times show higher values in the left IPS. Therefore, one would predict a left pituitary source of ACTH, in contradiction to the right-sided prediction by MRI.

Diagnosis: A right sided adenoma was removed at surgery. The IPSS therefore was incorrect as to the side. The venography during the study showed no venous anomalies or asymmetry. This shows the major limitation to IPSS, since it correctly lateralizes the lesion only about 70% of the time.[16]
Sample Patient C

	T: –10 min	T: –5 min	T: 0 min	T: 1 min	T: 3 min	T: 5 min	T: 10 min
R IPS	46	35	46	255	542	827	600
L IPS	141	157	201	477	1,185	1,416	1,419
Peripheral	12	11	14	14	24	41	77

All values are ACTH levels in ng/L; T, time; min, minutes before and after administration of CRH

Discussion: Consistently higher values are seen in either IPS compared to peripheral and left compared to right.

Diagnosis: A left-sided pituitary adenoma was removed and the patient's serum ACTH and cortisol returned to normal.

Cavernous Sinus Sampling

The results of cavernous sinus sampling are variable.
1) A study of 93 patients from an experienced endovascular group reported successful catheterization of the cavernous sinuses with zero complications and sampling successfully diagnosed a pituitary source of ACTH in 93% of cases pre-CRH and 100% post-CRH correctly predicting the side of the lesion in 83% of all cases, and 89% of those with symmetrical venous anatomy and good catheter position.[20]
    a) This is similar to the larger IPS sampling studies in terms of safety and accuracy, although cavernous sinus sampling seems better for lateralizing the lesion.
2) Another study of 90 patients from another experienced endovascular group also had no complications but showed accuracy of diagnosing Cushing's disease of 86% for cavernous sinus sampling compared to 97% for IPS sampling and 100% using both sites, but successful lateralization in only 62–68%.[29]
3) Cavernous sinus sampling accuracy suffers when CRH is not used[30,31] or if samples from each sinus are not obtained simultaneously.[32]
4) Transient sixth cranial nerve palsies have been reported in two cases.[33]
5) Most centers prefer IPS sampling since it is simpler, less invasive, and there is more experience with that technique.
6) The authors of this handbook use cavernous sinus sampling in selected cases when venous anatomic variants make IPS sampling more difficult or in cases in which IPS sampling results are equivocal.

Jugular Venous Sampling

In centers where there is limited experience with petrosal sinus catheterization, jugular venous catheterization is a much simpler and somewhat safer alternative.

1) A study comparing jugular sampling to IPS sampling found jugular venous sampling to have 83% sensitivity and 100% specificity, compared to sensitivity of 94% and specificity of 100% for IPS sampling.[34]
2) Consequently, if jugular venous sampling is positive for Cushing's disease, then the patient should respond to trans-sphenoidal surgery, and if the sampling results are negative or equivocal, the patient could be referred to a center with more experience in IPS or cavernous sinus sampling.

Venous Sampling in Suspected Ectopic ACTH Production

If the IPS:peripheral ACTH gradients is <2 pre-CRH or <3 post-CRH, the test is considered negative for a pituitary source (Cushing's disease) and an ectopic source of ACTH is then presumed.

1) The first step is to exclude a false negative test.
   a) The NIH group had 0.8% false negative IPSS results related to a hypoplastic IPS on the same side as a pituitary adenoma.[23]
   b) One should review the venograms obtained during the study, and, if there are venous anomalies, repeat the study with cavernous sinus sampling.
      i) Consider surgical exploration of the sella if there is elevation of ACTH in peripheral blood after CRH administration, and no other source of ACTH is found on body imaging.[35]
   c) If body imaging is not conclusive for an ectopic source of ACTH such as a bronchial carcinoid, sampling from various sites throughout the venous system may help focus the search for the lesion.
      i) The authors had a patient with a negative initial IPSS. A more extensive peripheral sampling procedure was then done, and samples from the jugular veins, facial veins, vertebral veins, subclavian veins, and vena cava showed high ACTH in only one jugular and the highest levels in the ipsilateral facial vein. This patient had a maxillary sinus mass that resembled a polyp on MRI, but at endoscopic surgery found to be a secretory adenoma producing ACTH.

Venous Sampling in Acromegaly

IPSS can also be used to measure growth hormone levels in patients suspected to have acromegaly, but who have equivocal laboratory and imaging studies.

1) IPSS made the diagnosis of acromegaly in a small group of patients with equivocal imaging studies.[36]
2) Side-to-side gradients of growth hormone have not proved to be reliable.[36,37]

Other Venous Sampling Procedures

Venous sampling has shown to be useful in locating secretory adenomas in cases of recurrent hyperparathyroidism after parathyroid surgery.[38] This procedure involves taking samples from various neck veins, including the internal and external jugular, the inferior thyroid veins, and brachiocephalic veins. Sampling of the internal thoracic and vertebral veins has been advocated to look for ectopic locations of parathyroid adenomas.[39] Other endocrine tumors can be localized by venous sampling, but those procedures are beyond the scope of this handbook.

12.5.   Transvenous Embolization

Background

Intracranial arteriovenous fistulas frequently usually consist of multiple arterial feeders converging on a single venous structure. Transvenous embolization can be more efficient and effective than transarterial embolization of a large number of individual arterial feeders. The safety and effectiveness of transvenous embolization for arteriovenous fistulas depends on a number of anatomic considerations:

1) The target venous structures must *not* be required for normal brain veins
   a) The shunt causes all flow to go away from, rather than toward the target vein.
   b) There should be adequate collaterals to drain the brain.
2) The target venous structure should be at the site of entry of all the arterial feeders.
3) For pial arteriovenous shunts, *there must not be an intervening arteriovenous malformation nidus* between the artery and vein to be occluded.
   a) Blocking veins of a true arteriovenous malformation prior to occluding the arterial feeders and nidus is a recipe for disaster with a high risk of hemorrhage from the nidus.
   b) Similarly, in direct arteriovenous fistulas that have aneurysms on the feeding arteries, occlusion of the draining vein risks aneurysm rupture as the pressure on the arterial side suddenly increases.
4) The venous target must be accessible.
   a) Pial arteriovenous fistulas often drain into a series of extremely tortuous cortical veins before draining into cavernous or transverse sinuses, making transvenous access to the fistula difficult, if not impossible.
   b) Dural arteriovenous fistula may be associated with considerable venous occlusive disease, often blocking direct venous access to the fistula.
      i) It is precisely those fistulas having occlusion of the primary venous outlets and reflux into tortuous cortical veins that are the most dangerous lesions requiring definitive occlusion.
5) Fistulas that are inaccessible via an endovascular route for transvenous therapy may still be treated using direct intraoperative access to the draining vein, allowing deposition of coils or liquid embolic agents to occlude the fistula.

Indications for Transvenous Embolization

1) Indirect carotid-cavernous arteriovenous fistulas
2) Direct carotid-cavernous fistula (CCF) patients who are poor candidates for transarterial embolization (e.g. Ehlers-Danlos or other connective tissue disorder, recent trauma, difficult arterial access, etc.)
3) Transverse, sigmoid, or superior sagittal sinus dural arteriovenous fistulas (dAVFs) draining into a sinus adjacent to a site of occlusion of that sinus.
4) Vein of Galen aneurysmal malformations of the typical mural-type *but with caveats* (see below)
5) Vertebral-venous fistulas (VVF)
6) Certain, rare direct pial fistulas
7) Certain, rare spinal fistulas

Complications of Transvenous Embolization

Informed consent prior to the procedure should include an estimate of the risk of complications.

Neurological Complications

1) Access-related complications may include perforation or rupture of intracranial venous structures, causing subarachnoid or subdural bleeding.
2) There is a risk of venous infarction and associated intraparenchymal hemorrhage if vital intracranial venous structures is occluded.
3) There can be worsening of symptoms of venous hypertension if a venous outlet is occluded and the arteriovenous fistula remains patent, redirecting flow into other venous pathways.
4) A risk of arterial-side complications can occur if a related arterial embolization is performed as part of the procedure.
5) Transvenous liquid acrylic embolization of an arteriovenous fistula risks reflux of glue into arterial feeders and further reflux into normal arterial territories if the injection is overly aggressive, or if it is done without optimal biplane fluoroscopic imaging.
6) Brain abscess has been reported after transvenous embolization.[40]
7) A series of 31 patients undergoing transvenous embolization found a 10% rate of neurological complications, with no permanent deficits.[41]
8) In a series of 135 cases of endovascular treatment of indirect carotid-cavernous fistulas, 6% had complications and 2% had permanent deficits, but an unspecified number of these cases underwent transarterial embolization along with, or instead of transvenous embolization.[42]
9) Even after successful transvenous embolization of a dural fistula, delayed development of a second fistula at a different site can occur.[43,44]

Non-neurological Complications

1) Coils or other embolic agents may migrate to the pulmonary circulation.
2) Anaphylactic reactions to iodinated contrast or any of the medications used can occur as with any endovascular procedure.
3) Similarly, groin hematomas can occur, but are less common and less severe compared to arterial punctures.
4) Venous thrombosis can occur anywhere along the catheter path or in the pulmonary circulation.
5) Anesthesia-related complications can occur.
6) Patients with Ehlers Danlos syndrome can experience a wide variety of complications related to their connective tissue fragility, including retroperitoneal hematoma and bowel perforation.[45,46]

Transvenous Embolization: Procedural Aspects

Venous Access Sheath

1. Transvenous embolization procedures are done using a femoral venous sheath, most commonly a 6F 25 cm sheath.
2. Alternatively, one can use a 5 or 6F 90 cm sheath, such as the Shuttle® sheath (Cook Inc., Bloomington, IN) which also acts as a guiding catheter.
3. In rare cases, to improve access to the intracranial sinuses, using ipsilateral retrograde jugular venous access may be considered.
   a. In that case, use a short, 10 cm 4 or 5F sheath for jugular access.

Anti-coagulation

Use of systemic heparin varies among practitioners of transvenous embolization, but jugular and femoral venous thrombosis has occurred in patients with fistulas embolized without systemic heparin.[41] The authors think it is prudent to use heparin in these procedures. During the procedure, after access is obtained, administer 50–70 units/kg intravenous heparin bolus.

Sedation/Anesthesia

Most commonly, transvenous embolization is performed with the patient under general anesthesia. Any catheterization above the skull base can often produce significant discomfort, and the procedure may take considerable time, so it is advisable to use general anesthesia. The lower systemic pressure attainable under general anesthesia also allows coil embolization with a lower risk of migration of coils from their intended destination. Intra-operative embolization also is usually done under general anesthesia.

Suggested Wires and Catheters for Transvenous Embolization

Access Wires
- Steerable hydrophilic wires like 0.035 or 0.038 in. angled Glidewire® (Terumo Medical, Somerset, NJ) can be used to advance a guiding catheter into the jugular vein.
- Softer, yet torquable wires such as the Headliner™ (Microvention, Tustin, CA) or Gold-tip Glidewire® (Terumo Medical, Somerset, NJ) can be helpful for navigating occasional pesky valves in the lower internal jugular.
- Soft-tip Transend™ or Synchro™ (Stryker Neurovascular, Fremont, CA) or other 0.014 in. wire is used to advance the microcatheter to the target vessel.
- If a170 cm microcatheter is used, a 200 cm microwire is necessary.

Guide Catheters
1) Supportive catheter, such as the 6F Northstar® Lumax® (Cook Medical, Inc., Bloomington, IN) is useful for transvenous embolization. However, it can be placed only as high as the jugular bulb for access.
2) Guide catheter position in the inferior petrosal sinus or transverse sinus requires a smaller, more flexible catheter, like the 4 or 5F Angled Glide-catheter® (Terumo Medical, Somerset, NJ) or 5F Guider Softip™ XF (Stryker Neurovascular, Fremont, CA).
3) A 6F 90 cm sheath (e.g., Shuttle® sheath, Cook Inc., Bloomington, IN) works very well as a guide catheter for transvenous embolizations. It provides extra stability.
   b) Consider using an intermediate catheter such as the DAC® (Stryker Neurovascular, Fremont, CA) advanced via the Shuttle into the intracral sinus for added support. The 038 and 044 systems come in lengths up to 136 cm., and will accept a microcatheter within it. Obviously one must be certain the microcatheter is long enough to extend beyond the end of the DAC.
4) The Neuron™ MAX 088 (Penumbra, Inc, Alameda, CA) can be as a guide catheter, and the smaller 6F Neuron can then be used as an intermediate catheter placed more distally.

Microcatheters
1) Larger-lumen microcatheters, like a RapidTransit® (Codman Neurovascular, Raynham, MA), or Excelsior® 1018® (Stryker Neurovascular, Fremont, CA) are helpful for transvenous embolization, since they accept a wide variety of microwires to facilitate access, and also allow use of various embolic agents, including pushable fibered platinum coils.
2) In cases with associated venous stenosis or tortuosity, it may be necessary to use a lower-profile microcatheter, such as the 1.7F Excelsior® SL-10® (Stryker, Fremont, CA) or Echelon™ 10 (ev3 Neurovascular, Irvine, CA) .
3) Access to the anterior superior sagittal sinus requires a 170 cm microcatheter (see Sect. 12.2). However, detachable coils are designed to be deployed via 150 cm microcatheters; this may limit the types of embolic materials that can be used with longer microcatheters.

Embolic Agents

- Detachable platinum coils:
  - Very controllable and allows repeated use of the microcatheter.
  - …however, a large number of coils are required to close high-flow fistulas.

- Detachable fibered coils:
  - Very controllable and more thrombogenic than bare platinum coils,
  - ...but they are quite stiff and they require a larger lumen microcatheter.
- Pushable fibered coils:
  - These coils promote thrombosis better than bare platinum coils,
  - ...but they are not easily retrievable if not properly positioned; they also require a larger-lumen microcatheter.
- Liquid embolic agents:
  - Injectable through a small microcatheter and achieves quick, secure occlusion,
  - ...but they are hard to control in high flow lesions and can potentially reflux into arterial structures.

Procedures

Venous Access

1) Depending on the size and type of stent being used, a sheath is placed in the right (or left) femoral vein.
   a) Usually a 6F, 90 cm Shuttle® sheath (Cook Inc., Bloomington, IN)
2) The 90 cm sheath is advanced into the dominant jugular vein, or other major vein draining the venous structure to be embolized.
3) Alternatively, the jugular vein can be used for access to the ipsilateral dural venous sinuses. Retrograde jugular puncture is performed using a small vessel access system, as discussed in the general venous access comments above.
4) When the needle is in the vein, the 0.018 in. platinum-tip wire is carefully advanced up the jugular vein, the needle removed, and the coaxial dilator inserted.
5) A 0.038 J-tip wire or Glidewire® (Terumo Medical, Somerset, NJ) is gently advanced into the jugular vein, as high as one can easily get it, to provide added support.
6) The tract may have to be dilated with a 5.5F dilator; wire access should not be lost and it must be ensured the wire does not traumatize the venous structure it is
7) A 10 cm long, 4 or 5F sheath is advanced to the upper jugular vein.

Arterial Access

With any transvenous embolization, an arterial catheter is helpful to allow for roadmap images and periodic arteriograms to monitor the progress of the embolization procedure:
1) Access the femoral artery contralateral to your venous access site.
2) Insert a 4F, 10 cm sheath into the artery.
3) Through the sheath, advance a 4F diagnostic arteriography catheter into the arterial system that supplies the fistula being treated.
4) Attach the catheter to a three-way stopcock for continuous infusion of heparinized saline.
5) Perform an arteriogram to determine the optimal site of transvenous embolization and optimal views to see the venous approach to the fistula.
6) Periodically inject contrast via the arterial catheter for roadmap imaging of the target vein and venous pathways emanating from it.
7) During the embolization, periodically perform arteriographic runs to ensure the embolization is progressing as planned, and to determine the endpoint of the embolization.

Intracranial Access

1) Through the venous sheath or guide catheter in the jugular vein, advance the desired large-lumen microcatheter, the RapidTransit® (Codman Neurovascular, Raynham, MA) over a wire, such as the 0.012 in. J-Tip Headliner™ (Terumo Medical, Somerset, NJ) or the 0.014 in. Soft-Tip Transend™ (Stryker Neurovascular, Fremont, CA) gently through the jugular into the intracranial venous sinuses and advance the catheter to the venous structure to be embolized.
2) The microwire may have to be removed periodically for microcatheter angiograms to confirm that the microcatheter is on the correct route to the target. On roadmaps made with an arterial catheter, closely aligned and parallel venous structures may all appear to be heading toward the target on roadmap images. However, these structures may really be heading in different directions.
3) Place the microcatheter within the venous structure to be embolized, and, if it has not already done, perform venography to confirm proper positioning of the catheter.
4) Be gentle with catheter and wire manipulation, and use *extreme caution* when catheterizing deep venous structures, cortical veins, or small venous structures. These are very fragile and deformable by stiff catheter systems.
5) Even if a venous sinus appears to be thrombosed on the angiogram, it may be possible to gently probe with a soft-tip wire and advance a low-profile microcatheter through the occlusion.
6) If a stenotic region or occlusion of a sinus is encountered, consider placing a stent to reduce venous hypertension, as is discussed in the Sect.12.7.

Coil Embolization

- As a general rule, deposit coils in the venous structure beginning from the area most distal to the point of endovascular access to the structure. Embolize from distal-to-proximal.
- Also, be sure to block any potential outlets into cortical or brainstem veins, so that one is certain that dangerous cerebral venous hypertension will be relieved, even if the procedure fails to completely cure the fistula.
- With high-flow fistulas, it is best to start with a detachable coil, oversized to the diameter of the vein being occluded. If it does not appear stable after positioning, *do not detach it*. Remove it and try a larger diameter coil or a 3-D configuration coil.
- Once the initial coil frames the vein and appears to be stable, detach it.
- Place additional detachable coils to further frame and fill the space. The softest possible coils work best to pack tightly into the space available.
- If the microcatheter has a large enough lumen, it is helpful to include fibered coils to induce thrombosis. Care may be taken not to displace the microcatheter with the stiffer coils or jam the coils in the microcatheter.
- If a 170 cm microcatheter is being used, pushable fibered coils (and not detachable coils, as they require a 150 cm catheter) can be used. Pushable coils can be deployed with a bolus injection of saline, although often the coil will not exit the catheter tip if the catheter takes a tortuous route or if the coil meets any resistance as it enters the vessel. A 180 cm or longer microwire can be used to push out the coil; one must use a big enough diameter wire is to certain that it cannot slide alongside the coil in the catheter.
- Continue to pack coils in the venous structure being occluded. Alternate between finishing coils to fill small spaces and fibered coils to promote thrombosis.
- Some operators advocate injection of 5 mm fragments of 2-O silk suture via the microcatheter to promote thrombosis[47] but these can jam in the catheter and are less predictable or controllable than pushable or detachable coils.
- For a large venous sinus or venous varix, it will take a number of coils to block flow. At times even 20–40 or more coils have been used in a case.
- Periodic arteriograms during the procedure will indicate when the arteriovenous shunting slows and finally stops.

Liquid Embolic Embolization

There are two different methods to using liquid embolic agents in the setting of transvenous embolization:
1) First packing of the venous outlet of an arteriovenous fistula with coils placed by a transvenous approach. Then, a catheter is placed in a dominant arterial feeder via a transarterial approach for injection of the liquid embolic material.
2) Direct injection of the liquid embolic agent via a transvenous catheter in the venous outlet of the fistula.

Transarterial n-BCA Injection

1) This technique is used most commonly in high flow fistulas to achieve quicker and more complete occlusion than transvenous coil embolization alone. Coils placed in the venous side of the fistula act like a filter to catch the embolic agent and prevent distal migration of embolic agent into the venous system.
2) Venous phase:
    a) Use a 5 or 6F guide catheter.
    b) Place coils via a transvenous route into the venous outlet of the fistula, as discussed above.
    c) When enough coils have been placed to create a filter within the vein, the tip of the transvenous microcatheter is then withdrawn from the coil mass, so that it does not get glued in place.
3) Arterial phase:
    a) Advance either a flow-directed or over-the-wire type microcatheter into the arterial feeder supplying the fistula.
    b) Position the microcatheter distal to any normal branches.
    c) Carefully pull back slightly on the microcatheter to remove any slack, and gradually loosen the RHV so that it just barely prevents back-flow of blood in the guiding catheter, without binding the microcatheter too tightly.
    d) Confirm proper catheter positioning with a contrast injection via the microcatheter for a superselective arteriogram. Select a projection that shows the microcatheter tip and its relationship to any curves in the arterial feeder distal to the catheter tip, any normal branches proximal to it, and the coil basket placed in the venous outlet.
    e) Study the microcatheter arteriogram carefully to schedule the arteriovenous transit time, and determine the morphology of the target arterial feeder and venous structure where the liquid agent will be deposited.
    f) Prepare the Trufill® n-BCA (Cordis Neurovascular, Miami Lakes, FL) with Ethiodol oil at a dilution appropriate for the velocity of flow through the fistula. Remember that as soon as the n-BCA contacts the coils, flow will start to slow, so the glue will need to be slightly more dilute than you might predict. With a fairly dense coil mass in the vein, a 4:1, oil:glue mix often works well.
    g) Attach a glue-compatible stopcock directly to your microcatheter. Cook Medical (Bloomington, IN) makes a high-pressure, white nylon plastic, and three-way stopcocks with Luer-lock fittings that hold up well during glue injections.
    h) Thoroughly flush the microcatheter with 5% dextrose solution. As the last milliliter of dextrose is being injected, close the stopcock to prevent blood backflow into the microcatheter.
    i) Holding the stopcock upright, fill the Luer-lock connection fully with dextrose.
    j) Create a blank roadmap mask to allow viewing the glue injection under digital subtraction.
    k) Attach a 3 mL syringe loaded with the prepared glue mixture.
    l) Slowly and steadily inject the glue using roadmap imaging, such that the glue column continuously moves forward.
    m) Fill the arterial feeder and the desired portions of the proximal part of the draining vein.
    n) Be alert for any signs of reflux of glue back along the catheter, passage of glue beyond the coil mass in the vein, or reflux of glue from the vein into other arterial branches feeding the fistula.

o) If any of these conditions occurs and one is using dilute glue, the injection may be briefly paused, then resumed cautiously. Sometimes the glue will find another pathway into the coil mass.

p) If there is any question that the glue is refluxing or going elsewhere, if one has finished filling the desired space with glue, stop injecting, aspirate the syringe to create negative pressure in the microcatheter, and swiftly withdraw the microcatheter completely from the patient and discard it.

q) Examine the RHV of the guide catheter for any retained droplets of glue, then aspirate and double flush the stopcock, rotating hemostatic valve, and guide catheter.

r) Once the guide catheter is thoroughly inspected and flushed, reinsert it to the arterial territory of interest, and perform a follow-up arteriogram to ensure that the goal is accomplished.

Transarterial Onyx® Injection

1) Have several vials of Onyx® (ev3, Irvine, CA) agitating in an automatic mixer for at least 30 min prior to the procedure.

2) Venous phase:
   a) Place coils are placed in the venous side of the fistula via a transvenous approach and then withdraw the venous microcatheter from the coil mass.

3) Arterial phase:

4) The transarterial technique is similar to the technique using n-BCA glue regarding the catheterization of the arterial feeder, except a dimethyl sulfoxide (DMSO)-compatible catheter must be used:
   a) Rebar® (ev3 Neurovascular, Irvine, CA)
   b) Marathon™ (ev3 Neurovascular, Irvine, CA)
   c) Echelon™ 14 (ev3 Neurovascular, Irvine, CA)

5) Confirm proper catheter positioning with a microcatheter angiogram. Select a projection that shows the microcatheter tip and its relationship to any curves in the arterial feeder distal to the catheter tip, any normal branches proximal to it, and the coil basket placed in the venous outlet.

6) Study the superselective arteriogram carefully assess the arteriovenous transit time and to determine the morphology of the target arterial feeder and venous structure where the Onyx® will be infused.

7) Select a premixed viscosity of the agent depending on the size of the feeder and degree of arteriovenous shunting. Big feeders with fast flow need Onyx® 34 and small feeders or slower shunting should be treated with Onyx® 18.

8) Use the proper syringe supplied by ev3, draw up 1 mL of DMSO. The technique for handling the Onyx syringes is illustrated in Fig. 7.3.

9) Using a blank roadmap, slowly inject the Onyx® under roadmap visualization at a rate of approximately 0.2 mL per min.

10) Continue injecting Onyx® as long as it is flowing forward into the desired areas.

11) If the Onyx® refluxes along the catheter, passes beyond the proximal part of the vein, or refluxes into other arterial feeders, pause the injection for 15 s, then resume injecting. If the Onyx® continues to flow in the wrong direction, pause again for 15–30 s, and then try again. If the Onyx® finds another, more desirable pathway, continue the slow injection.

12) When adequate filling of the desired vascular space has been achieved, or if the Onyx® repeatedly flows in the wrong direction, stop injecting, aspirate back on the syringe, and slowly, but steadily pull back on the microcatheter, disengage it from the deposited Onyx® and remove it. The heavy-duty catheters used for Onyx® can usually be pulled back on their own, without pulling the guide catheter as well.

13) After the microcatheter has been withdrawn from the guide catheter, examine the RHV of the guiding catheter for any retained droplets of Onyx®, then aspirate and double flush the stopcock, rotating hemostatic valve, and guide catheter.

14) Once the guide catheter is thoroughly inspected and flushed, do a follow-up arteriogram to ensure that all tasks have been accomplished.

Transvenous Embolization: Tips on Specific Disease Processes

1) Direct carotid-cavernous fistula (CCF)
   a) Indications:
      i) Transvenous approaches may be required when arterial access to the fistula is not feasible.[48]
      ii) Transvenous embolization should also be considered in patients with vessel wall fragility syndromes, such as Ehlers-Danlos, which can make transarterial embolization riskier.[45,49]
      iii) Due to lower pressures on the venous side, transvenous procedures decrease the likelihood of catastrophic bleeding.[46]
   b) Technique:
      i) Venous access to the cavernous sinus:
         (1) Transfemorally via the inferior petrosal sinus.[48]
         (2) Direct cut-down on the superior ophthalmic vein (SOV) in the orbit.[50]
         (3) Occasionally via the pterygoid plexus.[51]
         (4) Direct access to the cavernous sinus through surgical exposure can allow coiling of the cavernous sinus if all else fails.[52]
      ii) The general rule is to first occlude the parts of the sinus that drain to
         (1) Cortical veins (dangerous venous outlets)
         (2) Superior ophthalmic veins (symptomatic venous outlets)
      iii) Occlude from the region most distal to the venous access point first, and end with the region closest to the access point to the sinus.
      iv) When placing coils near the actual site of the fistula, be careful not to let the coils pass through the fistula into the arterial side. This can be difficult in a dilated cavernous sinus, with a large coil mass which may obscure the carotid artery.
      v) One can place a balloon such as a Hyperform™ (ev3 Neurovascular, Irvine, CA) in the carotid across the neck of the fistula, and inflate it periodically as coils are placed in the cavernous sinus. This will prevent the coils from prolapsing through the fistula into the artery.
         (1) Position the 0.010 in. balloon catheter microwire well within the middle cerebral artery to stabilize the balloon and prevent it from being sucked into the cavernous sinus by the high flow shunt. Have a tight J-shape curve on the wire to avoid getting into a small branch or perforating the vessel.
      vi) In some cases it helps to place a Neuroform™ stent (Stryker Neurovascular, Fremont, CA) in the carotid across the fistula, to assisting the balloon preventing coils from migrating from the cavernous sinus into the parent artery.

Cavernous Dural Arteriovenous Fistula (aka Indirect Carotid-Cavernous Fistula)

1) Cavernous dAVF treatment is routinely accomplished with transvenous embolization.[47]
2) Transvenous access to the cavernous sinus is most directly and effectively accomplished via the inferior petrosal sinus (IPS).
   a) This can be successful even when the IPS appears to be occluded or absent on angiographic studies.[47]
   b) Passage of a J-tip hydrophilic wire and low-profile microcatheter can be done safely if done gently and carefully.[53]
   c) Fistulas that drain into the contralateral cavernous sinus via the circular sinus may be accessible by catheterization of the contralateral posterior cavernous sinus via the IPS, with passage of the catheter across the intercavernous sinus to the sinus draining the fistula.

3) It is important to determine the exact site of the fistula before starting to deploy coils in the cavernous sinus.
    a) Avoid redirecting drainage into cortical or brainstem veins, or possibly worsen ocular venous hypertension if one blocks some of the venous outlets without fully occluding the fistula.
4) Some cavernous dAVFs are bilateral, with arteriovenous shunts involving both cavernous sinuses. This may require packing of both sinuses, but before doing that:
    a) Be absolutely sure there are bilateral shunts, rather than just drainage from one cavernous sinus to another.
    b) Have a plan of attack so that one does not inadvertently block access to one cavernous sinus as the other is coiled.
    c) Remember that after one cavernous sinus has been coiled, it will obscure the contralateral cavernous sinus on a straight lateral view.
    d) Try using some craniocaudal angulation on the lateral view to keep the two cavernous sinuses from overlapping and to get the coils in one cavernous sinus out of one's way for visualizing the contralateral sinus.
5) The SOV itself can be accessed:
    a) Via direct surgical exposure, passage of a detachable balloons[54] or coils[55] through a venotomy for embolization of the sinus[54]
        i) A series of 10 dAVF cases using this approach was successful in treating the fistula in 9 with no complications.[56]
        ii) The direct venotomy should be reserved for cases in which the more indirect endovascular approach has failed, since direct venotomy carries risk of local hematoma or nerve injury, especially if the vein is small.[57–59]
    b) Direct percutaneous direct puncture of the SOV deep in the orbit has been reported.[60]
    c) Access to the cavernous sinus via the SOV can also be done through the facial vein without using a direct cut-down.[61,62]
        (1) This approach requires good imaging systems and finesse to navigate a soft wire and low-profile microcatheter around the curves as the straight angular vein connects to the loopy eyelid veins and into the SOV.
    d) Various other access routes to the SOV can occasionally be done:
        i) Puncture of the jugular or facial veins to improve access.
        ii) Puncture of the frontal vein in the forehead.[63]
        iii) Puncture of superficial temporal vein in the temporal scalp.[64]
6) When transfemoral venous access via the IPS or cutdown to expose the SOV is not possible, other routes of entry may be required.
    a) Passage of a microcatheter from the jugular bulb and up the sigmoid sinus to the superior petrosal sinus may allow catheterization of the cavernous sinus in selected cases.[65]
    b) When everything else fails, direct surgical exposure of the cavernous sinus can be performed so that a microcatheter can be inserted via a cortical vein[66] or other tributary[67] into the cavernous sinus.
        i) The authors of this handbook have resorted to these open surgical approaches only in the case of dangerous fistulas with cortical venous drainage where less invasive endovascular approaches have been unsuccessful. These dangerous fistulas have a great deal of cortical venous congestion and considerable bleeding is possible during open surgery.
7) Most transvenous embolization of the cavernous sinus is done using coils.
8) Liquid embolic agents such as dilute n-butyl cyanoacryate glue[68] (Trufill® n-BCA, Codman Neurovascular, Raynham, MA) can be injected in the cavernous sinus slowly and carefully, with constant vigilance for signs of reflux into some of the arterial feeders of the fistula, which could reflux into the ophthalmic or carotid arteries and cause serious neurological complications.
    a) Advantages: adjustable polymerization time, can be used in a variety of catheter systems, and doesn't smell of DMSO like Onyx® does.
9) Onyx® (ev3 Neurovascular, Irvine, CA) can be injected via a transvenous catheter to cast the cavernous sinus and occlude the fistula.[69]
    a) Advantages: Onyx permits very slow and controlled deposition, and is non-adherent.
10) Another strategy is to inflate a balloon in the ipsilateral cavernous carotid during the liquid embolic injection, but that will not prevent reflux into the ophthalmic artery, which can blind the patient, or even to the contralateral cavernous carotid artery via parasellar and clival anastamoses from side to side.

11) These procedures should only be attempted by persons with considerable experience with either n-BCA or Onyx®.
12) Occasionally, a true intraorbital fistula may mimic a cavernous dural fistula clinically; even the angiographic studies may create the appearance of a cavernous dAVF if it drains both posteriorly toward the cavernous sinus and anteriorly to the SOV.
   a) These intraorbital fistulas are successfully treated by transvenous embolization[70,71] provided the site of the fistula is accurately determined.
   b) Orbital fistulas may connect directly to the SOV, so coils must be placed in that vessel at the site of the fistula, rather than in the cavernous sinus, as is usually done in cavernous dAVFs. This shows that it is always important to carefully evaluate high-quality angiographic studies before planning and executing a therapeutic procedure.

Transverse/Sigmoid Sinus dAVF

1) Dural AVFs involving the transverse and sigmoid sinuses have high cure rates with transvenous embolization of these lesions[72] and therefore this approach is usually the treatment of choice for these lesions.[73]
2) However, most of these lesions have a benign natural history, and occlusion of a major dural venous sinus is a drastic solution for benign disease.
3) Short-term symptoms of venous hypertension have been reported in small series after transvenous embolization[74] and long-term data on results of transvenous sinus occlusion is lacking.
4) Transvenous/sigmoid sinus occlusion is recommended only in the case of symptomatic fistulas or high risk lesions with reflux into cerebral cortical veins.
   a) As a rule in these situations, there is an occlusion of the normal drainage of the affected sinus, and transvenous embolization will only extend the occlusion to involve the site of the fistula.
   b) Transvenous embolization can be done in cases of apparently thrombosed access. Microcatheters may be passed through the thrombosed sinus for occlusion of the site of the fistula with coils.[75,76]
      i) The outlets into any cortical veins should always be occluded first; later the sinus at the site of the fistula should be taken.
      ii) When using liquid embolic agents, it is also helpful to follow this rule: Coils should be placed at the entry point of any cortical veins, and later the sinus should be filled with the liquid embolic; this will prevent n-BCA or Onyx® spreading out into cortical veins.
   c) Certain dangerous fistulas have arterial feeders that converge to an isolated segment of sinus which may not be accessible via a transvenous approach.
      i) The sinus is occluded on either side of the fistula and all drainage is by reflux into cerebral cortical veins.
      ii) In that situation, an option exists to perform open surgical exposure of the isolated sinus segment and insert a microcatheter either directly into the sinus or into one of the tributary vessels draining from the sinus.
      iii) Coils and/or liquid embolic agents can then be used to occlude the sinus segment and fistula.[72,77]
   d) dAVF development is thought to be the result of venous occlusive disease; it is ironic that the treatment involves occluding a venous sinus.
      i) A more physiological treatment would be to resolve the venous occlusive disease.
      ii) Stenting the affected sinus is proven to be effective in relieving symptoms and sometimes curing the fistula.[78]
      iii) Treatment of venous occlusion or stenosis for these dAVFs may make transvenous embolization a less commonly employed therapy. (See Sect. 12.7)

Superior Sagittal Sinus and Other Anterior Cranial Fossa dAVFs

1) Occlusion of the affected superior sagittal sinus itself is not recommended, except in its far anterior aspect. Consequently, transvenous embolization in

these cases is reserved for selected cases of anterior fossa dAVFs which first drain into a cortical vein before draining into the sinus. The cortical vein may be occluded at the site of the fistula.[79,80]

2) Fistulas draining into the anterior aspect of the sinus may require extra-long (170 cm) microcatheters to perform the transvenous embolization from a femoral venous access.

    a) The authors have had success with transvenous placement of coils at the site of the fistula in the cortical vein, followed by a transarterial glue embolization to cast the vein. The coils on the venous side prevent inadvertent spillage of glue into the superior sagittal sinus or beyond.

3) More posterior fistulas which drain directly into the superior sagittal sinus and are associated with stenosis of the sinus that produces cortical venous may respond to stenting of the stenotic sinus. (See Sect. 12.7)

Tentorial dAVFs

1) Tentorial fistulas have arterial feeders converging on a tentorial sinus or cortical vein above or below the tentorium and are often dangerous lesions that reflux into cortical veins, and may present with hemorrhage.[81] They may have numerous arterial feeders, but often the tentorial sinus or dilated cortical vein can be safely and effectively occluded by transvenous coil embolization.[82,83]

2) Access to the fistula is often via a circuitous pathway.

    a) This means that a very stable guide catheter in the jugular vein (at least 6F) is necessary along with a flexible, braided microcatheter that will not kink as it negotiates the turns, and a variety of soft microwires.

    b) The wire has to be treated gently, especially along curves, to avoid perforating veins.

    c) A useful microcatheter/microwire combination is the Echelon™ 10 (ev3, Irvine, CA) and 0.012 in. J-Tip Headliner™ (Terumo Medical, Somerset, NJ), but different cases may require different systems to facilitate access.

3) After depositing coils at the fistula site via transvenous access, transarterial glue injection into the coil mass may be required to fully occlude the fistula. The fistula must be completely closed for effective treatment.

4) Like other dAVFs, tentorial fistulas may be associated with venous occlusive disease. Endovascular treatment of the stenosis by transvenous stenting can be accomplished to reduce intracranial venous hypertension.[84] (See Sect. 12.7)

Vein of Galen Aneurysmal Malformations

Transtorcular coil embolization of the vein of Galen was originally developed as a life-saving measure to treat rapid arteriovenous shunting.[85] However, this approach requires craniotomy and direct puncture of the venous sinus. Transfemoral venous access to the vein of Galen is less traumatic for the patient and renders craniotomy unnecessary.[86] Transfemoral access to the vein of Galen also permits retrograde catheterization of larger arterial feeders, allowing coil occlusion of some of these feeders.[86] However, if transvenous embolization in VOGMs is used without regard for the arterial and venous anatomy, complications may occur. Any lesion with an associated arteriovenous nidus, as in Yasargil type IV lesions, should *never* undergo transvenous occlusion of the venous outlet.[87] Blind occlusion of the vein also impairs venous drainage of the brain when there is drainage of the deep veins into the vein.[88–90] Moreover, placement of a large number of coils in the vein creates a permanent mass that compresses the cerebral aqueduct contributing to hydrocephalus. Consequently, given currently available techniques for transarterial embolization of the fistulas in VOGM, transvenous embolization is rarely, if ever, required to treat these lesions.

Other Intracranial dAVFs

1) dAVFs at unusual sites amenable to transvenous embolization include:

    a) Superior petrosal sinus.[91]

    b) Inferior petrosal sinus.[92]

     c)   Anterior condylar vein.[93–95]
     d)   Jugular bulb.[96]
2) Successful treatment requires a thorough arteriogram and careful evaluation of drainage patterns of the fistula and normal venous drainage in the region. Then, it is only a matter of placing the microcatheter into venous side of the fistula for occlusion with coils.

Extracranial Head and Neck AVFs

Mandibular AVFs that converge on the inferior alveolar vein can result in problems of oral bleeding, tooth loss, and bone resorption, but may be effectively treated by transvenous coil embolization of the vein.[97–99] Usually, injection of transarterial glue may be needed to completely close the fistula, but the procedure can provide complete cure with restoration of resorbed bone in the mandible. The authors have also treated scalp and facial AVMs with direct percutaneous puncture of the venous outlet and injection of n-BCA glue. The venous outlets can be manually compressed during the glue injection to allow controlled retrograde filling of the AVM nidus without causing too much venous embolization.

Spinal AVFs

Transvenous embolization of spinal fistulas is extremely rare, due to the usual tortuosity of spinal venous structures. A high flow perimedullary fistulas was reportedly treated by direct, intraoperative access to the venous outlet and transvenous injection of glue.[100] Extradural fistulas may be more accessible to standard endovascular transvenous coil embolization techniques.[101]

12.6.   Venous Thrombolysis and Thrombectomy

Background

Cerebral venous thrombosis (CVT) is discussed in Chap. 16. Endovascular treatment may be helpful in the management of patients unresponsive to conventional medical therapy.

Indications for Venous Thrombolysis/Thrombectomy

1) Symptomatic CVT unresponsive to medical management (hydration, heparin, and ICP management).
2) CVT patients with contraindications to heparin (recent surgery, trauma, bleeding diathesis, anti-heparin antibodies).
3) CVT patients at higher risk of mortality (those with seizures, coma, disturbed consciousness, deep cerebral venous thrombosis, posterior fossa involvement, and progressive focal neurological deficits).[102]

Complications of Venous Thrombolysis/ Thrombectomy

Informed consent prior to the procedure should include an estimate of the risk of complications.

Neurological Complications

1) Development of, or worsening pre-existing intracerebral edema and/or hemorrhage from venous infarction.
2) Venous perforation by guidewires, stiff catheters, or retrieval devices may produce intracranial bleeding.
3) Rethrombosis of a revascularized venous structure may occur.
4) Good statistics on complications of cerebral venous revascularization procedures are lacking, since the series reported are small and the best results tend to get reported.

Non-neurological Complications

1) Anaphylactic reactions to iodinated contrast or any of the medications used can occur as with any endovascular procedure.
2) Groin hematomas can occur, especially if heparin, antiplatelet agents, and thrombolytic agents are administered.
3) Venous thrombosis can occur anywhere along the pathway of the catheter.
4) Mechanical clot disruption in the larger dural venous sinuses and jugular veins may result in pulmonary emboli.

Venous Thrombolysis and Thrombectomy: Technique

Vascular Access Sheath

Venous revascularization procedures are usually always done using a femoral venous sheath, most commonly a 6 or 7F Shuttle® sheath (Cook Inc., Bloomington, IN) which also acts as a guiding catheter. Large-lumen access to allow for more options, including microcatheters, balloon catheters, rheolytic catheters, etc. However, if direct puncture of the internal jugular vein is planned, a short, 10 cm 6 or 7F sheath is best.

Many venous revascularization cases can be assisted by obtaining arteriograms prior to and during the course of opening up occluded veins, in order to have a better visualization of the effects of the occlusion on brain perfusion. Consequently, femoral arterial access may also be obtained.

Suggested Wires and Catheters for Venous Thrombolysis and Thrombectomy

Access Wires
- Steerable hydrophilic wires such as the 0.035 or 0.038 in. angled Glidewire® (Terumo Medical, Somerset, NJ) can be used to advance the guide catheter into the jugular vein.
- Softer, yet torquable wires such as the Headliner™ (Microvention, Tustin, CA) or Gold-tip Glidewire® (Terumo Medical, Somerset, NJ) can be used navigate through the sometimes pesky valves in the lower internal jugular vein.
- Soft-tip Transend™ or Synchro™ (Stryker Neurovascular, Fremont, CA) or other 0.014 in. wire is used to advance the microcatheter to the target vessel.
- A good wire for passing through thrombus is the 0.012 in. J-Tip Headliner™ (Microvention, Tustin, CA), which is less likely to go into small branches and cause a perforation.
- Often, extra-support platinum-tipped, stainless steel coronary wires may be required to advance stiff rheolytic catheters.

Guide Catheters
1) Guide catheters used for these procedures should be supportive and have a large lumen to allow for a multimodal therapeutic approach.
2) A 90 cm sheath (e.g. Shuttle® sheath, Cook Inc., Bloomington, IN) works well.
3) An alternative approach includes standard 6 or 7F large-lumen gauge guide catheters, such as the 6F angle-tip Envoy® (Codman Neurovascular, Raynham,

MA) or 6F Northstar® Lumax® (Cook Medical, Inc., Bloomington, IN). Make sure that the internal lumen will accept the outer diameter of whatever devices (microcatheters, balloons, reperfusion catheters) are planned. The device package insert will indicate the recommended guide catheter size.

Microcatheters

Large-lumen microcatheters such as the RapidTransit® (Codman Neurovascular, Raynham, MA), are used for intracranial venous catheterization (see Sect. 12.2). If the thrombus is in the superior sagittal sinus, a 170 cm length microcatheter will be required. Occasionally a lower-profile system may to needed to penetrate firm thrombus or navigate beyond underlying venous sinus stenoses. Microcatheters with a 1.7F distal tip work well and include the Echelon-10™ (ev3, Irvine, CA), Excelsior® SL-10 (Boston Scientific, Natick, MA), or Prowler-10® (Codman Neurovascular, Raynham, MA).

Balloons for Venous Thrombolysis/Thrombectomy

1) Balloons *must* be sized smaller than the vessel being treated. As rule, begin with a small (say 2–3 mm) diameter balloon.
2) The best balloons for these procedures are over-the-wire, low-compliance angioplasty balloons which have an internal lumen through which one can infuse thrombolytic agents as well as use the balloon to disrupt clot.
3) The shaft of the balloon catheter must generally be 150 cm to reach the target vessel. The over-the-wire NC Ranger™ (Boston Scientific, Natick, MA) or NC Raptor™ (Cordis Endovascular, Miami, FL) are useful.
4) Soft flexible balloons, such as the 3.5 mm diameter Hyperglide™ (ev3, Irvine, CA) or Ascent® balloon (Codman Neurovascular, Raynham, MA) may be used to disrupt clot, but these very soft balloons only work on soft clot.

Thrombectomy Catheters

1) Penumbra Reperfusion catheters (Penumbra, Inc., Alameda, CA) come in 0.054, 0.041, 0.032, and 0.026 in lumen sizes. Each catheter comes with a matching separator wires to prevent clogging of the catheter by clot. It is best to use the 0.054 system if possible, to more efficiently remove clot. This Reperfusion catheter requires a 6F 90 cm. long sheath or a Neuron™ MAX 088 (Penumbra, Inc, Alameda, CA) as a guide catheter.
2) The AngioJet® XMI® catheter (Possis Medical, Minneapolis, MN) comes in both over-the-wire and rapid-exchange versions and the AngioJet® Spiroflex™ (Possis Medical, Minneapolis, MN) is a flexible rapid exchange system. These are 4F catheters that are compatible with 6F guide catheters and are flexible enough to reach the intracranial dural venous sinuses. These rheolytic catheters fragment and aspirate clot with a high-flow jet of saline that aspirates the clot using the Bernoulli principle, this requires the sterile connection set and pump console made specifically for this system. The drawback to these devices is that they can only aspirate small volumes of clot in a reasonable period of time. The company makes larger catheters for heavy-duty clot aspiration, but the larger systems are stiffer and harder to navigate through the sigmoid sinus.

Procedures

Venous Access

1) Prep and drape the groin area is bilaterally.
2) Palpate the femoral pulse at the inguinal crease, and infiltrate local anesthesia medial to the pulse, both by raising a wheal and injecting deeply toward the vein.
3) Make a 5 mm incision parallel to the inguinal crease with an 11-blade scalpel.
4) Attach an 18 gauge Potts needle to a 20 mL syringe. Advance the needle with the bevel facing upward while aspirating continuously. The needle is advanced at a 45 ° angle to the skin.

5) Aspiration of dark red blood confirms puncture of the femoral vein.
6) A 0.038 in. J-wire is advanced under fluoroscopic visualization into the inferior vena cava.
7) Depending on the size of the catheter being used, a sheath is placed in the right or left femoral vein.
8) In patients with intracranial venous thrombosis, it is not uncommon for there to also be femoral or iliac thrombosis, preventing access from that route. The other groin may be tried in that case.
9) If femoral venous access fails, direct jugular access can be done. Take care to avoid creating a neck hematoma, especially when using thrombolytics. Neck hematomas can compress the airway if they get too large.
10) If all else fails, a burr hole may be placed over the dural sinus to be treated with a rheolytic catheter[103] but this more invasive technique limits the options for using heparin and/or thrombolytic agents because of the risk of post-operative bleeding.

Catheter Manipulation

1) Attach all catheters to RHVs and use continuous infusion of saline containing 10,000 units heparin per liter.
2) Advance the guide catheter or 90 cm sheath over a steerable Glidewire® (Terumo Medical, Somerset, NJ) into the desired internal jugular vein.
3) If the venous structures being treated are more cephalad than the jugular bulb or IPS, advance a microcatheter coaxially through the rotating hemostatic valve of the guide catheter.
4) Warn awake patients that catheter manipulation may cause discomfort.
5) Carefully and gently advance the microcatheter over a soft-tip microwire into the venous sinus. The J-Tip Headliner™ (Microvention, Tustin, CA) is a good microwire to use to advance the microcatheter through the clot in an atraumatic fashion. Try to get the microcatheter tip as far as possible into the thrombus to allow for treatment of the largest volume of clot.
6) Perform a gentle test injection of 1–2 mL of contrast for a venogram, to confirm the presence of thrombus and to ensure that the microcatheter is in good position.
7) Cortical veins or deep veins like the internal cerebral veins should be very cautiously catheterized injected with only tiny volumes of contrast.
8) Do venograms with high quality DSA imaging systems using 2–4 frames per second.

Penumbra Reperfusion System

The Penumbra system uses suction and fragmentation to evacuate thrombus. It is discussed further in Chap. 9.
Technique:
1) Obtain femoral venous access and place a 90 cm. 6F sheath or a Neuron™ MAX 088 (Penumbra, Inc, Alameda, CA) in the internal jugular vein.
  a) Optional: park a diagnostic catheter in the ipsilateral internal carotid artery. Periodic angiograms during the procedure – with attention to the venous phase – allows evaluation of flow in the venous system and progress with the thrombectomy.
2) Estimate the size of the occlude vessel and choose an appropriately sized reperfusion catheter. For most venous occlusions, the Penumbra 054 system is best.
3) Give IV heparin (2,000 unit bolus and a 500 unit per hour infusion). A syringe containing protamine (50 mg) should be on the back table in case a hemorrhage occurs.
4) The guide catheter or sheath may be navigated directly into jugular vein over the hydrophilic wire. It is advantageous to use the right jugular in most cases, particularly if the superior sagittal sinus (SSS) is the target, because the right internal jugular is usually larger than the left, and because the SSS usually drains toward the right. Position the tip guide catheter as distally as possible.
5) The Reperfusion Catheter is then advanced over a microwire with a J-tip curve through the guide catheter and into the target vessel. The Reperfusion Catheter need only be navigated into a large vessel just proximal to the clot. A Reperfusion Catheter angiogram or an arterial angiogram can be done to confirm that the microcatheter tip is at the proximal face of the clot.

6) Larger Reperfusion Catheters (e.g. 041 or 054) are more easily advanced in a coaxial fashion over a smaller microcatheter (e.g. SL-10 or 032 catheters, respectively).
7) The Separator is then carefully positioned through the Reperfusion Catheter, until the gold radio-opaque marker on the Separator is visible just past the opaque tip of the microcatheter. There can be resistance advancing the Separator if the microcatheter passes through tortuous vasculature.
8) The Reperfusion Catheter RHV is then connected to the Aspiration Pump using the supplied sterile tubing. All tubing is flushed with sterile heparinized saline and connections are tightened.
9) Turn on the Aspiration Pump and gently move the Separator in and out of the Reperfusion Catheter to fragment clot and keep the tip of the catheter free of obstructing clot.
10) Be gentle with the Separator and keep in mind, that the tip of the Separator extends beyond the tip of the catheter and can injure the vessel, especially if it is advanced into a cortical vein or at a sharp curve.
11) Aspirate for 4–5 min periods at a time, and recheck with contrast injections via an arterial angiographic catheter to assess progress.
12) If a large quantity of liquid blood is aspirated, the Reperfusion Catheter tip may be too proximal.
13) If arterial catheter angiograms show incomplete venous recanalization, consider adding a thrombolytic agent and/or doing additional passes with the Penumbra system.
14) Several passes with the device may be required.
15) When firm clot that will not break up or be aspirated is encountered, a pass with a Merci retriever, a balloon, or a larger Penumbra Reperfusion Catheter may be helpful.

Thrombolysis

1) Draw up the thrombolytic agent and put it in specially marked 3 mL syringes. Most operators use tPA (Activase,® Genentech, South San Francisco, CA) mixed at a dilution of 1 mg mL and injected at a rate of approximately 1 mL/min.
2) Inject the tPA while slowly withdrawing and advancing the microcatheter through the thrombus to lace the clot with tPA.
3) Periodically use the soft microwire to gently probe the clot to create fissures in the thrombus to increase the surface area upon which the tPA can act.
4) A convenient technique is to use a large-lumen microcatheter, such as the Rapid Transit® (Codman Neurovascular, Raynham, MA), with a 0.012 in. J-Tip Headliner™ (Microvention, Tustin, CA) or other small wire to maintain wire access and continually probe the clot with the wire, since the tPA can be infused through the microcatheter around the wire.
5) Periodically (every 15 min or so) do a microcatheter angiogram to see if the thrombus is breaking up.
6) After every 10 mg of tPA infusion, advance the microcatheter to a new area of clot, and lace that region with tPA as well.
7) Do not exceed 0.9 mg tPA/kg body weight; a total of 30–40 mg is usually sufficient in the typical case.
8) Do not expect to get a complete resolution of the thrombus by the thrombolytic agent during the procedure. All that is required is a continuous channel through the clot, and the tPA and endogenous plasminogen activators will continue to work for hours after the procedure.
9) If, after about 30 min of tPA infusion and gentle guidewire probing, there is no significant improvement in flow through the vessel, the addition of balloon or catheter thrombectomy can be done to speed the process.
10) Although many hours of thrombolytic infusion to thoroughly clean out all the thrombus have been used in some cases, it is usually good enough to stop after achieving some flow through the sinus. This can usually be accomplished in an hour or two of treatment.
11) If, after restoration of flow in the vein, an underlying stenosis is seen, placement of a self-expanding stent to improve flow may be considered. (see Sect. 12.7)

Balloon-Assisted Thrombolysis

1) Use balloons only in the larger dural venous sinuses.
2) Begin by advancing a microcatheter and a soft-tip, 0.014 in. exchange-length microwire, such as a floppy-tip Transend™ or Synchro™ (Stryker Neurovascular, Fremont, CA) with a wire tip shaped in a tight J-shaped configuration.

3) Advance the microwire as distally as possible in the thrombosed venous sinus.
4) Exchange the microcatheter for a low-compliance, 2–3 mm diameter angioplasty balloon such as the NC Ranger™ (Boston Scientific, Natick, MA) or NC Raptor™ (Cordis Endovascular, Miami, FL).
   a) Alternatively, a compliant balloon catheter such as a Hyperglide™ (ev3, Irvine, CA) or Ascent® balloon (Codman Neurovascular, Raynham, MA) may work. These types of balloons are best advanced primarily from the guide catheter and into the clot.
5) Once the balloon is positioned in the thrombus, slowly inflate under low pressure to create a small channel. Keep the balloon positioned centrally in the sinus to avoid exerting pressure on the wall.
6) While maintaining microwire access in the sinus, slowly withdraw the uninflated balloon and perform repeated inflations and deflations as the balloon is pulled back through the clot.
7) When the balloon has reached the proximal end of the clot, either re-advance the balloon repeatedly with slightly larger volume inflations, or exchange it for a balloon with a slightly larger diameter. The goal is to slowly and gently dilate a channel though the full extent of the clot to restore flow.
8) If over-the-wire balloon is used, or the Ascent® balloon, further injections of thrombolytic agent can be made by either one can periodically removing the wire or by using a small 0.010 in. wire.
9) If an underlying stenosis is seen after restoration of flow in the vein, placement of a self-expanding stent to improve flow may be indicated (see Sect. 12.7.4).

Rheolytic Catheter Use

The main advantage rheolytic catheters is that they physically remove clot to quickly restore flow and decrease the likelihood of embolization of clot fragments to the lung. This technique works best when used in conjunction with thrombolytic therapy, since the thrombolytic aids in softening and fragmenting the clot into smaller pieces suitable for aspiration into the rheolytic catheter. However, rheolytic catheters can also be used without simultaneous use of thrombolytic drugs and they provide a treatment option for patients who have had recent trauma, surgery or extensive intracranial bleeding, making the use of thrombolytic agents contraindicated because of for hemorrhagic risk. The relatively stiff rheolytic catheters are only suitable for use in the larger dural venous sinuses, such as the sigmoid and transverse sinuses and the larger, posterior part of the superior sagittal sinus.
Technique
1) Use a large and stable guide catheter, such as a 6F Cook shuttle or a Neuron™ MAX 088 (Penumbra, Inc, Alameda, CA).
2) After obtaining microcatheter access to the intracranial venous sinuses, advance a 300 cm 0.014 in. microwire across the torcula, into the contralateral transverse and sigmoid sinus, and, preferably, down and into the contralateral internal jugular vein. This provides very stable wire support.
3) Remove the microcatheter, leaving the 0.014 in. exchange-length microwire in place.
4) Prepare the rheolytic catheter according to the manufacturer's recommendations. If the AngioJet® XMI® catheter (Possis Medical, Minneapolis, MN) is used, prepare the Drive Unit and Pump Set, according to the recommended set up procedures, to the letter. Skipping setps will cause the system to not work properly.
5) Advance the rheolytic catheter over the exchange-length microwire.
6) If resistance is encountered, the microwire should be gently pulled back, either by rotating the wire, or rapidly pushing forward and pulling back on the catheter a few millimeters at a time to reduce friction.
7) Monitor the guide catheter position continuously. If the guide catheter pushes back and buckles in the right atrium, it can cause arrhythmias.
8) If guide catheter stability is a problem, use a larger, stiffer system, or "Tower of Power," consisting of a 100 cm guide catheter within a 90 cm sheath.
9) Another option is to advance a relatively flexible guide catheter, like a 6F Neuron™ 070 Guide catheter (Penumbra, Inc., Alameda, CA) into the sigmoid sinus as distally as possible to bypass the curves in this region.
10) If microwire stability is a problem, use a stiffer, coronary exchange.
11) Once the rheolytic catheter is positioned within the thrombosed sinus, advance it through the clot as distal as possible.

12) Open the stopcocks be opened and operate the suction pump according to manufacturer's directions. Pass the catheter through the clot while aspirating while keeping the microwire in a stable position.

13) The catheter may be re-advanced into the clot for repeat aspiration as necessary until flow is restored.

14) If aspiration is not possible, the catheter may be clogged and will have to be removed and replaced.

15) If only pure blood appears to be aspirating, a channel in the clot may already have been created. Reposition the microwire in a different part of the clot, or use a larger catheter to aspirate a greater amount of thrombus and increase the size of the patent channel.

16) Do not attempt to remove every bit of thrombus, as too much blood is likely to be aspirated in the process.

17) If an underlying stenosis is found after aspiration of the thrombus, consider using a self-expanding stent to improve flow (see Sect. 12.7).

Post-procedure Care

After the procedure, patients will require close monitoring and intensive medical management. Intracranial pressure must be monitored and controlled. In extreme cases, this may require decompressive craniectomy and/or barbiturate coma induction.[104] Periodic CT scans should be done to confirm resolution of edema, and to look for hemorrhagic transformation or rethrombosis of the venous structures. The patient should be continued on systemic heparin, if possible, and later placed on warfarin therapy to prevent rethrombosis. Add an antiplatelet therapy with aspirin and clopidogril, if a stent was placed. Long term anticoagulation may be required, since recurrent CVT or other venous thrombosis may occur after 3–6 months later in 5.5–26% of these patients.[105]

12.7.   Transvenous Stenting

Background

Symptomatic intracranial venous sinus stenosis can be effectively treated with endovascular therapy. Unlike some arterial lesions, however, venous sinus stenosis rarely responds to balloon angioplasty alone, due to the elastic recoil of the walls of the sinus and the lack of adequate high pressure in the vessel to maintain patency. Therefore stent placement is required to ensure continued patency of the venous sinus. Another peculiarity of dural sinus stenosis is that the target vessel normal diameter is generally fairly large, requiring a stiff delivery system; yet the jugular bulb and sigmoid sinuses may be sharply angulated, making it advantageous to have a more flexible delivery system. The challenges of performing endovascular stenting of venous sinuses arise from this dilemma. Endovascular treatment of intracranial venous sinus stenosis is an emerging field with only a few isolated cases reports and small clinical series.

Indications for Venous Stenting

1) Symptoms of intracranial venous hypertension due to venous stenosis.
2) Intracranial venous hypertension in the setting of dAVFs.
3) Pulsatile tinnitus caused by venous stenosis, varix or jugular diverticulum.

Complications of Venous Stenting

Informed consent prior to the procedure should include an estimate of the risk of complications.

Neurological Complications

1) Transient headaches are very common. They are likely due to the stretching of the dural walls of the sinus by the self-expanding stent, and may last 1–3 weeks.
   a) Always carefully choose the size of the stent and avoid oversizing it, to limit the resultant headaches.
2) There is a risk of acute or delayed thrombosis of the venous structures catheterized, with resultant venous infarction.
3) Oversized stent placement or aggressive balloon angioplasty in intracranial vessels can rupture venous structures, potentially producing epidural, subdural, subarachnoid or intracerebral bleeding.
4) In-stent stenosis due to neointimal hyperplasia, with recurrent symptoms of venous hypertension has been reported.[106]
5) Statistics on complications of venous stenting are lacking, since it is an uncommon procedure.

Non-neurological Complications

1) Stenting or angioplasty of the jugular bulb or sigmoid sinus carries a risk of a profound vagal response, including bradycardia, hypotension, and even cardiac arrest.
2) Anaphylactic reactions to iodinated contrast or any of the medications used can occur as with any endovascular procedure.
3) Groin hematomas can occur, but are less common and less severe compared to arterial punctures
4) Deep vein thrombosis, pulmonary emboli, and other thrombotic events may occur.

Venous Stenting: Technique

Venous Access

Venous stenting procedures are usually done with a femoral vein 6 or 7F Shuttle® sheath (Cook Inc., Bloomington, IN). However, direct puncture of the internal jugular vein and placement of a 10 cm 6 or 7F sheath in the internal jugular vein is sometimes necessary.

Anti-thrombotic Medications

Any patient undergoing intracranial venous stenting should be treated with dual antiplatelet therapy (see Chap. 4). Do platelet function testing if desired (see Chap. 4). During the procedure, after access is obtained, administer 50–70 units/kg intravenous heparin bolus and hourly boluses as needed to keep the activated clotting times at least double the baseline value.

Wires and Catheters for Venous Stenting

Access Wires
- Steerable hydrophilic wires such as 0.035 or 0.038 in. angled Glidewire® (Terumo Medical, Somerset, NJ) can be used to advance the guide catheter into the jugular vein.
- Softer, yet torquable wires such as the Headliner™ (Microvention, Tustin, CA) or Gold-tip Glidewire® (Terumo Medical, Somerset, NJ) are helpful for navigating the sometimes pesky valves in the lower internal jugular.
- Soft-tip Transend™ or Synchro™ (Stryker Neurovascular, Fremont, CA) or other 0.014 in. wire is used to advance the stent delivery catheter to the target vessel.
- Often, extra-support platinum-tipped, stainless steel coronary wires may be required to advance the stiff stent delivery catheter.

Venography Catheters

Large-lumen microcatheters, such as the RapidTransit® (Cordis Neurovascular, Miami Lakes, FL), are used for intracranial venography prior to stent placement, and to allow wire access across the stenosis.

Stents for Venous Stenting

- Self-expanding stents allow for slow, atraumatic expansion of the stenosis.
- Nitinol (as opposed to stainless steel) stents cause limited artifact on MRI, allowing for follow-up brain imaging with MRA.
- The stent should be sized to cover the area of stenosis and have a diameter sized to the normal vessel on either side of the stenosis. Intracranial sinuses generally measure between 5 and 8 mm in diameter.
- Over-the-wire stent delivery catheters may require exchange length (300 cm) microwires. Over-the-wire systems can be awkward, but they navigate more easily through tight curves and stenotic regions compared to more convenient rapid-exchange versions of the stent systems.
- Precise® Stents (Cordis/Johnson and Johnson, Piscataway, NJ) come in sizes ranging from 5 to 10 mm diameter and have a relatively flexible delivery system. They can also accept up to a 0.018 in. guidewire for added support.
- The Acculink™ stent (Guidant, Santa Clara, CA) also comes in a variety of sizes and has a very smooth, tapered distal tip which crosses stenoses easily, but the delivery catheter is stiff, making it tricky to negotiate tight curves.
- Balloon-expandable stents are generally not recommended for venous stenting, since the rapid balloon dilation carries a risk of rupturing the vessel.

Procedures

Intracranial Access

1. Under roadmap guidance, advance the large-lumen microcatheter over the microwire gently through the internal jugular vein and into the intracranial venous sinuses and advance the catheter across the stenosis to be stented.
2. Periodically remove the microwire and inject contrast through the microcatheter to obtain roadmap images to help with navigation. Alternatively, a diagnostic angiography catheter, parked in the internal carotid artery, can also be used to make venous-phase roadmaps.
3. Advance the microcatheter across the region of stenosis, and do a venogram to confirm the presence and severity of stenosis, and do pressure measurements to confirm that the stenosis is hemodynamically significant (i.e., that there is at least 10 mmHg gradient across the stenosis).
4. Once the stenosis is localized, characterized and measured, select a stent that will cover the lesion sufficiently in length, and that has a nominal diameter of the normal vessel proximal and distal to the lesion.
5. Using the microcatheter, advance a 0.014 in., 300 cm wire as far as possible beyond the stenosis. If the region to be stented is in the transverse or sigmoid sinuses, advance the microwire across the torcular Herophili and into the contralateral internal jugular vein to obtain maximal microwire support.
6. If the stenosis is in the superior sagittal or straight sinus, choices for wire access are more limited. Make sure that the tip of the microwire is in a reasonably large and straight vein and not against the wall of the vein, to limit the risk of wire perforation.
7. Remove the microcatheter once the wire is appropriately positioned, being careful to leave the exchange-length microwire in good position.

Stent Placement

1. If, and only if, the stenosis measures less than the crossing diameter of the stent delivery system, one may have to pre-dilate with a small, low compliance angioplasty balloon. Usually a 3–4 mm balloon, *very slowly* inflated under low pressure, will dilate the stenotic area enough to get the stent in place.

2. After preparing the stent by flushing all lumens according to the manufacturer's instructions, attach an RHV and continuous heparinized saline drip to the lumen of the stent delivery catheter.
3. Advance the stent catheter over the microwire and position it across the stenosis.
4. Stent catheter navigation is rarely easy because tortuosity in the sigmoid sinus produces resistance.
5. Tips for getting the stent delivery catheter to advance beyond areas of resistance caused by tortuosity or stenosis:
    a. Optimal positioning of the guide catheter or Shuttle is critical. Advance the guide catheter as distally as possible.
        i. A triaxial system, using an intermediate catheter (a Neuron or DAC), can stabilize the guide catheter or sheath and help with distal navigation. Using a triaxial system, a Cook Shuttle can often be advanced into the sigmoid sinus.
    b. Rotate the microwire while advancing the stent catheter.
    c. Advance the stent catheter using rapid, jerky forward movements alternating with slight backward movements.
    d. Rotate the patient's head away from or toward the side of the lesion.
    e. Try a stiffer wire, such as a 0.014 in. stainless steel coronary support wire or a 0.018 in. wire, if the stent catheter will accommodate a wire that size.
    f. If possible, advance the wire across the torcula and down the contralateral jugular as far as possible, to provide further support.
    g. If one is using femoral venous access, switching to jugular venous access may be considered for greater pushability.
6. Position the stent across the region of stenosis. If it is not clear that the stent is appropriately positioned by using roadmap images or bony landmark, it may be necessary to perform an arterial injection for a roadmap, or, if an over-the-wire stent delivery system is being used, the microwire can be removed from the catheter and contrast injected through the central lumen of the stent delivery catheter to opacify the vein for a good roadmap. Do not forget to re-insert the microwire before deploying the stent to ensure proper stent deployment.
7. Deploy the self-expanding stent across the stenosis.
8. Remove the stent delivery system while leaving the wire in place.
9. If, and only if, there is still severe stenosis and the stent does not look like it will open the vessel, a gentle post-dilation may be performed with a low-compliance balloon shorter than the stent and undersized 20% less than the size of the normal vessel diameter within the lesion.
10. Otherwise, advance the large-lumen microcatheter through the stent and into the vessel beyond it.
11. Perform venograms and pressure measurements to see the results of the stent placement and check for any residual pressure gradient across the stent.
12. If the stent is appropriately sized, a gradual expansion of the stent will occur after deployment. Do not worry about moderate residual stenosis immediately after stent placement.

Postprocedure Care

Daily dual antiplatelet therapy, usually consisting of clopidogril and aspirin is to be continued for 90 days, followed by long-term aspirin. The authors obtain a follow-up CT venogram in 3–6 months, then annually, or as needed if symptoms do not resolve.

References

1. Ayanzen RH, Bird CR, Keller PJ, McCully FJ, Theobald MR, Heiserman JE. Cerebral MR venography: normal anatomy and potential diagnostic pitfalls. AJNR Am J Neuroradiol. 2000;21:74–8.

2. Henkes H, Felber SR, Wentz KU, et al. Accuracy of intravascular microcatheter pressure measurements: an experimental study. Br J Radiol. 1999;72:448–51.

3. Murayama Y, Massoud TF, Vinuela F. Transvenous hemodynamic assessment of experimental arteriovenous malformations. Doppler guidewire monitoring of embolotherapy in a swine model. Stroke. 1996;27:1365–72.

4. Sekhar LN, Pomeranz S, Janecka IP, Hirsch B, Ramasastry S. Temporal bone neoplasms: a report on 20 surgically treated cases. J Neurosurg. 1992;76:578–87.

5. Spetzler RF, Daspit CP, Pappas CT. The combined supra- and infratentorial approach for lesions of the petrous and clival regions: experience with 46 cases. J Neurosurg. 1992;76:588–99.

6. Schmid-Elsaesser R, Steiger HJ, Yousry T, Seelos KC, Reulen HJ. Radical resection of meningiomas and arteriovenous fistulas involving critical dural sinus segments: experience with intraoperative sinus pressure monitoring and elective sinus reconstruction in 10 patients. Neurosurgery. 1997;41:1005–16; discussion 16–8.

7. Houdart E, Saint-Maurice JP, Boissonnet H, Bonnin P. Clinical and hemodynamic responses to balloon test occlusion of the straight sinus: technical case report. Neurosurgery. 2002;51:254–6; discussion 6–7.

8. Doppman JL. There is no simple answer to a rare complication of inferior petrosal sinus sampling. AJNR Am J Neuroradiol. 1999;20:191–2.

9. Miller DL, Doppman JL, Peterman SB, Nieman LK, Oldfield EH, Chang R. Neurologic complications of petrosal sinus sampling. Radiology. 1992;185:143–7.

10. Sturrock ND, Jeffcoate WJ. A neurological complication of inferior petrosal sinus sampling during investigation for Cushing's disease: a case report. J Neurol Neurosurg Psychiatry. 1997;62:527–8.

11. Bonelli FS, Huston 3rd J, Meyer FB, Carpenter PC. Venous subarachnoid hemorrhage after inferior petrosal sinus sampling for adrenocorticotropic hormone. AJNR Am J Neuroradiol. 1999;20:306–7.

12. Lefournier V, Gatta B, Martinie M, et al. One transient neurological complication (sixth nerve palsy) in 166 consecutive inferior petrosal sinus samplings for the etiological diagnosis of Cushing's syndrome. J Clin Endocrinol Metab. 1999;84:3401–2.

13. Blevins Jr LS, Clark RV, Owens DS. Thromboembolic complications after inferior petrosal sinus sampling in patients with cushing's syndrome. Endocr Pract. 1998;4:365–7.

14. Refetoff S, Van Cauter E, Fang VS, Laderman C, Graybeal ML, Landau RL. The effect of dexamethasone on the 24-hour profiles of adrenocorticotropin and cortisol in Cushing's syndrome. J Clin Endocrinol Metab. 1985;60:527–35.

15. Van Cauter E, Refetoff S. Evidence for two subtypes of Cushing's disease based on the analysis of episodic cortisol secretion. N Engl J Med. 1985;312:1343–9.

16. Oldfield EH, Doppman JL, Nieman LK, et al. Petrosal sinus sampling with and without corticotropin-releasing hormone for the differential diagnosis of Cushing's syndrome. N Engl J Med. 1991;325:897–905.

17. Bonelli FS, Huston 3rd J, Carpenter PC, Erickson D, Young Jr WF, Meyer FB. Adrenocorticotropic hormone-dependent Cushing's syndrome: sensitivity and specificity of inferior petrosal sinus sampling. AJNR Am J Neuroradiol. 2000; 21:690–6.

18. Kaltsas GA, Giannulis MG, Newell-Price JD, et al. A critical analysis of the value of simultaneous inferior petrosal sinus sampling in Cushing's disease and the occult ectopic adrenocorticotropin syndrome. J Clin Endocrinol Metab. 1999;84:487–92.

19. Colao A, Faggiano A, Pivonello R, Pecori Giraldi F, Cavagnini F, Lombardi G. Inferior petrosal sinus sampling in the differential diagnosis of Cushing's syndrome: results of

20. Graham KE, Samuels MH, Nesbit GM, et al. Cavernous sinus sampling is highly accurate in distinguishing Cushing's disease from the ectopic adrenocorticotropin syndrome and in predicting intrapituitary tumor location. J Clin Endocrinol Metab. 1999;84:1602–10.

21. Oldfield EH, Girton ME, Doppman JL. Absence of intercavernous venous mixing: evidence supporting lateralization of pituitary microadenomas by venous sampling. J Clin Endocrinol Metab. 1985;61:644–7.

22. Manni A, Latshaw RF, Page R, Santen RJ. Simultaneous bilateral venous sampling for adrenocorticotropin in pituitary-dependent cushing's disease: evidence for lateralization of pituitary venous drainage. J Clin Endocrinol Metab. 1983;57:1070–3.

23. Doppman JL, Chang R, Oldfield EH, Chrousos G, Stratakis CA, Nieman LK. The hypoplastic inferior petrosal sinus: a potential source of false-negative results in petrosal sampling for Cushing's disease. J Clin Endocrinol Metab. 1999;84:533–40.

24. Mamelak AN, Dowd CF, Tyrrell JB, McDonald JF, Wilson CB. Venous angiography is needed to interpret inferior petrosal sinus and cavernous sinus sampling data for lateralizing adrenocorticotropin-secreting adenomas. J Clin Endocrinol Metab. 1996;81:475–81.

25. Kalogeras KT, Nieman LK, Friedman TC, et al. Inferior petrosal sinus sampling in healthy subjects reveals a unilateral corticotropin-releasing hormone-induced arginine vasopressin release associated with ipsilateral adrenocorticotropin secretion. J Clin Invest. 1996;97:2045–50.

26. Ratliff JK, Oldfield EH. Multiple pituitary adenomas in Cushing's disease. J Neurosurg. 2000;93:753–61.

27. Kim LJ, Klopfenstein JD, Cheng M, et al. Ectopic intracavernous sinus adrenocorticotropic hormone-secreting microadenoma: could this be a common cause of failed transsphenoidal surgery in Cushing disease? Case report. J Neurosurg. 2003; 98:1312–7.

28. Miller DL, Doppman JL, Nieman LK, et al. Petrosal sinus sampling: discordant lateralization of ACTH-secreting pituitary microadenomas before and after stimulation with corticotropin-releasing hormone. Radiology. 1990;176:429–31.

29. Liu C, Lo JC, Dowd CF, et al. Cavernous and inferior petrosal sinus sampling in the evaluation of ACTH-dependent Cushing's syndrome. Clin Endocrinol (Oxf). 2004;61:478–86.

30. Doppman JL, Nieman LK, Chang R, et al. Selective venous sampling from the cavernous sinuses is not a more reliable technique than sampling from the inferior petrosal sinuses in Cushing's syndrome. J Clin Endocrinol Metab. 1995;80:2485–9.

31. Fujimura M, Ikeda H, Takahashi A, Ezura M, Yoshimoto T, Tominaga T. Diagnostic value of super-selective bilateral cavernous sinus sampling with hypothalamic stimulating hormone loading in patients with ACTH-producing pituitary adenoma. Neurol Res. 2005;27:11–5.

32. Teramoto A, Nemoto S, Takakura K, Sasaki Y, Machida T. Selective venous sampling directly from cavernous sinus in Cushing's syndrome. J Clin Endocrinol Metab. 1993;76:637–41.

33. Lefournier V, Martinie M, Vasdev A, et al. Accuracy of bilateral inferior petrosal or cavernous sinuses sampling in predicting the lateralization of Cushing's disease pituitary microadenoma: influence of catheter position and anatomy of venous drainage. J Clin Endocrinol Metab. 2003;88:196–203.

34. Ilias I, Chang R, Pacak K, et al. Jugular venous sampling: an alternative to petrosal sinus sampling for the diagnostic evaluation of adrenocorticotropic hormone-dependent Cushing's syndrome. J Clin Endocrinol Metab. 2004;89:3795–800.

35. Swearingen B, Katznelson L, Miller K, et al. Diagnostic errors after inferior petrosal sinus sampling. J Clin Endocrinol Metab. 2004;89:3752–63.

36. Doppman JL, Miller DL, Patronas NJ, et al. The diagnosis of acromegaly: value of inferior petrosal sinus sampling. AJR Am J Roentgenol. 1990;154:1075–7.

37. Crock PA, Gilford EJ, Henderson JK, et al. Inferior petrosal sinus sampling in acromegaly. Aust N Z J Med. 1989; 19:244–7.

38. Miller DL, Doppman JL, Krudy AG, et al. Localization of parathyroid adenomas in patients who have undergone surgery. Part II. Invasive procedures. Radiology. 1987;162:138–41.

39. Chaffanjon PC, Voirin D, Vasdev A, Chabre O, Kenyon NM, Brichon PY. Selective venous sampling in recurrent and persistent hyperparathyroidism: indication, technique, and results. World J Surg. 2004;28:958–61.

40. Zurin AA, Ushikoshi S, Houkin K, Kikuchi Y, Abe H, Saitoh H. Cerebral abscess as an unusual complication of coil embolization in a dural arteriovenous fistula. Case report. J Neurosurg. 1997;87:109–12.

41. Klisch J, Huppertz HJ, Spetzger U, Hetzel A, Seeger W, Schumacher M. Transvenous treatment of carotid cavernous and dural arteriovenous fistulae: results for 31 patients and review of the literature. Neurosurgery. 2003;53:836–56; discussion 56–7.

42. Meyers PM, Halbach VV, Dowd CF, et al. Dural carotid cavernous fistula: definitive endovascular management and longterm follow-up. Am J Ophthalmol. 2002;134:85–92.

43. Nakagawa H, Kubo S, Nakajima Y, Izumoto S, Fujita T. Shifting of Dural arteriovenous malformation from the cavernous sinus to the sigmoid sinus to the transverse sinus after transvenous embolization. A case of left spontaneous carotidcavernous sinus fistula. Surg Neurol. 1992;37:30–8.

44. Yamashita K, Taki W, Nakahara I, Nishi S, Sadato A, Kikuchi H. Development of sigmoid dural arteriovenous fistulas after transvenous embolization of cavernous dural arteriovenous fistulas. AJNR Am J Neuroradiol. 1993;14:1106–8.

45. Horowitz MB, Purdy PD, Valentine RJ, Morrill K. Remote vascular catastrophes after neurovascular interventional therapy for type 4 Ehlers-Danlos syndrome. AJNR Am J Neuroradiol. 2000;21:974–6.

46. Chuman H, Trobe JD, Petty EM, et al. Spontaneous direct carotid-cavernous fistula in Ehlers-Danlos syndrome type IV: two case reports and a review of the literature. J Neuroophthalmol. 2002;22:75–81.

47. Halbach VV, Higashida RT, Hieshima GB, Hardin CW, Pribram H. Transvenous embolization of dural fistulas involving the cavernous sinus. AJNR Am J Neuroradiol. 1989; 10:377–83.

48. Goto K, Hieshima GB, Higashida RT, et al. Treatment of direct carotid cavernous sinus fistulae. Various therapeutic approaches and results in 148 cases. Acta Radiol Suppl. 1986;369:576–9.

49. Halbach VV, Higashida RT, Dowd CF, Barnwell SL, Hieshima GB. Treatment of carotid-cavernous fistulas associated with Ehlers-Danlos syndrome. Neurosurgery. 1990;26:1021–7.

50. Miller NR, Monsein LH, Debrun GM, Tamargo RJ, Nauta HJ. Treatment of carotid-cavernous sinus fistulas using a superior ophthalmic vein approach. J Neurosurg. 1995;83:838–42.

51. Chun GF, Tomsick TA. Transvenous embolization of a direct carotid cavernous fistula through the pterygoid plexus. AJNR Am J Neuroradiol. 2002;23:1156–9.

52. Barker 2nd FG, Ogilvy CS, Chin JK, Joseph MP, Pile-Spellman J, Crowell RM. Transethmoidal transsphenoidal approach for embolization of a carotid-cavernous fistula. Case report. J Neurosurg. 1994;81:921–3.

53. Benndorf G, Bender A, Lehmann R, Lanksch W. Transvenous occlusion of dural cavernous sinus fistulas through the thrombosed inferior petrosal sinus: report of four cases and review of the literature. Surg Neurol. 2000;54:42–54.

54. Monsein LH, Debrun GM, Miller NR, Nauta HJ, Chazaly JR. Treatment of dural carotid-cavernous fistulas via the superior ophthalmic vein. AJNR Am J Neuroradiol. 1991;12:435–9.

55. Quinones D, Duckwiler G, Gobin PY, Goldberg RA, Vinuela F. Embolization of dural cavernous fistulas via superior ophthalmic vein approach. AJNR Am J Neuroradiol. 1997;18:921–8.

56. Wolfe SQ, Cumberbatch NM, Aziz-Sultan MA, Tummala R, Morcos JJ. Operative approach via the superior ophthalmic vein for the endovascular treatment of carotid cavernous fistulas that fail traditional endovascular access. Neurosurgery. 2010;66:293–9; discussion 9.

57. Oishi H, Arai H, Sato K, Iizuka Y. Complications associated with transvenous embolisation of cavernous dural arteriovenous fistula. Acta Neurochir (Wien). 1999;141:1265–71.

58. Goldberg RA, Goldey SH, Duckwiler G, Vinuela F. Management of cavernous sinus-dural fistulas. Indications and techniques for primary embolization via the superior ophthalmic vein. Arch Ophthalmol. 1996;114:707–14.

59. Gupta N, Kikkawa DO, Levi L, Weinreb RN. Severe vision loss and neovascular glaucoma complicating superior ophthalmic vein approach to carotid-cavernous sinus fistula. Am J Ophthalmol. 1997;124:853–5.

60. Benndorf G, Bender A, Campi A, Menneking H, Lanksch WR. Treatment of a cavernous sinus dural arteriovenous fistula by deep orbital puncture of the superior ophthalmic vein. Neuroradiology. 2001;43:499–502.

61. Kohyama S, Kaji T, Tokumaru AM, Kusano S, Ishihara S, Shima K. Transfemoral superior ophthalmic vein approach via the facial vein for the treatment of carotid-cavernous fistulas–two case reports. Neurol Med Chir (Tokyo). 2002;42:18–22.

62. Biondi A, Milea D, Cognard C, Ricciardi GK, Bonneville F, van Effenterre R. Cavernous sinus dural fistulae treated by transvenous approach through the facial vein: report of seven cases and review of the literature. AJNR Am J Neuroradiol. 2003;24:1240–6.

63. Venturi C, Bracco S, Cerase A, et al. Endovascular treatment of a cavernous sinus dural arteriovenous fistula by transvenous embolisation through the superior ophthalmic vein via cannulation of a frontal vein. Neuroradiology. 2003;45:574–8.

64. Kazekawa K, Iko M, Sakamoto S, et al. Dural AVFs of the cavernous sinus: transvenous embolization using a direct superficial temporal vein approach. Radiat Med. 2003;21:138–41.

65. Mounayer C, Piotin M, Spelle L, Moret J. Superior petrosal sinus catheterization for transvenous embolization of a dural carotid cavernous sinus fistula. AJNR Am J Neuroradiol. 2002;23:1153–5.

66. Kuwayama N, Endo S, Kitabayashi M, Nishijima M, Takaku A. Surgical transvenous embolization of a cortically draining carotid cavernous fistula via a vein of the sylvian fissure. AJNR Am J Neuroradiol. 1998;19:1329–32.

67. Hara T, Hamada J, Kai Y, Ushio Y. Surgical transvenous embolization of a carotid-cavernous dural fistula with cortical drainage via a petrosal vein: two technical case reports. Neurosurgery. 2002;50:1380–3; discussion 3–4.

68. Wakhloo AK, Perlow A, Linfante I, et al. Transvenous n-butyl-cyanoacrylate infusion for complex dural carotid cavernous fistulas: technical considerations and clinical outcome. AJNR Am J Neuroradiol. 2005;26:1888–97.

69. Arat A, Cekirge S, Saatci I, Ozgen B. Transvenous injection of Onyx for casting of the cavernous sinus for the treatment of a carotid-cavernous fistula. Neuroradiology. 2004;46:1012–5.

70. Deguchi J, Yamada M, Ogawa R, Kuroiwa T. Transvenous embolization for a purely extraorbital arteriovenous fistula. Case report. J Neurosurg. 2005;103:756–9.

71. Caragine LP, Halbach Jr VV, Dowd CF, Higashida RT. Intraorbital arteriovenous fistulae of the ophthalmic veins treated by transvenous endovascular occlusion: technical case report. Neurosurgery. 2006;58:ONS-E170; discussion ONS-E170.

72. Halbach VV, Higashida RT, Hieshima GB, Mehringer CM, Hardin CW. Transvenous embolization of dural fistulas involving the transverse and sigmoid sinuses. AJNR Am J Neuroradiol. 1989;10:385–92.

73. Dawson 3rd RC, Joseph GJ, Owens DS, Barrow DL. Transvenous embolization as the primary therapy for arteriovenous fistulas of the lateral and sigmoid sinuses. AJNR Am J Neuroradiol. 1998;19:571–6.

74. Roy D, Raymond J. The role of transvenous embolization in the treatment of intracranial dural arteriovenous fistulas. Neurosurgery. 1997;40:1133–41; discussion 41–4.

75. Gobin YP, Houdart E, Rogopoulos A, Casasco A, Bailly AL, Merland JJ. Percutaneous transvenous embolization through the thrombosed sinus in transverse sinus dural fistula. AJNR Am J Neuroradiol. 1993;14:1102–5.

76. Naito I, Iwai T, Shimaguchi H, et al. Percutaneous transvenous embolisation through the occluded sinus for transverse-sigmoid dural arteriovenous fistulas with sinus occlusion. Neuroradiology. 2001;43:672–6.

77. Houdart E, Saint-Maurice JP, Chapot R, et al. Transcranial approach for venous embolization of dural arteriovenous fistulas. J Neurosurg. 2002;97:280–6.

78. Liebig T, Henkes H, Brew S, Miloslavski E, Kirsch M, Kuhne D. Reconstructive treatment of dural arteriovenous fistulas of the transverse and sigmoid sinus: transvenous angioplasty and stent deployment. Neuroradiology. 2005;47:543–51.

79. Defreyne L, Vanlangenhove P, Vandekerckhove T, et al. Transvenous embolization of a dural arteriovenous fistula of the anterior cranial fossa: preliminary results. AJNR Am J Neuroradiol. 2000;21:761–5.

80. Cloft HJ, Kallmes DF, Jensen JE, Dion JE. Percutaneous transvenous coil embolization of a type 4 sagittal sinus dural arteriovenous fistula: case report. Neurosurgery. 1997;41: 1191–3; discussion 3–4.

81. King WA, Martin NA. Intracerebral hemorrhage due to dural arteriovenous malformations and fistulae. Neurosurg Clin N Am. 1992;3:577–90.

82. Deasy NP, Gholkar AR, Cox TC, Jeffree MA. Tentorial dural arteriovenous fistulae: endovascular treatment with trans-venous coil embolisation. Neuroradiology. 1999;41:308–12.

83. Kallmes DF, Jensen ME, Cloft HJ, Kassell NF, Dion JE. Percutaneous transvenous coil embolization of a Djindjian type 4 tentorial dural arteriovenous malformation. AJNR Am J Neuroradiol. 1997;18:673–6.

84. Troffkin NA, Graham 3rd CB, Berkmen T, Wakhloo AK. Combined transvenous and transarterial embolization of a tentorial-incisural dural arteriovenous malformation followed by primary stent placement in the associated stenotic straight sinus. Case report. J Neurosurg. 2003;99:579–83.

85. Mickle JP, Quisling RG. The transtorcular embolization of vein of Galen aneurysms. J Neurosurg. 1986;64:731–5.

86. Dowd CF, Halbach VV, Barnwell SL, Higashida RT, Edwards MS, Hieshima GB. Transfemoral venous embolization of vein of Galen malformations. AJNR Am J Neuroradiol. 1990;11:643–8.

87. Lasjaunias P, Garcia-Monaco R, Rodesch G, et al. Vein of Galen malformation. Endovascular management of 43 cases. Childs Nerv Syst. 1991;7:360–7.

88. Lasjaunias P, Garcia-Monaco R, Rodesch G, Terbrugge K. Deep venous drainage in great cerebral vein (vein of Galen) absence and malformations. Neuroradiology. 1991;33:234–8.

89. Levrier O, Gailloud PH, Souei M, Manera L, Brunel H, Raybaud C. Normal galenic drainage of the deep cerebral venous system in two cases of vein of Galen aneurysmal malformation. Childs Nerv Syst. 2004;20:91–7; discussion 8–9.

90. Gailloud P, O'Riordan DP, Burger I, Lehmann CU. Confirmation of communication between deep venous drainage and the vein of galen after treatment of a vein of Galen aneurysmal malformation in an infant presenting with severe pulmonary hypertension. AJNR Am J Neuroradiol. 2006; 27:317–20.

91. Ng PP, Halbach VV, Quinn R, et al. Endovascular treatment for dural arteriovenous fistulae of the superior petrosal sinus. Neurosurgery. 2003;53:25–32; discussion 3.

92. Kato S, Fujii M, Tominaga T, Fujisawa H, Suzuki M. A case of dural arteriovenous fistula of the inferior petrosal sinus successfully treated by transarterial and transvenous embolizations. No Shinkei Geka. 2002;30:981–4.

93. Ernst R, Bulas R, Tomsick T, van Loveren H, Aziz KA. Three cases of dural arteriovenous fistula of the anterior condylar vein within the hypoglossal canal. AJNR Am J Neuroradiol. 1999;20:2016–20.

94. Kiyosue H, Tanoue S, Okahara M, Mori M, Mori H. Ocular symptoms associated with a dural arteriovenous fistula involving the hypoglossal canal: selective transvenous coil embolization. Case report. J Neurosurg. 2001;94:630–2.

95. Tanoue S, Goto K, Oota S. Endovascular treatment for dural arteriovenous fistula of the anterior condylar vein with unusual venous drainage: report of two cases. AJNR Am J Neuroradiol. 2005;26:1955–9.

96. Manabe H, Hasegawa S, Takemura A, Shafiqul IM, Ito C, Nagahata M. Contralateral inferior petrosal sinus approach for transvenous embolization of a dural arteriovenous fistula at isolated jugular bulb. Technical case report. Minim Invasive Neurosurg. 2003;46:366–8.

97. Beek FJ, ten Broek FW, van Schaik JP, Mali WP. Transvenous embolisation of an arteriovenous malformation of the mandible via a femoral approach. Pediatr Radiol. 1997;27:855–7.

98. Kiyosue H, Mori H, Hori Y, Okahara M, Kawano K, Mizuki H. Treatment of mandibular arteriovenous malformation by trans-venous embolization: a case report. Head Neck. 1999;21:574–7.

99. Kawano K, Mizuki H, Mori H, Yanagisawa S. Mandibular arteriovenous malformation treated by transvenous coil embolization: a long-term follow-up with special reference to bone regeneration. J Oral Maxillofac Surg. 2001;59:326–30.

100. Touho H, Monobe T, Ohnishi H, Karasawa J. Treatment of type II perimedullary arteriovenous fistulas by intraoperative transvenous embolization: case report. Surg Neurol. 1995;43:491–6.

101. Chul Suh D, Gon Choi C, Bo Sung K, Kim KK, Chul Rhim S. Spinal osseous epidural arteriovenous fistula with multiple small arterial feeders converging to a round fistular nidus as a target of venous approach. AJNR Am J Neuroradiol. 2004;25:69–73.

102. Ferro JM, Canhao P, Stam J, Bousser MG, Bacinagarrementeria F. Prognosis of cerebral vein and dural sinus thrombosis: results of the International Study on Cerebral Vein and Dural Sinus Thrombosis (ISCVT). Stroke. 2004;35:664–70.

103. Chahlavi A, Steinmetz MP, Masaryk TJ, Rasmussen PA. A transcranial approach for direct mechanical thrombectomy of dural sinus thrombosis. Report of two cases. J Neurosurg. 2004;101:347–51.

104. Smith AG, Cornblath WT, Deveikis JP. Local thrombolytic therapy in deep cerebral venous thrombosis. Neurology. 1997;48:1613–9.

105. van Nuenen BF, Munneke M, Bloem BR. Cerebral venous sinus thrombosis: prevention of recurrent thromboembolism. Stroke. 2005;36:1822–3.

106. Tsumoto T, Miyamoto T, Shimizu M, et al. Restenosis of the sigmoid sinus after stenting for treatment of intracranial venous hypertension: case report. Neuroradiology. 2003; 45:911–5.

Part 3. Specific Disease States

13. Intracranial Aneurysms and Subarachnoid Haemorrhage

An aneurysm is an abnormal dilatation of an artery. In layman terms, an aneurysm can be thought of as a weak spot in the wall of an artery, similar to a garden hose that has been filed down on one side; water under pressure inside the hose will make the weak spot bulge out. Intracranial aneurysms can be broadly classified as saccular, fusiform, or dissecting.

13.1.   Intracranial Aneurysms: Pathophysiology

Pathology of Intracranial Aneurysms

An aneurysm is, by definition, an arterial structure. Most saccular aneurysms share a common morphology.[1–3]
1) Mechanism of formation. Intracranial aneurysms appear to result from a complex series of factors including haemodynamic stress, sustained abnormal vascular remodeling, and inflammation.[4–7]
   a) Alterations in the expression of numerous genes in aneurysm walls have been identified.[8]
2) Saccular aneurysms are typically found at arterial branch points, where there is a gap in the media, although a significant percentage of aneurysms are not clearly associated with a branching vessel.
3) Gross anatomy:
   a) Unruptured aneurysms may appear uniformly pink, like adjacent arteries, or they may have red areas, representing nearly translucent regions of the aneurysm dome, through which blood can be seen. Aneurysms may also have thick, atheromatous areas as well.
   b) Ruptured aneurysms. Aneurysms typically rupture at the apex of the dome; a dense fibrin cap is usually found in this region during surgery.
4) Morphological features:
   a) Multiple lobes. Some 9% of unruptured aneurysms and 40% of ruptured aneurysms are multilobular.[9]
   b) Daughter sac. A daughter sac is found in 57% of ruptured aneurysms and 16% of unruptured aneurysms.[10] Also sometimes referred to as "Murphy's tit."
5) Site distribution (unruptured aneurysms in patients with no prior history of SAH).[11]
   a) Cavernous carotid artery, 16.9%.
      i) ICA, 24.8%.
   b) Anterior communicating or ACA, 10.0%.
   c) MCA, 22.7%.
   d) Posterior communicating artery, 13.9%.
   e) Vertebrobasilar or PCA, 6.6%.
   f) Basilar artery apex, 5.1%.
6) Single vs. multiple aneurysms:
   a) Two or more aneurysms are found in 15–30% of patients.[12–16]
   b) Risk factors for multiple aneurysms include female sex,[13–17] cigarette smoking,[13,14] hypertension,[14] a family history of cerebrovascular disease,[14] and postmenopausal state.[14]

M.R. Harrigan, J.P. Deveikis, *Handbook of Cerebrovascular Disease and Neurointerventional Technique*, DOI 10.1007/978-1-61779-946-4_13, © Springer Science+Business Media New York 2013

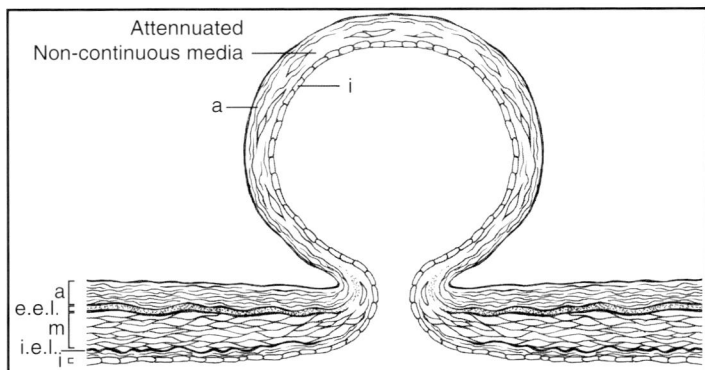

Fig. 13.1 Microscopic anatomy of an intracranial aneurysm. The internal elastic lamina is absent in the wall of the aneurysm, and the media is present but abnormal, being thin and discontinuous throughout the aneurysm dome. *a* adventitia, *m* media, *i* intima, *eel* external elastic lamina, *iel* internal elastic lamina.

7) Histopathology (Fig. 13.1):
   a) At the edge of the aneurysm neck, there is an abrupt termination of the tunica media and internal elastic lamina.
   b) The aneurysm sac is mostly composed of collagenous tissue and is frequently acellular.
   c) However, fibrin staining is present on the luminal side of the aneurysm wall in 50% of cases, and the aneurysm wall contains numerous polymorphonuclear leukocytes in 29% of cases; these findings may be a sign of "impending rupture" of the aneurysm.[10]
   d) Other "signs of impending rupture" include.[18]
      i) Unusually thin areas in the wall.
      ii) Daughter sacs.
      iii) Patchy fibrin infiltration.
      iv) Intraluminal thrombus.
      v) Inflammatory cells in the aneurysm wall.
      vi) Blood pigment containing macrophages and erythrocytes in the wall.

13.2. The Peculiar Infundibulum

An infundibulum is a conical dilatation at the origin of an artery (see Chap. 1). Infundibula are benign incidental findings. A small number of cases in which a P-comm infundibulum progressed to aneurysm formation and rupture have been reported. A total of 11 reports were analyzed by Marshman and colleagues in 1998.[19] In this review, there was a preponderance of women (female-to-male ratio, 9:1), left-sided lesions (left-to-right ratio, 9:2), and bilateral infundibula (60%).

Unruptured Intracranial Aneurysms

Prevalence

Prevalence of intracranial aneurysms in the general population:
1) A recent systematic review found that the prevalence of aneurysms for adults without SAH is approximately 3.2%:[20]

a) Sex distribution. The male/female ratio for aneurysms is approximately 1:1.3.
b) Age distribution. The prevalence of aneurysms increases with age, peaking in the 60–79 year age group.[21]
c) Prevalence is higher among patients with polycystic kidney disease, atherosclerosis, a brain tumour, and a family history of intracranial aneurysms.[20]

2) Unruptured aneurysms have been diagnosed at an increasing rate in recent years,[22] probably as a result of the improving quality and growing use of non-invasive imaging techniques.

Are Unruptured Aneurysms a Significant Cause of Headaches?
Possibly. Some 18–36% of patients presenting with unruptured aneurysms list headaches as their chief complaint.[11,23–25] Conventional thinking holds that most unruptured aneurysms are unrelated to the headaches.[26] However, a handful of studies have indicated that a significant percentage of patients' headaches improve after aneurysm treatment.[23,24] In a recent prospective study of patients undergoing either surgery or endovascular treatment, 92.45% of patients reported an improvement in their headaches by an average of 32.4 months after treatment.[26] There was no relationship between method of treatment (coiling versus clipping) and headache improvement.

Conditions Associated with Aneurysms

Familial Aneurysms

1) Definition of "familial aneurysm": When ≥2 first-degree relatives are affected.[27,28]
2) Aside from autosomal dominant polycystic kidney disease (ADPKD), a familial predisposition is the strongest risk factor for the development of intracranial aneurysms.[21]
3) Prevalence. Estimates of the frequency of familial intracranial aneurysms among all patients with aneurysms range from 7% to 20%.[28–31]
4) Inheritance patterns and features:
    a) In most pedigrees, the inheritance pattern is unclear, although autosomal dominant transmission is thought to be the most likely.[32,33]
    b) Familial aneurysms have a predilection for the middle cerebral artery.[33]
    c) Familial aneurysms are generally larger at the time of rupture and more likely to be multiple than sporadic aneurysms.[34]
    d) Subarachnoid haemorrhage tends to occur at a significantly younger age in patients with familial aneurysms compared to patients with sporadic aneurysms.[33]
    e) Patients with familial SAH have a greater risk of poor outcome than patients with sporadic SAH.[35]
5) A wide array of genes and chromosomal regions have been linked to intracranial aneurysms, of both sporadic and familial nature.[36–38]
    a) Interestingly, the Nordic Twin Cohort study, which analyzed 509 cases of SAH among it's subjects, concluded that SAH is mainly of nongenetic origin, and that familial SAHs can be mostly attributed to environmental risk factors.[39]
6) Screening in patients with familial intracranial aneurysms (Table 13.1)
    a) Controversial. A theoretical model concluded that routine screening is not advantageous, even in individuals with a history of ≥2 affected first-degree relatives with SAH.[40] The American Heart Association *Recommendations for the Management of Patients with Unruptured Intracranial Aneurysms* suggests that screening in patients at risk of familial intracranial aneurysms be done on an individual basis.[40]
    b) In most situations, the authors of this handbook prefer to use noninvasive imaging to screen patients with ≥2 first-degree relatives with aneurysms:
        i) This strategy will identify an aneurysm in 8–10% of individuals.[28,41–43]

Table 13.1 Yield of screening for asymptomatic intracranial aneurysms

Population	Risk of having an intracranial aneurysm (%)
General population	2–3
First-degree relatives in families with one affected member	2–4
First-degree relatives in families ≥2 affected members	10

Sources:[20,78]

7) The Familial Intracranial Aneurysm Study[44]
    a) Ongoing, international, multicenter study of families with a history of intracranial aneurysms.
    b) Families with at least two affected siblings are eligible.
    c) The study Web site is http://www.fiastudy.org and the toll free number 800-503-3427.

Connective Tissue Disorders

AUTOSOMAL DOMINANT POLYCYSTIC KIDNEY DISEASE

1) Most common life-threatening hereditary disease,[45] affecting 1 in 500 individuals in the United States and Europe:
    a) Expression is variable but penetrance reaches 100% by age 80.
    b) Two genes have been identified. Both are strongly expressed in vascular smooth muscle cells of normal adult arteries:
        i) *PKD1* is responsible for ~85% of ADPKD cases. It encodes polycystin 1, a membrane protein that mediates cell–cell and cell–matrix interactions.[46]
        ii) *PKD2*, responsible for most of the remaining cases of ADPKD, encodes polycystin 2, a membrane protein with homology to voltage-activated calcium channels, and is believed to interact with polycystin 1.[47]
        iii) Polycystins are involved in the functional interaction between arterial smooth muscle cells and adjacent elastic tissue or endothelial cells. Mutations in the genes for these proteins may disrupt this interaction and weaken the vessel wall.[48]
    c) ADPKD is a systemic disease:
        i) Cysts develop in the kidneys, liver, pancreas, spleen, ovaries, and seminal vesicles.
        ii) Systemic manifestations:[49] Hypertension (in 80% of patients), end-stage renal disease (in 45% of patients by age 60), and hepatic cysts (in 60% of adults). Other commonly associated conditions are pancreatic cysts, mitral valve prolapse and colonic diverticula.
    d) Neurological manifestations:
        i) Hypertensive intracerebral haemorrhage.
        ii) Ischemic stroke:
            (1) Hemorrhagic and ischemic stroke are the most common acute neurological events affecting patients with ADPKD.[50]
        iii) Intracranial aneurysms.
        iv) Cervicocephalic arterial dissections.[51]
        v) Intracranial dolichoectasia.[52]
        vi) Intracranial arachnoid cysts.[53]
        vii) Spinal meningeal diverticula.[54]
        viii) Chronic subdural hematomas.[55]
2) ADPKD and intracranial aneurysms:
    a) Estimates of the prevalence of intracranial aneurysms in patients with ADPKD: range from 4.0% to 40%:[56–59]
        i) Conversely, patients with ADPKD represent only a small fraction of patients with intracranial aneurysms.[28]
        ii) The risk of having an aneurysm in patients with ADPKD goes up with age.[59]
        iii) Most common location: ICA.[59]

b) The incidence of SAH in patients with ADPKD is estimated at approximately 1/2,000 person-years,[60] or about five times higher than the general population.[61] *However, a population-based study of the specific risk of SAH in patients with ADPKD and an unruptured aneurysm has not yet been published.*

c) The risk of having an intracranial aneurysm in a patient with ADPKD is strongly related to whether the patient has a family history of intracranial aneurysms or SAH:
   i) In three large prospective series of ADPKD, an intracranial aneurysm was found in 15.6% of patients with a family history of aneurysms versus 5.9% of patients without a family history of aneurysms.[56,57,62,63]

d) The average age of patients with ADPKD and SAH is 41, and 10% of patients are <21 years old.[64]

e) Patients with ADPKD and an aneurysm are prone to developing additional aneurysms. In an average follow-up period of 15.2 years, 25% of patients with known intracranial aneurysms were found to have at least one additional aneurysm:[65]
   i) Conversely, patients with ADPKD and no evidence of an intracranial aneurysm on radiographic imaging are unlikely to develop an aneurysm. At an average follow-up of 9.8 years, only 2.6% of patients were found to have an aneurysm on imaging.[66]

f) Screening for intracranial aneurysms in patients with ADPKD.[67]
   i) Routine screening is appropriate for:
      (1) Patients with a family history of aneurysms or SAH or,
      (2) Patients with a known aneurysm or a history of aneurysms or SAH.
   ii) Annual or biannual imaging with non-contrast MRA is adequate for screening.
   iii) Patients without a family or personal history of aneurysms are not routinely screened.

EHLERS-DANLOS SYNDROME (EDS) TYPE IV

1. Hereditary connective tissue disorder characterized by joint hypermobility, hyperelastic or fragile skin, easy bruising, and abnormal scarring. Ten subtypes have been described.

2. EDS Type IV, also known as *vascular EDS*, accounts for only 4% of EDS cases but is the most severe:
   (a) Prevalence: 1 in 50,000–100,000 persons.[67]
   (b) Characterized by a decrease or absence of type III collagen.
   (c) Autosomal dominant.
   (d) Median survival is 48 years.[68]
   (e) Vascular manifestations of EDS consist of spontaneous dissection, aneurysm formation, and rupture of large and medium arteries. Arterial rupture accounts for most deaths.
   (f) The most common neurovascular complication is spontaneous carotid-cavernous fistula, followed by ruptured intracranial aneurysms and spontaneous intracerebral haemorrhage, and carotid dissection:[69,70]
      • All vascular procedures in patients with EDS Type IV, including angiography, endovascular procedures, and surgery, are high risk, because of the friability of vessel walls. In a study of EDS Type IV patients undergoing angiography, major complications occurred in 22% and death in 5.6%.[71]
   (g) The utility of routine screening for intracranial aneurysms is controversial because of the high complication rates associated with treatment.[72]

α_1-ANTITRYPSIN DEFICIENCY

1. The major function of α_1-antitrypsin, a circulating antiprotease that is synthesized in the liver, is to protect the lungs against neutrophil elastase. α_1-Antitrypsin deficiency is characterized by damage to elastic tissue, most commonly emphysema. Inheritance follows an autosomal codominant pattern; the gene is located on chromosome 14, and a large number of allelic variants have been identified.[73]

2. Vascular disorders associated with α_1-antitrypsin deficiency include arterial aneurysms, spontaneous dissections, and fibromuscular dysplasia.

3. Both the heterozygous and homozygous α_1-antitrypsin deficiency states have been suspected to be genetic risk factors for intracranial aneurysms,[74] although other studies have found otherwise.[75–77]

4. Screening for asymptomatic intracranial aneurysms in individuals with α_1-antitrypsin deficiency is generally not recommended.[78]

MARFAN SYNDROME
1. Autosomal dominant disorder caused by mutations in the gene encoding fibrillin-1. Fibrillin-1 is a glycoprotein which is an important structural component of the extracellular matrix.
2. Vascular manifestations include aortic and mitral valve insufficiency, and aortic artery dissection and rupture.
3. Although a number of reports have associated Marfan syndrome with intracranial aneurysms, the weight of clinical evidence appears to indicate that Marfan syndrome is not associated with an increased prevalence of intracranial aneurysms.[79,80]

NEUROFIBROMATOSIS TYPE 1
1. Autosomal dominant disorder caused by mutations in the neurofibromatosis-1 gene, which encodes neurofibronin. Neurofibronin may have a regulatory role in the development of various connective tissues.
2. Vascular manifestations include stenosis, aneurysm or fistula formation, and rupture of large and medium size arteries.[78]
3. Firm evidence for an increased risk of intracranial aneurysms in patients with neurofibromatosis has not been shown.

PSEUDOXANTHOMA ELASTICUM
1. An inheritable connective tissue disorder in which the elastic fibers of the skin, eyes, and cardiovascular system become slowly calcified and characteristic skin lesions appear, which resemble xanthomas.
2. Prevalence is approximately 1 per 100,000.
3. Stroke caused by occlusive disease of the carotid and vertebral arteries is the most commonly reported neurovascular manifestation.[81]
4. An association between pseudoxanthoma elasticum and intracranial aneurysms has been reported,[82] although a study of 100 patients with the disorder found no history of "symptomatic intracranial aneurysms".[83] This association appears to be discussed in textbooks and reviews more often than it has actually been reported.

LOEYS-DIETZ SYNDROME
1) Autosomal dominant disorder characterized by the triad of:[84]
    a) Arterial tortuosity, aneurysms, or dissections
    b) Hypertelorism
    c) Bifid uvula or cleft palate
2) It is caused by mutations in the genes encoding transforming growth factor β 1 or 2.
3) Extracranial or intracranial aneurysms are present in 32–54% of patients.[85,86]
4) Arterial dissections are present in 12%.[86]
5) Other neurological manifestations include spinal instability, craniosynostosis, Chiari I malformation, hydrocephalus, and dural ectasia.[86]

ROBERTS/SC PHOCOMELIA SYNDROME
1) Autosomal recessive disorder characterized by microcephaly, mental retardation, hydrocephalus, and numerous other developmental defects.[87]
2) It is caused by a mutation of the *ESCO2* gene on 8p21.[88]
3) Roberts was the first to describe the syndrome in 1911.[89] The "S" and "C" refer to the surnames of two families with the afflictions described in 1969.[90] The term phocomelia refers to maldevelopment of the limbs and the syndrome has also been referred to as "pseudothalidomide syndrome.[90]"
4) A recent case report described a 10 year old girl with the syndrome and multiple intracranial aneurysms.[91]

Other Conditions Associated with Intracranial Aneurysms

ARTERIOVENOUS MALFORMATION
Up to 25% of patients with an arteriovenous malformation (AVM) have associated intracranial aneurysms.[92] About half of these aneurysms are present on a feeding vessel or on a major artery that participates in the arterial supply to the AVM, and most of the remaining are present within the AVM nidus. The effect of the presence of aneurysms in patients with an AVM on risk of hemorrhage is not clear, as some studies have found an increased risk of haemorrhage in this situation,[92–94] whilst others have not.[95,96]

FIBROMUSCULAR DYSPLASIA
A systematic review of 17 studies found a prevalence of intracranial aneurysms in patients with cervical carotid and/or vertebral artery fibromuscular dysplasia of about 7%.[97]

ABDOMINAL AORTIC ANEURYSMS

Intracranial aneurysms are associated with abdominal aortic aneurysms,[98] and first-degree relatives of patients with abdominal aortic aneurysms appear to be at a significantly increased risk of having an intracranial aneurysm (relative risk, 2.87–4.04).[99]

SICKLE CELL ANEMIA

Sickle cell anemia is associated with intracranial aneurysms. In a review of 44 reported cases of aneurysms in sickle cell patients, 57% of patients were found to have multiple aneurysms, and 31% of the aneurysms were located in the posterior circulation.[100]

SPONTANEOUS INTRACRANIAL HYPOTENSION

A retrospective case–control study found an incidence of intracranial aneurysms in patients with spontaneous intracranial hypotension of 8.6%, compared to 1.0% in the control group.[101]

BICUSPID AORTIC VALVE

Bicuspid aortic valve is a common congenital heart defect, affecting up to 2% of the population. A case–control study found that intracranial aneurysms are present in some 9.8% of patients with bicuspid aortic valves.[102]

Risk Factors for Aneurysm Formation and Subarachnoid Hemorrhage

A discussion of modifiable risk factors should be included in the management of any patient with an intracranial aneurysm. Of the following risk factors, cigarette smoking, hypertension and heavy drinking are the most significant.[103]

CIGARETTE SMOKING

Cigarette smoking appears to strongly influence intracranial aneurysms in a very meaningful way. The mechanism is unclear; however, an imbalance in the serum elastase/α_1-antitrypsin ratio or increased elastase activity in smokers likely contributes to aneurysm formation and SAH:[104]

1. Aneurysm formation. Smokers have a greater incidence of multiple aneurysms.[13,15]
2. Growth. Cigarette smoking was found to be strongly associated with growth of unruptured aneurysms.[105]
3. Rupture. Case–control studies have found the relative risk of aneurysmal SAH for smokers to be twice or more that of nonsmokers.[106,107] Other studies have confirmed that smoking is an independent risk factor for SAH.[76,108,109]
4. Vasospasm. Smokers have an increased incidence of symptomatic cerebral vasospasm after SAH.[110,111]
5. Recurrence. On follow-up imaging after coiling, smokers are more likely to have recurrent filling of the aneurysm, especially in women,[112] and also more likely to require additional treatment of the aneurysm.[113]

Smoking Cessation and Drugs to Help with It

Smoking is the single most important modifiable risk factor in patients with intracranial aneurysms. For patients who smoke, aneurysm management must include a discussion of the importance of smoking cessation and help, if needed. Two medications that can help patients stop smoking are varenicline and bupropion. Dosing and side effects are discussed in Chap. 17.

HYPERTENSION

Hypertension is a risk factor for SAH.[103,107,114,115]

ALCOHOL USE

Alcohol consumption (in most studies, >2 drinks per day) has been shown to increase the risk of SAH, independently of cigarette smoking, and history of hypertension.[76,103,116,117] Although epidemiological evidence suggests that there are health benefits to modest alcohol intake (1–2 drinks per day),[118] patients who drink more than their physician does should be advised to cut back on alcohol consumption.

ORAL CONTRACEPTIVES

There is evidence from systematic reviews both for[119] and against[120] oral contraceptives as a risk factor for SAH.

ATHEROSCLEROSIS
Increased serum cholesterol is a risk factor for SAH.[121]

COFFEE USE
Coffee consumption >5 cups per day is an independent risk factor for SAH.[114]

SEXUAL INTERCOURSE
Yes, even sex is associated with aneurysmal SAH.[122] See the review by Reynolds and colleagues for an in-depth discussion of the topic.[123]

WEATHER AND SEASON
Controversial. Although a number of studies have found an association between seasonal and weather patterns and spontaneous subarachnoid hemorrhage,[124-127] other studies,[128] including a recent study of 155 U.S. hospitals,[129] have found no such relationships.

Natural History

The natural history of unruptured intracranial aneurysms is unclear and controversial. The most prominent studies concerning natural history include a study by Juvela and colleagues of a Finnish population that featured a 100% follow-up averaging 18 years,[108] a meta-analysis of publications on the topic from 1955 to 1996,[21] a systematic review of the literature from Japan,[130] and the 800 pound gorilla in the field, the International Study of Unruptured Intracranial Aneurysms (ISUIA).[11,131] Each study has unique strengths and limitations. Two Japanese prospective studies are currently in progress, the Unruptured Cerebral Aneurysm Study in Japan[132] and the Small Unruptured Aneurysm Verification study.[133]

JUVELA 2000
1. Comprehensive cohort study of patients found to have unruptured intracranial aneurysms in Finland, from 1956 to 1978. The strengths of this study lay in the fact that prior to 1979, unruptured aneurysms were not surgically treated at the authors' center, which was the only neurosurgical center in Finland until the late 1960s. Also, the unique socioeconomic structure of Finland permitted longer and more complete follow-up than has been achieved in any other study.
2. A total of 142 patients were studied; mean follow-up was 18.1 years.
3. Annual rate of rupture according to:
    (a) Patient history:
        - Incidental aneurysm, no history of SAH, 1.0%.
        - Incidental aneurysm with a history of SAH, 1.3%.
        - Symptomatic aneurysm, 2.6%.
    (b) Aneurysm size:
        - 2–6 mm, 1.1%.
        - 7–9 mm, 2.3%.
        - 10–26 mm, 2.8%.
4. Mortality rate with rupture: 52%.
5. Limitations: Small total number of patients, homogeneous population, majority of patients (92%) had a history of SAH.

RINKEL 1998
1. Meta-analysis of nine studies, totaling 3,907 patient-years, found an overall risk of rupture of 1.9% per year, and an increased risk of rupture in women, older patients, symptomatic aneurysms, larger size, and posterior circulation location. Results are summarized in Table 13.2.
2. Limitations: The meta-analysis included retrospective studies and studies done prior to the CT-era.

MORITA 2005
1. Meta-analysis of 13 Japanese studies, totaling 3,801 patient-years, found an annual rupture rate of 2.7%. All studies were fairly recent (earliest was published in 1992).
2. The rate of rupture was increased by:
    (a) Diameter ≥10, relative risk (RR) 6.4.
    (b) Posterior circulation location, RR 2.3.
    (c) Symptomatic aneurysm, RR 2.1.
3. Evidence has accumulated in other studies to support the finding that Japanese patients with unruptured intracranial aneurysms are at higher risk of rupture compared to other ethnic groups. The rate of SAH in the Japanese population is nearly nine times higher than the incidence observed in Rochester, Minnesota,[134,135] while the prevalence of unruptured intracranial aneurysms is not significantly

Table 13.2 Systematic review: factors associated with rupture

Risk factor		Annual risk of rupture (%)
Overall		1.9
Sex	Male	1.3
	Female	2.6
Age	20–39	0
	40–59	3.5
	60–79	5.7
Type of aneurysm	Asymptomatic	0.8
	Asymptomatic, history of SAH	1.4
	Symptomatic	6.5
Site	ACA	1.1
	MCA	1.1
	ICA	1.2
	Posterior circulation	4.4
Size	≤10 mm	0.7
	>10 mm	4.0

From Rinkel et al.,[21] with permission

different,[21] and the prevalence of smoking and hypertension in Japanese adults is not higher than that of the US population.[136–138]

4. Limitations: The meta-analysis included retrospective studies; a single ethnic group.

International Study of Unruptured Intracranial Aneurysms

The ISUIA is the largest study of the natural history of unruptured intracranial aneurysms, involving a total of 4,060 patients at 53 centers in the United States, Canada, and Europe. The study began in 1991. Two reports have been published, in *The New England Journal of Medicine* in 1998 and in *Lancet* in 2003. The first paper, containing both retrospective and prospective data, generated controversy mainly because of the finding of a yearly rupture rate for small anterior circulation aneurysms of only 0.05%. The second report provided further evidence of a low rate of rupture for small anterior circulation aneurysms and also included more detailed data on treatment outcomes.

ISUIA FIRST STUDY

A total of 2,621 patients were included in the first ISUIA report.[11] The study had a retrospective component, in which the natural history of unruptured aneurysms was assessed, and a prospective component, which focused on surgical morbidity and mortality:

1. Retrospective component. A total of 1,449 patients with 1,937 intracranial aneurysms were divided into two groups: 727 individuals with no history of SAH (Group 1) and 722 with a history of SAH from a different aneurysm (Group 2). Mean duration of follow-up was 8.3 years:

   (a) Annual rupture rates:
   - Group 1:
     - Aneurysm diameter <10 mm: ~0.05%.
     - Aneurysm diameter ≥10 mm: ~1%.
   - Group 2:
     - Aneurysm diameter <10 mm: ~0.5%.
     - Aneurysm diameter ≥10 mm: ~1%.
   (b) Predictors of rupture:
   - Group 1. The only independent predictors of rupture were the size and location of the aneurysm:
     - Size. Relative risk of rupture for aneurysms 10–24 mm in diameter (compared to aneurysms <10 mm) was 11.6 ($p = 0.03$) and 59.0 for aneurysms ≥25 mm in diameter ($p < 0.001$).
     - Location. Compared to other locations, the relative risk of rupture of aneurysms at the basilar apex was 13.8 ($p = 0.001$), 13.6 for aneurysms of the vertebrobasilar or posterior cerebral artery ($p = 0.007$) and 8.0 for posterior communicating artery aneurysms ($p = 0.02$).

- Group 2. Relative risk of rupture was 5.1 for basilar apex aneurysms ($p = 0.004$) and 1.31 for "older age" patients ($p = 0.04$) (age was not defined).
2. Prospective component. Of 1,172 patients, 996 (85%) underwent surgery and the rest had endovascular treatment. Treatment-related results were reported for the surgical group only. Overall rates of morbidity and mortality:
   (a) Group 1 ($n = 798$):
      - 30 days: 17.5%.
      - 1 year: 15.7%.
   (b) Group 2 ($n = 197$):
      - 30 days: 13.6%.
      - 1 year: 13.1%.
   (c) The lower rates of morbidity and mortality in Group 2 were attributed to the selection of survivors of a first subarachnoid haemorrhage and craniotomy for clipping of an aneurysm.
3. Study conclusions:
   (a) The rate of rupture of anterior circulation aneurysms <10 mm in diameter is very low for patients without a history of SAH. Risk of rupture is substantially higher in patients with a history of SAH.
   (b) Surgery-related risks exceed the 7.5 year risk of rupture among patients without a history of SAH.

ISUIA SECOND STUDY

A total of 4,060 patients were included in the second ISUIA report.[131] The study was entirely prospective; 1,692 patients did not have treatment, 1,917 underwent surgery, and 451 had endovascular procedures. As in the first study, patients were divided into Group 1 (no history of SAH) and Group 2 (previous history of SAH from another lesion) (Tables 13.3 and 13.4)
1. Natural history. Mean follow-up was 4.1 years. A total of 51 patients (3%) in the untreated group had a confirmed aneurysmal SAH (mortality rate, 65%). As in the first study, patients were divided into Group 1 (no history of SAH) and Group 2 (previous history of SAH from another lesion). Patients in Group 1 had a lower rate of rupture for aneurysms <7 mm than patients in Group 2 ($p < 0.0001$); otherwise, rupture rates did not differ significantly between the groups (Table 13.3).
2. Treatment. Mean follow-up was 4.0 years for patients undergoing surgery and 3.7 years for patients who had endovascular treatment. Overall morbidity and mortality rates are reported in Table 13.4. Risk factors were assessed as potential predictors of outcome:
   (a) Surgical group. Age was found to be a strong predictor of outcome (Fig. 13.2). Asymptomatic patients age <50 years with unruptured aneurysms of the anterior circulation ≤24 mm in diameter have the lowest rate of surgical morbidity and mortality, 5.6% at 1 year. Factors predictive of a poor surgical outcome:
      - Age ≥50 years, relative risk, RR 2.4 ($p < 0.0001$).
      - Aneurysm diameter >12 mm, RR 2.6 ($p < 0.0001$).
      - Location in the posterior circulation, RR 1.6 ($p = 0.025$).
      - Previous ischemic cerebrovascular disease, RR 1.9 ($p = 0.01$).
      - Aneurysmal symptoms other than rupture, RR 1.59 ($p = 0.004$).
   (b) Endovascular group. Morbidity and mortality seemed to be less dependent on age in patients undergoing endovascular treatment. Poor outcome was associated with:
      - Aneurysm diameter >12 mm, RR 2.4 ($p < 0.03$).
      - Location in the posterior circulation, RR 2.25 ($p = 0.02$).

ISUIA ANOMALIES AND STUDY LIMITATIONS

The results of the ISUIA have been controversial because the low rates of rupture do not seem to match actual practice. Consider the following calculation. The prevalence of unruptured intracranial aneurysms is about 3%. If the population of the United States is 307 million, then approximately 9.1 million people are likely to have an aneurysm. If the average annual rupture rate is ~0.1%, as the ISUIA indicates for most aneurysms, then only about 9,100 cases of aneurysmal SAH should be seen in the US each year. However, some 21,000–33,000 cases of aneurysmal SAH occur in the US each year.[139] Moreover, the average size of ruptured aneurysms is 6–7 mm, well within the range estimated by ISUIA to have a benign natural history. One of the more colourful hypotheses to explain this is the "shrinking aneurysm theory," which holds that aneurysms become smaller after rupture.[140–142] This notion has been debunked by a series of 13 cases in which aneurysm imaging was available both before and after rupture; none of the aneurysms had a significant decrease in size after rupture.[143]

Table 13.3 ISUIA annual rupture rates according to location and size of unruptured aneurysm

	<7 mm (%)		7–12 mm (%)	13–24 mm (%)	≥25 mm (%)
	Group 1	Group 2			
Anterior communicating artery/MCA/ICA	0	0.3	0.52	2.9	8.0
Posterior circulation and posterior communicating artery	0.5	0.68	2.9	3.68	10
Cavernous ICA	0	0	0	0.6	1.28

Table 13.4 ISUIA outcomes after treatment

	Surgery (%)		Endovascular (%)	
	Group 1	Group 2	Group 1	Group 2
30-day morbidity and mortality	13.7	11.0	9.3	7.1
1-year morbidity and mortality	12.6	10.1	9.8	7.1

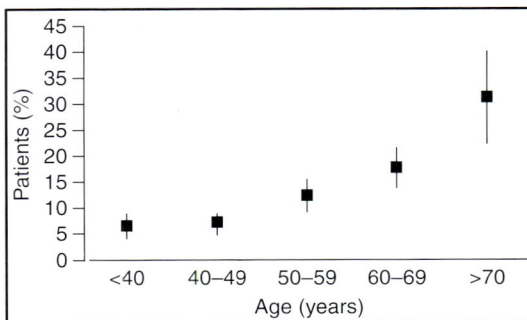

Fig. 13.2 ISUIA poor outcomes in the surgical cohort by age. Poor outcome is defined as death, a Rankin score between 3 and 5, or impaired cognitive status. *Bars* show 95% confidence interval (Reprinted from Wiebers and International Study of Unruptured Intracranial Aneurysms [131] © 2003 Elsevier Ltd., with permission).

Table 13.5 Life expectancy table and projected lifetime risk of aneurysm rupture

Age interval	Average no. of years remaining[a]	Estimated lifetime risk of rupture according to annual risk of rupture[b]				
		0.05%	0.50%	1%	2%	3%
20–24	58.2	0.06	0.25	0.44	0.69	0.83
25–29	53.5	0.05	0.24	0.42	0.66	0.8
30–34	48.7	0.05	0.22	0.39	0.63	0.77
35–39	44	0.04	0.2	0.36	0.59	0.74
40–44	39.3	0.04	0.18	0.33	0.55	0.7
45–49	34.8	0.03	0.16	0.3	0.5	0.65
50–54	30.3	0.03	0.14	0.27	0.46	0.6
55–59	26.1	0.03	0.12	0.23	0.41	0.55
60–64	22	0.02	0.1	0.2	0.36	0.49
65–69	18.2	0.02	0.09	0.17	0.31	0.43
70–74	14.7	0.01	0.07	0.14	0.26	0.36
75–79	11.5	0.01	0.06	0.11	0.21	0.3
80–84	8.8	0.01	0.04	0.08	0.16	0.24
85–89	6.5	0.01	0.03	0.06	0.12	0.18
90–94	4.8	0	0.02	0.05	0.09	0.14
95–99	3.6	0	0.02	0.04	0.07	0.1

[a]Average number of years of life remaining for beginning of age interval. Life expectancy data obtained from the United States Department of Health and Human Services [824]

[b]Annual rupture rates are approximated from the ISUIA.[131] Lifetime risk of rupture was calculated using the formula 1 – (risk of no hemorrhage)years remaining of life[825] Assumptions include a constant risk of rupture and no confounding factors

The most plausible explanation for these discrepancies is that the ISUIA results were affected by *selection* and *intervention bias*. The patients followed in the ISUIA were evaluated and counseled by cerebrovascular neurosurgeons, and a decision was made in each case to manage the patient expectantly. Patients already at lower risk of rupture may have been selected to be managed without intervention, and, once they were aware of their aneurysms, there is a distinct possibility that the patients and their physicians were successful in modifying risk factors for rupture, such as cigarette smoking and hypertension. Therefore, the results of ISUIA are applicable to some patients, but not necessarily to all patients, particularly if they are affected by confounding risk factors for haemorrhage. Management decisions for patients with unruptured aneurysms should be made on an individual basis, with careful consideration of life expectancy, risk factors for haemorrhage, and estimated risks associated with treatment (Table 13.5).

13.3.   Aneurysm Treatment

Conservative Management

The term "conservative management" is a bit of a misnomer, since it implies no treatment at all. However, it is prudent to follow patients with aneurysms that have not been treated, and modifiable risk factors should be addressed. Smoking cessation and management of hypertension take on new importance for patients with newly diagnosed unruptured aneurysms. Patients with unruptured aneurysms should be monitored for new onset headaches or cranial nerve palsies, which may be warning signs of impending rupture. Periodic imaging should be done since objective evidence of aneurysm growth is associated with an increased risk of rupture.[108] The authors of this handbook use annual CTA or MRA exams to follow asymptomatic patients with untreated intradural aneurysms. Growing or newly symptomatic aneurysms should be considered for more definitive treatment.

Treatment: Surgical Results

Microsurgery is the established "gold standard" for treatment of intracranial aneurysms. Successful surgery effectively excludes the aneurysm from the circulation, and recurrence is generally thought to be uncommon. Intraoperative or postoperative catheter angiography is necessary to check for residual aneurysm and to ensure that the parent vessels are preserved. Interpretation of surgical series is problematic, as publication bias can confound the results. For instance, in studies of surgery for unruptured aneurysms, single-center series generally report better results than multicenter or community-based studies.[144] As the largest multicenter trials to date, ISUIA and ISAT have provided the most reliable data for the treatment of unruptured and ruptured aneurysms.

Obliteration Rates, Recurrence, and Haemorrhage After Surgery

1. The frequency of residual aneurysm after clipping is 3.8–8%.[145–149]
2. Rupture or rerupture after clipping usually occurs when residual aneurysm is left behind after surgery:
   (a) In a surgical series of 715 patients with an average follow-up of 6 years, the chance of rebleeding from a residual aneurysm was 3.7%.[145] The chance of rehemorrhage for all patients was 0.14%.
   (b) Of a series of 12 cases with known residual aneurysm after surgery, two (16.7%) were found to have enlarged on follow-up angiography (mean follow-up, 4.4 years).[150]
3. Aneurysm recurrence after surgical obliteration:
   (a) In a surgical series of 220 cases, all of whom had postoperative angiography indicating complete obliteration of the aneurysm, three patients (1.4%) had SAH attributable to a recurrent aneurysm; two other patients were found to have unruptured recurrent aneurysms on angiography.[151] Mean follow-up was 9.9 years.
   (b) Of 135 clipped aneurysms shown to be obliterated on postoperative angiography, two (1.5%) were found to have recurred on follow-up angiography (mean follow-up, 4.4 years).[150]
   (c) In a cohort study involving nine centers and a total of 711 patients undergoing clipping after SAH, rerupture of the treated aneurysm did not occur during 2,666 person-years.[152]

Complication Rates with Surgery

1. Unruptured aneurysms:
   (a) A systematic review of 61 studies involving 2,460 patients having elective aneurysm surgery found a permanent morbidity rate of 10.9% and a mortality rate of 2.6%.[153]
   (b) In a state-wide analysis of patients undergoing surgery for unruptured aneurysms in California from 1990 to 1998, an adverse outcome (defined as an in-hospital death or discharge to a nursing home or rehab) occurred in 25% of cases, and death occurred in 3.5% of cases.[154]
   (c) ISUIA treatment results: The 30-day overall morbidity and mortality rate with surgery was 13.2%, and the mortality rate was 1.5%.[131] The 1-year morbidity and mortality rate was 12.2%, and the mortality rate was 2.3%.
   (d) Risk factors for complications with surgery for unruptured aneurysms include age >50 years, aneurysm size >12 mm, posterior circulation location, and complex anatomy.[131,155,156]
   (e) Post-operative seizures. Some 15.7% of patients have seizures after clipping of unruptured aneurysms.[157]
2. Ruptured aneurysms:
   (a) Surgical complication rates for ruptured aneurysms are confounded by the multiplicity of problems that affect patients with SAH.
   (b) Population-based studies have found a 30-day mortality rate of 13.4%, and 1-year mortality rates of 13.3–17.9%.[158,159]
   (c) ISAT: 1-year rate of death or dependency for surgical patients was 30.9%.

Treatment: Endovascular Results

Angiographic Results

Reports of angiographic results after endovascular treatment of intracranial aneurysms are confounded by differing definitions of angiographic findings as well as varying aneurysm locations and sizes, and whether the treated lesion was unruptured or ruptured (Table 13.6). An established graphic scheme for classifying anatomic results is illustrated in Fig. 13.3. A recent consensus grading scheme is in Fig. 13.4.

IMMEDIATE ANGIOGRAPHIC RESULTS
1. "Complete" aneurysm obliteration has been reported in approximately 50–60% of cases immediately after embolization, and "near complete" occlusion has been reported in about 90% of cases.[160–167]
2. Treatment failures (i.e., no embolization at all) have been reported in approximately 5% of cases,[164–166] although other reports have indicated higher rates.[168]
3. A systematic review of 48 studies found that initial occlusion rates were independent of aneurysm size, location, neck configuration, and whether the aneurysm was ruptured or unruptured.[160]

LONG-TERM ANGIOGRAPHIC RESULTS
1) By convention, initial follow-up imaging is typically done 3–6 months after treatment, then yearly after that, indefinitely.
2) *Aneurysm recurrence.* There are probably as many definitions of "aneurysm recurrence" after coiling as there are snowflakes, making comparisons between studies nearly impossible. The most meaningful definition of recurrence is *recanalization of a volume within the aneurysm large enough to permit retreatment with either endovascular or surgical means* (i.e., recanalizations classified as "major recurrences" by Raymond and colleagues):[169]
   i) Studies including cases mostly from the 1990s found significant recurrence rates of approximately 20% of cases in the first 12–18 months after treatment:
      (1) In a series of 466 patients treated from 1992 to 2002, the rate of major recurrences, defined as necessitating retreatment, occurred in 20.7% of patients and were found at a mean of 16.5 months.[169] Predictors of recurrence included treatment of a ruptured aneurysm, larger aneurysm size and neck width, suboptimal initial angiographic result, and length of follow-up.

Table 13.6 Comparison of various classification schemes for angiographic results after embolization

References	Complete occlusion	Dog ear (indicating a unilateral residual neck)	Residual neck	Aneurysm filling	Treatment failure
134	Grade I (totally occluded aneurysm with no lumen or visible neck remnant)	Grade II (90–99% obliteration, "subtotal")	Grade III (<90% obliteration "incomplete")		
135					
136	100%	95–99%	<95%		
137	Class I (complete obliteration)	Class II (residual neck)	Class III (residual or recurrent aneurysm)		
			Minor	Major (saccular and size large enough to permit retreatment with coils)	
130	Complete (no contrast filling of the dome, neck or body of aneurysm)	Neck remnant (residual filling of part of the neck of the aneurysm)	Incomplete (indicated by contrast within the body and dome of the aneurysm)	Attempted embolization (failure to deliver coils into aneurysm)	

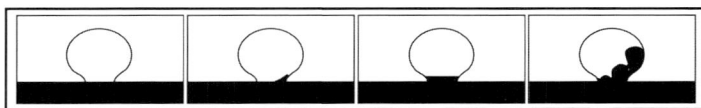

Fig. 13.3 Traditional graphical scheme for classification of angiographic results after aneurysm embolization. Complete occlusion indicates no filling of the aneurysm; "dog ear" indicates a unilateral residual neck; "residual neck" indicates that there is some filling of the neck of aneurysm for the entire length of the aneurysm neck; "aneurysm filling" indicates significant filling of the aneurysm; and "treatment failure" (not shown) indicates no embolization of the aneurysm (Adapted with permission from Roy et al.[821]).

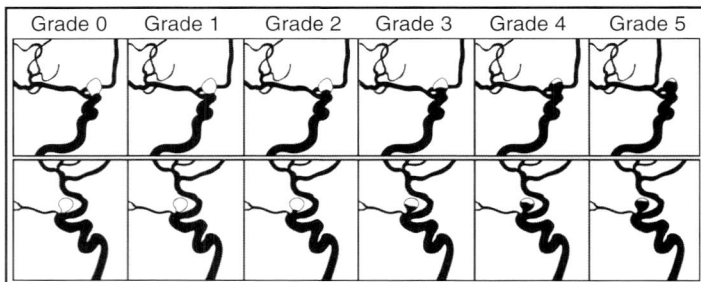

| Grade 0 | Grade 1 | Grade 2 | Grade 3 | Grade 4 | Grade 5 |

Fig. 13.4 Consensus grading scale for endovascular aneurysm occlusion. Grading scale for endovascular aneurysm occlusion is based on orthogonal images obtained in optimal projections to assess aneurysm dimensions: Grade 0, complete aneurysm occlusion; Grade 1, ≥90% aneurysm occlusion; Grade 2, 70–89% aneurysm occlusion; Grade 3, 50–69% aneurysm occlusion; Grade 4, 25–49% aneurysm occlusion; Grade 5, <25% aneurysm occlusion (Joint Writing Group of the Technology Assessment Committee, Society of Neurointerventional Surgery, Society of Interventional Radiology; Joint Section on Cerebrovascular Neurosurgery of the American Association of Neurological Surgeons and Congress of Neurological Surgeons; and Section of Stroke and Interventional Neurology of the American Academy of Neurology. Adapted with permission from Meyers et al. [822], with permission).

       (2) In a series of 818 patients treated at UCLA from 1990 to 2002, the overall rate of recanalization was 20.9%, at a mean follow-up of 11 months.[165] Recanalization was defined as >10% increase in contrast filling of the aneurysm. Factors contributing to recanalization included larger aneurysm size and wide necks. The authors also found a significant improvement in recurrence rates over time (26.1% in the first 5 years vs. 17.2% in the last 6 years), which they attributed to technical refinements.

       (3) More recent studies have found recurrence rates (including small recurrences and recanalization) of approximately 13–15% at 1 year,[170,171] and longer-term recurrence rates of about 20%.[171,172]

   3) Late recanalization. A study of 400 patients with MRA found evidence of recanalization after 6 months following treatment in 2.8%.[173] There were no late recanalizations of anterior communicating artery aneurysms.

   4) Predictors of recurrence include incomplete occlusion at the initial treatment, aneurysm size >10 mm, loose packing of the aneurysm:[169,171,174]

       a) Density of coil packing may correlate with occlusion durability.[174] Typically, only some 23–26% of the endosaccular volume is replaced by coils;[175] some studies have suggested that a volumetric percentage occlusion of at least 25–33% is necessary for durable occlusion.[174,176]

b) Aneurysm relationship with the parent vessel. Terminal aneurysms seem to recur at a higher rate compared to sidewall aneurysms. In a report of long-term results after coiling of 100 asymptomatic aneurysms rates of recanalization were 11% and for sidewall aneurysms and 38% for terminal aneurysms.[177]

Clinical Results with Embolization

COMPLICATION RATES

1) Overall complication rates with coiling tend to hover around 8–10%.[131,154,165,167] A systematic review of 48 studies totaling 1,383 patients found a rate of permanent complications with embolization of 3.7% (95% CI 2.7–4.9%).[160] An in-depth discussion of complications may be found in Chap. 5.
2) Complication rates are higher in certain situations:
   a) Stent-assisted coiling
      i) Morbidity and mortality rates are somewhat higher with stent-assisted coiling compared to primary coiling.
         (1) In a series of 1,109 aneurysm cases, stent-assisted coiling carried a 7.4% neurological morbidity versus 3.8% with primary coiling. Mortality was 4.6% versus 1.2%, respectively.[178]
   b) Very small aneurysms (≤3 mm).
      i) A systematic review found a procedural rupture rate of 8.3% and a combined rate of periprocedural morbidity and mortality of 7.3%.[179]

RUPTURE AFTER COILING

Rehemorrhage after coiling of ruptured aneurysms is uncommon, occurring in approximately 3% of cases.[151,161,180–189] Periprocedural rehemorrhages usually involve aneurysms that were incompletely occluded after the initial treatment.[190–192] The rate of periprocedural rerupture appears to have declined over the years; a recent multicenter study found a 30-day rerupture rate of 0.9%.[193] Later rehemorrhages tend to occur in aneurysms that have demonstrated some degree of recurrence, [161,185] underscoring the need for routine radiographic surveillance of coiled aneurysms.

In ISAT, a total of 35 (3.3%) rebleeds after treatment occurred in patients after coiling within 1 year of treatment.[194] Of the patients in whom coils were placed in the aneurysm, 15 (1.5%) had a rehemorrhage after the initial procedure and before 30 days postprocedure.[195] Among these 15 patients, 7 had incomplete occlusion of the aneurysm, 3 had complete occlusion, and 5 received thrombolytic therapy to treat thromboembolic complications after the initial endovascular treatment.

Selected Studies Comparing Coiling and Clipping

UNRUPTURED ANEURYSMS, RETROSPECTIVE STUDIES

1. In a cohort study of 2,357 surgical cases and 255 endovascular cases at 60 university hospitals, adverse outcomes were significantly more common in surgical cases (18.5%) compared to endovascular cases (10.6%) ($p = 0.002$).[196] In-hospital mortality was higher for surgical cases (2.3% vs. 0.4%; $p = 0.039$). The length of stay and hospital charges were also significantly greater for surgical cases ($p < 0.0001$ for each).
2. In a state-wide analysis of patients undergoing surgery for unruptured aneurysms in California from 1990 to 1998, an adverse outcome (defined as an in-hospital death or discharge to a nursing home or rehab) occurred in 10% of endovascular cases, compared to 25% of surgical cases ($p < 0.001$).[154] In-hospital death occurred in 0.5% of endovascular cases and 3.5% of surgical cases ($p < 0.001$). Adverse outcomes declined from 1991 to 1998 in patients treated with endovascular therapy but not in those who underwent surgery ($p < 0.005$).
3. An aggregate analysis of 1,829 endovascular patients and 10,541 surgical patients found a cumulative adverse outcome rate of 8.8% (95% CI 7.6–10.1%) for coiling and 17.8% (95% CI 17.2–18.6%) for clipping.[197]

Table 13.7 Nationwide inpatient sample analysis of coiling versus clipping in patients with unruptured intracranial aneurysms

		Coiling (%)	Clipping (%)	
Age < 50	Morbidity	3.5	8.1	P < 0.0001
	Mortality	0.6	0.6	P = 0.72
Age 50–64	Morbidity	4.0	13.7	P < 0.0001
	Mortality	0.5	1.1	P < 0.0001
Age 65–79	Morbidity	6.9	26.8	P < 0.0001
	Mortality	0.8	2.0	P < 0.0001
Age ≥ 80	Morbidity	9.8	33.5	P < 0.0001
	Mortality	2.4	21.4	P < 0.0001

From Brinjikji et al. [198], with permission

4. A study of the Nationwide Inpatient Sample from 2001 to 2008 (Table 13.7) found lower rates of morbidity and mortality with coiling compared to clipping, and that these differences became more pronounced with age.[198] These results are similar to the ISUIA results, and serve to confirm the ISUIA findings. Another study of the Nationwide Inpatient Sample also found lower lengths of hospital stay, mortality, and periprocedural complications with unruptured aneurysm coiling compared to clipping.[199]

UNRUPTURED ANEURYSMS, PROSPECTIVE STUDIES
1. ISUIA: 1,917 patients underwent surgery and 451 patients had endovascular treatment. Overall morbidity and mortality at 1 year was 12.2% for the surgical group and 9.5% for the endovascular group. ISUIA is discussed in detail above.

RUPTURED ANEURYSMS, PROSPECTIVE STUDIES
1. A single-center randomized 109 patients with SAH to either surgery ($n = 52$) or coiling ($n = 57$).[190] Better angiographic results were obtained after surgery in patients with ACA aneurysms ($p = 0.005$), and after coiling in patients with posterior circulation aneurysms ($p = 0.045$). Clinical outcome was not significantly different at 3 months.
2. Long-term rerupture rates were evaluated in an "ambidirectional" cohort study of 711 surgical cases and 299 endovascular cases at nine centers.[152] The mean length of follow-up was 4.4 years for surgical patients and 8.9 years for endovascular patients. Rerupture of the index aneurysm after 1 year occurred in one patient treated with coil embolization during 904 person-years of follow-up (annual rate 0.11%) and in no surgical patients during 2,666 person-years ($p = 0.11$). Aneurysm retreatment after 1 year was more frequent in patients treated with coiling ($p < 0.0001$), but major complications during retreatment were rare.
3. ISAT: Randomized trial of coiling versus clipping in 2,143 patients with SAH.[194] The 1-year rate of death and dependency was lower in the endovascular group compared to the surgical group (23.5% vs. 30.9%; $p = 0.0001$). The ISAT is discussed in detail below.
4. CONSCIOUS-1: Randomized trial of 413 patients with SAH to evaluate clazosentan for vasospasm prophylaxis.[200] The trial included 199 clipping patients and 214 coiling patients. Coiling was associated with a significantly reduced risk of angiographic vasospasm and delayed ischemic neurological deficit compared to coiling.[201] Rates of cerebral infarction and clinical outcome were not significantly different between the groups.

What Should Patients Expect with Aneurysm Coiling?
The authors prefer to quote a risk of complications with coiling of approximately 10%, and a chance of aneurysm recurrence (necessitating retreatment) of about 20% over several years. The actual rates may be lower, but it is often wise to err on the conservative side when helping patients and their families formulate expectations about treatment. A tendency to err on the conservative side is also important when discussing alternatives, including surgical clipping, as well.

Table 13.8 Patient selection for coiling or clipping

Relative indications	Relative contraindications
Endovascular treatment	
Poor surgical candidate	Elongated aortic arch or otherwise difficult vascular access
Favorable aneurysm anatomy	Cervical or cranial vessel disease (e.g., occlusion, dissection, fibromuscular dysplasia, friable atherosclerotic plaque)
Favorable vascular access anatomy	Giant aneurysms
Previous contralateral cranial surgery or hemispheric injury	Aortic or femoral artery occlusion
Need for long-term anticoagulation (e.g., warfarin therapy for atrial fibrillation)	Intraluminal thrombus
High risk for anesthesia complications	Intolerance to iodinated contrast
Posterior circulation aneurysms	Intolerance to heparin and/or antiplatelet agents (if stent-assisted coiling is anticipated)
Vascular neurosurgeon unavailable	Patient unable or unwilling to have routine radiographic follow-up
Surgical treatment	
Younger patient	Advanced age
Few medical conditions	Multiple medical conditions
No previous cranial surgery	Previous cranial surgery
Middle cerebral artery aneurysms	Giant aneurysms
Symptoms attributable to aneurysm mass affect	Specialized neurosurgical care unavailable
Surgically accessible	Calcification or significant atherosclerosis of the aneurysm neck

Treatment Decision-Making: Clip or Coil?

Both surgery and endovascular treatment are valid for many aneurysms. Patient-specific factors are summarized in Table 13.8. Operator-specific factors include the background and comfort level of the physician in handling any particular case.

Flow Diversion

Flow diverters disrupt flow into the aneurysm, leading to thrombosis of the aneurysm with preservation of normal flow in the parent vessel and its branches, and eventual endothelialization across the neck of the aneurysm. Although the introduction of several different flow diverters in the last several years represent a paradigm shift in the endovascular treatment of aneurysms, global experience is still extremely limited. The present time is still only the dawn of the flow diversion era, and numerous refinements in device design and technique in years to come can be expected.

Concept and Experimental Data

Flow diversion, in its present state, is based on the placement of a wire mesh stent within the parent vessel across the neck of the aneurysm. The wire mesh has the effect of reducing flow into the aneurysm without interfering with flow in normal arterial branches that the stent also crosses. Existing flow diverters have 30–35% surface area coverage[202–204] (compared to, say, the Neuroform stent, which as 6–9% coverage). Exclusion of the aneurysm occurs in three phases:[205]
  1) Mechanical
     a) Placement of a physical barrier redirects the flow of blood away from the aneurysm and into the lumen of the parent vessel.

2) Physiological
   a) Reduction of flow into the aneurysm leads to thrombosis within the aneurysm. The rate of formation of the clot is variable, and may take days to months.
   b) Symptoms, such as headaches or cranial nerve problems, may appear during this time.
3) Biological
   a) Endothelialization of the stent and thrombus resorption occurs, which takes months.

Computational fluid dynamics studies have demonstrated that low-porosity stents disrupt flow into aneurysms,[206,207] and that flow reduction is greater in side-wall aneurysms compared to aneurysms located on a curved parent vessel.[208,209]

A key feature of flow diversion with wire mesh stents is the ability to maintain flow into branches of the parent vessel that are covered by the stent. Flow into arterial branches is driven by a pressure gradient between the parent vessel and the lower-pressure branches. Because of this pressure gradient, more than 50% occlusion of the luminal surface area of the branch vessel ostium is necessary before flow begins to diminish significantly.[210,211] Histological evaluation of Pipeline devices implanted into rabbit aorta showed a homogenous sheet of neoendothelium and growing across the stent struts, interrupted only by the ostia of the branch vessels.[202]

Devices

See Chap. 5 for more detail about the devices.
1) Pipeline™ embolization device (PED) (ev3, Irvine, CA). Oldest device in current clinical use. Presently both FDA and CE mark-approved.
2) Silk (Balt Extrusion, Montmorency, France)
3) Willis covered stent (Micro-Port, Shanghai, China). Balloon-expandable stent with a polytetrafluoroethylene membrane.
4) Surpass (Surpass Medical, Tel-Aviv, Israel)[204,212]

Flow Diverter Grading Scale

O'Kelly and colleagues developed a grading scale for flow diverters (Fig. 13.5).

Flow Diverter Clinical Studies

1) *Pipeline*
   a) *Pipeline for the Intracranial Treatment of Aneurysms (PITA)* [213]
      i) Prospective study of 31 patients with mostly sidewall aneurysms, mean size 11.5 mm.
         (1) Pipeline placement was successful in 30 cases (96.8%)
         (2) One stent was used in 18 (58%) cases and two stents were used in 11(35%).
            (a) Pipeline was used alone in 15 (48%) cases; coils were used along with Pipeline in 16 (52%) of cases.
         (3) Two patients (6.5%) had a major stroke.
         (4) Of 30 patients who had 6-month angiographic follow-up, 28 (93%) were angiographically cured.
   b) Buenos Aires experience[214]
      i) Retrospective study of 63 mostly anterior circulation aneurysms in 53 patients treated with Pipeline.
      ii) Pipeline deployment was successful in 70 of 72 attempts (97%)
         (1) One stent was used for 44 (70%) of the aneurysms, two stents were used for 17 (27%), and three stents were used for two (3%).
         (2) Pipeline was used alone in 15 (48%) cases; coils were used along with Pipeline in 16 (52%) of cases.
      iii) No strokes or deaths occurred within 30 days. Minor complication rate was 11%.

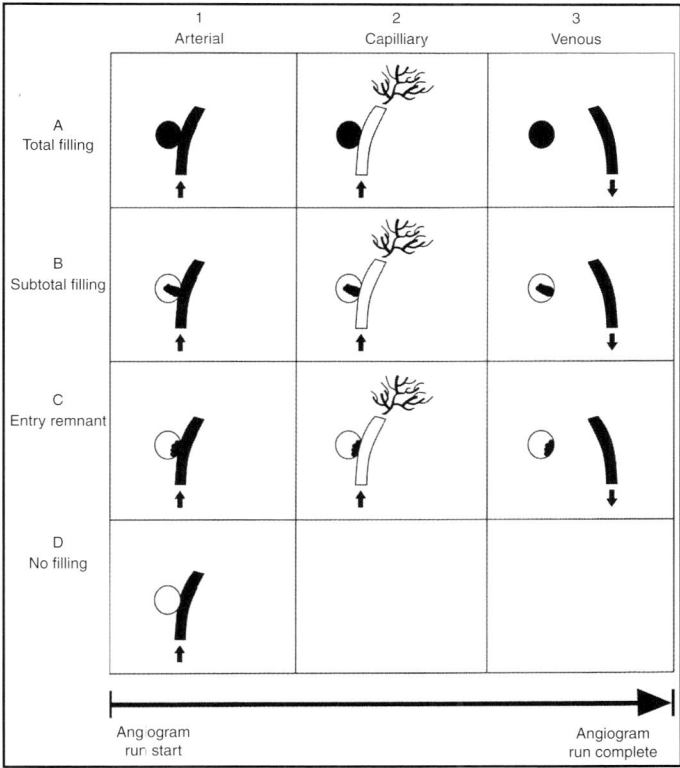

Fig. 13.5 OKM scale for flow diversion. The O'Kelly-Marotta (OKM) grading scale for aneurysms treated by flow diversion. An angiogram extending into the venous phase is necessary for this scale. The aneurysm is assigned a grade according to the initial degree of filling (*A, B, C* or *D*) and the degree of stasis (1, 2 or 3). The degree of initial filling is defined as the percentage of the aneurysm that is filled with contrast during the arterial phase. The degree of stasis depends on how rapidly the contrast clears from the aneurysm: (1) no stasis (clearance within the arterial phase, prior to the capillary phase) (2) moderate stasis (clearance prior to the venous phase) (3) significant stasis (contrast persists in aneurysm into the venous phase and beyond) (Reprinted from O'Kelly et al.[823] © 2010 Centauro, with permission).

    iv) Angiographic follow-up:
        (1) Immediate occlusion was seen in only 5 (8%) of the aneurysms. All of these were small aneurysms.
        (2) At 6 months, 26 (93%) of 28 aneurysms imaged with angiography at that time had progressed to complete occlusion.
        (3) At 12 months, 17 (94.4%) of 18 aneurysms imaged at that time had progressed to complete occlusion.
        (4) The presence of a pre-existing stent impaired adequate wall apposition of the Pipeline stent and was a factor contributing to delayed incomplete aneurysm occlusion.

2) *Budapest experience*[215]
   a) Prospective study of 19 wide-necked aneurysms were treated in 18 patients.
   b) Pipeline deployment was successful in 39 of 41 cases (95%). Ten aneurysms were treated with Pipeline and coils, and nine were treated with Pipeline alone.
      i) One stent was used for five aneurysms, two stents were used for four, and three stents were used for one.
      ii) Pipeline was used alone in nine cases; coils were used along with Pipeline in ten cases.
   c) Complications occurred in four cases (22%).
      i) Overall morbidity: 17%
      ii) Overall mortality: 6%
   d) Angiographic follow-up: 18 of 19 (95%) aneurysms with 6-month angiographic follow-up were found to be completely occluded.
3) *Stuttgart experience*[216]
   a) Retrospective study of 88 patients with 101 intracranial aneurysms (n = 96) or dissections (n = 5).
   b) Pipeline deployment was successful in 100 (99%).
   c) One stent was used for 34 (34%) of the aneurysms. The median number of stents was 3.0 (range 2–18).
   d) Periprocedural adverse events occurred in 5 of 84 procedures (6%). However, the majority of the adverse events (four of them) occurred in cases in which the Pipeline device was deployed inside of a previously placed stent.
      i) Overall morbidity: 4%
      ii) Overall mortality: 2%
   e) Angiographic follow-up:
      i) At 3 months, 47 of 90 lesions (52%) were occluded.
      ii) At 10 months, 36 of 49 lesions (74%) were occluded.
4) *Ongoing studies*:
   a) Complete Occlusion of Coilable Aneurysms Using Pipeline Embolization Device (COCOA)
      i) Randomized trial of Pipeline reconstruction versus coiling for ICA aneurysms. Study results have not yet been published.
   b) Pipeline Embolization Device for Uncoilable or Failed Aneurysms (PUFS)[217]
      i) Single arm study of Pipeline treatment of large and giant wide-necked or fusiform aneurysms.
5) *Silk*
   a) *Lubicz and colleagues*[218]
      i) Prospective study of 29 patients treated with the Silk device.
      ii) Silk deployment was successful in 26 (90%) of cases.
      iii) Complications
         (1) Overall complication rate was 38%
         (2) Morbidity: 15%
         (3) Mortality: 4%
      iv) Angiographic follow-up
         (1) Overall, 69% of the aneurysms were completely occluded at 3–6 months.
         (2) Some 33% of follow-up angiograms showed significant parent vessel stenosis, usually in cases in which the distal end of the stent had been placed within an artery that had significantly smaller diameter than the proximal one.
   b) *Byrne and colleagues*[219]
      i) Prospective study of 70 patients treated with the Silk device at 18 centers.
      ii) Silk deployment was successful in 67 (96%) of cases.
         (1) The Silk device was used alone in 57 (81%) cases; coils were used along with Silk in 10 (14%) of cases.
         (2) Difficulties in Silk deployment (such as poor deployment or positioning or parent vessel thrombosis) were reported in 15 (21%) of cases, and parent artery thrombosis occurred in 8 (11%) of cases.
      iii) Complication rates:
         (1) Early complications: 1.4%
         (2) Late complications: 4%

        (3) Mortality: 8%
        (4) Aneurysm rupture: 2%
     iv) Angiographic follow-up:
        (1) Immediate occlusion was seen in 10% of cases.
        (2) Follow-up interval of 20–40 weeks: 50% of aneurysms were
            occluded.
        (3) Follow-up interval of 40–60 weeks: 100% of aneurysms were
            occluded.
  c) *Basilar artery aneurysm study*[220]
     i) Retrospective study of 12 patients with basilar artery aneurysms
        treated with Silk.
     ii) Silk deployment was successful in all cases.
        (1) A single device was used in all but one case.
     iii) During a mean follow-up period of 16 weeks, there were four (33%)
        symptomatic neurological events:
        (1) One basilar artery occlusion within hours of the procedure,
            likely due to incomplete stent opening.
        (2) Three perforator infarctions (two thalamic and one pontine)
            presenting weeks after the procedure. Rate of branch occlu-
            sion: 3/12 (25%).
     iv) Angiographic occlusion rate at a mean follow-up period of 16 weeks:
        7 of 12 (58%).
6) *Flow diversion-specific adverse events*
  a) Aneurysm rupture
     i) Incidence: 0–4%[213–215,219,221]
     ii) Hypothesized mechanisms (controversial):
        (1) Intra-aneurysmal thrombosis.[222,223]
            (a) In some cases, intraluminal thrombus may cause
                degradation of the aneurysm wall via a cascade of
                physiological effects, including de-endothelialization,
                and inflammation of the aneurysm wall.
        (2) Hemodynamic theory.[224]
            (a) Flow diversion may cause an increase in pressure
                within the aneurysm, possibly via a ball-valve effect.
     iii) Prevention (also controversial)
        (1) Combine coiling with flow diversion in large and giant aneu-
            rysms to minimize the volume of thrombosis within the
            aneurysm.
        (2) Avoid using flow diverters in aneurysms that may have a
            high risk of post-treatment rupture due to hemodynamic
            stress, such as aneurysms associated with a proximal par-
            ent artery stenosis or parent vessels that are extremely
            tortuous.[224]
  b) Parent vessel or branch artery occlusion
     i) Incidence: 0–33% Lylyk, 2009 #1323}[213,215,219–221]
     ii) Branch vessel occlusion has been reported for both the Pipeline[225]
        and Silk devices,[220] although it seems to be more common with Silk
        than with Pipeline. Several cases of vessel occlusion have been
        linked to insufficient antiplatelet therapy.[216,220]

Summary of Clinical Data

The Silk device[218–220] appears to be associated with higher complication rates compared to the Pipeline.[213–216] A recent review of prospective studies of flow diversion
found:[226]
1) Overall occlusion rates:
  a) 3 months: 56%[214]
  b) 6 months: 49–95%[213–215,219]
  c) 12 months: 95%[214]
2) Early complication rates: 0–7.6%[213–215,219,221]
3) Late complications: 0–7.6%[213–215,219,221]
4) Mortality: 0–8%[213–215,219,221]
5) Aneurysm rupture: 0–4%[213–215,219,221]

Other Flow Diverters

1) Willis covered stent (Micro-Port, Shanghai, China)
   a) Balloon-expandable stent consisting of a cobalt chromium stent and an expandable polytetrafluoroethylene membrane.[227–229]
   b) Report of 37 aneurysms treated with the Willis covered stent in 33 patients:[230]
      i) Stent deployment was successful in 42 of 43 attempts (98%).
      ii) One stent was used for 28 aneurysms, three aneurysms were treated with two stents, and two aneurysms were treated with three stents.
      iii) Adverse events:
         (1) Morbidity: none.
         (2) Mortality: two patients (6%)
      iv) Angiographic follow-up, mean 17.5 months:
         (1) Complete occlusion: 94%
         (2) Incomplete occlusion: 6%
2) LEO (Balt Extrusion, Montmorency, France)
   a) The LEO stent, which is designed for stent-assisted aneurysm coiling,[231] has somewhat greater surface area coverage than the Neuroform stent and has been used for flow diversion.[232]

Intracranial Aneurysms by Type or Location

Unruptured Intracranial Aneurysms Presenting with Mass Effect

1. Solomon and colleagues found that the proportion of patients without hemorrhage presenting with mass effect from an intracranial aneurysm to be 8%,[233] although currently, the proportion is likely to be lower because of an increase in noninvasive imaging detection of intracranial aneurysms. Cranial nerve palsies are a typical feature of unruptured aneurysms presenting with mass effect;[234] oculomotor palsy related to impingement on the third cranial nerve from a P-comm aneurysm is the most frequent scenario. Oculomotor palsies are a presenting feature in some 7.2–94% of patients with small unruptured aneurysms.[235,236] Cranial nerve palsies have traditionally thought to be due to mechanical compression of the nerve, although transmission of pulsations is likely to be a significant component as well:[237]
   (a) Endovascular treatment of aneurysms with mass effect: Some degree of improvement has been reported in up to 75% of patients,[234,238,239] although overall rates of complete symptom resolution with coiling are 32–50%.[234,238]
   (b) Dampening of pulsations is likely to be the primary mechanism of improvement of symptoms with coiling. Interestingly, symptoms improved in three out of four patients who underwent coiling of aneurysms for cranial nerve dysfunction, despite a significant increase in aneurysm volume after coiling.[237]
   (c) The shorter the duration of symptoms, the higher the likelihood of recovery, for both surgery and endovascular treatment; one series found that treatment within 5 days of symptom onset was associated with complete resolution of symptoms.
2. Posterior communicating artery aneurysms. In a retrospective comparison of clipping vs. coiling for patients with P-comm aneurysm-induced oculomotor palsy, 6 out of 7 patients (86%) recovered completely, compared with 2 out of 6 patients (33%) treated with coiling.[240] Other studies have reported complete recovery in 48–92% of patients undergoing clipping:[241–243]
   (a) The presence or absence of a pupillary reflex is a prototypical feature that can help distinguish a third nerve palsy due to a compressive lesion, such as a P-comm aneurysm, from an intrinsic lesion affecting the nerve, such as diabetes-associated oculomotor palsy. A diminished pupillary reaction to light results from involvement of parasympathetic fibers that are in a superficial position within the nerve, and are thus vulnerable to compression. The mnemonic, "If the pupil is involved, we're involved! (i.e., we = neurointerventionalist or neurosurgeon)" applies.

- Conversely, third nerve dysfunction in diabetic patients typically results from small vessel ischemia to the nerve. Since the microvascular blood supply to the nerve is oriented from outside-to-inside, the central parts of the nerve are more susceptible to ischemic injury, and the outer parasympathetic fibers are more likely to be spared. Thus, pupil sparing third nerve palsy is *less* likely to be related to extrinsic compression by a P-comm aneurysm.
  (b) Recovery of oculomotor function after surgery follows a predictable course. Ptosis is typically the first symptom to improve, but complete recovery can take months.
  (c) The presence of diabetes, older age, delayed intervention, and complete oculomotor palsy are poor prognostic factors for recovery of function after coiling.[243]
3. Cavernous segment ICA aneurysms:
  (a) See below.[168,244–247]
4. The authors favor surgical treatment of intradural aneurysms with symptoms of mass effect for younger patients who are good surgical candidates, and reserve coiling for older patients at higher risk for surgical complications.

Cavernous ICA Aneurysms

Approximately 4% of all intracranial aneurysms arise from the cavernous segment of the ICA. Many are discovered incidentally; symptomatic cavernous aneurysms can present with diplopia, pain, or a carotid-cavernous fistula. There is a strong female preponderance, with women accounting for up to 92% of patients with cavernous aneurysms:[245]
1. Radiographic appearance and anatomy:
  (a) The cavernous segment of the ICA extends from the petrous carotid to the distal dural ring. Most cavernous aneurysms are easy to identify and are clearly proximal to the distal dural ring.
  (b) Aneurysms involving the cavernous segment can be difficult to distinguish from intradural aneurysms. A useful landmark on CTA in distinguishing cavernous aneurysms from intradural aneurysms is the optic strut, seen on coronal CTA images (Fig. 13.6).[248] Aneurysms that arise proximal to the optic strut are within the cavernous sinus, and aneurysms that arise distal to the optic strut are intradural.
  (c) *Transitional* aneurysms involve both the cavernous segment and the intradural space. A focal narrowing, or waist, of the aneurysm dome on angiography is an indication of subarachnoid extension.[249]
  (d) The position of several cranial nerves within the cavernous sinus, including the third, fourth, and sixth cranial nerves as well as the V1 and V2 divisions of the trigeminal nerve, makes them vulnerable to compressive injury by large cavernous aneurysms, or a carotid-cavernous fistula.
2. Symptoms and physical findings:
  (a) Unruptured cavernous aneurysms:
    - Cavernous aneurysms typically produce symptoms by interfering with cranial nerve function. Involvement of the trigeminal nerve can produce severe pain and numbness in the face. The pain may be constant and burning, or it may include a lancinating component evocative of trigeminal neuralgia.
    - The most common symptoms at presentation are diplopia (65%) and pain (59%).[245] In patients with diplopia, all three oculomotor nerves are involved most commonly (18% of patients); an isolated sixth cranial nerve palsy is present in 17%, and an isolated third cranial nerve palsy is found in 12%.[245] Other physical findings include a reduced or absent corneal reflex, fifth cranial nerve dysesthesias, Horner's pupil, and compressive optic neuropathy.
    - In contrast to third nerve dysfunction due to P-comm aneurysm, cavernous aneurysms can produce a *pupil sparing* third nerve palsy.
  (b) Ruptured cavernous aneurysms:
    - In a recent series of 185 patients with cavernous aneurysms, ruptured aneurysms accounted for 6.5%. In a series of symptomatic cavernous aneurysms treated with endovascular techniques, ruptured aneurysms accounted for 24.4% of cases.[250]

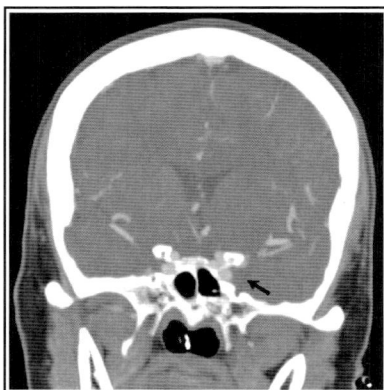

Fig. 13.6 The optic strut and carotid aneurysms. Coronal CTA maximum intensity projection (MIP). The optic strut is clearly seen on the left (*arrow*). An intradural, paraclinoid "carotid cave" aneurysm arises from the medial aspect of the vessel.

- Ruptured cavernous aneurysms often produce a spontaneous carotid-cavernous fistula. In a series of ten patients with ruptured cavernous aneurysms, all had an audible pulsatile bruit. Exophthalmos, ophthalmoplegia, and diminished vision were common features. Importantly, five patients were found to have cortical venous drainage, indicating some degree of risk of intracranial hemorrhage.
- Epistaxis[250] and SAH[251–253] are rare sequelae of cavernous aneurysm rupture.

3. Natural history:
   (a) The risk of rupture of small cavernous segment aneurysms is extremely low.[251] In the ISUIA, with a mean follow-up of 4.1 years, no cavernous aneurysms <13 mm ruptured.[131] The annual rupture risk for cavernous aneurysms 13–24 and ≥25 mm was 0.6% and 1.28%, respectively.
   (b) Transitional and giant cavernous aneurysms carry a risk of SAH.[253]
   (c) The natural history of *symptomatic* cavernous aneurysms is variable.[254] Symptoms may progress, or even spontaneously disappear.[251,254] In an analysis of 125 untreated cavernous aneurysms manifesting with pain or diplopia, pain resolved or improved spontaneously in 56% of cases, and diplopia resolved, improved, or became unnoticed in 56% as well.[245]

4. Treatment (more discussion of this topic is in Appendix: direct carotid-cavernous fistulas):
   (a) Coil embolization or balloon test occlusion, followed by therapeutic sacrifice of the ICA is the primary treatment option. Detachable balloons were traditionally used for the carotid sacrifice, but are not currently available in the US. Acta Vascular Systems, Santa Clara, CA, is working on getting FDA approval of detachable balloons.
   (b) Treatment should be reserved for cavernous aneurysms with extension into the subarachnoid space, and for selected symptomatic aneurysms:
      - In a systematic review of nine clinical series totaling 69 patients who underwent coil embolization for cavernous aneurysms causing diplopia, diplopia was improved in 96% and unchanged or increased in 3.6%.[255] After coiling, 80% of aneurysms were occluded by >90%.

- Pain may be more responsive to treatment than diplopia. In a single-center retrospective review, diplopia was resolved, improved or became unnoticed in 61% of patients undergoing endovascular treatment; this was not significantly different from the results in patients who did not have treatment (56% had the same result).[245] In contrast, pain was resolved or improved in 96% of patients having treatment, compared to 56% of patients who did not have treatment ($p = 0.002$).

   (c) Complications:
   - In a systematic review, none of the 68 patients treated with coil embolization had a complication.[255] In a large single-center series, stroke occurred in 5% of patients and TIAs occurred in 5%, although the authors pointed out that all of these cases were done before 1993 and suggested that improved technique and devices led to a reduction in ischemic complications[245]

   (d) A dilemma that occurs in the management of symptomatic cavernous aneurysms is that, whereas a significant percentage of symptoms will improve without intervention, the chance of symptomatic improvement, particularly when vision or oculomotor function is affected, is best when treatment is undertaken soon after the onset of symptoms.

5. The authors of this handbook favor coiling of unruptured cavernous aneurysms with extension into the subarachnoid space, and for ruptured cavernous aneurysms in patients with a bothersome bruit, cortical venous drainage, or significant diplopia or pain. Selected patients with symptomatic unruptured cavernous aneurysms are also candidates for endovascular treatment, depending on the clinical situation.

Paraclinoid ICA Aneurysms

Intradural aneurysms arising from the ICA between the distal dural ring and the P-comm artery are classified as paraclinoid aneurysms because of their proximity to the anterior clinoid process.

Bilateral aneurysms are not uncommon, being present in some 23% of cases[256] Numerous terms and classification systems exist for aneurysms in this region, which has created considerable confusion. Two main types of aneurysms in this region are named for the branch of the ICA they are associated with, the ophthalmic artery and the superior hypophyseal artery. Much less common aneurysms arising from this segment of the ICA are not clearly associated with an arterial branch and include "carotid cave" and "lateral paraclinoid" aneurysms.

OPHTHALMIC SEGMENT ANEURYSMS

Ophthalmic aneurysms arise at the distal aspect of the origin of the ophthalmic artery and project in a superior and medial direction. They comprise 33% of paraclinoid aneurysms:[257]

1. *Presentation*. About half of symptomatic ophthalmic aneurysms present with visual symptoms, and the remaining present with SAH[258] As the aneurysm enlarges, distortion of the optic nerve can occur, which may be clinically silent despite significant involvement of the nerve. Impingement of the lateral aspect of the optic nerve can produce a monocular superior nasal quadrantanopia (although the patient may not notice it), and in advanced cases complete ipsilateral visual loss may be present. Visual symptoms are almost always attributable to giant (≥2.5 cm) aneurysms. Although giant ophthalmic aneurysms have been reported to cause a *contralateral* superior temporal quadrantanopia, due to involvement of the "anterior knee of Wilbrand" (nasal retinal fibers which travel in an anterior direction for a short distance within the contralateral optic nerve after they decussate),[259] more recent data suggests that the "anterior knee of Wilbrand" does not actually exist.[260]

2. *Surgical considerations*. Surgical access to ophthalmic aneurysms usually requires removal of the anterior clinoid process. Visual loss can occur from manipulation from the optic nerve or disruption of optic nerve perforating vessels during aneurysm exposure, and occurs in some 4–8.7% of cases.[256,261] A preoperative CT should be checked for the presence of calcification of the neck;

significant calcification can make clipping difficult. The ophthalmic artery should be preserved whenever possible, however some patients will tolerate occlusion of this vessel without ischemic injury to the retina thanks to collateral circulation from the external carotid artery branches.

3. *Endovascular treatment.* Coiling is an attractive option for treatment of ophthalmic aneurysms because of the risk of visual loss with surgery. Morbidity with endovascular treatment of paraclinoid aneurysms is 1.4–8.3%.[261–263] However, ophthalmic aneurysms are prone to recurrence after coiling. Strictly speaking, ophthalmic aneurysms are sidewall aneurysms; however their location along the bend of the ICA as it arches up from the cavernous sinus may create a hemodynamic effect that is similar to that experienced by end-artery aneurysms. Relatively high recurrence rates have been reported after coiling, occurring in 18.9–53% of cases.[261,264,265] Because of this, methodical radiographic follow-up after coiling of ophthalmic aneurysms is mandatory.

SUPERIOR HYPOPHYSEAL ARTERY ANEURYSMS

Some 47% of paraclinoid aneurysms are associated with the origin of the superior hypophyseal artery.[257] These aneurysms arise from the inferomedial aspect of the ICA and project inferiorly and medially. Most aneurysms of this type are incidental findings or present with SAH. Rarely, superior hypophyseal aneurysms can become large enough to compress the pituitary stalk and the optic chiasm. Surgical access to these aneurysms is technically challenging because the aneurysm is located on the opposite side of the ICA as the vessel is approached via a pterional craniotomy, and the aneurysm dome may be adherent to the parasellar dura.

SUPERIOR HYPOPHYSEAL ARTERY ANEURYSMS

Some 20% of paraclinoid aneurysms are not associated with a branch of the ICA.[257] Most of these are arise from the ICA in either a medial or lateral direction:

1. *Medial clinoidal segment aneurysms* (aka *carotid cave* aneurysms). The term "carotid cave" refers to a space inferior to a redundant fold of dura, which extends from the medial aspect of the distal dural ring,[266] and is present in some 68–77% of cases.[257] Aneurysms extending into the carotid cave are usually small and project medially in the AP plane (Fig. 13.6). They are distinguished from superior hypophyseal aneurysms by their more proximal location and the absence of an associated branching artery.

2. *Lateral paraclinoid aneurysms.* These aneurysms project in a superior and lateral direction and are uncommon, accounting for only 8.2% of paraclinoid aneurysms.[257] They can present with SAH.

Supraclinoid ICA Aneurysms

Aneurysms arising from the ICA between the P-comm artery and the carotid terminus are classified as supraclinoid aneurysms and account for 50% of all intracranial aneurysms.[268]

POSTERIOR COMMUNICATING ARTERY ANEURYSMS

P-comm aneurysms usually arise just distal to the origin of the posterior communicating artery, and project inferiorly and laterally. Both surgery and endovascular treatment of P-comm aneurysms are often relatively uncomplicated, and therefore each approach is generally valid. Some 25% of the aneurysms randomized in ISAT were P-comm aneurysms:[195]

1. *Presentation.* Unruptured P-comm aneurysms are a common cause of acute third cranial nerve palsy and are discussed above, in Sect. 13.3.7.1. P-comm aneurysms are also a common cause of SAH; blood on CT is usually concentrated in the lateral suprasellar and ambient cisterns.

2. *Surgical considerations.* The standard approach for P-comm aneurysms is a pterional craniotomy; resection of the anterior clinoid process can improve access to the proximal ICA. P-comm aneurysms have a tendency to rupture or rerupture during surgery at a higher rate than other aneurysms,[269] particularly with retraction of the temporal lobe.[270]

3. *Endovascular treatment.* Endovascular access and coiling P-comm aneurysms is usually uncomplicated, although P-comm aneurysms seem to have a tendency to be relatively wide-necked. Sometimes these aneurysms arise at a bizarre reverse angle from the parent vessel, requiring the use of sharply curved, pre-shaped microcatheters to access the lesion. Stent-assisted coiling is appropriate for unruptured wide-necked P-comm aneurysms. In patients with SAH due to a wide-necked P-comm aneurysm, capping of the dome with coils can protect

against rerupture in the acute phase after SAH, with more definitive stent-assisted coiling of the remnant at a later date.

ANTERIOR CHOROIDAL ARTERY ANEURYSMS

Anterior choroidal artery aneurysms account for 4% of all intracranial aneurysms. They tend to be small (average size in one series was 4 mm),[271] and project in an inferior and posterior direction. In most cases they arise near or adjacent to the origin of the anterior choroidal artery, although in 18% of patients the aneurysm originates entirely or in part from the anterior choroidal artery itself.[272] In treatment of these aneurysms, preservation of the anterior choroidal artery is critical, as the vessel is notorious for having poor collateral circulation to the proximal territory of the anterior choroidal, which, unfortunately, is just that part of this vessel that supplies the internal capsule. Ischemic stroke from occlusion of the anterior choroidal artery, described as *Anterior Choroidal Syndrome*, can cause contralateral hemiplegia, hemianesthesia, and hemianopia, although in a series of ischemic complications with surgery for anterior choroidal aneurysms, sensory and visual changes were less consistent than motor deficits:[272]

1. *Presentation.* Most anterior choroidal artery aneurysms present with SAH or are incidental findings. Much less commonly, they can present with acute third cranial nerve palsy or cerebral ischemic symptoms from embolization of the intraluminal thrombus.
2. *Surgical considerations.* Anterior choroidal aneurysms are accessible via a pterional craniotomy. The greatest technical challenge occurs because the aneurysm usually appears on the side of the ICA opposite to the surgeon's approach, and visualization of the anterior choroidal artery origin can be problematic. In a series of 50 patients undergoing surgery for anterior choroidal aneurysms, 16% of patients had anterior choroidal territory ischemic strokes.[272] Most of these strokes occurred in a delayed fashion, 6–36 h after surgery.
3. *Endovascular treatment.* The small size of anterior choroidal aneurysms and the orientation of the aneurysm, at a right angle to the axis of the ICA, can make coiling these lesions tricky. Published results, however, are encouraging. In a series of 18 patients undergoing coiling of anterior choroidal aneurysms, the overall complication rate was 11%.[271] There was one treatment-related death due to aneurysm perforation, and another patient developed a transient contralateral hemiparesis. No rehemorrhages occurred during an average follow-up of 14 months.

CAROTID BIFURCATION ANEURYSMS

The internal carotid bifurcation is the location of some 5% of all intracranial aneurysms, and men and women appear to be affected equally.[273] Some data suggest that these aneurysms hemorrhage at a lower age than aneurysms in other locations.[273] These aneurysms tend to arise on the side of A1 at an average distance of 1.6 mm between the midline of the ICA and the midline of the aneurysm neck.[274]

Anterior Cerebral Artery Aneurysms

Together, the ACA and A-comm are the most common location for intracranial aneurysms, accounting for some 39% of all ruptured aneurysms.[275]

ANTERIOR COMMUNICATING ARTERY ANEURYSMS

The A-comm is the single most common site of aneurysms presenting with SAH. Like P-comm aneurysms, both surgery and endovascular treatment of A-comm aneurysms are often relatively straightforward, and therefore each approach is generally valid. Some 45% of the aneurysms randomized in ISAT were A-comm aneurysms:[195]

1. *Presentation.* On CT there is typically a clot in the interhemispheric fissure. Intraventricular hemorrhage is present in 79% of cases, and acute hydrocephalus occurs in 25% of patients.[276] Hyponatremia occurs more frequently in patients with ruptured A-comm aneurysms (51%) than in patients with ruptured aneurysms in other location, presumably because of the proximity of the A-comm complex to the hypothalamus.[277] Another common consequence of SAH due to a ruptured A-comm aneurysm is cognitive dysfunction, occasionally referred to as the "A-comm Syndrome." Features of this syndrome include short-term memory impairment, personality changes, and confabulation, and are attributed to injury to the basal forebrain.[278] Some data suggests that surgical patients have higher chance of memory and frontal lobe executive function deficits compared to patients treated with endovascular means.[279]
2. *Surgical considerations.* The standard surgical approach for A-comm aneurysms is a pterional craniotomy. Opening of the Sylvian fissure and partial

resection of the gyrus rectus are maneuvers that can enhance access to the A-comm region. The orientation of the aneurysm strongly affects the ease of surgery; larger, inferiorly directed aneurysms can make surgical access to the contralateral A1 – necessary for proximal control – challenging.

3. *Endovascular treatment.* Several studies of endovascular treatment of A-comm aneurysms have been published.[188,280,281] Technical factors that can limit endovascular treatment are the acute angle formed by the A1 segment relative to the ICA (which can make catheter access difficult), the relative small size of A-comm aneurysms, and the difficulty, in some cases, of adequate fluoroscopic visualization of the A-comm complex during the procedure. A recent analysis of 123 patients with A-comm aneurysms reported that successful embolization was accomplished in 70% of patients.[281] Embolization was attempted but not successful in 9.8% of patients. At a mean follow-up of 8.6 months, some degree of recanalization was observed in 33.3% of cases. Anteriorly projecting aneurysms were more likely to be successfully coiled than either inferiorly or posteriorly/superiorly directed aneurysms, and inferiorly projecting aneurysms and wide-necked aneurysms had significantly higher rates of recanalization.

4. The authors of this handbook prefer surgery in younger patients, and endovascular treatment in older patients, and in those with complex or inferiorly directed aneurysm anatomy.

DISTAL ANTERIOR CEREBRAL ARTERY ANEURYSMS

Anterior cerebral artery aneurysms arising distally to the A-comm artery comprise about 5% of all intracranial aneurysms.[282] Most are located at the A2–A3 junction (usually referred to as pericallosal artery aneurysms); however aneurysms are also often located on the A2 and A3 segments. Some 41% of patients with distal ACA aneurysms have one or more additional intracranial aneurysms.[282] Although an azygous A2 is found in <1% of the general population,[283] the anatomical variant is strongly associated with aneurysms; some 41% of azygous A2 segments have a terminal aneurysm.[284] The distal ACA is also a common site for traumatic aneurysms; some 25–30% of traumatic aneurysms are located on the distal ACA:[285,286]

1. *Presentation.* Ruptured distal ACA aneurysms appear with an intracerebral hematoma in 50% of cases[287,288] or an interhemispheric subdural hematoma. Patients with a ruptured distal ACA aneurysm tend to present at a poorer grade compared to patients with aneurysms at other locations; some 60–63% of patients present with a Hunt and Hess grade of 3 or higher.[288,289]

2. *Surgical considerations.* The surgical approach depends on the location of the aneurysm. Aneurysms <1 cm distal to the A-comm aneurysm may be approached via a pterional craniotomy. Aneurysms in the proximity of the genu of the corpus callosum usually require a bicoronal skin incision, frontal craniotomy, and interhemispheric approach. More distal aneurysms ("supracallosal" aneurysms) can be approached with a horseshoe skin flap and a posterior frontal craniotomy.

3. *Endovascular treatment.* Distal ACA aneurysms are typically small and located some distance along the ACA, making endovascular treatment challenging in some cases.[290] Pericallosal aneurysms, particularly those associated with an azygous A2, are the most accessible (Fig. 1.31).

MIDDLE CEREBRAL ARTERY ANEURYSMS

Middle cerebral artery aneurysms constitute about 20% of all intracranial aneurysms and are the third most common cause of aneurysmal SAH.[291,292] Mirror MCA aneurysms occur in up to 11% of patients, and patients with MCA aneurysms also have an increased incidence of pericallosal artery aneurysms.[293] Some 85% of MCA aneurysms arise at the bifurcation, 10–15% are located along the M1 segment,[291] and the remaining MCA aneurysms, appearing on the M2–4 segments, are more likely to be infectious or inflammatory in origin.[294] The anatomy of the MCA makes the vessel somewhat unique compared to other common aneurysm locations. The MCA trunk forms a true bifurcation, giving rise to two M2 divisions, in about 80% of cases; in 12% of cases there is a trifurcation, and in the remaining cases there are multiple branches.[295] MCA aneurysms project laterally in 45% of cases and inferiorly in 38% of cases:[293]

1. *Presentation.* Unruptured MCA aneurysms are less likely to be symptomatic than aneurysms at other locations.[25] Cerebral ischemic phenomena such as TIAs and stroke are more likely to occur with MCA aneurysms than with others. Patients with seizure disorders attributable to an unruptured MCA aneurysm have been reported.[296–298] Ruptured MCA aneurysms are commonly associated with intracerebral hematomas, which are found in nearly 40% of cases.[299]

2. *Surgical considerations.* There are three surgical approaches to MCA aneurysms. The medial transsylvian approach provides early access to the ICA for proximal control, and is often favored for surgery on ruptured MCA aneurysms. The lateral transsylvian approach is advantageous because it minimizes frontal and temporal lobe retraction and is useful for distal aneurysms, for aneurysms that project in an anterior direction, and for cases with a long MCA trunk.[300] The superior temporal gyrus approach is the preferred approach when evacuation of an intracerebral hematoma is required.[301]

3. *Endovascular treatment.* Aneurysms at the M1 segment terminus are typically wide-necked and eccentric toward one division, and the aneurysm neck may incorporate one or more branches. Coil embolization can be difficult to accomplish without risk of stenosis or occlusion of at least one division. In an early report, published in 1999, coil embolization was attempted but unsuccessful in 85% of cases.[302] Improved technique, better case selection, and the advent of 3D angiographic imaging has led to better results in recent reports.[172,303] A recent systematic review found an overall rate of complete or near-complete occlusion of 82.4%, with permanent procedure-related morbidity and mortality of 5.1% and 6.0% for unruptured and ruptured MCA aneurysms, respectively.[304]

4. Doerfler and colleagues reported complete occlusion in 33 of 38 MCA aneurysms treated with coiling.[303] Thromboembolic occlusion occurred in five patients (13%), although recanalization of the occluded vessel was obtained in four of these patients with thrombolytic treatment.[303] In a series of 154 MCA aneurysms treated with coiling, thromboembolic complications occurred in 13.4% of cases, and recanalization was found on follow-up angiography in 20% (mean follow-up 15 months).[172] The advent of 3D angiographic imaging during endovascular treatment of complex MCA aneurysms has greatly improved the ability to safely treat these aneurysms.

Unruptured Aneurysms and Epilepsy
Unruptured aneurysms are a rare cause of seizures. A surgical series identified nine (2.6%) patients with seizures attributable to the aneurysm among 347 undergoing craniotomy and clipping.[298] All of the aneurysms were in the anterior circulation; six of them were surrounded by gliosis evidence on MRI FLAIR imaging, and six of them were in contact with anterior temporomedial structures. Seven of the six patients underwent clipping, with or without resection of the gliotic tissue, and all patients were seizure-free after surgery. Two case reports have also described improvement in seizures after endovascular aneurysm treatment in this setting as well.[305,306]

POSTERIOR CIRCULATION ANEURYSMS
Posterior circulation aneurysms comprise about 15% of all intracranial aneurysms.

BASILAR APEX ANEURYSMS
Some 50% of all posterior circulation aneurysms are located at the basilar apex. In a systematic review of endovascular treatment of posterior circulation aneurysms, 82% were basilar apex aneurysms[307]:

1. *Presentation.* If large enough, unruptured basilar apex aneurysms can cause a third cranial nerve palsy or brainstem compression, or, rarely, interference with the optic chiasm.[308] The pattern of blood seen on the CT after SAH can be similar to that seen with some anterior circulation ruptured aneurysms and perimesencephalic aneurysmsal SAH.

2. *Surgical considerations.* Surgery of the basilar apex is challenging because of the location, the presence of brainstem perforating vessels, and the difficulty of obtaining proximal control:

   (a) Approach. An array of approaches to the basilar apex exist and selection of the surgical approach usually depends on the height of the aneurysm relative to the posterior clinoid process. The transsylvian approach is typically employed for relatively "high" basilar apex aneurysms, originating between the midlevel of the sella turcica and about 1 cm superior to the posterior clinoid. A subtemporal approach provides better access to low-lying and posteriorly projecting aneurysms. An orbitozygomatic osteotomy and division of the tentorium are maneuvers that can enhance access to the basilar apex. Intraoperative hypothermic cardiac arrest is another strategy that can reduce the chance of ischemic injury, particularly with large and giant aneurysms. A major priority of surgery of the basilar artery is preservation of the numerous brainstem perforating vessels that arise in this region.

(b) Complications. Postoperative third cranial nerve palsy is common, occurring 32–52.8% of cases;[309,310] however complete resolution of the palsy occurs in 80% of patients within 6 months.[310] Younger patients and posteriorly pointing aneurysms are risk factors for third cranial nerve palsy.

3. *Endovascular treatment.* Because of the technical difficulty with surgery, and the relative ease of catheter access, coiling has become the treatment of choice for basilar apex aneurysms in most centers. Randomized data is not available; in ISAT, only 17 (0.7%) of the cases were at the basilar apex.[195] In a review of six basilar apex aneurysm coiling series, the procedural morbidity was 6.6% and the procedural mortality was 1.3% (both ruptured and unruptured aneurysms were included in these figures).[311] In a study of 316 coiled basilar apex aneurysms, a 90–100% occlusion was obtained in 86% of cases, and the overall complication rate was 19%.[311] The end-artery position of basilar apex aneurysms may make them more vulnerable to recurrence after coiling. At a mean follow-up period of 19 months, coil compaction was evident in 24% of cases.[311]

How Many Names Can There Be?
Aneurysms at the basilar apex have been called by a variety of names, including *basilar summit* [17], *basilar top* [312], *basilar tip* [313], *basilar terminus* [314], and *basilar bifurcation*. Although the authors of this handbook consider terms such as "summit" and "top" to be quaint, they prefer the term basilar apex aneurysm.

POSTERIOR CEREBRAL ARTERY ANEURYSMS

PCA aneurysms are uncommon, comprising some 1% of all intracranial aneurysms.[315–317] They have a predilection for the P1 and P2 segments [318] and they are frequently discovered at an earlier age than aneurysms in other anatomic sites.[315] In addition, they are more likely to be large or giant compared to aneurysms at other locations,[319] and have a relatively high incidence of coexisting vascular dysplasias.[318]

1. *Presentation.* Most PCA aneurysms present with SAH. Approximately 25% of patients present with hemianopia or oculomotor disturbances.[318,320] Giant aneurysms of the P3 segment can cause memory loss due to compression of the hippocampus.[318]

2. *Surgical considerations.* P1 aneurysms can be approached via a pterional craniotomy.[321] Most aneurysms of the P2 segment can be approached subtemporally. P2 aneurysms that are superior to the tentorium may be reached transcortically and via the temporal horn of the lateral ventricle and the choroidal fissure.[322] P3 aneurysms may be reached through the occipital interhemispheric fissure. A recent series of occipital artery-to-posterior cerebral artery bypass cases for distal PCA aneurysms noted a relatively high rate of complications, and led the authors to recommend against the operation for most patients.[323]

3. *Endovascular treatment.* Endovascular strategies include coil embolization or sacrifice of the parent vessel. In a series of 20 patients with PCA aneurysms treated with endovascular techniques, 66% were treated with preservation of the parent vessel and in the remaining 33% the parent vessel was occluded.[318] The overall permanent morbidity rate was 10% with no mortality. Endovascular occlusion of the PCA should be done distal to the P1 segment, to preserve important brainstem and thalamic perforators. It is often well tolerated due to well-developed collateral circulation between the distal PCA and the anterior circulation and other branches of the vertebrobasilar system. In a series of nine P2 segment aneurysms cases which were treated with occlusion of the parent vessel, no neurologic deficits occurred after treatment.[324]

SUPERIOR CEREBELLAR ARTERY ANEURYSMS

Most superior cerebellar artery aneurysms arise from the lateral basilar artery wall, in the crotch between the origins of the PCA and SCA. Many surgical series grouped SCA aneurysms together with basilar apex aneurysms. Because of the lateral position of these aneurysms, surgery for SCA aneurysms is somewhat more straight-forward than surgery for basilar apex aneurysms. Moreover, the approach is similar and the risk of postoperative third cranial nerve palsy (39%) is also comparable.[310] SCA aneurysms are typically small and arise from the basilar artery at a 90° angle, characteristics that can make endovascular treatment challenging. In a series of 12 SCA aneurysms treated with coiling, complete occlusion was obtained in 50%, and procedural morbidity was limited to one SCA territory infarct with good recovery.[325]

DISTAL SUPERIOR CEREBELLAR ARTERY ANEURYSMS

Distal SCA aneurysms are rare and usually present with SAH or fourth cranial nerve dysfunction.[326–328] They are also frequently associated with an AVM or are traumatic in origin.[326,329]

Distal SCA aneurysms can be treated effectively with endovascular parent vessel sacrifice,[330–332] particularly since the collateral circulation between the SCA and the AICA and PICA, and even the proximal PCA is generally well developed.

BASILAR TRUNK ANEURYSMS

Aneurysms of the basilar artery trunk are rare, comprising <1% of all intracranial aneurysms, and 8% of vertebrobasilar aneurysms.[333] Approximately twice as many are located in the upper basilar artery as there are in the lower part of the vessel:[334]

1. *Presentation.* Basilar trunk aneurysms typically present with SAH; large and giant aneurysms may present with brainstem or cranial nerve symptoms.
2. *Surgical considerations.* Surgery in this region is impaired by the petrous bone, which interferes with direct surgical access to this region. Surgical series reports complete aneurysm occlusion rates ranging from 34% to 91%.[335–337]
3. *Endovascular treatment.* Coil embolization of basilar trunk aneurysms is preferred in most centers because of the difficulty with surgery and because catheter access to this region is relatively easy. The technical ease of endovascular treatment was illustrated by a series in which the average procedure time was only 61 min.[338] A number of endovascular series have reported generally favorable results, although basilar trunk aneurysms may tend to recur after coiling. In a report of 14 cases of coiling of basilar trunk aneurysms with an average follow-up of 20 months, recanalization occurred in 4 (28.6%).[339] An alternative strategy is parent vessel sacrifice. Surgical.[340] or endovascular basilar trunk occlusion can be relatively safe and effective in carefully selected patients.[341] The authors of this handbook caution that management of patients after basilar artery occlusion can be challenging.

ANTERIOR INFERIOR CEREBELLAR ARTERY ANEURYSMS

Aneurysms of the anterior inferior cerebellar artery (AICA) usually arise at the origin of the vessel. In a series of 3,500 aneurysms treated with surgery, AICA aneurysms comprised 1.3%.[342] Most surgical series group AICA aneurysms together with basilar trunk aneurysms. AICA aneurysms typically present with SAH, although brainstem compression is a feature in some 20% of cases.[342] Like SCA aneurysms, AICA aneurysms can be associated with an AVM.[343] Surgical strategies include the retrosigmoid, transpetrosal, far lateral, and subtemporal-transtentorial approach. Possibly because of their infrequency, relatively few reports of endovascular treatment of AICA origin aneurysms have been published so far. Of four basilar artery/AICA aneurysms treated with coiling, complete occlusion was obtained in two and excellent or good outcomes were had by all.[339]

Distal AICA aneurysms are rare, and usually arise from the rostral branch of the vessel.[342] They typically present with SAH, and hearing loss may be present due to involvement of the internal auditory artery.[344] Endovascular occlusion of the parent vessel distal to the origin of the internal auditory artery is feasible for treatment of these aneurysms because the collateral circulation in this region is usually well developed.[345]

VERTEBROBASILAR JUNCTION ANEURYSMS

Vertebrobasilar junction aneurysms arise at the confluence of the vertebral arteries, and are very uncommon, accounting for some 3–4% of all posterior circulation aneurysms.[334] They are frequently associated with vertebrobasilar fenestrations.[346] Dissecting aneurysms have a tendency to appear in this location.[347] Surgical access to this region is limited. Endovascular options include primary coiling, stenting and stent-assisted coiling, and parent vessel sacrifice. Because aneurysms at this location may be filled from both vertebral arteries the resulting hemodynamic stress may lead to a relatively high risk of recanalization after coiling. In one study, three of five VBJ aneurysms required permanent occlusion of one or both vertebral arteries.[339] A potential hazard is occlusion of brainstem perforators or the anterior spinal artery; in a series of basilar artery aneurysms, 2 out of 3 ischemic complications occurred in VBJ aneurysms.[339]

DISTAL VERTEBRAL/PROXIMAL PICA ANEURYSMS

Aneurysms of the vertebral artery at the origin of the PICA comprise about 2% of all intracranial aneurysms, and 80% of aneurysms involving the PICA.[348] They tend to be relatively small (<12.5 mm).[348] Fusiform, nonsaccular aneurysms are more common in the distal vertebral artery than at other locations, and dissecting aneurysms are also more common, accounting for 28% of intracranial vertebral artery aneurysms in one series:[349]

1. *Presentation.* The most frequent presentation of PICA origin aneurysms is SAH, and intraventricular hemorrhage along with acute hydrocephalus are present in >95% of these cases.[350] Some 9–12% of distal vertebral or PICA origin aneurysms present with symptoms of mass effect or ischemia.[351]
2. *Surgical considerations.* Aneurysms at the PICA–vertebral junction usually occur at least 1 cm above the foramen magnum and arise distally to the PICA origin in the angle between the two vessels. A far lateral suboccipital craniotomy usually provides adequate access. When clipping of the aneurysm with preservation of the PICA is not feasible, a PICA–PICA bypass is an option.[352]
3. *Endovascular treatment.* Recent reports of endovascular treatment of PICA aneurysms are encouraging. In a series of 31 patients treated with coiling for proximal PICA aneurysms, angiographic occlusion was achieved in 30 (97%) patients.[353] Procedural complications occurred in three (10%) patients, including one aneurysm rupture during coiling, one minor PICA ischemic stroke, and one temporary femoral neuropathy. No recanalizations were observed at a mean angiographic follow-up of 9 months.

DISTAL PICA ANEURYSMS

Distal PICA aneurysms account for ≤1% of all intracranial aneurysms.[348,354,355] They may arise from any segment of the PICA but typically occur at branching sites and at curves in the vessel and project in the direction in which flow would have continued if the curve had not been present.[348] They are commonly associated with AVMs and other vascular abnormalities, such as dural AV fistulas.[354,356] Unlike distal aneurysms in other vascular territories, which are often mycotic or traumatic, distal PICA aneurysms are usually sporadic and are almost never related to an infectious etiology. Men and women are affected equally.[354,357] Most authors recommend treatment of unruptured distal PICA aneurysms of any size, as a significant percentage of ruptured distal PICA aneurysms are <5 mm in size:[354,358]

1. *Presentation.* The majority of distal PICA aneurysms present with hemorrhage, and intraventricular hemorrhage and acute hydrocephalus are common.[354,356]
2. *Surgical considerations.* The surgical approach depends on the location of the aneurysm; aneurysms arising from the most distal part of the PICA, the telovelotonsillar and cortical segments can be approached via a midline suboccipital craniectomy. More proximal PICA aneurysms, of the anterior and lateral medullary segments, usually require a far lateral suboccipital approach. Sacrifice of the PICA is a valid strategy for the treatment of distal PICA aneurysms, and is generally agreed to be safe when it is done distally to the portion of the PICA that gives rise to important perforating vessels (i.e., distal to the choroidal point, or the top of the cranial loop).[358] For aneurysms of the proximal segments of the PICA that cannot be clipped with preservation of the parent vessel, trapping with a PICA–PICA bypass is an option.[352]
3. *Endovascular treatment.* Endovascular treatment can be problematic due to the difficulty of navigating a catheter into the distal PICA, and because distal PICA aneurysms tend to be relatively wide-necked. Therefore, parent vessel occlusion, when possible, is usually the most feasible endovascular approach.[332] Very distal aneurysms may require treatment with liquid embolic materials, rather than coils, if a soft, flow-directed microcatheter must be used to catheterize the distal vessel.

A Brief History of Endovascular Treatment of Intracranial Aneurysms

The first successful case of the treatment of an intracranial aneurysm by "electrothrombosis" was reported in 1941.[359] For the treatment of an ICA aneurysm, "thirty feet of No. 34 gauge coin silver enamel wire was introduced into the aneurysm through a special needle" advanced through the orbit, and the wire was "heated to an average temperature of 80°C for a total of 40 s. The aneurysm no longer bled when the needle was cleared at the end of the operation." Further attempts to treat intracranial aneurysms by electrothrombosis via the stereotactic insertion of a needle passed through a burr hole and into the aneurysm were reported by Sean Mullan and colleagues in 1965.[360]

Several creative approaches to aneurysm treatment were explored in the 1960s and 1970s. The "pilojection" technique involved the forcible injection of hog hairs or horse hairs into the aneurysm with a pneumatic gun.[361] Stereotactic magnetically guided embolization of aneurysms with iron particles was also investigated.[362]

Alfred Luessenhop and A.C. Velasquez published the first report of an endovascular attempt at the treatment of an intracranial aneurysm in 1964.[363] They described an effort to occlude a supraclinoid aneurysm with a silicone balloon. Inspired by watching helium balloons on tethers during a May Day celebration in Moscow in 1959, Fedor Serbinenko, a Russian neurosurgeon, developed silicone and latex balloon catheters, initially intended for diagnostic procedures. The balloon at the end of the catheter was used for flow-directed navigation and temporary diagnostic occlusion of major cerebral arteries. Serbinenko accomplished his first successful detachable balloon embolization for sacrifice of an ICA to treat a carotid-cavernous fistula in 1969; the technique involved filling a balloon when it was positioned at the target site with silicone polymer and detaching it by severing the catheter with the cutting edge of an arterial introduction needle.[364] Later, technical refinements in the balloon detachment mechanism permitted placement of the detachable balloons within intracranial aneurysms.[365]

Although balloon embolization of intracranial lesions was popularized in the late 1970s and 1980s,[366,367] the technique had several drawbacks. Placement of balloons inside aneurysms was problematic because no guidewire could be used, and the preformed spherical or oval shapes of balloons limited their usefulness in aneurysms with complex shapes. In addition, a balloon placed inside an aneurysm could have a ball-valve effect, leading to an accumulation of blood inside the aneurysm, recanalization, and rupture.[368] Because of these problems and the later introduction of detachable coils, balloon embolization of intracranial lesions has trailed off; the last manufacturer of detachable balloons in the US, Boston Scientific, Inc., stopped selling them in the US because of low demand and regulatory issues with the FDA. Detachable balloons continue to be available in other countries, and will likely eventually be reintroduced into the US, although it is doubtful that they will ever return as a potential treatment for aneurysms, except as a method for achieving large vessel parent artery occlusion.

Therapeutic arterial occlusion with endovascular "pushable" metal coils was originated for the treatment of lesions in the peripheral vasculature.[369] Although some operators (including the authors of this handbook) have in days long ago used pushable coils for the treatment of intracranial aneurysms,[370,371] pushable coils were severely hampered by their stiffness, and by an inability to manipulate the coil inside the aneurysm and to retrieve each coil, if necessary, after it is deployed. Continued experimentation with electrothrombosis eventually lead to the development of detachable coils. Guido Guglielmi, an Italian neurosurgeon, conceived of detachable coils serendipitously in the early 1980s. During the treatment of an experimental aneurysm with a stainless steel electrode to promote electrothrombosis, accidental detachment of the electrode tip occurred. Later, working with engineers at Target Therapeutics, Inc., he developed the Guglielmi detachable coil (GDC, Stryker Neurovascular, Fremont, CA). The GDC coil system permits placement of a platinum alloy coil inside the aneurysm, through a microcatheter; the coil remains attached to the pusher wire until it is in a satisfactory position. The operator then detaches the coil from the wire by applying a low-amplitude electrical current to the pusher wire, which causes electrolysis of the connection between the wire and the coil. Clinical use of GDC coils began in 1991, and in 1995 the FDA granted approval of GDC coils for the treatment of high-risk, inoperable, or ruptured intracranial aneurysms.

A number of technical refinements in the design of aneurysm coils have occurred over the last decade. An array of shapes and sizes of coils have been introduced. *Stretch resistant* coils contain a filament inside the coil to bind the distal end of the coil and resist stretching of the coil when tension is applied. Alternative detachment systems have been introduced, some of which (including TruFill DCS, Cordis Neurovascular, Miami Lakes, FL) are hydraulic rather than electrolytic.

The greatest drawback to the coiling of aneurysms has been the occurrence of recanalization in a significant percentage of treated aneurysms over time, occurring in as many as approximately 20% of coiled aneurysms in 5 years.[165] *Augmented coils (aka bioactive coils)* have attracted much interest, as a means of enhancing thrombosis and eventual fibrosis within the aneurysm to reduce the likelihood of recanalization. Augmented coils include the Matrix™ (Stryker Neurovascular, Fremont, CA) and Cerecyte™ (Codman Neurovascular, Raytham, MA) systems, both of which contain polyglycolic–polylactic acid (PGLA), and the HydroCoil® system (Terumo Medical/MicroVention, Inc., Tustin, CA), in which the coils are treated with a gel that swells upon contact with water and occupies space within the aneurysm. The latest addition to this niche market is the Axium™ MicroFX™ PGLA-treated coil (ev3, Irvine, CA). Interest in PGLA-treated coils has faded since the completion of the Cerecyte trial and the Matrix And Platinum Science (MAPS) trials; both studies failed to show a benefit with PGLA-treated coils compared to bare platinum coils.

The treatment of wide-necked aneurysms is problematic, and several techniques and devices have evolved to facilitate coiling of these lesions. Balloon remodeling, a technique popularized by Jacques Moret,[372] involves the positioning of a temporary balloon in the parent vessel adjacent to the aneurysm neck. The balloon is inflated and permits the placement of a nest of coils within the aneurysm, which are stable once the balloon is deflated and removed. Stent-assisted coiling involves the deployment of a thin wire mesh stent in the parent vessel across the neck of the aneurysm; a microcatheter is then guided through the interstices of the stent for coil deployment. The stent acts as a scaffold to prevent the coils from prolapsing into the parent vessel. The Neuroform™ stent (Stryker Neurovascular, Fremont, CA), designed specifically for the treatment of wide-necked aneurysms, is currently in its third generation. Another stent for the treatment of aneurysms, the Enterprise™ Vascular Reconstruction Device (Codman Neurovascular, Raynham, MA) received an FDA Humanitarian Device Exemption in 2007. Unfortunately, neither Stryker nor Codman have invested the resources necessary to obtain full FDA approval for their stents, and now, more than a decade after the introduction of the Neuroform stent and after sales of tens of thousands of the devices world wide, they are still available only on a "humanitarian exemption" basis.

The International Subarachnoid Aneurysm Trial (ISAT) (see below) was the first multicenter, randomized trial to compare surgery to coiling in patients with ruptured aneurysms. The results of the trial, which demonstrated a significant advantage to coiling in 1-year outcomes, led to greater acceptance of the use of coils in all types of intracranial aneurysms. In the United States following the publication of the ISAT results, there was a significant increase in endovascular treatment of ruptured aneurysms and a corresponding decrease in in-hospital mortality due to SAH.[373]

Flow diversion is shaping up to the next paradigm shift in the endovascular treatment of aneurysms. After initial favorable experience in Europe with the Pipeline Embolization Device (ev3, Irvine, CA), the device received CE mark approval in Europe in 2008 and FDA approval in 2011. Another flow-diversion stent, currently with CE mark approval in Europe, is the Silk (Balt Extrusion, Montmorency, France).

13.4.   Subarachnoid Hemorrhage

This section will focus on aneurysmal SAH, which accounts for approximately 80% of all nontraumatic SAH cases.[374] Angiographic work-up is negative in approximately in some 15–20% of patients with spontaneous SAH.[375] Traumatic SAH is considered separately below. The remaining ~20% of spontaneous SAH:

1) *Perimesencephalic nonaneurysmal subarachnoid hemorrhage (PMSAH)* – a distinct entity with characteristic clinical and imaging features and an excellent prognosis:
   a) Overall incidence: 0.5 per 100,000 persons age ≥18,[376] representing approximately 5% of all SAH.
   b) Diagnosis:
      i) Patients typically present as HH 1 or 2.
      ii) Usual CT appearance: Hemorrhage is centered anterior to the pons (Fig. 13.7), although a posterior variant has been described, with the hemorrhage primarily in the in the quadrigeminal cistern.[377]
      iii) Radiographic work-up is negative for an aneurysm.

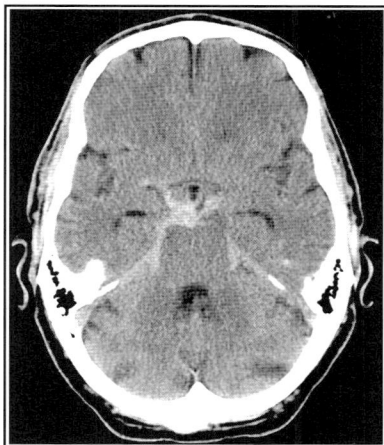

Fig. 13.7 CT appearance of perimesencephalic nonaneurysmal subarachnoid hemorrhage. In patients with perimesencephalic nonaneurysmal subarachnoid hemorrhage, the pattern of blood is frequently asymmetric and includes the ambient cisterns.

    c) Mechanism is unknown, although a venous source is suspected. PMSAH is associated with a pattern of primitive venous drainage directly into dural sinuses, instead of via the vein of Galen, as is seen in most patients with SAH.[378]Outcome: Excellent. In a series of 24 patients with this syndrome, only one had a neurological change (and it was transient), and no rebleeds occurred.[55]

2) Reversible Cerebrovascular Constriction Syndrome (aka Call-Fleming Syndrome)[379]
    a) See also Chap. 17 for discussion of this syndrome as a cause of ischemic stroke.
    b) Presentation:
        i) Thunderclap headache is common.
        ii) Some 20–30% have SAH,[380,381] although the CT scan is normal in the majority of patients.
    c) Epidemiology:
        i) Peak incidence between age 20 and 50; mean 42 years.[382] Patients are most often women.
    d) Diagnosis:
        i) "Segmental vasoconstriction" on cerebral angiography (DSA or MRA) is pathognomonic.
    e) Management:
        i) Calcium channel blockers (e.g., nimodipine) are the most commonly reported medications used.[383]
    f) Prognosis: Overall very good. Symptoms and angiographic changes usually resolve after a week. Recurrence is uncommon.[384]

3) Other causes of SAH:[385]
    a) Intracranial arterial dissection
    b) AVM
    c) Dural AVF
    d) Infectious aneurysms
    e) Infectious endocarditis
    f) Trauma
    g) Coagulation disorders

h) Cocaine
i) Cervical origin of the hemorrhage (e.g., spinal AVM or fistula)
j) Cavernous malformations
k) Vasculitis or other vasculopathy
l) Intracranial tumor
m) Sickle cell disease and syndrome
n) Pituitary apoplexy
o) Intracranial venous sinus thrombosis

Aneurysmal Subarachnoid Hemorrhage

Incidence

1. Global annual incidence of aneurysmal SAH is approximately 10/100,000[386-388]
2. Some 21,000–33,000 new cases of SAH occur in the US each year.[139]
3. Mean age at presentation: 55 years.[389]
4. Risk of SAH for women is 1.6 times that of men, and compared to Caucasians, the risk for African Americans and for Hispanics is higher by a factor of 1.6 and 1.3, respectively.[388] Other risk factors for SAH, such as connective tissue disorders and smoking, are discussed above.

Diagnosis

PRESENTATION
It is typically described as the "worst headache of my life." Nausea and vomiting, meningismus, diminished level of consciousness, focal neurological findings, and the presence of risk factors for SAH should raise suspicion of aneurysmal SAH. The Hunt-Hess scale is in Table 13.9.

1) Loss of consciousness at the time of onset is highly predictive of aneurysmal rupture.[390]
2) Vomiting occurs in up to 70% of patients with aneurysmal SAH.[391]
3) A history of "sentinel headache" is present in 10–43% of patients, and may be the only presenting symptom of SAH.[392]
4) Intraocular hemorrhage occurs in approximately 17% of patients with SAH:[393,394]
   a) *Terson Syndrome*, i.e., hemorrhage in the vitreous humor, has been seen in 8–17%, and is associated with a significantly elevated mortality rate.[394,395]
   b) Subhyaloid (i.e., preretinal) hemorrhage is seen in 11–33% of cases, and appears fundoscopically as bright red blood near the optic disc that obscures the retinal vessels.[396]
5) Seizures with the onset of SAH occur in approximately 6% of patients.[397]

RADIOGRAPHIC WORK-UP
1) The characteristic appearance of aneurysmal SAH on CT is hyperdense blood in the cisterns and fissures. The Fisher system is in Table 13.10.

Table 13.9 Hunt–Hess scale

Grade	Description
1	Asymptomatic, mild headache, slight nuchal rigidity
2	Moderate-to-severe headache, nuchal rigidity, no neurological deficit other than cranial nerve palsy
3	Drowsiness/confusion and/or mild focal neurological deficit
4	Stupor, moderate-to-severe hemiparesis
5	Coma, decerebrate posturing

From Honda et al.,[321] with permission

Table 13.10 Fisher grading system for SAH

Fisher grade	Appearance of blood on CT
1	No subarachnoid blood visualized
2	Diffuse or thin sheets (vertical layers <1 mm thick)
3	Localized clot and/or vertical layers (≥1 mm thick)
4	Diffuse or no SAH, but with intraventricular or intraparenchymal clot

From Seoane et al. [322]

2) CT is falsely negative in some 2.5–7% of aneurysmal SAH cases.[398] Because blood can be cleared from CSF spaces relatively rapidly, the sensitivity of CT drops to 50% at 7 days.[399]
   a) When the clinical suspicion for SAH is high but CT is negative, lumbar puncture (LP) is indicated, to detect blood in the CSF:
      i) Optimal results are obtained if at least 6 h, and preferably 12, have elapsed between the onset of the headache and the LP, to permit lysis of the red blood cells and the appearance of xanthochromia (a yellow tinge after centrifugation).[400]
      ii) Lumbar puncture technique: Collect four sequential specimens of CSF. Send the first and fourth tubes for cell count and differential. The specimens should be examined for the presence of xanthochromia.
      iii) True LP evidence of SAH can be distinguished by the presence of xanthochromia (a yellow tinge after centrifugation) and by a significant drop (defined as ≥25% in one study)[401] in the red blood cell count between the first and fourth tube.
3) CT angiography (CTA) is rapidly replacing catheter angiography as the first-line study in the work up of spontaneous SAH:
   a) CTA has sensitivity in the detection of intracranial aneurysms that is comparable or even superior to angiography.[402,403]
   b) CTA carries less risk and expense than angiography, and has the additional advantage of demonstrating bony anatomy, which is helpful in surgical planning.
   c) The era of the late-night angiogram for patients with SAH, in anticipation of surgery or coiling the next morning, has ended.
4) Catheter angiography remains the "gold standard" for imaging the intracranial vasculature and is indicated for cases in which the CTA does not explain the hemorrhage.
5) Angiogram-negative SAH:
   a) A brain and cervical-spine MRI is an option. Causes of SAH that may not be detected on a cerebral angiogram include cavernous malformations, vasculitis, and spinal vascular malformations or tumors. MR imaging revealed abnormalities in 14% of patients with angiographically negative SAH, and resulted in a significant change in management in 6% of patients.[404] However, a recent analysis of 179 cases of angiogram-negative SAH concluded that MRI of the brain and neck provided no additional benefit, and that the costs of such studies exceeded their value.[405]
   b) A repeat angiogram may be needed. An aneurysm can be obscured on the initial angiogram because of thrombosis or vasospasm. The combined result of a second angiogram in eight reported series was 30 aneurysms in 177 patients (17%).[406]
      i) The yield of a repeat angiogram depends on the appearance of the initial haemorrhage on CT.[405]
         (1) Perimesencephalic pattern: Repeat angiogram showed the bleeding source in 2.0% of cases.
         (2) Non-perimesencephalic pattern: Repeat angiogram showed the bleeding source in 9.8% of cases.

MORTALITY, MORBIDITY AND OUTCOMES
1. SAH accounts for 4.4% of stroke mortality but 27.3% of all stroke-related years of potential life lost before age 65.[407]
2. Mortality:
   (a) The in-hospital mortality rate is 26.3%,[408] and the 30-day case fatality rate is 16–38%.[409-411]

(b) Prospective studies, which include deaths occurring prior to hospital admission, have shown consistently higher mortality rates, ranging from 56% to 86%.[131,412,413]
3. Most deaths occur within 2 weeks of the initial hemorrhage, with 61% occurring within 48 h of the event.[414]
4. Patients with posterior circulation aneurysms are three times more likely to die before reaching the hospital or within the first 48 h after SAH than patients with anterior circulation aneurysms.[415]
5. Some 10–20% of SAH survivors remain dependent.[416]

REBLEEDING AND TIMING OF TREATMENT
1) Rebleeding prior to treatment:
    a) The peak rate of rehemorrhage occurs in the first 24 h[417] – the "spike of death" – and ranges as high as 17–19%.[418–420]
    b) The rebleed rate appears to be approximately 20% within the first 2 weeks of the ictus,[418,421,422a] 40% at 1 month, and 50% at 6 months.[422b]
        i) The rate of rebleeding is roughly 2–3% per day.
    c) Patients with higher Hunt and Hess grades and larger aneurysms are at higher risk of rebleeding.[423]
    d) Rebleeding after SAH carries a mortality rate of up to 74%.[424,425]
2) Antifibrinolytic therapy:
    a) Epsilon-aminocaproic acid (Amicar®, Wyeth-Ayerst, Carolina, PR) and tranexamic acid are synthetic lysine analogues, which block lysine binding sites on plasminogen molecules, inhibiting plasmin formation and thereby inhibiting fibrinolysis.[426]
    b) Prolonged administration of each agent has been shown to protect against recurrent hemorrhage,[427–431] although overall outcome did not improve due to aggravated vasospasm and delayed ischemia caused by these agents.[428,431] In addition, some studies have reported a 24–48 h lag in the effectiveness of epsilon-aminocaproic acid.[432,433]
    c) There has been a revival in interest in the use of antifibrinolytic agents, specifically to protect against rebleeding in the short term, from the time of diagnosis to treatment of the aneurysm.[434–436]
        i) Leipzig and colleagues circumvented the drawbacks to epsilon-aminocaproic acid by using a loading dose – to overcome the lag in effectiveness – and limited administration of the drug to a brief course, prior to early surgical intervention.[437] The overall rebleed rate of 1.3% compared favorably to historical controls.
        ii) Another recent single center study of epsilon-aminocaproic acid reported an overall rebleeding rate of 1.4% and a rate of rehemorrhage per 24-h period of 0.71%.[435]
        iii) A multicenter randomized trial of immediate administration of tranexamic acid, prior to early clipping or coiling of the aneurysm, showed a reduction in the rebleeding rate from 10.8% to 2.4% ($p < 0.01$) and an 80% reduction in the mortality rate from early rebleeding ($p < 0.05$).[438]
        iv) Adverse effects:
            (1) Hydrocephalus. The rate of shunting was 42.3% in patients treated with epsilon-aminocaproic acid,[435] compared to a shunt rate of 20% in patients at the same center who had not been treated with epsilon-aminocaproic acid.[439]
            (2) Deep venous thrombosis. There was a significant 8-fold increase in deep venous thrombosis in patients treated with epsilon-aminocaproic acid but no increase in pulmonary embolism.[434] Another recent study found no such association.[436]
3) Timing of treatment:
    a) Several large-scale studies in the 1970s and 1980s showed that outcomes are better the earlier surgery is done for ruptured aneurysms in most patients.[440–442]
    b) A more recent study showed a significant reduction in patients dead or dependant if treated within 24 h of SAH.[443] The relative risk reduction for a bad outcome was much greater when the treatment was coiling.
4) The primary rationale for early treatment of ruptured aneurysms is to minimize the risk of rehemorrhage and to undertake the procedure (surgery or coiling) prior to the onset of vasospasm, when the risk of complications from treatment may be greater.

5) Long-term risk of recurrent SAH after aneurysm clipping:
    a) In the first 10 years after the initial SAH, the cumulative risk of recurrent SAH after clipping is 3.2%, with an incidence of 286 per 100,000 patient-years.[109] This is 22 times higher than expected in the general population.

HYDROCEPHALUS

1. Some degree of ventricular enlargement is common in SAH, occurring in about 20% of patients.[444-447] Often the ventricles, especially the temporal horns, will "flare" in the first day or two after the ictus, then return to normal:
    (a) 50% of patients who have clinical hydrocephalus recover spontaneously within the first 24 h.[446]
2. Hydrocephalus causing a depressed level of consciousness occurs in some 8% of patients.[448]
3. Risk factors for acute hydrocephalus after SAH:
    (a) Intraventricular hemorrhage, diminished level of consciousness, increasing age, posterior circulation aneurysm site, and a larger volume of subarachnoid blood.[449]
4. Ventriculostomy prior to protection of the ruptured aneurysm should be reserved *only* for patients with a diminished level of consciousness and ventriculomegaly.
    (a) *Important*: In patients with ventriculostomy, care should be taken to avoid overdrainage of CSF, to prevent an abrupt change in intracranial pressure – and transmural aneurysm pressure – that may increase the risk of rehemorrhage:
        • Placement of a ventriculostomy is associated with an increased incidence of rebleeding.[448,450]
    (b) The ICP after ventriculostomy should be maintained at or above 20–25 mmHg, because lower values have been associated with higher incidence of rebleeding.[451]
    (c) For patients undergoing craniotomy for clipping, a ventriculostomy done at the time of surgery can produce brain relaxation and help with exposure.
5. Chronic hydrocephalus:
    (a) Reports vary widely, with rates of shunt-dependent post-SAH hydrocephalus ranging from 10% to 63.4%.[447,452-454]
        • The indications for shunt placement typically include persistent or progressive ventriculomegaly, chronic headaches, and a lack of neurological improvement after SAH.
    (b) In a randomized trial, gradual weaning was not found to lead to a lower rate of shunting compared to rapid weaning.[452]
    (c) The authors' preference is to routinely obtain a head CT 1 month after SAH to check for progressive hydrocephalus.

SEIZURES

1. Seizures after SAH occur in some about 8% of patients, and 90% occur in the first 24 h after aneurysm rupture.[455-457]
2. Any patient who has a seizure after SAH should be evaluated with a CT to rule out recurrent hemorrhage.
3. Prophylactic anticonvulsant treatment was routine in many centers until recently. Seizure prevention, usually with phenytoin, was felt to be necessary to minimize the risks of rebleeding and chronic seizure disorder. Accumulating evidence suggests that routine seizure prophylaxis is not advantageous, for the following reasons:
    (a) In a multivariate model, seizures were not found to be associated with an increased risk of rebleeding.[423]
    (b) The majority of seizures occur prior to hospitalization and are uncommon after 7 days of hospitalization.[457]
    (c) Phenytoin exposure is associated with functional and cognitive disability after SAH.[458]
    (d) Early seizures (within 1 week of SAH) are not a risk factor for late epilepsy.[456,459]
    (e) The authors of this handbook prefer to reserve anticonvulsants for patients who have had, or are suspected to have had, a seizure.
4. Treatment of seizures after SAH:
    (a) An active seizure can usually be controlled with lorazepam, 1–2 mg IV.
    (b) Load with phenytoin, 1 g (or 17 mg/kg) IV, then maintenance dose of 100 mg PO/NG/IV TID.

(c) Levetiracetam (Keppra®, UCB Pharma, Inc., Brussels, Belgium) is a recently introduced anticonvulsant with a favorable side effect profile. Although the drug has not been studied in patients with seizures after SAH, it appears to be a good alternative to phenytoin. Typical starting dose is 500 mg PO/NG BID; can be increased to a total of 1,500 mg BID if necessary to control seizures. An IV form of levetiracetam is now available and the dosing is the same as for the oral form: 500 mg BID. Serum levels cannot be monitored; dosing is titrated to clinical effect (seizure elimination). Primary side effect is drowsiness, and the principle drawback is that it is expensive compared to phenytoin and valproic acid.

(d) By convention, patients who have seizures after SAH should be maintained on an anticonvulsant for at least 6 months and then weaned off, depending on how the patient is doing.

(e) In most states, patients with a history of seizure after SAH must be seizure-free for 6 months before being allowed to resume driving an automobile.

5. The incidence of epilepsy after SAH (defined as ≥2 seizures at least 1 week after SAH) is 3–8%.[459–461]

(a) In ISAT, there were significantly fewer seizures in patients treated with coiling compared to craniotomy and clipping (see below).[194]

Associated Medical Problems

Medical problems are a major source of morbidity in patients with SAH. In a study of 457 patients with SAH, 40% of patients had at least one life-threatening medical complication, and 23% of all deaths were attributable to medical complications.[462] The occurrence of fevers, anemia, hyperglycemia, and acute hypoxia and hypotension related to neurogenic cardiac injury each have a significant impact on mortality and functional outcome.[463] There is a growing recognition that optimal medical management of SAH patients includes tight control of serum glucose and electrolyte levels and fluid volume. Recent data indicates that immunodepression is observed early after aneurysmal SAH, and is associated with a high risk of pneumonia.[464]

Hyperglycemia

Hyperglycemia is common in patients with SAH, occurring in some 30% of patients and is an independent predictor of a poor outcome.[465–467] Hyperglycemia in this setting is presumably due to a catecholamine surge and generalized stress response.[468,469] Ischemic injury to the insula is also associated with hyperglycemia.[470]

Hyperglycemia exacerbates cerebral ischemic injury.[471,472] Hyperglycemia appears to worsen cerebral acidosis, leads to free radical production,[473] and has direct cerebrovascular effects that can worsen ischemia.[474] In severely ill patients in a surgical ICU, intensive insulin therapy to maintain serum glucose at or below 110 mg/dL, even in patients without diabetes, was shown to reduce morbidity and mortality.[475] A preliminary trial of glucose and insulin infusions to maintain serum glucose within a target range of 5.0–7.0 mmol/L (90–125 mg/dL) in SAH indicates that this strategy is safe, although larger trials to evaluate the benefit of this strategy are needed.

Serum Electrolyte Derangements

HYPONATREMIA

Hyponatremia occurs in as many as 30–43% of patients with SAH.[476–478] Although hyponatremia typically appears within days of SAH, it appears >7 days following SAH in 21.4% of patients.[479] Hyponatremia is strongly associated with cerebral vasospasm (84% of patients with hyponatremia have symptomatic vasospasm),[480] and may be a causative factor.[481] Hyponatremia is also associated with raised intracranial pressure.[482]

1. Risk factors for hyponatremia after SAH:

(a) Aneurysmsal SAH (compared to angiogram-negative spontaneous SAH).[479] Hyponatremia occurs significantly more often in patients with ruptured anterior communicating artery aneurysms (51%) compared to patients with aneurysms in other locations.[277]

(b) Third ventricular enlargement.[483]

(c) Diabetes, congestive heart failure, cirrhosis, and adrenal insufficiency.

2. Cerebral salt wasting (CSW) is defined as the renal loss of sodium during intracranial disease leading to hyponatremia and a decrease in extracellular fluid volume. CSW must be distinguished from the syndrome of inappropriate ADH secretion (SIADH) because the primary treatment for SIADH, water restriction, will exacerbate hypovolemia in patients with CSW and may place them at risk of cerebral ischemia.

3. CSW appears to occur *as frequently or more frequently* than SIADH in neurosurgical patients.[484] A decrease in plasma volume of >10% occurs in some 50% of patients with aneurysmal SAH;[485] this finding supports the notion that volume depletion – and thus CSW, when hyponatremia appears with volume depletion – is relatively common in SAH.

4. The mechanism of CSW has not been clearly elucidated. Intracranial pathology is thought to lead to a release of one or more natriuretic factors, causing natriuresis and diuresis. Although early reports implicated atrial natriuretic factor (ANP) as the primary natriuretic factor, more recent data has linked an increase in serum levels of brain natriuretic factor (BNP) with cerebral salt wasting.[486] Serum levels of BNP are consistently elevated in patients with SAH.[487,488] BNP is released by the cardiac ventricles; sympathetic stimulation during SAH,[489] and during vasospasm,[490] may cause release of BNP. BNP has also been localized to the hypothalamus,[491] and may be released when that part of the brain is injured.[487]

5. Diagnosis:
   (a) The critical feature distinguishing CSW from SIADH is volume status; patients with CSW are hypovolemic, as evidenced by a negative water balance and diminished weight, and central venous pressure. Serum osmolality, blood urea nitrogen concentration, and hematocrit may be elevated. In contrast, SIADH is invariably a normovolemic or hypervolemic state.
   (b) Urine sodium concentration may be elevated in both CSW and SIADH and therefore is not useful in this setting. Similarly, serum ADH and ANP levels are also not helpful in distinguishing CSW from SIADH.

6. Management:
   (a) CSW is treated with volume replacement and maintenance of a positive salt balance. IV hydration should be undertaken with 0.9% NaCl (at least 100 mL/h or at a rate sufficient to match fluid losses). For most cases of mild and moderate cases of hyponatremia attributable to CSW, sodium repletion with NaCl tablets, 2 g PO/NG TID is sufficient. For symptomatic CSW and a serum sodium level <130 mEq/L, a 3% NaCl IV infusion may be necessary.
   (b) Overcorrection should be avoided. Rapid correction of hyponatremia is associated with central pontine myelinolysis. Elevation of the serum sodium level should not be faster than 0.7 mEq L/h, for a maximum total daily change not to exceed 20 mEq/L.

HYPERNATREMIA

Some degree of hypernatremia (serum sodium >150 mmol/L) has been found in 20% of patients[466] and is an independent predictor of a poor outcome.[478] Hypernatremia typically arises in patients with SAH as the result of mannitol administration, diabetes insipidus, or widespread brain injury. Diabetes insipidus has been reported in some 0.04% of subarachnoid patients.[492] Treatment of hypernatremia consists of replacement of fluid losses with hypotonic IV fluids and desmopressin, a synthetic analogue of ADH that is usually given as 1–2 mcg IV, SQ, or intranasal doses.

HYPOKALEMIA

Some 27% of patients with SAH have hypokalemia.[493] Hypokalemia can lead to QTc prolongation and serious ventricular arrhythmias.[494] Women are at higher risk of hypokalemia after SAH,[495] and female sex and hypokalemia are independent risk factors for severe QTc prolongation in patients with SAH.[496] In a literature review of 1,139 patients with SAH, there were five cases of torsade de pointes, and all of these patients were hypokalemic.[497] Serum potassium levels should be checked daily and repleted as necessary to maintain the serum potassium level ≥3 mmol/L (7.3 mg/dL).

HYPOMAGNESEMIA

Hypomagnesemia (<0.70 mmol/L or 1.7 mg/dL) occurs in nearly 40% of patients with SAH.[493,498] Hypomagnesemia at admission is associated with more blood on CT and a greater severity of illness,[498] and is also associated with EKG changes in patients with SAH.[493] Although some authors have found an association between hypomagnesemia and cerebral ischemic injury in patients with SAH,[498] others have not.[499] Some centers use magnesium sulfate infusion for prophylaxis of vasospasm, although published data about this is inconsistent (see discussion of Sect. 13.4.2.5.4).

Cardiac Abnormalities

EKG CHANGES

EKG changes are common after SAH. Changes in the ST segment (15–51% of patients), T waves (12–92%), the appearance of U waves (4–47%), QT prolongation (11–66%), and sinus dysrhythmias are the most frequent changes.[500,501] Although EKG abnormalities correlate with the severity of SAH,[502] they usually disappear within a day with no change in the neurological or cardiac condition,[494,503] and are generally not predictors of serious cardiac complications.[176,500,504]

CARDIAC ARRHYTHMIAS

Serious cardiac arrhythmias occur in some 1–4% of patients with SAH,[462,494] with malignant ventricular arrhythmias (i.e., torsade de pointes and ventricular flutter or fibrillation) reported in 4.3%; these patients also had QTc prolongation and hypokalemia.[494] An increased frequency of arrhythmias was found on the day of, and on the day after, aneurysm surgery.[462] Increased sympathetic tone and electrolyte alterations appear to be the primary causative factors; the insula and injury to this region of the brain have also been linked to the occurrence of cardiac arrhythmias.[505,506]v Continuous EEG monitoring in the acute phase after SAH is essential.[507]

REVERSIBLE CARDIOMYOPATHY

A syndrome of reversible cardiomyopathy, described as "stunned myocardium," occurs in a significant percentage of patients with SAH. Left ventricular dysfunction occurs in about 10% of patients,[504,508] and 20% of patients with SAH develop cTI >1.0 μg/L.[509] Cardiac dysfunction is believed to be due to massive sympathetic nervous activation that occurs after SAH;[509–512] coronary vasospasm has also been implicated:[513]

1. Risk factors:
   (a) Hunt–Hess score >2, female sex, larger body surface area and left ventricular mass, lower systolic blood pressure, and higher heart rate are independent predictors of troponin elevation.[509]
2. Management implications:
   (a) Cardiac troponin I elevation after SAH is associated with an increased risk of cardiopulmonary complications, delayed cerebral ischemia, and death or poor functional outcome at discharge.[514,515]
   (b) In most cases, the cardiac changes are reversible.[516,517]
   (c) The optimal management of severely affected patients is unclear.[518] Low cardiac output in these patients may exacerbate cerebral ischemia and inotropic agents such as dobutamine may be beneficial.[504,516,519] In patients with profound cardiac dysfunction and cerebral vasospasm, an intra-aortic balloon pump may augment cerebral perfusion and assist cardiac function.[520]
   (d) Aggressive hyperdynamic therapy should be avoided in patients with cardiac complications and symptomatic vasospasm. In these patients, angioplasty may be more beneficial than hyperdynamic therapy in the treatment of vasospasm.[517]

Neurogenic Pulmonary Edema

Pulmonary complications are common in patients with SAH. The incidence of acute pulmonary edema in SAH is 20–27%,[462,521,522] with some 6% of patients having severe pulmonary edema.[462] The incidence of pneumonia is 20%.[466] The syndrome of neurogenic pulmonary edema is likely to be due to sustained elevated sympathetic tone, leading to a catecholamine-induced increase in pulmonary capillary permeability and pulmonary vasoconstriction.[523] Diastolic dysfunction may also contribute to pulmonary edema.[524] Risk factors include symptomatic vasospasm,[521] severity of illness, clinical grade of hemorrhage, red blood cell transfusions, and sepsis.[522] Neurogenic pulmonary edema appears most often on days 3–7 after SAH,[462] although it has been observed at any time from day 1 to day 14:

1. Management:
   (a) Intubate if necessary. Mechanical ventilation parameters should be chosen to minimize positive end-expiratory pressure (PEEP), and maintain PaO_2 >96%.[525]
   (b) *Judicious* use of diuretics, while maintaining normovolemia, may improve pulmonary function without compromising cerebral perfusion.
   (c) Dobutamine infusion may also be a useful adjunctive measure; this drug has the advantage of not impairing cerebral perfusion.[526]

Vasospasm

Cerebral vasospasm is defined as narrowing of large or small intracranial arteries after SAH. Symptomatic vasospasm (aka *clinical vasospasm*, or *delayed ischemic neurological deficit*) is the leading cause of death and disability in patients with SAH. The pathogenesis of vasospasm is not well understood. Arterial hemorrhage surrounding the major cerebral arteries in the subarachnoid space appears to initiate a series of changes in the arterial walls that results, several days after the hemorrhage, in narrowing of the vessel lumen. Sustained smooth muscle cell contraction appears to be the primary mechanism of vasospasm,[527] although inflammatory, immune-mediated, and proliferative processes have also been implicated.[528] Red blood cells are necessary for vasospasm to occur, and the 3–5 day time course of red cell lysis corresponds to the onset of clinical vasospasm. An array of vasoconstrictive mediators have also been identified which appear to have a role in vasospasm; these include oxyhemoglobin and other erythrocyte breakdown products, free radicals, eicosanoids, nitric oxide, endothelin, and various neurogenic factors.

FREQUENCY AND TIME COURSE
1) Some degree of vasospasm is seen on approximately 70% of angiograms done during the second week after SAH.[529,530]
2) Symptomatic vasospasm occurs in 20–25% of patients:[531,532]
   a) Symptoms of vasospasm probably do not appear unless there is at least a 50% reduction in arterial caliber.[533]
   b) Angiographic vasospasm with >50% reduction in arterial caliber is seen in 23–30% of patients.[534–536]
3) Onset of vasospasm rarely occurs prior to day 3 after SAH. Vasospasm is maximal at days 6–8, and is significantly reduced or gone in most patients within 2 weeks.[537,538]
   a) Fewer than 4% of cases occur after day 12 after SAH.[530]
   b) The onset of symptomatic vasospasm has been reported to appear as long as 35 days after SAH.[539]

RISK FACTORS
1) The best predictor of vasospasm is the amount of blood seen on the initial head CT scan, which correlates with the frequency and severity of vasospasm.[540–542]
2) Other risk factors for symptomatic vasospasm include age <50 years, hyperglycemia, history of hypertension, larger aneurysm size, intraventricular hemorrhage, and cocaine use.[543]
   a) However, more recent data indicates that age is not a significant predictor for vasospasm.[544]
3) The question of whether vasospasm is more likely after clipping or coiling is unresolved, as each modality has been found by various authors to be associated with a lesser incidence of vasospasm.[545,546]

CLINICAL FEATURES AND DIAGNOSIS
1. Symptomatic vasospasm typically presents as confusion and a decline in the level of consciousness. Focal neurological deficits may appear as well.
2. The onset of symptoms may be sudden or insidious.[537]
3. Neurological change is the best indicator of symptomatic vasospasm, and therefore frequent neurological exams are essential in patients with SAH.
   (a) Daily interruption of sedation was found to reduce ICU length of stay and the incidence of complications of in-patients in a medical intensive care unit.[547]
4. Autoregulation is impaired.[548]
5. Radiographic evaluation:
   (a) Catheter angiography:
      • Gold standard for diagnosis of cerebral vasospasm.
      • Significant vasospasm is indicated by a reduction in arterial caliber by 25–50% or more.
   (b) CTA:
      • CTA is relatively accurate for ruling in (90.7%) or ruling out (99.5%) hemodynamically significant vasospasm affecting large intracranial vessels.[549] It is less accurate for evaluating distal vessels and for detecting mild or moderate vasospasm. Sources of error in CTA in this setting include over-windowing and an excessive delay in scanning after administration of the contrast dose.
   (c) CT perfusion:
      • CT perfusion can detect reductions in regional CBF indicative of symptomatic vasospasm. CT perfusion using the deconvolution

technique has significant drawbacks including the necessity of selecting a reference artery and a dependence on hemispheric asymmetry to identify ischemia, when cerebral vasospasm can be a global phenomenon. The authors have had satisfactory results with CT perfusion using the maximum slope model.[550] Deconvolution CT perfusion is less satisfactory than and appears to be most useful in this setting when combined with CTA.[551] See also the Appendix 1: primer on imaging in stroke.

(d) Transcranial Doppler (TCD) ultrasonography:
- Flow velocity within a vessel is directly proportional to the volume of blood flow and inversely proportional to the square of the diameter of the vessel. Therefore, TCD velocity changes can be nonspecific and can reflect either vasospasm or an *increase* in CBF.[552] TCD measurements are also notoriously vulnerable to operator technique.
- The MCA is the most reliable vessel to assess,[553] and mean flow velocities >200 cm/s are highly suggestive of significant vasospasm, whereas velocities <100 cm/s are not.[554]
  - Most studies have defined an MCA flow velocity of >120 cm/s as evidence of some degree of vasospasm.[555,556]
  - Velocities ≥130 and ≥110 cm/s are indicative of ACA and PCA vasospasm, respectively.[557]
  - Velocities in the vertebral artery of ≥80 cm/s or the basilar artery of ≥95 cm/s have been found to indicate posterior circulation vasospasm.[558]
  - TCD seems to be more useful in *ruling in* vasospasm than ruling it out. A systematic review found the positive predictive value of MCA velocity changes in the diagnosis of vasospasm to be 97%, and the negative predictive value to be 78%.[553]
- Lindegaard ratio: Attempts to correct for changes in CBF by calculating the ratio between the MCA velocity and the ICA velocity.[559] A ratio of <3 is normal and a ratio >6 is highly suggestive of vasospasm; intermediate values are indeterminate:
  - A "modified Lindegaard ratio" for basilar artery vasospasm: the ratio between the basilar artery velocity and the extracranial vertebral artery ratio. A ratio >2 had 100% sensitivity in identification of patients with basilar artery vasospasm.[560]
- The authors of this handbook use TCD examinations selectively. A baseline TCD examination is done on all patients on admission, to create a baseline, and then TCD values are obtained on a daily basis for surveillance in patients for whom it is difficult to rely on a change in the neurological exam to identify vasospasm, such as high-grade SAH patients, or patients on a mechanical ventilator.

PREVENTION OF ISCHEMIC INJURY DUE TO VASOSPASM

Standard management of all patients with SAH should include adequate hydration, maintenance of normonatremia, and ventricular drainage, if needed. Both hypovolemia and hyponatremia have been shown to increase the risk of cerebral ischemia in patients with SAH.[476] Nimodipine is firmly established as a prophylactic measure in patients with SAH. Recent evidence also indicates that statin therapy may be significantly beneficial as well. Some evidence has also suggested that magnesium infusion and lumbar drainage may lower the incidence of symptomatic vasospasm. Although prophylactic hyperdynamic therapy may reduce the risk of vasospasm, it carries an increased risk of complications, and most clinicians reserve hyperdynamic therapy for the treatment of vasospasm, rather than prophylaxis:

1) Nimodipine:
   a) Nimodipine is a voltage-gated calcium channel antagonist and reduces calcium entry into smooth muscle cells and neurons. Nicardipine is another dihydropyridine calcium channel blocker that has been studied in patients with SAH, but much less extensively than nimodipine. Nimodipine has been shown in a total of eight randomized trials to have a modest but statistically significant effect on outcome in patients (*not angiographic vasospasm*) with aneurysmal SAH.[561–567]
   b) The largest trial was the British Aneurysm Nimodipine Trial (BRANT).[567] A total of 554 patients with SAH were randomized to receive either placebo or nimodipine, 60 mg PO Q 4 h for 21 days. Treatment was begun within 96 h of the ictus:

   i) The 3-month incidence of cerebral infarction:
    (1) 33% in the placebo group.
    (2) 22% in the nimodipine group ($p = 0.003$).
   ii) The 3-month rate of poor outcomes (death, vegetative state, or severe disability):
    (1) 33% in the placebo group.
    (2) 20% in the nimodipine group ($p < 0.001$).
 c) A systematic review of three randomized trials of oral nimodipine showed a significant benefit with nimodipine, demonstrating a relative risk of death or dependence 0.70 ($p = 0.0002$).[568]
 d) Both PO/NG and IV nimodipine have been evaluated, although the IV formulation is not available in North America. The most common side effect of oral nimodipine is transient hypotension; this can be mitigated by administering the drug 30 mg Q 2 h instead of 60 mg Q 4 h.
 e) The mechanism of nimodipine's beneficial effect is not clear, as the oral formulation has not been found to decrease the rate of vasospasm.[567] Nimodipine may function as a direct neuroprotectant or enhance cerebral microcirculation by causing arteriolar dilation.[569]
 f) Although the duration of treatment in BRANT was 21 days, it seems reasonable to discontinue nimodipine earlier in good-grade patients who are beyond the standard risk period for vasospasm.[533,570] A retrospective study of 90 patients with Hunt–Hess I–III SAH who were treated with nimodipine for 15 days or less found no evidence of a delayed neurological deficit.[570] In addition, nimodipine is expensive and not available in all pharmacies. The authors prefer to stop nimodipine treatment upon discharge from the hospital for patients who are neurologically intact.

2) Statins:
 a) Hydroxymethylglutaryl coenzyme A reductase inhibitors (statins) have surprisingly emerged as beneficial to patients with SAH. One retrospective study[571] and two prospective randomized trials[572–575] have supported the use of statins in the prevention and management of vasospasm.
 b) The larger of the two trials was conducted at Addenbrooke's Hospital in the United Kingdom.[573–575] A total of 80 patients with SAH were randomized to receive either placebo or pravastatin, 40 mg PO QD. Treatment was begun within 72 h of ictus and continued for up to 14 days or until discharge:
   i) The incidence of vasospasm:[573]
    (1) 62.5% in the placebo group.
    (2) 42.5% in the pravastatin group ($p = 0.006$).
   ii) The incidence of vasospasm-related delayed ischemic deficits:[573]
    (1) 30.0% in the placebo group.
    (2) 5.0% in the pravastatin group ($p < 0.001$).
   iii) Mortality:[573]
    (1) 20.0% in the placebo group.
    (2) 5.0% in the pravastatin group ($p < 0.037$).
   iv) Multivariate analysis showed that pravastatin reduced unfavorable outcomes at discharge by 73% ($p = 0.041$) and by 71% at 6 months ($p = 0.063$).[574]
 c) Pravastatin adverse effects. Although myalgia, myopathy, and hepatotoxicity are commonly associated with statin use, a large-scale prospective study found no difference in the rates of these symptoms in patients taking pravastatin 40 mg QD compared to patients taking a placebo.[576] In the British pravastatin study, no adverse events attributable to pravastatin were reported; alanine aminotransferase (ALT) elevations were similar in the drug and placebo patients:
   i) Myalgia occurs in 2% of all patients treated with pravastatin.[577] Reversible with pravastatin discontinuation.
   ii) Myopathy with creatine phosphokinase (CPK) elevations >10× normal occurs in <0.1% of all patients treated with pravastatin.[577]
   iii) Hepatotoxicity. ALT elevation (>3× normal) (1.4%).[576]
 d) Mechanism. Numerous potential mechanisms have been invoked to explain the beneficial effect of statins in SAH, including effects independent of the cholesterol-lowering effects such as improved cerebral vasomotor reactivity and a reduction in cytokine responses to cerebral ischemia.[578,579] Recent data suggests that cerebrovascular protection may also function through cholesterol-dependent mechanisms as well.[575]
 e) Clazosentan (Actelion Pharmaceuticals, Allschwil, Switzerland)

e) Endothelin receptor antagonist. Two phase 2 trials showed significant efficacy against angiographic vasospasm in patients with SAH.[200,580] Clazonsentan produced a dose-dependent reduction in moderate or severe angiographic vasospasm with a 65% relative risk reduction with the highest dose.[580]

f) CONSCIOUS-2, a phase 3 randomized, double-blinded, placebo-controlled trial of clazonsentan (5 mg/h) in patients with SAH secured by clipping, found no significant benefit with the drug in terms of mortality, vasospasm-related morbidity, or functional outcome.[581]

g) CONSCIOUS-3 is a phase 3 trial of clazonsentan in patients with SAH treated by coiling.[582] The trial is currently in progress.

3) Lumbar drainage:

a) Continuous lumbar drainage in patients with SAH is based on the idea that enhanced evacuation of the cisternal blood may reduce the risk of vasospasm. Two retrospective studies have reported a benefit with lumbar drainage in patients with SAH.[583,584] However, lumbar drainage carries a risk of overdrainage (14% in one series[585]) and should be used with caution in this setting.

4) Magnesium infusion:

a) Hypomagnesemia is common among SAH patients and may be associated with cerebral ischemia and poor outcomes.[498] Magnesium supplementation reverses vasospasm and reduces infarct volume in experimental SAH.[586–588] Magnesium supplementation is well established in obstetrics and cardiology,[589] and is inexpensive and readily available. Magnesium may exert beneficial effects by inhibition of the release of excitatory amino acids and blockade of the N-methyl-D-aspartate-glutamate receptor.[590,591] Magnesium is also a voltage-gated calcium channel antagonist and has a cerebral vasodilatory effect.[592]

b) Initial clinical data suggested that magnesium supplementation may improve outcomes after SAH.[593] More recent data, however, has cast doubt on whether magnesium supplementation is helpful in this setting. The Intravenous Magnesium Sulfate for Aneurysmal Subarachnoid Hemorrhage (IMASH) trial, a randomized, double-blinded multicenter trial, did not find an improvement in clinical outcomes with magnesium infusion.[594] Post hoc analyses of two trials have actually indicate worse outcomes with higher plasma magnesium concentrations.[595,596]

c) The authors of this handbook do not recommend routine magnesium infusion in SAH patients for vasospasm prophylaxis unless further data confirms a benefit.

5) Prophylactic hyperdynamic therapy:

a) Hyperdynamic therapy, also known as "Triple H" therapy, consists of the maintenance of hypervolemia, hypertension, and hemodilution, to improve the rheologic properties of blood, to enhance cerebral perfusion. Prophylactic hyperdynamic therapy can raise CBF in patients after SAH.[597]

b) A systematic review of four prospective studies with a total of 488 patients found a decreased risk of symptomatic vasospasm and death with prophylactic hyperdynamic therapy, but no significant change in the incidence of delayed ischemic neurological deficits.[598] However, only one of these studies was randomized.[599] The paucity of information and limitations in the design of the studies lead the authors of this review article to conclude that the efficacy of prophylaxis is undecided and that recommendations for the use of prophylactic hyperdynamic therapy cannot be made.[598] Similarly, two other systematic reviews of hypervolemic therapy identified only two randomized studies and found no sound evidence for the use of this technique in patients with SAH.[600,601]

c) One randomized trial found no increase in CBF with prophylactic hypervolemia;[599] the authors of this study surmised that any beneficial effects of prophylactic volume expansion were likely to be due to avoidance of hypovolemia, rather than any direct benefit of additional fluid volume.

d) Because of a lack of proven efficacy[602,603] and an established increase in the risk of complications with hyperdynamic therapy (see below), the authors of this handbook prefer to use hyperdynamic therapy only in patients with evidence of symptomatic vasospasm.

6) Other preventative measures:

a) Clot evacuation and lysis:

   i) Surgical clot removal.

   ii) Thrombolysis.

      (1) Intraventricular tPA infusion.[604]

b) Dantrolene[605]
c) Hypertonic saline infusion has been reported to improve cerebral blood flow and brain tissue oxygen in patients with poor-grade SAH.[606]

Treatment of Vasospasm

Blood flow in large vessels is described by the Hagen–Poiseuille equation:

$$Q = \Delta P \pi r^4 / 8 L \eta$$

where Q is the blood flow, ΔP is the pressure gradient, r is the vessel radius, L is the length, and η is the viscosity. Theoretically, flow in cerebral vessels affected by vasospasm can be increased by increasing the pressure gradient (by induced hypertension or hypervolemia), by decreasing the viscosity (by hemodilution), or by expanding the vessel radius (by angioplasty).

HYPERDYNAMIC THERAPY

"Triple H" therapy (hypertension, hypervolemia, and hemodilution) is first-line therapy in the treatment of symptomatic vasospasm, and should be reserved for patients who have undergone treatment of the ruptured aneurysm.[607] Hypertension and hypervolemia *do not* appear to increase the risk of hemorrhage from untreated, unruptured aneurysms in patients with SAH.[608] To avoid promoting cerebral edema or hemorrhagic transformation, hyperdynamic therapy should not be used in patients with a significant brain edema or a large infarction; hyperdynamic therapy should be discontinued as soon as the ischemic deficit resolves.[609]

Of the three components of hyperdynamic therapy, blood pressure elevation appears to be the most beneficial;[610–612] volume expansion seems to be useful mostly as a measure to avoid hypovolemia, which can exacerbate delayed ischemic injury.[599] Specific endpoints and methods of hyperdynamic therapy vary widely; no particular quantitative endpoint (e.g., SBP vs. CPP vs. PCWP) has been shown convincingly to be superior to others. The most important endpoint is clinical improvement.

1) Hypertension:
   a) Induced hypertension has been found to reverse deficits in patients with symptomatic vasospasm.[607,613–615]
   b) Endpoints:
      i) Systolic blood pressure (SBP):
         (1) A radial arterial catheter is helpful for blood pressure monitoring.
         (2) Giannotta and colleagues reported a significant improvement in 88% of patients with symptomatic vasospasm managed in the following way: CVP was elevated to 8–10 cm water (~6–7 mmHg) with blood and plasma transfusions and albumin; for patients who did not improve and whose SBP remained <140 mmHg, dopamine or phenylephrine was used to raise SBP to 150–170 mmHg.[613]
         (3) Awad and coworkers reported a reversal of deficits in 60% of patients treated first with aggressive hypervolemic therapy (10–12 mmHg; ~14–16 cm water), and then with hypertension if the deficits did not improve.[614] Phenylephrine or dopamine was used to elevate blood pressure until the deficits cleared or to a maximum of 200 mmHg.
      ii) Cerebral perfusion pressure (CPP):
         (1) Obviously CPP requires intracranial pressure monitoring.
         (2) Moderate hypertension (CPP 90–120 mmHg, CVP 5–10 mmHg, Hct 25–40) led to a greater increase in brain tissue PO_2 compared to hypervolemia (CVP 10–15 mmHg) or more aggressive hypertension (CPP >120 mmHg).[610]
      iii) Pulmonary capillary wedge pressure (PCWP):
         (1) Requires placement of a Swan–Ganz catheter.
         (2) Recommended target values for PCWP range from 12 to 15 mmHg[616] to 16–18 mmHg.[617]
   c) Methods to induce hypertension:
      i) Volume expansion first, with isotonic saline and 5% albumin.
      ii) Inotropes, such as dobutamine and dopamine, increase cardiac output and are the most commonly reported hypertensive agents in hyperdynamic therapy. An increase in cardiac output, without changes in mean arterial pressure, can elevate CBF in patients

with vasospasm.[618] Inotropes are also preferred over vasoconstrictors such as phenylephrine and levophed because of the potential for systemic ischemic complications with vasoconstrictors.

    (1) Dobutamine dose: 2.5–10 mcg/kg/min, up to 40 mcg/kg/min as needed.

    (2) Dopamine dose: 5 mcg/kg/min, up to 20–50 mcg/kg/min as needed.

    (3) Phenylephrine dose: 0.1 mcg/kg/min, up to 4 mcg/kg/min as needed.

d) The authors of this handbook use SBP as the primary quantitative endpoint for blood pressure management during treatment of symptomatic vasospasm. SBP is a simple, straightforward measurement that can be assessed in all patients, whereas CPP requires intracranial pressure monitoring and PCWP requires use of a Swan–Ganz catheter. In all patients with SAH and a treated ruptured aneurysm, SBP is allowed to rise as high as 200 mmHg; in patients with symptomatic vasospasm, volume expansion and inotropes are used to maintain SBP >160 mmHg.

2) Hypervolemia:

a) A central venous pressure (CVP) catheter should be placed in all patients with aneurysmal SAH.

b) Target parameters range from 6 to 12 mmHg (8–16 cm water).[613,614,619]

c) IV fluids: 0. 9% normal saline at 100–140 mL/h.

d) 5% albumin (250 mL TID) can be used for additional volume expansion.

    i) Infusion of 5% albumin (250 mL IV every 2 h as needed for CVP ≤8 mmHg) has been found to be effective in maintaining CVP >8 mmHg in patients with SAH.[619]

e) Dextran and hetastarch should be avoided because of potential effects on coagulation.

f) A systematic review found no sound evidence for or against the use of volume expansion in patients with SAH.[600] The authors view moderate hypervolemia as a method to ensure that the patient is well hydrated and to facilitate hypertensive therapy, if needed.

3) Hemodilution:

a) Some degree of "hemodilution" occurs with volume expansion.

b) No clinical data exist to support *deliberate* hemodilution in the setting of SAH:[533]

c) Controlled, isovolemic hemodilution to a hematocrit of 28% in patients with vasospasm produced an increase in global CBF but a pronounced reduction in oxygen delivery capacity.[620]

d) A systematic review found no net benefit with hemodilution in patients with acute ischemic stroke.[621]

e) The authors of this handbook maintain the hematocrit at about 30%. A hematocrit of 30% has been found to be the optimal hematocrit for reducing cerebral infarction in some animal models, and hematocrit >30% has been found to be associated with reduced perfusion and tissue survival in patients with acute ischemic stroke.[622]

4) Complications of hyperdynamic therapy:

a) Numerous complications are associated with hyperdynamic therapy; overall complication rates are 24–30%.[462,623] Pulmonary edema is the most frequent complication.

b) Intracranial complications include hemorrhagic transformation of infarcts, increased intracranial pressure, aneurysm rebleeding, and hypertensive encephalopathy.[607,624]

c) Extracranial complications include pulmonary edema in 17% of patients,[617] myocardial infarction (2%), coagulopathy, hemothorax.[607] Complications in patients with Swan–Ganz catheters were detailed by Rosenwasser and colleagues and include sepsis (13%), congestive heart failure (2%), subclavian vein thrombosis (1.3%), pneumothorax (1%) and hemothorax.[625]

5) Authors' protocol for symptomatic vasospasm:

a) Use isotonic saline and 5% albumin to maintain the CVP 8–10 cm water. Maintain SBP ≥160 mmHg with an inotrope if needed (dobutamine or dopamine). Modify these endpoints as needed, depending on the clinical situation, to minimize the risk of complications (e.g., the parameters are lowered if significant pulmonary or brain edema is already present). Discontinue hyperdynamic therapy once the clinical deficit clears, or the theoretic risk period for vasospasm has been passed (i.e., >12 days after the hemorrhage).

ANGIOPLASTY

1. Balloon angioplasty is an option for symptomatic vasospasm affecting intracranial arteries >1.5 mm in diameter,[626] such as the intracranial ICA, the M1, A1, and the vertebral and basilar arteries and P1 segments. Technique is discussed in Chap. 11.

2. Angioplasty stretches and thins the internal elastic lamina and smooth muscle cells.[627] Dilation of the vessel segments is essentially "permanent" for the duration of the clinical vasospasm; vasospasm generally does not recur after angioplasty.

3. Results:
   (a) Reversal of neurological deficits with angioplasty has been reported in 30–70% of patients who fail Triple H therapy.[628–631]
   (b) Clinical improvement appears to be strongly dependent on the timing of the procedure, with significantly better results reported with angioplasty done within 24 h,[630] and within 2 h[632] of the neurological change.

4. Complications:
   (a) Overall complication rates are ~5–10%.[628,633]
   (b) Complications include rupture of the vessel, wire perforation, ischemic stroke, vessel dissection, femoral artery injury, retroperitoneal hemorrhage, and failure to improve symptoms.

5. Strategies:
   (a) Some authors advocate attempting a trial of hyperdynamic therapy for vasospasm prior to performing angioplasty,[533] whereas others prefer to do angioplasty first on an emergent basis.[632]
   (b) Angioplasty in combination with aneurysm coiling has been used successfully for patients presenting with SAH and symptomatic vasospasm.[634] Alternatively, surgery to clip the aneurysm can be followed by immediate postoperative angioplasty.[635]
   (c) Some operators are reluctant to perform angioplasty when the affected cerebral region shows evidence of infarction on CT, because of a concern for the possibility of hemorrhagic transformation. However, in a series of 17 cases in which angioplasty was done despite a CT scan showing a new hypodensity, there were no hemorrhages or worsening of symptoms.[636] There was resolution of the CT hypodensities in 5 of the 17 patients and the majority of the patients improved clinically.
   (d) Prophylactic angioplasty for vasospasm was studied in a single-center trial; however, one patient in the trial died as the result of vessel rupture during the procedure.[637]

INTRA-ARTERIAL PHARMACOLOGIC TREATMENT

Intra-arterial (IA) infusion of antispasmodic medications can supplement angioplasty, and can be used for the endovascular treatment of vasospasm of arteries that are too small for balloon angioplasty. Although IA papaverine used to be popular, it has fallen out of favor in recent years because its effect is short-lived and because of side effects such as dramatic ICP elevation, decreased brain oxygenation, and increased cases of ischemic infarction in territories infused. Preliminary reports of IA infusion of calcium channel blockers have been encouraging.

1) IA calcium channel blockers:
   a) Nicardipine:
      i) In a series of 18 patients treated with IA nicardipine, all arteries that were treated demonstrated angiographic improvement, and neurologic improvement occurred in 42% of patients. Transient ICP elevation occurred in 28% of patients and sustained ICP, requiring mannitol infusion, occurred in one patient (6%):[638]
      ii) Regimen: Nicardipine (Cardene IV; ESP Pharma, Inc., Edison, NJ) was diluted in 0.9% NaCl to a concentration of 0.1 mg/mL and administered in 1 mL aliquots through a microcatheter to a maximal dose of 5 mg per vessel. Dose per vessel was based on the angiographic effect observed.
   b) Nimodipine:
      i) In a series of 25 patients treated with IA nimodipine, clinical improvement was observed in 76% of patients and notable vascular dilation was observed in 43% of the procedures:[639]
      ii) Regimen: A 25% dilution of nimodipine in saline was made. Slow infusion of the solution at a rate of 2 mL/min was done with an electric pump. Each infusion lasted 10–30 min per vessel. The total dose per vessel was 1–3 mg and the total dose per patient was ≤5 mg.
      iii) Note: Parenteral nimodipine is not available in the United States.

c) Verapamil:
   i) In a series of 17 patients treated with IA verapamil alone, five patients (29%) experienced neurologic improvement.[640] The average increase in vessel diameter was $44 \pm 9\%$, and no patients had ICP elevation:
   ii) Regimen: On average, the total dose of verapamil per patient was 3 mg and two vessels were treated in each patient. The average dose per vessel was 2 mg and the largest single dose per vessel was 8 mg.
      (1) A study of high-dose IA verapamil (median dose 23 mg) reported increases in ICP and reductions in CPP.[641] These changes persisted for up to 6 h after the procedure.
2) IA papaverine:
   a) Papaverine is an alkaloid that causes vasodilation of cerebral arteries through a direct inhibitory effect on smooth muscle contraction. IA papaverine infusion reverses angiographic vasospasm.[642,643]
   b) The effect of papaverine is short-lived, lasting less than 3 h.[644]
   c) Papaverine has significant adverse effects, including increased ICP,[645] seizures,[646] paradoxical worsening of vasospasm,[647] diminished brain oxygen during infusion,[648] and permanent gray matter damage.[644,649]
   d) In a comparison of IA papaverine and balloon angioplasty, angioplasty was found to have a more sustained favorable effect.[650]
   e) IA papaverine is no longer used in most centers.
3) Nitroglycerin
   a) In an animal model, intravenous nitroglycerine was shown to improve the caliber of cerebral vessels.[651,652]
   b) Intra-thecal infusions have also been successful in preventing vasospasm in an animal model.[653]
   c) Scattered small reports of successful management of EC-IC bypass-graft vasospasm with intra-arterial[654] or transdermal[655] nitroglycerin have been published.[654]
   d) In clinical practice, many operators use IA nitroglycerine (in 30 mcg individual doses) in cases in which an angioplasty balloon cannot be navigated into position (e.g., the A1 segment in some patients). However, scant evidence supports the practice.
   e) The agent is not without risk, since nitroglycerin causes hypotension and has been shown to increase intracranial pressure.[656]
4) Best options: IA nicardipine or verapamil infusion for the endovascular treatment of diffuse, small vessel vasospasm (e.g., vasospasm affecting the M2 segments or beyond, despite treatment of the M1 segment).

Subarachnoid Hemorrhage Management Protocol

1) Standard orders are listed in Table 13.11.
2) Procedures
   a) Place an arterial line and a central line on admission.
   b) Ventriculostomy is placed only for symptomatic hydrocephalus.
3) All SAH patients are kept well hydrated. Full-blown hyperdynamic therapy ("H3") is initiated only when a diagnosis of symptomatic cerebral vasospasm is made.
4) Any neurologic change should prompt a standard work-up, including review of electrolytes, vital signs, and a head CT if indicated. If this work-up is negative, a presumptive diagnosis of symptomatic vasospasm may be made.

The International Subarachnoid Aneurysm Trial (ISAT)

Randomized, prospective, multicenter trial of endovascular coiling vs. surgical clipping for selected patients with ruptured intracranial aneurysms deemed suitable for either therapy. The study began in 1994 and continued enrollment through 2002.[194,195,657]

1) A total of 9,559 patients were screened, and 2,143 (22.4%) were randomly assigned to either surgery ($n = 1,070$) or endovascular treatment ($n = 1,073$).

Table 13.11 SAH management protocol

Admission orders	Comments and references
Admit to the Neuro-ICU	A dedicated neurocritical care team was associated with reduced in-hospital mortality and length of stay in Neuro-ICU patients [826]
Diagnosis: SAH	
Condition: critical	
Allergies:	
Vital signs: Q 1 h with neurochecks	Meticulous monitoring of the patient's neurologic status will identify changes that require prompt treatment, such as aneurysm rehemorrhage, vasospasm, or hydrocephalus [827]
Activity: bedrest	
Nursing: SAH Precautions (low light, minimal stimulation, etc.), record CVP and UOP hourly	
NPO except meds until management plan for the aneurysm is decided	
Enteral feeding is begun as soon as feasible (diet is advanced as tolerated); a nasogastric feeding tube (Dobhoff tube) is placed and tube feeding is begun for intubated patients or those unable to eat	Nutritional needs are elevated by SAH, due to a profound stress response and increased catabolism [828]
IVF: 0.9 N.S. with 20 mEq KCl/L at 120 mL/h	Aggressive hydration with isotonic fluids is meant to minimize risk of hypovolemia and hyponatremia, both of which have been shown to increase the risk of cerebral ischemia after SAH [476,480]
5% Albumin 250 mL IV Q 6 h, hold for CVP >12	Volume expansion with albumin is a method to prevent hypovolemia. Retrospective data suggests 5% albumin may improve outcome and reduce hospital costs in SAH patients [829]
Nimodipine 60 mg PO/NG Q 4 h for 21 days	Nimodipine is associated with improved outcomes in patients with aneurysmal SAH [561–567]
Pravastatin, 40 mg PO QD up to 14 days or until discharge	Begin pravastatin after admission labs (liver function tests and CK) are checked and are normal. Pravastatin is associated with lower rates of vasospasm and spasm-related cerebral ischemia [572,573]
Morphine 2–6 mg IV Q 1 h PRN (any other IV narcotic is acceptable)	
Esomeprazole 40 mg PO/IV QD (any other stress ulcer prophylactic medication is acceptable)	GI prophylaxis is recommended for all SAH patients [830]
MgSO$_4$ gtt (prepare 40 g in 1,000 mL sterile water; infuse at a rate of 17 mL/h). Discontinue when the patient is transferred out of the NICU	A randomized trial of magnesium in SAH found a trend toward a significant benefit with treatment without major side effects [593]
Labetalol 5–20 mg IV Q 20 min PRN SBP > 160 (BP parameters are liberalized when the aneurysm is treated, i.e., SBP up to 200 is okay)	Early rebleeding was found to correlate with SBP ≥160 mmHg [55], and extremes of blood pressure on admission (MAP > 130 or <70 mmHg) are associated with poor outcome after SAH [598]
Ondansetron 4 mg IV Q 4–6 h PRN (most other antiemetics are acceptable)	
Amicar 5 g IV load given over 1 h, then infusion at 1 g IV Q 1 h (24 g in 1 L of 0.5 N.S. at 42 mL/h). *Amicar is discontinued when the aneurysm is treated*	Short-term antifibrinolytic treatment may reduce the risk of rebleeding without an associated increase in risk of ischemic complications or hydrocephalus [437] Tranexamic acid, an antifibrinolytic that is not available in the US, was shown in a randomized trial to reduce the risk of rehemorrhage [438]

(continued)

Table 13.11 (continued)

Admission orders	Comments and references
Avoid warfarin, clopidogrel, ticlopidine, LMWH, especially when patient has had craniotomy, ventriculostomy, or intracerebral hemorrhage	
External pneumatic compression devices on lower extremities at all times	External pneumatic calf compression reduces deep venous thrombosis in patients with SAH [831]
Admission labs: CBC, serum electrolytes, coagulation parameters, toxicology screen, liver function tests, CK, CK-MB	
Daily labs: CBC, serum electrolytes, only (unless a question requiring a specific lab arises)	Surveillance for electrolyte disorders and infection
12 Lead EKG and chest X-ray on admission	
TCDs: obtain one baseline study on day of admission or day after admission. HH 4 and 5 patients: obtain TCDs daily	TCDs are useful for surveillance for symptomatic vasospasm, particularly in high-grade SAH patients with depressed mental status, in whom subtle neurologic changes are difficult to ascertain

2) Clinical outcomes were assessed at 2 months and 1 year. Recruitment was stopped after an interim analysis showed a significant advantage of endovascular therapy:
    a) Patients dead or dependent at 1 year:
        i) 23.5% in the endovascular group.
        ii) 30.9% in the surgical group:
        iii) Absolute risk reduction of 7.4% ($p = 0.0001$).
        iv) The early survival advantage was maintained for up to 7 years and was significant ($p = 0.03$).
    b) Subgroup analyses showed significant benefits with endovascular therapy for patients age 50–69; all Fisher grades; aneurysm lumen size ≤10 mm; and ICA aneurysm location. No subgroup showed a significant benefit with surgery.
    c) The number of patients with confirmed rebleeding from the target aneurysm at 1 year was slightly greater in the endovascular group:
        i) 45 in the endovascular group.
        ii) 39 in the surgical group:
            (1) However, 28 of the rebleeds in the surgical group occurred prior to treatment, vs. only 17 in the endovascular group. This may be partly explained by the fact that the mean interval to treatment was 1.7 days in the surgical group, and 1.1 days in the endovascular group. Not counting rebleeds occurring prior to first treatment, total 1-year rebleeds were:
                (a) 35 in the endovascular group.
                (b) 13 in the surgical group.
        iii) Late rebleeding (>1 year) was higher in the endovascular group:
            (1) 7 in the endovascular group.
            (2) 2 in the surgical group.
    d) There was a significant reduction in seizures with endovascular treatment, from hospital discharge to 1 year:
        i) 27 in the endovascular group.
        ii) 44 in the surgical group.
        iii) Relative risk of seizures with endovascular treatment compared to surgery: 0.52 (95% CI 0.37–0.74).
    e) Endovascular patients had better cognitive outcomes compared to surgical patients. [658]
3) ISAT long term follow-up (mean 9 years): [657]
    a) Rebleeding from the treated aneurysm >1 year after treatment:
        i) 10 in the endovascular group
        ii) 3 in the surgical group

b) 5-year mortality:
    i) 11% in the endovascular group
    ii) 14% in the surgical group (P = 0.03)
c) Proportion of survivors who were independent at 5 years:
    i) 83% in the endovascular group
    ii) 82% in the surgical group (P = 0.61)
4) Study limitations and controversies:
    a) The study results are applicable only to aneurysms that are treatable with either surgery or coiling. Of the 9,559 patients eligible for inclusion, 69% were excluded because the aneurysm could not be treated by either procedure.
    b) Most of the centers in the study were located in Europe, and therefore the results may not be applicable to patients in the US, where the degree of subspecialization and experience of neurovascular surgeons may be different.[659]
    c) Although clinical outcomes at 1 year were superior in the endovascular group, the rebleeding rate after treatment was higher. Over a longer term, the effect of rebleeding may reduce the early benefit of coiling.

13.5. Intracranial Aneurysms: Special Situations

Pediatric Aneurysms

Pediatric intracranial aneurysms are uncommon but have a number of features that are distinct from aneurysms found in adults.

Epidemiology and Characteristic Features

1. Pediatric cases account for about <1% of all intracranial aneurysm cases:[660–662]
    (a) To date, only approximately 700 cases have been reported in the literature.[663]
    (b) It is estimated that most academic centers typically see one case per year.[664]
2. About twice as many boys are affected than girls.[661]
3. Age at presentation is bimodal:[660]
    (a) Birth to age 6 years, and peaking at 6 months.
    (b) Age 8 to adolescence.
4. Aneurysms in children are more likely than adults to be at the ICA or MCA bifurcations or in the posterior circulation:
    (a) A review of all cases reported by 2004 found the most common locations to be the ICA bifurcation (26%), A-comm (19%), MCA bifurcation (17%), and posterior circulation (17%).[661]
    (b) Pediatric intracranial aneurysms are also more likely than adult aneurysms to be located in the peripheral vasculature,[665] possibly reflecting the higher incidence of traumatic aneurysms in children, which are typically located in the periphery.
    (c) A systematic review of reports of aneurysms occurring in children <1 year of age found that a prevalence of aneurysms on the MCA is nearly three times higher than on any other vessel, and did not find that boys are more frequently affected, as has been reported for other age groups.[666]
5. Etiology and pathophysiology:
    (a) A number of conditions are associated with pediatric aneurysms (Table 13.12):
        • Some authors recommend routine noninvasive screening for intracranial aneurysms for children with aortic coarctation, polycystic kidney disease, and Ehlers–Danlos syndrome.[660]

Table 13.12 Conditions associated with pediatric intracranial aneurysms

Bacterial endocarditis
Brain tumors
Cardiac myxoma
Closed or penetrating head injury
Ehlers–Danlos syndrome
Fibromuscular dysplasia
G-6-PD deficiency
Human immunodeficiency virus
Irradiation
Marfan syndrome
Moyamoya disease
Polycystic kidney disease
Pseudoxanthoma elasticum
Sickle cell anemia
Syphilis
Thalassemia
Tuberous sclerosis
Type IV collagenopathy
Vascular anomalies

      (b) Idiopathic pediatric aneurysms are pathologically distinct from adult aneurysms. Some characteristic features of adult aneurysms, such as atherosclerotic changes and an abrupt termination of the internal elastic lamina at the aneurysm neck, were not found in an autopsy series of pediatric aneurysms.[667]

      (c) Pediatric aneurysms are more likely to be complex than adult aneurysms;[668] fusiform and dolichoectatic aneurysms comprised 51% of the aneurysms in one series.[663]

      (d) Traumatic aneurysms, arising after closed or penetrating head injury, comprise 14–39% of all pediatric aneurysms.[669]

      (e) Some 20% of pediatric aneurysms are giant.[661]

6. Clinical features:

      (a) Pediatric aneurysms are usually symptomatic at the time of presentation.

      (b) SAH is the most common mode of presentation; aneurysms in children are four times as likely to present with SAH than not.[661]

      (c) Children with SAH appear to have a lesser incidence [668] and a greater tolerance[660] for cerebral vasospasm:

         • Vasospasm was found in 53% of children undergoing angiography between the 4th and 16th day after SAH.[670]

      (d) Mortality after SAH is lower than in adults, ranging from 10% to 20%.[671]

Management

    Intracranial aneurysms in children are fundamentally different from adult aneurysms, and therefore clinical data from adult series cannot be extrapolated to the pediatric population. Interpretation of literature about the treatment of pediatric aneurysms is impaired by the infrequency of these lesions, and the fact that endovascular therapy has evolved considerably in recent years; some series report cases extending back to the infancy of neurointervention (i.e., the 1970s):[663]

    1) Surgical series have generally reported favorable results, although direct clipping of the aneurysm has been accomplished only 30–46% of cases.[660,663] Adjunctive surgical techniques such as trapping, large vessel occlusion, or bypass are frequently required.

    2) Endovascular series have also reported good results.[671]

3) A recent single-center retrospective review found complete obliteration rates of 94% for surgical patients and 82% for endovascular patients, with no deaths and similar rates of new neurological deficits (7.7% for surgery and 6.3% for endovascular treatment).[663]
4) A multidisciplinary approach is important, with participation of pediatric neurosurgeons, vascular neurosurgeons, and neurointerventionalists, decision making and management.
5) *Meticulous life-long follow-up is mandatory after both surgery and endovascular treatment*:
   a) Recurrence after treatment occurs at a higher rate in children compared to adults:
      i) In a series of 35 pediatric aneurysms treated with surgery, there was an annual recurrence rate 2.6%[672]
         (1) This recurrence rate is six times higher than for adult aneurysms.[150]
   b) De novo aneurysms occur in up 19% of pediatric patients after treatment.[663,672]
   c) Follow-up imaging with MRA should be done at regular intervals indefinitely.[663,672]

Pregnancy and Intracranial Aneurysms

Unruptured Aneurysms and Pregnancy

The risk of SAH in pregnant patients with an unruptured aneurysm is five times that of nonpregnant women in the same age group.[673,674] The risk of rupture increases with advancing maternal age[673–675] and as gestation progresses.[673] These observations, combined with the considerable risk of SAH to the mother and the fetus, support treatment of unruptured aneurysms before patients become pregnant.

Evaluation

1. Head CT and cerebral angiography can both be performed safely during pregnancy. Recommendations for radiation exposure of the fetus include a maximum dose of 0.5 rem (roentgen-equivalent-man).[676] By shielding the uterus with a lead apron, the maximum dose to the fetus during a head CT is less than 0.05 rem.[677]
2. Catheter angiography in pregnant patients is discussed in Chap. 2. The diagnostic yield of angiography in aneurysmal SAH during pregnancy is believed to be superior to that of the general population.

Subarachnoid Hemorrhage in Pregnant Patients

CLINICAL FEATURES
1. The incidence of spontaneous SAH during pregnancy is 0.01–0.05% of all pregnancies.[673,678,679]
2. The risk of hemorrhage increases with advancing gestational age, peaking at 30–34 weeks.[678]
3. The overall mortality rate is 35%, comparable to that of the nonpregnant population.[678]
4. The effect of parity on subarachnoid hemorrhage is unclear. The most recent data suggest that primigravidae are at higher risk than multiparous woman.[678,680]
5. The clinical features of aneurysmal subarachnoid hemorrhage in pregnant patients are similar to those of nonpregnant patients.[678] "The worst headache of my life" is the most common presenting complaint. A history of a sentinel headache may be present in 50% of cases.[681]
6. Hypertension is a risk factor for SAH during pregnancy, occurring in 29% of patients with antepartum aneurysmal hemorrhage and in 67% of patients with postpartum aneurysmal hemorrhage.[673]

DIFFERENTIAL DIAGNOSIS

1. As with SAH in the general population, trauma is the most common cause of SAH in pregnant patients.[673]
2. SAH must be distinguished from *preeclampsia* and *eclampsia*, which are more common than SAH in pregnant women and can appear with features similar to those of spontaneous SAH. In addition, aneurysmal SAH can precipitate preeclampsia:
   (a) Preeclampsia is defined as the presence of hypertension in pregnant patients accompanied by proteinuria, edema, or both. Preeclampsia typically occurs after the 24th week of pregnancy and usually in primiparas. Severe preeclampsia can include a sharp increase in blood pressure, hyperreflexia, neurologic changes and visual disturbances.
   (b) Eclampsia is defined as the occurrence of seizures in a preeclamptic patient not attributable to other causes and can cause intracranial hemorrhage. Of patients with fatal eclampsia, 40% exhibit subarachnoid hemorrhage or intraparenchymal hemorrhage on autopsy [682,683], although the incidence in nonfatal cases is unknown.[678] Typical CT findings in eclampsia are multiple subcortical petechial hemorrhages or a single, large intracerebral hematoma.[678]
3. The next most common cause of spontaneous intracranial hemorrhage during pregnancy after eclamptic disorders and aneurysmal SAH is a ruptured AVM. In a study of 154 cases of intracranial hemorrhage during pregnancy, aneurysms were the cause in 77% of patients and AVMs in 23%.[678]
4. Other causes of spontaneous SAH during pregnancy include disseminated intravascular coagulopathy,[684] sickle cell anemia,[684] anticoagulation therapy,[685] cocaine abuse,[686] metastatic choriocarcinoma,[687] Moyamoya disease,[688] and spinal vascular anomalies.[673]

NEUROVASCULAR MANAGEMENT

1. Standard medical management of a pregnant patient with SAH includes:
   (a) Placement of an arterial line to permit continuous monitoring of blood pressure and treatment of hypertension and hypotension:
      • Hypotension should be avoided because the fetus is passively dependent on maternal blood pressure for adequate perfusion and is vulnerable to maternal hypotension.
   (b) Continuous fetal heart rate monitoring.
   (c) Adequate analgesia, sedation, and antiemetics should be provided.
   (d) Medication selection should be done in consultation with a pharmacist with consideration of the possible effects of each drug on the fetus.
2. Treatment to prevent rebleeding is recommended:
   (a) Rehemorrhage without surgical or endovascular treatment during the pregnancy occurs in 33–50% of cases and is associated with a maternal mortality rate of 50–68%.[678,689–691]
   (b) In a study of 118 pregnant patients with aneurysmal SAH, surgical treatment of the ruptured aneurysm was associated with significantly lower maternal and fetal mortality rates than conservative treatment:[678]
      • The maternal mortality rate in patients undergoing surgery for the ruptured aneurysm prior to delivery (11%) was significantly lower than for patients not undergoing surgery (63%). The fetal mortality rate was significantly better after surgery (5%) compared with patients not undergoing surgery (27%).[678]
   (c) The decision to treat the aneurysm should be based on neurosurgical criteria, and the method of delivery should be based on obstetric considerations:
      • Obstetrical issues should take priority over neurosurgical concerns during active labor (which can be triggered by SAH), eclampsia, or fetal distress. In these cases, delivery should be performed promptly by cesarean section, followed as soon as possible by neurosurgical treatment.[673,692]
3. Both surgery[678] and endovascular techniques[693–695] are valid options for treatment of the aneurysm during pregnancy.

OBSTETRICAL MANAGEMENT

1. Method of delivery. Delivery should be undertaken in most situations according to obstetric rather than neurosurgical criteria. Both vaginal delivery and cesarean section are reasonable, and neither method seems to offer a significant advantage for patients with SAH. The risk of bleeding during vaginal delivery is not significantly different from that during cesarean section.[675] Mortality

rates also appear to be similar after vaginal delivery or cesarean section for pregnant patients with vascular disorders:[678,680,696,697]

    (a) Obstetric methods to minimize bleeding during vaginal delivery include caudal or epidural anesthesia, shortening of the second stage of labor, and low forceps delivery.

    (b) Cesarean delivery can be used for fetal salvage when the mother is moribund and in the third trimester.[698]

2. Fetal monitoring. Patients should be followed before, during, and after neurosurgical procedures with continuous fetal monitoring. If persistent fetal distress appears and is not reversed by changes in oxygenation, positioning, or blood pressure, emergent cesarean delivery should be performed:

    (a) If labor begins and delivery becomes imminent during craniotomy, the intracranial procedure should be suspended, the bone flap temporarily replaced if possible, and the child delivered vaginally or by cesarean section according to obstetric indications. The intracranial procedure should be resumed after delivery.

3. Oxytocin is used to control uterine bleeding after delivery. The safety of oxytocin in patients with SAH is not clear. However, oxytocin can cause maternal hypertension, and it does appear to have effects on cerebral vasoconstrictive effects.[699,700] Therefore, the use of oxytocin in patients with SAH when possible, particularly if the ruptured aneurysm has not yet been treated or if the patient is felt to be at significant risk of vasospasm. A neonatologist or a pediatric intensivist should be available for care of the anesthetized infant.[675,678]

OUTCOMES

Dias and Sekhar found the overall maternal mortality rate from aneurysmal subarachnoid hemorrhage to be 35%,[678] which is similar to that of the nonpregnant population. The fetal mortality rate was 17%.

Elderly Patients with Aneurysms

Elderly patients are defined by most authors as those who are ≥70 years of age.

Unruptured Aneurysms in the Elderly

1) As life expectancy increases and noninvasive imaging becomes less expensive and more widespread, unruptured aneurysms are being identified in greater numbers of older patients.

2) Surgical outcomes are related to age.[701] Although a systematic review of surgical series published between 1966 and 1996 did not find a significant relationship between age and surgical outcomes,[153] other studies have found advanced age to be a predictor of poor outcome after surgery for unruptured aneurysms.[155] ISUIA found that poor outcomes in patients having surgery for unruptured aneurysms increased in frequency with each decade of life beginning at age 50.[131] For patients with an age ≥70, poor outcome (death, a Rankin score between 3 and 5, or impaired cognitive status) occurred in about 30% of patients:

    a) In a single-center series of elderly patients being treated for unruptured aneurysms, 6-month outcomes were: excellent, 70%; good, 15%; fair, 5%; poor, 7.5%; and death, 2.5%.[702]

3) Endovascular treatment is better tolerated by elderly patients than surgery. Single-center series of endovascular treatment of unruptured aneurysms in elderly patients have reported outcomes that are comparable to outcomes in younger patients.[703,704] In a study of 22 elderly endovascular patients, 20 (91%) had excellent outcomes (modified Rankin Scale score 0 or 1):[704]

    a) Although an effect of age similar to that of surgery was not found in the endovascular group in ISUIA, the size of the endovascular cohort (451 patients) was much smaller than the surgical group (1,917 patients), and therefore the size of the group may have been too small to detect a statistically significant effect.

    b) An advantage of treating elderly patients with endovascular techniques is that long-term outcome may be less important than in younger patients, given a shorter overall life expectancy.[703]

4) Decision making in elderly patients with an unruptured aneurysm should take into account the life expectancy of the patient (see Table 13.5), a realistic

estimate of the risk of rupture, and an estimate of morbidity and mortality with treatment. Good results can be obtained both with surgery and with endovascular treatment in carefully selected patients.[702] The authors of this handbook favor endovascular treatment when possible and reserve serious consideration of treatment of unruptured aneurysms in elderly patients to those who are relatively healthy, with an aneurysm that is large, symptomatic, in the posterior circulation, or found to be enlarging on serial imaging.

Subarachnoid Hemorrhage in the Elderly

1. Increasing life expectancy in recent years has translated into a larger percentage of SAH patients who are elderly.[705,706]
2. Outcome is strongly related to age in patients with SAH:[703,707,708]
   (a) In a series consisting of both surgical and endovascularly treated SAH patients, 21% of elderly patients were independent at discharge.[709]
   (b) In a study of case fatality rates over time, improvements in survival among younger patients with SAH were offset by increasing numbers of elderly patients, who have not experienced a similar improvement in outcome.[705]
   (c) Interestingly, Japanese studies have consistently reported better results in elderly patients, even among patients age ≥80.[708,710,711]
3. Among the elderly, poor-grade patients (Hunt–Hess 4 or 5) do very poorly:[708,709,712]
   (a) In recent studies of elderly patients treated with endovascular techniques, 77% of poor-grade patients had a very poor outcome (modified Rankin Scale score, 4–5). Similarly, in another series, 62% of patients were severely disabled or dead.[713]
4. In endovascular series, a significant percentage of good-grade elderly patients with SAH have had good outcomes. In one study, 89% of the patients with low-grade SAH (Hunt and Hess Grade 1 or 2) achieved excellent outcomes (modified Rankin Scale score, 0–1).[704]
5. The authors favor endovascular treatment for good-grade elderly patients with SAH. Poor-grade patients are candidates for endovascular treatment provided that the patient's family understands that the chance of a good outcome is low.

Infectious Aneurysms

The first report of an infectious intracranial aneurysm appeared in 1869 and described a 13-year-old boy with mitral valve endocarditis.[714] Although *mycotic* is synonymous with *fungal*, the term *mycotic aneurysm* is a colloquialism for all infectious aneurysms and is attributed to William Osler, who used it to refer to an aortic aneurysm that arose in the setting of bacterial endocarditis.[715]

Epidemiology and Etiology

1. In autopsy series, infectious aneurysms comprise some 2.6–6% of all intracranial aneurysms in adults,[716] although a recent report from a busy cerebrovascular center found that infectious aneurysms accounted for less than 1% of all treated aneurysms.[717] Infectious aneurysms seem to be somewhat more common in children, comprising some 2–10% of reported cases of intracranial aneurysms in children.[661,718]
2. Some 65–80% of patients with intracranial infectious aneurysms have endocarditis:[717,719]
   (a) Conversely, infectious aneurysms occur in 3–15% of patients with infectious endocarditis.[720,721]
   (b) Other predisposing medical conditions are meningitis, cavernous sinus thrombophlebitis, osteomyelitis of the skull, and sinus infections.[722]
3. Some 75% of infectious aneurysms present with rupture, and 70% are found in the middle cerebral artery territory.[717] Multiple lesions are found in 20% of patients.[723]
4. *Streptococcal* species are the most common cause of infectious aneurysms, and *staphylococcus* species are the second most common cause. In a recent series, blood cultures identified *Streptococcus viridans* in 37.5% and *Staphylococcus*

aureus in 18.7%.[721] Other pathogens include enterococci, *Pseudomonas*, and corynebacteria. An organism is not identified in some 12–19% of cases:[723,724]

   (a) Most bacterially infectious aneurysms occur as the result of intravascular seeding. The infection appears to begin in the adventitia and move inward, toward the intimal surface. This pattern has lead to speculation that infectious dissemination begins in the Virchow–Robin spaces of small penetrating vessels.[725]

   (b) Infectious aneurysms are typically friable, fusiform in shape, and difficult to separate from surrounding brain parenchyma.

5. Intracranial fungal aneurysms are rare, and usually occur in immunocompromised patients. *Aspergillus* is the most common fungal pathogen, followed by Phycomycetes and *Candida albicans*. Aspergillosis of the intracranial space can occur by direct extension from the paranasal sinuses or by hematogenous spread from the lungs.[726]

Management

An algorithm for the management of infectious aneurysms is provided in Fig. 13.8.

1. Antibiotic therapy is first-line treatment for most unruptured infectious aneurysms, and for patients with hemorrhage who do not require urgent surgery.

2. Specimens for blood culture should be obtained prior to the initiation of antibiotic therapy, to permit later speciation and modification of the antibiotic regimen:

   (a) CSF cultures are usually *not* helpful in identifying pathogens in patients with infectious aneurysms caused by hematogenous spread, as they are often negative despite an active infection.[721,727]

3. The diagnosis can usually be made based on CT findings and the clinical situation. Catheter angiography is necessary to affirm the diagnosis, clarify anatomy, and to look for other possible lesions.

4. A prolonged course of antibiotics is usually necessary, for at least 4–6 weeks:

   (a) Infectious aneurysms may continue to decrease in size after discontinuation of antibiotic therapy.[728]

5. Surgery:

   (a) Surgery should be reserved for hemorrhagic lesions that are surgically accessible, or for lesions that persist or enlarge with conservative management.

   (b) A course of antibiotic therapy will permit fibrosis of the aneurysm wall to occur and may make surgery more feasible.[729]

   (c) The surgical strategy can consist of trapping and resection, trapping and bypass, clipping, or wrapping.[717]

6. Endovascular therapy for intracranial infectious aneurysms has been reported. Reported strategies include embolization of the aneurysm, or provocative testing followed by endovascular occlusion of the parent vessel.[730,731] Endovascular treatment is appropriate for lesions that are poorly accessible by surgery, or for patients who are poor surgical candidates. The fragility of these aneurysms and the adjacent vessels may increase the risk of endovascular techniques.[731] A theoretical drawback to endovascular treatment is the threat of trapping, or sequestering bacteria within the lesion, making them less accessible to systemic antibiotic therapy, although this phenomenon has not been reported.

7. Radiographic follow-up. Infectious aneurysms may shrink, stabilize, or enlarge despite antibiotic therapy and even surgery, necessitating routine radiographic follow-up. Some authors have recommended serial angiography as frequently as 7 days, 14 days, 1 month, 3 months, and 1 year after the initiation of therapy.[724] The authors of this handbook prefer to use noninvasive imaging, such as CTA, for surveillance imaging after treatment, with at least one follow-up catheter angiogram after completion of treatment to ensure resolution of the lesion.

Outcomes

1. Historical mortality rates have approached 40%.[724]

2. Recent series have reported an overall mortality rate of 10–18.7%,[717,721] with good outcomes occurring in 80% of cases.[717]

   (a) Infectious aneurysms of the cavernous segment of the ICA seem to carry the best prognosis, only one death and one poor outcome have been reported in a series of 18 patients.[724,732]

3. Fungal aneurysms carry a worse prognosis, with mortality rates of 85–90%.[726]

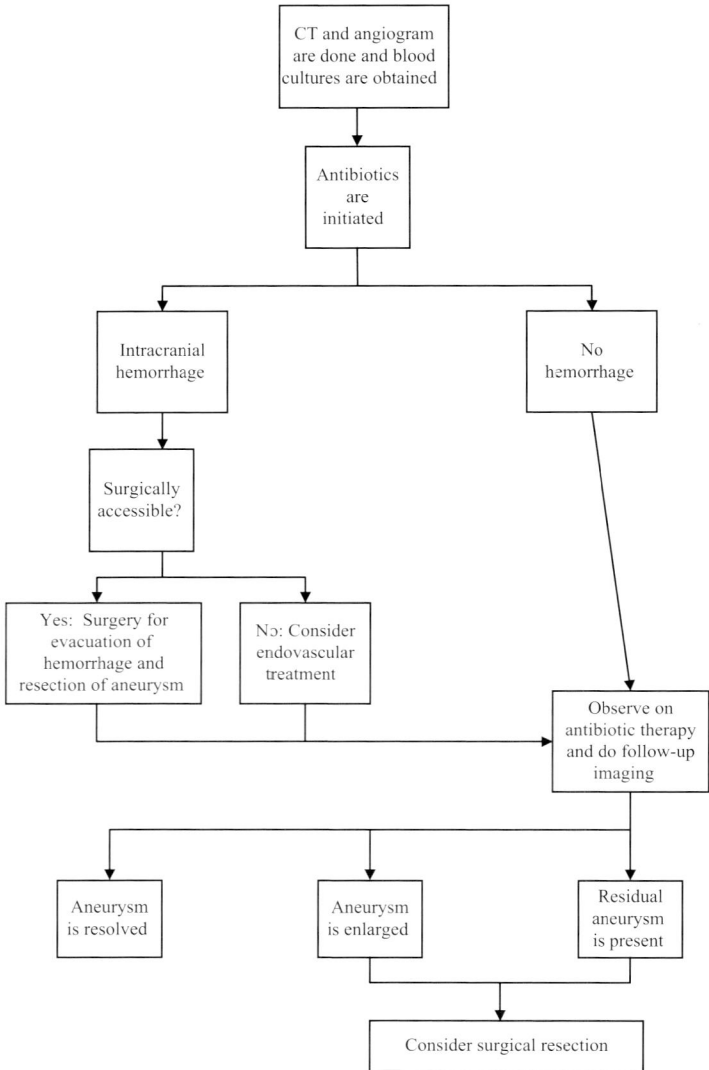

Fig. 13.8 Treatment algorithm for infectious intracranial aneurysms (Adapted from Phuong et al.[721] © 2002 Lippincott Williams & Wilkins, with permission).

Giant Aneurysms

By definition giant intracranial aneurysms are ≥25 mm in diameter. The first report of a giant aneurysm was in 1875; the lesion was diagnosed by an audible bruit.[733] Giant aneurysm morphology may be saccular or fusiform, and the lesions seem to have a propensity for the posterior circulation, occurring in the vertebrobasilar system in about a third of cases.[734] The presence of intraluminal thrombus is common. Giant aneurysms are thought to form via several different mechanisms. In smaller aneurysms destined to become giant ones, damage to the endothelium and internal elastic lamina and stagnant flow may induce mural thrombus formation, followed by scarring and further weakening of the wall. The presence of a thrombus may exacerbate turbulent flow, cause further damage to the aneurysm wall and increase wall shear stress. These aneurysms may also grow because of recurrent hemorrhage within the wall of the aneurysm; the highly vascular wall of a giant aneurysm may behave like a growing encapsulated chronic subdural hematoma.[735,736] In addition, intrathrombotic capillary channels may also be an important factor in the growth of thrombosed giant aneurysms.[737]

Epidemiology

1. Giant aneurysms comprise ~5% of all intracranial aneurysms.[738,739]
2. They are typically diagnosed in the fifth to seventh decade of life.[738,740]
3. They are slightly more common in women.[738]

Presentation

1. Approximately one third to one half of patients with giant aneurysms present with SAH.[738,741,742]
2. Some 50–70% of patients present with mass effect or brain edema caused by intraluminal thrombosis.[738,742,743]
   (a) It is important to note that an acute thrombus within an aneurysm can promote vasogenic edema in surrounding brain tissue just like an intracerebral hematoma.
3. About 8% of patients present with thromboembolic symptoms from an intraluminal thrombus.[738]
4. Hypothalamic[744] or frontal lobe dysfunction[745] is also present in some patients.
5. Most giant aneurysms arise from the ICA, MCA, or vertebrobasilar system. Giant aneurysms of the ACA are rare.
   (a) In a series of 18 patients with giant ACA aneurysms, dementia was present in patients with aneurysms ≥3.5 cm in diameter, and was caused by direct brain compression rather than hydrocephalus.[746] Optic apparatus compression was seen with smaller giant aneurysms (2.7–3.2 cm) when they pointed inferiorly.

Evaluation

1. CT and CTA can identify the dimensions of the lesion, the presence of intraluminal thrombus, calcification of the aneurysm wall, surrounding brain edema, as well as pertinent skull base anatomy, should surgery be anticipated.
2. Catheter angiography is complimentary to CTA and can demonstrate precise vascular anatomy, collateral circulation, and information about blood flow dynamics.

Natural History

1. Risk of rupture:
   (a) ISUIA: The annual risk of rupture for giant aneurysms is relatively high:[131]
      - Anterior communicating artery/MCA/ICA: 8.0%.
      - Posterior circulation and P-comm: 10%.
      - Cavernous ICA: 1.28%.
   (b) Early series of patients with untreated giant aneurysms reported mortality rates of 75–100% within 2–5 years.[747,748]
   (c) The risk of rehemorrhage after an initial SAH may be similar to that of smaller aneurysms; in a recent series the cumulative risk of rebleeding was 18.4% within 14 days of admission.[422a] Of those, one third died during the hospitalization.
2. In patients with SAH due to a ruptured giant aneurysm, the mortality rate is >50%.[749]

Management

1) Medical management, consisting of blood pressure management, smoking cessation, and antiplatelet therapy – if symptoms attributable to intraluminal thrombosis are present – is appropriate for patients who are at high risk of complications with surgical or endovascular treatment. Elderly patients or those with significant comorbidities or extremely complex lesions may be better off with a conservative approach.
2) Surgery. An array of surgical strategies exist for giant aneurysms, including clipping, trapping with or without a bypass, proximal occlusion, and surgical occlusion of the common carotid artery to reduce flow to the lesion and promote thrombosis.[750] Additional surgical techniques include hypothermic cardiac arrest and various skull base approaches.
   a) Endovascular techniques:
      i) Parent vessel sacrifice.[751,752] Endovascular sacrifice of the vessel is an established approach for the treatment of giant aneurysms. A balloon test occlusion is necessary for carotid lesions.
         (1) Caution: Vessel sacrifice increases hemodynamic stress on the other cerebral artery, which can cause new aneurysms to form. New aneurysms have been found in up to 20% patients after carotid sacrifice.[753]
      ii) Primary coiling.[742,751,754] Occlusion of a giant aneurysm by coil embolization is an option but is typically problematic, particularly for very large aneurysms or when intraluminal thrombus is present. Giant aneurysms require a large number of coils for complete embolization, larger aneurysms are prone to recur after coiling, and, if a thrombus is present, the coil mass can sink into the clot following embolization like a Cadillac parked in the sand at the beach.
      iii) Most operators recommend parent vessel sacrifice over primary coiling as the first endovascular option for giant aneurysms. In two endovascular series, hemorrhage occurred after coiling in 33%[755] and 6.4%[742] of patients, whereas no hemorrhages occurred after parent vessel sacrifice.
      iv) Stent-assisted coiling.[756] Some wide-necked giant saccular aneurysms and fusiform aneurysms can be treated with stent-assisted coiling.
      v) Covered stent.[757] Covered stents (also known as "stent-grafts") have been used for the treatment of giant and fusiform aneurysms.

Dissecting Intracranial Aneurysms

Spontaneously dissecting aneurysms are uncommon (traumatic dissecting aneurysms are considered separately below), but are distinctly different from more common saccular aneurysms. Dissecting aneurysms also have specific characteristics that distinguish them from lesions that may have similar radiographic features, such as fusiform and dolichoectatic aneurysms. The majority of literature about dissecting aneurysms is from Japan, although it is not clear whether these lesions are actually more common among the Japanese population, or just more often written about.

Clinical Features

1. In contrast to saccular aneurysms, dissecting aneurysms have a strong male preponderance.[758]
2. Also in distinction to saccular aneurysms, the vast majority of dissecting aneurysms occur in the vertebrobasilar circulation rather than the anterior circulation. In a Japanese nationwide study of 322 dissecting aneurysms, 93% were vertebrobasilar lesions and 7% were in the anterior circulation:[758]
    (a) Among anterior circulation cases, ACA lesions are more common than MCA.[759]
3. *Presentation*:
    (a) In contrast to most fusiform and dolichoectatic aneurysms, the evolution and presentation of a dissecting aneurysm is an acute and progressive process.[760]
    (b) The most common presentation is SAH, occurring in 53% of patients in the Japanese nationwide study.[758]
    (c) Cerebral ischemia or infarction is also a common mode of presentation. In a series of patients with lateral medullary infarction (Wallenberg syndrome), 18% were attributable to intracranial vertebral artery dissection.[761] In anterior circulation cases, presentation with ischemic symptoms are more common than hemorrhage.[758,759]
4. *Radiographic appearance*:
    (a) Dissecting aneurysms often arise from an arterial trunk, such as the vertebral or basilar arteries or the ICA, in contrast to saccular aneurysms, which usually arise from arterial branch points.
    (b) Dissecting aneurysms are typically irregular structures, often including a narrow tapered parent vessel lumen associated with proximal or distal focal dilatation ("pearl and string" sign). Arterial occlusion, an intimal flap, a double lumen, extension of the aneurysm into distal branches, and retention of contrast material into the late venous phase are also angiographic features of dissecting aneurysms[351,762]
    (c) The single pathognomonic sign of a dissecting aneurysm is a double lumen.[763]
    (d) On MRI, enhancement of the dissecting aneurysm with gadolinium is seen in 95% of cases.[764]
5. *Pathogenesis*:
    (a) Dissecting aneurysms result primarily by a sudden disruption of the internal elastic media.[765]
    (b) Compared to the extradural arteries, normal intradural arteries have a thin media and adventitia with relatively few elastic fibers, making them more vulnerable to dissection, hemorrhage, and pseudoaneurysm formation.[766] Also, intracranial arteries have diminished vasa vasorum, which may limit healing.[767]
    (c) Dissecting aneurysms are dynamic lesions, with evolution of the angiographic appearance characteristically occurring over 2–3 months.
    (d) Most spontaneous dissecting aneurysms are idiopathic, although associated risk factors include atherosclerosis, hypertension, a history of tumor resection, aneurysm clipping, or head injury, mucoid degeneration of the media, syphilis, migraines, fibromuscular dysplasia, homocystinuria, strenuous physical exertion, periarteritis nodosa, moyamoya disease, Guillain–Barré syndrome, and Marfan syndrome.[759,768]

Management

1. Hemorrhagic dissecting aneurysms:
    (a) The risk of rebleeding for ruptured dissecting aneurysms is significant, and may be higher than that for saccular aneurysms. In a series of 31 patients with ruptured vertebrobasilar dissecting aneurysms managed either with or without surgery, the rate of rebleeding was 71.4%, with an associated mortality rate of 46.7%.[769]

(b) Treatment of dissecting aneurysms is controversial; although most agree that either surgery or endovascular treatment to prevent rebleeding is critical. In a study of ruptured dissecting aneurysms, the mortality rate in the treated group was 20%, whereas that in the untreated group was 50%:[347]

- Surgical techniques include proximal occlusion of the parent vessel, trapping of the lesion, and wrapping. When sacrifice of a portion of a vessel with critical branches is anticipated, surgical bypass may be necessary. Clipping of the aneurysm at the neck, as is done with saccular aneurysms, is generally not feasible.
- Primary endovascular options include proximal occlusion and parent vessel occlusion.[347,770] Stent placement for the treatment of dissecting aneurysms has also been reported:[771,772]
  - Recent endovascular series have reported favorable results. A recent series of 29 patients reported overall morbidity and mortality rates of 13.8% and 17.2%, respectively.[770]

2. Nonhemorrhagic dissecting aneurysms:
  (a) For symptomatic dissecting aneurysms without hemorrhage, conservative management may be the best option. In the Japanese nationwide study, the majority of nonhemorrhagic dissecting aneurysms were managed without surgery or intervention, and a good recovery (by Glasgow outcome scale) was achieved in 79% of patients.[758]

Dolichoectatic, Fusiform and Serpentine Aneurysms

Dolichoectatic and fusiform aneurysms are uncommon, accounting for <2% of all intracranial aneurysms.[773–775] The term *serpentine aneurysm* generally refers to giant dolichoectatic aneurysms filled largely with thrombus;[776] these lesions are also very uncommon. One school of thought holds that small fusiform aneurysms and giant serpentine aneurysms are part of a spectrum of the same pathological process, although this notion is controversial. Common to all of these aneurysms is a nonsaccular shape and the pathological involvement of a length of artery with separate inflow and outflow sites.[777] The carotid and vertebrobasilar systems appear to be affected almost equally.[774,775,777] Hypertension is strongly associated with these lesions.[778,779]

Presentation

Symptoms may arise from compression of neural structures, cerebral ischemia, or rupture.[777] Compression and ischemia are the most common causes of symptoms.[778,780–782] Cranial nerve dysfunction appears in multiple reports, as do symptoms from brainstem compression. In a series of 132 patients with "megadolichovertebrobasilar anomaly," 31% of patients had symptoms attributable to brainstem or cerebellar compression.[783] Hydrocephalus can occur in patients with basilar artery dolichoectasia.[778,784] Ischemic symptoms occurred in 25% of patients in one series,[777] and can result from obstruction of perforating vessels or embolization of intraluminal thrombus. Compared to saccular aneurysms, rupture is relatively uncommon as a presenting symptom, occurring in 18–40% of patients.[773,777,778,780]

Pathogenesis

Intracranial fusiform aneurysms can be divided into two types: acute dissecting aneurysms and chronic fusiform or dolichoectatic aneurysms.[785] Arterial dissection is thought to be a factor in the formation of a significant percentage of fusiform intracranial aneurysms, particularly those without elongation or tortuosity of the parent vessel.[766,786,787] An acute dissection may be the inciting event in the pathogenesis of chronic fusiform aneurysms.[775] A series of four cases of dolichoectasia were found on MRI imaging to be dissections with aneurysmal dilation.[788]

Atherosclerosis, formerly thought to be an important factor in dolichoectasia, may not be a common feature of these lesions. Pathological studies of dolichoectatic aneurysms have found atherosclerosis to be absent or not a significant finding.[785,789] However, defects in the internal elastic lamina are a consistent pathological finding in most dolichoectatic aneurysms.[777,789–791] Chronic fusiform and dolichoectatic aneurysms may actually be progressive lesions that begin with fragmentation of the internal elastic lamina, followed by neoangiogenesis within a thickened intima, intramural thrombus formation, and repetitive intramural hemorrhage from newly formed vessels within the thrombus.[785]

Natural History

Most natural history data pertain to vertebrobasilar dolichoectasia. A cohort study of 45 patients with vertebrobasilar dolichoectasia found an increased risk of stroke in affected patients (OR = 3.6, p = 0.018).[792] In a prospective study of 159 patients with vertebrobasilar fusiform aneurysms or dolichoectasia, the 1-, 5-, and 10-year risk of cerebral infarction due to the vertebral artery lesion was 2.7%, 11.3%, and 15.9%, respectively.[782] The risk of recurrent ischemic symptoms was 6.7% per patient year. Median survival was 7.8 years and death was most commonly due to ischemia. In a prospective study of hemorrhage risk with a mean follow-up 4.4 years, the annual rupture rate was 0.9% overall and 2.3% in those with transitional or fusiform aneurysm subtypes.[779] Evidence of aneurysm enlargement was a significant predictor of lesion rupture.

Management

Surgery or endovascular treatment is indicated for select patients with symptomatic lesions who are good candidates for a major intracranial procedure. Surgery of fusiform and dolichoectatic aneurysms can be complex. In some cases, the parent vessel can be reconstructed with a series of stacked fenestrated clips. Wrapping of fusiform aneurysms with cotton or some other material is of unclear benefit. Surgical trapping or proximal occlusions, with or without a bypass, and with or without debulking of the aneurysm are other options. Trapping is superior to proximal occlusion when possible. Because of the rarity of these lesions, endovascular reports are limited to case reports and small series. Good results have been obtained with endovascular parent vessel occlusion[752,793] and intravascular stenting combined with coiling.[756] Flow diversion may be an even better option, but results are preliminary. For cases that are managed conservatively, some authors advocate anticoagulation[775] or antiplatelet therapy to minimize the risk of ischemic symptoms.[778]

Traumatic Aneurysms and Traumatic Subarachnoid Hemorrhage

Traumatic Aneurysms

1. Traumatic aneurysms comprise <1% of all intracranial aneurysms,[794,795] however they account for up to one third of all pediatric intracranial aneurysms.[669]
2. Presentation:
   (a) Traumatic aneurysms are commonly found after the appearance of delayed SAH after head injury, or unexplained neurological deterioration, epistaxis, cranial nerve palsy, or unexplained cortical bleeding.[286,796,797]
   (b) Traumatic aneurysms usually require a period of time to develop, ranging from 2[797] to 3 weeks[798] after the initial injury.
3. Diagnosis:
   (a) A history of head injury is the main criterion for diagnosis.
   (b) Typical angiographic features include a location in the peripheral vasculature, delayed filling and emptying of the aneurysm, an irregular contour, no visible neck, and a location separate from common arterial branch points.[661,795,799]
4. Traumatic aneurysms can be divided into those arising from nonpenetrating head injury and those arising from penetrating head injury. Nonpenetrating head injury is a more common cause of traumatic aneurysms than penetrating injury.

(a) Nonpenetrating head injury:
- Traumatic aneurysms due to nonpenetrating head injury usually result from rapid deceleration, causing sudden brain movement and vessel wall injury from stationary structures. Injury to the pericallosal artery by the edge of the falx accounts for the finding that distal ACA is the most common location for traumatic aneurysms in children.[669]
- The majority of traumatic aneurysms are found in the anterior circulation. A review published in 2002 found only 21 reports of posterior circulation traumatic aneurysms in the English language literature.[800]
- Skull fractures are a harbinger of traumatic aneurysms, and are present in some 90% of traumatic intracranial aneurysms.[795] Cortical traumatic aneurysms may appear adjacent to calvarial fractures,[801] and traumatic aneurysms of the petrous or cavernous ICA are almost always associated with basilar skull fractures:[797,802,803]
  - In a study of 55 patients with carotid canal fractures, ICA injury was found in six cases, two of which were traumatic aneurysms.[804]

(b) Penetrating head injury:
- Traumatic aneurysms due to penetrating injury may appear as early as 2 h after the injury, and appear most frequently on peripheral branches of the middle cerebral artery, and less often on the pericallosal artery.[805] Posterior circulation aneurysms are rare, probably because penetrating trauma to that part of the head is often fatal.
- Some 20% of these lesions are multiple.[805]

5. Management:
(a) Obliteration of the aneurysm or sacrifice of the parent vessel is recommended for traumatic intracranial aneurysms. Conservative management is associated with a mortality rate of nearly 50%,[669,795,806] and death is three times less likely if a traumatic aneurysm is identified before a hemorrhage has occurred, compared with diagnosis after rupture.[307]
(b) Clinical series of endovascular test occlusion followed by sacrifice of the parent vessel have reported favorable results.[797,807]
(c) Both surgical and endovascular techniques can be necessary for the management of aneurysms due to penetrating trauma.[808]

Traumatic Subarachnoid Hemorrhage

Trauma is the single most common cause of SAH. Subarachnoid hemorrhage occurs in 33–60% of patients with traumatic brain injury[809–811] and is associated with worse outcomes.[810,812] However, it is not clear whether the finding of traumatic SAH on CT is an independent risk factor for poor outcome, as good outcomes have been reported in >90% of patients with *mild* head injury and SAH on CT.[813,814] Although some data from angiography, TCD measurements, and CBF studies indicate that vasospasm occurs in patients with head injury less frequently or as frequently as patients with aneurysmal SAH,[815,816] other studies indicate that the incidence of vasospasm in head injury patients is low and does not lead to ischemic brain injury.[817,818] Moreover, assessment of the effects of vasospasm in head injury is confounded by the array of brain injuries attributable to the trauma itself. Several trials have evaluated the efficacy of calcium channel blockers in traumatic brain injury. A systematic review of six randomized controlled trials of calcium channel blockers in this setting found a benefit in terms of a lower rate of unfavorable outcomes (odds ratio 0.67, 95% CI 0.46–0.98),[819] although increased adverse reactions in the treated groups may offset the benefit. Published endovascular management of vasospasm after traumatic SAH is limited to a case report describing papaverine infusion in this setting.[820]

References

1. Abruzzo T, Shengelaia GG, Dawson 3rd RC, Owens DS, Cawley CM, Gravanis MB. Histologic and morphologic comparison of experimental aneurysms with human intracranial aneurysms. AJNR Am J Neuroradiol. 1998;19: 1309–14.

2. Walker AE, Allegre GW. The pathology and pathogenesis of cerebral aneurysms. J Neuropathol Exp Neurol. 1954;13:248–59.

3. Suzuki J, Ohara H. Clinicopathological study of cerebral aneurysms. Origin, rupture, repair, and growth. J Neurosurg. 1978;48:505–14.

4. Krings T, Piske RL, Lasjaunias PL. Intracranial arterial aneurysm vasculopathies: targeting the outer vessel wall. Neuroradiology. 2005;47:931–7.

5. Hashimoto T, Meng H, Young WL. Intracranial aneurysms: links among inflammation, hemodynamics and vascular remodeling. Neurol Res. 2006;28:372–80.

6. Aoki T, Kataoka H, Shimamura M, et al. NF-kappaB is a key mediator of cerebral aneurysm formation. Circulation. 2007;116:2830–40.

7. Pera J, Korostynski M, Krzyszkowski T, et al. Gene expression profiles in human ruptured and unruptured intracranial aneurysms: what is the role of inflammation? Stroke. 2010;41:224–31.

8. Kurki MI, Hakkinen SK, Frosen J, et al. Upregulated signaling pathways in ruptured human saccular intracranial aneurysm wall: an emerging regulative role of toll-like receptor signaling and nuclear factor-kappaB, hypoxia-inducible factor-1A, and ETS transcription factors. Neurosurgery. 2011;68:1667–76.

9. Hademenos GJ, Massoud TF, Turjman F, Sayre JW. Anatomical and morphological factors correlating with rupture of intracranial aneurysms in patients referred for endovascular treatment. Neuroradiology. 1998;40:755–60.

10. Crompton MR. Mechanism of growth and rupture in cerebral berry aneurysms. Br Med J. 1966;5496:1138–42.

11. International Study of Unruptured Intracranial Aneurysms Investigators. Unruptured intracranial aneurysms – risk of rupture and risks of surgical intervention. N Engl J Med. 1998;339:1725–33.

12. Bjorkesten G, Halonen V. Incidence of intracranial vascular lesions in patients with subarachnoid hemorrhage investigated by four-vessel angiography. J Neurosurg. 1965;23:29–32.

13. Qureshi AI, Suarez JI, Parekh PD. Risk factors for multiple intracranial aneurysms. Neurosurgery. 1998;43:22–6; discussion 6–7.

14. Ellamushi HE, Grieve JP, Jager HR, Kitchen ND. Risk factors for the formation of multiple intracranial aneurysms. J Neurosurg. 2001;94:728–32.

15. Juvela S. Risk factors for multiple intracranial aneurysms. Stroke. 2000;31:392–7.

16. Kaminogo M, Yonekura M, Shibata S. Incidence and outcome of multiple intracranial aneurysms in a defined population. Stroke. 2003;34:16–21.

17. Nehls DG, Flom RA, Carter LP, Spetzler RF. Multiple intracranial aneurysms: determining the site of rupture. J Neurosurg. 1985;63:342–8.

18. Stehbens W. Pathology of the cerebral blood vessels. St. Louis: Mosby; 1972. p. 351–470.

19. Marshman LA, Ward PJ, Walter PH, Dossetor RS. The progression of an infundibulum to aneurysm formation and rupture: case report and literature review. Neurosurgery. 1998;43:1445–8; discussion 8–9.

20. Vlak MH, Algra A, Brandenburg R, Rinkel GJ. Prevalence of unruptured intracranial aneurysms, with emphasis on sex, age, comorbidity, country, and time period: a systematic review and meta-analysis. Lancet Neurol. 2011;10:626–36.

21. Rinkel GJE, Djibuti M, Algra A, van Gijn J. Prevalence and risk of rupture of intracranial aneurysms: a systematic review. Stroke. 1998;29:251–6.

22. Gabriel RABS, Kim HP, Sidney S, et al. Ten-year detection rate of brain arteriovenous malformations in a large, multiethnic, defined population. Stroke. 2010;41:21–6.

23. Qureshi AI, Suri MF, Kim SH, et al. Effect of endovascular treatment on headaches in patients with unruptured intracranial aneurysms. Headache. 2003;43:1090–6.

24. Kong DS, Hong SC, Jung YJ, Kim JS. Improvement of chronic headache after treatment of unruptured intracranial aneurysms. Headache. 2007;47:693–7.

25. Raps EC, Rogers JD, Galetta SL, et al. The clinical spectrum of unruptured intracranial aneurysms. Arch Neurol. 1993;50:265–8.

26. Choxi AA, Durrani AK, Mericle RA. Both surgical clipping and endovascular embolization of unruptured intracranial aneurysms are associated with long-term improvement in self-reported quantitative headache scores. Neurosurgery. 2011;69:128–34.

27. Lozano AM, Leblanc R. Familial intracranial aneurysms. J Neurosurg. 1987;66:522–8.

28. Ronkainen A, Hernesniemi J, Puranen M, et al. Familial intracranial aneurysms. Lancet. 1997;349:380–4.

29. De Braekeleer M, Perusse L, Cantin L, Bouchard JM, Mathieu J. A study of inbreeding and kinship in intracranial aneurysms in the Saguenay Lac-Saint-Jean region (Quebec, Canada). Ann Hum Genet. 1996;60(Pt 2):99–104.

30. Norrgard O, Angquist KA, Fodstad H, Forsell A, Lindberg M. Intracranial aneurysms and heredity. Neurosurgery. 1987; 20:236–9.

31. Schievink WI, Schaid DJ, Michels VV, Piepgras DG. Familial aneurysmal subarachnoid hemorrhage: a community-based study. J Neurosurg. 1995;83:426–9.

32. Schievink WI, Schaid DJ, Rogers HM, Piepgras DG, Michels VV. On the inheritance of intracranial aneurysms. Stroke. 1994; 25:2028–37.

33. Bromberg JE, Rinkel GJ, Algra A, et al. Familial subarachnoid hemorrhage: distinctive features and patterns of inheritance. Ann Neurol. 1995;38:929–34.

34. Ruigrok YM, Rinkel GJE, Algra A, Raaymakers TWM, van Gijn J. Characteristics of intracranial aneurysms in patients with familial subarachnoid hemorrhage. Neurology. 2004;62:891–4.

35. Bromberg JE, Rinkel GJ, Algra A, Limburg M, van Gijn J. Outcome in familial subarachnoid hemorrhage. Stroke. 1995;26:961–3.

36. Yamada S, Utsunomiya M, Inoue K, et al. Genome-wide scan for Japanese familial intracranial aneurysms: linkage to several chromosomal regions. Circulation. 2004;110:3727–33.

37. Ruigrok YM, Seitz U, Wolterink S, Rinkel GJE, Wijmenga C, Urban Z. Association of polymorphisms and haplotypes in the elastin gene in Dutch patients with sporadic aneurysmal subarachnoid hemorrhage. Stroke. 2004;35:2064–8.

38. Schievink WI. Genetics of intracranial aneurysms. Neurosurgery. 1997;40:651–62; discussion 62–3.

39. Korja M, Silventoinen KP, McCarron P, et al. Genetic epidemiology of spontaneous subarachnoid hemorrhage: Nordic twin study. Stroke. 2010;41:2458–50.

40. Bederson JB, Awad IA, Wiebers DO, et al. Recommendations for the management of patients with unruptured intracranial aneurysms: a statement for healthcare professionals from the Stroke Council of the American Heart Association. Stroke. 2000;31:2742–50.

41. Brown BM, Soldevilla F. MR angiography and surgery for unruptured familial intracranial aneurysms in persons with a family history of cerebral aneurysms. AJR Am J Roentgenol. 1999;173:133–8.

42. Ronkainen A, Puranen MI, Hernesniemi JA, et al. Intracranial aneurysms: MR angiographic screening in 400 asymptomatic individuals with increased familial risk. Radiology. 1995; 195:35–40.

43. Raaymakers TW, Rinkel GJ, Ramos LM. Initial and follow-up screening for aneurysms in families with familial subarachnoid hemorrhage. Neurology. 1998;51:1125–30.

44. Broderick JP, Sauerbeck LR, Foroud T, et al. The Familial Intracranial Aneurysm (FIA) study protocol. BMC Med Genet. 2005;6:17.

45. Iglesias CG, Torres VE, Offord KP, Holley KE, Beard CM, Kurland LT. Epidemiology of adult polycystic kidney disease, Olmsted County, Minnesota: 1935–1980. Am J Kidney Dis. 1983;2:630–9.

46. Hughes J, Ward CJ, Peral B, et al. The polycystic kidney disease 1 (PKD1) gene encodes a novel protein with multiple cell recognition domains. Nat Genet. 1995;10:151–60.

47. Mochizuki T, Wu G, Hayashi T, et al. PKD2, a gene for polycystic kidney disease that encodes an integral membrane protein. Science. 1996;272:1339–42.

48. Arnaout MA. The vasculopathy of autosomal dominant polycystic kidney disease: insights from animal models. Kidney Int. 2000;58:2599–610.

49. Badani KK, Hemal AK, Menon M. Autosomal dominant polycystic kidney disease and pain – a review of the disease from aetiology, evaluation, past surgical treatment options to current practice. J Postgrad Med. 2004;50:222–6.

50. Chapman AB, Johnson AM, Gabow PA. Intracranial aneurysms in patients with autosomal dominant polycystic kidney disease: how to diagnose and who to screen. Am J Kidney Dis. 1993;22:526–31.

51. Bobrie G, Brunet-Bourgin F, Alamowitch S, et al. Spontaneous artery dissection: is it part of the spectrum of autosomal dominant polycystic kidney disease? Nephrol Dial Transplant. 1998;13:2138–41.

52. Schievink WI, Torres VE, Wiebers DO, Huston 3rd J. Intracranial arterial dolichoectasia in autosomal dominant polycystic kidney disease. J Am Soc Nephrol. 1997;8:1298–303.

53. Schievink WI, Huston 3rd J, Torres VE, Marsh WR. Intracranial cysts in autosomal dominant polycystic kidney disease. J Neurosurg. 1995;83:1004–7.

54. Schievink WI, Torres VE. Spinal meningeal diverticula in autosomal dominant polycystic kidney disease. Lancet. 1997; 349:1223–4.

55. Widjicks EFM. Aneurysmal subarachnoid hemorrhage. In: The clinical practice of critical care neurology. 2nd ed. Oxford: Oxford University Press; 2003. p. 185–220.

56. Chapman AB, Rubinstein D, Hughes R, et al. Intracranial aneurysms in autosomal dominant polycystic kidney disease. N Engl J Med. 1992;327:916–20.

57. Huston 3rd J, Torres VE, Sulivan PP, Offord KP, Wiebers DO. Value of magnetic resonance angiography for the detection of intracranial aneurysms in autosomal dominant polycystic kidney disease. J Am Soc Nephrol. 1993;3: 1871–7.

58. Fehlings MG, Gentili F. The association between polycystic kidney disease and cerebral aneurysms. Can J Neurol Sci. 1991;18:505–9.

59. Xu HW, Yu SQ, Mei CL, Li MH. Screening for intracranial aneurysm in 355 patients with autosomal-dominant polycystic kidney disease. Stroke. 2011;42:204–6.

60. Schievink WI, Torres VE, Piepgras DG, Wiebers DO. Saccular intracranial aneurysms in autosomal dominant polycystic kidney disease. J Am Soc Nephrol. 1992;3:88–95.

61. Schievink WI. Intracranial aneurysms. N Engl J Med. 1997;336:28–40.

62. Ruggieri PM, Poulos N, Masaryk TJ, et al. Occult intracranial aneurysms in polycystic kidney disease: screening with MR angiography. Radiology. 1994;191:33–9.

63. Pirson Y, Chauveau D, Torres V. Management of cerebral aneurysms in autosomal dominant polycystic kidney disease. J Am Soc Nephrol. 2002;13:269–76.

64. Chauveau D, Pirson Y, Verellen-Dumoulin C, Macnicol A, Gonzalo A, Grunfeld JP. Intracranial aneurysms in autosomal dominant polycystic kidney disease. Kidney Int. 1994;45: 1140–6.

65. Belz MM, Fick-Brosnahan GM, Hughes RL, et al. Recurrence of intracranial aneurysms in autosomal-dominant polycystic kidney disease. Kidney Int. 2003;63:1824–30.

66. Schrier RW, Belz MM, Johnson AM, et al. Repeat imaging for intracranial aneurysms in patients with autosomal dominant polycystic kidney disease with initially negative studies: a prospective ten-year follow-up. J Am Soc Nephrol. 2004; 15:1023–8.

67. Byers PH. Ehlers-Danlos type IV: a genetic disorder in many guises. J Invest Dermatol. 1995;105:311–3.

68. Germain DP. Clinical and genetic features of vascular Ehlers-Danlos syndrome. Ann Vasc Surg. 2002;16:391–7.

69. North KN, Whiteman DA, Pepin MG, Byers PH. Cerebrovascular complications in Ehlers-Danlos syndrome type IV. Ann Neurol. 1995;38:960–4.

70. Mitsuhashi T, Miyajima M, Saitoh R, Nakao Y, Hishii M, Arai H. Spontaneous carotid-cavernous fistula in a patient with Ehlers-Danlos syndrome type IV–case report. Neurol Med Chir (Tokyo). 2004;44:548–53.

71. Freeman RK, Swegle J, Sise MJ. The surgical complications of Ehlers-Danlos syndrome. Am Surg. 1996;62: 869–73.

72. Schievink WI, Piepgras DG, Earnest Ft, Gordon H. Spontaneous carotid-cavernous fistulae in Ehlers-Danlos syndrome Type IV. Case report. J Neurosurg. 1991;74:991–8.

73. DeMeo DL, Silverman EK. {alpha}1-Antitrypsin deficiency {middle dot 2}: genetic aspects of {alpha}1-antitrypsin deficiency: phenotypes and genetic modifiers of emphysema risk. Thorax. 2004;59:259–64.

74. Schievink WI, Katzmann JA, Piepgras DG, Schaid DJ. Alpha-1-antitrypsin phenotypes among patients with intracranial aneurysms. J Neurosurg. 1996;84:781–4.

75. St Jean P, Hart B, Webster M. Alpha-1-antitrypsin deficiency in aneurysmal disease. Hum Hered. 1996;46:92–7.

76. Kissela BM, Sauerbeck L, Woo D, et al. Subarachnoid hemorrhage: a preventable disease with a heritable component. Stroke. 2002;33:1321–6.

77. Yoneyama T, Kasuya H, Akagawa H, et al. Absence of Alpha-1 Antitrypsin Deficiency Alleles (S and Z) in Japanese and Korean patients with aneurysmal subarachnoid hemorrhage. Stroke. 2004;35:e376–8.

78. Schievink WI. Genetics of intracranial aneurysms. In: Winn HR, editor. Youmans neurological surgery. 5th ed. Philadelphia: Saunders; 2004. p. 1769–79.

79. van den Berg JSP, Limburg M, Hennekam RCM. Is Marfan syndrome associated with symptomatic intracranial aneurysms? Stroke. 1996;27:10–2.

80. Conway JE, Hutchins GM, Tamargo RJ. Marfan syndrome is not associated with intracranial aneurysms. Stroke. 1999;30: 1632–6.

81. Iqbal A, Alter M, Lee SH. Pseudoxanthoma elasticum: a review of neurological complications. Ann Neurol. 1978;4:18–20.

82. Munyer TP, Margulis AR. Pseudoxanthoma elasticum with internal carotid artery aneurysm. AJR Am J Roentgenol. 1981;136:1023–4.

83. van den Berg JS, Hennekam RC, Cruysberg JR, et al. Prevalence of symptomatic intracranial aneurysm and ischaemic stroke in pseudoxanthoma elasticum. Cerebrovasc Dis. 2000;10:315–9.

84. Loeys BL, Chen J, Neptune ER, et al. A syndrome of altered cardiovascular, craniofacial, neurocognitive and skeletal development caused by mutations in TGFBR1 or TGFBR2. Nat Genet. 2005;37:275–81.

85. Loeys BL, Schwarze U, Holm T, et al. Aneurysm syndromes caused by mutations in the TGF-beta receptor. N Engl J Med. 2006;355:788–98.

86. Rodrigues VJ, Elsayed S, Loeys BL, Dietz HC, Yousem DM. Neuroradiologic manifestations of Loeys-Dietz syndrome type 1. AJNR Am J Neuroradiol. 2009;30:1614–9.

87. Van Den Berg DJ, Francke U. Roberts syndrome: a review of 100 cases and a new rating system for severity. Am J Med Genet. 1993;47:1104–23.

88. Vega H, Waisfisz Q, Gordillo M, et al. Roberts syndrome is caused by mutations in ESCO2, a human homolog of yeast ECO1 that is essential for the establishment of sister chromatid cohesion. Nat Genet. 2005;37:468–70.

89. Robers JB. A child with double cleft of lip and palate, protrusion of the intermaxillary portion of the upper jaw and imperfect development of the bones of the four extremities. Ann Surg. 1919;70:252–3.

90. Herrman J, Feingold M, Tuffli GA, Opitz JM. A familial dysmorphogenetic syndrome of limb deformities, characteristic facial appearance and associated anomalies: the "Pseudothalidomide" or SC-syndrome. In: Paul NW, editor. Cumulative index birth defects: original article series. New York: Alan R. Liss; 1982. p. 81–9.

91. Wang AC, Gemmete JJ, Keegan CE, et al. Spontaneous intracranial hemorrhage and multiple intracranial aneurysms in a patient with Roberts/SC phocomelia syndrome. J Neurosurg Pediatr. 2011;8:460–3.

INTRACRANIAL ANEURYSMS AND SUBARACHNOID HAEMORRHAGE

92. Stapf C, Mohr JP, Pile-Spellman J, et al. Concurrent arterial aneurysms in brain arteriovenous malformations with haemorrhagic presentation. J Neurol Neurosurg Psychiatry. 2002;73:294–8.

93. Brown Jr RD, Wiebers DO, Forbes GS. Unruptured intracranial aneurysms and arteriovenous malformations: frequency of intracranial hemorrhage and relationship of lesions. J Neurosurg. 1990;73:859–63.

94. Redekop G, TerBrugge K, Montanera W, Willinsky R. Arterial aneurysms associated with cerebral arteriovenous malformations: classification, incidence, and risk of hemorrhage. J Neurosurg. 1998;89:539–46.

95. Meisel HJ, Mansmann U, Alvarez H, Rodesch G, Brock M, Lasjaunias P. Cerebral arteriovenous malformations and associated aneurysms: analysis of 305 cases from a series of 662 patients. Neurosurgery. 2000;46:793–800; discussion 800–2.

96. Mansmann U, Meisel J, Brock M, Rodesch G, Alvarez H, Lasjaunias P. Factors associated with intracranial hemorrhage in cases of cerebral arteriovenous malformation. Neurosurgery. 2000;46:272–9; discussion 9–81.

97. Cloft HJ, Kallmes DF, Kallmes MH, Goldstein JH, Jensen ME, Dion JE. Prevalence of cerebral aneurysms in patients with fibromuscular dysplasia: a reassessment. J Neurosurg. 1998;88:436–40.

98. Norrgard O, Angqvist KA, Fodstad H, Forssell A, Lindberg M. Co-existence of abdominal aortic aneurysms and intracranial aneurysms. Acta Neurochir (Wien). 1987;87:34–9.

99. Kanai H, Umezu M, Koide K, Hato M. Ruptured intracranial aneurysm associated with unruptured abdominal aortic aneurysm – case report. Neurol Med Chir (Tokyo). 2001;41:260–3.

100. Preul MC, Cendes F, Just N, Mohr G. Intracranial aneurysms and sickle cell anemia: multiplicity and propensity for the vertebrobasilar territory. Neurosurgery. 1998;42:971–7; discussion 7–8.

101. Schievink WI, Maya MM. Frequency of intracranial aneurysms in patients with spontaneous intracranial hypotension. J Neurosurg. 2011;115:113–5.

102. Schievink WI, Raissi SS, Maya MM, Velebir A. Screening for intracranial aneurysms in patients with bicuspid aortic valve. Neurology. 2010;74:1430–3.

103. Feigin VL, Rinkel GJE, Lawes CMM, et al. Risk factors for subarachnoid hemorrhage: an updated systematic review of epidemiological studies. Stroke. 2005;36:2773–80.

104. Baker CJ, Fiore A, Connolly Jr ES, Baker KZ, Solomon RA. Serum elastase and alpha-1-antitrypsin levels in patients with ruptured and unruptured cerebral aneurysms. Neurosurgery. 1995;37:56–61; discussion 61–2.

105. Juvela S, Poussa K, Porras M. Factors affecting formation and growth of intracranial aneurysms: a long-term follow-up study. Stroke. 2001;32:485–91.

106. Morris KM, Shaw MD, Foy PM. Smoking and subarachnoid haemorrhage: a case control study. Br J Neurosurg. 1992;6:429–32.

107. Canhao P, Pinto AN, Ferro H, Ferro JM. Smoking and aneurysmal subarachnoid haemorrhage: a case–control study. J Cardiovasc Risk. 1994;1:155–8.

108. Juvela S, Porras M, Poussa K. Natural history of unruptured intracranial aneurysms: probability of and risk factors for aneurysm rupture. J Neurosurg. 2000;93:379–87.

109. Wermer MJH, Greebe P, Algra A, Rinkel GJE. Incidence of recurrent subarachnoid hemorrhage after clipping for ruptured intracranial aneurysms. Stroke. 2005;36:2394–9.

110. Lasner TM, Weil RJ, Riina HA, et al. Cigarette smoking-induced increase in the risk of symptomatic vasospasm after aneurysmal subarachnoid hemorrhage. J Neurosurg. 1997;87:381–4.

111. Weir BK, Kongable GL, Kassell NF, Schultz JR, Truskowski LL, Sigrest A. Cigarette smoking as a cause of aneurysmal subarachnoid hemorrhage and risk for vasospasm: a report of the Cooperative Aneurysm Study. J Neurosurg. 1998;89:405–11.

112. Ortiz R, Stefanski M, Rosenwasser R, Veznedaroglu E. Cigarette smoking as a risk factor for recurrence of aneurysms treated by endosaccular occlusion. J Neurosurg. 2008;108:672–5.

113. Veznedaroglu E, Koebbe CJ, Siddiqui A, Rosenwasser RH. Initial experience with bioactive cerecyte detachable coils:

114. Isaksen J, Egge A, Waterloo K, Romner B, Ingebrigtsen T. Risk factors for aneurysmal subarachnoid haemorrhage: the Tromso study. J Neurol Neurosurg Psychiatry. 2002;73:185–7.

115. Rinkel GJ. Intracranial aneurysm screening: indications and advice for practice. Lancet Neurol. 2005;4:122–8.

116. Juvela S, Hillbom M, Numminen H, Koskinen P. Cigarette smoking and alcohol consumption as risk factors for aneurysmal subarachnoid hemorrhage. Stroke. 1993;24:639–46.

117. Longstreth Jr WT, Nelson LM, Koepsell TD, van Belle G. Cigarette smoking, alcohol use, and subarachnoid hemorrhage. Stroke. 1992;23:1242–9.

118. Doll R, Peto R, Boreham J, Sutherland I. Mortality in relation to alcohol consumption: a prospective study among male British doctors. Int J Epidemiol. 2005;34:199–204.

119. Johnston SC, Colford Jr JM, Gress DR. Oral contraceptives and the risk of subarachnoid hemorrhage: a meta-analysis. Neurology. 1998;51:411–8.

120. Teunissen LL, Rinkel GJ, Algra A, van Gijn J. Risk factors for subarachnoid hemorrhage: a systematic review. Stroke. 1996;27:544–9.

121. Adamson J, Humphries SE, Ostergaard JR, Voldby B, Richards P, Powell JT. Are cerebral aneurysms atherosclerotic? Stroke. 1994;25:963–6.

122. Ferro JM, Pinto AN. Sexual activity is a common precipitant of subarachnoid hemorrhage. Cerebrovasc Dis. 1994;4:375.

123. Reynolds MR, Willie JT, Zipfel GJ, Dacey RG. Sexual intercourse and cerebral aneurysmal rupture: potential mechanisms and precipitants. J Neurosurg. 2011;114:969–77.

124. Chyatte D, Chen TL, Bronstein K, Brass LM. Seasonal fluctuation in the incidence of intracranial aneurysm rupture and its relationship to changing climatic conditions. J Neurosurg. 1994;81:525–30.

125. Inagawa T, Takechi A, Yahara K, et al. Primary intracerebral and aneurysmal subarachnoid hemorrhage in Izumo City, Japan. Part I: incidence and seasonal and diurnal variations. J Neurosurg. 2000;93:958–66.

126. Abe T, Ohde S, Ishimatsu S, et al. Effects of meteorological factors on the onset of subarachnoid hemorrhage: a time-series analysis. J Clin Neurosci. 2008;15:1005–10.

127. Buxton N, Liu C, Dasic D, Moody P, Hope DT. Relationship of aneurysmal subarachnoid hemorrhage to changes in atmospheric pressure: results of a prospective study. J Neurosurg. 2001;95:391–2.

128. Beseoglu K, Hanggi D, Stummer W, Steiger HJ. Dependence of subarachnoid hemorrhage on climate conditions: a systematic meteorological analysis from the Dusseldorf metropolitan area. Neurosurgery. 2008;62:1033–8; discussion 8–9.

129. Cowperthwaite MC, Burnett MG. The association between weather and spontaneous subarachnoid hemorrhage: an analysis of 155 US hospitals. Neurosurgery. 2011;68:132–9.

130. Morita A, Fujiwara S, Hashi K, Ohtsu H, Kirino T. Risk of rupture associated with intact cerebral aneurysms in the Japanese population: a systematic review of the literature from Japan. J Neurosurg. 2005;102:601–6.

131. Wiebers DO, Whisnant JP, Huston 3rd J, et al. Unruptured intracranial aneurysms: natural history, clinical outcome, and risks of surgical and endovascular treatment. Lancet. 2003;362:103–10.

132. Morita A. On-line outcome study of unruptured cerebral aneurysm in Japan (UCAS Japan). Rinsho Shinkeigaku. 2002;42:1188–90.

133. Yonekura M. Small unruptured aneurysm verification (SUAVe Study, Japan) – interim report. Neurol Med Chir (Tokyo). 2004;44:213–4.

134. Kiyohara Y, Ueda K, Hasuo Y, et al. Incidence and prognosis of subarachnoid hemorrhage in a Japanese rural community. Stroke. 1989;20:1150–5.

135. Ingall TJ, Whisnant JP, Wiebers DO, O'Fallon WM. Has there been a decline in subarachnoid hemorrhage mortality? Stroke. 1989;20:718–24.

136. Burt VL, Whelton P, Roccella EJ. Prevalence of hypertension in the US adult population. Results from the third national health and nutrition examination survey, 1988–1991. Hypertension. 1995;25:305–13.

137. Patterson JM, Eberly LE, Ding Y, Fargreaves M. Associations of smoking prevalence with individual and area level social cohesion. J Epidemiol Community Health. 2004;58:692–7.

138. Ministry of Health LaW. Current status of nutrition in Japanese population (survey in 1998). Tokyo: Daiichi Shuppan; 2000.

139. Association AH. Heart disease and stroke statistics – 2005 update. Dallas: American Heart Association. 2005.

140. Wiebers DO, Whisnant JP, Sundt Jr TM, O'Fallon WM. The significance of unruptured intracranial saccular aneurysms. J Neurosurg. 1987;66:23–9.

141. Forget Jr TR, Benitez R, Veznedaroglu E. A review of size and location of ruptured intracranial aneurysms. Neurosurgery. 2001;49:1322–5; discussion 5–6.

142. Beck J, Rohde S, Berkefeld J, Seifert V, Rache A. Size and location of ruptured and unruptured intracranial aneurysms measured by 3-dimensional rotational angiography. Surg Neurol. 2006;65:18–25; discussion 25–7.

143. Rahman M, Ogilvy CS, Zipfel GJ, et al. Unruptured cerebral aneurysms do not shrink when they rupture: multicenter collaborative aneurysm study group. Neurosurgery. 2011;68:155–61.

144. Yoshimoto Y. Publication bias in neurosurgery: lessons from series of unruptured aneurysms. Acta Neurochir (Wien). 2003;145:45–8.

145. Feuerberg I, Lindquist C, Lindqvist M, Steiner L. Natural history of postoperative aneurysm rests. J Neurosurg. 1987;66:30–4.

146. Macdonald RL, Wallace MC, Kestle JR. Role of angiography following aneurysm surgery. J Neurosurg. 1993;79:826–32.

147. Thornton J, Bashir Q, Aletich VA, Debrun GM, Ausman JI, Charbel FT. What percentage of surgically clipped intracranial aneurysms have residual necks? Neurosurgery. 2000; 46:1294–8; discussion 8–300.

148. Sindou M, Acevedo JC, Turjman F. Aneurysmal remnants after microsurgical clipping: classification and results from a prospective angiographic study (in a consecutive series of 305 operated intracranial aneurysms). Acta Neurochir (Wien). 1998;140:1153–9.

149. Le Roux PD, Elliott JP, Eskridge JM, Cohen W, Winn HR. Risks and benefits of diagnostic angiography after aneurysm surgery: a retrospective analysis of 597 studies. Neurosurgery. 1998;42:1248–54; discussion 54–5.

150. David CA, Vishteh AG, Spetzler RF, Lemole M, Lawton MT, Partovi S. Late angiographic follow-up review of surgically treated aneurysms. J Neurosurg. 1999;91:395–401.

151. Tsutsumi K, Ueki K, Usui M, Kwak S, Kirino T. Risk of recurrent subarachnoid hemorrhage after complete obliteration of cerebral aneurysms. Stroke. 1998;29:2511–3.

152. The CI. Rates of delayed rebleeding from intracranial aneurysms are low after surgical and endovascular treatment. Stroke. 2006;37:1437–42.

153. Raaymakers TW, Rinkel GJ, Limburg M, Algra A. Mortality and morbidity of surgery for unruptured intracranial aneurysms: a meta-analysis. Stroke. 1998;29:1531–8.

154. Johnston SC, Zhao S, Dudley RA, Berman MF, Gress DR. Treatment of unruptured cerebral aneurysms in California. Stroke. 2001;32:597–605.

155. Khanna RK, Malik GM, Qureshi N. Predicting outcome following surgical treatment of unruptured intracranial aneurysms: a proposed grading system. J Neurosurg. 1996; 84:49–54.

156. Ogilvy CS, Carter BS. Stratification of outcome for surgically treated unruptured intracranial aneurysms. Neurosurgery. 2003;52:82–7; discussion 7–8.

157. Rabinowicz AL, Ginsburg DL, DeGiorgio CM, Gott PS, Giannotta SL. Unruptured intracranial aneurysms: seizures and antiepileptic drug treatment following surgery. J Neurosurg. 1991;75:371–3.

158. Ronkainen A, Niskanen M, Rinne J, Koivisto T, Hernesniemi J, Vapalahti M. Evidence for excess long-term mortality after treated subarachnoid hemorrhage. Stroke. 2001;32:2850–3.

159. Britz GW, Salem L, Newell DW, Eskridge J, Flum DR. Impact of surgical clipping on survival in unruptured and ruptured cerebral aneurysms: a population-based study. Stroke. 2004;35:1399–403.

160. Brilstra EH, Rinkel GJ, van der Graaf Y, van Rooij WJ, Algra A. Treatment of intracranial aneurysms by embolization with coils: a systematic review. Stroke. 1999;30:470–6.

161. Byrne JV, Sohn MJ, Molyneux AJ, Chir B. Five-year experience in using coil embolization for ruptured intracranial aneurysms: outcomes and incidence of late rebleeding. J Neurosurg. 1999;90:656–63.

162. Cognard C, Weill A, Spelle L, et al. Long-term angiographic follow-up of 169 intracranial berry aneurysms occluded with detachable coils. Radiology. 1999;212: 348–56.

163. Raftopoulos C, Mathurin P, Boscherini D, Billa RF, Van Boven M, Hantson P. Prospective analysis of aneurysm treatment in a series of 103 consecutive patients when endovascular embolization is considered the first option. J Neurosurg. 2000;93:175–82.

164. Ng P, Khangure MS, Phatouros CC, Bynevelt M, ApSimon H, McAuliffe W. Endovascular treatment of intracranial aneurysms with Guglielmi detachable coils: analysis of midterm angiographic and clinical outcomes. Stroke. 2002; 33:210–7.

165. Murayama Y, Nien YL, Duckwiler G, et al. Guglielmi detachable coil embolization of cerebral aneurysms: 11 years' experience. J Neurosurg. 2003;98:959–66.

166. Gonzalez N, Murayama Y, Nien YL, et al. Treatment of unruptured aneurysms with GDCs: clinical experience with 247 aneurysms. AJNR Am J Neuroradiol. 2004;25:577–83.

167. Pouratian N, Oskouian Jr RJ, Jensen ME, Kassell NF, Dumont AS. Endovascular management of unruptured intracranial aneurysms. J Neurol Neurosurg Psychiatry. 2006;77:572–8.

168. Goddard AJ, Annesley-Williams D, Gholkar A. Endovascular management of unruptured intracranial aneurysms: does outcome justify treatment? J Neurol Neurosurg Psychiatry. 2002;72:485–90.

169. Raymond J, Guilbert F, Weill A, et al. Long-term angiographic recurrences after selective endovascular treatment of aneurysms with detachable coils. Stroke. 2003;34:1398–403.

170. Gallas S, Pasco A, Cottier J-P, et al. A multicenter study of 705 ruptured intracranial aneurysms treated with Guglielmi detachable coils. AJNR Am J Neuroradiol. 2005;26:1723–31.

171. Li MH, Gao BL, Fang C, et al. Angiographic follow-up of cerebral aneurysms treated with Guglielmi detachable coils: an analysis of 162 cases with 173 aneurysms. AJNR Am J Neuroradiol. 2006;27:1107–12.

172. Iijima A, Piotin M, Mounayer C, Spelle L, Weill A, Moret J. Endovascular treatment with coils of 149 middle cerebral artery berry aneurysms. Radiology. 2005;237:611–9.

173. Ferns SP, Sprengers MES, van Rooij WJ, et al. Late reopening of adequately coiled intracranial aneurysms: frequency and risk factors in 400 patients with 440 aneurysms. Stroke. 2011;42:1331–7.

174. Tamatani S, Ito Y, Abe H, Koike T, Takeuchi S, Tanaka R. Evaluation of the stability of aneurysms after embolization using detachable coils: correlation between stability of aneurysms and embolized volume of aneurysms. AJNR Am J Neuroradiol. 2002;23:762–7.

175. Szikora I, Wakhloo AK, Guterman LR, et al. Initial experience with collagen-filled Guglielmi detachable coils for endovascular treatment of experimental aneurysms. AJNR Am J Neuroradiol. 1997;18:667–72.

176. Zaroff JG, Rordorf GA, Newell JB, Ogilvy CS, Levinson JR. Cardiac outcome in patients with subarachnoid hemorrhage and electrocardiographic abnormalities. Neurosurgery. 1999;44:34–9; discussion 9–40.

177. Soeda A, Sakai N, Sakai H, Iihara K, Nagata I. Endovascular treatment of asymptomatic cerebral aneurysms: anatomic and technical factors related to ischemic events and coil stabilization. Neurol Med Chir (Tokyo). 2004;44:456–65; discussion 66.

178. Piotin M, Blanc R, Spelle L, et al. Stent-assisted coiling of intracranial aneurysms: clinical and angiographic results in 216 consecutive aneurysms. Stroke. 2010;41: 110–5.

179. Brinjikji W, Lanzino G, Cloft HJ, Rabinstein A, Kallmes DF. Endovascular treatment of very small (3 mm or smaller) intracranial aneurysms: report of a consecutive series and a meta-analysis. Stroke. 2010;41:116–21.

180. Graves VB, Strother CM, Duff TA, Perl 2nd J. Early treatment of ruptured aneurysms with Guglielmi detachable coils: effect on subsequent bleeding. Neurosurgery. 1995;37: 640–7; discussion 7–8.

181. Friedman JA, Nichols DA, Meyer FB, et al. Guglielmi detachable coil treatment of ruptured saccular cerebral aneurysms: retrospective review of a 10-year single-center experience. AJNR Am J Neuroradiol. 2003;24: 526–33.

182. Lempert TE, Malek AM, Halbach VV, et al. Endovascular treatment of ruptured posterior circulation cerebral aneurysms. Clinical and angiographic outcomes. Stroke. 2000;31:100–10.

183. Kuether TA, Nesbit GM, Barnwell SL. Clinical and angiographic outcomes, with treatment data, for patients with cerebral aneurysms treated with Guglielmi detachable coils: a single-center experience. Neurosurgery. 1998;43: 1016–25.

184. Nichols DA, Brown Jr RD, Thielen KR, Meyer FB, Atkinson JL, Piepgras DG. Endovascular treatment of ruptured posterior circulation aneurysms using electrolytically detachable coils. J Neurosurg. 1997;87:374–80.

185. Uda K, Goto K, Ogata N, Izumi N, Nagata S, Matsuno H. Embolization of cerebral aneurysms using Guglielmi detachable coils – problems and treatment plans in the acute stage after subarachnoid hemorrhage and long-term efficiency. Neurol Med Chir (Tokyo). 1998;38:143–52; discussion 52–4.

186. Raymond J, Roy D. Safety and efficacy of endovascular treatment of acutely ruptured aneurysms. Neurosurgery. 1997;41:1235–45; discussion 45–6.

187. Eskridge JM, Song JK. Endovascular embolization of 150 basilar tip aneurysms with Guglielmi detachable coils: results of the food and drug administration multicenter clinical trial. J Neurosurg. 1998;89:81–6.

188. Elias T, Ogungbo B, Connolly D, Gregson B, Mendelow AD, Gholkar A. Endovascular treatment of anterior communicating artery aneurysms: results of clinical and radiological outcome in Newcastle. Br J Neurosurg. 2003;17:278–86.

189. Plowman RS, Clarke A, Clarke M, Byrne JV. Sixteen-year single-surgeon experience with coil embolization for ruptured intracranial aneurysms: recurrence rates and incidence of late rebleeding. J Neurosurg. 2011;114:863–74.

190. Vanninen R, Koivisto T, Saari T, Hernesniemi J, Vapalahti M. Ruptured intracranial aneurysms: acute endovascular treatment with electrolytically detachable coils – a prospective randomized study. Radiology. 1999;211:325–36.

191. Cognard C, Weill A, Castaings L, Rey A, Moret J. Intracranial berry aneurysms: angiographic and clinical results after endovascular treatment. Radiology. 1998;206:499–510.

192. Sluzewski M, van Rooij WJ, Rinkel GJ, Wijnalda D. Endovascular treatment of ruptured intracranial aneurysms with detachable coils: long-term clinical and serial angiographic results. Radiology. 2003;227:720–4.

193. Fleming JB, Hoh BL, Simon SD, et al. Rebleeding risk after treatment of ruptured intracranial aneurysms. J Neurosurg. 2011;114:1778–84.

194. Molyneux AJ, Kerr RS, Yu LM, et al. International subarachnoid aneurysm trial (ISAT) of neurosurgical clipping versus endovascular coiling in 2143 patients with ruptured intracranial aneurysms: a randomised comparison of effects on survival, dependency, seizures, rebleeding, subgroups, and aneurysm occlusion. Lancet. 2005;366:809–17.

195. Molyneux A, Kerr R, Stratton I, et al. International Subarachnoid Aneurysm Trial (ISAT) of neurosurgical clipping versus endovascular coiling in 2143 patients with ruptured intracranial aneurysms: a randomised trial. Lancet. 2002;360:1267–74.

196. Johnston SC, Dudley RA, Gress DR, Ono L. Surgical and endovascular treatment of unruptured cerebral aneurysms at university hospitals. Neurology. 1999;52:1799–805.

197. Lee T, Baytion M, Sciacca R, Mohr JP, Pile-Spellman J. Aggregate analysis of the literature for unruptured intracranial aneurysm treatment. AJNR Am J Neuroradiol. 2005; 26:1902–8.

198. Brinjikji W, Rabinstein AA, Lanzino G, Kallmes DF, Cloft HJ. Effect of age on outcomes of treatment of unruptured cerebral aneurysms: a study of the national inpatient sample 2001–2008. Stroke. 2011;42:1320–4.

199. Alshekhlee A, Mehta S, Edgell RC, et al. Hospital mortality and complications of electively clipped or coiled unruptured intracranial aneurysm. Stroke. 2010;41:1471–6.

200. Vajkoczy P, Meyer B, Weidauer S, et al. Clazosentan (AXV-034343), a selective endothelin A receptor antagonist, in the prevention of cerebral vasospasm following severe aneurysmal subarachnoid hemorrhage: results of a randomized, double-blind, placebo-controlled, multicenter phase IIa study. J Neurosurg. 2005;103:9–17.

201. Dumont AS, Crowley RW, Monteith SJ, et al. Endovascular treatment or neurosurgical clipping of ruptured intracranial aneurysms: effect on angiographic vasospasm, delayed ischemic neurological deficit, cerebral infarction, and clinical outcome. Stroke. 2010;41:2519–24.

202. Kallmes DF, Ding YH, Dai D, Kadirvel R, Lewis DA, Cloft HJ. A new endoluminal, flow-disrupting device for treatment of saccular aneurysms. Stroke. 2007;38:2346–52.

203. Fiorella D, Woo HH, Albuquerque FC, Nelson PK. Definitive reconstruction of circumferential, fusiform intracranial aneurysms with the pipeline embolization device. Neurosurgery. 2008;62:1115–20; discussion 20–1.

204. Sadasivan C, Cesar L, Seong J, Wakhloo AK, Lieber BB. Treatment of rabbit elastase-induced aneurysm models by flow diverters: development of quantifiable indexes of device performance using digital subtraction angiography. IEEE Trans Med Imaging. 2009;28:1117–25.

205. Fiorella D, Lylyk P, Szikora I, et al. Curative cerebrovascular reconstruction with the pipeline embolization device: the emergence of definitive endovascular therapy for intracranial aneurysms. J Neurointerv Surg. 2009;1:56–65.

206. Aenis M, Stancampiano AP, Wakhloo AK, Lieber BB. Modeling of flow in a straight stented and nonstented side wall aneurysm model. J Biomech Eng. 1997;119: 206–12.

207. Kim YH, Xu X, Lee JS. The effect of stent porosity and strut shape on saccular aneurysm and its numerical analysis with lattice Boltzmann method. Ann Biomed Eng. 2010;38:2274–92.

208. Kim M, Taulbee DB, Tremmel M, Meng H. Comparison of two stents in modifying cerebral aneurysm hemodynamics. Ann Biomed Eng. 2008;36:726–41.

209. Meng H, Wang Z, K m M, Ecker RD, Hopkins LN. Saccular aneurysms on straight and curved vessels are subject to different hemodynamics: implications of intravascular stenting. AJNR Am J Neuroradiol. 2006;27:1861–5.

210. Wakhloo AK, Tio FO, Lieber BB, Schellhammer F, Graf M, Hopkins LN. Self-expanding nitinol stents in canine vertebral arteries: hemodynamics and tissue response. AJNR Am J Neuroradiol. 1995;16:1043–51.

211. Lopes DK, Ringer AJ, Boulos AS. Fate of branch arteries after intracranial stenting. Neurosurgery. 2003;52:1275–8; discussion 8–9.

212. Sadasivan C, Cesar L, Seong J, et al. An original flow diversion device for the treatment of intracranial aneurysms: evaluation in the rabbit elastase-induced model. Stroke. 2009;40:952–8.

213. Nelson PK, Lylyk P, Szikora I, Wetzel SG, Wanke I, Fiorella D. The pipeline embolization device for the intracranial treatment of aneurysms trial. AJNR Am J Neuroradiol. 2011;32:34–40.

214. Lylyk P, Miranda C, Ceratto R. Curative endovascular reconstruction of cerebral aneurysms with the pipeline embolization device: the Buenos Aires experience. Neurosurgery. 2009;64:632–42; discussion 42–3; quiz N6.

215. Szikora I, Berentei Z, Kulcsar Z, et al. Treatment of intracranial aneurysms by functional reconstruction of the parent artery: the Budapest experience with the pipeline embolization device. AJNR Am J Neuroradiol. 2010;31:1139–47.

216. Fischer S, Vajda Z, Aguilar Perez M, et al. Pipeline embolization device (PED) for neurovascular reconstruction: initial experience in the treatment of 101 intracranial aneurysms and dissections. Neuroradiology. 2012;54(4):369–82.

217. Pipeline for Uncoilable or Failed Aneurysms (PUFS). U.S. National Institutes of Health. 2011. http://clinicaltrials.gov/ct2/show/NCT00777088. Accessed 8 Sept 2011.

218. Lubicz B, Collignon L, Raphaeli G, et al. Flow-diverter stent for the endovascular treatment of intracranial aneurysms: a prospective study in 29 patients with 34 aneurysms. Stroke. 2010;41:2247–53.

219. Byrne JV, Beltechi R, Yarnold JA, Birks J, Kamran M. Early experience in the treatment of intra-cranial aneurysms by endovascular flow diversion: a multicentre prospective study. PLoS One. 2010;5(9):1–8.

220. Kulcsár Z, Ernemann U, Wetze SG, et al. High-profile flow diverter (silk) implantation in the basilar artery: efficacy in the treatment of aneurysms and the role of the perforators. Stroke. 2010;41:1690–6.

221. Lubicz B, Lefranc F, Levivier M, et al. Endovascular treatment of intracranial aneurysms with a branch arising from the sac. AJNR Am J Neuroradiol. 2006;27:142–7.

222. Kulcsár Z, Houdart E, Bonafe A, et al. Intra-aneurysmal thrombosis as a possible cause of delayed aneurysm rupture after flow-diversion treatment. AJNR Am J Neuroradiol. 2011;32:20–5.

223. Turowski B, Macht S, Kulcsar Z, Hanggi D, Stummer W. Early fatal hemorrhage after endovascular cerebral aneurysm treatment with a flow diverter (SILK-Stent): do we need to rethink our concepts? Neuroradiology. 2011;53:37–41.

224. Cebral JR, Mut F, Raschi M, et al. Aneurysm rupture following treatment with flow-diverting stents: computational hemodynamics analysis of treatment. AJNR Am J Neuroradiol. 2011;32:27–33.

225. van Rooij WJ, Sluzewski M. Perforator infarction after placement of a pipeline flow-diverting stent for an unruptured A1 aneurysm. AJNR Am J Neuroradiol. 2010;31:E43–4.

226. D'Urso PI, Lanzino G, Cloft HJ, Kallmes DF. Flow diversion for intracranial aneurysms: a review. Stroke. 2011;42:2363–8.

227. Li MH, Li YD, Gao BL, et al. A new covered stent designed for intracranial vasculature: application in the management of pseudoaneurysms of the cranial internal carotid artery. AJNR Am J Neuroradiol. 2007;28:1579–85.

228. Li MH, Li YD, Tan HQ, Luo QY, Cheng YS. Treatment of distal internal carotid artery aneurysm with the Willis covered stent: a prospective pilot study. Radiology. 2009;253:470–7.

229. Li MH, Zhu YQ, Fang C, et al. The feasibility and efficacy of treatment with a Willis covered stent in recurrent intracranial aneurysms after coiling. AJNR Am J Neuroradiol. 2008;29:1395–400.

230. Tan H-Q, Li M-H, Zhang P-L, et al. Reconstructive endovascular treatment of intracranial aneurysms with the Willis covered stent: medium-term clinical and angiographic follow-up. J Neurosurg. 2011;114:1014–20.

231. Pumar JM, Blanco M, Vazquez F, Castineira JA, Guimaraens L, Garcia-Allut A. Preliminary experience with Leo self-expanding stent for the treatment of intracranial aneurysms. AJNR Am J Neuroradiol. 2005;26:2573–7.

232. Pumar JM, Lete I, Pardo MI, Vazquez-Herrero F, Blanco M. LEO stent monotherapy for the endovascular reconstruction of fusiform aneurysms of the middle cerebral artery. AJNR Am J Neuroradiol. 2008;29:1775–6.

233. Solomon RA, Fink ME, Pile-Spellman J. Surgical management of unruptured intracranial aneurysms. J Neurosurg. 1994;80:440–6.

234. Malisch TW, Guglielmi G, Vinuela F. Unruptured aneurysms presenting with mass effect symptoms: response to endosaccular treatment with Guglielmi detachable coils. Part I. Symptoms of cranial nerve dysfunction. J Neurosurg. 1998;89:956–61.

235. Friedman JA, Piepgras DG, Pichelmann MA, Hansen KK, Brown Jr RD, Wiebers DO. Small cerebral aneurysms presenting with symptoms other than rupture. Neurology. 2001;57:1212–6.

236. Yanaka K, Matsumaru Y, Mashiko R, Hyodo A, Sugimoto K, Nose T. Small unruptured cerebral aneurysms presenting with oculomotor nerve palsy. Neurosurgery. 2003;52:553–7; discussion 6–7.

237. Rodriguez-Catarino M, Frisen L, Wikholm G, Elfverson J, Quiding L, Svendsen P. Internal carotid artery aneurysms, cranial nerve dysfunction and headache: the role of deformation and pulsation. Neuroradiology. 2003;45:236–40.

238. Halbach VV, Higashida RT, Dowd CF, et al. The efficacy of endosaccular aneurysm occlusion in alleviating neurological deficits produced by mass effect. J Neurosurg. 1994;80:659–66.

239. Kazekawa K, Tsutsumi M, Aikawa H, et al. Internal carotid aneurysms presenting with mass effect symptoms of cranial

nerve dysfunction: efficacy and imitations of endosaccular embolization with GDC. Radiat Med. 2003;21:80–5.

240. Chen PR, Amin-Hanjani S, Albuquerque FC, McDougall C, Zabramski JM, Spetzler RF. Outcome of oculomotor nerve palsy from posterior communicating artery aneurysms: comparison of clipping and coiling. Neurosurgery. 2006;58:1040–6; discussion 1040–6.

241. Feely M, Kapoor S. Third nerve palsy due to posterior communicating artery aneurysm: the importance of early surgery. J Neurol Neurosurg Psychiatry. 1987;50:1051–2.

242. Giombini S, Ferraresi S, Pluchino F. Reversal of oculomotor disorders after intracranial aneurysm surgery. Acta Neurochir (Wien). 1991;112:19–24.

243. Ahn JY, Han IB, Yoon PH, et al. Clipping vs. coiling of posterior communicating artery aneurysms with third nerve palsy. Neurology. 2006;66:121–3.

244. van der Schaaf IC, Brilstra EH, Buskens E, Rinkel GJE. Endovascular treatment of aneurysms in the cavernous sinus: a systematic review on balloon occlusion of the parent vessel and embolization with coils. Stroke. 2002;33:313–8.

245. Stiebel-Kalish H, Kalish Y, Bar-On RH. Presentation, natural history, and management of carotid cavernous aneurysms. Neurosurgery. 2005;57:850–7; discussion 850–7.

246. Field M, Jungreis CA, Chengelis N, Kromer H, Kirby L, Yonas H. Symptomatic cavernous sinus aneurysms: management and outcome after carotid occlusion and selective cerebral revascularization. AJNR Am J Neuroradiol. 2003;24:1200–7.

247. Bavinzski G, Killer M, Ferraz-Leite H, Gruber A, Gross CE, Richling B. Endovascular therapy of idiopathic cavernous aneurysms over 11 years. AJNR Am J Neuroradiol. 1998;19:559–65.

248. Gonzalez LF, Walker MT Zabramski JM, Partovi S, Wallace RC, Spetzler RF. Distinction between paraclinoid and cavernous sinus aneurysms with computed tomographic angiography. Neurosurgery. 2003;52:1131–7; discussion 8–9.

249. White JA, Horowitz ME, Samson D. Dural waisting as a sign of subarachnoid extension of cavernous carotid aneurysms: a follow-up case report. Surg Neurol. 1999;52:607–9; discussion 9–10.

250. van Rooij WJ, Sluzewski M, Beute GN. Ruptured cavernous sinus aneurysms causing carotid cavernous fistula: incidence, clinical presentation, treatment, and outcome. AJNR Am J Neuroradiol. 2006;27:185–9.

251. Kupersmith MJ, Hurst E, Berenstein A, Choi IS, Jafar J, Ransohoff J. The benign course of cavernous carotid artery aneurysms. J Neurosurg. 1992;77:690–3.

252. Lee AG, Mawad ME, Baskin DS. Fatal subarachnoid hemorrhage from the rupture of a totally intracavernous carotid artery aneurysm: case report. Neurosurgery. 1996;38:596–8; discussion 8–9.

253. Hamada H, Endo S, Fukuda O, Ohi M, Takaku A. Giant aneurysm in the cavernous sinus causing subarachnoid hemorrhage 13 years after detection: a case report. Surg Neurol. 1996;45:143–6.

254. Linskey ME, Sekhar LN, Hirsch Jr WL, Yonas H, Horton JA. Aneurysms of the intracavernous carotid artery: natural history and indications for treatment. Neurosurgery. 1990;26:933–7; discussion 7–8.

255. van der Schaaf I, Algra A, Wermer M, et al. Endovascular coiling versus neurosurgical clipping for patients with aneurysmal subarachnoid haemorrhage. Cochrane Database Syst Rev. 2005:CD003085.

256. De Jesus O, Sekhar LN, Riedel CJ. Clinoid and paraclinoid aneurysms: surgical anatomy, operative techniques, and outcome. Surg Neurol. 1999;51:477–88.

257. Tanaka Y, Hongo K, Tada T, et al. Radiometric analysis of paraclinoid carotid artery aneurysms. J Neurosurg. 2002;96:649–53.

258. Day AL. Aneurysms of the ophthalmic segment. A clinical and anatomical analysis. J Neurosurg. 1990;72:677–91.

259. Berson EL, Freeman MI, Gay AJ. Visual field defects in giant suprasellar aneurysms of internal carotid. Report of three cases. Arch Ophthalmol. 1966;76:52–8.

260. Lee JH, Tobias S, Kwon J-T, Sade B, Kosmorsky G. Wilbrand's knee: does it exist? Surg Neurol. 2006;66:11–7.

261. Yadla S, Campbell PG, Grobelny BBA, et al. Open and endovascular treatment of unruptured carotid-ophthalmic aneurysms:

clinical and radiographic outcomes. Neurosurgery. 2011;68: 1434–43.

262. Iihara K, Murao K, Sakai N, et al. Unruptured paraclinoid aneurysms: a management strategy. J Neurosurg. 2003;99:241–7.

263. Park HK, Horowitz M, Jungreis C. Endovascular treatment of paraclinoid aneurysms: experience with 73 patients. Neurosurgery. 2003;53:14–23; discussion 4.

264. Hoh BL, Carter BS, Budzik RF, Putman CM, Ogilvy CS. Results after surgical and endovascular treatment of paraclinoid aneurysms by a combined neurovascular team. Neurosurgery. 2001;48:78–89; discussion 89–90.

265. Boet R, Wong GK, Poon WS, Lam JM, Yu SC. Aneurysm recurrence after treatment of paraclinoid/ophthalmic segment aneurysms – a treatment-modality assessment. Acta Neurochir (Wien). 2005;147:611–6; discussion 6.

266. Kobayashi S, Kyoshima K, Gibo H, Hegde SA, Takemae T, Sugita K. Carotid cave aneurysms of the internal carotid artery. J Neurosurg. 1989;70:216–21.

267. Kim JM, Romano A, Sanan A, van Loveren HR, Keller JT. Microsurgical anatomic features and nomenclature of the paraclinoid region. Neurosurgery. 2000;46:670–80; discussion 80–2.

268. Sundt Jr TM, Whisnant JP. Subarachnoid hemorrhage from intracranial aneurysms. Surgical management and natural history of disease. N Engl J Med. 1978;299:116–22.

269. Leipzig TJ, Morgan J, Horner TG, Payner T, Redelman K, Johnson CS. Analysis of intraoperative rupture in the surgical treatment of 1694 saccular aneurysms. Neurosurgery. 2005;56:455–68; discussion 455–68.

270. Lawton MT, Du R. Effect of the neurosurgeon's surgical experience on outcomes from intraoperative aneurysmal rupture. Neurosurgery. 2005;57:9–15; discussion 9.

271. Piotin M, Mounayer C, Spelle L, Williams MT, Moret J. Endovascular treatment of anterior choroidal artery aneurysms. AJNR Am J Neuroradiol. 2004;25:314–8.

272. Friedman JA, Pichelmann MA, Piepgras DG, et al. Ischemic complications of surgery for anterior choroidal artery aneurysms. J Neurosurg. 2001;94:565–72.

273. Miyazawa N, Nukui H, Horikoshi T, Yagishita T, Sugita M, Kanemaru K. Surgical management of aneurysms of the bifurcation of the internal carotid artery. Clin Neurol Neurosurg. 2002;104:103–14.

274. Sakamoto S, Ohba S, Shibukawa M. Characteristics of aneurysms of the internal carotid artery bifurcation. Acta Neurochir (Wien). 2006;148:139–43; discussion 43.

275. Locksley HB. Natural history of subarachnoid hemorrhage, intracranial aneurysms and arteriovenous malformations. Based on 6368 cases in the cooperative study. J Neurosurg. 1966;25:219–39.

276. Yock Jr DH, Larson DA. Computed tomography of hemorrhage from anterior communicating artery aneurysms, with angiographic correlation. Radiology. 1980;134: 399–407.

277. Sayama T, Inamura T, Matsushima T, Inoha S, Inoue T, Fukui M. High incidence of hyponatremia in patients with ruptured anterior communicating artery aneurysms. Neurol Res. 2000;22:151–5.

278. DeLuca J. Cognitive dysfunction after aneurysm of the anterior communicating artery. J Clin Exp Neuropsychol. 1992;14:924–34.

279. Fontanella M, Perozzo P, Ursone R, Garbossa D, Bergui M. Neuropsychological assessment after microsurgical clipping or endovascular treatment for anterior communicating artery aneurysm. Acta Neurochir (Wien). 2003;145: 867–72; discussion 72.

280. Moret J, Pierot L, Boulin A, Castaings L, Rey A. Endovascular treatment of anterior communicating artery aneurysms using Guglielmi detachable coils. Neuroradiology. 1996;38:800–5.

281. Birknes JK, Hwang SK, Pandey AS. Feasibility and limitations of endovascular coil embolization of anterior communicating artery aneurysms: morphological considerations. Neurosurgery. 2006;59:43–52; discussion 43–52.

282. Steven DA, Ferguson GG. Distal anterior cerebral artery aneurysms. In: Winn HR, editor. Youmans neurological surgery. Philadelphia: Saunders; 2004. p. 1945–57.

283. Baptista AG. Studies on the arteries of the brain. Ii. The anterior cerebral artery: some anatomic features and their clinical implications. Neurology. 1963;13:825–35.

284. Huber P, Braun J, Hirschmann D, Agyeman JF. Incidence of berry aneurysms of the unpaired pericallosal artery: angiographic study. Neuroradiology. 1980;19:143–7.

285. Asari S, Nakamura S, Yamada O, Beck H, Sugatani H. Traumatic aneurysm of peripheral cerebral arteries. Report of two cases. J Neurosurg. 1977;46:795–803.

286. Fleischer AS, Patton JM, Tindall GT. Cerebral aneurysms of traumatic origin. Surg Neurol. 1975;4:233–9.

287. Inci S, Erbengi A, Ozgen T. Aneurysms of the distal anterior cerebral artery: report of 14 cases and a review of the literature. Surg Neurol. 1998;50:130–9; discussion 9–40.

288. Snyckers FD, Drake CG. Aneurysms of the distal anterior cerebral artery. A report on 24 verified cases. S Afr Med J. 1973;47:1787–91.

289. Hernesniemi J, Tapaninaho A, Vapalahti M, Niskanen M, Kari A, Luukkonen M. Saccular aneurysms of the distal anterior cerebral artery and its branches. Neurosurgery. 1992;31:994–8; discussion 8–9.

290. Pierot L, Boulin A, Castaings L, Rey A, Moret J. Endovascular treatment of pericallosal artery aneurysms. Neurol Res. 1996;18:49–53.

291. Sundt Jr TM, Kobayashi S, Fode NC, Whisnant JP. Results and complications of surgical management of 809 intracranial aneurysms in 722 cases. Related and unrelated to grade of patient, type of aneurysm, and timing of surgery. J Neurosurg. 1982;56:753–65.

292. Kassell NF, Torner JC, Haley Jr EC, Jane JA, Adams HP, Kongable GL. The International Cooperative Study on the timing of aneurysm surgery. Part 1: overall management results. J Neurosurg. 1990;73:18–36.

293. Rinne J, Hernesniemi J, Niskanen M, Vapalahti M. Analysis of 561 patients with 690 middle cerebral artery aneurysms: anatomic and clinical features as correlated to management outcome. Neurosurgery. 1996;38:2–11.

294. Stoodley MA, Macdonald RL, Weir BK. Surgical treatment of middle cerebral artery aneurysms. Neurosurg Clin N Am. 1998;9:823–34.

295. Friedman J, Piepgras D. Middle cerebral artery aneurysms. In: Winn HR, editor. Youmans neurological surgery. Philadelphia: Saunders; 2004. p. 1959–70.

296. Tanaka K, Hirayama K, Hattori H, et al. A case of cerebral aneurysm associated with complex partial seizures. Brain Dev. 1994;16:233–7.

297. Miele VJ, Bendok BR, Batjer HH. Unruptured aneurysm of the middle cerebral artery presenting with psychomotor seizures: case study and review of the literature. Epilepsy Behav. 2004;5:420–8.

298. Hänggi D, Winkler PA, Steiger H-J. Primary epileptogenic unruptured intracranial aneurysms: incidence and effect of treatment on epilepsy. Neurosurgery. 2010;66:1161–5.

299. Tokuda Y, Inagawa T, Katoh Y, Kumano K, Ohbayashi N, Yoshioka H. Intracerebral hematoma in patients with ruptured cerebral aneurysms. Surg Neurol. 1995;43:272–7.

300. Pritz MB, Chandler WF. The transsylvian approach to middle cerebral artery bifurcation/trifurcation aneurysms. Surg Neurol. 1994;41:217–9; discussion 9–20.

301. Ogilvy CS, Crowell RM, Heros RC. Surgical management of middle cerebral artery aneurysms: experience with transsylvian and superior temporal gyrus approaches. Surg Neurol. 1995;43:15–22; discussion 22–4.

302. Regli L, Uske A, de Tribolet N. Endovascular coil placement compared with surgical clipping for the treatment of unruptured middle cerebral artery aneurysms: a consecutive series. J Neurosurg. 1999;90:1025–30.

303. Doerfler A, Wanke I, Goericke SL, et al. Endovascular treatment of middle cerebral artery aneurysms with electrolytically detachable coils. AJNR Am J Neuroradiol. 2006;27:513–20.

304. Brinjikji W, Lanzino G, Cloft HJ, Rabinstein A, Kallmes DF. Endovascular treatment of middle cerebral artery aneurysms: a systematic review and single-center series. Neurosurgery. 2011;68:397–402.

305. Patankar T, Hughes D. Resolution of temporal lobe epilepsy and MRI abnormalities after coiling of a cerebral aneurysm. AJR Am J Roentgenol. 2005;185:1664–5.

306. Kuba R, Krupa P, Okacova L, Rektor I. Unruptured intracranial aneurysm as a cause of focal epilepsy: an excellent postoperative outcome after intra-arterial treatment. Epileptic Disord. 2004;6:41–4.

307. Lozier AP, Connolly Jr ES, Lavine SD, Solomon RA. Guglielmi detachable coil embolization of posterior circulation aneurysms: a systematic review of the literature. Stroke. 2002;33:2509–18.

308. Drake CG. The treatment of aneurysms of the posterior circulation. Clin Neurosurg. 1979;26:96–144.

309. Horikoshi T, Nukui H, Yagishita T, Nishigaya K, Fukasawa I, Sasaki H. Oculomotor nerve palsy after surgery for upper basilar artery aneurysms. Neurosurgery. 1999;44:705–10; discussion 10–1.

310. Al-Khayat H, Al-Khayat H, White J, Manner D, Samson D. Upper basilar artery aneurysms oculomotor outcomes in 163 cases. J Neurosurg. 2005;102:482–8.

311. Henkes H, Fischer S, Mariushi W, et al. Angiographic and clinical results in 316 coil-treated basilar artery bifurcation aneurysms. J Neurosurg. 2005;103:990–9.

312. Kwon OK, Kim SH, Kwon BJ, et al. Endovascular treatment of wide-necked aneurysms by using two microcatheters: techniques and outcomes in 25 patients. AJNR Am J Neuroradiol. 2005;26:894–900.

313. Benndorf G, Claus B, Strother CM, Chang L, Klucznik RP. Increased cell opening and prolapse of struts of a neuroform stent in curved vasculature: value of angiographic computed tomography: technical case report. Neurosurgery. 2006;58:ONS-E380; discussion ONS-E.

314. Josephson SA, Dillon WP, Dowd CF, Malek R, Lawton MT, Smith WS. Continuous bleeding from a basilar terminus aneurysm imaged with CT angiography and conventional angiography. Neurocrit Care. 2004;1:103–6.

315. Ferrante L, Acqui M, Trillo G, Lunardi P, Fortuna A. Aneurysms of the posterior cerebral artery: do they present specific characteristics? Acta Neurochir (Wien). 1996;138: 840–52.

316. Gerber CJ, Neil-Dwyer G. A review of the management of 15 cases of aneurysms of the posterior cerebral artery. Br J Neurosurg. 1992;6:521–7.

317. Sakata S, Fujii K, Matsushima T. Aneurysm of the posterior cerebral artery: report of eleven cases – surgical approaches and procedures. Neurosurgery. 1993;32:163–7; discussion 7–8.

318. Ciceri EF, Klucznik RP, Grossman RG, Rose JE, Mawad ME. Aneurysms of the posterior cerebral artery: classification and endovascular treatment. AJNR Am J Neuroradiol. 2001;22:27–34.

319. Hamada J, Morioka M, Yano S, Todaka T, Kai Y, Kuratsu J. Clinical features of aneurysms of the posterior cerebral artery: a 15-year experience with 21 cases. Neurosurgery. 2005;56:662–70; discussion 662–70.

320. Pia HW, Fontana H. Aneurysms of the posterior cerebral artery. Locations and clinical pictures. Acta Neurochir (Wien). 1977;38:13–35.

321. Honda M, Tsutsumi K, Yokoyama H, Yonekura M, Nagata I. Aneurysms of the posterior cerebral artery: retrospective review of surgical treatment. Neurol Med Chir (Tokyo). 2004;44:164–8; discussion 9.

322. Seoane ER, Tedeschi H, de Oliveira E, Siqueira MG, Calderon GA, Rhoton Jr AL. Management strategies for posterior cerebral artery aneurysms: a proposed new surgical classification. Acta Neurochir (Wien). 1997;139:325–31.

323. Chang SW, Abla AA, Kakarla UK, et al. Treatment of distal posterior cerebral artery aneurysms: a critical appraisal of the occipital artery-to-posterior cerebral artery bypass. Neurosurgery. 2010;67:16–26.

324. Hallacq P, Piotin M, Moret J. Endovascular occlusion of the posterior cerebral artery for the treatment of P2 segment aneurysms: retrospective review of a 10-year series. AJNR Am J Neuroradiol. 2002;23:1128–36.

325. Haw C, Willinsky R, Agid R, TerBrugge K. The endovascular management of superior cerebellar artery aneurysms. Can J Neurol Sci. 2004;31:53–7.

326. Gacs G, Vinuela F, Fox AJ, Drake CG. Peripheral aneurysms of the cerebellar arteries. Review of 16 cases. J Neurosurg. 1983;58:63–8.

327. Papo I, Caruselli G, Salvolini U. Aneurysm of the superior cerebellar artery. Surg Neurol. 1977;7:15–7.

328. Collins TE, Mehalic TF, White TK, Pezzuti RT. Trochlear nerve palsy as the sole initial sign of an aneurysm of the superior cerebellar artery. Neurosurgery. 1992;30:258–61.

329. Proust F, Callonec F, Bellow F, Laquerriere A, Hannequin D, Freger P. Tentorial edge traumatic aneurysm of the superior cerebellar artery. Case report. J Neurosurg. 1997;87: 950–4.

330. Danet M, Raymond J, Roy D. Distal superior cerebellar artery aneurysm presenting with cerebellar infarction: report of two cases. AJNR Am J Neuroradiol. 2001;22: 717–20.

331. Chaloupka JC, Putman CM, Awad IA. Endovascular therapeutic approach to peripheral aneurysms of the superior cerebellar artery. AJNR Am J Neuroradiol. 1996;17:1338–42.

332. Eckard DA, O'Boynick PL, McPherson CM, et al. Coil occlusion of the parent artery for treatment of symptomatic peripheral intracranial aneurysms. AJNR Am J Neuroradiol. 2000;21:137–42.

333. Drake CG, Peerless SJ, Hernesniemi JA. Surgery of vertebrobasilar aneurysms: London, Ontario, experience on 1767 patients. Vienna: Springer; 1996.

334. Peerless SJ, Drake CG. Posterior circulation aneurysms. In: Wilkins RH, Rengachary SS, editors. Neurosurgery. New York: McGraw-Hill; 1996. p. 2341–56.

335. Mizoi K, Yoshimoto T, Takahashi A, Ogawa A. Direct clipping of basilar trunk aneurysms using temporary balloon occlusion. J Neurosurg. 1994;80:230–6.

336. Peerless SJ, Hernesniemi JA, Gutman FB, Drake CG. Early surgery for ruptured vertebrobasilar aneurysms. J Neurosurg. 1994;80:643–9.

337. Seifert V. Direct surgery of basilar trunk and vertebrobasilar junction aneurysms via the combined transpetrosal approach. Neurol Med Chir (Tokyo). 1998;38(Suppl):86–92.

338. Van Rooij WJ, Sluzewski M, Menovsky T, Wijnalda D. Coiling of saccular basilar trunk aneurysms. Neuroradiology. 2003;45:19–21.

339. Uda K, Murayama Y, Gobin YP, Duckwiler GR, Vinuela F. Endovascular treatment of basilar artery trunk aneurysms with Guglielmi detachable coils: clinical experience with 41 aneurysms in 39 patients. J Neurosurg. 2001;95:624–32.

340. Steinberg GK, Drake CG, Peerless SJ. Deliberate basilar or vertebral artery occlusion in the treatment of intracranial aneurysms. Immediate results and long-term outcome in 201 patients. J Neurosurg. 1993;79:161–73.

341. Wenderoth JD, Khangure MS, Phatouros CC, ApSimon HT. Basilar trunk occlusion during endovascular treatment of giant and fusiform aneurysms of the basilar artery. AJNR Am J Neuroradiol. 2003;24:1226–9.

342. Gonzalez LF, Alexander MJ, McDougall CG, Spetzler RF. Anteroinferior cerebellar artery aneurysms: surgical approaches and outcomes – a review of 34 cases. Neurosurgery. 2004;55:1025–35.

343. Akyuz M, Tuncer R. Multiple anterior inferior cerebellar artery aneurysms associated with an arteriovenous malformation: case report. Surg Neurol. 2005;64 Suppl 2:S106–8.

344. Spallone A, De Santis S, Giuffre R. Peripheral aneurysms of the anterior inferior cerebellar artery. Case report and review of literature. Br J Neurosurg. 1995;9:537–41.

345. Suzuki K, Meguro K, Wada M, Fujita K, Nose T. Embolization of a ruptured aneurysm of the distal anterior inferior cerebellar artery: case report and review of the literature. Surg Neurol. 1999;51:509–12.

346. Yoon SM, Chun YI, Kwon Y, Kwun BD. Vertebrobasilar junction aneurysms associated with fenestration: experience of five cases treated with Guglielmi detachable coils. Surg Neurol. 2004;61:248–54.

347. Rabinov JD, Hellinger FR, Morris PP, Ogilvy CS, Putman CM. Endovascular management of vertebrobasilar dissecting aneurysms. AJNR Am J Neuroradiol. 2003;24:1421–8.

348. Hudgins RJ, Day AL, Quisling RG, Rhoton Jr AL, Sypert GW, Garcia-Bengochea F. Aneurysms of the posterior inferior cerebellar artery. A clinical and anatomical analysis. J Neurosurg. 1983;58:381–7.

349. Yamaura A, Watanabe Y, Saeki N. Dissecting aneurysms of the intracranial vertebral artery. J Neurosurg. 1990;72:183–8.

350. Kallmes DF, Lanzino G, Dix JE, et al. Patterns of hemorrhage with ruptured posterior inferior cerebellar artery aneurysms: CT findings in 44 cases. AJR Am J Roentgenol. 1997;169:1169–71.

351. Yamaura A. Diagnosis and treatment of vertebral aneurysms. J Neurosurg. 1988;69:345–9.

352. Lemole Jr GM, Henn J, Javedan S, Deshmukh V, Spetzler RF. Cerebral revascularization performed using posterior inferior cerebellar artery-posterior inferior cerebellar artery bypass. Report of four cases and literature review. J Neurosurg. 2002;97:219–23.

353. Mericle RA, Reig AS, Burry MV, Eskioglu E, Firment CS, Santra S. Endovascular surgery for proximal posterior inferior cerebellar artery aneurysms: an analysis of Glasgow Outcome Score by Hunt-Hess Grades Neurosurgery. 2006;58:619–25; discussion 619–25.

354. Lewis SB, Chang DJ, Peace DA, Lafrentz PJ, Day AL. Distal posterior inferior cerebellar artery aneurysms: clinical features and management. J Neurosurg. 2002;97: 756–66.

355. Horiuchi T, Tanaka Y, Hongo K, Nitta J, Kusano Y, Kobayashi S. Characteristics of distal posteroinferior cerebellar artery aneurysms. Neurosurgery. 2003;53:589–95; discussion 95–6.

356. Orakcioglu B, Schuknecht B, Otani N, Khan N, Imhof HG, Yonekawa Y. Distal posterior inferior cerebellar artery aneurysms: clinical characteristics and surgical management. Acta Neurochir (Wien). 2005;147:1131–9.

357. Dernbach PD, Sila CA, Little JR. Giant and multiple aneurysms of the distal posterior inferior cerebellar artery. Neurosurgery. 1988;22:309–12.

358. Heros RC. Posterior inferior cerebellar artery. J Neurosurg. 2002;97:747–8; discussion 8.

359. Werner S, Blakemore A, King B. Aneurysm of the internal carotid artery within the skull: wiring and electrothermic coagulation. JAMA. 1941;116:578–82.

360. Mullan S, Raimondi AJ, Dobben G, Vailati G, Hekmatpanah J. Electrically induced thrombosis in intracranial aneurysms. J Neurosurg. 1965;22:539–47.

361. Gallagher JP. Obliteration of intracranial aneurysms by pilojection. JAMA. 1963;183:231–6.

362. Alksne JF, Fingerhut AG. Magnetically controlled metallic thrombosis of intracranial aneurysms. A preliminary report. Bull Los Angeles Neurol Soc. 1965;30:153–5.

363. Luessenhop AJ, Velasquez AC. Observations on the tolerance of the intracranial arteries to catheterization. J Neurosurg. 1964;21:85–91.

364. Teitelbaum GP, Larsen DW, Zelman V, Lysachev AG, Likhterman LB. A tribute to Dr. Fedor A. Serbinenko, founder of endovascular neurosurgery. Neurosurgery. 2000;46:462–9; discussion 9–70.

365. Serbinenko FA. Balloon catheterization and occlusion of major cerebral vessels. J Neurosurg. 1974;41:125–45.

366. Debrun G, Lacour P, Caron JP, Hurth M, Comoy J, Keravel Y. Detachable balloon and calibrated-leak balloon techniques in the treatment of cerebral vascular lesions. J Neurosurg. 1978;49:635–49.

367. Hieshima GB, Grinnell VS, Mehringer CM. A detachable balloon for therapeutic transcatheter occlusions. Radiology. 1981;138:227–8.

368. Kwan ES, Heilman CB, Shucart WA, Klucznik RP. Enlargement of basilar artery aneurysms following balloon occlusion – "water-hammer effect". Report of two cases. J Neurosurg. 1991;75:963–8.

369. Gianturco C, Anderson JH, Wallace S. Mechanical devices for arterial occlusion. Am J Roentgenol Radium Ther Nucl Med. 1975;124:428–35.

370. Higashida RT, Halbach VV, Dowd CF, Barnwell SL, Hieshima GB. Interventional neurovascular treatment of a giant intracranial aneurysm using platinum microcoils. Surg Neurol. 1991;35:64–8.

371. Hilal SK, Solomon RA. Endovascular treatment of aneurysms with coils. J Neurosurg. 1992;76:337–9.

372. Moret J, Cognard C, Weill A, Castaings L, Rey A. Reconstruction technic in the treatment of wide-neck intracranial aneurysms. Long-term angiographic and clinical results. Apropos of 56 cases. J Neuroradiol. 1997;24: 30–44.

373. Qureshi AI, Vazquez G, Tariq N, Suri MFK, Lakshminarayan K, Lanzino G. Impact of international subarachnoid aneurysm trial results on treatment of ruptured intracranial aneurysms in the United States. J Neurosurg. 2011;114:834–41.

374. Adams Jr HP, Gordon DL. Nonaneurysmal subarachnoid hemorrhage. Ann Neurol. 1991;29:461–2.

375. Stranjalis G, Korfias S, Vemmos KN, Sakas DE. Spontaneous subarachnoid haemorrhage in the era of transition from surgery to embolization. A study of the overall outcome. Br J Neurosurg. 2005;19:389–94.

376. Flaherty ML, Haverbusch M, Kissela B, et al. Perimesencephalic subarachnoid hemorrhage: incidence, risk factors, and outcome. J Stroke Cerebrovasc Dis. 2005;14:267–71.

377. Schwartz TH, Mayer SA. Quadrigeminal variant of perimesencephalic nonaneurysmal subarachnoid hemorrhage. Neurosurgery. 2000;46:584–8.

378. van der Schaaf IC, Velthuis BK, Gouw A, Rinkel GJ. Venous drainage in perimesencephalic hemorrhage. Stroke. 2004;35:1614–8.

379. Call GK, Fleming MC, Sealfon S, Levine H, Kistler JP, Fisher CM. Reversible cerebral segmental vasoconstriction. Stroke. 1988;19:1159–70.

380. Edlow BL, Kasner SE, Hurst RW, Weigele JB, Levine JM. Reversible cerebral vasoconstriction syndrome associated with subarachnoid hemorrhage. Neurocrit Care. 2007;7:203–10.

381. Ducros A, Fiedler U, Porcher R, Boukobza M, Stapf C, Bousser MG. Hemorrhagic manifestations of reversible cerebral vasoconstriction syndrome: frequency, features, and risk factors. Stroke. 2010;41:2505–11.

382. Ducros A. Reversible cerebral vasoconstriction syndrome. Presse Med. 2010;39:312–22.

383. Chen SP, Fuh JL, Lirng JF, Chang FC, Wang SJ. Recurrent primary thunderclap headache and benign CNS angiopathy: spectra of the same disorder? Neurology. 2006;67:2164–9.

384. Hajj-Ali RA, Furlan A, Abou-Chebel A, Calabrese LH. Benign angiopathy of the central nervous system: cohort of 16 patients with clinical course and long-term followup. Arthritis Rheum. 2002;47:662–9.

385. Rinkel GJ, van Gijn J, Wijdicks EF. Subarachnoid hemorrhage without detectable aneurysm. A review of the causes. Stroke. 1993;24:1403–9.

386. Linn FHH, Rinkel GJE, Algra A, van Gijn J. Incidence of subarachnoid hemorrhage: role of region, year, and rate of computed tomography: a meta-analysis. Stroke. 1996;27:625–9.

387. Menghini VV, Brown Jr RD, Sicks JD, O'Fallon WM, Wiebers DO. Incidence and prevalence of intracranial aneurysms and hemorrhage in Olmsted county, Minnesota, 1965 to 1995. Neurology. 1998;51:405–11.

388. Labovitz DL, Halim AX, Brent B, Boden-Albala B, Hauser WA, Sacco RL. Subarachnoid hemorrhage incidence among whites, blacks and Caribbean Hispanics: the northern Manhattan study. Neuroepidemiology. 2006;26:147–50.

389. Mayberg MR, Batjer HH, Dacey R. Guidelines for the management of aneurysmal subarachnoid hemorrhage. A statement for healthcare professionals from a special writing group of the Stroke Council, American Heart Association. Stroke. 1994;25:2315–28.

390. Dupont SA, Lanzino G, Wijdicks EFM, Rabinstein AA. The use of clinical and routine imaging data to differentiate between aneurysmal and nonaneurysmal subarachnoid hemorrhage prior to angiography. J Neurosurg. 2010;113:790–4.

391. van Gijn J, Rinkel GJE. Subarachnoid haemorrhage: diagnosis, causes and management. Brain. 2001;124:249–78.

392. Polmear A. Sentinel headaches in aneurysmal subarachnoid haemorrhage: what is the true incidence? A systematic review. Cephalalgia. 2003;23:935–41.

393. Frizzell RT, Kuhn F, Morris R, Quinn C, Fisher 3rd WS. Screening for ocular hemorrhages in patients with ruptured cerebral aneurysms: a prospective study of 99 patients. Neurosurgery. 1997;41:529–33; discussion 33–4.

394. Pfausler B, Belcl R, Metzler R, Mohsenipour I, Schmutzhard E. Terson's syndrome in spontaneous subarachnoid hemorrhage: a prospective study in 60 consecutive patients. J Neurosurg. 1996;85:392–4.

395. McCarron MO, Alberts MJ, McCarron P. A systematic review of Terson's syndrome: frequency and prognosis after subarachnoid haemorrhage. J Neurol Neurosurg Psychiatry. 2004;75:491–3.

396. Tsementzis SA, Williams A. Ophthalmological signs and prognosis in patients with a subarachnoid haemorrhage. Neurochirurgia (Stuttg). 1984;27:133–5.

397. Pinto AN, Canhao P, Ferro JM. Seizures at the onset of subarachnoid haemorrhage. J Neurol. 1996;243:161–4.

398. Edlow JA, Wyer PC. Evidence-based emergency medicine/ clinical question. How good is a negative cranial computed tomographic scan result in excluding subarachnoid hemorrhage? Ann Emerg Med. 2000;36:507–16.

399. Bambakidis N, Selman W. Subarachnoid hemorrhage. In: Suarez JI, editor. Critical care neurology and neurosurgery. Totowa: Humana Press; 2004. p. 365–77.

400. Vermeulen M, van Gijn J. The diagnosis of subarachnoid haemorrhage. J Neurol Neurosurg Psychiatry. 1990;53: 365–72.

401. Heasley DC, Mohamed MA, Yousem DM. Clearing of red blood cells in lumbar puncture does not rule out ruptured aneurysm in patients with suspected subarachnoid hemorrhage but negative head CT findings. AJNR Am J Neuroradiol. 2005;26:820–4.

402. Villablanca JP, Jahan R, Hooshi P, et al. Detection and characterization of very small cerebral aneurysms by using 2D and 3D helical CT angiography. AJNR Am J Neuroradiol. 2002;23:1187–98.

403. Jayaraman MV, Mayo-Smith WW, Tung GA, et al. Detection of intracranial aneurysms: multi-detector row CT angiography compared with DSA. Radiology. 2004;230:510–8.

404. Rogg JM, Smeaton S, Doberstein C, Goldstein JH, Tung GA, Haas RA. Assessment of the value of MR imaging for examining patients with angiographically negative subarachnoid hemorrhage. AJR Am J Roentgenol. 1999;172:201–6.

405. Maslehaty H, Petridis AK, Barth H, Mehdorn HM. Diagnostic value of magnetic resonance imaging in perimesencephalic and nonperimesencephalic subarachnoid hemorrhage of unknown origin. J Neurosurg. 2011;114:1003–7.

406. Suarez JI, Tarr RW, Selman WR. Aneurysmal subarachnoid hemorrhage. N Engl J Med. 2006;354:387–96.

407. Johnston SC, Selvin S, Gress DR. The burden, trends, and demographics of mortality from subarachnoid hemorrhage. Neurology. 1998;50:1413–8.

408. Qureshi AI, Suri MF, Nasar A. Trends in hospitalization and mortality for subarachnoid hemorrhage and unruptured aneurysms in the United States. Neurosurgery. 2005;57: 1–8; discussion 1–8.

409. Fischer T, Johnsen SP, Pedersen L, Gaist D, Sorensen HT, Rothman KJ. Seasonal variation in hospitalization and case fatality of subarachnoid hemorrhage – a nationwide Danish study on 9,367 patients. Neuroepidemiology. 2005;24:32–7.

410. Stegmayr B, Eriksson M, Asplund K. Declining mortality from subarachnoid hemorrhage: changes in incidence and case fatality from 1985 through 2000. Stroke. 2004;35:2059–63.

411. Biotti D, Jacquin A, Boutarbouch M, et al. Trends in case-fatality rates in hospitalized nontraumatic subarachnoid hemorrhage: results of a population-based study in Dijon, France, from 1985 to 2006. Neurosurgery. 2010;66:1039–43.

412. Juvela S, Porras M, Heiskanen O. Natural history of unruptured intracranial aneurysms: a long-term follow-up study. J Neurosurg. 1993;79:174–82.

413. Tsutsumi K, Ueki K, Morita A, Kirino T. Risk of rupture from incidental cerebral aneurysms. J Neurosurg. 2000; 93:550–3.

414. Broderick JP, Brott TG, Duldner JE, Tomsick T, Leach A. Initial and recurrent bleeding are the major causes of death following subarachnoid hemorrhage. Stroke. 1994;25:1342–7.

415. Schievink WI, Wijdicks EF, Piepgras DG, Chu CP, O'Fallon WM, Whisnant JP. The poor prognosis of ruptured intracranial aneurysms of the posterior circulation. J Neurosurg. 1995;82:791–5.

416. Hop JW, Rinkel GJ, Algra A. van Gijn J. Case-fatality rates and functional outcome after subarachnoid hemorrhage: a systematic review. Stroke. 1997;28:660–4.

417. Kassell NF, Torner JC. Aneurysmal rebleeding: a preliminary report from the Cooperative Aneurysm Study. Neurosurgery. 1983;13:479–81.

418. Inagawa T, Kamiya K, Ogasawara H, Yano T. Rebleeding of ruptured intracranial aneurysms in the acute stage. Surg Neurol. 1987;28:93–9.

419. Fujii Y, Takeuchi S, Sasaki O, Minakawa T, Koike T, Tanaka R. Ultra-early rebleeding in spontaneous subarachnoid hemorrhage. J Neurosurg. 1996;84:35–42.

420. Brilstra EH, Rinkel GJ, Algra A, van Gijn J. Rebleeding, secondary ischemia, and timing of operation in patients with subarachnoid hemorrhage. Neurology. 2000;55:1656–60.

421. Steiger HJ, Fritschi J, Seiler RW. Current pattern of inhospital aneurysmal rebleeds. Analysis of a series treated with individually timed surgery and intravenous nimodipine. Acta Neurochir (Wien). 1994;127:21–6.

422a. Khurana VG, Piepgras DG, Whisnant JP. Ruptured giant intracranial aneurysms. Part I. A study of rebleeding. J Neurosurg. 1998;88:425–9.

422b. Jane JA, Kassell NF, Torner JC, Winn HR. The natural history of aneurysms and arteriovenous malformations. J Neurosurg 1985;62:321–3.

423. Naidech AM, Janjua N, Kreiter KT, et al. Predictors and impact of aneurysm rebleeding after subarachnoid hemorrhage. Arch Neurol. 2005;62:410–6.

424. Hijdra A, Vermeulen M, van Gijn J, van Crevel H. Rerupture of intracranial aneurysms: a clinicoanatomic study. J Neurosurg. 1987;67:29–33.

425. Juvela S. Rebleeding from ruptured intracranial aneurysms. Surg Neurol. 1989;32:323–6.

426. Dunn CJ, Goa KL. Tranexamic acid: a review of its use in surgery and other indications. Drugs. 1999;57:1005–32.

427. Fodstad H, Liliequist B. Schannong M, Thulin CA. Tranexamic acid in the preoperative management of ruptured intracranial aneurysms. Surg Neurol. 1978;10:9–15.

428. Kassell NF, Torner JC, Adams Jr HP. Antifibrinolytic therapy in the acute period following aneurysmal subarachnoid hemorrhage. Preliminary observations from the Cooperative Aneurysm Study. J Neurosurg. 1984;61:225–30.

429. Mullan S. Dawley J. Antifibrinolytic therapy for intracranial aneurysms. J Neurosurg. 1968;28:21–3.

430. Vermeulen M, Lindsay KW, Murray GD, et al. Antifibrinolytic treatment in subarachnoid hemorrhage. N Engl J Med. 1984;311:432–7.

431. Vermeulen M, van Gijn J, Hijdra A, van Crevel H. Causes of acute deterioration in patients with a ruptured intracranial aneurysm. A prospective study with serial CT scanning. J Neurosurg. 1984;60:935.

432. Burchiel KJ, Hoffman JM, Bakay RA. Quantitative determination of plasma fibrinolytic activity in patients with ruptured intracranial aneurysms who are receiving epsilon-aminocaproic acid: relationship of possible complications of therapy to the degree of fibrinolytic inhibition. Neurosurgery. 1984;14:57–63.

433. Fodstad H, Pilbrant A, Schannong M, Stromberg S. Determination of tranexamic acid (AMCA) and fibrin/fibrinogen degradation products in cerebrospinal fluid after aneurysmal subarachnoid haemorrhage. Acta Neurochir (Wien). 1981;58:1–13.

434. Starke RM, Kim GH, Fernandez A, et al. Impact of a protocol for acute antifibrinolytic therapy on aneurysm rebleeding after subarachnoid hemorrhage. Stroke. 2008;39:2617–21.

435. Harrigan MR, Rajneesh KF, Ardelt AA, Fisher 3rd WS. Short-term antifibrinolytic therapy before early aneurysm treatment in subarachnoid hemorrhage: effects on rehemorrhage, cerebral ischemia, and hydrocephalus. Neurosurgery. 2010;67:935–9; discussion 9–40.

436. Hui FK, Schuette AJ, Lieber M, et al. Epsilon aminocaproic acid in angiographically negative subarachnoid hemorrhage patients is safe: a retrospective review of 83 consecutive patients. Neurosurgery. 2012;70(3):702–5.

437. Leipzig TJ, Redelman K, Horner TG. Reducing the risk of rebleeding before early aneurysm surgery: a possible role for antifibrinolytic therapy. J Neurosurg. 1997;86:220–5.

438. Hillman J, Fridriksson S, Nilsson O, Yu Z, Saveland H, Jakobsson KE. Immediate administration of tranexamic acid and reduced incidence of early rebleeding after aneurysmal subarachnoid hemorrhage: a prospective randomized study. J Neurosurg. 2002;97:771–8.

439. Vale FL, Bradley EL, Fisher 3rd WS. The relationship of subarachnoid hemorrhage and the need for postoperative shunting. J Neurosurg. 1997;86:462–6.

440. Haley Jr EC, Kassell NF, Torner JC. The International Cooperative Study on the timing of aneurysm surgery. The North American experience. Stroke. 1992;23:205–14.

441. Ohman J, Heiskanen O. Timing of operation for ruptured supratentorial aneurysms: a prospective randomized study. J Neurosurg. 1989;70:55–60.

442. Chyatte D, Fode NC, Sundt Jr TM. Early versus late intracranial aneurysm surgery in subarachnoid hemorrhage. J Neurosurg. 1988;69:326–31.

443. Phillips TJ, Dowling RJ, Yan B, Laidlaw JD, Mitchell PJ. Does treatment of ruptured intracranial aneurysms within 24 hours improve clinical outcome? Stroke. 2011;42: 1936–45.

444. van Gijn J, Hijdra A, Wijdicks EF, Vermeulen M, van Crevel H. Acute hydrocephalus after aneurysmal subarachnoid hemorrhage. J Neurosurg. 1985;63:355–62.

445. Hasan D, Tanghe HL. Distribution of cisternal blood in patients with acute hydrocephalus after subarachnoid hemorrhage. Ann Neurol. 1992;31:374–8.

446. Suarez-Rivera O. Acute hydrocephalus after subarachnoid hemorrhage. Surg Neurol. 1998;49:563–5.

447. Dehdashti AR, Rilliet B, Rufenacht DA, de Tribolet N. Shunt-dependent hydrocephalus after rupture of intracranial aneurysms: a prospective study of the influence of treatment modality. J Neurosurg. 2004;101:402–7.

448. Hasan D, Vermeulen M, Wijdicks EF, Hijdra A, van Gijn J. Management problems in acute hydrocephalus after subarachnoid hemorrhage. Stroke. 1989;20:747–53.

449. Graff-Radford NR, Torner J, Adams Jr HP, Kassell NF. Factors associated with hydrocephalus after subarachnoid hemorrhage. A report of the Cooperative Aneurysm Study. Arch Neurol. 1989;46:744–52.

450. Pare L, Delfino R, Leblanc R. The relationship of ventricular drainage to aneurysmal rebleeding. J Neurosurg. 1992; 76:422–7.

451. Voldby B, Enevoldsen EM. Intracranial pressure changes following aneurysm rupture. Part 3: recurrent hemorrhage. J Neurosurg. 1982;56:784–9.

452. Klopfenstein JD, Kim LJ, Feiz-Erfan I, et al. Comparison of rapid and gradual weaning from external ventricular drainage in patients with aneurysmal subarachnoid hemorrhage: a prospective randomized trial. J Neurosurg. 2004;100:225–9.

453. O'Kelly CJ, Kulkarni AV, Austin PC, Urbach D, Wallace MC. Shunt-dependent hydrocephalus after aneurysmal subarachnoid hemorrhage: incidence, predictors, and revision rates. Clinical article. J Neurosurg. 2009;111:1029–35.

454. Komotar RJ, Hahn DK, Kim GH, et al. Efficacy of lamina terminalis fenestration in reducing shunt-dependent hydrocephalus following aneurysmal subarachnoid hemorrhage: a systematic review. Clinical article. J Neurosurg. 2009; 111:147–54.

455. Hasan D, Schonck RS, Avezaat CJ, Tanghe HL, van Gijn J, van der Lugt PJ. Epileptic seizures after subarachnoid hemorrhage. Ann Neurol. 1993;33:286–91.

456. Baker CJ, Prestigiacomo CJ, Solomon RA. Short-term perioperative anticonvulsant prophylaxis for the surgical treatment of low-risk patients with intracranial aneurysms. Neurosurgery. 1995;37:863–70; discussion 70–1.

457. Rhoney DH, Tipps LB, Murry KR, Basham MC, Michael DB, Coplin WM. Anticonvulsant prophylaxis and timing of seizures after aneurysmal subarachnoid hemorrhage. Neurology. 2000;55:258–65.

458. Naidech AM, Kreiter KT, Janjua N, et al. Phenytoin exposure is associated with functional and cognitive disability after subarachnoid hemorrhage. Stroke. 2005;36:583–7.

459. Sbeih I, Tamas LB, O'Laoire SA. Epilepsy after operation for aneurysms. Neurosurgery. 1986;19:784–8.

460. Claassen J, Peery S, Kreiter KT, et al. Predictors and clinical impact of epilepsy after subarachnoid hemorrhage. Neurology. 2003;60:208–14.

461. Lin CL, Dumont AS, Lieu AS, et al. Characterization of perioperative seizures and epilepsy following aneurysmal subarachnoid hemorrhage. J Neurosurg. 2003;99:978–85.

462. Solenski NJ, Haley Jr EC, Kassell NF. Medical complications of aneurysmal subarachnoid hemorrhage: a report of the multicenter, cooperative aneurysm study. Participants of the multicenter cooperative aneurysm study. Crit Care Med. 1995;23:1007–17.

463. Wartenberg KE, Mayer SA. Medical complications after subarachnoid hemorrhage: new strategies for prevention and management. Curr Opin Crit Care. 2006;12:78–84.

464. Sarrafzadeh A, Schlenk F, Meisel A, Dreier J, Vajkoczy P, Meisel C. Immunodepression after aneurysmal subarachnoid hemorrhage. Stroke. 2011;42:53–8.

465. Dorhout Mees SM, van Dijk GW, Algra A, Kempink DRJ, Rinkel GJE. Glucose levels and outcome after subarachnoid hemorrhage. Neurology. 2003;61:1132–3.

466. Wartenberg KE, Schmidt JM, Claassen J. Impact of medical complications on outcome after subarachnoid hemorrhage. Crit Care Med. 2006;34:617–23; quiz 24.

467. Frontera JA, Fernandez A, Claassen J, et al. Hyperglycemia after SAH: predictors, associated complications, and impact on outcome. Stroke. 2006;37:199–203.

468. Woo E, Ma JT, Robinson JD, Yu YL. Hyperglycemia is a stress response in acute stroke. Stroke. 1988;19:1359–64.

469. Capes SE, Hunt D, Malmberg K, Pathak P, Gerstein HC. Stress hyperglycemia and prognosis of stroke in nondiabetic and diabetic patients: a systematic overview. Stroke. 2001;32:2426–32.

470. Allport LE, Butcher KS, Baird TA, et al. Insular cortical ischemia is independently associated with acute stress hyperglycemia. Stroke. 2004;35:1886–91.

471. Parsons MW, Barber PA, Desmond PM, et al. Acute hyperglycemia adversely affects stroke outcome: a magnetic resonance imaging and spectroscopy study. Ann Neurol. 2002;52:20–8.

472. Baird TA, Parsons MW, Phanh T, et al. Persistent poststroke hyperglycemia is independently associated with infarct expansion and worse clinical outcome. Stroke. 2003; 34:2208–14.

473. Ste-Marie L, Hazell AS, Bemeur C, Butterworth R, Montgomery J. Immunohistochemical detection of inducible nitric oxide synthase, nitrotyrosine and manganese superoxide dismutase following hyperglycemic focal cerebral ischemia. Brain Res. 2001;918:10–9.

474. Kawai N, Keep RF, Betz AL, Dietrich WD. Hyperglycemia and the vascular effects of cerebral ischemia. Stroke. 1997;28:149–54.

475. Van den Berghe G, Wouters P, Weekers F, et al. Intensive insulin therapy in critically ill patients. N Engl J Med. 2001;345:1359–67.

476. Hasan D, Wijdicks EF, Vermeulen M. Hyponatremia is associated with cerebral ischemia in patients with aneurysmal subarachnoid hemorrhage. Ann Neurol. 1990;27: 106–8.

477. Kurokawa Y, Uede T, Ishiguro M. Pathogenesis of hyponatremia following subarachnoid hemorrhage due to ruptured cerebral aneurysm. Surg Neurol. 1996;46:500–7; discussion 7–8.

478. Qureshi AI, Suri MF, Sung GY. Prognostic significance of hypernatremia and hyponatremia among patients with aneurysmal subarachnoid hemorrhage. Neurosurgery. 2002;50:749–55; discussion 55–6.

479. Sherlock M, O'Sullivan E, Agha A, et al. The incidence and pathophysiology of hyponatraemia after subarachnoid haemorrhage. Clin Endocrinol (Oxf). 2006;64:250–4.

480. Morinaga K, Hayashi S, Matsumoto Y, et al. Hyponatremia and cerebral vasospasm in patients with aneurysmal subarachnoid hemorrhage. No To Shinkei. 1992;44:629–32.

481. Moro N, Katayama Y, Kojima J, Mori T, Kawamata T. Prophylactic management of excessive natriuresis with hydrocortisone for efficient hypervolemic therapy after subarachnoid hemorrhage. Stroke. 2003;34:2807–11.

482. Nelson RJ, Roberts J, Rubin C, Walker V, Ackery DM, Pickard JD. Association of hypovolemia after subarachnoid hemorrhage with computed tomographic scan evidence of raised intracranial pressure. Neurosurgery. 1991;29:178–82.

483. Wijdicks EF, Vandongen KJ, Vangijn J, Hijdra A, Vermeulen M. Enlargement of the third ventricle and hyponatraemia in aneurysmal subarachnoid haemorrhage. J Neurol Neurosurg Psychiatry. 1988;51:516–20.

484. Harrigan MR. Cerebral salt wasting syndrome. Crit Care Clin. 2001;17:125–38.

485. Wijdicks EF, Vermeulen M, ten Haaf JA, Hijdra A, Bakker WH, van Gijn J. Volume depletion and natriuresis in patients with a ruptured intracranial aneurysm. Ann Neurol. 1985; 18:211–6.

486. McGirt MJ, Blessing R, Nimjee SM. Correlation of serum brain natriuretic peptide with hyponatremia and delayed ischemic neurological deficits after subarachnoid hemorrhage. Neurosurgery. 2004;54:1369–73; discussion 73–4.

487. Berendes E, Walter M, Cullen P, et al. Secretion of brain natriuretic peptide in patients with aneurysmal subarachnoid haemorrhage. Lancet. 1997;349:245–9.

---

488. Tomida M, Muraki M, Uemura K, Yamasaki K. Plasma concentrations of brain natriuretic peptide in patients with subarachnoid hemorrhage. Stroke. 1998;29:1584–7.

489. Tung PP, Olmsted E, Kopelnik A, et al. Plasma B-type natriuretic peptide levels are associated with early cardiac dysfunction after subarachnoid hemorrhage. Stroke. 2005; 36:1567–9.

490. Sviri GE, Feinsod M, Soustiel JF. Brain natriuretic peptide and cerebral vasospasm in subarachnoid hemorrhage: clinical and TCD correlations. Stroke. 2000;31:118–22.

491. Takahashi K, Totsune K, Sone M, et al. Human brain natriuretic peptide-like immunoreactivity in human brain. Peptides. 1992;13:121–3.

492. Takaku A, Shindo K, Tanaka S, Mori T, Suzuki J. Fluid and electrolyte disturbances in patients with intracranial aneurysms. Surg Neurol. 1979;11:349–56.

493. van den Bergh WM, Algra A, Rinkel GJE. Electrocardiographic abnormalities and serum magnesium in patients with subarachnoid hemorrhage. Stroke. 2004;35:644–8.

494. Andreoli A, di Pasquale G, Pinel i G, Grazi P, Tognetti F, Testa C. Subarachnoid hemorrhage: frequency and severity of cardiac arrhythmias. A survey of 70 cases studied in the acute phase. Stroke. 1987;18:558–64.

495. Fukui S, Otani N, Katoh H, et al. Female gender as a risk factor for hypokalemia and QT prolongation after subarachnoid hemorrhage. Neurology. 2002;59:134–6.

496. Fukui S, Katoh H, Tsuzuki N, et al. Multivariate analysis of risk factors for QT prolongation following subarachnoid hemorrhage. Crit Care. 2003;7:R7–R12.

497. Machado C, Baga JJ, Kawasaki R, Reinoehl J, Steinman RT, Lehmann MH. Torsade de pointes as a complication of subarachnoid hemorrhage: a critical reappraisal. J Electrocardiol. 1997;30:31–7.

498. van den Bergh WM, Algra A. van der Sprenkel JW, Tulleken CA, Rinkel GJ. Hypomagnesemia after aneurysmal subarachnoid hemorrhage. Neurosurgery. 2003;52: 276–81; discussion 81–2.

499. Collignon FP, Friedman JA, Piepgras DG, et al. Serum magnesium levels as related to symptomatic vasospasm and outcome following aneurysmal subarachnoid hemorrhage. Neurocrit Care. 2004;1:441–8.

500. Brouwers PJ, Wijdicks EF, Hasan D, et al. Serial electrocardiographic recording in aneurysmal subarachnoid hemorrhage. Stroke. 1989;20:1162–7.

501. Marion DW, Segal R, Thompson ME. Subarachnoid hemorrhage and the heart. Neurosurgery. 1986;18:101–6.

502. Manninen PH, Ayra B, Gelb AW, Pelz D. Association between electrocardiographic abnormalities and intracranial blood in patients following acute subarachnoid hemorrhage. J Neurosurg Anesthesiol. 1995;7:12–6.

503. Kuroiwa T, Morita H, Tanabe H, Ohta T. Significance of ST segment elevation in electrocardiograms in patients with ruptured cerebral aneurysms. Acta Neurochir (Wien). 1995;133:141–6.

504. Mayer SA, Lin J, Homma S, et al. Myocardial injury and left ventricular performance after subarachnoid hemorrhage. Stroke. 1999;30:780–6.

505. Svigelj V, Grad A, Tekavcic I, Kiauta T. Cardiac arrhythmia associated with reversible damage to insula in a patients with subarachnoid hemorrhage. Stroke. 1994;25:1053–5.

506. Fink JN, Selim MH, Kumar S, Voetsch B. Fong WC, Caplan LR. Insular cortex infarction in acute middle cerebral artery territory stroke: predictor of stroke severity and vascular lesion. Arch Neurol. 2005;62:1081–5.

507. Lanzino G, Kongable GL, Kassell NF. Electrocardiographic abnormalities after nontraumatic subarachnoid hemorrhage. J Neurosurg Anesthesiol. 1994;6 156–62.

508. Kono T, Morita H, Kuroiwa T, Onaka H, Takatsuka H, Fujiwara A. Left ventricular wall motion abnormalities in patients with subarachnoid hemorrhage: neurogenic stunned myocardium. J Am Coll Cardiol 1994;24: 636–40.

509. Tung P, Kopelnik A, Banki N, et al. Predictors of neurocardiogenic injury after subarachnoid hemorrhage. Stroke. 2004;35:548–51.

510. Sato N, Masuda T, Izumi T. Subarachnoid hemorrhage and myocardial damage clinical and experimental studies. Jpn Heart J. 1999;40:683–701.

511. Naredi S, Lambert G, Eden E, et al. Increased sympathetic nervous activity in patients with nontraumatic subarachnoid hemorrhage. Stroke. 2000;3 :901–6.

512. Banki NM, Kopelnik A, Dae MW, et al. Acute neurocardiogenic injury after subarachnoid hemorrhage. Circulation. 2005;112:3314–9.

513. Yuki K, Kodama Y, Onda J, Enoto K, Morimoto T, Uozumi T. Coronary vasospasm following subarachnoid hemorrhage as a cause of stunned myocardium. Case report. J Neurosurg. 1991;75:308–11.

514. Naidech AM, Kreiter KT, Janjua N, et al. Cardiac troponin elevation, cardiovascular morbidity, and outcome after subarachnoid hemorrhage. Circulation. 2005;112:2851–6.

515. Schuiling WJ, Dennesen PJW Tans JTJ, Kingma LM, Algra A, Rinkel GJE. Troponin I in predicting cardiac or pulmonary complications and outcome in subarachnoid haemorrhage. J Neurol Neurosurg Psychiatry. 2005;76:1565–9.

516. Parr MJA, Finfer SR, Morgan MK. Lesson of the week: reversible cardiogenic shock complicating subarachnoid haemorrhage. BMJ. 1996;3 3:681–3.

517. Jain R, Deveikis J, Thompson BG. Management of patients with stunned myocardium associated with subarachnoid hemorrhage. AJNR Am J Neuroradiol. 2004;25:126–9.

518. Naval NS, Stevens RD, Mirski MA, Bhardwaj A. Controversies in the management of aneurysmal subarachnoid hemorrhage. Crit Care Med. 2006;34:511–24.

519. Levy ML, Rabb CH, Zelman V, Giannotta SL. Cardiac performance enhancement from dobutamine in patients refractory to hypervolemic therapy for cerebral vasospasm. J Neurosurg. 1993;79:494–9.

520. Apostolides PJ, Greene KA. Zabramski JM, Fitzgerald JW, Spetzler RF. Intra-aortic baloon pump counterpulsation in the management of concomitant cerebral vasospasm and cardiac failure after subarachnoid hemorrhage: technical case report. Neurosurgery. 1996; 8:1056–9; discussion 9–60.

521. Friedman JA, Pichelmann MA, Piepgras DG. Pulmonary complications of aneurysmal subarachnoid hemorrhage. Neurosurgery. 2003;52:1025–31; discussion 31–2.

522. Kahn JM, Caldwell EC, Deem S, Newell DW, Heckbert SR, Rubenfeld GD. Acute lung njury in patients with subarachnoid hemorrhage: incidence, risk factors, and outcome. Crit Care Med. 2006;34:196–202.

523. Smith WS, Matthay MA. Evidence for a hydrostatic mechanism in human neurogenic pulmonary edema. Chest. 1997;111:1326–33.

524. Kopelnik A, Fisher L, Miss JC, et al. Prevalence and implications of diastolic dysfunction after subarachnoid hemorrhage. Neurocrit Care. 2005;3:132–8.

525. Macmillan CS, Grant IS, Andrews PJ. Pulmonary and cardiac sequelae of subarachnoid haemorrhage: time for active management? Intensive Care Med. 2002;28:1012–23.

526. Knudsen F, Jensen HP, Petersen PL. Neurogenic pulmonary edema: treatment with dobutamine. Neurosurgery. 1991;29: 269–70.

527. Vorkapic P, Bevan JA, Bevan RD. Longitudinal in vivo and in vitro time-course study of chronic cerebrovasospasm in the rabbit basilar artery. Neurosurg Rev. 1991;14:215–9.

528. Findley JM. Cerebral vasospasm. In: Winn HR, editor. Youmans neurological surgery. Philadelphia: Saunders; 2004. p. 1839–67.

529. Kassell NF, Sasaki T, Colohan AR, Nazar G. Cerebral vasospasm following aneurysmal subarachnoid hemorrhage. Stroke. 1985;16:562–72.

530. Dorsch NW, King MT. A review of cerebral vasospasm in aneurysmal subarachnoid hemorrhage: incidence and effects. J Clin Neurosci. 1994;1:19–26.

531. Murayama S, Malisch T, Guglielmi G, et al. Incidence of cerebral vasospasm after endovascular treatment of acutely ruptured aneurysms: report on 69 cases. J Neurosurg. 1997;87:830–5.

532. Charpentier C, Audibert G, Guillemin F, et al. Multivariate analysis of predictors of cerebral vasospasm occurrence after aneurysmal subarachnoid hemorrhage. Stroke. 1999; 30:1402–8.

533. Macdonald RL. Management of cerebral vasospasm. Neurosurg Rev. 2006;29(3+:179–93.

534. Findlay JM, Kassell NF, Weir BK. A randomized trial of intraoperative, intracisternal tissue plasminogen activator

for the prevention of vasospasm. Neurosurgery. 1995;37: 168–76; discussion 77–8.

535. Haley Jr EC, Kassell NF, Appersor-Hansen C, Maile MH, Alves WM. A randomized, double-blind, vehicle-controlled trial of tirilazad mesylate in patients with aneurysmal subarachnoid hemorrhage: a cooperative study in North America. J Neurosurg. 1997;86:467–74.

536. Kassell NF, Haley Jr EC, Apperson-Hansen C, Alves WM. Randomized, double-blind, vehicle-controlled trial of tirilazad mesylate in patients with aneurysmal subarachnoid hemorrhage: a cooperative study in Europe, Australia, and New Zealand. J Neurosurg. 1996;84:221–8.

537. Fisher CM, Roberson GH, Ojemann RG. Cerebral vasospasm with ruptured saccular aneurysm – the clinical manifestations. Neurosurgery. 1977;1:245–8.

538. Weir B, Grace M, Hansen J, Rothberg C. Time course of vasospasm in man. J Neurosurg. 1978;48:173–8.

539. Yamaguchi M, Bun T, Kuwahara T, Kitamura S. Very lateonset symptomatic cerebral vasospasm caused by a large residual aneurysmal subarachnoid hematoma – case report. Neurol Med Chir (Tokyo). 1999;39:677–80.

540. Kistler JP, Crowell RM, Davis KR, et al. The relation of cerebral vasospasm to the extent and ocation of subarachnoid blood visualized by CT scan: a prospective study. Neurology. 1983;33:424–36.

541. Hijdra A, van Gijn J, Nagelkerke NJ, Vermeulen M, van Crevel H. Prediction of delayed cerebral ischemia, rebleeding, and outcome after aneurysmal subarachnoid hemorrhage. Stroke. 1988;19:1250–6.

542. Claassen J, Bernardini GL, Kreiter K, et al. Effect of cisternal and ventricular blood on risk of delayed cerebral ischemia after subarachnoid hemorrhage: the fisher scale revisited. Stroke. 2001;32:2012–20.

543. Conway JE, Tamargo RJ. Cocaine use is an independent risk factor for cerebral vasospasm after aneurysmal subarachnoid hemorrhage. Stroke. 2001:32:2338–43.

544. Ryttlefors M, Enblad P, Ronne-Engstrom E, Persson L, Ilodigwe D, Macdonald RL. Patient age and vasospasm after subarachnoid hemorrhage. Neurosurgery. 2010;67:911–7.

545. Hoh BL, Topcuoglu MA, Singhal AB. Effect of clipping, craniotomy, or intravascular coiling on cerebral vasospasm and patient outcome after aneurysmal subarachnoid hemorrhage. Neurosurgery. 2004;55:779–86; discussion 86–9.

546. Rabinstein AA, Pichelmann MA, Friedman JA, et al. Symptomatic vasospasm and outcomes following aneurysmal subarachnoid hemorrhage: a comparison between surgical repair and endovascular coil occlusion. J Neurosurg. 2003;98:319–25.

547. Schweickert WD, Gehlbach BK, Pohlmar AS, Hall JB, Kress JP. Daily interruption of sedative infusions and complications of critical illness in mechanically ventilated patients. Crit Care Med. 2004;32:1272–6.

548. Handa Y, Hayashi M, Takeuchi H, Kubota T, Kobayashi H, Kawano H. Time course of the impairment of cerebral autoregulation during chronic cerebral vasospasm after subarachnoid hemorrhage in primates. J Neurosurg. 1992;76:493–501.

549. Yoon DY, Choi CS, Kim KH, Cho BM. Multidetector-row CT angiography of cerebral vasospasm after aneurysmal subarachnoid hemorrhage: comparison of volume-rendered images and digital subtraction angiography. AJNR Am J Neuroradiol. 2006;27:370–7.

550. Harrigan MR, Leonardo J, Gibbens KJ, Guterman LR, Hopkins LN. CT perfusion cerebral blood flow imaging in neurological critical care. Neurocrit Care. 2005;2:352–66.

551. Wintermark M, Ko NU, Smith WS, Liu S, Higashida RT, Dillon WP. Vasospasm after subarachnoid hemorrhage: utility of perfusion CT and CT angiography on diagnosis and management. AJNR Am J Neuroradiol. 2006;27:26–34.

552. Clyde BL, Resnick DK, Yonas H, Smith HA, Kaufmann AM. The relationship of blood velocity as measured by transcranial Doppler ultrasonography to cerebral blood flow as determined by stable xenon computed tomographic studies after aneurysmal subarachnoid hemorrhage. Neurosurgery. 1996;38:896–904; discussion 904–5.

553. Lysakowski C, Walder B, Costanza MC, Tramer MR. Transcranial Doppler versus angiography in patients with vasospasm due to a ruptured cerebral aneurysm: a systematic review. Stroke. 2001;32:2292–8.

554. Aaslid R, Huber P, Nornes H. Evaluation of cerebrovascular spasm with transcranial Doppler ultrasound. J Neurosurg. 1984;60:37–41.

555. Burch CM, Wozniak MA, Sloan MA, et al. Detection of intracranial internal carotid artery and middle cerebral artery vasospasm following subarachnoid hemorrhage. J Neuroimaging. 1996;6:8–15.

556. Kyoi K, Hashimoto H, Tokunaga H, et al. Time course of blood velocity changes and clinical symptoms related to cerebral vasospasm and prognosis after aneurysmal surgery. No Shinkei Geka. 1989;17:21–30.

557. Wozniak MA, Sloan MA, Rothman MI. Detection of vasospasm by transcranial Doppler sonography. The challenges of the anterior and posterior cerebral arteries. J Neuroimaging. 1996;6:87–93.

558. Sloan MA, Burch CM, Wozniak MA, et al. Transcranial Doppler detection of vertebrobasilar vasospasm following subarachnoid hemorrhage. Stroke. 1994;25:2187–97.

559. Lindegaard KF, Nornes H, Bakke SJ, Sorteberg W, Nakstad P. Cerebral vasospasm after subarachnoid haemorrhage investigated by means of transcranial Doppler ultrasound. Acta Neurochir Suppl (Wien). 1988;42:81–4.

560. Soustiel JF, Shik V, Shreiber R, Tavor Y, Goldsher D, Muizelaar JP. Basilar vasospasm diagnosis: investigation of a modified "Lindegaard Index" based on imaging studies and blood velocity measurements of the basilar artery * editorial comment: investigation of a modified "Lindegaard Index" based on imaging studies and blood velocity measurements of the basilar artery. Stroke. 2002;33:72–8.

561. Allen GS, Ahn HS, Preziosi TJ, et al. Cerebral arterial spasm – a controlled trial of nimodipine in patients with subarachnoid hemorrhage. N Engl J Med. 1983;308: 619–24.

562. Barker 2nd FG, Ogilvy CS. Efficacy of prophylactic nimodipine for delayed ischemic deficit after subarachnoid hemorrhage: a metaanalysis. J Neurosurg. 1996;84:405–14.

563. Mee E, Dorrance D, Lowe D, Neil-Dwyer G. Controlled study of nimodipine in aneurysm patients treated early after subarachnoid hemorrhage. Neurosurgery. 1988;22:484–91.

564. Ohman J, Heiskanen O. Effect of nimodipine on the outcome of patients after aneurysmal subarachnoid hemorrhage and surgery. J Neurosurg. 1988;69:683–6.

565. Petruk KC, West M, Mohr G. Nimodipine treatment in poorgrade aneurysm patients. Results of a multicenter doubleblind placebo-controlled trial. J Neurosurg. 1988;68: 505–17.

566. Philippon J, Grob R, Dagreou F, Guggiari M, Rivierez M, Viars P. Prevention of vasospasm in subarachnoid haemorrhage. A controlled study with nimodipine. Acta Neurochir (Wien). 1986;82:110–4.

567. Pickard JD, Murray GD, Illingworth R, et al. Effect of oral nimodipine on cerebral infarction and outcome after subarachnoid haemorrhage: British aneurysm nimodipine trial. BMJ. 1989;298:636–42.

568. Rinkel GJ, Feigin VL, Algra A, van den Bergh WM, Vermeulen M, van Gijn J. Calcium antagonists for aneurysmal subarachnoid haemorrhage. Cochrane Database Syst Rev. 2005:CD000277.

569. Wong MC, Haley Jr EC. Calcium antagonists: stroke therapy coming of age. Stroke. 1990;21:494–501.

570. Toyota BD. The efficacy of an abbreviated course of nimodipine in patients with good-grade aneurysmal subarachnoid hemorrhage. J Neurosurg. 1999;90:203–6.

571. Parra A, Kreiter KT, Williams S. Effect of prior statin use on functional outcome and delayed vasospasm after acute aneurysmal subarachnoid hemorrhage: a matched controlled cohort study. Neurosurgery. 2005;56:476–84; discussion 476–84.

572. Lynch JR, Wang H, McGirt MJ, et al. Simvastatin reduces vasospasm after aneurysmal subarachnoid hemorrhage: results of a pilot randomized clinical trial. Stroke. 2005; 35:2024–6.

573. Tseng MY, Czosnyka M, Richards H, Pickard JD, Kirkpatrick PJ. Effects of acute treatment with pravastatin on cerebral vasospasm, autoregulation, and delayed ischemic deficits after aneurysmal subarachnoid hemorrhage: a phase II randomized placebo-controlled trial. Stroke. 2005;36:1627–32.

574. Tseng MY, Hutchinson PJ, Czosnyka M, Richards H, Pickard JD, Kirkpatrick PJ. Effects of acute pravastatin treatment on intensity of rescue therapy, length of inpatient stay, and 6-month outcome in patients after aneurysmal subarachnoid hemorrhage. Stroke. 2007;38:1545–50.

575. Tseng MY, Hutchinson PJ, Turner CL, et al. Biological effects of acute pravastatin treatment in patients after aneurysmal subarachnoid hemorrhage: a double-blind, placebo-controlled trial. J Neurosurg. 2007;107:1092–100.

576. Pfeffer MA, Keech A, Sacks FM, et al. Safety and tolerability of pravastatin in long-term clinical trials: prospective pravastatin pooling (PPP) project. Circulation. 2002;105:2341–6.

577. Hunninghake DB, Knopp RH, Schonfeld G, et al. Efficacy and safety of pravastatin in patients with hypercholesterolemia. Atherosclerosis. 1990;85:81–9.

578. McGirt MJ, Pradilla G, Legnani FG. Systemic administration of simvastatin after the onset of experimenta. subarachnoid hemorrhage attenuates cerebral vasospasm. Neurosurgery. 2006;58:945–51; discussion 945–51.

579. Sterzer P, Meintzschel F, Rosler A, Lanfermann H, Steinmetz H, Sitzer M. Pravastatin improves cerebral vasomotor reactivity in patients with subcortical small-vessel disease. Stroke. 2001;32:2817–20.

580. Macdonald RL, Kassell NF, Mayer S, et al. Clazosentan to overcome neurological ischemia and infarction occurring after subarachnoid hemorrhage (CONSCIOUS-1): randomized, double-blind, placebo-controlled phase 2 dose-finding trial. Stroke. 2008;39:3015–21.

581. Macdonald RL, Higashida RT, Keller E, et al. Clazosentan, an endothelin receptor antagonist, in patients with aneurysmal subarachnoid haemorrhage undergoing surgical clipping: a randomised, double-blind, placebo-controlled phase 3 trial (CONSCIOUS-2). Lancet Neurol. 2011;10:618–25.

582. Roux S. CONSCIOUS-3 Clazosentan in aneurysmal subarachnoid hemorrhage. 2011. http://www.strokecenter.org/trials/TrialDetail.aspx?tid=1013. Accessed 12 Aug 2011.

583. Klimo Jr P, Kestle JR, MacDonald JD, Schmidt RH. Marked reduction of cerebral vasospasm with lumbar drainage of cerebrospinal fluid after subarachnoid hemorrhage. J Neurosurg. 2004;100:215–24.

584. Kwon OY, Kim YJ, Cho CS, Lee SK, Cho MK. The utility and benefits of external lumbar CSF drainage after endovascular coiling on aneurysmal subarachnoid hemorrhage. J Korean Neurosurg Soc. 2008;43:281–7.

585. Staykov D, Speck V, Volbers B, et al. Early recognition of lumbar overdrainage by lumboventricular pressure gradient. Neurosurgery. 2011;68:1187–91.

586. Marinov MB, Harbaugh KS, Hoopes FJ, Pikus HJ, Harbaugh RE. Neuroprotective effects of preischemia intraarterial magnesium sulfate in reversible focal cerebral ischemia. J Neurosurg. 1996;85:117–24.

587. van den Bergh WM, Zuur JK, Kamerling NA, et al. Role of magnesium in the reduction of ischemic depolarization and lesion volume after experimental subarachnoid hemorrhage. J Neurosurg. 2002;97:416–22.

588. Ram Z, Sadeh M, Shacked I, Sahar A, Hadani M. Magnesium sulfate reverses experimental delayed cerebral vasospasm after subarachnoid hemorrhage in rats. Stroke. 1991;22:922–7.

589. Fawcett WJ, Haxby EJ, Male DA. Magnesium: physiology and pharmacology. Br J Anaesth. 1999;83:302–20.

590. Johnson JW, Ascher P. Voltage-dependent block by intracellular Mg2+ of N-methyl-D-aspartate-activated channels. Biophys J. 1990;57:1085–90.

591. Rothman S. Synaptic release of excitatory amino acid neurotransmitter mediates anoxic neuronal death. J Neurosci. 1984;4:1884–91.

592. Euser AG, Cipolla MJ. Resistance artery vasodilation to magnesium sulfate during pregnancy and the postpartum state. Am J Physiol Heart Circ Physiol. 2005:288:H1521–5.

593. van den Bergh WM, on behalf of the MSG. Magnesium sulfate in aneurysmal subarachnoid hemorrhage: a randomized controlled trial. Stroke. 2005;36:1011–5.

594. Wong GK, Poon WS, Chan MT, et al. Intravenous magnesium sulphate for aneurysmal subarachnoid hemorrhage (IMASH): a randomized, double-blinded, placebo-controlled, multicenter phase III trial. Stroke. 2010;41:921–6.

595. Wong GKCF, Poon WSFF, Chan MTVF, et al. Plasma magnesium concentrations and clinical outcomes in aneurysmal subarachnoid hemorrhage patients: post hoc analysis of intravenous magnesium sulphate for aneurysmal subarachnoid hemorrhage trial. Stroke. 2010;41:1841–4.

596. Dorhout Mees SM, van den Bergh WM, Algra A, Rinkel GJ. Achieved serum magnesium concentrations and occurrence of delayed cerebral ischaemia and poor outcome in aneurysmal subarachnoid haemorrhage. J Neurol Neurosurg Psychiatry. 2007;78:729–31.

597. Origitano TC, Wascher TM, Reichman OH, Anderson DE. Sustained increased cerebral blood flow with prophylactic hypertensive hypervolemic hemodilution ("triple-H" therapy) after subarachnoid hemorrhage. Neurosurgery. 1990; 27:729–39; discussion 39–40.

598. Treggiari MM, Walder B, Suter PM, Romand JA. Systematic review of the prevention of delayed ischemic neurological deficits with hypertension, hypervolemia, and hemodilution therapy following subarachnoid hemorrhage. J Neurosurg. 2003;98:978–84.

599. Lennihan L, Mayer SA, Fink ME, et al. Effect of hypervolemic therapy on cerebral blood flow after subarachnoid hemorrhage: a randomized controlled trial. Stroke. 2000; 31:383–91.

600. Feigin VL, Rinkel GJ, Algra A, van Gijn J. Circulatory volume expansion for aneurysmal subarachnoid hemorrhage. Cochrane Database Syst Rev. 2000:CD000483.

601. Rinkel GJ, Feigin VL, Algra A, van Gijn J. Circulatory volume expansion therapy for aneurysmal subarachnoid haemorrhage. Cochrane Database Syst Rev. 2004:CD000483.

602. Egge A, Waterloo K, Sjoholm H, Solberg T, Ingebrigtsen T, Romner B. Prophylactic hyperdynamic postoperative fluid therapy after aneurysmal subarachnoid hemorrhage: a clinical, prospective, randomized, controlled study. Neurosurgery. 2001;49:593–605; discussion 605–6.

603. Raabe A, Beck J, Berkefeld J, et al. Recommendations for the management of patients with aneurysmal subarachnoid hemorrhage. Zentralbl Neurochir. 2005;66:79–91.

604. Ramakrishna R, Sekhar LN, Ramanathan D, et al. Intraventricular tissue plasminogen activator for the prevention of vasospasm and hydrocephalus after aneurysmal subarachnoid hemorrhage. Neurosurgery. 2010;67:110–7.

605. Muehlschlegel SM, Rordorf G, Sims J. Effects of a single dose of dantrolene in patients with cerebral vasospasm after subarachnoid hemorrhage: a prospective pilot study. Stroke. 2011;42:1301–6.

606. Al-Rawi PGB, Tseng M-YP, Richards HKP, et al. Hypertonic saline in patients with poor-grade subarachnoid hemorrhage improves cerebral blood flow, brain tissue oxygen, and pH. Stroke. 2010;41:122–8.

607. Kassell NF, Peerless SJ, Durward QJ, Beck DW, Drake CG, Adams HP. Treatment of ischemic deficits from vasospasm with intravascular volume expansion and induced arterial hypertension. Neurosurgery. 1982;11:337–43.

608. Hoh BL, Carter BS, Ogilvy CS. Risk of hemorrhage from unsecured, unruptured aneurysms during and after hypertensive hypervolemic therapy. Neurosurgery. 2002;50: 1207–11; discussion 11–2.

609. Shimoda M, Oda S, Tsugane R, Sato O. Intracranial complications of hypervolemic therapy in patients with a delayed ischemic deficit attributed to vasospasm. J Neurosurg. 1993;78:423–9.

610. Raabe A, Beck J, Keller M, Vatter H, Zimmermann M, Seifert V. Relative importance of hypertension compared with hypervolemia for increasing cerebral oxygenation in patients with cerebral vasospasm after subarachnoid hemorrhage. J Neurosurg. 2005;103:974–81.

611. Harrigan MR. Hypertension may be the most important component of hyperdynamic therapy in cerebral vasospasm. Crit Care. 2010;14:151.

612. Dankbaar JW, Slooter AJ, Rinkel GJ, Schaaf IC. Effect of different components of triple-H therapy on cerebral perfusion in patients with aneurysmal subarachnoid haemorrhage: a systematic review. Crit Care. 2010;14:R23.

613. Giannotta SL, McGillicuddy JE, Kindt GW. Diagnosis and treatment of postoperative cerebral vasospasm. Surg Neurol. 1977;8:286–90.

614. Awad IA, Carter LP, Spetzler RF, Medina M, Williams Jr FC. Clinical vasospasm after subarachnoid hemorrhage: response to hypervolemic hemodilution and arterial hypertension. Stroke. 1987;18:365–72.

615. Kosnik EJ, Hunt WE. Postoperative hypertension in the management of patients with intracranial arterial aneurysms. J Neurosurg. 1976;45:148–54.

616. Rosenwasser RH, Delgado TE, Buchheit WA, Freed MH. Control of hypertension and prophylaxis against vasospasm in cases of subarachnoid hemorrhage: a preliminary report. Neurosurgery. 1983;12:658–61.

617. Corsten L, Raja A, Guppy K. Contemporary management of subarachnoid hemorrhage and vasospasm: the UIC experience. Surg Neurol. 2001;56:140–8; discussion 8–50.

618. Joseph M, Ziadi S, Nates J, Dannenbaum M, Malkoff M. Increases in cardiac output can reverse flow deficits from vasospasm independent of blood pressure: a study using xenon computed tomographic measurement of cerebral blood flow. Neurosurgery. 2003;53:1044–51; discussion 12–3.

619. Mayer SA, Solomon RA, Fink ME. Effect of 5% albumin solution on sodium balance and blood volume after subarachnoid hemorrhage. Neurosurgery. 1998;42:759–67; discussion 67–8.

620. Ekelund A, Reinstrup P, Ryding E. Effects of iso- and hypervolemic hemodilution on regional cerebral blood flow and oxygen delivery for patients with vasospasm after aneurysmal subarachnoid hemorrhage. Acta Neurochir (Wien). 2002;144:703–12; discussion 12–3.

621. Asplund K, Israelsson K, Schampi I. Haemodilution for acute ischaemic stroke. Cochrane Database Syst Rev. 2000:CD000103.

622. Allport LE, Parsons MW, Butcher KS, et al. Elevated hematocrit is associated with reduced reperfusion and tissue survival in acute stroke. Neurology. 2005;65:1382–7.

623. Macdonald RL. Cerebral vasospasm. Neurosurg Q. 1995;5:73–97.

624. Amin-Hanjani S, Schwartz RB, Sathi S, Stieg PE. Hypertensive encephalopathy as a complication of hyperdynamic therapy for vasospasm: report of two cases. Neurosurgery. 1999;44:1113–6.

625. Rosenwasser RH, Jallo JI, Getch CC, Liebman KE. Complications of Swan-Ganz catheterization for hemodynamic monitoring in patients with subarachnoid hemorrhage. Neurosurgery. 1995;37:872–5; discussion 5–6.

626. American Society of Interventional and Therapeutic Neuroradiology. Mechanical and pharmocologic treatment of vasospasm. AJNR Am J Neuroradiol. 2001;22: 26S–7.

627. Zubkov AY, Lewis AI, Scalzo D, Bernanke DH, Harkey HL. Morphological changes after percutaneous transluminal angioplasty. Surg Neurol. 1999;51:399–403.

628. Eskridge JM, Newell DW, Winn HR. Endovascular treatment of vasospasm. Neurosurg Clin N Am. 1994;5:437–47.

629. Coyne TJ, Montanera WJ, Macdonald RL, Wallace MC. Percutaneous transluminal angioplasty for cerebral vasospasm after subarachnoid hemorrhage. Can J Surg. 1994;37: 391–6.

630. Bejjani GK, Bank WO, Olan WJ, Sekhar LN. The efficacy and safety of angioplasty for cerebral vasospasm after subarachnoid hemorrhage. Neurosurgery. 1998;42:979–86; discussion 86–7.

631. Fujii Y, Takahashi A, Yoshimoto T. Effect of balloon angioplasty on high grade symptomatic vasospasm after subarachnoid hemorrhage. Neurosurg Rev. 1995;18:7–13.

632. Rosenwasser RH, Armonda RA, Thomas JE, Benitez RP, Gannon PM, Harrop J. Therapeutic modalities for the management of cerebral vasospasm: timing of endovascular options. Neurosurgery. 1999;44:975–9; discussion 9–80.

633. Higashida RT, Halbach VV, Cahan LD, et al. Transluminal angioplasty for treatment of intracranial arterial vasospasm. J Neurosurg. 1989;71:648–53.

634. Murayama Y, Song JK, Uda K, et al. Combined endovascular treatment for both intracranial aneurysm and symptomatic vasospasm. AJNR Am J Neuroradiol. 2003;24:133–9.

635. Le Roux PD, Newell DW, Eskridge J, Mayberg MR, Winn HR. Severe symptomatic vasospasm: the role of immediate postoperative angioplasty. J Neurosurg. 1994;80:224–9.

636. Jabbour P, Veznedaroglu E, Liebman K, Rosenwasser RH. Is radiographic ischemia a contraindication for angioplasty in subarachnoid hemorrhage? In: AANS annual meeting. San Francisco: American Association of Neurological Surgeons; 2006.

637. Muizelaar JP, Zwienenberg M, Rudisill NA, Hecht ST. The prophylactic use of transluminal balloon angioplasty in patients with fisher grade 3 subarachnoid hemorrhage: a pilot study. J Neurosurg. 1999;91:51–8.

638. Badjatia N, Topcuoglu MA, Pryor JC, et al. Preliminary experience with intra-arterial nicardipine as a treatment for cerebral vasospasm. AJNR Am J Neuroradiol. 2004;25:819–26.

639. Biondi A, Ricciardi GK, Puybasset L, et al. Intra-arterial nimodipine for the treatment of symptomatic cerebral vasospasm after aneurysmal subarachnoid hemorrhage: preliminary results. AJNR Am J Neuroradiol. 2004;25:1067–76.

640. Feng L, Fitzsimmons B-F, Young WL, et al. Intraarterially administered verapamil as adjunct therapy for cerebral vasospasm: safety and 2-year experience. AJNR Am J Neuroradiol. 2002;23:1284–90.

641. Stuart RM, Helbok R, Kurtz P, et al. High-dose intra-arterial verapamil for the treatment of cerebral vasospasm after subarachnoid hemorrhage: prolonged effects on hemodynamic parameters and brain metabolism. Neurosurgery. 2011;68:337–45.

642. Kassell NF, Helm G, Simmons N, Phillips CD, Cail WS. Treatment of cerebral vasospasm with intra-arterial papaverine. J Neurosurg. 1992;77:848–52.

643. Kaku Y, Yonekawa Y, Tsukahara T, Kazekawa K. Superselective intra-arterial infusion of papaverine for the treatment of cerebral vasospasm after subarachnoid hemorrhage. J Neurosurg. 1992;77:842–7.

644. Vajkoczy P, Horn P, Bauhuf C, et al. Effect of intra-arterial papaverine on regional cerebral blood flow in hemodynamically relevant cerebral vasospasm. Stroke. 2001;32: 498–505.

645. McAuliffe W, Townsend M, Eskridge JM, Newell DW, Grady MS, Winn HR. Intracranial pressure changes induced during papaverine infusion for treatment of vasospasm. J Neurosurg. 1995;83:430–4.

646. Carhuapoma JR, Qureshi AI, Tamargo RJ, Mathis JM, Hanley DF. Intra-arterial papaverine-induced seizures: case report and review of the literature. Surg Neurol. 2001;56: 159–63.

647. Barr JD, Mathis JM, Horton JA. Transient severe brain stem depression during intraarterial papaverine infusion for cerebral vasospasm. AJNR Am J Neuroradiol. 1994;15:719–23.

648. Stiefel MF, Spiotta AM, Udoetuk JD, et al. Intra-arterial papaverine used to treat cerebral vasospasm reduces brain oxygen. Neurocrit Care. 2006;4:113–8.

649. Smith WS, Dowd CF, Johnston SC, et al. Neurotoxicity of intra-arterial papaverine preserved with chlorobutanol used for the treatment of cerebral vasospasm after aneurysmal subarachnoid hemorrhage. Stroke. 2004;35:2518–22.

650. Elliott JP, Newell DW, Lam DJ, et al. Comparison of balloon angioplasty and papaverine infusion for the treatment of vasospasm following aneurysmal subarachnoid hemorrhage. J Neurosurg. 1998;88:277–84.

651. Kistler JP, Lees RS, Candia G, Zervas NT, Crowell RM, Ojemann RG. Intravenous nitroglycerin in experimental cerebral vasospasm. A preliminary report. Stroke. 1979;10:26–9.

652. Fathi AR, Pluta RM, Bakhtian KD, Qi M, Lonser RR. Reversal of cerebral vasospasm via intravenous sodium nitrite after subarachnoid hemorrhage in primates. J Neurosurg. 2011;115(6):1213–20.

653. Fathi AR, Marbacher S, Graupner T. Continuous intrathecal glyceryl trinitrate prevents delayed cerebral vasospasm in the single-SAH rabbit model in vivo. Acta Neurochir (Wien). 2011;153:1669–75; discussion 75.

654. Qanwash OM, Alaraj A, Aletich V, Charbel FT, Amin-Hanjani S. Safety of early endovascular catheterization and intervention through extracranial-intracranial bypass grafts. J Neurosurg. 2012;116(1):201–7.

655. Natarajan SK, Hauck EF, Hopkins LN, Levy EI, Siddiqui AH. Endovascular management of symptomatic spasm of radial artery bypass graft: technical case report. Neurosurgery. 2010;67:794–8; discussion 8.

656. Ghani GA, Sung YF, Weinstein MS, Tindall GT, Fleischer AS. Effects of intravenous nitroglycerin on the intracranial pressure and volume pressure response. J Neurosurg. 1983;58:562–5.

657. Molyneux AJ, Kerr RS, Birks J, et al. Risk of recurrent subarachnoid haemorrhage, death, or dependence and standardised mortality ratios after clipping or coiling of an intracranial aneurysm in the International Subarachnoid Aneurysm Trial (ISAT): long-term follow-up. Lancet Neurol. 2009;8:427–33.

658. Scott RBP, Eccles FD, Molyneux AJV, Kerr RSCMS, Rothwell PMF, Carpenter KDP. Improved cognitive outcomes with endovascular coiling of ruptured intracranial aneurysms: neuropsychological outcomes from the international subarachnoid aneurysm trial (ISAT). Stroke. 2010;41:1743–7.

659. Harbaugh RE, Heros RC, Hadley MN. More on ISAT. Lancet. 2003;361:783–4; author reply 4.

660. Khoo LT, Levy ML. Intracerebral aneurysms. In: Albright AL, Pollack IF, Adelson PD, editors. Principles and practice of pediatric neurosurgery. New York Thieme Medical Publishers; 1999.

661. Huang J, McGirt MJ, Gailloud P, Tamargo RJ. Intracranial aneurysms in the pediatric population: case series and literature review. Surg Neurol. 2005;63:424–32; discussion 32–3.

662. Fulkerson DH, Voorhies JM, Payner TD, et al. Middle cerebral artery aneurysms in children: case series and review. J Neurosurg Pediatr. 2011;8:79–89.

663. Sanai N, Quinones-Hinojosa A, Gupta NM, et al. Pediatric intracranial aneurysms: durability of treatment following microsurgical and endovascular management. J Neurosurg. 2006;104:82–9.

664. Laughlin S, terBrugge KG, Willinsky RA, Armstrong DC, Montanera WJ, Humphreys RP. Endovascular management of paediatric intracranial aneurysms. Intervent Neuroradiol. 1997;3:205–14.

665. Kanaan I, Lasjaunias P, Coates R. The spectrum of intracranial aneurysms in pediatrics. Minim Invasive Neurosurg. 1995;38:1–9.

666. Buis DR, van Ouwerkerk WJ, Takahata H, Vandertop WP. Intracranial aneurysms in children under 1 year of age: a systematic review of the literature. Childs Nerv Syst. 2006;22(11):1395–409.

667. Batnitzky S, Muller I. Infantile and juvenile cerebral aneurysms. Neuroradiology. 1978;16:61–4.

668. Aryan HE, Giannotta SL, Fukushima T, Park MS, Ozgur BM, Levy ML. Aneurysms in children: review of 15 years experience. J Clin Neurosci. 2006;13:188–92.

669. Ventureyra EC, Higgins MJ. Traumatic intracranial aneurysms in childhood and adolescence. Case reports and review of the literature. Childs Nerv Syst. 1994;10:361–79.

670. Ostergaard JR, Voldby B. Intracranial arterial aneurysms in children and adolescents. J Neurosurg. 1983;58:832–7.

671. Lasjaunias P, Wuppalapati S, Alvarez H, Rodesch G, Ozanne A. Intracranial aneurysms in children aged under 15 years: review of 59 consecutive children with 75 aneurysms. Childs Nerv Syst. 2005;21:437–50.

672. Kakarla UK, Beres EJ, Ponce FA. Microsurgical treatment of pediatric intracranial aneurysms: long-term angiographic and clinical outcomes. Neurosurgery. 2010;67:237–49; discussion 50.

673. Sawin P. Spontaneous subarachnoid hemorrhage in pregnancy and the puerperium. In: Loftus C, editor. Neurosurgical aspects of pregnancy. Park Ridge: American Association of Neurological Surgeons; 1996. p. 85–99.

674. Wiebers DO. Subarachnoid hemorrhage in pregnancy. Semin Neurol. 1988;8:226–9.

675. Robinson JL, Hall CJ, Sedzimir CB. Subarachnoid hemorrhage in pregnancy. J Neurosurg. 1972;36:27–33.

676. Measurements NCoRPa, editors. Recommendations on limits for exposure to ionizing radiation. NCRP Report No. 91. Bethesda: National Council on Radiation Protection; 1987.

677. Piper J. Fetal toxicity of common neurosurgical drugs. In: Loftus C, editor. Neurosurgical aspects of pregnancy. Park Ridge: American Association of Neurological Surgeons; 1996. p. 1–20.

678. Dias MS, Sekhar LN. Intracranial hemorrhage from aneurysms and arteriovenous malformations during pregnancy

and the puerperium. Neurosurgery. 1990;27:855–65; discussion 65–6.

679. Maymon R, Fejgin M. Intracranial hemorrhage during pregnancy and puerperium. Obstet Gynecol Surv. 1990;45:157–9.

680. Barrett JM, Van Hooydonk JE, Boehm FH. Pregnancy-related rupture of arterial aneurysms. Obstet Gynecol Surv. 1982;37:557–66.

681. Verweij RD, Wijdicks EF, van Gijn J. Warning headache in aneurysmal subarachnoid hemorrhage. A case–control study. Arch Neurol. 1988;45:1019–20.

682. Donnelly JF, Lock FR. Causes of death in five hundred thirty-three fatal cases of toxemia of pregnancy. Am J Obstet Gynecol. 1954;68:184–90.

683. Schwartz J. Pregnancy complicated by subarachnoid hemorrhage. Am J Obstet Gynecol. 1951;62:539–47.

684. Barno A, Freeman DW. Maternal deaths due to spontaneous subarachnoid hemorrhage. Am J Obstet Gynecol. 1976; 125:384–92.

685. Hirsh J, Cade JF, Gallus AS. Anticoagulants in pregnancy: a review of indications and complications. Am Heart J. 1972;83:301–5.

686. Henderson CE, Torbey M. Rupture of intracranial aneurysm associated with cocaine use during pregnancy. Am J Perinatol. 1988;5:142–3.

687. Salcman M. Choriocarcinoma in pregnancy. In: Loftus C, editor. Neurosurgical aspects of pregnancy. Park Ridge: American Association of Neurological Surgeons; 1996. p. 147–55.

688. Enomoto H, Goto H. Moyamoya disease presenting as intracerebral hemorrhage during pregnancy: case report and review of the literature. Neurosurgery. 1987;20:33–5.

689. Botterell EH, Cannell DE. Subarachnoid hemorrhage and pregnancy. Am J Obstet Gynecol. 1956;72:844–55.

690. Daane TA, Tandy RW. Rupture of congenital intracranial aneurysm in pregnancy. Obstet Gynecol. 1960;15:305–14.

691. Pool JL. Treatment of intracranial aneurysms during pregnancy. JAMA. 1965;192:209–14.

692. Lennon RL, Sundt Jr TM, Gronert GA. Combined cesarean section and clipping of intracerebral aneurysm. Anesthesiology. 1984;60:240–2.

693. Meyers PM, Halbach VV, Malek AM, et al. Endovascular treatment of cerebral artery aneurysms during pregnancy: report of three cases. AJNR Am J Neuroradiol. 2000;21: 1306–11.

694. Piotin M, de Souza Filho CB, Kothimbakam R, Moret J. Endovascular treatment of acutely ruptured intracranial aneurysms in pregnancy. Am J Obstet Gynecol. 2001; 185:1261–2.

695. Kizilkilic O, Albayram S, Adaletli I, et al. Endovascular treatment of ruptured intracranial aneurysms during pregnancy: report of three cases. Arch Gynecol Obstet. 2003;268:325–8.

696. Srinivasan K. Cerebral venous and arterial thrombosis in pregnancy and puerperium. A study of 135 patients. Angiology. 1983;34:731–46.

697. Pedowitz P, Perell A. Aneurysms complicated by pregnancy. II. Aneurysms of the cerebral vessels. Am J Obstet Gynecol. 1957;73:736–49.

698. Heikkinen JE, Rinne RI, Alahuhta SM, et al. Life support for 10 weeks with successful fetal outcome after fatal maternal brain damage. Br Med J (Clin Res Ed). 1985;290: 1237–8.

699. Stolz-Born G, Widder B, Born J. Vascular effects of oxytocin on human middle cerebral artery determined by transcranial Doppler sonography. Regul Pept. 1996;62:37–9.

700. Suzuki Y, Satoh S, Kimura M, et al. Effects of vasopressin and oxytocin on canine cerebral circulation in vivo. J Neurosurg. 1992;77:424–31.

701. Barker FG, Amin-Hanjani S, Butler WE. Age-dependent differences in short-term outcome after surgical or endovascular treatment of unruptured intracranial aneurysms in the United States, 1996–2000. Neurosurgery. 2004;54:18–28; discussion 28–30.

702. Chung RY, Carter BS, Norbash A, Budzik R, Putnam C, Ogilvy CS. Management outcomes for ruptured and unruptured aneurysms in the elderly. Neurosurgery. 2000;47:827–32; discussion 32–3.

703. Bradac GB, Bergui M, Fontanella M. Endovascular treatment of cerebral aneurysms in elderly patients. Neuroradiology. 2005;47:938–41.

704. Cai Y, Spelle L, Wang H. Endovascular treatment of intracranial aneurysms in the elderly: single-center experience in 63 consecutive patients. Neurosurgery. 2005;57:1096–102; discussion 1096–102.

705. Inagawa T. Trends in incidence and case fatality rates of aneurysmal subarachnoid hemorrhage in Izumo City, Japan, between 1980–1989 and 1990–1998. Stroke. 2001;32: 1499–507.

706. Shimamura N, Munakata A, Ohkuma H. Current management of subarachnoid hemorrhage in advanced age. Acta Neurochir Suppl. 2011;110:151–5.

707. Lanzino G, Kassell NF, Germanson TP, et al. Age and outcome after aneurysmal subarachnoid hemorrhage: why do older patients fare worse? J Neurosurg. 1996;85:410–8.

708. Sedat J, Dib M, Lonjon M, et al. Endovascular treatment of ruptured intracranial aneurysms in patients aged 65 years and older: follow-up of 52 patients after 1 year. Stroke. 2002;33:2620–5.

709. Nieuwkamp DJ, Rinkel GJE, Silva R, Greebe P, Schokking DA, Ferro JM. Subarachnoid haemorrhage in patients older than 75 years: clinical course, treatment and outcome. J Neurol Neurosurg Psychiatry. 2006;77:933–7.

710. Takeuchi J. Aneurysm surgery in patients over the age of 80 years. Br J Neurosurg. 1993;7:307–9.

711. Lan Q, Ikeda H, Jimbo H, Izumiyama H, Matsumoto K. Considerations on surgical treatment for elderly patients with intracranial aneurysms. Surg Neurol. 2000;53: 231–8.

712. Ferch R, Pasqualin A, Barone G, Pinna G, Bricolo A. Surgical management of ruptured aneurysms in the eighth and ninth decades. Acta Neurochir (Wien). 2003;145: 439–45; discussion 45.

713. Jain R, Deveikis J, Thompson BG. Endovascular management of poor-grade aneurysmal subarachnoid hemorrhage in the geriatric population. AJNR Am J Neuroradiol. 2004;25:596–600.

714. Church W. Aneurysm of the right cerebral artery in a boy of thirteen. Trans Pathol Soc Lond. 1869;20:109.

715. Osler W. Gulstonian lectures on malignant endocarditis. Lancet. 1885;1:415–8, 508–8.

716. Clare CE, Barrow DL. Infectious intracranial aneurysms. Neurosurg Clin N Am. 1992;3:551–66.

717. Chun JY, Smith W, Halbach VV, Higashida RT, Wilson CB, Lawton MT. Current multimodality management of infectious intracranial aneurysms. Neurosurgery. 2001;48: 1203–13; discussion 13–4.

718. Herman JM, Rekate HL, Spetzler RF. Pediatric intracranial aneurysms: simple and complex cases. Pediatr Neurosurg. 1991;17:66–72; discussion 3.

719. Bohmfalk GL, Story JL, Wissinger JP, Brown Jr WE. Bacterial intracranial aneurysm. J Neurosurg. 1978;48: 369–82.

720. Lerner PI. Neurologic complications of infective endocarditis. Med Clin North Am. 1985;69:385–98.

721. Phuong LK, Link M, Wijdicks E. Management of intracranial infectious aneurysms: a series of 16 cases. Neurosurgery. 2002;51:1145–51; discussion 51–2.

722. Yao KC, Bederson JB. Infectious intracranial aneurysms. In: Winn HR, editor. Youmans neurological surgery. Philadelphia: Saunders; 2004. p. 2101–6.

723. Ojemann RG. Surgical management of bacterial intracranial aneurysms. In: Schmidek HH, Sweet WH, editors. Operative neurosurgical techniques. New York: Grune & Stratton; 1988. p. 997–1001.

724. Kojima Y, Saito A, Kim I. The role of serial angiography in the management of bacterial and fungal intracranial aneurysms – report of two cases and review of the literature. Neurol Med Chir (Tokyo). 1989;29:202–16

725. Molinari GF, Smith L, Goldstein MN, Satran R. Pathogenesis of cerebral mycotic aneurysms. Neurology. 1973;23:325–32.

726. Hurst RW, Judkins A, Bolger W, Chu A, Loevner LA. Mycotic aneurysm and cerebral infarction resulting from fungal sinusitis: imaging and pathologic correlation. AJNR Am J Neuroradiol. 2001;22:858–63.

727. Pruitt AA, Rubin RH, Karchmer AW, Duncan GW. Neurologic complications of bacterial endocarditis. Medicine (Baltimore). 1978;57:329–43.

728. Morawetz RB, Karp RB. Evolution and resolution of intracranial bacterial (mycotic) aneurysms. Neurosurgery. 1984; 15:43–9.

729. Barrow DL, Prats AR. Infectious intracranial aneurysms: comparison of groups with and without procedures. Neurosurgery. 1990;27:562–72; discussion 72–3.

730. Cloft HJ, Kallmes DF, Jensen ME, Lanzino G, Dion JE. Endovascular treatment of ruptured, peripheral cerebral aneurysms: parent artery occlusion with short Guglielmi detachable coils. AJNR Am J Neuroradiol. 1999;20: 308–10.

731. Frizzell RT, Vitek JJ, Hill DL, Fisher 3rd WS. Treatment of a bacterial (mycotic) intracranial aneurysm using an endovascular approach. Neurosurgery. 1993;32:852–4.

732. Rout D, Sharma A, Mohan PK, Rao VR. Bacterial aneurysms of the intracavernous carotid artery. J Neurosurg. 1984;60:1236–42.

733. Hutchinson J. Aneurysms of the internal carotid within the skull diagnosed 11 years before the patient's death: spontaneous cure. Trans Clin Soc (Lond). 1987;8:127.

734. Choi IS, David C. Giant intracranial aneurysms: development, clinical presentation and treatment. Eur J Radiol. 2003;46:178–94.

735. Schubiger O, Valavanis A, Wichmann W. Growth-mechanism of giant intracranial aneurysms; demonstration by CT and MR imaging. Neuroradiology. 1987;29:266–71.

736. Koyama S, Kotani A, Sasaki J. Giant basilar artery aneurysm with intramural hemorrhage and then disastrous hemorrhage: case report. Neurosurgery. 1996;39:174–7; discussion 7–8.

737. Nagahiro S, Takada A, Goto S, Kai Y, Ushio Y. Thrombosed growing giant aneurysms of the vertebral artery: growth mechanism and management. J Neurosurg. 1995;82: 796–801.

738. Lawton MT, Spetzler RF. Surgical strategies for giant intracranial aneurysms. Neurosurg Clin N Am. 1998;9: 725–42.

739. Lemole JGM, Henn JS, Spetzler RF, Riina HA. Giant aneurysms. In: Winn HR, editor. Youmans neurological surgery. Philadelphia: Saunders; 2004. p. 2079–99.

740. Pia HW, Zierski J. Giant cerebral aneurysms. Neurosurg Rev. 1982;5:117–48.

741. Ausman JI, Diaz FG, Sadasivan B, Gonzeles-Portillo Jr M, Malik GM, Deopujari CE. Giant intracranial aneurysm surgery: the role of microvascular reconstruction. Surg Neurol. 1990;34:8–15.

742. Gruber A, Killer M, Bavinzski G, Richling B. Clinical and angiographic results of endosaccular coiling treatment of giant and very large intracranial aneurysms: a 7-year, single-center experience. Neurosurgery. 1999;45:793–803; discussion 803–4.

743. Drake CG, Peerless SJ. Giant fusiform intracranial aneurysms: review of 120 patients treated surgically from 1965 to 1992. J Neurosurg. 1997;87:141–62.

744. Raymond LA, Tew J. Large suprasellar aneurysms imitating pituitary tumour. J Neurol Neurosurg Psychiatry. 1978;41:83–7.

745. Bokemeyer C, Frank B, Brandis A, Weinrich W. Giant aneurysm causing frontal lobe syndrome. J Neurol. 1990; 237:47–50.

746. Lownie SP, Drake CG, Peerless SJ, Ferguson GG, Pelz DM. Clinical presentation and management of giant anterior communicating artery region aneurysms. J Neurosurg. 2000;92:267–77.

747. Michael WF. Posterior fossa aneurysms simulating tumours. J Neurol Neurosurg Psychiatry. 1974;37:218–23.

748. Kodama N, Suzuki J. Surgical treatment of giant aneurysms. Neurosurg Rev. 1982;5:155–60.

749. Barrow DL, Alleyne C. Natural history of giant intracranial aneurysms and indications for intervention. Clin Neurosurg. 1995;42:214–44.

750. Elhammady MS, Wolfe SQ, Farhat H, Ali Aziz-Sultan M, Heros RC. Carotid artery sacrifice for unclippable and uncoilable aneurysms: endovascular occlusion vs. common carotid artery ligation. Neurosurgery. 2010;67:1431–7.

751. Gobin YP, Vinuela F, Gurian JH, et al. Treatment of large and giant fusiform intracranial aneurysms with Guglielmi detachable coils. J Neurosurg. 1996;84:55–62.

752. Otsuka G, Miyachi S, Handa T, et al. Endovascular trapping of giant serpentine aneurysms by using Guglielmi detachable coils: successful reduction of mass effect. Report of two cases. J Neurosurg. 2001;94:836–40.

753. Briganti F, Cirillo S, Caranci F, Esposito F, Maiuri F. Development of "de novo" aneurysms following endovascular procedures. Neuroradiology. 2002;44:604–9.

754. Ross IB, Weill A, Piotin M, Moret J. Endovascular treatment of distally located giant aneurysms. Neurosurgery. 2000;47:1147–52; discussion 52–3.

755. Malisch TW, Guglielmi G, Vinuela F, et al. Intracranial aneurysms treated with the Guglielmi detachable coil: mid-term clinical results in a consecutive series of 100 patients. J Neurosurg. 1997;87:176–83.

756. Higashida RT, Smith W, Gress D. Intravascular stent and endovascular coil placement for a ruptured fusiform aneurysm of the basilar artery. Case report and review of the literature. J Neurosurg. 1997;87:944–9.

757. Islak C, Kocer N, Albayram S, Kizilkilic O, Uzma O, Cokyuksel O. Bare stent-graft technique: a new method of endoluminal vascular reconstruction for the treatment of giant and fusiform aneurysms. AJNR Am J Neuroradiol. 2002;23:1589–95.

758. Yamaura A, Ono J, Hirai S. Clinical picture of intracranial non-traumatic dissecting aneurysm. Neuropathology. 2000;20:85–90.

759. Kurino M, Yoshioka S, Ushio Y. Spontaneous dissecting aneurysms of anterior and middle cerebral artery associated with brain infarction: a case report and review of the literature. Surg Neurol. 2002;57:428–36; discussion 36–8.

760. Mizutani T, Kojima H. Clinicopathological features of non-atherosclerotic cerebral arterial trunk aneurysms. Neuropathology. 2000;20:91–7.

761. Okuchi K, Watabe Y, Hiramatsu K, et al. Dissecting aneurysm of the vertebral artery as a cause of Wallenberg's syndrome (in Japanese with English abstract). No Shinkei Geka. 1990;18:721–7.

762. Ojemann RG, Fisher CM, Rich JC. Spontaneous dissecting aneurysm of the internal carotid artery. Stroke. 1972; 3:434–40.

763. Bhattacharya RN, Menon G, Nair S. Dissecting intracranial vertebral artery aneurysms. Neurol India. 2001;49:391–4.

764. Nagahiro S, Hamada J, Sakamoto Y, Ushio Y. Follow-up evaluation of dissecting aneurysms of the vertebrobasilar circulation by using gadolinium-enhanced magnetic resonance imaging. J Neurosurg. 1997;87:385–90.

765. Mizutani T, Kojima H, Asamoto S, Miki Y. Pathological mechanism and three-dimensional structure of cerebral dissecting aneurysms. J Neurosurg. 2001;94:712–7.

766. Sasaki O, Ogawa H, Koike T, Koizumi T, Tanaka R. A clinicopathological study of dissecting aneurysms of the intracranial vertebral artery. J Neurosurg. 1991;75:874–82.

767. Clower BR, Sullivan DM, Smith RR. Intracranial vessels lack vasa vasorum. J Neurosurg. 1984;61:44–8.

768. Tuna M, Gocer AI, Ozel S, Bagdatoglu H, Zorludemir S, Haciyakupoglu S. A giant dissecting aneurysm mimicking serpentine aneurysm angiographically. Case report and review of the literature. Neurosurg Rev. 1998;21:284–9.

769. Mizutani T, Aruga T, Kirino T, Miki Y, Saito I, Tsuchida T. Recurrent subarachnoid hemorrhage from untreated ruptured vertebrobasilar dissecting aneurysms. Neurosurgery. 1995;36:905–11; discussion 12–3.

770. Yuki I, Murayama Y, Vinuela F. Endovascular management of dissecting vertebrobasilar artery aneurysms in patients presenting with acute subarachnoid hemorrhage. J Neurosurg. 2005;103:649–55.

771. Benndorf G, Herbon U, Sollmann WP, Campi A. Treatment of a ruptured dissecting vertebral artery aneurysm with double stent placement: case report. AJNR Am J Neuroradiol. 2001;22:1844–8.

772. Chiaradio JC, Guzman L, Padilla L, Chiaradio MP. Intravascular graft stent treatment of a ruptured fusiform dissecting aneurysm of the intracranial vertebral artery: technical case report. Neurosurgery. 2002;50:213–6; discussion 6–7.

773. Hayes WT, Bernhardt H, Young JM. Fusiform arteriosclerotic aneurysm of the basilar artery. Five cases including two ruptures. Vasc Surg. 1967;1:171–8.

774. Housepian EM, Pool JL. A systematic analysis of intracranial aneurysms from the autopsy file of the Presbyterian Hospital, 1914 to 1956. J Neuropathol Exp Neurol. 1958;17:409–23.

775. Yu YL, Moseley IF, Pullicino P, McDonald WI. The clinical picture of ectasia of the intracerebral arteries. J Neurol Neurosurg Psychiatry. 1982;45:29–36.

776. Segal HD, McLaurin RL. Giant serpentine aneurysm. Report of two cases. J Neurosurg. 1977;46:115–20.

777. Anson JA, Lawton MT, Spetzler RF. Characteristics and surgical treatment of dolichoectatic and fusiform aneurysms. J Neurosurg. 1996;84:185–93.

778. Nishizaki T, Tamaki N, Takeda N, Shirakuni T, Kondoh T, Matsumoto S. Dolichoectatic basilar artery: a review of 23 cases. Stroke. 1986;17:1277–81.

779. Flemming KD, Wiebers DO, Brown Jr RD, et al. Prospective risk of hemorrhage in patients with vertebrobasilar nonsaccular intracranial aneurysm. J Neurosurg. 2004;101:82–7.

780. Little JR, St Louis P, Weinstein M, Dohn DF. Giant fusiform aneurysm of the cerebral arteries. Stroke. 1981;12:183–8.

781. Suzuki S, Takahashi T, Ohkuma H, Shimizu T, Fujita S. Management of giant serpentine aneurysms of the middle cerebral artery–review of literature and report of a case successfully treated by STA-MCA anastomosis only. Acta Neurochir (Wien). 1992;117:23–9.

782. Flemming KD, Wiebers DO, Brown Jr RD, et al. The natural history of radiographically defined vertebrobasilar nonsaccular intracranial aneurysms. Cerebrovasc Dis. 2005;20:270–9.

783. Resta M, Gentile MA, Di Cuonzo F, Vinjau E, Brindicci D, Carella A. Clinical-angiographic correlations in 132 patients with megadolichovertebrobasilar anomaly. Neuroradiology. 1984;26:213–6.

784. Rozario RA, Levine HL, Scott RM. Obstructive hydrocephalus secondary to an ectatic basilar artery. Surg Neurol. 1978;9:31–4.

785. Nakatomi H, Segawa H, Kurata A, et al. Clinicopathological study of intracranial fusiform and dolichoectatic aneurysms: insight on the mechanism of growth. Stroke. 2000;31:896–900.

786. Shimoji T, Bando K, Nakajima K, Ito K. Dissecting aneurysm of the vertebral artery. Report of seven cases and angiographic findings. J Neurosurg. 1984;61:1038–46.

787. Caplan LR, Baquis GD, Pessin MS, et al. Dissection of the intracranial vertebral artery. Neurology. 1988;38:868–77.

788. Mizutani T, Aruga T. "Dolichoectatic" intracranial vertebrobasilar dissecting aneurysm. Neurosurgery. 1992;31: 765–73; discussion 73.

789. Sacks JG, Lindenburg R. Dolicho-ectatic intracranial arteries: symptomatology and pathogenesis of arterial elongation and distention. Johns Hopkins Med J. 1969;125: 95–106.

790. Nijensohn DE, Saez RJ, Reagan TJ. Clinical significance of basilar artery aneurysms. Neurology. 1974;24:301–5.

791. Hegedus K. Ectasia of the basilar artery with special reference to possible pathogenesis. Surg Neurol. 1985;24:463–9.

792. Ubogu EE, Zaidat OO. Vertebrobasilar dolichoectasia diagnosed by magnetic resonance angiography and risk of stroke and death: a cohort study. J Neurol Neurosurg Psychiatry. 2004;75:22–6.

793. Mawad ME, Klucznik RP. Giant serpentine aneurysms: radiographic features and endovascular treatment. AJNR Am J Neuroradiol. 1995;16:1053–60.

794. Benoit BG, Wortzman G. Traumatic cerebral aneurysms. Clinical features and natural history. J Neurol Neurosurg Psychiatry. 1973;36:127–38.

795. Parkinson D, West M. Traumatic intracranial aneurysms. J Neurosurg. 1980;52:11–20.

796. Giannotta SL, Gruen P. Vascular complications of head trauma. In: Barrow DL, editor. Complications and sequelae of head injury. Park Ridge American Association of Neurological Surgeons; 1992. p. 31–49.

797. Uzan M, Cantasdemir M, Seckin MS. Traumatic intracranial carotid tree aneurysms. Neurosurgery. 1998;43:1314–20; discussion 20–2.

798. Aarabi B. Management of traumatic aneurysms caused by high-velocity missile head wounds. Neurosurg Clin N Am. 1995;6:775–97.

799. Steinmetz H, Heiss E, Mironov A. Traumatic giant aneurysms of the intracranial carotid artery presenting long after head injury. Surg Neurol. 1988;30:305–10.

800. Nishioka T, Maeda Y, Tomogane Y, Nakano A, Arita N. Unexpected delayed rupture of the vertebral-posterior inferior cerebellar artery aneurysms following closed head injury. Acta Neurochir (Wien). 2002;144:839–45; discussion 45.

801. Buckingham MJ, Crone KR, Ball WS, Tomsick TA, Berger TS, Tew Jr JM. Traumatic intracranial aneurysms in childhood: two cases and a review of the literature. Neurosurgery. 1988;22:398–408.

802. Sadar ES, Jane JA, Lewis LW, Adelman LS. Traumatic aneurysms of the intracranial circulation. Surg Gynecol Obstet. 1973;137:59–67.

803. Teal JS, Bergeron RT, Rumbaugh CL, Segall HD. Aneurysms of the petrous or cavernous portions of the internal carotid artery associated with nonpenetrating head trauma. J Neurosurg. 1973;38:568–74.

804. Resnick DK, Subach BR, Marion DW. The significance of carotid canal involvement in basilar cranial fracture. Neurosurgery. 1997;40:1177–81.

805. Haddad FS, Haddad GF, Taha J. Traumatic intracranial aneurysms caused by missiles: their presentation and management. Neurosurgery. 1991;28:1–7.

806. Holmes B, Harbaugh RE. Traumatic intracranial aneurysms: a contemporary review. J Trauma. 1993;35:855–60.

807. Luo C-B, Teng MM-H, Chang F-C, Lirng J-F, Chang C-Y. Endovascular management of the traumatic cerebral aneurysms associated with traumatic carotid cavernous fistulas. AJNR Am J Neuroradiol. 2004;25:501–5.

808. Horowitz MB, Kopitnik TA, Landreneau F, et al. Multidisciplinary approach to traumatic intracranial aneurysms secondary to shotgun and handgun wounds. Surg Neurol. 1999;51:31–42.

809. Eisenberg HM, Gary Jr HE, Aldrich EF. Initial CT findings in 753 patients with severe head injury. A report from the NIH Traumatic Coma Data Bank. J Neurosurg. 1990;73:688–98.

810. Kakarieka A, Braakman R, Schakel EH. Clinical significance of the finding of subarachnoid blood on CT scan after head injury. Acta Neurochir (Wien). 1994;129:1–5.

811. Mattioli C, Beretta L, Gerevini S, et al. Traumatic subarachnoid hemorrhage on the computerized tomography scan obtained at admission: a multicenter assessment of the accuracy of diagnosis and the potential impact on patient outcome. J Neurosurg. 2003;98:37–42.

812. Servadei F, Murray GD, Teasdale GM. Traumatic subarachnoid hemorrhage: demographic and clinical study of 750 patients from the European brain injury consortium survey of head injuries. Neurosurgery. 2002;50:261–7; discussion 7–9.

813. Gomez PA, Lobato RD, Ortega JM, De La Cruz J. Mild head injury: differences in prognosis among patients with a Glasgow Coma Scale score of 13 to 15 and analysis of factors associated with abnormal CT findings. Br J Neurosurg. 1996;10:453–60.

814. Shackford SR, Wald SL, Ross SE, et al. The clinical utility of computed tomographic scanning and neurologic examination in the management of patients with minor head injuries. J Trauma. 1992;33:385–94.

815. Macpherson P, Graham DI. Correlation between angiographic findings and the ischaemia of head injury. J Neurol Neurosurg Psychiatry. 1978;41:122–7.

816. Oertel M, Boscardin WJ, Obrist WD, et al. Posttraumatic vasospasm: the epidemiology, severity, and time course of an underestimated phenomenon: a prospective study performed in 299 patients. J Neurosurg. 2005;103:812–24.

817. Fukuda T, Hasue M, Ito H. Does traumatic subarachnoid hemorrhage caused by diffuse brain injury cause delayed ischemic brain damage? Comparison with subarachnoid hemorrhage caused by ruptured intracranial aneurysms. Neurosurgery. 1998;43:1040–9.

818. Macmillan CS, Wild JM, Wardlaw JM, Andrews PJ, Marshall I, Easton VJ. Traumatic brain injury and subarachnoid haemorrhage: in vivo occult pathology demonstrated by magnetic resonance spectroscopy may not be "ischaemic". A primary study and review of the literature. Acta Neurochir (Wien). 2002;144:853–62; discussion 62.

819. Langham J, Goldfrad C, Teasdale G, Shaw D, Rowan K. Calcium channel blockers for acute traumatic brain injury. Cochrane Database Syst Rev. 2003:CD000565.

820. Cairns CJ, Finfer SR, Harrington TJ, Cook R. Papaverine angioplasty to treat cerebral vasospasm following traumatic subarachnoid haemorrhage. Anaesth Intensive Care. 2003;31:87–91.

821. Roy D, Raymond J, Bouthillier A, Bojanowski MW, Moumdjian R, L'Esperance G. Endovascular treatment of ophthalmic segment aneurysms with Guglielmi detachable coils. AJNR Am J Neuroradiol. 1997;18:1207–15.

822. Meyers PM, Schumacher HC, Higashida RT, et al. Reporting standards for endovascular repair of saccular intracranial cerebral aneurysms. J Neurointerv Surg. 2010;2:312–23.

823. O'Kelly CJ, Krings T, Fiorella D, Marotta TR. A novel grading scale for the angiographic assessment of intracranial aneurysms treated using flow diverting stents. Interv Neuroradiol. 2010;16:133–7.

824. Arias E. United States life tables, 2002. Natl Vital Stat Rep. 2004;53:1–38.

825. Kondziolka D, McLaughlin MR, Kestle JR. Simple risk predictions for arteriovenous malformation hemorrhage. Neurosurgery. 1995;37:851–5.

826. Suarez JI, Zaidat OO, Suri MF, et al. Length of stay and mortality in neurocritically ill patients: impact of a specialized neurocritical care team. Crit Care Med. 2004;32:2311–7.

827. Finn SS, Stephensen SA, Miller CA, Drobnich L, Hunt WE. Observations on the perioperative management of aneurysmal subarachnoid hemorrhage. J Neurosurg. 1986;65:48–62.

828. Kasuya H, Kawashima A, Namiki K, Shimizu T, Takakura K. Metabolic profiles of patients with subarachnoid hemorrhage treated by early surgery. Neurosurgery. 1998;42:1268–74; discussion 74–5.

829. Suarez JI, Shannon L, Zaidat OO, et al. Effect of human albumin administration on clinical outcome and hospital cost in patients with subarachnoid hemorrhage. J Neurosurg. 2004;100:585–90.

830. Flemming KD, Brown Jr RD, Wiebers DO. Subarachnoid hemorrhage. Curr Treat Options Neurol. 1999;1:97–112.

831. Black PM, Crowell RM, Abbott WM. External pneumatic calf compression reduces deep venous thrombosis in patients with ruptured intracranial aneurysms. Neurosurgery. 1986;18:25–8.

14. Arteriovenous Malformations

Arteriovenous malformations (AVMs) are congenital vascular lesions that may appear throughout the central nervous system. They consist of direct connections between arteries and veins, without an intervening capillary bed. They about one-tenth as common as intracranial aneurysms. Spinal AVMs are discussed in Chap. 20. Vein of Galen malformations are a separate entity and are discussed in the Appendix to this chapter.

14.1.   Pathophysiology

Pathology

1. Gross appearance
   (a) Intracranial AVMs often resemble a ball of red and blue noodles, described by Cushing and Bailey as a *snarl* of tangled vessels.[1]
   (b) AVMs are frequently pyramidal-shaped lesions, with the base at and parallel to the cortical surface and the apex directed toward the ventricle.
   (c) The nidus may be compact or diffuse, and range in size from several millimeters to an entire hemisphere.
   (d) The adjacent brain parenchyma may be haemosiderin-stained from previous haemorrhage, and the overlying meninges may be thickened and fibrotic.[2] Extensive gliosis, fibrosis, and calcification may be present.
2. Histopathological features
   (a) Arteries
      • AVM arteries are abnormally dilated, with marked thinning in some regions and degeneration or absence of the media and elastic lamina.[3] Degenerative changes are present, presumably due to wall shear stress caused by high flow.[2] These include irregular thickening of the vessel wall in some regions, endothelial proliferation, medial hypertrophy, and multilaminated, thickened basal laminae.[4]
   (b) Nidus
      • Nidal vessels may contain a hypertrophic media, blurring the distinction between arteries and veins.
      • Aneurysms and islands of sclerotic tissue may be present within the nidus.
   (c) Veins
      • "Arterialized" veins may exhibit thickening of the vein wall due to cellular proliferation.[2]
      • Although thickened AVM veins may grossly resemble arteries, they lack an organized elastic lamina and therefore are not truly arterial structures.
   (d) Functional brain tissue is usually not present within an AVM, although in diffuse lesions, AVM vessels may be separated by normal tissue.

Etiology

1. AVMs are assumed to appear during fetal development between the 4th and 8th weeks of life.
   a) However, some evidence suggests that AVMs may develop later in life, as AVMs are rarely detected in utero[5] or found in infants.[6] One hypothesis maintains that AVMs first appear in utero but then continue to grow after birth.[5]

M.R. Harrigan, J.P. Deveikis, *Handbook of Cerebrovascular Disease and Neurointerventional Technique*, DOI 10.1007/978-1-61779-946-4_14, © Springer Science+Business Media New York 2013

2. The precise etiology of AVMs is unclear. Some theories:
    (a) AVMs represent persistent direct connections between arteries and veins within the primitive vascular plexus.
    (b) AVMs are dynamic and result from a derangement in vessel growth, i.e., a "proliferative capillaropathy".[7]
    (c) AVMs result from a dysfunction of the remodeling process at the junction between capillaries and veins.[8]
    (d) AVMs may represent fistualized cerebral venous angiomas.[9]

Physiology

1. Haemodynamic characteristics
    (a) AVMs are typically high-flow, low-resistance systems.[10]
    (b) *Steal phenomenon.* In some cases, high-flow diversion of blood flow through an unruptured AVM is believed to produce symptoms by reducing perfusion in adjacent normal brain tissue.[11] Steal, as a mechanism of symptoms, is thought to be very rare or nonexistent.
        • Regional CBF surrounding the lesion may be reduced.[12]
        • Adaptive changes in autoregulation in peri-lesional brain tissue may occur.[13]
        • *Evidence against steal phenomenon*: In a prospective study of 152 patients with unruptured AVMs, only 2 (1.3%) had focal neurological symptoms possibly attributable to steal phenomenon.[14] TCD examinations showed no relation between feeding artery pressure or flow velocities and neurological deficits; the authors took these findings as evidence against steal as a pathophysiological mechanism in most patients.
    (c) Increased pressure in feeding arteries and in draining veins (i.e., outflow restriction) is associated with haemorrhage.[12,15]
2. Functional displacement. Development of an AVM within the brain appears to lead to reorganization and displacement of functional tissue.[16,17]

14.2.   Clinical Features

Epidemiology

1. Prevalence
    (a) Estimates of the prevalence of brain AVMs in the general population range from 0.005% to 0.6%.[18–22]
    (b) In contrast to unruptured intracranial aneurysms, which have been diagnosed at an increasing rate in recent years, there has been a decline in the rate of detection of brain AVMs in recent years.[23]
2. Incidence of AVM-related haemorrhage
    a) New York Islands Arteriovenous Malformation Study.[24,25] Incidence of first-ever AVM haemorrhage: 0.51 per 100,000 person-years.
3. Slightly more common in men (55% of all cases).[24,26]
4. Mean age at diagnosis: 31.2 years.[26]

Anatomic Features

1. Location
    (a) Equally distributed between the left and right sides.[22,27,28]
    (b) About 65% of lesions involve the cerebral hemispheres.[29]; 15% involve deep midline structures, and 20% are in the posterior fossa.[30]
    (c) Eloquent tissue (sensorimotor, language, or visual cortex; hypothalamus or thalamus; internal capsule; brainstem; cerebellar peduncles, or cerebellum) is involved in up to 71% of the cases.[31]

2. Feeding vessels
   a) Feeding arteries have been divided into three types:[32]
      • Terminal: Arteries which may supply normal tissue proximally but terminate within the AVM.
      • Pseudo-terminal: Feeders that supply normal brain distal to their supply to the AVM.
      • Indirect (aka *en passage*): feeders that typically arise at right angles from larger normal arteries.
3. Multiplicity
   (a) Up to 9% of patients have multiple AVMs.[33]
   (b) Most patients with multiple AVMs frequently have an associated vascular syndrome, such as hereditary haemorrhagic telangiectasia (see below).[34]

Conditions Associated with AVMs

Familial Intracranial AVMs

Most intracranial AVMs are sporadic. "Familial" AVMs are rare; only 53 cases in 25 families have been reported.[35] A systematic review of reported cases found:[35]
1. Mean age at diagnosis: 27 years, which was younger than in patients with sporadic AVMs.
2. Patients with familial AVMs did not differ from the reference populations with respect to sex and mode of presentation.
3. In families with familial AVMs in successive generations, the age of the child at diagnosis was younger than the age of the parent at diagnosis, which suggests clinical anticipation.

Hereditary Haemorrhagic Telangiectasia

Hereditary haemorrhagic telangiectasia (aka Rendu-Osler-Weber syndrome) is group of autosomal dominant disorders of vascular structure, affecting the brain as well as the nose, skin, lungs, and gastrointestinal tract. Similar cases were independently reported by Rendu,[36] Osler,[37] and Weber[38] around the beginning of the last century.
1. Diagnosis is based on four primary clinical features:[39]
   (a) Spontaneous recurrent nosebleeds
   (b) Muco-cutaneous telangiectasia
   (c) Visceral involvement
   (d) An affected first-degree relative
      • *Definite*: three criteria are present
      • *Suspected*: two criteria are present
      • *Unlikely*: one criterion is present
2. Epidemiology
   (a) Prevalence is 1 in 5,000–8,000.[40–42]
   (b) Men and women are affected equally.[43]
   (c) Wide distribution across ethnic groups but Caucasians appear to be affected primarily.[43]
3. Clinical features
   a) Central nervous system
      • Cerebrovascular abnormalities associated with Rendu-Osler-Weber syndrome include AVMs, telangiectasias, cavernous malformations, and aneurysms.[44,45]
         – An MRI screening study found a prevalence of cerebrovascular lesions of 23%[46]
      • AVMs are the most common vascular lesions. Intracranial or spinal AVMs are present in some 10–15% of patients.[43,47–49]
         – The presence of pulmonary AVMs is a risk factor for having brain AVMs.[48]
         – Brain AVMs are mostly low-grade (Spetzler–Martin Grade I or II) and are frequently multiple.[34,48]
      • The incidence of haemorrhage in patients with an AVM and Rendu-Osler-Weber syndrome is comparable to (or less than) the incidence in the non-Rendu-Osler-Weber population, although haemorrhage is six times more common among women.[48,49]

- Cerebral ischaemic events and brain abscesses may be attributable to right-to-left shunting due to pulmonary AVMs.[50]
- *Screening* for brain AVMs in patients with Rendu-Osler-Weber syndrome is recommended by some authors.[47,49,51]
  - CTA is not optimal for screening due to false negative results.[48]
  (b) Epistaxis
  - Spontaneous epistaxis from telangiectasias of the nasal mucosa is the most common clinical manifestation; in 80% of cases epistaxis is the first clinical symptom of the disease.[52]
  - More than 50% of patients have recurrent epistaxis before the age of 20.[53]
  - Epistaxis occurs in a biphasic 24-h pattern, with a primary peak in the morning and a smaller second peak in the evening.[54]
  (c) Skin
  - Cutaneous and mucocutaneous telangiectasias are present in 50–80% of cases.[43]
  (d) Lungs
  - Pulmonary AVMs are present in 14–33% of patients.[47,55,56]
  - Embolization to the brain is a risk of endovascular treatment of pulmonary AVMs.[57]
  (e) GI tract
  - Recurrent gastrointestinal haemorrhage occurs in a minority of cases.[43]
4. Pathophysiology
  a) The initial morphologic change of hereditary haemorrhagic telangiectasia consists of focal dilatations of postcapillary venules accompanied by a diminishing capillary network.[43,58] As the venules enlarge over time, they become tortuous and connected to enlarging arterioles, eventually forming direct arteriovenous fistulae.
5. Genetics
  (a) Autosomal dominant.
  (b) Affected patients are heterozygous; homozygous forms are lethal.[59]
  (c) Two genes have been identified:
  - Endoglin (*ENG*), on chromosome 9q.[60,61]
  - Activin-receptor-like kinase (*ALK1*), on chromosome 12q.[62]

Wyburn-Mason Syndrome

Wyburn-Mason syndrome (aka unilateral retinocephalic vascular malformation or Bonnet-Dechaume-Blanc syndrome) is a rare condition characterized by the presence of AVMs in the brain and retina. Roger Wyburn-Mason published the first English language analysis of this syndrome in London in 1943.[63] Théron and colleagues published an analysis of 25 cases.[64]
1. Wyburn-Mason syndrome is congenital, nonhereditary, and without sex or race predilection.
2. The initial diagnosis of the syndrome is usually made when a retinal AVM is detected.
3. The associated intracranial vascular lesion is unilateral, related to the optic pathway, and frequently involves the optic nerve, chiasm, optic tract, and basal ganglia.[64] In some cases the AVM may extend to the occipital lobe.

Sturge-Weber Syndrome

Sturge-Weber syndrome (aka encephalotrigeminal angiomatosis) is a neurocutaneous disorder. Patients typically present with angiomas involving the leptomeninges, retina, and the dermatomes (port wine stains) of the face. The leptomeningeal venous angioma consists of numerous small tortuous, thin-walled vessels lying in the pia and adjacent hemisphere, typically in the posterior parietal and anterior occipital lobes. Associated intracranial AVMs have been reported.[65,66]

Moyamoya Syndrome Associated with AVM

Numerous case reports show that AVMs may be seen in patients with the occlusive changes in moyamoya.[67–69] The chronic ischaemia in moyamoya syndrome results in an environment of high levels of angiogenic factors to improve development of collaterals (see Chap 19). Interestingly, there have been reports of *de novo* appearance of AVMs in pediatric patients being followed with moyamoya syndrome.[70,71] The process of angiogenesis in the development of AVMs may be similar to the angiogenesis that produces the collateral vessels in moyamoya.[72] On the other hand, there has also been a report of *de novo* development of the bilateral stenotic changes of moyamoya 9 months after radiosurgery for a right temporal AVM.[73]

Natural History

Natural history data comes from numerous retrospective studies and several prospective studies. Estimates of the annual rate of haemorrhage from an AVM range from <2% to 17.8%.[28,74–79] The risk of haemorrhage from an AVM depends strongly on whether there has been a previous haemorrhage.

1. *With* a previous haemorrhage
   (a) The most commonly reported incidence of rebleeding in the first year after haemorrhage is approximately 7%.[28,75,79–82]
      - Other studies: 3.9%,[77] 10.4%,[85] 17.9%,[81] 17.8%.[78]
      - Risk decreases to baseline after 3–5 years.[75,81]
2. *Without* a previous haemorrhage
   (a) Most studies: 2–4% per year.[28,74,77,83–85]
3. Spontaneous regression
   (a) Rare. In a review of 700 cases, a total of six cases (0.9%) of angiographically documented lesions disappeared on follow-up angiograms.[86] Three of these cases occurred in patients that had undergone partial resection of the lesion.

Lifetime Risk of Haemorrhage

Assuming a constant annual risk of haemorrhage of 2–4%, the lifetime risk of haemorrhage can be estimated by the following formula:[87]

Lifetime risk = 1 – (Risk of no haemorrhage)$^{\text{Years remaining of life}}$

Alternative method. Assuming a 3% annual risk, lifetime risk can be approximated as follows:[88]

Lifetime risk (%) = 105 – The patient's age in years (Table 14.1).

Risk Factors for Haemorrhage

Risk of haemorrhage is not uniform across the population of patients with AVM,[89] and appears to vary widely according to a number of patient characteristics. *However, data about risk factors for haemorrhage must be interpreted with caution. For nearly every factor that has been associated with AVM haemorrhage, there is at least one other study that has not found a significant association.*[90]
1. Prior haemorrhage is a strong predictor of haemorrhage.[79,83,91,92]
2. AVM size – controversial
   (a) Increased bleeding risk has been associated with small AVM.[15,28,93–97]
   (b) In contrast, other studies have found a lower risk of haemorrhage for smaller AVMs[84,98] or a higher risk for large AVMs.[99]
   (c) Yet other studies have not found a relationship between size and haemorrhage risk.[74,81,84]
3. Deep venous drainage.[92,96]
4. Presence of only a single draining vein.[83,97]
5. Impaired venous drainage (i.e., venous stenosis or venous reflux).[15,100]
6. Infratentorial location.[30]
7. Deep brain location.[83,92,101]
8. Periventricular location.[102,103]
9. Presence of intracranial aneurysms.[84,103,104]
10. Presence of MCA perforator feeding vessels.[104]

Table 14.1 Life expectancy table and projected lifetime risk of AVM haemorrhage

Age interval	Average no. of years remaining[a]	Estimated lifetime risk of rupture according to annual risk of rupture[b]		
		2%	3%	4%
5–9	72.9	0.77	0.89	0.95
10–14	67.9	0.75	0.87	0.94
15–19	63.0	0.72	0.85	0.92
20–24	58.2	0.69	0.83	0.91
25–29	53.5	0.66	0.8	0.89
30–34	48.7	0.63	0.77	0.86
35–39	44	0.59	0.74	0.83
40–44	39.3	0.55	0.7	0.8
45–49	34.8	0.5	0.65	0.76
50–54	30.3	0.46	0.6	0.71
55–59	26.1	0.41	0.55	0.66
60–64	22	0.36	0.49	0.59
65–69	18.2	0.31	0.43	0.52
70–74	14.7	0.26	0.36	0.45
75–79	11.5	0.21	0.3	0.37
80–84	8.8	0.16	0.24	0.3
85–89	6.5	0.12	0.18	0.23
90–94	4.8	0.09	0.14	0.18
95–99	3.6	0.07	0.1	0.14

[a]Average number of years of life remaining for beginning of age interval. Life expectancy data obtained from the United States Department of Health and Human Services.[301]

[b]Annual rupture rates are based on studies of patients without a previous haemorrhage.[28,74,77,84] Lifetime risk of rupture was calculated using the formula 1 − (risk of no haemorrhage) years remaining of life.[87] Assumptions include a constant risk of rupture and no confounding factors

11. Presence of non-intranidal aneurysms.[76]
12. Increasing age.[27,28,74,89,92]
13. Female sex and of reproductive age.[98]
14. Hypertension.[96]
15. Hispanic ethnicity.[105]
16. A polymorphism in the inflammatory cytokine IL6 (i.e., patients homozygous for the interleukin (IL)-6-174 G allele).[106]

Outcome After Haemorrhage

The overall morbidity of AVM haemorrhage is lower than it is for intracranial haemorrhage due to other causes,[91] possibly because AVMs are thought to be congenital lesions, and the adjacent brain is adapted to the presence of the lesion.[107]
1. Mortality with haemorrhage
    (a) 5–30%[27,28,74,77,78,80–82,84,108,109]
2. Morbidity with haemorrhage
    (a) 20–30%[27,28,74,77,78,80–82,84,108,109]

Presentation

1. Haemorrhage
    (a) Most common symptom at presentation, occurring in some 53% of patients at initial diagnosis.[26]

2. Seizures
    (a) After haemorrhage, seizures are the second most common presenting symptom of intracranial AVMs, occurring in 20–25% of cases.[84,108,110]
    (b) The annual incidence of epilepsy in patients with AVMs is 1–4%.[28,74]
    (c) Lesion location in the temporal and parietal lobes is more associated with seizure disorders than in other locations.[74,111]
    (d) Seizures associated with parietal lobe AVMs are typically focal, whereas seizures due to frontal lobe AVMs are frequently generalized.[108]
3. Headaches
    (a) Headache complaints are more common among patients with AVMs than the general population,[112] suggesting that unruptured AVMs may cause headaches.
    (b) Various reports have described an association between AVMs and migraine and other headache syndromes.[112–114]
4. Developmental learning disorders
    (a) Patients with AVMs are more likely to have developmental learning disorders than patients with other intracranial disorders, even many years prior to the diagnosis of the AVM.[115] This may be due to subtle injury to the brain by the AVM, displacement of functional tissue by the AVM, or steal phenomenon.

Special Section: Cerebral Proliferative Angiopathy

This important clinical entity (aka diffuse cerebral angiomatosis[116] or diffuse AVM)[117] was termed cerebral proliferative angiopathy (CPA) by Lasjaunias and colleagues in *Stroke* in 2008.[118] CPA (Fig. 14.2) is a vascular malformation that can be confused with a brain AVM, but has several important features that distinguish it from classic brain AVMs. These lesions comprise some 3.4% of brain AVMs.[118] The existing literature on the topic consists mostly of Lasjaunias' series of 49 patients and several case reports.[119–121]

1) Features that distinguish cerebral proliferative angiopathy from brain AVMs:[118]
    a) Large size (usually lobar or hemispheric)
    b) Absence of dominant feeders or flow-related aneurysms
    c) Presence of transdural supply (which is unusual in classic brain AVMs)
    d) Presence of proximal stenosis on feeding arteries
    e) Absence of large, early-draining veins
    f) Normal brain tissue is intermingled between the vessels
2) Epidemiology and presentation
    a) Some 67% of patients are female (compared to 48% of patients with brain AVMs)
    b) Mean age at diagnosis: 22 years
    c) Presenting symptom:
        i) Seizures (45%)
        ii) Severe headaches (41%)
        iii) Haemorrhage (12%)
        iv) Stroke, TIA or other neurological deficit (16%)
    d) Associated with haemangioma of the face and tongue.[120]
3) Pathophysiology
    a) Unlike brain AVMs, CPA vessels appear to be proliferative, which may be a response to cerebral ischaemia. Angiogenesis and neovascularization is evidenced by meningeal arterial involvement,[122] which is not typical of brain AVMs. Perfusion-weighted imaging has demonstrated evidence of cortical ischaemia,[123] and stenosis of feeding vessels is present in 39% of cases.[118] Taken together, the evidence suggests that cerebral ischaemia may drive the formation of CPA lesions.
4) Imaging
    a) CPA lesions tend to be large and diffuse, with normal brain parenchyma intermingled with the vascular elements.
    b) Catheter angiography should include imaging of the external carotid arteries because of the frequent presence of meningeal feeders.
    c) Draining veins are not conspicuous and early draining veins are usually not present.

5) Management
   a) Treatment with surgery, radiosurgery, and embolization is problematic because of the large size of CPA lesions and the presence of normal brain tissue among the vessels.
      i) Selective embolization of "fragile areas" in patients presenting with haemorrhage has been advocated.[124]
   b) Burr hole encephalodurosynangiosis procedures provided improvement in headaches in two patients in Lasjaunias' series.[118]
   c) For patients presenting with seizures without haemorrhage, treatment limited to medical anticonvulsant therapy may be the most prudent option.

Imaging

1. CT/CTA
   (a) CT is still the best imaging technique to check for an acute haemorrhage.
   (b) A noncontrast CT of an unruptured AVM may appear normal; sensitivity can be increased by using IV contrast or doing a CTA.
      CT findings with AVMs:
      – Heightened vascularity.
      – Serpentine, enlarged veins.
      – In some cases, perilesional atrophy and/or hydrocephalus.
   (c) CTA: AVMs are typically best seen on MIP images.
2. MRI
   (a) More sensitive than CT in identifying subtle lesions.
   (b) Permits precise anatomic localization of lesions.
   (c) Detection of associated aneurysms is limited, particularly intranidal aneurysms and aneurysms <5 mm in size.[125,126]
3. Angiography
   (a) Catheter angiography provides information about AVMs that is superior to complimentary compared to other imaging techniques. Advantages include:
      • Greater sensitivity.
      • Able to clarify anatomy of feeding vessels and draining veins (e.g., distinguishes between ACA and MCA contributions to a cerebral convexity lesion).
      • Best imaging technique to identify intranidal aneurysms.
      • Able to determine arteriovenous transit times.
   b) Angiography remains the gold standard for the evaluation of AVMs, and the authors of this handbook believe that it should be considered for every patient with an intracranial AVM, or an intracerebral haemorrhage that may be due to an AVM.
      • *Yield of angiography* in patients with spontaneous ICH (i.e., the chance of finding an underlying vascular abnormality:[127]
         – Patients age ≤45 years: 50%
         – Patients age >45 years: 18%
         – Patients without a history of hypertension: 44%
         – Patients with a history of hypertension: 9%
   (c) *Complications*: A systematic review found that the risk of complications of angiography in patients with AVMs (0.3–0.8%) is significantly lower than for patients being evaluated for TIA or stroke (3.0–3.7%).[128]

Special Section: AVM mimics

A number of cerebrovascular lesions can masquerade as brain AVMs on imaging (Figs. 14.1, 14.2, 14.3, and 14.4).

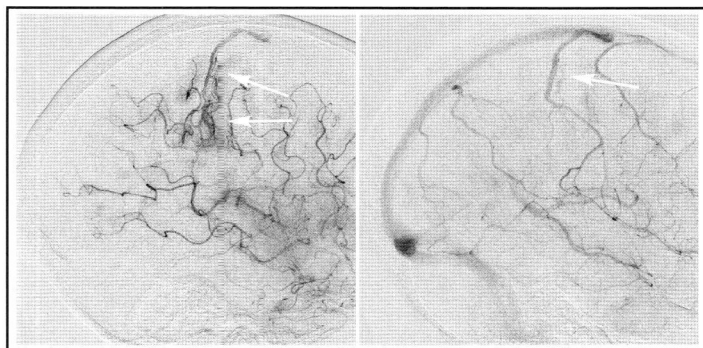

Fig. 14.1 Ischaemic stroke with arteriovenous shunting. This patient had an embolic stroke. Several days after the event, the arterial phase angiogram shows heightened vascularity and an early draining vein in the affected territory (*arrows, right*). The venous phase angiogram shows the early-appearing vein to be a normal cortical vein (*arrow, left*).

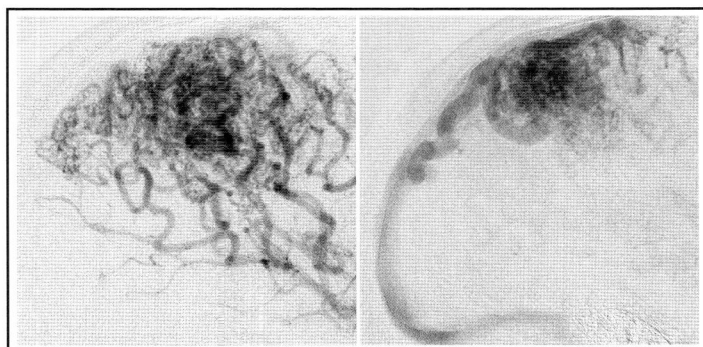

Fig. 14.2 Cerebral proliferative angiopathy.[118] Seventeen year old boy who presented with a seizure. Note the typical features of cerebral proliferative angiopathy that distinguish it from an AVM, such as large, diffuse nidus and absence of early draining veins. Lateral view, right parietal area, arterial phase (*left*) and venous phase (*right*).

14.3.   Management

Management options for patients with an AVM are
1. Expectant management
2. Surgery
3. Radiosurgery

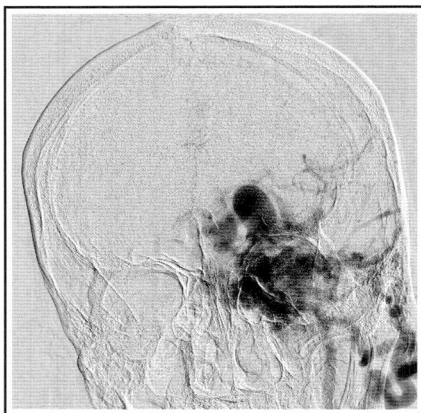

Fig. 14.3 Intracranial dural arteriovenous fistula. This patient, with a large Borden 3 left transverse/sigmoid sinus dAVF, was originally misdiagnosed as having a brain AVM. Frontal view with injection into the left CCA.

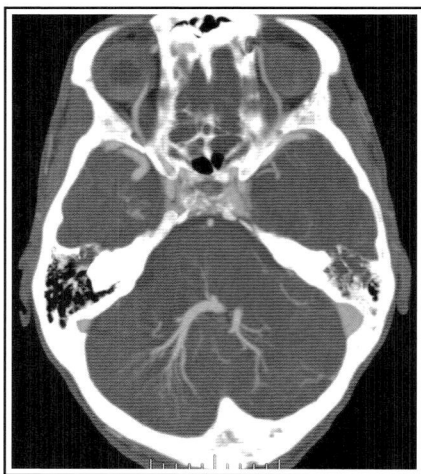

Fig. 14.4 Large developmental venous anomaly. This patient, with a large posterior fossa DVA, was originally misdiagnosed as having a brain AVM. Axial MIP image from a CTA.

4. Embolization
5. A combination of embolization, radiosurgery, and/or surgery

Obviously, AVMs and patients with them vary greatly, and so the management strategy for any given patient must be highly individualized. Mainstream thinking presently favours surgery or radiosurgery for most patients;[129] embolization is usually most useful as a preparatory step prior to surgery or radiosurgery. Conservative management is gaining favour for large or difficult-to-treat lesions, and for patients at high risk of complications.[130]

Table 14.2 Spetzler–Martin scale

Lesion characteristic		Number of points
Size	Small (<3 cm)	1
	Medium (3–6 cm)	2
	Large (>6 cm)	3
Location	Non-eloquent site	0
	Eloquent site (sensorimotor, language, or visual cortex; hypothalamus or thalamus; internal capsule; brainstem; cerebellar peduncles, or cerebellum)	1
Pattern of venous drainage	Superficial only	0
	Any deep	1

From Spetzler and Martin,[31] with permission
This grading system was developed to predict surgical risk, not prognosis. Size indicates maximum diameter

Expectant Management

Non-surgical and non-interventional management of some patients with AVMs is appropriate. Some authors, considering the natural history of asymptomatic AVMs and the relative low morbidity associated with haemorrhage of some lesions, argue against the routine treatment of asymptomatic lesions.[131] An ongoing NIH-sponsored multi-center study, A Randomized Trial of Unruptured Brain Arteriovenous Malformations (ARUBA), is comparing treatment of unruptured lesions with conservative management (http://www.arubastudy.org).[132] Large AVMs may also warrant conservative management, considering the difficulty and morbidity of treatment.

Surgery

Surgical resection of brain AVMs is the "gold standard" for the treatment of small, accessible lesions.[129,133,134] Decision making in most cases begins with stratification according to the Spetzler–Martin grading system (Table 14.2), which is currently the most commonly used system. A decision analysis model suggested that surgical resection of small, asymptomatic AVMs, assuming a risk of major neurological morbidity and mortality <6.8%, offers the greatest overall quality of life over time compared to observation or radiosurgery.[135]

Surgical Outcomes

1. Obliteration rates.
   (a) Spetzler–Martin grades I–III: 94–100%.[136–142]
       Grades I–III lesions account for ~60–80% of AVMs.[136,143]
   (b) Spetzler–Martin grades IV–V: There is a paucity of data on angiographic obliteration rates after surgery for high grade AVMs, partly because multimodality treatment strategies are frequently used. Separate discussions of *Large AVMs* and *Multimodality Treatment* appear below.
   (c) For a discussion of surgery compared to radiosurgery, see below.
2. Complications. A systematic review of 25 reports, including 2,425 patients, found an overall rate of post-operative mortality of 3.3% and permanent morbidity of 8.6%.[142]
   (a) Spetzler–Martin grades I—III:
       • Permanent morbidity 0–5%.[137,139–141,144]
       • Mortality 0–3.9%.[137,141,144,145]
   (b) Spetzler–Martin grades IV–V:
       • Morbidity 12.2–21.9%.[136,138]
       • Mortality 11.1–38.4%.[136,145]
3. Effects on patients with seizures
   (a) After surgery, 43.6–81% of patients with a history of seizures are seizure-free.[136,146,147]

Surgery: Practical Issues

1. *Timing of surgery*. AVMs do not carry the same high rehaemorrhage risk that ruptured aneurysms do; therefore, timing of surgery depends on several factors other than rehaemorrhage risk. Most authors recommend that surgery be done on an elective basis,[129,148,149] days to weeks after the ictus, to allow the patient to recover from the initial event and to allow the clot to liquefy. Others advocate earlier surgery in most cases.[150]
   (a) *Early surgery* is indicated when
       • The clot has significant mass effect and the patient will benefit from evacuation of the hematoma.
       • The lesion is surgically accessible.
   (b) *Late surgery* (several weeks or more after the haemorrhage) is indicated when:
       • The clot burden is relatively low.
       • The patient is relatively poor surgical candidate soon after the initial haemorrhage.
       • Imaging studies do not show the AVM clearly, and a delayed, detailed angiogram may show the lesion more clearly.
2. *Surgery combined with embolization or radiosurgery*. See the sections below on *Radiosurgery* and *Embolization*.
3. *Intraoperative and postoperative angiography*: Either intraoperative or postoperative angiography is *always* indicated, to ensure complete obliteration of the lesion.
   (a) *Intraoperative angiography*
       • Advantages: Allows for detection, and removal, of residual AVM during the operation.
       • Disadvantages: Adds time to the operation; angiography in the OR is usually lower-quality than biplane angiography in a dedicated neuro-angio suite.
       • Results: A review of published reports of intraoperative angiography found that the results of the intraoperative angiogram altered the management of the case in an average of 15% of the time (range: 5.6–57%).[151]
           – When the intraoperative angiogram was compared to a post-op angiogram, a false negative result was found in 4.4% cases, and a false positive result occurred in 1.7% of cases.[151]
           – The reported technical failure rate was 2.5% and the complication rate was 3.1%.[151]
   (b) *Post-op angiography*
       • Results: In a series of 324 patients undergoing post-op angiography craniotomy for AVM resection, 1.8% were found to have residual lesions.[152]
4. *Surgical complications*
   (a) *Seizures*
       • New-onset seizures occur in 6.5–22% of patients after AVM treatment.[153]
           – Some authors recommend routine antiseizure prophylaxis for patients undergoing AVM surgery.[134 154]
   (b) *Cerebral oedema*
       • Perioperative cerebral oedema occurs in ≤3% of cases[136,155–158] and may first occur in the operating room or up to 11 days after surgery.[155] Cerebral oedema may occur after AVM surgery or embolization.[159]
       • Post-treatment cerebral oedema is believed to be attributable in most cases to (1) *normal perfusion pressure breakthrough* or (2) *occlusive hyperaemia*.
           – *Normal perfusion pressure breakthrough*.[160] This theory maintains that the tissue around an AVM is subject to chronic steal because of diversion of flow into the AVM, resulting in sustained dilation and loss of autoregulation. Presumably, in some cases the vessels in this tissue are unable to autoregulate when normal perfusion is reestablished after resection of the AVM, resulting in oedema and haemorrhage.
           – *Occlusive hyperaemia*.[155,159] According to this theory, brain oedema after AVM resection is due to obstruction of venous outflow, with associated vascular engorgement, and to sluggish flow in former arterial feeders with subsequent hypoperfusion and ischaemia.

Management
- Standard measures to control cerebral oedema in this setting include:[161]
  (a) Head CT to exclude haemorrhage (*obviously*).
  (b) The head and neck should be maintained in a neutral position to minimize jugular vein compression and obstruction of CSF outflow.
  (c) IV mannitol.
  (d) Ventriculostomy.
  (e) Intubation and mechanical ventilation if the patient's neurological status is diminished; judicious hyperventilation may be helpful, as cerebrovascular reactivity to CO_2 remains intact after AVM resection.[162,163]
  (f) Decompressive craniectomy (or removal of the bone flap).
  (g) High-dose barbiturate anesthesia.

(c) *Rehaemorrhage*
  • Overall incidence of early rehaemorrhage after surgery (≤1 week) is 2%.[164] Risk factors for rehaemorrhage include higher grade AVMs and the presence of lenticulostriate feeders.[164]
  • Often attributable to residual AVM.
  • Aggressive post-operative blood pressure control can minimize risk of rehaemorrhage.

(d) *Vasospasm*
  • Symptomatic vasospasm, attributable to extensive dissection and exposure of major intracranial arteries, occurs in <1% of cases.[7]

(e) *Intracranial thrombosis*
  • Retrograde thrombosis of an arterial feeder, with recanalization of the vessel with IA urokinase, has been reported.[165]
  • Delayed venous thrombosis and infarction after AVM resection has also been reported.[166]

Radiosurgery

Radiosurgery involves the administration of multiple beams of radiation; each beam is delivered from a different direction, and all beams converge on the target, or isocenter. The radiation dose in the isocenter is high but the radiation dose received by non-targeted structures is relatively low. Advantages of radiosurgery are that it is minimally invasive, relatively low-risk, and useful for treatment of surgically inaccessible lesions. Disadvantages include a latency period (usually 2–3 years) until AVM obliteration occurs, and that it is most effective for smaller lesions.

Radiosurgery Techniques

1. Gamma knife.
   (a) Most widely used platform for AVM radiosurgery.
   (b) Two hundred and one gamma ray beams from cobalt-60 sources pass through holes (collimators) in a helmet and converge on the isocenter. Dosing is controlled by determining the size of the collimators and the exposure time.[167]
2. Linear accelerator (LINAC).
   (a) LINACs use microwaves to accelerate electrons that then collide with a target to generate high energy photons. The LINAC is mounted on a gantry that rotates through an arc and concentrates radiation energy on the isocenter. Dosing is controlled by using multiple intersecting arcs and beam weight adjustment. Current LINAC devices include Novalis® (BrainLAB, Helmstetten, Germany), X-Knife™ (Radionics, Burlington MA), Trilogy™ (Varian Medical Systems, Palo Alto, CA), and CyberKnife® (Accuray, Sunnyvale, CA).
3. Particle beam.
   (a) Charged particles are delivered rather than photons. The theoretical advantage of particle beam treatment over photon beam radiosurgery is that the energy deposition is more concentrated (and tissue exposure

outside of the target is lessened) due to the Bragg peak effect. Another theoretical advantage is that the relative biological effectiveness is higher compared to other techniques. Both protons and helium nuclei have been used to treat AVMs.[168,169] Disadvantage is that particle beam radiosurgery requires a relatively expensive cyclotron or synchrotron.

Mechanism of AVM Obliteration in Radiosurgery

The earliest and primary effect of radiosurgery is damage to AVM endothelial cells. Progressive occlusion of the vessel lumen occurs during a sequence of events that is similar to wound healing.[170] Endothelial damage induces the proliferation of smooth muscle cells and myofibroblasts and an accumulation of extracellular collagen, causing stenosis and occlusion of the nidus.[170,171] A chronic inflammatory response also contributes to the formation of granulation tissue in the region of the AVM.

Radiosurgery Outcomes

1. Obliteration rates. Rates of angiographic cure depend primarily on lesion size. Most of the following results are at 2–5 year follow-up.
    (a) Lesion diameter ≤3 cm: 75–95%[146,168,172–177]
    (b) Lesion diameter ≥3 cm: ≤70%[174,176]
    (c) Brainstem AVMs. These lesions represent a special case because of the high morbidity of rupture and because of the need for excellent three-dimension dose conformality, to minimize injury to adjacent vital structures. In a recent series of 44 patients with brainstem AVMs treated with radiosurgery, the obliteration rate was 52% at 5 years; disease-specific survival was 86% at 10 years after treatment.[178]
2. Effect on haemorrhage risk
    (a) Risk of haemorrhage persists during the latency period between radiosurgery and AVM obliteration, but may be reduced compared to the risk of haemorrhage prior to radiosurgery.[179] One study found the annual risk of haemorrhage during the 2-year latency period to be 4.8%;[180] more recent studies found annual risk of haemorrhage after radiosurgery to be 1.8–2.8%.[83,181]
    (b) The presence of an unsecured proximal aneurysm is associated with an increased risk of haemorrhage during the latency period.[180]
    (c) Even with complete angiographic obliteration, the risk of haemorrhage may not be zero; Shin and colleagues estimated the risk of rebleeding after complete nidus obliteration to be 0.3% per year.[182]
3. Effect on patients with seizures
    (a) Radiosurgery can be effective in patients with seizures attributable to an AVM. Seizure-free rates after radiosurgery are 51–80%.[183–186]
4. Complications. Pooled data from 1,255 patients:[187]
    (a) Overall rate of neurological complications (transient or permanent neurologic deficits): 8%
    (b) Permanent neurologic deficits: 4.8%
    (c) Complications:
        • Radiation injury to brain parenchyma (6.4%)
        • Cranial nerve injury (1%)
        • New or worsened seizures (0.8%)
        • Death (0.2%)

Radiosurgery: Practical Issues

1) Dosing and treatment strategy
    a) Dose
        i) The applied radiation dose is inversely proportional to the irradiated volume. To determine the dose of radiation, a dose/volume curve is used.
        ii) Dose–response studies have found meaningful responses up to 25 Gy.[188] Above this point, there is minimal incremental increase in obliteration rates but a significant increase in complications.

iii) The volume of tissue that receives 12 Gy (the 12 Gy volume) correlates with complications of radiation treatment.[189–191] Lower success rates for treatment of large AVMs with radiosurgery are believed to be due to lower doses used for those cases in an effort to minimize the 12 Gy volume.[192]

b) Fractionation
  i) Fractionation (e.g., two or more separate target volumes are planned, with the treatments separated in time) has been used for large AVMs.
    (1) A hypofractionation scheme (dose of 25–30 Gy in 5–6 daily fractions) used for large AVMs (>5 cm) resulted in a reduction of AVM volume by 44% per year.[193]

2) Complication management
  a) Transient brain oedema is a source of headaches and neurologic deficits in some patients after radiosurgery. Some operators use low-dose oral dexamethasone therapy for 2 weeks after treatment.[174] Delayed symptoms attributable to brain oedema usually respond to a short course (2–3 days) of IV dexamethasone.

3) Follow-up imaging
  a) Follow-up catheter angiography is necessary in all patients 2–3 years after radiosurgery for an AVM, because of the significant (5–25%) chance of residual and because complete lesion obliteration is necessary to minimize haemorrhage risk.[194]

4) Repeat radiosurgery
  a) When complete obliteration of the lesion is not obtained within 3 years after treatment, repeat radiosurgery is an option. Repeat radiosurgery is associated with a 62–70% chance of cure.[193,195–197]

Surgery Compared to Radiosurgery

Several reports have compared surgery to radiosurgery, with the expected results. Surgery is associated with a higher cure rate with a lower rehaemorrhage risk, while radiosurgery is less morbid.

1. Pikus and colleagues compared a surgical series to published radiosurgery reports and found advantages in surgery in terms of angiographic cure rates and rehaemorrhage risk, although surgery had a significantly higher rate of neurological complications.[139]

2. Nataf and coworkers compared two series of patients with lesions that were considered equally suitable for treatment by surgery or radiosurgery.[198] Although the rate of cure was similar for both groups of patients, neurological morbidity was higher after surgery and recurrent bleeding was more frequent after radiosurgery.

Embolization

A Brief History of Embolization of Intracranial AVMs

The first report of embolization of a brain AVM appeared in 1960.[199] A patient with a large left Sylvian fissure AVM underwent surgical exposure of the cervical carotid artery, and four spheres of methyl methacrylate, measuring between 2.5 and 4.2 mm in diameter, were embolized into the lesion. Angiography showed near total occlusion of the lesion and good filling of normal vessels. This technique evolved into a strictly endovascular process with placement of a large-bore catheter in the femoral artery.[200] The spheres were then injected one-by-one through the catheter into the cerebral circulation. The appearance of the spheres traveling through the vessels on fluoroscopy was strangely fascinating, and can be compared to watching a pinball at an arcade. An element of chance was always involved, and one could never be certain where they would land. Still, because of preferential flow to the AVM, most would end up in the feeding arteries to the lesion.

Limited further progress was made with AVM embolization during the 1960s, largely because of the absence of useful catheters and embolic agents. Flow-directed particulate embolization,[201] balloon embolization,[202] and delivery of embolic material through a punctured microballoon (the "calibrated leak balloon" technique)[203,204] were reported in the 1970s.

An array of embolic agents were used in the 1970s and early 1980s, including silk threads, alcohol, polyvinyl alcohol (PVA) and isobutyl-2-cyanoacrylate (i-BCA). Reports of toxicity and carcinogenicity with i-BCA in animal studies[205,206] led to the withdrawal of this material from the market and the introduction of N-butyl-2-cyanoacrylate (n-BCA).[207]

Advancements in catheter design in the 1980s permitted selective catheterization of AVM pedicles. The introduction of the flow-directed Magic catheter was a major breakthrough.[208] With the additional availability of 0.010-in. wires and the addition of hydrophilic coating to the catheters, intranidal catheterization was possible.[209]

During the 1990s, n-BCA and polyvinyl alcohol emerged as the most popular embolization materials for AVMs. FDA approval of n-BCA (Trufill, Codman Neurovascular, Raynham, MA), was granted in 2000. While the principal advantage of n-BCA is its resistance to recanalization, compared to PVA (which is prone to recanalization),[210] the adhesive properties of n-BCA require great care during injection to minimize the risk of catheter retention. A randomized trial comparing n-BCA to PVA for preoperative embolization of AVMS found no difference and also that the two agents were equivalent in terms of percentage of nidus reduction and number of feeding pedicles embolized.[211] Interestingly, although the overall rates of procedural complications were similar in both groups, patients treated with PVA had a significantly higher rate of post-resection haemorrhage compared to patients treated with n-BCA (17.8% vs. 4.8%).

Ethylene vinyl alcohol copolymer in dimethyl sulfoxide solution (Onyx, Micro Therapeutics, Inc., Irvine, CA) was introduced in 1990. Although Onyx was originally conceived of as an embolic agent for intracranial aneurysms, somewhat disappointing results in a North American randomized trial of the material for aneurysms[212] were followed by encouraging initial results with the use of the agent for the treatment of AVMs.[213] Onyx received FDA approval for presurgical embolization of AVMs in 2005.

Embolization Results

AVM embolization techniques and strategies are discussed in detail in Chap. 7, *Intracranial Embolization*.
1) Cure rates
   a) Complete AVM obliteration has been reported in some 5–10% of cases.[214–219]
   b) The relatively low cure rate with embolization alone is probably due to the fact that only a minority of AVMs have a single pedicle, or several pedicles, that can be safely catheterized.
2) Palliation
   a) Embolization to improve symptoms attributable to "steal phenomenon" has been reported.[220,221]
3) Embolization combined with surgery or radiosurgery (or both). Numerous reports of presurgical[31,136,214,215,222–227] and pre-radiosurgical[210,217,228–230] embolization have been published.
   a) Pre-surgery embolization.
      i) The goals of pre-surgery embolization are to reduce the volume of the nidus and to occlude deep and difficult-to-reach feeders when possible.
      ii) Embolization has been reported to shorten operative time and blood loss.[31,136,214,215,222–227,231]
      iii) In a series comparing AVM surgery patients with presurgical embolization to those without it, complication rates and the proportion of patients with good or excellent outcomes were similar in both groups, despite the fact that the embolization group had higher grade lesions.[222]
      iv) Vinuela and colleagues suggested that occlusion of >75% of the AVM nidus facilitates surgical resection, while elimination of <50% does little to facilitate surgery.[232]

Table 14.3 Estimation of AVM volume based on diameter[a]

Diameter (cm)	Volume (cm³)
1	0.51
2	4.19
3	14.14
4	33.51
5	65.45
6	113.09

[a]Assumes that the lesion is a sphere: volume = $(4/3)\pi r^3$

b) Pre-radiosurgery embolization
   i) Controversial! Embolization prior to radiosurgery may reduce the effectiveness of radiosurgery
   ii) The aim of pre-radiosurgery embolization is to reduce the volume of the nidus.
   iii) Older reports indicated improved rates of AVM obliteration have been found when the volume is reduced with embolization to <10 cm.[3,210,217] Volume – diameter relationships are listed in Table 14.3.
   iv) However, more recent data from multiple centers suggests that embolization before radiosurgery reduces the obliteration rate of AVMs[233–235]
      (1) Possible mechanisms:
         (a) Radio-opaque embolic material may reduce the delivered radiation dose.[236]
            (i) On the other hand, an *in-vitro* study calculating dose in the presence of either glue or Onyx showed <0.01 – 0.2% reduction in dose to the AVM when using the high-energy cobalt source.[237]
         (b) Embolization may increase angiogenic activity of AVM tissue by inducing local hypoxia.[238,239]
         (c) When using non-adhesive agents, recanalization of occluded vessels may occur.
4) Complications. A systematic review of 25 reports, including 2,425 patients, found an overall rate of permanent morbidity associated with pre-surgical embolization of 4–8.9%.[142]
   a) Overall permanent morbidity: 2–14%.[211,218,219,223,231,240,241]
   b) Mortality: 1.2–3.7%.[211,218,219,223,231,240,241]

Specific Considerations

Associated Aneurysms

Most reports indicate that intracranial aneurysms are found in some 15–25% of patients with AVMs.[242,243] One study of superselective angiography reported an incidence of associated aneurysms of 58%.[103]
1. Classification and incidence of AVM-associated aneurysms
   (a) Feeding artery aneurysms
      • Attributable to wall-shear stress caused by high flow through AVM feeding arteries.
      • Incidence: 11.2–17%.[242,243]
         – Approximately twice as common as intranidal aneurysms.[242,243]
   (b) Intranidal aneurysms
      • True intranidal aneurysms
         – True aneurysms in the AVM nidus can be distinguished from venous varices by their early appearance during the arterial phase on angiography.[244]
         – Incidence: 5.5–8%.[242,243]
         Intranidal *pseudoaneurysms*
            – Uncommon lesions that can only be firmly diagnosed by histopathology. An intranidal pseudoaneurysm

may be identified as a new finding on a follow-up angiogram.[245] Found in 8% of angiograms of patients with an AVM.[245] Differentiation between true- and pseudo-intranidal aneurysms is academic and has no therapeutic implications.[246]

(c) Incidental aneurysms
  • Aneurysms not related to the AVM seem to occur in AVM patients at about the same rate as aneurysms in the general population (0.8%).[212]

2. Risk of haemorrhage
  (a) Patients with an AVM and an associated aneurysm (feeding artery *or* intranidal) are at increased risk of haemorrhage compared to patients with an AVM only.[243]
    • Annual risk of haemorrhage: 7%.[76]
  (b) Feeding artery aneurysm
    • Presence of a feeding artery aneurysm is an independent risk factor for haemorrhage in AVM patients, although only 6% of the attributable risk is due to the aneurysm (i.e., only 6% of haemorrhages could be prevented by eliminating the feeding artery aneurysm).[243]
  (c) Intranidal aneurysm
    • Annual risk of haemorrhage 9.8%.[242]

3. Management
  (a) No consensus exists for the management of associated aneurysms. Some authors advocate treatment of the aneurysm first,[247–249] whereas others recommend treatment of the AVM first,[242] or treatment of both lesions simultaneously.[250–252]
  (b) Effect of AVM treatment on feeding vessel aneurysms:
    • Some feeding vessel aneurysms may regress with treatment of the AVM. In a report of 23 AVMs with feeding vessel aneurysms, 18 were unchanged after treatment, four were smaller, and 1 disappeared completely.[242]
    • Feeding vessel aneurysm rupture has been reported immediately after AVM resection[248] or within 3 weeks after AVM treatment.[247]
    • The presence of an unsecured proximal aneurysm is a risk factor for post-radiosurgery haemorrhage.[180]
  (c) The authors of this handbook recommend the following strategy:
    • For patients who present with haemorrhage, treat the lesion that caused the haemorrhage first (*obviously*).
    • For patients who present without haemorrhage, treat the feeding vessel or intranidal aneurysm first, if feasible.

Large and Giant AVMs

Large AVMs are variously defined as Spetzler–Martin IV–V lesions, or lesions with a diameter >3 cm or volume >10–15 cm³. Giant AVMs are lesions with a diameter >6 cm. These AVMs are problematic because they are difficult to treat and the natural history is murky. *Important! Large AVMs must be distinguished from cerebral proliferative angiopathy lesions (see above).*

1) Natural history
  (a) Natural history studies have reported widely divergent haemorrhage rates for patients with Grade IV and V AVMs.
    • One retrospective study found an annual haemorrhage risk of 1.5%,[253] while another found an annual pretreatment haemorrhage rate of 10.4% for all patients (13.9% for patients presenting with haemorrhage and 7.3% for patients without haemorrhage at presentation).[254]
    • A prospective study of 301 patients with AVMs found that lesion diameter >3 cm was an independent risk factor for haemorrhage (odds ratio 2.5, $P < 0.0001$).[99]
  (b) Although some evidence has suggested that larger AVMs may be at a lower risk of haemorrhage than smaller lesions,[15,28,74,93–97] estimates of higher risk for larger AVMs,[99,254] seem plausible, given that larger lesions are more likely to contain other anatomic features, aside from size, that are established risk factors for haemorrhage, such as deep location or deep venous drainage.[254]

2. Surgery
   (a) Morbidity and mortality with surgery of Grade IV–V lesions runs as high as 21.9 and 38.4%, respectively.[136,145]
3. Radiosurgery
   (a) Complete obliteration rates for large AVMs with single-treatment radiosurgery are very low.[255–257]
      - Obliteration rates for AVMs ≥ 15 cm^3 are 25%.[256,257]
      - A study of staged volume radiosurgery for AVMs >15 cm^3 reported obliteration in 50% of cases.[258] In these cases, two or three separate anatomic compartments were irradiated at a 3- to 8-month intervals. Fourteen percent of patients had a haemorrhage after radiosurgery, 14% developed peri-AVM imaging changes requiring steroid treatment, and neurological worsening occurred in 4%.
4. Effects of partial treatment
   (a) Most authors agree that maximal protection against haemorrhage risk is obtained only with complete obliteration of the lesion.
   (b) Han and colleagues found an increased annual risk of haemorrhage with partial treatment, compared to no treatment (10.4% vs. 1.5%).[253]
   (c) Conversely, Meisel and coworkers found a decreased risk of haemorrhage with partial embolization.[240]
5. Multimodality strategies
   (a) A combination of embolization, radiosurgery, and surgery may be effective in some cases.
   (b) In a series of 53 patients with giant (>6 cm) AVMs undergoing multimodality treatment, 36% were completely cured of the AVM.[259] The patients were treated with surgery (51%), embolization (98%), and/or radiosurgery (89%). Long-term treatment-related morbidity was 15%. At a mean follow-up of 37 months, clinical results were excellent in 51%, good in 28%, poor in 6%, and 15% were dead.
6. Management recommendations
   (a) No consensus exists for the management of large AVMs. Some prominent authors have recently recommended conservative management in most patients,[253,260] while others have advocated treatment, particularly of patients who present with haemorrhage.[254]
   (b) "Palliative" treatment does not appear to reduce the risk of haemorrhage (and may actually increase it); therefore, any treatment of large AVMs should be directed toward eventual obliteration of the lesion.

AVMs in Children

Pediatric patients with intracranial AVMs differ from adults in important ways: AVM recurrence after treatment is more frequent in children and prognosis after haemorrhage is better.
1. Prevalence of AVMs among children
   (a) About 10–20% of newly diagnosed brain AVMs are in children.[261,262]
   (b) Overall prevalence in children is 0.014–0.028%.[263]
2. Risk of haemorrhage
   (a) Although anecdotal reports have suggested that children are at higher risk of haemorrhage from AVMs than adults, a recent study found the annual risk of haemorrhage for children (age <20) and adults to be similar, 2.0 and 2.2%, respectively.[85]
3. Presentation
   (a) Up to 75% of children with AVMs present with haemorrhage, and 15% present with seizures.[261]
4. Haemorrhage
   (a) Any child with a spontaneous intracranial haemorrhage should be presumed to have an underlying AVM until proven otherwise.[264]
   (b) Children may be more likely than adults to present with haemorrhage
      - Haemorrhage is the presenting symptom in 63% of children and seizures are the presenting symptom in 13.4%.[265]
   (c) Outcomes after haemorrhage
      - Seventeen percent have fair or poor outcomes.[265]
      - Among pediatric AVM patients who present in a coma, mortality is 40%, however, >50% have a good functional outcome.[266]

5. Management
   (a) Surgery
      - Obliteration rates: 90–95%[265,267]
      - Complications:
         - Perioperative morbidity: 19%[265];
         - Perioperative mortality: ≤5%[265,268]
   (b) Radiosurgery
      - Obliteration rates: 68–95%.[177,269]
      - Permanent neurological complications: <3%[177,269]
6. AVM recurrence after treatment
   (a) Unlike adults, AVMs in children have a tendency to recur after treatment in a small percentage of patients.[265,270,271]
      - In a series of 808 patients who had undergone complete surgical resection of an AVM, five patients (0.6%) were found to have recurrent AVMs after negative postoperative angiography, and they were all in the pediatric age group.[270]
      - A recent series reported a recurrence rate of 5.6%.[265]
   (b) Follow-up surveillance imaging
      - Because of the possibility of recurrence, most authors recommend continued follow-up imaging in children, even after complete obliteration.[264]

Pregnancy and AVMs

1. AVM haemorrhage during pregnancy.
   (a) Relatively common cause of ICH in pregnant woman. An AVM is the cause of haemorrhage in 21–48% of ICH cases during pregnancy and the puerperium.[272–275]
   (b) Mean gestational age at time of haemorrhage is 30 weeks.[273]
   (c) Hypertension is present in 17% of pregnant patients with an AVM haemorrhage.[273]
   (d) Outcomes are worse in pregnant women compared to nonpregnant AVM patients.[276]
      - Some 57% of pregnant patients are stuperous or comatose at presentation.[273]
      - Maternal mortality rates range from 0% to 28%.[273,275,277,278]
      - Fetal mortality rate is 14%.[273]
   (e) Rehaemorrhage is more frequent in pregnant patients; 25–30% of pregnant patients rebleed during the same pregnancy.[272,275,278,279]
   (f) Neurosurgical Management
      - Given the relatively high rate of rebleeding and high morbidity associated with haemorrhage, treatment of the AVM to prevent further haemorrhage is usually prudent.
      - Most authors recommend surgery, when feasible, and that the decision to operate should be based on neurosurgical criteria.[273,274,279] Embolization may be an option for selected, small lesions that can be safely and completely obliterated with a single procedure. Radiosurgery and, in most cases, embolization are not able to quickly reduce the risk of rehaemorrhage and are not appropriate for pregnant patients.
      - Conservative management may be appropriate for cases in which surgery would be risky or difficult. Dias and Sekhar did not find a significant advantage for surgery compared with nonsurgical management in terms of maternal or fetal mortality rates.[273]
   (g) Obstetrical Management
      - The choice of delivery method should be based on obstetric rather than neurosurgical criteria, as there does not seem to be a significant advantage for either cesarean or vaginal delivery.[273]
   (h) Reasonable efforts should be taken to minimize radiation dose to the fetus during both diagnostic imaging and any interventional procedure.

2. Unruptured AVMs in pregnant patients and in women anticipating becoming pregnant.
    (a) Although pregnancy does not appear to confer an increased risk of haemorrhage in women with an AVM,[276] outcomes after haemorrhage during pregnancy are significantly worse than in nonpregnant patients.[273]
        • The risk of first haemorrhage for pregnant women with an unruptured AVM is 3.5%,[276] which is comparable to the annual risk of bleeding among all patients with an AVM.
    (b) Pregnancy should be deferred until AVM treatment is completed.
    (c) In pregnant patients with an unruptured AVM, assiduous blood pressure control may reduce the risk of haemorrhage, given that hypertension is associated with haemorrhage in this setting.[273]

14.4.   Appendix: Vein of Galen Malformations

Vein of Galen malformations are congenital abnormalities that are distinct from other intracranial vascular malformations. They have a spectrum of severity and may present at birth, during infancy, or during later childhood. They are rare, and are believed to comprise ≤1% of intracranial vascular malformations.[156] Management of these lesions is presently handled primarily by pediatric neurosurgeons and neurointerventionalists.

Angiographic Classification

Lasjaunias and colleagues divided congenital vein of Galen lesions into three types[280]:
1. Choroidal. Network of feeders, resembling a nidus, supplied primarily by the choroidal arteries.
2. Mural. One or more arterial feeders connected to a dilated vein of Galen.
3. Secondary. Enlargement of the vein of Galen due to an adjacent vascular malformation, fistula, or venous outlet obstruction.

Yasargil introduced the following classification scheme[281]:
1. Type I. Relatively few feeders, arising principally from the pericallosal and posterior cerebral arteries.
2. Type II. Feeders arise mainly from the thalamoperforators and posterior cerebral arteries.
3. Type III (aka true, or choroidal type). *Most common type.* Mixed pattern of feeders, arising from the pericallosal arteries, thalamoperforators, and posterior cerebral arteries.
4. Type IV (aka secondary type). Aneurysmal dilatation (i.e., varix) of the vein of Galen resulting from shunting from adjacent parenchymal AVM or dural AV fistula, or outlet obstruction in the straight sinus.

Development, Anatomy and Pathophysiology

Embryology

The embryonic precursor to the normal vein of Galen is the median prosencephalic vein, which has arteriovenous fistulous connections within the primitive vascular bed. The fistulous connections normally involute between the 5th and 7th weeks of development,[282] and by 3 months of development, the posterior part of the median prosencephalic vein joins the internal cerebral veins and the basal veins to form the vein of Galen. Persistence of the median prosencephalic vein and its primitive arteriovenous connections leads to a true vein of Galen malformation. The sump effect of the high flow, low resistance venous drainage leads to the recruitment and enlargement of feeding arteries.

Anatomy

Vein of Galen malformations are midline structures, extending from the interventricular foramen to the choroidal fissure, and laterally to the atria.[280]

1. Arterial supply is usually bilateral and symmetrical.[283]
   (a) Choroidal arteries. In most cases all of the choroidal arteries contribute feeders.
   (b) Subependymal arterial network arising from the posterior circle of Willis.
   (c) Thalamoperforators – rare.
2. Venous drainage is into a dilated median vein of the prosencephalon, which drains into a falcine sinus and then into the superior sagittal sinus or the posterior venous sinuses.
   (a) The straight sinus is absent in most patients.[284]
   (b) Venous outlet obstruction may be present.
   (c) There is preferential drainage away from the deep cerebral venous system.
       • Because of this, deep brain structures tend to use alternative drainage pathways, which typically includes thalamic and subtemporal or lateral mesencephalic veins, which have an epsilon shape on a lateral angiogram.

Clinical Features

The clinical manifestations of patients with vein of Galen malformations can be divided into cardiac and neurological problems. Patients may be divided into three age groups:[285] (1) neonates.birth to 2 months of age, (2) infants.age 2 months to 2 years, and (3) older children and adults. Neonates typically appear with cardiac failure; infants usually present with hydrocephalus and head enlargement;[286] older patients frequently present with hydrocephalus, headaches, and developmental delay.

1. High output cardiac failure.
   (a) The intracranial AV shunt can be haemodynamically significant, resulting in dilatation of the right chambers of the heart,[287] pulmonary hypertension, and left heart failure.
   (b) A loud, machine-like bruit may be present over the head and chest.[285]
   (c) May be diagnosed by prenatal ultrasound; 22% of children with a prenatal diagnosis have irreversible brain damage at birth and die.[283]
   (d) The severity of cardiac symptoms vary widely, from asymptomatic cardiomegaly to cardiogenic shock.
       • In some cases, a brief (3-day) period of relative stability occurs after birth, followed by acute decompensation.[283]
       • Some patients require emergent embolization of the intracranial lesion, whereas others may be medically stabilized for a while, and undergo embolization later in life.
2. Neurological manifestations.
   (a) Neurological symptoms are attributable to:
       • Intracranial venous hypertension, resulting from AV shunting and venous outflow obstruction.
       • Heart failure, which may cause pre- and post-natal brain damage. MRI may show white matter lesions or diffuse brain destruction (i.e., *melting brain syndrome*).[288]
       • Hydrocephalus.
         – The intracranial venous system normally possesses a pressure gradient that facilitates absorption of CSF. Intracranial venous hypertension interferes with this process.

Natural History and Overall Prognosis

Although many publications about vein of Galen malformations include a discussion of the "natural history" of these lesions, a firm understanding of the prognosis of untreated patients is nearly impossible to obtain. The rarity of these lesions, the wide spectrum of severity at presentation, and the variety of treatment approaches currently in use (treatment vs. no treatment, arterial vs. venous embolization, ventricular shunting vs. no shunting) make it difficult to generalize about outcome. Clinical results reported below are from large series published by the Hopital de Bicêtre in France and the Hospital for Sick Children in Toronto.

1. Overall, the survival rate for neonates with vein of Galen malformations is 50–76.9%.[285,289]
2. Spontaneous thrombosis of a vein of Galen malformation is rare, and has been reported to occur in some 2.5% of patients (with half of them neurologically normal).[283]

Management and Outcomes

Most authors agree that patients at the two ends of the spectrum of severity, those with profound symptoms and multisystem failure, and those with completely asymptomatic lesions may be followed expectantly.[285]

Neonates

Lasjaunias and colleagues have developed scoring system to help with decision-making (Table 14.4).[290]

1. Score <8 is associated with a poor systemic or neurological outcome and may be an indication to withhold therapy.
2. Score 8–12 is associated with normal neurological status by medically-refractory heart failure, and emergent embolization should be considered.
3. Score >12 indicates that the patient may be stable enough to delay embolization until the child is at least 5 months of age.

Treatment in Neonates

1. Evaluation of neonates with vein of Galen malformations should include the following:[284]
   (a) Weight and head circumference
   (b) Renal and liver function tests
   (c) Cranial and cardiac ultrasound exams
   (d) Brain MRI, to provide information about lesion anatomy and the status of myelination.
       • Catheter angiography is *not indicated* unless embolization is planned.
2. The optimal age for embolization is ≥5 months.[283] Treatment should be delayed until then when possible.
3. The interventional strategy consists of arterial embolization to reduce the shunt.
   (a) Venous embolization in neonates is associated with higher morbidity[291-294] and should be used only as a last resort when an arterial route is not available.[283]
   (b) Glue (e.g., n-BCA) is the preferred agent for embolization because it is more resistant to recanalization than particles or coils.
4. Reduction of 30% of shunt volume is sufficient to improve cardiac function and permit weaning of the ventilator.[283]
   (a) An angiographic cure is of the lesion is not necessary to control symptoms and allow the brain to develop normally.

Outcomes in Neonates

Of 23 neonates treated at the Hopital de Bicêtre, death occurred despite or because of embolization in 52%; of the survivors, 36.4% were neurologically normal and 63.6% had moderate or severe retardation.[284]

Table 14.4 Bicêtre neonatal evaluation score

Points	Cardiac function	Cerebral function	Respiratory function	Hepatic function	Renal function
5	Normal	Normal	Normal	–	–
4	Overload, no medical treatment	Subclinical, isolated EEG abnormalities	Tachypnea, finishes bottle	–	–
3	Failure; stable with medical treatment	Nonconvulsive intermittent neurological signs	Tachypnea, does not finish bottle	No hepatomegaly, normal hepatic function	Normal
2	Failure; not stable with medical treatment	Isolated convulsion	Assisted ventilation, normal saturation FIO_2 <25%	Hepatomegaly, normal hepatic function	Transient anuria
1	Ventilation necessary	Seizures	Assisted ventilation, normal saturation FIO_2 >25%	Moderate or transient hepatic insufficiency	Unstable diuresis with treatment
0	Resistant to medical therapy	Permanent neurological signs	Assisted ventilation, desaturation	Abnormal coagulation, elevated enzymes	Anuria

Reproduced from Lasjaunias [290] © 1997 Springer Science and Business Media with permission
EEG electroencephalogram, *FIO_2* fraction of inspired oxygen. Maximum score = 21

Infants

1. Hydrocephalus in vein of Galen malformation patients is due to intracranial venous hypertension, and frequently responds to treatment of the lesion.
2. CSF shunting should be reserved until after endovascular treatment has been undertaken.[283,286]
   (a) Less than 50% of patients with hydrocephalus go on to require a shunt.[285]
   (b) CSF shunting can be problematic in these patients. Shunting may contribute to venocongestive brain oedema,[295] and carries a risk of subdural hematoma development.
   (c) Endoscopic third ventriculostomy is an acceptable alternative to ventricular shunting in selected patients.[283]

Outcomes in Infants

Of 153 infants treated at the Hopital de Bicêtre, death occurred despite or because of embolization in 7.2%; of the survivors, 78.9% were neurologically normal and 21.1% had moderate or severe retardation.[284]

Children and Adults

Developmental delay is part of the natural history of untreated symptomatic vein of Galen malformations,[284] because of sustained, long-term intracranial venous hypertension and hydrocephalus.
1. Elevated intracranial venous pressures are well-documented in patients with vein of Galen malformations.[296]
2. Some authors argue strenuously that embolization should be done to normalize venous pressure, and treat hydrocephalus, prior to CSF shunt placement.[284]
3. Adults: Very rare.[297–300]

Outcomes in Children

Of 40 children treated, no deaths occurred, 67.5% were neurologically normal and 32.5% had moderate or severe retardation.[284]

Complications of Embolization Procedures

At Hopital de Bicêtre, total of 196 patients, 1981–2002:[284]
1. Transient neurological disability: 1.6%
2. Permanent neurological disability: 2.1%
3. Nondisabling nonneurological complications: 6.7%
4. Haemorrhage: 5.6%

References

1. Cushing H, Bailey P. Tumors arising from the blood vessels of the brain: angiomatous malformations and hemangioblastomas. Springfield: Charles C. Thomas; 1928. p. 9–102.

2. Challa VR, Moody DM, Brown WR. Vascular malformations of the central nervous system. J Neuropathol Exp Neurol. 1995;54:609–21.

3. Mandybur TI, Nazek M. Cerebral arteriovenous malformations. A detailed morphological and immunohistochemical study using actin. Arch Pathol Lab Med. 1990;114:970–3.

4. Zabramski JM, Henn JS, Coons S. Pathology of cerebral vascular malformations. Neurosurg Clin N Am. 1999;10:395–410.

5. Mullan S, Mojtahedi S, Johnson DL, Macdonald RL. Embryological basis of some aspects of cerebral vascular fistulas and malformations. J Neurosurg. 1996;85:1–8.

6. Suh DC, Alvarez H, Bhattacharya JJ, Rodesch G, Lasjaunias PL. Intracranial haemorrhage within the first two years of life. Acta Neurochir (Wien). 2001;143:997–1004.

7. Yaşargil MG. AVM of the brain, history, embryology, pathological considerations, hemodynamics, diagnostic studies, microsurgical anatomy. Stuttgart: George Thieme Verlag; 1988.

8. Lasjaunias P. A revised concept of the congenital nature of cerebral arteriovenous malformations. Interv Neuroradiol. 1997;3:275–81.

9. Mullan S, Mojtahedi S, Johnson DL, Macdonald RL. Cerebral venous malformation-arteriovenous malformation transition forms. J Neurosurg. 1996;85:9–13.

10. Iwama T, Hayashida K, Takahashi JC, Nagata I, Hashimoto N. Cerebral hemodynamics and metabolism in patients with cerebral arteriovenous malformations: an evaluation using positron emission tomography scanning. J Neurosurg. 2002;97:1314–21.

11. Kader A, Young WL. The effects of intracranial arteriovenous malformations on cerebral hemodynamics. Neurosurg Clin N Am. 1996;7:767–81.

12. Todaka T, Hamada J, Kai Y, Morioka M, Ushio Y. Analysis of mean transit time of contrast medium in ruptured and unruptured arteriovenous malformations: a digital subtraction angiographic study. Stroke. 2003;34:2410–4.

13. Young WL, Pile-Spellman J, Prohovnik I, Kader A, Stein BM. Evidence for adaptive autoregulatory displacement in hypotensive cortical territories adjacent to arteriovenous malformations. Columbia University AVM Study Project. Neurosurgery. 1994;34:601–10; discussion 10–11.

14. Mast H, Mohr JP, Osipov A, et al. 'Steal' is an unestablished mechanism for the clinical presentation of cerebral arteriovenous malformations. Stroke. 1995;26:1215–20.

15. Duong DH, Young WL, Vang MC, et al. Feeding artery pressure and venous drainage pattern are primary determinants of hemorrhage from cerebral arteriovenous malformations. Stroke. 1998;29:1167–76.

16. Burchiel KJ, Clarke H, Ojemann GA, Dacey RG, Winn HR. Use of stimulation mapping and corticography in the excision of arteriovenous malformations in sensorimotor and language-related neocortex. Neurosurgery. 1989;24:322–7.

17. Alkadhi H, Kollias SS, Crelier GR, Golay X, Hepp-Reymond MC, Valavanis A. Plasticity of the human motor cortex in patients with arteriovenous malformations: a functional MR imaging study. AJNR Am J Neuroradiol. 2000;21:1423–33.

18. McCormick WF. The pathology of vascular ("arteriovenous") malformations. J Neurosurg. 1966;24:807–16.

19. Courville CB. Intracranial tumors. Notes upon a series of three thousand verified cases with some current observations pertaining to their morbidity. Bull Los Angeles Neurol Soc. 1967;32 Suppl 2:1–80.

20. Jellinger K. Vascular malformations of the central nervous system: a morphological overview. Neurosurg Rev. 1986;9:177–216.

21. Sarwar M, McCormick WF. Intracerebral venous angioma. Case report and review. Arch Neurol. 1978;35:323–5.

22. Brown Jr RD, Wiebers DO, Torner JC, O'Fallon WM. Incidence and prevalence of intracranial vascular malformations in Olmsted County, Minnesota, 1965 to 1992. Neurology. 1996;46:949–52.

23. Gabriel RABS, Kim HP, Sidney SMDMPH, et al. Ten-year detection rate of brain arteriovenous malformations in a large, multiethnic, defined population. Stroke. 2010;41:21–6.

24. Stapf C, Mast H, Sciacca RR, et al. The New York Islands AVM Study: design, study progress, and initial results. Stroke. 2003;34:e29–33.

25. Stapf C, Labovitz DL, Sciacca RR, Mast H, Mohr JP, Sacco RL. Incidence of adult brain arteriovenous malformation hemorrhage in a prospective population-based stroke survey. Cerebrovasc Dis. 2002;13:43–5.

26. Hofmeister C, Stapf C, Hartmann A, et al. Demographic, morphological, and clinical characteristics of 1289 Patients with brain arteriovenous malformation. Stroke. 2000; 31:1307–10.

27. ApSimon HT, Reef H, Phadke RV, Popovic EA. A population-based study of brain arteriovenous malformation: long-term treatment outcomes. Stroke. 2002;33:2794–800.

28. Graf CJ, Perret GE, Torner JC. Bleeding from cerebral arteriovenous malformations as part of their natural history. J Neurosurg. 1983;58:331–7.

29. McCormick WF, Rosenfield DB. Massive brain hemorrhage: a review of 144 cases and an examination of their causes. Stroke. 1973;4:946–54.

30. Khaw AV, Mohr JP, Sciacca RR, et al. Association of infratentorial brain arteriovenous malformations with hemorrhage at initial presentation. Stroke. 2004;35:660–3.

31. Spetzler RF, Martin NA. A proposed grading system for arteriovenous malformations. J Neurosurg. 1986;65:476–83.

32. Valavanis A. The role of angiography in the evaluation of cerebral vascular malformations. Neuroimaging Clin N Am. 1996;6:679–704.

33. Willinsky RA, Lasjaunias P, Terbrugge K, Burrows P. Multiple cerebral arteriovenous malformations (AVMs). Review of our experience from 203 patients with cerebral vascular lesions. Neuroradiology. 1990;32:207–10.

34. Putman CM, Chaloupka JC, Fulbright RK, Awad IA, White Jr H, Fayad PB. Exceptional multiplicity of cerebral arteriovenous malformations associated with hereditary hemorrhagic telangiectasia (Osler-Weber-Rendu syndrome). AJNR Am J Neuroradiol. 1996;17: 1733–42.

35. van Beijnum J, van der Worp HB, Schippers HM, et al. Familial occurrence of brain arteriovenous malformations: a systematic review. J Neurol Neurosurg Psychiatry. 2007;78(11):1213–7.

36. Rendu HJLM. Épistaxis répétées chez un sujet porteur de petits angiomes cutanés et muqueux. Bull Soc Med Hop. 1896;13:731–3.

37. Osler W. On family form of recurring epistaxis, associated with multiple telangiectasias of skin and mucous membranes. Bull Johns Hopkins Hosp. 1901;12:333–7.

38. Weber EP. Multiple hereditary developmental angiomata (telangiectasia) of the skin and mucous membranes associated with recurring hemorrhages. Lancet. 1907;2:160–2.

39. Shovlin CL, Guttmacher AE, Buscarini E, et al. Diagnostic criteria for hereditary hemorrhagic telangiectasia (Rendu-Osler-Weber syndrome). Am J Med Genet. 2000;91:66–7.

40. Bideau A, Plauchu H, Brunet G, Robert J. Epidemiological investigation of Rendu-Osler disease in France: its geographical distribution and prevalence. Popul. 1989;44:3–22.

41. Kjeldsen AD, Vase P, Green A. Hereditary haemorrhagic telangiectasia: a population-based study of prevalence and mortality in Danish patients. J Intern Med. 1999;245:31–9.

42. Dakeishi M, Shioya T, Wada Y, et al. Genetic epidemiology of hereditary hemorrhagic telangiectasia in a local community in the northern part of Japan. Hum Mutat. 2002;19:140–8.

43. Sadick H, Sadick M, Gotte K, et al. Hereditary hemorrhagic telangiectasia: an update on clinical manifestations and diagnostic measures. Wien Klin Wochenschr. 2006;118:72–80.

44. Roman G, Fisher M, Perl DP Poser CM. Neurological manifestations of hereditary hemorrhagic telangiectasia (Rendu-Osler-Weber disease): report of 2 cases and review of the literature. Ann Neurol. 1978;4:130–44.

45. Waller JD, Greenberg JH, Lewis CW. Hereditary hemorrhagic telangiectasia with cerebrovascular malformations. Arch Dermatol 1976;112 49–52.

46. Fulbright RK, Chaloupka JC, Putman CM, et al. MR of hereditary hemorrhagic telangiectasia: prevalence and spectrum of cerebrovascular malformations. AJNR Am J Neuroradiol. 1998;19:477–84.

47. Haitjema T, Disch F, Overtoom TT, Westermann CJ, Lammers JW. Screening family members of patients with hereditary hemorrhagic telangiectasia. Am J Med. 1995;99: 519–24.

48. Willemse RB, Mager JJ, Westermann CJ, Overtoom TT, Mauser H, Wolbers JG. Bleeding risk of cerebrovascular malformations in hereditary hemorrhagic telangiectasia. J Neurosurg. 2000;92:779–84.

49. Easey AJ, Wallace GM, Hughes JM, Jackson JE, Taylor WJ, Shovlin CL. Should asymptomatic patients with hereditary haemorrhagic telangiectasia (HHT) be screened for cerebral vascular malformations? Data from 22,061 years of HHT patient life. J Neurol Neurosurg Psychiatry. 2003;74:743–8.

50. Burke CM, Safai C, Nelson DP, Raffin TA. Pulmonary arteriovenous malformations: a critical update. Am Rev Respir Dis. 1986;134:334–9.

51. Jessurun GA, Kamphuis DJ, van der Zande FH, Nossent JC. Cerebral arteriovenous malformations in The Netherlands Antilles. High prevalence of hereditary hemorrhagic telangiectasia-related single and multiple cerebral arteriovenous malformations. Clin Neurol Neurosurg. 1993;95:193–8.

52. Romer W, Burk M, Schneider W. Hereditary hemorrhagic telangiectasia (Osler's disease). Dtsch Med Wochenschr. 1992;117:669–75.

53. Haitjema T, Balder W, Disch FJ, Westermann CJ. Epistaxis in hereditary haemorrhagic telangiectasia. Rhinology. 1996;34:176–8.

54. Sadick H, Fleischer I, Goessler U, Hormann K, Sadick M. Twenty-four-hour and annual variation in onset of epistaxis in Osler disease. Caronobiol Int. 2007;24:357–64.

55. White Jr RI, Lynch-Nyhan A, Terry P, et al. Pulmonary arteriovenous malformations: techniques and long-term outcome of embolotherapy. Radiology. 1988;169:663–9.

56. Vase P, Holm M, Arendrup H. Pulmonary arteriovenous fistulas in hereditary hemorrhagic telangiectasia. Acta Med Scand. 1985;218:105–9.

57. Mager HJ, Overtoom TT, Mauser HW, Westermann KJ. Early cerebral infarction after embolotherapy of a pulmonary arteriovenous malformation. J Vasc Interv Radiol. 2001;12:122–3.

58. Guttmacher AE, Marchuk DA, White Jr RI. Hereditary hemorrhagic telangiectasia. N Engl J Med. 1995;333:918–24.

59. Snyder LH, Doan CA. Clinical and experimental studies in human inheritance Is the homozygous form of multiple telangiectasia lethal? J Lab Clin Med. 1944;29:1211–32.

60. Shovlin CL, Hughes JM, Tuddenham EG, et al. A gene for hereditary haemorrhagic telangiectasia maps to chromosome 9q3. Nat Genet. 1994;6:205–9.

61. McDonald MT, Papenberg KA, Ghosh S, et al. A disease locus for hereditary haemorrhagic telangiectasia maps to chromosome 9q33-34. Nat Genet. 1994;6:197–204.

62. Johnson DW, Berg JN, Gallione CJ, et al. A second locus for hereditary hemorrhagic telangiectasia maps to chromosome 12. Genome Res. 1995;5:21–8.

63. Wyburn-Mason R. Arteriovenous aneurysm of midbrain and retina, facial naevi and mental changes. Brain. 1943;66:163–203.

64. Théron J, Newton TH, Hoyt WF. Unilateral retinocephalic vascular malformations. Neuroradiology. 1974;7:185–96.

65. Mizutani T, Tanaka H, Aruga T. Multiple arteriovenous malformations located in the cerebellum, posterior fossa, spinal cord, dura, and scalp with associated port-wine stain and supratentorial venous anomaly. Neurosurgery. 1992;31:137–40; discussion 140–1.

66. Laufer L, Cohen A. Sturge-Weber syndrome associated with a large left hemispheric arteriovenous malformation. Pediatr Radiol. 1994;24:272–3.

67. Kayama T, Suzuki S, Sakurai Y, Nagayama T, Ogawa A, Yoshimoto T. A case of moyamoya disease accompanied by an arteriovenous malformation. Neurosurgery. 1986;18:465–8.

68. Okada T, Kida Y, Kinomoto T, Sakurai T, Kobayashi T. Arteriovenous malformation associated with moyamoya disease–case report. Neurol Med Chir (Tokyo). 1990;30:945–8.

69. Somasundaram S, Thamburaj K, Burathoki S, Gupta AK. Mcyamoya disease with cerebral arteriovenous malformation presenting as primary subarachnoid hemorrhage. J Neuroimaging. 2007;17:251–4.

70. Schmit BP, Burrows PE, Kuban K, Goumnerova L, Scott RM. Acquired cerebral arteriovenous malformation in a child with moyamoya disease. Case report. J Neurosurg. 1996;84: 677–80.

71. O'Shaughnessy BA, DiPatri Jr AJ, Parkinson RJ, Batjer HH. Development of a de novo cerebral arteriovenous malformation in a child with sickle cell disease and moyamoya arteriopathy. Case report. J Neurosurg. 2005;102:238–43.

72. Lim M, Cheshier S, Steinberg GK. New vessel formation in the central nervous system during tumor growth, vascular malformations, and Moyamoya. Curr Neurovasc Res. 2006;3:237–45.

73. Wu TC, Guo WY, Wu HM, Chang FC, Shiau CY, Chung WY. The rare association of moyamoya disease and cerebral arteriovenous malformations: a case report. Korean J Radiol. 2008;9(Suppl):S65–7.

74. Crawford PM, West CR, Chadwick DW, Shaw MD. Arteriovenous malformations of the brain: natural history in unoperated patients. J Neurol Neurosurg Psychiatry. 1986;49:1–10.

75. Itoyama Y, Uemura S, Ushio Y, et al. Natural course of unoperated intracranial arteriovenous malformations: study of 50 cases. J Neurosurg. 1989;71:805–9.

76. Brown Jr RD, Wiebers DO, Forbes GS. Unruptured intracranial aneurysms and arteriovenous malformations: frequency of intracranial hemorrhage and relationship of lesions. J Neurosurg. 1990;73:859–63.

77. Ondra SL, Troupp H, George ED, Schwab K. The natural history of symptomatic arteriovenous malformations of the brain: a 24-year follow-up assessment. J Neurosurg. 1990;73:387–91.

78. Mast H, Young WL, Koennecke HC, et al. Risk of spontaneous haemorrhage after diagnosis of cerebral arteriovenous malformation. Lancet. 1997;350:1065–8.

79. Halim AX, Johnston SC, Singh V, et al. Longitudinal risk of intracranial hemorrhage in patients with arteriovenous malformation of the brain within a defined population. Stroke. 2004;35:1697–702.

80. Forster DM, Steiner L, Hakanson S. Arteriovenous malformations of the brain. A long-term clinical study. J Neurosurg. 1972;37:562–70.

81. Fults D, Kelly Jr DL. Natural history of arteriovenous malformations of the brain: a clinical study. Neurosurgery. 1984;15:658–62.

82. Cho JH, Mast H, Sciacca RR, et al. Clinical outcome after first and recurrent hemorrhage in patients with untreated brain arteriovenous malformation. Stroke. 2006;37:1243–7.

83. Yen C-PMD, Sheehan JPMDP, Schwyzer LMD, Schlesinger DP. Hemorrhage risk of cerebral arteriovenous malformations before and during the latency period after gamma knife radiosurgery. Stroke. 2011;42:1691–6.

84. Brown Jr RD, Wiebers DO, Forbes G, et al. The natural history of unruptured intracranial arteriovenous malformations. J Neurosurg. 1988;68:352–7.

85. Fullerton HJ, Achrol AS, Johnston SC, et al. Long-term hemorrhage risk in children versus adults with brain arteriovenous malformations. Stroke. 2005;36:2099–104.

86. Abdulrauf SI, Malik GM, Awad IA. Spontaneous angiographic obliteration of cerebral arteriovenous malformations. Neurosurgery. 1999;44:280–7; discussion 287–8.

87. Kondziolka D, McLaughlin MR, Kestle JR. Simple risk predictions for arteriovenous malformation hemorrhage. Neurosurgery. 1995;37:851–5.

88. Brown Jr RD. Simple risk predictions for arteriovenous malformation hemorrhage. Neurosurgery. 2000;46:1024.

89. Stapf C, Khaw AV, Sciacca RR, et al. Effect of age on clinical and morphological characteristics in patients with brain arteriovenous malformation. Stroke. 2003;34:2664–9.

90. Choi JH, Mohr JP. Brain arteriovenous malformations in adults. Lancet Neurol. 2005;4:299–308.

91. Hartmann A, Mast H, Mohr JP, et al. Morbidity of intracranial hemorrhage in patients with cerebral arteriovenous malformation. Stroke. 1998;29:931–4.

92. Stapf C, Mast H, Sciacca RR, et al. Predictors of hemorrhage in patients with untreated brain arteriovenous malformation. Neurology. 2006;66:1350–5.

93. Waltimo O. The change in size of intracranial arteriovenous malformations. J Neurol Sci. 1973;19:21–7.

94. Guidetti B, Delitala A. Intracranial arteriovenous malformations. Conservative and surgical treatment. J Neurosurg. 1980;53:149–52.

95. Spetzler RF, Hargraves RW, McCormick PW, Zabramski JM, Flom RA, Zimmerman RS. Relationship of perfusion pressure and size to risk of hemorrhage from arteriovenous malformations. J Neurosurg. 1992;76:918–23.

96. Langer DJ, Lasner TM, Hurst RW, Flamm ES, Zager EL, King Jr JT. Hypertension, small size, and deep venous drainage are associated with risk of hemorrhagic presentation of cerebral arteriovenous malformations. Neurosurgery. 1998;42:481–6; discussion 487–9.

97. Albert P, Salgado H, Polaina M, Trujillo F, Ponce de Leon A, Durand F. A study on the venous drainage of 150 cerebral arteriovenous malformations as related to haemorrhagic risks and size of the lesion. Acta Neurochir (Wien). 1990;103:30–4.

98. Karlsson B, Lindquist C, Johansson A, Steiner L. Annual risk for the first hemorrhage from untreated cerebral arteriovenous malformations. Minim Invasive Neurosurg. 1997;40:40–6.

99. Stefani MA, Porter PJ, ter Brugge KG, Montanera W, Willinsky RA, Wallace MC. Large and deep brain arteriovenous malformations are associated with risk of future hemorrhage. Stroke. 2002;33:1220–4.

100. Nataf F, Meder JF, Roux FX, et al. Angioarchitecture associated with haemorrhage in cerebral arteriovenous malformations: a prognostic statistical model. Neuroradiology. 1997;39:52–8.

101. Fleetwood IG, Marcellus ML, Levy RP, Marks MP, Steinberg GK. Deep arteriovenous malformations of the basal ganglia and thalamus: natural history. J Neurosurg. 2003;98:747–50.

102. Drummond JC, Patel PM. Cerebral physiology and the effects of anesthetics and techniques. In: Miller RD, editor. Anesthesia. 5th ed. Philadelphia: Churchill Livingstone; 2000.

103. Turjman F, Massoud TF, Vinuela F, Sayre JW, Guglielmi G, Duckwiler G. Correlation of the angioarchitectural features of cerebral arteriovenous malformations with clinical presentation of hemorrhage. Neurosurgery. 1995;37:856–60; discussion 860–2.

104. Miyasaka Y, Yada K, Ohwada T, Kitahara T, Kurata A, Irikura K. An analysis of the venous drainage system as a factor in hemorrhage from arteriovenous malformations. J Neurosurg. 1992;76:239–43.

105. Kim H, Sidney S, McCulloch CE, et al. Racial/ethnic differences in longitudinal risk of intracranial hemorrhage in brain arteriovenous malformation patients. Stroke. 2007;38:2430–7.

106. Pawlikowska L, Tran MN, Achrol AS, et al. Polymorphisms in genes involved in inflammatory and angiogenic pathways and the risk of hemorrhagic presentation of brain arteriovenous malformations. Stroke. 2004;35:2294–300.

107. Stapf C, Mohr JP, Pile-Spellman J, Solomon RA, Sacco RL, Connolly Jr ES. Epidemiology and natural history of arteriovenous malformations. Neurosurg Focus. 2001;11:e1.

108. Wilkins RH. Natural history of intracranial vascular malformations: a review. Neurosurgery. 1985;16:421–30.

109. Perret G, Nishioka H. Report on the cooperative study of intracranial aneurysms and subarachnoid hemorrhage. Section VI. Arteriovenous malformations. An analysis of 545 cases of cranio-cerebral arteriovenous malformations and fistulae reported to the cooperative study. J Neurosurg. 1966;25:467–90.

110. Yeh HS, Kashiwagi S, Tew Jr JM, Berger TS. Surgical management of epilepsy associated with cerebral arteriovenous malformations. J Neurosurg. 1990;72:216–23.

111. Parkinson D, Bachers G. Arteriovenous malformations. Summary of 100 consecutive supratentorial cases. J Neurosurg. 1980;53:285–99.

112. Monteiro JM, Rosas MJ, Correia AP, Vaz AR. Migraine and intracranial vascular malformations. Headache. 1993;33:563–5.

113. Haas DC. Migraine and intracranial vascular malformations. Headache. 1994;34:287.

114. Obermann M, Gizewski ER, Limmroth V, Diener HC, Katsarava Z. Symptomatic migraine and pontine vascular malformation: evidence for a key role of the brainstem in the pathophysiology of chronic migraine. Cephalalgia. 2006;26:763–6.

115. Lazar RM, Connaire K, Marshall RS, et al. Developmental deficits in adult patients with arteriovenous malformations. Arch Neurol. 1999;56:103–6.

116. Schreiber SJ, Doepp F, Bender A, Schmierer K, Valdueza JM. Diffuse cerebral angiomatosis. Neurology. 2003;60:1216–8.

117. Chin LS, Raffel C, Gonzalez-Gomez I, Giannotta SL, McComb JG. Diffuse arteriovenous malformations: a clinical, radiological, and pathological description. Neurosurgery. 1992;31:863–89; discussion 8–9.

118. Lasjaunias PL, Landrieu P, Rodesch G, et al. Cerebral proliferative angiopathy: clinical and angiographic description of an entity different from cerebral AVMs. Stroke. 2008;39:878–85.

119. Vargas MC, Castillo M. Magnetic resonance perfusion imaging in proliferative cerebral angiopathy. J Comput Assist Tomogr. 2011;35:33–8.

120. Hong KS, Lee JI, Hong SC. Neurological picture. Cerebral proliferative angiopathy associated with haemangioma of the face and tongue. J Neurol Neurosurg Psychiatry. 2010;81: 36–7.

121. Lv X, Wu Z, Jiang C, Li Y. Illustrative case: a patient with cerebral proliferative angiopathy. Eur J Radiol. 2011;78: e67–70.

122. Soderman M, Rodesch G, Lasjaunias P. Transdural blood supply to cerebral arteriovenous malformations adjacent to the dura mater. AJNR Am J Neuroradiol. 2002;23: 1295–300.

123. Ducreux D, Meder JF, Fredy D, Bittoun J, Lasjaunias P. MR perfusion imaging in proliferative angiopathy. Neuroradiology. 2004;46:105–12.

124. Berenstein A, Lasjaunias PL, TerBrugge KG. Surgical neuroangiography. 2nd ed. Heidelberg/Berlin: Springer Verlag; 2004.

125. Korogi Y, Takahashi M, Mabuchi N, et al. Intracranial aneurysms: diagnostic accuracy of three-dimensional, Fourier transform, time-of-flight MR angiography. Radiology. 1994;193:181–6.

126. 3rd Huston J, Rufenacht DA, Ehman RL, Wiebers DO. Intracranial aneurysms and vascular malformations: comparison of time-of-flight and phase-contrast MR angiography. Radiology. 1991;181:721–30.

127. Zhu XL, Chan MS, Poon WS. Spontaneous intracranial hemorrhage: which patients need diagnostic cerebral angiography? A prospective study of 206 cases and review of the literature. Stroke. 1997;28:1406–9.

128. Cloft HJ, Joseph GJ, Dion JE. Risk of cerebral angiography in patients with subarachnoid hemorrhage, cerebral aneurysm, and arteriovenous malformation: a meta-analysis. Stroke. 1999;30:317–20.

129. Ogilvy CS, Stieg PE, Awad I, et al. AHA Scientific statement: recommendations for the management of intracranial arteriovenous malformations: a statement for healthcare professionals from a special writing group of the Stroke Council, American Stroke Association. Stroke. 2001;32: 1458–71.

130. Cockroft KM. Unruptured cerebral arteriovenous malformations: to treat or not to treat. Stroke. 2006;37:1148–9.

131. Stapf C, Mohr JP, Choi JH, Hartmann A, Mast H. Invasive treatment of unruptured brain arteriovenous malformations is experimental therapy. Curr Opin Neurol. 2006;19:63–8.

132. Mohr JP, Moskowitz AJ, Stapf C, et al. The ARUBA trial. Stroke. 2010;41:e537–40.

133. Fleetwood IG, Steinberg GK. Arteriovenous malformations. Lancet. 2002;359:863–73.

134. Baskaya MK, Jea A, Heros RC, Javahary R, Sultan A. Cerebral arteriovenous malformations. Clin Neurosurg. 2006;53:114–44.

135. McInerney J, Gould DA, Birkmeyer JD, Harbaugh RE. Decision analysis for small, asymptomatic intracranial arteriovenous malformations. Neurosurg Focus. 2001;11:e7.

136. Heros RC, Korosue K, Diebold PM. Surgical excision of cerebral arteriovenous malformations: late results. Neurosurgery. 1990;26:570–7; discussion 7–8.

137. Sisti MB, Kader A, Stein BM. Microsurgery for 67 intracranial arteriovenous malformations less than 3 cm in diameter. J Neurosurg. 1993;79:653–60.

138. Hamilton MG, Spetzler RF. The prospective application of a grading system for arteriovenous malformations. Neurosurgery. 1994;34:2–6; discussion –7.

139. Pikus HJ, Beach ML, Harbaugh RE. Microsurgical treatment of arteriovenous malformations: analysis and comparison with stereotactic radiosurgery. J Neurosurg. 1998;88:641–6.

140. Pik JH, Morgan MK. Microsurgery for small arteriovenous malformations of the brain: results in 110 consecutive patients. Neurosurgery. 2000;47:571–5; discussion 5–7.

141. Lawton MT. Spetzler-Martin Grade III arteriovenous malformations: surgical results and a modification of the grading scale. Neurosurgery. 2003;52:740–8; discussion 8–9.

142. Castel JP, Kantor G. Postoperative morbidity and mortality after microsurgical exclusion of cerebral arteriovenous malformations. Current data and analysis of recent literature Neurochirurgie. 2001;47:369–83.

143. Schaller C, Schramm J, Haun D. Significance of factors contributing to surgical complications and to late outcome after elective surgery of cerebral arteriovenous malformations. J Neurol Neurosurg Psychiatry. 1998;65:547–54.

144. Morgan MK, Rochford AM, Tsahtsarlis A, Little N, Faulder KC. Surgical risks associated with the management of Grade I and II brain arteriovenous malformations. Neurosurgery. 2004;54:832–7; discussion 7–9.

145. Russell SM, Woo HH, Joseffer SS, Jafar JJ. Role of frameless stereotaxy in the surgical treatment of cerebral arteriovenous malformations: technique and outcomes in a controlled study of 44 consecutive patients. Neurosurgery. 2002;51:1108–16; discussion 16–8.

146. Steiner L, Lindquist C, Adler JR, Torner JC, Alves W, Steiner M. Clinical outcome of radiosurgery for cerebral arteriovenous malformations. J Neurosurg. 1992;77:1–8.

147. Hoh BL, Chapman PH, Loeffler JS, Carter BS, Ogilvy CS. Results of multimodality treatment for 141 patients with brain arteriovenous malformations and seizures: factors associated with seizure incidence and seizure outcomes. Neurosurgery. 2002;51:303–9; discussion 9–11.

148. Martin NA, Wilson CB. Preoperative and postoperative care: Management of intracranial hemorrhage. In: Wilson CB, Stein BM, editors. Intracranial arteriovenous malformations. Baltimore: Williams & Wilkins; 1984. p. 121–9.

149. Solomon RA, Stein BM Management of deep supratentorial and brain stem arteriovenous malformations. In: Barrow DL, editor. Intracranial vascular malformations. Park Ridge: American Association of Neurological Surgeons; 1990. p. 125–41.

150. Jafar JJ, Rezai AR. Acute surgical management of intracranial arteriovenous malformations. Neurosurgery. 1994;34:8–12; discussion –3.

151. Lefkowitz MA, Vinuela F, Martin N. Critical Care Management. In: Stieg PE, Batjer HH, Samson D, editors. Intracranial arteriovenous malformations. New York: Informa; 2007. p. 329–42.

152. Hoh BL, Carter BS, Ogilvy CS. Incidence of residual intracranial AVMs after surgical resection and efficacy of immediate surgical re-exploration. Acta Neurochir (Wien). 2004;146:1–7; discuss on 7.

153. Morcos JJ, Heros RC. Supratentorial arteriovenous malformations. In: Carter LP, Spetzler RF, Hamilton MG, editors. Neurovascular surgery New York: McGraw-Hill; 1995. p. 979–1004.

154. Harrigan MR, Thompson BG. Critical care management. In: Stieg PE, Batjer HH, Samson D, editors. Intracranial arteriovenous malformations. New York: Informa; 2007. p. 383–92.

155. al-Rodhan NR, Sundt Jr TM, Piepgras DG, Nichols DA, Rufenacht D, Stevens LN. Occlusive hyperemia: a theory for the hemodynamic complications following resection of intracerebral arteriovenous malformations. J Neurosurg. 1993;78:167–75.

156. Drake CG. Cerebral arteriovenous malformations: considerations for and experience with surgical treatment in 166 cases. Clin Neurosurg. 1979;26:145–208.

157. Kader A, Young WL. Arteriovenous malformations: Considerations for perioperative critical care monitoring. In: Batjer H, editor. Cerebrovascular disease. Philadelphia: Lippencott-Raven; 1997.

158. Morgan MK, Johnston IH, Hallinan JM, Weber NC. Complications of surgery for arteriovenous malformations of the brain. J Neurosurg. 1993;78:176–82.

159. Wilson CB, Hieshima G. Occlusive hyperemia: a new way to think about an old problem. J Neurosurg. 1993;78:165–6.

160. Spetzler RF, Wilson CB, Weinstein P, Mehdorn M, Townsend J, Telles D. Normal perfusion pressure breakthrough theory. Clin Neurosurg. 1978;25:651–72.

161. Day AL, Friedman WA, Sypert GW, Mickle JP. Successful treatment of the normal perfusion pressure breakthrough syndrome. Neurosurgery. 1982;11:625–30.

162. Batjer HH, Devous Sr MD. The use of acetazolamide-enhanced regional cerebral blood flow measurement to predict risk to arteriovenous malformation patients. Neurosurgery. 1992;31:213–7. discussion 7–8.

163. Young WL, Prohovnik I, Ornstein E, et al. The effect of arteriovenous malformation resection on cerebrovascular reactivity to carbon dioxide. Neurosurgery. 1990;27:257–66; discussion 66–7.

164. Morgan MK, Winder M, Little NS, Finfer S, Ritson E. Delayed hemorrhage following resection of an arteriovenous malformation in the brain. J Neurosurg. 2003;99:967–71.

165. Sipos EP, Kirsch JR, Nauta HJ, Debrun G, Ulatowski JA, Bell WR. Intra-arterial urokinase for treatment of retrograde thrombosis following resection of an arteriovenous malformation. Case report. J Neurosurg. 1992;76:1004–7.

166. Miyasaka Y, Yada K, Ohwada T, et al. Hemorrhagic venous infarction after excision of an arteriovenous malformation: case report. Neurosurgery. 1991;29:265–8.

167. Yamamoto M. Gamma Knife radiosurgery: technology, applications, and future directions. Neurosurg Clin N Am. 1999;10:181–202.

168. Steinberg GK, Fabrikant JI, Marks MP, et al. Stereotactic helium ion Bragg peak radiosurgery for intracranial arteriovenous malformations. Detailed clinical and neuroradiologic outcome. Stereotact Funct Neurosurg. 1991;57:36–49.

169. Kjellberg RN. Stereotactic Bragg peak proton beam radiosurgery for cerebral arteriovenous malformations. Ann Clin Res. 1986;18 Suppl 47:17–9.

170. Schneider BF, Eberhard DA, Steiner LE. Histopathology of arteriovenous malformations after gamma knife radiosurgery. J Neurosurg. 1997;87:352–7.

171. Szeifert GT, Kemeny AA, Timperley WR, Forster DM. The potential role of myofibroblasts in the obliteration of arteriovenous malformations after radiosurgery. Neurosurgery. 1997;40:61–5; discussion 65–6.

172. Lunsford LD, Kondziolka D, Flickinger JC, et al. Stereotactic radiosurgery for arteriovenous malformations of the brain. J Neurosurg. 1991;75:512–24.

173. Colombo F, Pozza F, Chierego G, Casentini L, De Luca G, Francescon P. Linear accelerator radiosurgery of cerebral arteriovenous malformations: an update. Neurosurgery. 1994;34:14–20; discussion 20–1.

174. Friedman WA, Bova FJ, Mendenhall WM. Linear accelerator radiosurgery for arteriovenous malformations: the relationship of size to outcome. J Neurosurg. 1995;82:180–9.

175. Yamamoto Y, Coffey RJ, Nichols DA, Shaw EG. Interim report on the radiosurgical treatment of cerebral arteriovenous malformations. The influence of size, dose, time, and technical factors on obliteration rate. J Neurosurg. 1995;83:832–7.

176. Schlienger M, Atlan D, Lefkopoulos D, et al. Linac radiosurgery for cerebral arteriovenous malformations: results in 169 patients. Int J Radiat Oncol Biol Phys. 2000;46:1135–42.

177. Shin M, Kawamoto S, Kurita H, et al. Retrospective analysis of a 10-year experience of stereotactic radio surgery for arteriovenous malformations in children and adolescents. J Neurosurg. 2002;97:779–84.

178. Koga TMD, Shin MMDP, Terahara AMDP, Saito NMDP. Outcomes of radiosurgery for brainstem arteriovenous malformations. Neurosurgery. 2011;69:45–52.

179. Maruyama K, Kawahara N, Shin M, et al. The risk of hemorrhage after radiosurgery for cerebral arteriovenous malformations. N Engl J Med. 2005;352:146–53.

180. Pollock BE, Flickinger JC, Lunsford LD, Bissonette DJ, Kondziolka D. Hemorrhage risk after stereotactic radiosurgery of cerebral arteriovenous malformations. Neurosurgery. 1996;38:652–9; discussion 9–61.

181. Karlsson B, Lax I, Soderman M. Risk for hemorrhage during the 2-year latency period following gamma knife radiosurgery for arteriovenous malformations. Int J Radiat Oncol Biol Phys. 2001;49:1045–51.

182. Shin M, Kawahara N, Maruyama K, Tago M, Ueki K, Kirino T. Risk of hemorrhage from an arteriovenous malformation confirmed to have been obliterated on angiography after stereotactic radiosurgery. J Neurosurg. 2005;102:842–6.

183. Kurita H, Kawamoto S, Suzuki I, et al. Control of epilepsy associated with cerebral arteriovenous malformations after radiosurgery. J Neurol Neurosurg Psychiatry. 1998;65:648–55.

184. Eisenschenk S, Gilmore RL, Friedman WA, Henchey RA. The effect of LINAC stereotactic radiosurgery on epilepsy associated with arteriovenous malformations. Stereotact Funct Neurosurg. 1998;71:51–61.

185. Schauble B, Cascino GD, Pollock BE, et al. Seizure outcomes after stereotactic radiosurgery for cerebral arteriovenous malformations. Neurology. 2004;63:643–7.

186. Lim YJ, Lee CY, Koh JS, Kim TS, Kim GK, Rhee BA. Seizure control of Gamma Knife radiosurgery for non-hemorrhagic arteriovenous malformations. Acta Neurochir Suppl. 2006;99:97–101.

187. Flickinger JC, Kondziolka D, Lunsford LD, et al. A multi-institutional analysis of complication outcomes after arteriovenous malformation radiosurgery Int J Radiat Oncol Biol Phys. 1999;44:67–74.

188. Flickinger JC, Kondziolka D, Maitz AH, Lunsford LD. An analysis of the dose–response for arteriovenous malformation radiosurgery and other factors affecting obliteration. Radiother Oncol. 2002;63:347–54.

189. Friedman WA, Bova FJ, Bollampally S, Bradshaw P. Analysis of factors predictive of success or complications in arteriovenous malformation radiosurgery. Neurosurgery. 2003;52:296–307; discussion 307–8.

190. Flickinger JC, Kondziolka D, Pollock BE, Maitz AH, Lunsford LD. Complications from arteriovenous malformation radiosurgery: multivariate analysis and risk modeling. Int J Radiat Oncol Biol Phys. 1997;38:485–90.

191. Korytko T, Radivoyevitch T, Colussi V, et al. 12 Gy gamma knife radiosurgical volume is a predictor for radiation necrosis in non-AVM intracranial tumors. Int J Radiat Oncol Biol Phys. 2006;64:419–24.

192. Pannullo SC, Abbott J, Allbright R. Radiosurgical principles. In: Stieg PE, Batjer HH, Samson D, editors. Intracranial arteriovenous malformations. New York: Informa; 2007. p. 177–88.

193. Xiao FMD, Gorgulho AAMDM, Lin C-SMD, et al. Treatment of giant cerebral arteriovenous malformation: hypofractionated stereotactic radiation as the first stage. Neurosurgery. 2010;67:1253–9.

194. Guo WY, Karlsson B, Ericson K, Lindqvist M. Even the smallest remnant of an AVM constitutes a risk of further bleeding. Case report. Acta Neurochir (Wien). 1993;121:212–5.

195. Karlsson B, Kihlstrom L, Lindquist C, Steiner L. Gamma knife surgery for previously irradiated arteriovenous malformations. Neurosurgery. 1998;42:1–5; discussion 5–6.

196. Liscak R, Vladyka V, Simonova G et al. Arteriovenous malformations after Leksell gamma knife radiosurgery: rate of obliteration and complications. Neurosurgery. 2007;60:1005–14; discussion 15–6.

197. Yen CP, Jain S, Haq IU, et al. Repeat gamma knife surgery for incompletely obliterated cerebral arteriovenous malformations. Neurosurgery. 2010;67:55–64.

198. Nataf F, Schlienger M, Bayram M, Ghossoub M, George B, Roux FX. Microsurgery or radiosurgery for cerebral arteriovenous malformations? A study of two paired series. Neurosurgery. 2007;61:39–49; discussion –50.

199. Luessenhop AJ, Spence WT. Artificial embolization of cerebral arteries. Report of use in a case of arteriovenous malformation. JAMA. 1960;172:1153–5.

200. Wolpert SM, Stein BM. Catheter embolization of intracranial arteriovenous malformations as an a d to surgical excision. Neuroradiology. 1975;10:73–85.

201. Djindjian R, Houdart R, Rey A. Place of embolization in the investigation and therapy of cerebral and spinal malformations and vascular tumors. (Apropos of 50 cases). Ann Med Interne (Paris). 1973;124:365–75.

202. Serbinenko FA. Balloon catheterization and occlusion of major cerebral vessels. J Neurosurg. 1974;41:125–45.

203. Kerber C. Balloon catheter with a calibrated leak. A new system for superselective angiography and occlusive catheter therapy. Radiology. 1976;120:547–50.

204. Pevsner PH. Micro-balloon catheter for superselective angiography and therapeutic occlusion. AJR Am J Roentgenol. 1977;128:225–30.

205. Ciapetti G, Stea S, Cenni E, et al. Toxicity of cyanoacrylates in vitro using extract dilution assay on cell cultures. Biomaterials. 1994;15:92–6.

206. Vinters HV, Galil KA, Lundie MJ, Kaufmann JC. The histotoxicity of cyanoacrylates. A selective review. Neuroradiology. 1985;27:279–91.

207. Brothers MF, Kaufmann JC, Fox AJ, Deveikis JP. n-Butyl 2-cyanoacrylate–substitute for IBCA in interventional neuroradiology: histopathologic and polymerization time studies. AJNR Am J Neuroradiol. 1989;10:777–86.

208. Dion JE, Duckwiler GR, Lylyk P, Vinuela F, Bentson J. Progressive suppleness pursil catheter: a new tool for superselective angiography and embolization. AJNR Am J Neuroradiol. 1989;10:1068–70.

209. Aletich VA, Debrun GM, Koenigsberg R, Ausman JI, Charbel F, Dujovny M. Arteriovenous malformation nidus catheterization with hydrophilic wire and flow-directed catheter. AJNR Am J Neuroradiol. 1997;18:929–35.

210. Mathis JA, Barr JD, Horton JA, et al. The efficacy of particulate embolization combined with stereotactic radiosurgery for treatment of large arteriovenous malformations of the brain. AJNR Am J Neuroradiol. 1995;16:299–306.

211. The n BCATI. N-Butyl cyanoacrylate embolization of cerebral arteriovenous malformations: results of a prospective, randomized. multi-center trial. AJNR Am J Neuroradiol. 2002;23:748–55.

212. Neurological Devices Panel of the Medical Devices Advisory Committee, FDA. Statistical review for PMA P030004, Onyx Liquid Embolic System. http://www.fda.gov/ohrms/dockets/ac/03/briefing/3975b1.htm (Accessed 3 Oct 2007)

213. Jahan R, Murayama Y, Gobin YP, Duckwiler GR, Vinters HV, Vinuela F. Embolization of arteriovenous malformations with Onyx: clinicopathological experience in 23 patients. Neurosurgery. 2001;48:984–95; discussion 95–7.

214. Deruty R, Pelissou-Guyotat I, Mottolese C, Bascoulergue Y, Amat D. The combined management of cerebral arteriovenous malformations. Experience with 100 cases and review of the literature. Acta Neurochir (Wien). 1993;123:101–12.

215. Fournier D, TerBrugge KG, Willinsky R, Lasjaunias P, Montanera W. Endovascular treatment of intracerebral arteriovenous malformations: experience in 49 cases. J Neurosurg. 1991;75:228–33.

216. Wikholm G, Lundqvist C, Svendsen P. Embolization of cerebral arteriovenous malformations: part I–technique, morphology, and complications. Neurosurgery. 1996;39:448–57; discussion 57–9.

217. Gobin YP, Laurent A, Merienne L, et al. Treatment of brain arteriovenous malformations by embolization and radiosurgery. J Neurosurg. 1996;85:19–28.

218. Valavanis A, Yaşargil MG. The endovascular treatment of brain arteriovenous malformations. Adv Tech Stand Neurosurg. 1998;24:131–214.

219. Frizzel RT, 3 rd Fisher WS. Cure, morbidity, and mortality associated with embolization of brain arteriovenous malformations: a review of 1246 patients in 32 series over a 35-year period. Neurosurgery. 1995;37:1031–9; discussion 9–40.

220. Sugita M, Takahashi A, Ogawa A, Yoshimoto T. Improvement of cerebral blood flow and clinical symptoms associated with embolization of a large arteriovenous malformation: case report. Neurosurgery. 1993;33:748–51; discussion 52.

221. Fox AJ, Girvin JP, Vinuela F, Drake CG. Rolandic arteriovenous malformations: improvement in limb function by

IBC embolization. AJNR Am J Neuroradiol. 1985;6:
575–82.

222. Jafar JJ, Davis AJ, Berenstein A, Choi IS, Kupersmith MJ.
The effect of embolization with N-butyl cyanoacrylate prior
to surgical resection of brain arteriovenous malformations. J Neurosurg. 1993;78:60–9.

223. Debrun GM, Aletich V, Ausman JI, Charbel F, Dujovny M.
Embolization of the nidus of brain arteriovenous malformations
with n-butyl cyanoacrylate. Neurosurgery. 1997;40:112–20;
discussion 20–1.

224. DeMeritt JS, Pile-Spellman J, Mast H, et al. Outcome
analysis of preoperative embolization with N-butyl cyanoacrylate in cerebral arteriovenous malformations. AJNR
Am J Neuroradiol. 1995;16:1801–7.

225. Grzyska U, Westphal M, Zanella F, Freckmann N,
Herrmann HD, Zeumer H. A joint protocol for the neurosurgical and neuroradiologic treatment of cerebral arteriovenous malformations: indications, technique, and results
in 76 cases. Surg Neurol. 1993;40:476–84.

226. Pasqualin A, Scienza R, Cioffi F, et al. Treatment of cerebral arteriovenous malformations with a combination of
preoperative embolization and surgery. Neurosurgery.
1991;29:358–68.

227. Pelz DM, Fox AJ, Vinuela F, Drake CC, Ferguson GG.
Preoperative embolization of brain AVMs with isobutyl-2
cyanoacrylate. AJNR Am J Neuroradiol. 1988;9:757–64.

228. Deruty R, Pelissou-Guyotat I, Amat D, et al.
Multidisciplinary treatment of cerebral arteriovenous malformations. Neurol Res. 1995;17:169–77.

229. Hurst RW, Berenstein A, Kupersmith MJ, Madrid M,
Flamm ES. Deep central arteriovenous malformations of
the brain: the role of endovascular treatment. J Neurosurg.
1995;82:190–5.

230. Lundqvist C, Wikholm G, Svendsen P. Embolization of cerebral arteriovenous malformations: part II–aspects of complications and late outcome. Neurosurgery. 1996;39:460–7;
discussion 7–9.

231. Taylor CL, Dutton K, Rappard G, et al. Complications of
preoperative embolization of cerebral arteriovenous malformations. J Neurosurg. 2004;100:810–2.

232. Vinuela F, Dion JE, Duckwiler G, et al. Combined endovascular embolization and surgery in the management of cerebral arteriovenous malformations: experience with 101
cases. J Neurosurg. 1991;75:856–64.

233. Andrade-Souza YM, Ramani M, Scora D, Tsao MN, terBrugge
K, Schwartz ML. Embolization Before Radiosurgery Reduces the
Obliteration Rate of Arteriovenous Malformations. Neurosurgery.
2007;60:443–52. doi:10.1227/01.NEU.0000255347.25959.D0.

234. Back AG, Vollmer D, Zeck O, Shkedy C, Shedden PM.
Retrospective analysis of unstaged and staged Gamma
Knife surgery with and without preceding embolization for
the treatment of arteriovenous malformations. J Neurosurg.
2008;109(Suppl):57–64.

235. Sure U, Surucu O, Engenhart-Cabillic R. Embolization
before radiosurgery reduces the obliteration rate of arteriovenous malformations. Neurosurgery. 2008;63:E376;
author reply E.

236. Andrade-Souza YM, Ramani M, Beachey DJ, et al. Liquid
embolisation material reduces the delivered radiation dose: a
physical experiment. Acta Neurochir (Wien). 2008;150:161–
4; discussion 4.

237. Mamalui-Hunter M, Jiang T, Rich KM, Derdeyn CP,
Drzymala RE. Effect of liquid embolic agents on Gamma
Knife surgery dosimetry for arteriovenous malformations.
Clinical article. J Neurosurg. 2011;115:364–70.

238. Sure U, Butz N, Siegel AM, Mennel HD, Bien S,
Bertalanffy H. Treatment-induced neoangiogenesis in cerebral arteriovenous malformations. Clin Neurol Neurosurg.
2001;103:29–32.

239. Akakin A, Ozkan A, Akgun E, et al. Endovascular treatment increases but gamma knife radiosurgery decreases
angiogenic activity of arteriovenous malformations: an
in vivo experimental study using a rat cornea model.
Neurosurgery. 2010;66:121–9; discussion 9–30.

240. Meisel HJ, Mansmann U, Alvarez H, Rodesch G, Brock M,
Lasjaunias P. Effect of partial targeted N-butyl-cyano-
acrylate embolization in brain AVM. Acta Neurochir
(Wien). 2002;144:879–87; discussion 88.

241. Hartmann A, Pile-Spellman J, Stapf C, et al. Risk of endovascular treatment of brain arteriovenous malformations.
Stroke. 2002;33:1816–20.

242. Redekop G, TerBrugge K, Montanera W, Willinsky R.
Arterial aneurysms associated with cerebral arteriovenous
malformations: classification, incidence, and risk of hemorrhage. J Neurosurg. 1998;89:539–46.

243. Stapf C, Mohr JP, Pile-Spellman J, et al. Concurrent arterial
aneurysms in brain arteriovenous malformations with haemorrhagic presentation. J Neurol Neurosurg Psychiatry.
2002;73:294–8.

244. Marks MP, Lane B, Steinberg GK, Snipes GJ. Intranidal
aneurysms in cerebral arteriovenous malformations: evaluation and endovascular treatment. Radiology. 1992;183:
355–60.

245. Garcia-Monaco R, Rodesch G, Alvarez H, Iizuka Y, Hui F,
Lasjaunias P. Pseudoaneurysms within ruptured intracranial
arteriovenous malformations: diagnosis and early endovascular management. AJNR Am J Neuroradiol. 1993;14:
315–21.

246. Murray RA, Russell EJ. Radiographic Diagnosis. In: Stieg
PE, Batjer HH, Samson D, editors. Intracranial
arteriovenous malformations. New York: Informa; 2007.
p. 95–113.

247. Thompson RC, Steinberg GK, Levy RP, Marks MP. The
management of patients with arteriovenous malformations
and associated intracranial aneurysms. Neurosurgery.
1998;43:202–11; discussion 11–2.

248. Batjer H, Suss RA, Samson D. Intracranial arteriovenous
malformations associated with aneurysms. Neurosurgery.
1986;18:29–35.

249. Piotin M, Ross IB, Weill A, Kothimbakam R, Moret J.
Intracranial arterial aneurysms associated with arteriovenous malformations: endovascular treatment. Radiology.
2001;220:506–13.

250. Suzuki J, Onuma T. Intracranial aneurysms associated
with arteriovenous malformations. J Neurosurg. 1979;50:
742–6.

251. Kondziolka D, Nixon BJ, Lasjaunias P, Tucker WS,
TerBrugge K, Spiegel SM. Cerebral arteriovenous malformations with associated arterial aneurysms: hemodynamic
and therapeutic considerations. Can J Neurol Sci. 1988;15:
130–4.

252. Deruty R, Mottolese C, Soustiel JF, Pelissou-Guyotat I.
Association of cerebral arteriovenous malformation and
cerebral aneurysm. Diagnosis and management. Acta
Neurochir (Wien). 1990;107:133–9.

253. Han PP, Ponce FA, Spetzler RF. Intention-to-treat analysis of
Spetzler-Martin grades IV and V arteriovenous malformations: natural history and treatment paradigm. J Neurosurg.
2003;98:3–7.

254. Jayaraman MV, Marcellus ML, Do HM, et al. Hemorrhage
rate in patients with Spetzler-Martin grades IV and V arteriovenous malformations: is treatment justified? Stroke.
2007;38:325–9.

255. Kjellberg RN, Hanamura T, Davis KR, Lyons SL, Adams
RD. Bragg-peak proton-beam therapy for arteriovenous
malformations of the brain. N Engl J Med. 1983;309:
269–74.

256. Miyawaki L, Dowd C, Wara W, et al. Five year results of
LINAC radiosurgery for arteriovenous malformations: outcome for large AVMS. Int J Radiat Oncol Biol Phys.
1999;44:1089–106.

257. Pan DH, Guo WY, Chung WY, Shiau CY, Chang YC, Wang
LW. Gamma knife radiosurgery as a single treatment
modality for large cerebral arteriovenous malformations.
J Neurosurg. 2000;93 Suppl 3:113–9.

258. Sirin S, Kondziolka D, Niranjan A, Flickinger JC, Maitz
AH, Lunsford LD. Prospective staged volume radiosurgery
for large arteriovenous malformations: indications and outcomes in otherwise untreatable patients. Neurosurgery.
2006;58:17–27; discussion 17–27.

259. Chang SD, Marcellus ML, Marks MP, Levy RP, Do HM,
Steinberg GK. Multimodality treatment of giant intracranial
arteriovenous malformations. Neurosurgery. 2003;53:1–11;
discussion –3.

260. Heros RC. Spetzler-Martin grades IV and V arteriovenous
malformations. J Neurosurg. 2003;98:1–2; discussion.

261. Celli P, Ferrante L, Palma L, Cavedon G. Cerebral arterio-venous malformations in children. Clinical features and outcome of treatment in children and in adults. Surg Neurol. 1984;22:43–9.

262. Millar C, Bissonnette B, Humphreys RP. Cerebral arterio-venous malformations in children. Can J Anaesth. 1994;41:321–31.

263. Garza-Mercado R, Cavazos E, Tamez-Montes D. Cerebral arteriovenous malformations in children and adolescents. Surg Neurol. 1987;27:131–40.

264. Greenfield JP, Souweidane MM. Diagnosis and manage-ment of pediatric arteriovenous malformations. In: Stieg PE, Batjer HH, Samson D, editors. Intracranial arteriovenous malformations. New York: Informa; 2007. p. 359–69.

265. Bristol RE, Albuquerque FC, Spetzler RF, Rekate HL, McDougall CG, Zabramski JM. Surgical management of arteriovenous malformations in children. J Neurosurg. 2006;105:88–93.

266. Meyer PG, Orliaguet GA, Zerah M, et al. Emergency man-agement of deeply comatose children with acute rupture of cerebral arteriovenous malformations. Can J Anaesth. 2000;47:758–66.

267. Hoh BL, Ogilvy CS, Butler WE, Loeffler JS, Putman CM, Chapman PH. Multimodality treatment of nongalenic arte-riovenous malformations in pediatric patients. Neurosurgery. 2000;47:346–57; discussion 57–8.

268. Fong D, Chan ST. Arteriovenous malformation in children. Childs Nerv Syst. 1988;4:199–203.

269. Cohen-Gadol AA, Pollock BE. Radiosurgery for arteriovenous malformations in children. J Neurosurg. 2006;104:388–91.

270. Kader A, Goodrich JT, Sonstein WJ, Stein BM, Carmel PW, Michelsen WJ. Recurrent cerebral arteriovenous malforma-tions after negative postoperative angiograms. J Neurosurg. 1996;85:14–8.

271. Ali MJ, Bendok BR, Rosenblatt S, Rose JE, Getch CC, Batjer HH. Recurrence of pediatric cerebral arteriovenous malformations after angiographically documented resec-tion. Pediatr Neurosurg. 2003;39:32–8.

272. Sawin P. Spontaneous subarachnoid hemorrhage in preg-nancy and the puerperium. In: Loftus C, editor. Neurosurgical aspects of pregnancy. Park Ridge: American Association of Neurological Surgeons; 1996. p. 85–99.

273. Dias MS, Sekhar LN. Intracranial hemorrhage from aneu-rysms and arteriovenous malformations during pregnancy and the puerperium. Neurosurgery. 1990;27:855–65; dis-cussion 65–6.

274. Amias AG. Cerebral vascular disease in pregnancy. I. Haemorrhage. J Obstet Gynaecol Br Commonw. 1970;77: 100–20.

275. Robinson JL, Hall CS, Sedzimir CB. Arteriovenous malfor-mations, aneurysms, and pregnancy. J Neurosurg. 1974;41:63–70.

276. Horton JC, Chambers WA, Lyons SL, Adams RD, Kjellberg RN. Pregnancy and the risk of hemorrhage from cerebral arteriovenous malformations. Neurosurgery. 1990;27:867–71; discussion 71–2.

277. Schwartz J. Pregnancy complicated by subarachnoid hem-orrhage. Am J Obstet Gynecol. 1951;62:539–47.

278. Majewski T, Liebert W, Nowak S. Smol S.Conservative treatment of cerebral arteriovenous malformations. Follow-up study of 31 cases Neurol Neurochir Pol. 1998;32:573–9.

279. Sadasivan B, Malik GM, Lee C, Ausman JI. Vascular mal-formations and pregnancy. Surg Neurol. 1990;33:305–13.

280. Lasjaunias P, Terbrugge K, Piske R, Lopez Ibor L, Manelfe C. Dilatation of the vein of Galen Anatomoclinical forms and endovascular treatment apropos of 14 cases explored and/or treated between 1983 and 1986 Neurochirurgie. 1987;33:315–33.

281. Yaşargil MG. AVM of the brain, clinical considerations, general and specific operative techniques, surgical results,

nonoperated cases, cavernous and venous angiomas, neuroanesthesia. In: Microneurosurgery. Stuttgart: Georg Thieme; 1988. p. 317–96.

282. Raybaud CA, Strother CM, Hald JK. Aneurysms of the vein of Galen: embryonic considerations and anatomical fea-tures relating to the pathogenesis of the malformation. Neuroradiology. 1989;31:109–28.

283. Alvarez H, Garcia Monaco R, Rodesch G, Sachet M, Krings T, Lasjaunias P. Vein of galen aneurysmal malfor-mations. Neuroimaging Clin N Am. 2007;17:189–206.

284. Lasjaunias PL, Chng SM, Sachet M, Alvarez H, Rodesch G, Garcia-Monaco R. The management of vein of Galen aneurysmal malformations. Neurosurgery. 2006;59:S184–94; discussion S3-13.

285. Mickle JP, Mericle RA, Burry MV, Shon Williams L. Vein of Galen malformations. In: Winn HR, editor. Youmans neurological surgery. Philadelphia: Saunders; 2004. p. 3433–46.

286. Zerah M, Garcia-Monaco R, Rodesch G, et al. Hydrodynamics in vein of Galen malformations. Childs Nerv Syst. 1992;8:111–7; discussion 7.

287. Chevret L, Durand P, Alvarez H, et al. Severe cardiac failure in newborns with VGAM. Prognosis significance of hemodynamic parameters in neonates presenting with severe heart failure owing to vein of Galen arte-riovenous malformation. Intensive Care Med. 2002;28: 1126–30.

288. Lasjaunias P, Rodesch G, Terbrugge K, Taylor W. Arterial and venous angioarchitecture in cerebral AVMs in adults. Rivista di Neuroradiologica. 1994;7:35–9.

289. Li AH, Armstrong D, ter Brugge KG. Endovascular treat-ment of vein of Galen aneurysmal malformation: manage-ment strategy and 21-year experience in Toronto. J Neurosurg Pediatr. 2011;7:3–10.

290. Lasjaunias P. Neonatal evaluation score (Bicêtre). In: Vascular diseases in neonates, infants and children: inter-ventional neuroradiology management. Berlin: Springer; 1997. p. 49.

291. Mickle JP, Quisling RG. The transtorcular embolization of vein of Galen aneurysms. J Neurosurg. 1986;64:731–5.

292. Dowd CF, Halbach VV, Barnwell SL, Higashida RT, Edwards MS, Hieshima GB. Transfemoral venous embo-lization of vein of Galen malformations. AJNR Am J Neuroradiol. 1990;11:643–8.

293. Charafeddine L, Numaguchi Y, Sinkin RA. Disseminated coagulopathy associated with transtorcular embolization of vein of Galen aneurysm in a neonate. J Perinatol. 1999;19:61–3.

294. Lylyk P, Vinuela F, Dion JE, et al. Therapeutic alternatives for vein of Galen vascular malformations. J Neurosurg. 1993;78:438–45.

295. Andeweg J. Intracranial venous pressures, hydrocephalus and effects of cerebrospinal fluid shunts. Childs Nerv Syst. 1989;5:318–23.

296. Quisling RG, Mickle JP. Venous pressure measurements in vein of Galen aneurysms. AJNR Am J Neuroradiol. 1989;10:411–7.

297. Abe T, Matsumoto K, Kiyota K, Tanaka H. Vein of Galen aneurysmal malformation in an adult: a case report. Surg Neurol. 1996;45:39–43.

298. Mylonas C, Booth AE. Vein of Galen aneurysm presenting in middle age. Br J Neurosurg. 1992;6:491–4.

299. Hassan T, Timofeev EV, Ezura M, et al. Hemodynamic analysis of an adult vein of Galen aneurysm malformation by use of 3D image-based computational fluid dynamics. AJNR Am J Neuroradiol. 2003;24:1075–82.

300. Marques RM, Lobao CA, Sassaki VS, Aguiar LR. Vein of Galen aneurysm in an adult: case report. Arq Neuropsiquiatr. 2006;64:862–4.

301. Arias E. United States life tables, 2002. Natl Vital Stat Rep. 2004;53:1–38.

15. Dural Arteriovenous Fistulas

Intracranial dural AV fistulas (dAVF, aka dural AV fistulas, dural arteriovenous fistulous malformation)[1] are acquired lesions that usually involve one of the intracranial venous sinuses. They comprise ≤10% of all intracranial vascular malformations.[2] Typically, numerous branches of the ECA, ICA, and/or vertebral artery form direct connections to a venous sinus and/or intracranial veins. Any intracranial venous sinus may be involved. Clinical features, natural history and management options depend upon the location and anatomy of the lesion. Lesions causing arterialization of intradural veins (aka retrograde leptomeningeal cortical venous flow) are classically associated with intracranial haemorrhage. Spinal dural AV fistulas are discussed in Chap. 20.

15.1.   Pathophysiology

Anatomy and Classification

All intracranial dAVFs consist of one or more meningeal feeding arteries that drain directly into a venous sinus or intracranial vein. Two classification systems are in common usage and both have been validated as predictive of risk of haemorrhage.[3] Borden and colleagues:[1]

1. Type I. Dural AVFs that drain directly into a dural venous sinus or meningeal vein.
2. Type II. Dural AVFs that drain into a dural venous sinus with retrograde drainage into subarachnoid veins.
3. Type III. Dural AVFs that drain directly into subarachnoid veins.
4. Further classification into subtypes *a* and *b* indicate single or multiple fistulas, respectively.

Cognard and coworkers:[4]

1. Type I. Drainage is into a sinus, with normal antegrade flow.
2. Type II. Dural AVFs with reflux.
   - (a) IIa Reflux into the sinus.
   - (b) IIb Reflux into cortical veins.
   - (c) IIa + b Reflux into both.
3. Type III. Direct cortical venous drainage without venous ectasia.
4. Type IV. Direct cortical venous drainage with venous ectasia larger than 5 mm in diameter and three times larger than the diameter of the draining vein.
5. Type V. Drainage occurs into spinal perimedullary veins.

Etiology

Several lines of evidence have lead to a three-stage hypothesis for the formation of dAVFs (Fig. 15.1).[5–7]

1. Stage 1. Venous sinus thrombosis is the initial event,[8] possibly combined with other anatomic features that limit venous outflow, such as venous sinus stenosis.
2. Stage 2. Nascent microscopic fistulas within the wall of the venous sinus, connecting vaso vasorum to tiny venous tributaries, enlarge. This process may be the result of a build-up of back pressure in the venous system, inflammatory changes in response to the thrombosis, and/or via an increase in angiogenic factor expression.[7,9–13]
3. Stage 3. Recanalization of the thrombosed venous sinus occurs. If only partial recanalization appears, or if there is some other venous sinus outflow obstruction (like venous sinus stenosis), arterial flow is diverted into the subarachnoid venous system (i.e., retrograde leptomeningeal flow occurs).

M.R. Harrigan, J.P. Deveikis, *Handbook of Cerebrovascular Disease and Neurointerventional Technique*, DOI 10.1007/978-1-61779-946-4_15, © Springer Science+Business Media New York 2013

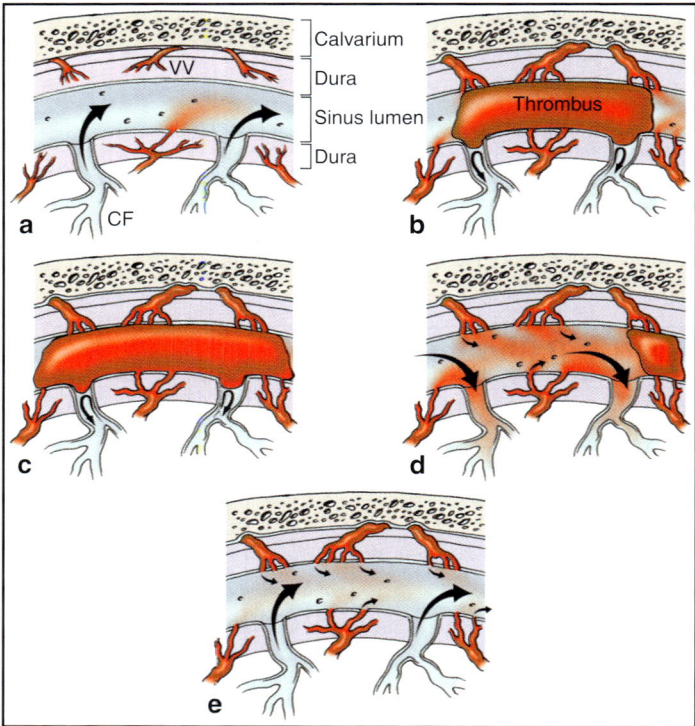

Fig. 15.1 Stages in the formation of dural arteriovenous fistulas. (**a**) Normal anatomy of the dural venous sinus. (**b**) Stage 1. Thrombosis of the venous sinus occurs, leading to diversion of flow in the entering venous tributaries. (**c**) Stage 2. Thrombosis of the venous sinus provides an impetus to the enlargement and expansion of nascent connections between vaso vasorum and fistulas between vaso vasorum and nearby arteries within the wall of the venous sinus. Over time, as dural arteries enlarge, grooves in the adjacent bone develop. (**d**) Stage 3-Partial recanalizaton. Incomplete recanalization of the thrombosed sinus occurs, (or some other venous outflow-limiting factor exists, such as venous sinus stenosis), leading to diversion of arterial flow into subarachnoid veins. (**e**) Stage 3-Complete recanalization. Normal venous outflow resumes, and AV fistulas may or may not continue to be patent.

Evidence in Favor of the Three Stage Hypothesis

1. Microscopic fistulas between meningeal arteries and veins are normal and present throughout the dura.[14–17]
   - Also, the dura has an elaborate network of arterial anastomoses[15] which explains why fistulas apparently supplied only by ECA branches can promptly recruit blood supply from ICA branches after embolization.[18]
2. Development of abnormal communications between dural arteries and veins appears to be an essential factor in the development of dAVFs.[19]

3. Dural AV fistulas are usually located either in the wall of dural venous sinuses.[20] or within a centimeter or so of a dural venous sinus.[17]
4. Venous sinus thrombosis is strongly associated with intracranial dAVFs.[5,8,11,21]
   - Experimental models have also reproduced venous thrombosis- or venous hypertension-associated dAVFs.[10,22,23]
5. Venous sinus thrombosis can redirect arterial blood into subarachnoid veins.[24]
6. Progressive thrombosis can transform Type I malformations into Type II malformations.

15.2. Clinical Features

1) Most patients with dAVFs are adults; dAVFs in children are rare but have been reported.[25]
2) Benign dAVFs are most common among women,[26,27] whereas dAVFs with cortical venous drainage appear to be most common among men.[28,29]
3) Multiple intracranial dAVFs are present in 6.7% of patients.[30]
4) *Presentation*. Symptoms and physical findings are highly variable, and depend on the location and anatomy of the lesion (see below for discussion of dAVFs by location).
   a) Overall, pulsatile tinnitus is the most common symptom and is present in about 60% of patients.[31] See section on Pulsatile Tinnitus below.
   b) A bruit is present in about 50% of patients.[31]
   c) Hydrocephalus may be present and is attributable to venous hypertension in the superior sagittal sinus, interfering with CSF absorption.[24]
5) Significant symptoms from dAVFs are generally divided into those attributable to haemorrhage or "non-haemorrhagic neurological defects,"[32,33] which are usually due to intracranial venous hypertension.
   a) *Haemorrhage.*
      i) In a prospective study of intracranial haemorrhage due to an intracranial vascular malformation (brain AVM, cavernoma, or dAVF), a dAVF was the underlying cause in 6.4% of cases.[34]
      ii) Risk factors for haemorrhage:[5,24,35]
         (1) Leptomeningeal venous drainage
         (2) Variceal or aneurysmal venous dilatations
         (3) Galenic drainage
         (4) Stenosis or occlusion of associated venous sinuses
         (5) Location in the anterior fossa, middle fossa, or tentorial incisura
      iii) Case fatality rate with haemorrhage: 20%[31,32]
   b) *Intracranial venous hypertension* The intracranial venous system is valveless and so elevated pressure within arterialized venous sinuses and/or intracranial veins may be transmitted throughout the intracranial venous system. Diffuse white matter changes on MRI due to venous congestion may be seen.[36,37] Decreased apparent diffusion coefficient (ADC) is observed in the brain tissue affected by retrograde cortical venous flow and is associated with brain dysfunction.[38]
      i) Neurological symptoms attributable to elevated intracranial venous pressure include:
         (1) Progressive dementia (aka venous hypertensive encephalopathy, venous congestive encephalopathy, or progressive cognitive impairment).[24,39–42]
         (2) Pseudotumor cerebri.[43]
         (3) Parkinsonism.[44]
         (4) Cervical myelopathy.[45]

Pulsatile Tinnitus: What Does It Mean?

Some 4% of all patients with tinnitus have pulsatile tinnitus (aka pulse-synchronous tinnitus).[46] Pulsatile tinnitus is usually caused by vibrations from turbulent blood flow. Dural AV fistulas are the single most common cause of pulsatile tinnitus, followed by carotid-cavernous fistulas and atherosclerotic carotid stenosis.[47] In a series of 24 patients with Borden Type I dAVFs of the transverse-sigmoid region, pulsatile tinnitus was the presenting symptom in all patients.[27] A vascular disorder is present in 42% of patients with pulsatile tinnitus; a non-vascular disorder is the cause of pulsatile tinnitus in 14% of patients.[47]

1. Vascular causes
    (a) dAVF
    (b) ICA stenosis or occlusion
    (c) Carotid dissection
    (d) Fibromuscular dysplasia
    (e) Persistent stapedial artery
    (f) Aberrant or lateralized ICA
    (g) Intracranial venous hypertension
    (h) High-riding internal jugular vein.[48]
    (i) Venous sinus stenosis.[49]
    (j) Turbulent flow through a dominant internal jugular vein
    (k) Vertebral artery-venous fistula
2. Non-vascular causes of pulsatile tinnitus
    (a) Middle ear disorders (otitis media, glomus tympanicum, cholesteatoma)
    (b) Labyrinth disorders (otospongiosis)
    (c) High cardiac output disorders (anemia, thyrotoxicosis, valvular heart disease)
    (d) Skull base tumors
3. Work-up for pulsatile tinnitus
    (a) Pulsatile tinnitus is either *objective* (a bruit on the skull or mastoid process can be heard by the examiner) or *subjective* (only the patient can perceive it). Objective tinnitus should raise a high suspicion of an underlying vascular abnormality and a catheter angiogram is frequently indicated.
    (b) Imaging
        • CT is insensitive in the assessment of pulsatile tinnitus
        • MRI is more sensitive than CT
            – In patients with subjective pulsatile tinnitus, MRI/MRA defined anatomical abnormalities that may contribute to pulsatile tinnitus in 63% of patients.[50]
    (c) In the absence of objective pulsatile tinnitus, MRI/MRA is an appropriate initial diagnostic step.[50]

Imaging

Angiography

Catheter angiography is the best technique for the diagnosis of an intracranial dAVF.[51,52]

1. Technique
    (a) A complete 6-vessel cerebral angiogram is necessary, as some lesions may have feeding arteries from both sides, as well as from the ICA or vertebral arteries as well as the ECAs. For example, it is not uncommon for a transverse/sigmoid sinus fistula to receive feeders from both middle meningeal arteries.
    (b) Each angiogram should be carried well into the venous phase, to assess intracranial vein and venous sinus anatomy.

2. Pertinent findings
  (a) The single most important goal of angiography in patients with a dAVF is to look for retrograde leptomeningeal venous drainage.
    • Good visualization of the venous phase is essential.
    • Tortuous, engorged veins seen during the venous phase is termed *pseudophlebitic pattern* and is a sign of venous congestion.[53] A pseudophlebitic pattern was seen in 81% with retrograde leptomeningeal venous drainage and in only 8% of dAVF patients with drainage into a venous sinus only.[53]
    • Subtle findings seen during the venous phase include drainage via pial or medullary collateral veins, focal regions of delayed circulation and venous rerouting to the orbit or to transosseous veins.[53]
  (b) The arterial feeders must be characterized.
    • Occasionally, a dAVF may have only a single (or two or three) endovascularly accessible arterial pedicles and thus be a prospect for curative arterial embolization.
  (c) Venous outflow obstruction should be checked for (e.g., venous sinus stenosis or thrombosis).

MRI

MRI may not show some dAVFs and should not be used instead of catheter angiography to exclude the presence of a dAVF. *Remember: a normal MRI does not exclude the presence of a dAVF.*
1. MRI findings in patients with dAVFs:
  (a) Preliminary experience with MRA assessment of dAVFs has been reported.[54]
  (b) A surplus of pial vessels suggests the presence of a dAVF with cortical venous drainage.[36]
  (c) Enhanced MRI is superior to non-enhanced MRI in assessing retrograde venous drainage in intracranial dAVFs.
2. MRI may provide complementary information that is not available with catheter angiography:
  (a) MRI evidence of white matter edema (diffuse T2 hyperintensity in the white matter) is evidence of venous congestion.[36]
  (b) Evaluation for hydrocephalus.
  (c) Quantitative assessment of cerebral blood volume by dynamic susceptibility contrast MRI can provide quantitative information about retrograde cortical venous drainage.[55]
  (d) Decreased apparent diffusion coefficient (ADC) can be seen with retrograde cortical venous flow and is associated with brain dysfunction.[38]

CTA

Like MRI, CTA may not show some dAVFs,[56] and should not be used instead of catheter angiography.
1. CTA can identify some dAVFs, particularly those with enlarged intracranial veins.[57]

Natural History

Intracranial dAVFs are dynamic. In a study of 112 patients with dAVFs who were managed conservatively, 12.5% showed spontaneous occlusion of the fistula (most commonly transverse and cavernous sinus locations) and 4.0% showed conversion to a higher grade dAVF.[58]

Risk of Haemorrhage

The overall annual risk of haemorrhage in patients with intracranial dAVFs is 1.8%, with a case fatality rate of 20% with haemorrhage.[31] However, the natural history of dAVFs depends strongly on the pattern of venous drainage. Most Borden Type I lesions (aka Cognard Type I or IIa) are "benign" whereas higher grade lesions are "aggressive."

Borden Type I dAVFs: Most Are Benign

1. In a series of 112 patients with Borden Type I lesions followed for median time of 27.9 months, observation and/or palliative therapy resulted in a benign and tolerable level of disease in 98.2% of cases.[26]
   (a) Palliation consisted of embolization to reduce symptoms without obliteration of the lesion.
   (b) In 2% of cases conversion to a higher grade lesion occurred, with progressive thrombosis of venous outlets.
2. A previous study reported on a group of 54 patients with Borden Type I lesions.[59] During a mean follow-up period of 33 months, 53 (98%) patients had good outcomes (i.e., symptoms were resolved, improved, or unchanged). One death was reported; this patient had a complex torcular dAVF and his death was attributed to venous hypertension and elevated intracranial pressure.
3. Cognard and colleagues reported on a group of seven patients with Type I lesions, followed for a mean time of 7 years, all of whom developed a worsening in both the venous drainage pattern and clinical symptoms.[60] The authors did not indicate the number of patients with Type I lesions in the entire group, so an incidence of worsening cannot be calculated from this paper.

Borden Type II and III dAVFs: Aggressive

Patients with high grade dAVFs are at significant risk of haemorrhage or neurological problems because of intracranial venous hypertension.

1. Risk of haemorrhage or non-haemorrhagic neurological deficit.
   (a) van Dijk and colleagues reported on 20 patients with Borden Type II or III lesions who were either partially treated or not treated at all and followed for a mean period of 4.3 years.[33]
   * The annual rate of haemorrhage was 8.1% and the annual rate of a non-haemorrhagic neurological deficit was 6.9%, yielding an annual event rate of 15%.
   (b) Davies and coworkers reported on 14 patients with Borden Type II or III lesions who were followed for a mean period of 25 months without or prior treatment.[32]
   * The annual rate of haemorrhage was 19.2% and the annual rate of a non-haemorrhagic neurological deficit was 10.9%. The overall annual mortality rate was 19.3%.
2. Risk of rehaemorrhage.
   (a) In a series of patients with dAVFs with cortical venous drainage presenting with haemorrhage, rebleeding occurred in 35% within 2 weeks of the initial haemorrhage.[61]

15.3.   Management

Management options for patients with a dAVF:
1. Conservative management
2. Endovascular techniques

3. Surgery
4. Radiosurgery
5. A combination of endovascular treatment, radiosurgery, and/or surgery

Conservative Management

Conservative management (i.e., no endovascular or surgical procedure, with or without surveillance imaging) is reasonable in certain situations. Asymptomatic or minimally symptomatic Borden Type I lesions without evidence of cortical venous drainage may be managed expectantly. It is well established that spontaneous regression of dAVFs occurs in some cases. This is particularly true of cavernous sinus dAVFs,[62,63] in which spontaneous regression has been reported in up to 73% of cases.[64–66] Intermittent manual compression is also effective for some patients with cavernous sinus or transverse-sigmoid lesions.[67,68]

Endovascular Treatment

Generally the most effective treatment of dAVFs is occlusion of the draining vein.[7] In most cases, obliteration of the lesion can only be accomplished by treatment of the venous side of the lesion. Transvenous techniques appear to carry the highest success rates among endovascular techniques. Even successful arterial embolization usually occurs only when the microcatheter is positioned well within or adjacent to the nidus, so that embolic material can be pushed through the nidus into the venous side. If only feeding arteries are occluded and not the draining vein, collateral vessels usually develop and the fistula will recur. Conversely, it is equally important to ensure that normal venous drainage is preserved after embolization to avoid exacerbated venous hypertension and risk of haemorrhage.

Embolization of the arterial feeders alone is usually only palliative. Embolization of feeders proximal to the nidus will nearly invariably be followed by recruitment of a new arterial supply and possibly the redirection of the venous outflow with an increased risk of haemorrhage.

Surgery

Surgery for intracranial dAVFs has evolved considerably over the last three decades from simple ligature of feeding vessels (which produced success rates of only 0–8%),[69] to blood-soaked fistula resection and packing of the venous sinus,[70] or to more elegant interruption of the draining vein when the anatomy is favorable.[71] Although endovascular techniques are presently first-line treatments for many dAVFs, surgery remains standard for anterior fossa dAVFs.[69] A variety of hybrid surgical/endovascular procedures have evolved as well, including surgical exposure of the superior ophthalmic vein for embolization of the cavernous sinus[72,73] and craniectomy with direct puncture of a venous sinus.[74]

Radiosurgery

Preliminary reports of radiosurgery for intracranial dAVFs are encouraging.[75,76] In many cases embolization is combined with radiosurgery.[77] Overall rates of lesion obliteration are 58–83%.[76,78–81] Interestingly, a single report indicated a higher obliteration rate with embolization followed by radiosurgery (83%) compared to radiosurgery alone (67%),[81] which is the opposite of the situation with radiosurgery for brain AVMs.[82–84]

15.4.   Dural AVFs by Location

In North American and European series, the transverse-sigmoid sinus region is the most common location for dAVFs;[31,35] in a Korean report, the cavernous sinus was the most common location, accounting for 64% of cases (Fig. 15.2).[85]

Most common locations for dAVFs are.[86]

1. Transverse-sigmoid sinus 35%
2. Cavernous sinus 35%
3. Tentorium/Superior petrosal sinus 5%
4. Superior sagittal sinus 5%
5. Anterior fossa 5%

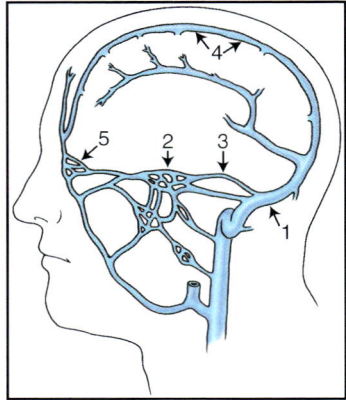

Fig. 15.2 Most common locations of dural arteriovenous fistulas.

Transverse-Sigmoid Sinus dAVFs

The transverse-sigmoid sinus (aka lateral sinus) is the most common location for intracranial dAVFs, comprising 38% of all intracranial dAVFs.[86]

Clinical Features

1. Women are affected more than men and the lesion is present most often on the left.[5,87]
2. Borden Type I dAVFs of the transverse-sigmoid sinus (analysis of 24 cases):[27]
   (a) Seventy-nine percent women; median age at onset of symptoms: 54 years.
   (b) Unilateral pulsatile tinnitus was the presenting symptom (and a bruit could be heard) in all patients.
   (c) MRI was normal in all patients.
3. May be associated with meningiomas.[88]
4. Anatomy
   (a) Feeders – may be bilateral
       • ECA branches are most common: occipital, posterior auricular, ascending pharyngeal, middle meningeal, accessory meningeal and superficial temporal arteries.
       • ICA branches: meningohypophyseal trunk, inferolateral trunk.
       • Vertebral artery branches: posterior meningeal artery, cerebellar falcine and muscular branches.
   (b) Venous drainage
       • The transverse or sigmoid sinus is stenotic or occluded in a significant percentage of cases.[5]
       • Retrograde venous flow, when present, may be into occipital and parietal cortical veins.
5. Presentation
   (a) Haemorrhage or intracranial venous hypertension
       • Patients with transverse-sigmoid dAVFs present with haemorrhage or other serious symptoms in only 11% of cases.[51]

(b) Symptoms without haemorrhage may include.[87]
- Pulsatile tinnitus (most common symptom)
- Headache
- Visual disturbance
- Mastoid pain/otalgia
- Dizziness
- Hydrocephalus
- Trigeminal neuralgia.[89]

Management

Relative to dAVFs in other locations, theses lesions are often benign and frequently require treatment only to alleviate symptoms such as pulsatile tinnitus. Lesions with aggressive characteristics, such as retrograde venous flow and/or venous hypertension, should be treated.

Selection of the treatment strategy involves weighing several different factors. Paramount among these is the venous anatomy; other considerations include the clinical gravity of the situation, the arterial anatomy and the patient's ability to undergo endovascular and/or surgical procedures. A systematic review in 1997 found that combined therapy (endovascular plus surgical treatment) was significantly more effective than either therapy alone ($P < 0.01$).[69]

1. Manual compression
   (a) Technique: Instruct the patient to compress the pulsatile occipital artery with either hand for 30 min TID.
   (b) Results: In 25% of cases complete thrombosis may occur within 4–6 weeks.[68] Occipital artery compression may also provide transient relief from dAVF-associated headaches.[68]
2. Surgery
   (a) Early surgical technique consisted of complete excision coupled with packing of the sigmoid sinus, a procedure associated with significant blood loss.[70] More recently, good results have been obtained with surgical disconnection of the draining vein or veins.[29,90]
3. Embolization
   (a) Venous embolization
      - Venous embolization, or venous embolization combined with arterial embolization, results in significantly higher cure rates compared to arterial embolization alone. Successful venous embolization depends upon identifying patients with favorable anatomy for this approach; occlusion of a sinus that freely communicates with normal venous structures can cause a venous infarction and haemorrhage.
      - Suitable venous anatomy:
         – The affected sinus is compromised and no longer contributes to the drainage of normal tissue.[1,91,92]
         – *Parallel venous channel.* Caragine and colleagues reported on ten patients with dAVF consisting of arterial feeders converging on a "parallel venous channel," that was separate from, but in communication with the transverse or sigmoid sinus.[93] Embolization of the venous channel and cure of the fistula, with preservation of the venous sinuses, was achieved in all patients.
      - Venous approaches
         – Femoral venous access is the most commonly reported route; alternatives include direct puncture of the internal jugular vein and craniectomy with direct puncture of a venous sinus.[74]
   (b) Arterial embolization
      - Arterial embolization is rarely curative and should be reserved for palliation or as an adjunct to venous embolization.[94] or surgery.
   (c) Embolization results
      - Most published series of transverse-sigmoid dAVF embolizations employed a combination venous/arterial strategy in some patients and venous embolization only in others.
      - Angiographic cure rates: 55–87.5%.[91,92,95,96]
      - Symptom improvement or resolution: 90–96%[91,92,95]
      - Transient complications: 10–15%[91,95]
      - Permanent complications: 0–5%[91,92,95]

4. Venous sinus angioplasty and stenting
    (a) Treatment of a transverse sinus dAVF by sinus recanalization, angioplasty and stent placement has been reported.[97]
5. Radiosurgery
    (a) Two reports dedicated specifically to radiosurgery transverse-sigmoid dAVFs of a total of 45 patients:[77,79]
        • Angiographic cure rates: 55–87.5%
        • Symptom improvement or resolution: 74–96%
        • No neurologic complications were reported.

Cavernous Sinus dAVFs

Carotid-cavernous fistulas (CC fistulas) may be direct or indirect. *Direct* CC fistulas (aka high flow CCFs) consist of a defect in the wall of the ICA, causing a shunt between the ICA and the cavernous sinus (e.g., traumatic CCF or ruptured cavernous segment aneurysm). *Indirect* CC fistulas (aka low flow CC fistulas) are equivalent to dAVFs of the cavernous sinus; they comprise about 35% of all dAVFs.[86] Barrow and colleagues established the following classification scheme:[65]

1. Type A. Direct shunt between ICA and cavernous sinus (e.g., traumatic CCF or ruptured cavernous segment aneurysm). Direct CC fistulas are discussed separately in the Appendix.
2. Type B. Indirect fistula between branches of the ICA and the cavernous sinus.
3. Type C. Indirect fistula between branches of the ECA and the cavernous sinus.
4. Type D. Indirect fistula between branches of both the ICA and ECA and the cavernous sinus.
    (a) Type D1: Unilateral.[98]
    (b) Type D2: Bilateral

Indirect CC Fistulas: Clinical Features

1. Most patients are women in the sixth or seventh decade of life.
    (a) Men comprise 27% of cases.[98]
2. Barrow Type D is most common.[99]
3. Slight propensity for the left.[100]
4. Anatomy
    (a) Feeders
        • May be bilateral.
        • ECA: Branches of the internal maxillary, middle meningeal, accessory meningeal, ascending pharyngeal.
        • ICA: Cavernous segment branches.
    (b) Venous drainage
        • Highly variable.
        • Impaired venous drainage is typical and enlargement of the superior ophthalmic vein is a frequent finding.
        • Cortical venous drainage is present in 31–34% of cases.[100]
    (c) *Inferior petrosal sinus dAVF*
        • A variant of cavernous dAVFs; accounts for some 3% of intracranial dAVFs.[101]
        • Presentation is similar to cavernous dAVFs.[102]
5. Presentation
    (a) Termed "Red-eyed shunt syndrome" by some authors.[64]
    (b) Most common findings:[100]
        • Chemosis (94%)
        • Exophthalmos (87%)
        • Cranial nerve palsy (54%)
        • Increased intraocular pressure (60%)
        • Diplopia (51%)
        • Impaired vision (28%)
        • Pulsatile tinnitus.[103]
    (c) A bruit is present in >50% of patients.[68]

(d) So-called "white-eye" CC fistulas occur when posterior venous drainage predominates and a painful ocular motor nerve palsy develops without congestive orbital features.[104]

6. Imaging
   (a) CT: Typical findings include proptosis and superior ophthalmic vein enlargement.
   (b) MRA: May show an enlarged superior ophthalmic vein.
   (c) A catheter angiogram remains the gold standard for a complete evaluation of an indirect CC fistula.[105] Angiography is most important for assessing the presence of retrograde cortical venous flow, as well as delineating feeders and the precise pattern of venous drainage; all of these critical anatomic features of any given CC fistula are poorly seen with noninvasive imaging.

Indirect CC Fistulas: Management

Spontaneous resolution of an indirect fistula is not uncommon, with reported rates of spontaneous remission ranging from 5.6%[63] to 73%.[64–66] Some authors, like the senior author of this handbook, prefer to attempt conservative management of most patients with indirect CC fistulas, whereas the junior author offers intervention to most patients with bothersome symptoms. Barrow and colleagues proposed the following indications for treatment:[65] (1) Visual deterioration; (2) Obtrusive diplopia; (3) Intolerable bruit or headache; and (4) "Malignant" proptosis with untreatable corneal exposure. The presence of retrograde cortical venous drainage is also a good indication for treatment.

Selection of technique: Venous occlusion is the most reliable method to treat indirect CC fistulas. A systematic review in 1997 found overall success rates of 78% for transvenous approaches and 62% for transarterial approaches.[69]

1. Manual compression
   (a) Technique:[67] Instruct the patient to use the opposite hand to locate the pulse of the carotid artery in the mid-neck region just lateral to the trachea. Gradual y increasing pressure is applied until the palpable pulse is stopped. The opposite hand is used in case hemispheric ischemia develops. Compression is maintained for 10–15 s at a time, 2–3 times an hour.
      • Contraindications: Cervical carotid artery disease (atherosclerosis, dissection), sick sinus syndrome, poor patient compliance.
   (b) Results: In 30% of cases closure occurred within a mean of 41 days (range, several minutes to 6 months).[67]
2. Embolization
   (a) Venous: Most effective technique. Several different routes to the cavernous sinus may be used; the most commonly used are the inferior petrosal sinus and the superior ophthalmic vein.
      • Femoral vein/Inferior petrosal sinus.[100,106–108]
         – Successful embolization of the cavernous sinus via the femoral vein and inferior petrosal sinus reported in 64% of cases.[109]
         – A thrombosed inferior petrosal sinus can be traversed in some cases.[106,110,111]
         – A 0.035″ guidewire may be used to gently probe through and open a recently occluded interior petrosal sinus.[100]
      • Superior ophthalmic vein.[72,73]
         – Surgical exposure is obtained through the upper eyelid.
            (a) Percutaneous puncture of the superior ophthalmic vein has been reported.[112]
         – Success rate (92–100%)[72,73] is higher compared to transfemoral venous routes.
      • Alternative techniques for access:
         – Direct puncture of the internal jugular vein.[113]
         – Transfemoral facial vein approach.[113]
         – Superior petrosal sinus.[114]
         – Sylvian vein.[115]
         – Pterygoid plexus.[116]
         – Frontal vein.[117]
      • Coil placement should begin in the posterior part of the superior ophthalmic vein and extend into the cavernous sinus, when approaching from a posterior route.[100]

(b) Arterial: Embolization of arterial feeders is rarely curative and should be used only for palliation in select cases.
(c) Embolic material. Detachable coils are the most commonly used material; recent reports have described good results with NBCA either alone or in combination with coils.[118,119] Onxy embolization has also been reported.[120]
(d) Endovascular results. Overall results in two large recent series are very favorable:
  • Complete cure: 90–94.5% of cases.[100,107]
    – Fistula closure will usually result in normalization of intraocular pressure.[121] Improvement in vision may take longer and is less certain, as several different mechanisms may contribute to vision loss (e.g., optic neuropathy, keritis and corneal ulceration, vitreous haemorrhage, retinal ischemia, or retinal detachment).
  • Procedure-related permanent morbidity: 0–2.3%[100,107]
3. Radiosurgery
(a) Several reports have been published on the use of radiosurgery for the treatment of cavernous CC fistulas.[75,78,122,123] Although the results are generally favorable, with obliteration rates >80%, the wide variety of techniques used (dosing, use of embolization, lesion anatomy) make it difficult to make firm conclusions about the usefulness of radiosurgery in this setting.

Tentorial dAVFs

Tentorial dAVFs (aka superior petrosal dAVFs)[101,124] comprise about 5% of all intracranial dAVFs.[86] Although in most cases, the lesion is located on the petrous ridge and involves the superior petrosal sinus, most publications refer to them as "tentorial" dAVFs.[71,125–127] These lesions are thought to be prone to haemorrhage and are difficult to treat by surgery and by embolization. All, or nearly all, tentorial dAVFs are Borden Type II or III lesions.[32,125] Picard and colleagues classified tentorial dAVFs:[128]
1. Tentorial marginal type, located along the free edge of the tentorium.
2. Tentorial lateral type, located adjacent to the lateral venous sinuses.
3. Tentorial medial type, located adjacent to the straight sinus and torcula.

Clinical Features

1. Anatomy
(a) Feeders. Majority are bilateral.[129]
  • Typically, multiple fine feeders arise from (in order of frequency):[127]
    – Middle meningeal artery
    – Meningohypophyseal trunk
    – Posterior cerebral artery
    – Occipital artery
    – Posterior meningeal artery
    – Superior cerebellar artery
(b) Venous drainage
  • Drainage is retrograde in all cases.[127]
    – Cerebral and/or cerebellar veins
    – Basal vein of Rosenthal
    – Pontine and paramesencephalic veins
    – Cervical paramedullary spinal veins
2. Presentation
(a) Some 80–90% of patients present with haemorrhage or a history of haemorrhage.[130]
(b) Symptoms from unruptured lesions may include pulsatile tinnitus,[131] hemi-facial spasm,[132] myelopathy visual problems,[133] trigeminal neuralgia,[134] or hemisensory disturbance.[135]
3. Imaging.[127]
(a) CT: Haemorrhage centered in the ambient cistern or posterior fossa
(b) MRI: High signal on T2-weighted images indicating edema in the thalamus, midbrain, and cerebellum

Management

Tentorial dAVFs are aggressive lesions and should be obliterated when feasible. Incomplete treatment should be avoided, as recruitment of new feeders and redirection of venous outflow may occur.[136] No single treatment strategy is ideal; selection of surgery and/or embolization depends on the clinical situation (vascular anatomy, patient age and health status, etc.). Because of the aggressive nature of these lesions, late (1–2 years post-treatment) follow-up catheter angiography should be done, even in cases in which an angiographic cure is obtained.

1. Surgery
   (a) Surgery is most effective for patients who are good candidates for a craniotomy and who have a lesion with a single, surgically accessible draining vein.
   (b) Technique: Surgical technique for tentorial dAVFs has evolved considerably in recent years.[71,125,126] In most cases, resection of the nidus is not necessary: obliteration of the lesion can be accomplished by coagulation and division of the arterialized draining vein or veins, when the anatomy is suitable.[71,126] Interruption of the draining vein may be effective when no other pathway for venous drainage exists.[71] Lewis and coworkers, however, emphasized the importance of surgical interruption of the arterial supply, rather than the draining veins.[129] The route of cranial access (e.g., suboccipital versus subtemporal craniotomy) depends on where the arterialized veins are located. Pre-operative arterial embolization may facilitate surgery.[125,127]
   (c) Surgical results: Several small recent series have reported angiographic cures with no mortality.[71,125,127]
2. Embolization
   (a) Venous embolization
      - In most cases, tortuous retrograde leptomeningeal drainage is not connected to a venous sinus, making transvenous embolization difficult or impossible. Some patients, however, have anatomy that is favorable for a transfemoral venous approach.
      - Venous embolization should be done only when a venous drainage pouch that is separate from veins draining normal brain tissue can be identified and accessed with a microcatheter.[125] When embolization is limited to the venous outlet immediately adjacent to the nidus, with preservation of functional drainage, venous embolization with platinum coils can provide adequate treatment.[137]
   (b) Arterial embolization
      - Arterial embolization can lead to an angiographic cure only when the microcatheter tip is placed close enough to the nidus to permit placement of embolic material across the nidus to the venous side.[124,125] NBCA has been the agent of choice,[125] because of its resistance to recanalization. Onyx may be a good alternative.[138]
      - van Rooj and coworkers recommend temporary balloon-occlusion of the ICA when a microcatheter is placed in the tentorial artery, to stabilize the microcatheter, obtain flow-arrest during the injection of embolic agent and to prevent reflux into the ICA.[131]
      - Brief, reversible asystole due to a trigeminocardiac reflex during arterial embolization has been reported.[138]
3. Radiosurgery
   (a) Some authors argue strenuously against the use of radiosurgery for treatment of tentorial dAVFs, given the latency period of radiosurgery, <100% obliteration rate, and risk of injury to adjacent structures such as the brainstem and cranial nerves.[125,127] On the other hand, successful obliteration has been reported,[75–77,139,140] and in two dAVF radiosurgery series, tentorial dAVFs were the most common kind of lesion treated.[76,78]

Superior Sagittal Sinus dAVFs

Comprise 5% of intracranial dAVFs.[35]

Clinical Features

1. Men and women are equally affected.[141]
2. Anatomy. These lesions are typically located in the midportion of the sagittal sinus and feeding arteries are bilateral in the majority of cases.
   (a) Feeders (listed in descending order of frequency):[141]
      - Middle meningeal artery
      - Occipital artery
      - Superficial temporal artery
      - Vertebral artery
      - Posterior auricular artery
      - Anterior falx artery
   (b) Venous drainage
      - Two patterns: directly into the sagittal sinus (majority of cases) or into cortical veins.[142]
      - Sagittal sinus may or may not be occluded.
3. Presentation
   (a) Over a third of patients present with haemorrhage.[141]
      - Subarachnoid haemorrhage, intraparenchymal haemorrhage, or subdural haemorrhage may be present.
   (b) Symptoms without haemorrhage may include those attributable to venous hypertension (e.g., mental status changes, headache).
   (c) May be misdiagnosed as acute sagittal sinus thrombosis.

Management

Lesion obliteration is indicated in patients with haemorrhage or symptoms attributable to the fistula. Sagittal sinus dAVFs associated with a downstream venous sinus occlusion are believed to be at highest risk of haemorrhage or venous hypertension.
1. Surgery
   (a) Surgery is usually fairly straightforward and effective in achieving complete obliteration of the lesion. Surgical techniques include skeletonization of the superior sagittal sinus (i.e., disconnection of arterialized veins) and surgical exposure followed by direct puncture for embolization of the sinus.[143]
   (b) Surgical occlusion of the superior sagittal sinus should be avoided or only done if the affected portion is within the anterior third of the superior sagittal sinus, to minimize risk of venous infarction.[144]
2. Embolization
   (a) Venous embolization
      - Successful transcranial venous embolization of sagittal sinus dAVFs has been reported.[74]
   (b) Arterial embolization
      - The "angiographically remote" location of these lesions can make them difficult to reach from a transfemoral approach. The multiplicity (and bilaterality) of feeders in many cases further impairs endovascular attempts at a cure.
         – Direct cervical carotid puncture (with the patient adequately sedated or under general anesthesia) may facilitate arterial access to the nidus.
      - Case reports and small series report an angiographic cure in about 50% of cases.[145]
      - Arterial embolization has been successfully combined with surgery and radiosurgery.[146]
3. Radiosurgery
   (a) Successful radiosurgery of superior sagittal sinus dAVFs has been reported.[76,78,147]

Anterior Fossa dAVFs

Anterior fossa dAVFs (aka ethmoidal dAVFs, cribriform dAVFs) comprise about 5% of all intracranial dAVFs.[86] These lesions are unique for two reasons:

1. They always have retrograde leptomeningeal venous drainage.
   (a) Because of this, they are at high risk of haemorrhage.
2. They are frequently supplied by a fine tuft of feeders arising from anterior ethmoidal branches of the ophthalmic arteries.
   (a) Because of this, they are difficult to treat with embolization because it is difficult to embolize the feeders without also embolizing the distal ophthalmic artery and retina.

Clinical Features

1. Men are more commonly affected than women.[148–150]
2. Anatomy. Typically, numerous arteries converge on the dura of the anterior cranial fossa floor and falx and merge into a single dilated draining vein.
   (a) Feeders
       - Supply is via the anterior ethmoidal branches of the ophthalmic artery in 84% of cases.[148]
       - Bilateral in 50% of cases.[149]
       - Other feeders may arise from the internal maxillary artery, middle meningeal artery[151] and superficial temporal artery.
       - Rarely, additional feeders from the anterior cerebral artery may be present.[151,152]
   (b) Venous drainage
       - Drainage is into intradural frontal veins in all cases.[149]
3. Presentation
   (a) Most patients present with haemorrhage.[148,149]
       - A review of reported cases found a history of haemorrhage in 62% of all cases of anterior fossa dAVFs, compared to about 15% for all intracranial dAVFs.[148]
   (b) Symptoms without haemorrhage may include
       - Visual loss, presumably from diversion of flow from the ophthalmic artery.[153]
       - Proptosis and chemosis.[154]
       - Diminished olfactory sensation and taste.[149]
       - Intracranial venous hypertension and dementia.[154]

Management

The natural history of anterior fossa dAVFs is not known. However, the fact that >80% of patients present with haemorrhage or have a history of haemorrhage, combined with the invariable retrograde venous drainage pattern seen with these lesions, lead most authors to agree that they are aggressive lesions that should be obliterated when feasible.[149,150,154]

1. Surgery
   (a) Surgery is first-line treatment for most patients, given the high haemorrhage risk of these lesions and the difficulties associated with embolization.[149,155]
   (b) Technique: A pterional or low-frontal craniotomy provides access to the floor of the frontal fossa. The key maneuver is interruption of the fistulous connection between the arteries perforating the dura around the cribriform plate and the draining vein or veins.[149] Coagulation and division of the connecting vein is usually all that is necessary for obliteration of the lesion; excision of the dura, or entry into the orbit for excision of the nidus are not necessary.[149,156]
   (c) Surgical results: A systematic review found a rate of obliteration with surgery of 95%.[69] Lawton and colleagues reported on 15 patients undergoing surgery; occlusion of the fistula was obtained in all patients.[149] No surgical complications were reported and a good outcome was described in all patients except one, who presented initially in a coma.
2. Embolization
   (a) Venous embolization
       - Successful transvenous embolization by direct puncture of the internal jugular vein has been reported.[157]

(b) Arterial embolization.
- The proximity of the central retinal artery to the anterior ethmoidal branches makes arterial embolization of anterior fossa dAVFs problematic. Nevertheless, successful arterial embolization of these lesions has been reported by several authors.[150,154] Embolization may be a reasonable option for symptomatic palliation and for patients who are poor surgical candidates.
- The microcatheter tip should be positioned distal to the origin of the central retinal artery, for obvious reasons.
- Provocative testing with amytal and lidocaine prior to embolization is critical.
- Use of embolic particles >400 μm in size (the average diameter of the central retinal artery)[158] may minimize risk of retinal ischemia.
3. Radiosurgery
(a) Successful radiosurgery of anterior fossa dAVFs has been reported.[76]

15.5. Appendix: Direct Carotid-Cavernous Fistulas

Direct CC Fistulas: Clinical Features

1. Causes
   (a) Trauma (most common cause)
   (b) Ruptured cavernous segment ICA aneurysm (cause of ≤20% of direct CC fistulas)[159–161]
   (c) Ehlers-Danlos Type IV.[162] (see separate discussion below)
   (d) Fibromuscular dysplasia.[163]
   (e) Pseudoxanthoma elasticum
   (f) Iatrogenesis:
   - Endoscopic sinus surgery.
   - Transsphenoidal pituitary surgery.
   - Trigeminal balloon microcompression gangliolysis.[164]
   - Perforation of the meningohypophyseal trunk during embolization of a meningioma.[165]
   (g) Fungal arteritis associated with:
   - Osteogenesis imperfecta.[166]
2. Anatomy
   (a) ICA defect:
   - Most direct fistulas are a single hole measuring 2–6 mm in diameter.[167]
   - Most common location the defect in traumatic cases is the horizontal cavernous segment.[167]
   - May consist of more than one defect in the ICA (e.g., "double-hole" fistula) or a complete transection of the ICA.
   (b) Bilateral traumatic CC fistulas are present in 1–2% of cases.[160,168]
   (c) Venous drainage:
   - Cavernous sinus.
   - Retrograde intracranial venous flow is present in 9% of patients.[169]
3. Presentation
   (a) Classic description: Pulsating exophthalmos.[170,171]
   (b) Most frequent presentation: Exophthalmia with pulsating conjunctival hyperhemia and vascular murmur.[159]
   (c) Severity of symptoms depends on the cause of fistula and the severity of the ICA lesion. Common findings include injection and chemosis, proptosis, elevated intraocular pressure, ophthalmoplegia, and a periorbital bruit.
   - The sixth cranial nerve is most commonly affected.[121]
   - A third cranial nerve palsy, when present, may or may not be pupil-sparing (in contrast to third cranial nerve palsies due to a

posterior communicating artery aneurysm, which nearly invariably has pupillary involvement).
- Rarely, seventh cranial nerve dysfunction is present.[172]
(d) A bruit is present in 80% of cases.[160]
(e) Cerebral ischemia of the ipsilateral hemisphere can occur if the ICA flow is diverted into the cavernous sinus (i.e., a *functional* ICA occlusion is present, even if the vessel is physically patent) and collateral circulation is insufficient. A direct CC fistula may also act as a sump and divert flow from major intracranial arteries such as the p-comm.[169]
4. Imaging
   (a) CT
      - In traumatic cases, a fine-cut head CT should be obtained to assess for skull fractures.
         - Skull fractures are present in 7–17% of traumatic CC fistula cases.
      - CTA may show occlusion of the ICA or engorgement of the cavernous sinus.
   (b) MRA: Elliptical centric time-resolved imaging of contrast kinetics (EC-TRICKS) has provided good imaging of a direct CC fistula.[173]
   (c) Angiography
      - A catheter angiogram remains the gold standard for a complete evaluation of a direct CC fistula.[105]
         - Contralateral carotid and vertebral injections should be done to assess collateral circulation.
      - The anatomy of high-flow fistulas are difficult to discern, particularly if all of the contrast is diverted into the cavernous sinus. Helpful angiographic techniques:
         - Mehringer–Hieshima maneuver:[174] Low-rate injection (2–3 mL/s) into the ipsilateral ICA while manual compression is applied to the ipsilateral CCA. Flow through the fistula is reduced to make it easier to see.
         - Huber maneuver:[175] Selective injection of the dominant vertebral artery while manual compression is applied to the ipsilateral CCA. The fistula will opacify by retrograde flow.

Direct CC Fistulas: Management

Spontaneous closure of direct CC fistulas occurs, but it is rare.[161] Some small asymptomatic direct fistulas can be left untreated, but most do require intervention. Further discussion of the management of cavernous segment ICA aneurysms is in Chap. 13.
1. Manual compression
   (a) Technique: The patient is instructed to use the opposite hand to locate the pulse of the carotid artery in the mid-neck region just lateral to the trachea. Gradually increasing pressure is applied until the palpable pulse is stopped. The opposite hand is used in case hemispheric ischemia develops. Compression is maintained for 10–15 s at a time, 2–3 times an hour.
      - Contraindications: Cervical carotid artery disease (atherosclerosis, dissection), sick sinus syndrome, poor patient compliance.
   (b) Results: 17% of patients with a direct CC fistula had complete closure of the fistula with no recurrence either clinically or at angiography done 1 year later.[67]
2. Cavernous sinus embolization
   (a) Transarterial
      - Detachable balloons
         - Cavernous sinus embolization with detachable balloons is associated with a fistula occlusion rate of ~90% with preservation of the ICA in 60–88% of cases.[65,167,168,176] Detachable balloons are not currently available in the United States, but they are still in use in other countries.[177,178]
      - Coils.[179,180]
         - Coil embolization is most useful for the treatment of direct CC fistulas due to a ruptured cavernous segment aneurysm.[178] Transarterial embolization of traumatic CC fistulas can be problematic, particularly when the defect in the wall of the ICA is large. An initial closure of the fistula may be obtained, but the coils may migrate within the cavernous sinus over time,

leading to a recurrence of the fistula. The authors of this handbook have witnessed this scenario repeatedly.
- Coils or balloons + liquid embolics
  - Transarterial embolization of the cavernous sinus with coils, combined with glue (n-BCA) or Onyx, can be effective in select cases.[177]
- Access to the cavernous sinus can even be reached through the vertebral artery.[181]
(b) Transvenous
- Transvenous embolization with coils alone seems to be more effective than transarterial embolization with coils alone, likely because better microcatheter positioning is possible and tighter packing of the cavernous sinus can be achieved.[179,180]
- Superior ophthalmic vein approach.[72]
3. Stenting
  (a) Stent-assisted embolization.[182]
  (b) Covered stent repair of the ICA.[183–185]
4. Carotid sacrifice
  (a) Parent vessel occlusion is a valid option, but should be preceded by balloon test occlusion

Ehlers-Danlos Type IV

Ehlers-Danlos Type IV (aka vascular type) is rare autosomal dominant collagen-vascular disorder. Type IV accounts for 4% of all Ehlers-Danlos cases and is the most severe form of the disease.
1. Diagnosis
  (a) Four clinical criteria:[186]
    - Easy bruising
    - Thin skin with visible veins
    - Characteristic facial features
    - Rupture of arteries, uterus, or intestines
  (b) Confirmation of diagnosis:
    - Cultured fibroblasts synthesize abnormal type III procollagen molecules or identification of a mutation in the gene for type III procollagen.[187]
2. Pathophysiology
  (a) Type III collagen is decreased or absent.
  (b) The vessels in affected patients have reduced total collagen content and have thin walls with irregular elastic fibrils and reduced cross-sectional area.
3. Epidemiology
  (a) Very rare. Prevalence is unknown.
4. Clinical features
  (a) Hypermobility of large joints and hyperextensibility of the skin, features of the more common forms of Ehlers-Danlos syndrome are unusual in Type IV.
  (b) Median life expectancy is 48 years.[187]
    - Complications are rare in childhood; 25% of patients have a first complication by the age of 20 years and more than 80% have at least one complication by the age of 40.[187]
    - Most deaths result from arterial dissection or rupture.[187]
  (c) *Cerebrovascular manifestations*
    - About 10% of patients have an arterial problem affecting the central nervous system.[187]
      - Direct CC fistulas
      - Most common cerebrovascular complication.
      - Patients are predominantly female.[188]
      - May be bilateral.[189]
      - Endovascular treatment of direct CC fistulas in patients with Ehlers Danlos IV is very hazardous because of the fragility of the vessels.[162,189,190]
      - A review of published reports of diagnostic cerebral angiography in patients with Elhers-Danlos IV, the overall morbidity was 36% and mortality was 12%.[191] In another report, two of four patients died due to remote vascular injuries around the time of their neurointerventional procedures.[190]

References

1. Borden JA, Wu JK, Shucart WA. A proposed classification for spinal and cranial dural arteriovenous fistulous malformations and implications for treatment. J Neurosurg. 1995;82:166–79.
2. Al-Shahi R, Bhattacharya JJ, Currie DG, et al. Prospective, population-based detection of intracranial vascular malformations in adults: the Scottish Intracranial Vascular Malformation Study (SIVMS). Stroke. 2003;34:1163–9.
3. Davies MA, TerBrugge K, Willinsky R, Coyne T, Saleh J, Wallace MC. The validity of classification for the clinical presentation of intracranial dural arteriovenous fistulas. J Neurosurg. 1996;85:830–7.
4. Cognard C, Gobin YP, Pierot L, et al. Cerebral dural arteriovenous fistulas: clinical and angiographic correlation with a revised classification of venous drainage. Radiology. 1995;194:671–80.
5. Houser OW, Campbell JK, Campbell RJ, Sundt Jr TM. Arteriovenous malformation affecting the transverse dural venous sinus – an acquired lesion. Mayo Clin Proc. 1979;54:651–61.
6. Piton J, Guilleux MH, Guibert-Tranier F, Caille JM. Fistulae of the lateral sinus. J Neuroradiol. 1984;11:143–59.
7. Mullan S. Reflections upon the nature and management of intracranial and intraspinal vascular malformations and fistulae. J Neurosurg. 1994;80:606–16.
8. Chaudhary MY, Sachdev VP, Cho SH, Weitzner Jr I, Puljic S, Huang YP. Dural arteriovenous malformation of the major venous sinuses: an acquired lesion. AJNR Am J Neuroradiol. 1982;3:13–9.
9. Terada T, Tsuura M, Komai N, et al. The role of angiogenic factor bFGF in the development of dural AVFs. Acta Neurochir (Wien). 1996;138:877–83.
10. Lawton MT, Jacobowitz R, Spetzler RF. Redefined role of angiogenesis in the pathogenesis of dural arteriovenous malformations. J Neurosurg. 1997;87:267–74.
11. Uranishi R, Nakase H, Sakaki T. Expression of angiogenic growth factors in dural arteriovenous fistula. J Neurosurg. 1999;91:781–6.
12. Tirakotai W, Bian LG, Bertalanffy H, Siegfried B, Sure U. Immunohistochemical study in dural arteriovenous fistula and possible role of ephrin-B2 for development of dural arteriovenous fistula. Chin Med J (Engl). 2004;117:1815–20.
13. Klisch J, Kubalek R, Scheufler KM, Zirrgiebel U, Drevs J, Schumacher M. Plasma vascular endothelial growth factor and serum soluble angiopoietin receptor sTIE-2 in patients with dural arteriovenous fistulas: a pilot study. Neuroradiology. 2005;47:10–7.
14. Arkhipovich AA. The functional significance of the arteriovenous anastomoses of the cerebral dura mater. Vopr Neirokhir. 1974;0:37–42.
15. Rowbotham GF, Little E. The circulations and reservoir of the brain. Br J Surg. 1962;50:244–50.
16. Kerber CW, Newton TH. The macro and microvasculature of the dura mater. Neuroradiology. 1973;6:175–9.
17. Ishikawa T, Sato S, Sasaki T, et al. Histologic study of arteriovenous shunts in the normal dura mater adjacent to the transverse sinus. Surg Neurol. 2007;68:272–6.
18. Djindjian R, Cophignon J, Rey A, Theron J, Merland JJ, Houdart R. Superselective arteriographic embolization by the femoral route in neuroradiology. Study of 50 cases. II. Embolization in vertebromedullary pathology. Neuroradiology. 1973;6:132–42.
19. Hamada Y, Goto K, Inoue T, et al. Histopathological aspects of dural arteriovenous fistulas in the transverse-sigmoid sinus region in nine patients. Neurosurgery. 1997;40:452–6; discussion 6–8.
20. Nishijima M, Takaku A, Endo S, et al. Etiological evaluation of dural arteriovenous malformations of the lateral and sigmoid sinuses based on histopathological examinations. J Neurosurg. 1992;76:600–6.
21. Handa J, Yoneda S, Handa H. Venous sinus occlusion with a dural arteriovenous malformation of the posterior fossa. Surg Neurol. 1975;4:433–7.
22. Herman JM, Spetzler RF, Bederson JB, Kurbat JM, Zabramski JM. Genesis of a dural arteriovenous malformation in a rat model. J Neurosurg. 1995;83:539–45.
23. Terada T, Higashida RT, Halbach VV, et al. Development of acquired arteriovenous fistulas in rats due to venous hypertension. J Neurosurg. 1994;80:884–9.
24. Lasjaunias P, Chiu M, ter Brugge K, Tolia A, Hurth M, Bernstein M. Neurological manifestations of intracranial dural arteriovenous malformations. J Neurosurg. 1986;64:724–30.
25. Kincaid PK, Duckwiler GR, Gobin YP, Vinuela F. Dural arteriovenous fistula in children: endovascular treatment and outcomes in seven cases. AJNR Am J Neuroradiol. 2001;22:1217–25.
26. Satomi J, van Dijk JM, Terbrugge KG, Willinsky RA, Wallace MC. Benign cranial dural arteriovenous fistulas: outcome of conservative management based on the natural history of the lesion. J Neurosurg. 2002;97:767–70.
27. Raupp S, van Rooij WJ, Sluzewski M, Tijssen CC. Type I cerebral dural arteriovenous fistulas of the lateral sinus: clinical features in 24 patients. Eur J Neurol. 2004;11:489–91.
28. van Rooij WJ, Sluzewski M, Beute GN. Dural arteriovenous fistulas with cortical venous drainage: incidence, clinical presentation, and treatment. AJNR Am J Neuroradiol. 2007; 28:651–5.
29. van Dijk JM, TerBrugge KG, Willinsky RA, Wallace MC. Selective disconnection of cortical venous reflux as treatment for cranial dural arteriovenous fistulas. J Neurosurg. 2004;101:31–5.
30. Barnwell SL, Halbach VV, Dowd CF, Higashida RT, Hieshima GB, Wilson CB. Multiple dural arteriovenous fistulas of the cranium and spine. AJNR Am J Neuroradiol. 1991;12:441–5.
31. Brown Jr RD, Wiebers DO, Nichols DA. Intracranial dural arteriovenous fistulae: angiographic predictors of intracranial hemorrhage and clinical outcome in nonsurgical patients. J Neurosurg. 1994;81:531–8.
32. Davies MA, ter Brugge K, Willinsky R, Wallace MC. The natural history and management of intracranial dural arteriovenous fistulae. Part 2: aggressive lesions. Interv Neuroradiol. 1997;3:303–11.
33. van Dijk JMC, terBrugge KG, Willinsky RA, Wallace MC. Clinical course of cranial dural arteriovenous fistulas with long-term persistent cortical venous reflux. Stroke. 2002;33:1233–6.
34. Cordonnier C, Al-Shahi Salman R, Bhattacharya JJ, et al. Differences between intracranial vascular malformation types in their presenting haemorrhages: prospective, population-based study. J Neurol Neurosurg Psychiatry. 2008;79:47–51.
35. Awad IA, Little JR, Akarawi WP, Ahl J. Intracranial dural arteriovenous malformations: factors predisposing to an aggressive neurological course. J Neurosurg. 1990;72:839–50.
36. Willinsky R, Terbrugge K, Montanera W, Mikulis D, Wallace MC. Venous congestion: an MR finding in dural arteriovenous malformations with cortical venous drainage. AJNR Am J Neuroradiol. 1994;15:1501–7.
37. Yamakami I, Kobayashi E, Yamaura A. Diffuse white matter changes caused by dural arteriovenous fistula. J Clin Neurosci. 2001;8:471–5.
38. Sato K, Shimizu H, Fujimura M, Inoue T, Matsumoto Y, Tominaga T. Compromise of brain tissue caused by cortical venous reflux of intracranial dural arteriovenous fistulas: assessment with diffusion-weighted magnetic resonance imaging. Stroke. 2011;42:998–1003.
39. Hirono N, Yamadori A, Komiyama M. Dural arteriovenous fistula: a cause of hypoperfusion-induced intellectual impairment. Eur Neurol. 1993;33:5–8.
40. Cognard C, Casasco A, Toevi M, Houdart E, Chiras J, Merland J-J. Dural arteriovenous fistulas as a cause of intracranial hypertension due to impairment of cranial venous outflow. J Neurol Neurosurg Psychiatry. 1998;65:308–16.

41. Hurst RW, Bagley LJ, Galetta S, et al. Dementia resulting from dural arteriovenous fistulas: the pathologic findings of venous hypertension encephalopathy. AJNR Am J Neuroradiol. 1998;19:1267–73.
42. Hasumi T, Fukushima T, Haisa T, Yonemitsu T, Waragai M. Focal dural arteriovenous fistula (DAVF) presenting with progressive cognitive impairment including amnesia and alexia. Intern Med. 2007;46:1317–20.
43. Silberstein P, Kottos P, Worner C, et al. Dural arteriovenous fistulae causing pseudotumour cerebri syndrome in an elderly man. J Clin Neurosci. 2003;10:242–3.
44. Lee PH, Lee JS, Shin DH, Kim BM, Huh K. Parkinsonism as an initial manifestation of dural arteriovenous fistula. Eur J Neurol. 2005;12:403–6.
45. Kim N-H, Cho K-T, Seo HS. Myelopathy due to intracranial dural arteriovenous fistula: a potential diagnostic pitfall. J Neurosurg. 2011;114:830–3.
46. Stouffer JL, Tyler RS. Characterization of tinnitus by tinnitus patients. J Speech Hear Disord. 1990;55:439–53.
47. Waldvogel D, Mattle HP, Sturzenegger M, Schroth G. Pulsatile tinnitus – a review of 84 patients. J Neurol. 1998;245:137–42.
48. Adler JR, Ropper AH. Self-audible venous bruits and high jugular bulb. Arch Neurol. 1986:43:257–9.
49. Russell EJ, De Michaelis BJ, Wiet R, Meyer J. Objective pulse-synchronous "essential" tinnitus due to narrowing of the transverse dural venous sinus. Int Tinnitus J. 1995;1: 127–37.
50. Shin EJ, Lalwani AK, Dowd CF. Role of angiography in the evaluation of patients with pulsatile tinnitus. Laryngoscope. 2000;110:1916–20.
51. Cawley CM, Barrow DL, Dion JE. Treatment of lateral-sigmoid and sagittal sinus dural arteriovenous malformations. In: Winn HR, editor. Youmans neurological surgery. Philadelphia: Saunders; 2004. p. 2283–91.
52. van Rooij WJ, Sluzewski M, Beute GN. Intracranial dural fistulas with exclusive perimedullary drainage: the need for complete cerebral angiography for diagnosis and treatment planning. AJNR Am J Neuroradiol. 2007;28:348–51.
53. Willinsky R, Goyal M, terBrugge K, Montanera W. Tortuous, engorged pial veins in intracranial dural arteriovenous fistulas: correlations with presentation, location, and MR findings in 122 patients. AJNR Am J Neuroradiol. 1999;20: 1031–6.
54. Coley SC, Romanowski CA, Hodgson TJ, Griffiths PD. Dural arteriovenous fistulae: noninvasive diagnosis with dynamic MR digital subtraction angiography. AJNR Am J Neuroradiol. 2002;23:404–7.
55. Noguchi K, Kubo M, Kuwayama N, et al. Intracranial dural arteriovenous fistulas with retrograde cortical venous drainage: assessment with cerebral blood volume by dynamic susceptibility contrast magnetic resonance imaging. AJNR Am J Neuroradiol. 2006;27:1252–6.
56. Hashimoto Y, Kin S, Haraguchi K, Niwa J. Pitfalls in the preoperative evaluation of subarachnoid hemorrhage without digital subtraction angiography: report on 2 cases. Surg Neurol. 2007;68:344–8.
57. Coskun O, Hamon M, Catroux G, Gosme L, Courtheoux P, Theron J. Carotid-cavernous fistulas: diagnosis with spiral CT angiography. AJNR Am J Neuroradiol. 2000;21:712–6.
58. Kim DJ, terBrugge K, Krings T, Willinsky R, Wallace C. Spontaneous angiographic conversion of intracranial dural arteriovenous shunt: long-term follow-up in nontreated patients. Stroke. 2010;41:1489–94.
59. Davies MA, Saleh J, ter Brugge K, Willinsky R, Wallace MC. The natural history and management of intracranial dural arteriovenous fistulae. Part 1: benign lesions. Interv Neuroradiol. 1997;3:295–302.
60. Cognard C, Houdart E, Casascc A, Gabrillargues J, Chiras J, Merland JJ. Long-term changes in intracranial dural arteriovenous fistulae leading to worsening in the type of venous drainage. Neuroradiology. 1997;39:59–66.
61. Duffau H, Lopes M, Janosevic V, et al. Early rebleeding from intracranial dural arteriovenous fistulas: report of 20 cases and review of the literature. J Neurosurg. 1999;90:78–84.
62. Olutola PS, Eliam M, Molot M, Talalla A. Spontaneous regression of a dural arteriovenous fistula. Neurosurgery. 1983;12:687–90.

63. Hamby WB. Signs and symptoms of carotid-cavernous fistula. In: Carotid cavernous fistula. Charles C. Thomas: Springfield; 1966.
64. Phelps CD, Thompson HS, Ossoinig KC. The diagnosis and prognosis of atypical carotid-cavernous fistula (red-eyed shunt syndrome). Am J Ophthalmol. 1982;93:423–36.
65. Barrow DL, Spector RH, Braun IF, Landman JA, Tindall SC, Tindall GT. Classification and treatment of spontaneous carotid-cavernous sinus fistulas. J Neurosurg. 1985;62:248–56.
66. Sasaki H, Nukui H, Kaneko M, et al. Long-term observations in cases with spontaneous carotid-cavernous fistulas. Acta Neurochir (Wien). 1988;90:117–20.
67. Higashida RT, Hieshima GB, Halbach VV, Bentson JR, Goto K. Closure of carotid cavernous sinus fistulae by external compression of the carotid artery and jugular vein. Acta Radiol Suppl. 1986;369:580–3.
68. Halbach VV, Higashida RT, Hieshima GB, Goto K, Norman D, Newton TH. Dural fistulas involving the transverse and sigmoid sinuses: results of treatment in 28 patients. Radiology. 1987;163:443–7.
69. Lucas CP, Zabramski JM, Spetzler RF, Jacobowitz R. Treatment for intracranial dural arteriovenous malformations: a meta-analysis from the English language literature. Neurosurgery. 1997;40:1119–30; discussion 30–2.
70. Sundt Jr TM, Piepgras DG. The surgical approach to arteriovenous malformations of the lateral and sigmoid dural sinuses. J Neurosurg. 1983;59:32–9.
71. Thompson BG, Doppman JL, Oldfield EH. Treatment of cranial dural arteriovenous fistulae by interruption of leptomeningeal venous drainage. J Neurosurg. 1994;80:617–23.
72. Miller NR, Monsein LH, Debrun GM, Tamargo RJ, Nauta HJ. Treatment of carotid-cavernous sinus fistulas using a superior ophthalmic vein approach. J Neurosurg. 1995;83:838–42.
73. Quinones D, Duckwiler G, Gobin PY, Goldberg RA, Vinuela F. Embolization of dural cavernous fistulas via superior ophthalmic vein approach. AJNR Am J Neuroradiol. 1997;18: 921–8.
74. Houdart E, Saint-Maurice JP, Chapot R, et al. Transcranial approach for venous embolization of dural arteriovenous fistulas. J Neurosurg. 2002;97:280–6.
75. Koebbe CJ, Singhal D, Sheehan J, et al. Radiosurgery for dural arteriovenous fistulas. Surg Neurol. 2005;64:392–8; discussion 8–9.
76. Soderman M, Edner G, Ericson K, et al. Gamma knife surgery for dural arteriovenous shunts: 25 years of experience. J Neurosurg. 2006;104:867–75.
77. Friedman JA, Pollock BE, Nichols DA, Gorman DA, Foote RL, Stafford SL. Results of combined stereotactic radiosurgery and transarterial embolization for dural arteriovenous fistulas of the transverse and sigmoid sinuses. J Neurosurg. 2001;94:886–91.
78. O'Leary S, Hodgson TJ, Coley SC, Kemeny AA, Radatz MW. Intracranial dural arteriovenous malformations: results of stereotactic radiosurgery in 17 patients. Clin Oncol (R Coll Radiol). 2002;14:97–102.
79. Pan DH, Chung WY, Guo WY, et al. Stereotactic radiosurgery for the treatment of dural arteriovenous fistulas involving the transverse-sigmoid sinus. J Neurosurg. 2002;96:823–9.
80. Cifarelli CP, Kaptain G, Yen C-P, Schlesinger D, Sheehan JP. Gamma knife radiosurgery for dural arteriovenous fistulas. Neurosurgery. 2010;67:1230–5.
81. Yang H-C, Kano H, Kondziolka D, et al. Stereotactic radiosurgery with or without embolization for intracranial dural arteriovenous fistulas. Neurosurgery. 2010;67:1276–85.
82. Andrade-Souza YM, Ramani M, Scora D, Tsao MN, ter-Brugge K, Schwartz ML. Embolization before radiosurgery reduces the obliteration rate of arteriovenous malformations. Neurosurgery. 2007;60:443–52. doi:10.1227/01.NEU.0000255347.25959.D0.
83. Back AG, Vollmer D, Zeck O, Shkedy C, Shedden PM. Retrospective analysis of unstaged and staged Gamma Knife surgery with and without preceding embolization for the treatment of arteriovenous malformations. J Neurosurg. 2008;109(Suppl):57–64.
84. Sure U, Surucu O, Engenhart-Cabillic R. Embolization before radiosurgery reduces the obliteration rate of arteriovenous malformations. Neurosurgery. 2008;63:E376; author reply E.

85. Kim MS, Han DH, Kwon OK, Oh C-W, Han MH. Clinical characteristics of dural arteriovenous fistula. J Clin Neurosci. 2002;9:147–55.

86. McDougall CG, Halbach VV, Higashida RT, et al. Treatment of dural arteriovenous fistulas. Neursurg Q. 1997;7:110–34.

87. Lalwani AK, Dowd CF, Halbach VV. Grading venous restrictive disease in patients with dural arteriovenous fistulas of the transverse/sigmoid sinus. J Neurosurg. 1993;79:11–5.

88. Horinaka N, Nonaka Y, Nakayama T, Mori K, Wada R, Maeda M. Dural arteriovenous fistula of the transverse sinus with concomitan ipsilateral meningioma. Acta Neurochir (Wien). 2003; 145:501–4;discussion 4.

89. de Paula Lucas C, Zabramski JM. Dural arteriovenous fistula of the transverse-sigmoid sinus causing trigeminal neuralgia. Acta Neurochir (Wien). 2007;149:1249–53.

90. Collice M, D'Aliberti G, Talamonti G, et al. Surgical interruption of leptomeningeal drainage as treatment for intracranial dural arteriovenous fistulas without dural sinus drainage. J Neurosurg. 1996;84:810–7.

91. Urtasun F, Biondi A, Casaco A, et al Cerebral dural arteriovenous fistulas: percutaneous transvenous embolization. Radiology. 1996;199:209–17.

92. Roy D, Raymond J. The role of transvenous embolization in the treatment of intracranial dural arteriovenous fistulas. Neurosurgery. 1997;40:1133–41; discussion 41–4.

93. Caragine LP, Halbach VV, Dowd CF Ng PP, Higashida RT. Parallel venous channel as the recipient pouch in transverse/ sigmoid sinus dural fistulae. Neurosurgery. 2003;53:1261– 6; discussion 6–7.

94. Dawson 3rd RC, Joseph GJ, Owens DS, Barrow DL. Transvenous embolization as the primary therapy for arteriovenous fistulas of the lateral and sigmoid sinuses. AJNR Am J Neuroradiol. 1998; :9:571–6.

95. Halbach VV, Higashida RT, Hieshima GB, Christopher FD. Endovascular therapy of dural fistulas. In: Vinuela F, Halbach VV, Dion JE, editors. Interventional neuroradiology: endovascular therapy of the central nervous system. New York: Raven; 1992. p. 29–50.

96. Olteanu-Nerbe V, Uhl E, Steiger HJ Yousry T, Reulen HJ. Dural arteriovenous fistulas including the transverse and sigmoid sinuses: results of treatment in 30 cases. Acta Neurochir (Wien). 1997;139:307–18

97. Murphy KJ, Gailloud P, Venbrux A Deramond H, Hanley D, Rigamonti D. Endovascular treatment of a grade IV transverse sinus dural arteriovenous fistula by sinus recanalization, angioplasty, and stent placement: technical case report. Neurosurgery. 2000;46:497–500; discussion –1.

98. Tomsick TA. Etiology, prevalence, and natural history. In: Tomsick TA, editor. Carotid cavernous fistula. Cincinnati: Digital Educational Publishing; 1997. p. 59–73.

99. Ernst RJ, Tomsick TA. Classification and angiography of carotid cavernous fistulas. In: Tomsick TA, editor. Carotid cavernous fistula. Cincinnati: Digital Educational Publishing; 1997. p. 13–21.

100. Kirsch M, Henkes H, Liebig T, et al. Endovascular management of dural carotid-cavernous sinus fistulas in 141 patients. Neuroradiology. 2006;48:486–90.

101. Malek AM, Halbach VV, Higashida RT, Phatouros CC, Meyers PM, Dowd CF. Treatment of dural arteriomalformations and fistulas. In: Rosenwasser RH, editor. Neuroendovascular surgery. Philadelphia: W.B. Saunders; 2000. p. 147–66.

102. Barnwell SL, Halbach VV, Dowd CF, Higashida RT, Hieshima GB. Dural arteriovenous fistulas involving the inferior petrosal sinus: angiographic findings in six patients. AJNR Am J Neuroradiol. 1990;11:5 1–6.

103. Mohyuddin A. Indirect carotid cavernous fistula presenting as pulsatile tinnitus. J Laryngol Otol. 2000;114:788–9.

104. Acierno MD, Trobe JD, Cornblath WT, Gebarski SS. Painful oculomotor palsy caused by posterior-draining dural carotid cavernous fistulas Arch Ophthalmol. 1995;113:1045–9.

105. Phatouros CC, Meyers PM, Dowd CF, Halbach VV, Malek AM, Higashida RT. Carotid artery cavernous fistulas. In: Rosenwasser RH, editor. Neuroendovascular surgery. Philadelphia: W.B. Saunders; 2000. . 67–84.

106. Yamashita K, Taki W, Nishi S, et al. Transvenous embolization of dural caroticocavernous fistulae: technical considerations. Neuroradiology. 1993;35:475–9.

107. Meyers PM, Halbach VV, Dowd CF, et al. Dural carotid cavernous fistula: definitive endovascular management and long-term follow-up. Am J Ophthalmol. 2002;134:85–92.

108. Kinugasa K, Tokunaga K, Kamata I, et al. Selection and combination of techniques for treating spontaneous carotid-cavernous sinus fistulas. Neurol Med Chir (Tokyo). 1994;34:597–606.

109. Kim DJ, Kim DI, Suh SH, et al. Results of transvenous embolization of cavernous dural arteriovenous fistula: a single-center experience with emphasis on complications and management. AJNR Am J Neuroradiol. 2006;27:2078–82.

110. Halbach VV, Higashida RT, Hieshima GB, Hardin CW, Pribram H. Transvenous embolization of dural fistulas involving the cavernous sinus. AJNR Am J Neuroradiol. 1989;10:377–83.

111. Benndorf G, Bender A, Lehmann R, Lanksch W. Transvenous occlusion of dural cavernous sinus fistulas through the thrombosed inferior petrosal sinus: report of four cases and review of the literature. Surg Neurol. 2000;54:42–54.

112. Benndorf G, Bender A, Campi A, Menneking H, Lanksch WR. Treatment of a cavernous sinus dural arteriovenous fistula by deep orbital puncture of the superior ophthalmic vein. Neuroradiology. 2001;43:499–502.

113. Agid R, Willinsky RA, Haw C, Souza MP, Vanek IJ, ter-Brugge KG. Targeted compartmental embolization of cavernous sinus dural arteriovenous fistulae using transfemoral medial and lateral facial vein approaches. Neuroradiology. 2004;46:156–60.

114. Mounayer C, Piotin M, Spelle L, Moret J. Superior petrosal sinus catheterization for transvenous embolization of a dural carotid cavernous sinus fistula. AJNR Am J Neuroradiol. 2002;23:1153–5.

115. Kuwayama N, Endo S, Kitabayashi M, Nishijima M, Takaku A. Surgical transvenous embolization of a cortically draining carotid cavernous fistula via a vein of the sylvian fissure. AJNR Am J Neuroradiol. 1998;19:1329–32.

116. Jahan R, Gobin YP, Glenn B, Duckwiler GR, Vinuela F. Transvenous embolization of a dural arteriovenous fistula of the cavernous sinus through the contralateral pterygoid plexus. Neuroradiology. 1998;40:189–93.

117. Venturi C, Bracco S, Cerase A, et al. Endovascular treatment of a cavernous sinus dural arteriovenous fistula by transvenous embolisation through the superior ophthalmic vein via cannulation of a frontal vein. Neuroradiology. 2003;45:574–8.

118. Wakhloo AK, Perlow A, Linfante I, et al. Transvenous n-butyl-cyanoacrylate infusion for complex dural carotid cavernous fistulas: technical considerations and clinical outcome. AJNR Am J Neuroradiol. 2005;26:1888–97.

119. Shaibani A, Rohany M, Parkinson R, et al. Primary treatment of an indirect carotid cavernous fistula by injection of N-butyl cyanoacrylate in the dural wall of the cavernous sinus. Surg Neurol. 2007;67:403–8; discussion 8.

120. Suzuki S, Lee DW, Jahan R, Duckwiler GR, Vinuela F. Transvenous treatment of spontaneous dural carotid-cavernous fistulas using a combination of detachable coils and Onyx. AJNR Am J Neuroradiol. 2006;27:1346–9.

121. Kupersmith MJ, Berenstein A. Flamm E, Ransohoff J. Neuroophthalmologic abnormalities and intravascular therapy of traumatic carotid cavernous fistulas. Ophthalmology. 1986;93:906–12.

122. Guo WY, Pan DH, Wu HM, et al. Radiosurgery as a treatment alternative for dural arteriovenous fistulas of the cavernous sinus. AJNR Am J Neuroradiol. 1998;19:1081–7.

123. Pollock BE, Nichols DA, Garrity JA, Gorman DA, Stafford SL. Stereotactic radiosurgery and particulate embolization for cavernous sinus dural arteriovenous fistulae. Neurosurgery. 1999;45:459–66; discussion 66–7.

124. Ng PP, Halbach VV, Quinn R, et al. Endovascular treatment for dural arteriovenous fistulae of the superior petrosal sinus. Neurosurgery. 2003;53:25–32; discussion –3.

125. Tomak PR, Cloft HJ, Kaga A, Cawley CM, Dion J, Barrow DL. Evolution of the management of tentorial dural arteriovenous malformations. Neurosurgery. 2003;52:750–60; discussion 60–2.

126. Grisoli F, Vincentelli F, Fuchs S, et al. Surgical treatment of tentorial arteriovenous malformations draining into the subarachnoid space. Report of four cases. J Neurosurg. 1984;60:1059–66.

127. Zhou L-F, Chen L, Song D-L, Gu Y-X, Leng B. Tentorial dural arteriovenous fistulas. Surg Neurol. 2007;67:472–81.

128. Picard L, Bracard S, Islak C, et al. Dural fistulae of the tentorium cerebelli. Radioanatomical, clinical and therapeutic considerations. J Neuroradiol. 1990;17:161–81.

129. Lewis AI, Rosenblatt SS, Tew Jr JM. Surgical management of deep-seated dural arteriovenous malformations. J Neurosurg. 1997;87:198–206.

130. King WA, Martin NA. Intracerebral hemorrhage due to dural arteriovenous malformations and fistulae. Neurosurg Clin N Am. 1992;3:577–90.

131. van Rooij W, Sluzewski M, Beute GN. Tentorial artery embolization in tentorial dural arteriovenous fistulas. Neuroradiology. 2006;48:737–43.

132. Deshmukh VR, Maughan PH, Spetzler RF. Resolution of hemifacial spasm after surgical obliteration of a tentorial arteriovenous fistula: case report. Neurosurgery. 2006;58: E202; discussion E.

133. Benndorf G, Schmidt S, Sollmann WP, Kroppenstedt SN. Tentorial dural arteriovenous fistula presenting with various visual symptoms related to anterior and posterior visual pathway dysfunction: case report. Neurosurgery. 2003;53:222–6; discussion 6–7.

134. Matsushige T, Nakaoka M, Ohta K, Yahara K, Okamoto H, Kurisu K. Tentorial dural arteriovenous malformation manifesting as trigeminal neuralgia treated by stereotactic radiosurgery: a case report. Surg Neurol. 2006;66:519–23; discussion 23.

135. Iwamuro Y, Nakahara I, Higashi T, et al. Tentorial dural arteriovenous fistula presenting symptoms due to mass effect on the dilated draining vein: case report. Surg Neurol. 2006;65:511–5.

136. Detwiler PW, Lucas CP, Zabramski JM, McDougall CG. Cranial dural arteriovenous malformations. BNI Quarterly. 2000;16:24–32.

137. Kallmes DF, Jensen ME, Cloft HJ, Kassell NF, Dion JE. Percutaneous transvenous coil embolization of a Djindjian type 4 tentorial dural arteriovenous malformation. AJNR Am J Neuroradiol. 1997;18:673–6.

138. Lv X, Li Y, Lv M, Liu A, Zhang J, Wu Z. Trigeminocardiac reflex in embolization of intracranial dural arteriovenous fistula. AJNR Am J Neuroradiol. 2007;28:1769–70.

139. Lewis AI, Tomsick TA, Tew Jr JM. Management of tentorial dural arteriovenous malformations: transarterial embolization combined with stereotactic radiation or surgery. J Neurosurg. 1994;81:851–9.

140. Shin M, Kurita H, Tago M, Kirino T. Stereotactic radiosurgery for tentorial dural arteriovenous fistulae draining into the vein of Galen: report of two cases. Neurosurgery. 2000;46:730–3; discussion 3–4.

141. Kurl S, Saari T, Vanninen R, Hernesniemi J. Dural arteriovenous fistulas of superior sagittal sinus: case report and review of literature. Surg Neurol. 1996;45:250–4.

142. Barnwell SL, Halbach VV. Dowd CF, Higashida RT, Hieshima GB, Wilson CB. A variant of arteriovenous fistulas within the wall of dural sinuses. Results of combined surgical and endovascular therapy. J Neurosurg. 1991;74:199–204.

143. Pierot L, Visot A, Boulin A, Dupuy M. Combined neurosurgical and neuroradiological treatment of a complex superior sagittal sinus dural fistula: technical note. Neurosurgery. 1998;42:194–7.

144. Jaeger R. Observations on resection of the superior longitudinal sinus at and posterior to the rolandic venous inflow. J Neurosurg. 1951;8:103–9.

145. Halbach VV, Higashida RT, Hieshima GB, Rosenblum M, Cahan L. Treatment of dural arteriovenous malformations involving the superior sagittal sinus. AJNR Am J Neuroradiol. 1988;9:337–43.

146. Bertalanffy A, Dietrich W, Krtz K, Bavinzski G. Treatment of dural arteriovenous fistulae (dAVF's) at the superior sagittal sinus (SSS) using embolisation combined with microor radiosurgery. Minim Invasive Neurosurg. 2001;44:205–10.

147. Maruyama K, Shin M, Kurita H, Tago M, Kirino T. Stereotactic radiosurgery for dural arteriovenous fistula involving the superior sagittal sinus. Case report. J Neurosurg. 2002;97:481–3.

148. Gliemroth J, Nowak G, Arnold H. Dural arteriovenous malformation in the anterior cranial fossa. Clin Neurol Neurosurg. 1999;101:37–43.

149. Lawton MT, Chun J, Wilson CB, Halbach VV. Ethmoidal dural arteriovenous fistulae: an assessment of surgical and endovascular management. Neurosurgery. 1999;45:805–10; discussion 10–1.

150. Lefkowitz M, Giannotta SL, Hieshima G, et al. Embolization of neurosurgical lesions involving the ophthalmic artery. Neurosurgery. 1998;43:1298–303.

151. Newton TH, Cronqvist S. Involvement of dural arteries in intracranial arteriovenous malformations. Radiology. 1969;93:1071–8.

152. Martin NA, King WA, Wilson CB, Nutik S, Carter LP, Spetzler RF. Management of dural arteriovenous malformations of the anterior cranial fossa. J Neurosurg. 1990;72: 692–7.

153. Tiyaworabun S, Vonofakos D, Lorenz R. Intracerebral arteriovenous malformation fed by both ethmoidal arteries. Surg Neurol. 1986;26:375–82.

154. Abrahams JM, Bagley LJ, Flamm ES, Hurst RW, Sinson GP. Alternative management considerations for ethmoidal dural arteriovenous fistulas. Surg Neurol. 2002;58:410–6.

155. Halbach VV, Higashida RT, Hieshima GB, Wilson CB, Barnwell SL, Dowd CF. Dural arteriovenous fistulas supplied by ethmoidal arteries. Neurosurgery. 1990;26: 816–23.

156. Im S-H, Oh CW, Han DH. Surgical management of an unruptured dural arteriovenous fistula of the anterior cranial fossa: natural history for 7 years. Surg Neurol. 2004;62: 72–5.

157. Defreyne L, Vanlangenhove P, Vandekerckhove T, et al. Transvenous embolization of a dural arteriovenous fistula of the anterior cranial fossa: preliminary results. AJNR Am J Neuroradiol. 2000;21:761–5.

158. Tsutsumi S, Rhoton Jr AL. Microsurgical anatomy of the central retinal artery. Neurosurgery. 2006;59:870–8; discussion 8–9.

159. Desal H, Leaute F, Auffray-Calvier E, et al. Direct carotid-cavernous fistula. Clinical, radiologic and therapeutic studies. Apropos of 49 cases. J Neuroradiol. 1997;24:141–54.

160. Lewis AI, Tomsick TA, Tew Jr JM. Management of 100 consecutive direct carotid-cavernous fistulas: results of treatment with detachable balloons. Neurosurgery. 1995;36: 239–44; discussion 44–5.

161. Debrun GM, Vinuela F, Fox AJ, Davis KR, Ahn HS. Indications for treatment and classification of 132 carotid-cavernous fistulas. Neurosurgery. 1988;22:285–9.

162. Desal HA, Toulgoat F, Raoul S, et al. Ehlers-Danlos syndrome type IV and recurrent carotid-cavernous fistula: review of the literature, endovascular approach, technique and difficulties. Neuroradiology. 2005;47:300–4.

163. Numaguchi Y, Higashida RT, Abernathy JM, Pisarello JC. Balloon embolization in a carotid-cavernous fistula in fibromuscular dysplasia. AJNR Am J Neuroradiol. 1987;8: 380–2.

164. Kuether TA, O'Neill OR, Nesbit GM, Barnwell SL. Direct carotid cavernous fistula after trigeminal balloon microcompression gangliolysis: case report. Neurosurgery. 1996; 39:853–5; discussion 5–6.

165. Barr JD, Mathis JM, Horton JA. Iatrogenic carotid-cavernous fistula occurring after embolization of a cavernous sinus meningioma. AJNR Am J Neuroradiol. 1995;16: 483–5.

166. de Campos JM, Ferro MO, Burzaco JA, Boixados JR. Spontaneous carotid-cavernous fistula in osteogenesis imperfecta. J Neurosurg. 1982;56:590–3.

167. Debrun G, Lacour P, Vinuela F, Fox A, Drake CG, Caron JP. Treatment of 54 traumatic carotid-cavernous fistulas. J Neurosurg. 1981;55:678–92.

168. Higashida RT, Halbach VV, Tsai FY, et al. Interventional neurovascular treatment of traumatic carotid and vertebral artery lesions: results in 234 cases. AJR Am J Roentgenol. 1989;153:577–82.

169. Halbach VV, Hieshima GB, Higashida RT, Reicher M. Carotid cavernous fistulae: indications for urgent treatment. AJR Am J Roentgenol. 1987;149:587–93.

170. Dandy WE, Follis RH. On the pathology of carotid-cavernous aneurysms (pulsating exophthalmos). Am J Ophthalmol. 1941;24:365–85.

171. Sugar HS, Meyer SJ. Pulsating exophthalmos. Arch Ophthalmol. 1940;64:1288–321

172. Kapur A, Sanghavi NG, Parikh NK, Amin SK. Spontaneous carotid-cavernous fistula with ophthalmoplegia and facial palsy. Postgrad Med J. 1982;58:773–5.

173. Vattoth S, Cherian J, Pandey T. Magnetic resonance angiographic demonstration of carotid-cavernous fistula using elliptical centric time resolved imaging of contrast kinetics (EC-TRICKS). Magn Reson Imaging. 2007;25:1227–31.

174. Mehringer CM, Hieshima GB, Grinnell VS, Tsai F, Pribram HF. Improved localization of carotid cavernous fistula during angiography. AJNR Am J Neuroradiol. 1982;3:82–4.

175. Huber P. A technical contribution of the exact angiographic localization of carotid cavernous fistulas. Neuroradiology. 1976;10:239–41.

176. Goto K, Hieshima GB, Higashida RT, et al. Treatment of direct carotid cavernous sinus fistulae. Various therapeutic approaches and results in 148 cases. Acta Radiol Suppl. 1986;369:576–9.

177. Luo CB, Teng MMH, Chang FC, Chang CY. Transarterial balloon-assisted n-butyl-2-cyanoacrylate embolization of direct carotid cavernous fistulas. AJNR Am J Neuroradiol. 2006;27:1535–40.

178. van Rooij WJ, Sluzewski M, Beute GN. Ruptured cavernous sinus aneurysms causing carotid cavernous fistula: incidence, clinical presentation, treatment, and outcome. AJNR Am J Neuroradiol. 2006;27: 85–9.

179. Nesbit GM, Barnwell SL. The use of electrolytically detachable coils in treating high- low arteriovenous fistulas. AJNR Am J Neuroradiol. 1998;19: 565–9.

180. Jansen O, Dorfler A, Forsting M, et al. Endovascular therapy of arteriovenous fistulae with electrolytically detachable coils. Neuroradiology. 1999 41:951–7.

181. Debrun GM, Ausman JI, Charbel FT, Aletich VA. Access to the cavernous sinus through the vertebral artery: technical case report. Neurosurgery. 1995;37:144–6; discussion 6–7.

182. Moron FE, Klucznik RP, Mawad ME, Strother CM. Endovascular treatment of high-flow carotid cavernous fistulas by stent-assisted coil placement. AJNR Am J Neuroradiol. 2005;26:1399–404.

183. Kocer N, Kizilkilic O, Albayram S, Adaletli I, Kantarci F, Islak C. Treatment of iatrogenic internal carotid artery laceration and carotid cavernous fistula with endovascular stent-graft placement. AJNR Am J Neuroradiol. 2002;23: 442–6.

184. Archondakis E, Pero G, Valvassori L, Boccardi E, Scialfa G. Angiographic follow-up of traumatic carotid cavernous fistulas treated with endovascular stent graft placement. AJNR Am J Neuroradiol. 2007;28:342–7.

185. Gomez F, Escobar W, Gomez AM, Gomez JF, Anaya CA. Treatment of carotid cavernous fistulas using covered stents: midterm results in seven patients. AJNR Am J Neuroradiol. 2007;28:1762–8.

186. Beighton P, De Paepe A, Steinmann B, Tsipouras P, Wenstrup RJ. Ehlers-Danlos syndromes: revised nosology, Villefranche, 1997. Ehlers-Danlos National Foundation (USA) and Ehlers-Danlos Support Group (UK). Am J Med Genet. 1998;77:31–7.

187. Pepin M, Schwarze U, Superti-Furga A, Byers PH. Clinical and genetic features of Ehlers-Danlos syndrome type IV, the vascular type. N Engl J Med. 2000;342: 673–80.

188. Mitsuhashi T, Miyajima M, Saitoh R, Nakao Y, Hishii M, Arai H. Spontaneous carotid-cavernous fistula in a patient with Ehlers-Danlos syndrome type IV – case report. Neurol Med Chir (Tokyo). 2004;44:548–53.

189. Halbach VV, Higashida RT, Dowd CF, Barnwell SL, Hieshima GB. Treatment of carotid-cavernous fistulas associated with Ehlers-Danlos syndrome. Neurosurgery. 1990;26:1021–7.

190. Horowitz MB, Purdy PD, Valentine RJ, Morrill K. Remote vascular catastrophes after neurovascular interventional therapy for type 4 Ehlers-Danlos syndrome. AJNR Am J Neuroradiol. 2000;21:974–6.

191. Schievink WI, Piepgras DG, Earnest Ft, Gordon H. Spontaneous carotid-cavernous fistulae in Ehlers-Danlos syndrome type IV. Case report. J Neurosurg. 1991;74: 991–8.

16. Venous Disease and Cavernous Malformations

This chapter covers the gamut of intracranial venous issues, ranging from the most common entity – developmental venous anomalies – to the nonexistent: "chronic cerebrospinal venous insufficiency."

16.1.　Developmental Venous Anomalies

Developmental venous anomalies (DVA) (aka venous angiomas, venous malformations, venous anomalies, medullary venous malformations, or caput medusae) are a normal variant of intraparenchymal medullary veins, being larger and more visible on imaging than most medullary veins (Fig. 16.1).[1] They are usually found in white matter and are associated with cavernous malformations.[2] They are characterized histologically by a complex of sometimes thickened and hyalinized veins with interspersed normal neural parenchyma.[3]

The most important thing to know about DVAs is that they are usually incidental findings on imaging, and with rare exception, are completely benign.[4–6] When associated with a cavernous malformation, they may be erroneously identified as the source of symptoms.[7] They may also be confused with AVMs and other aggressive lesions by the uninitiated. The authors of this handbook wish they had a dollar for every patient referred to them with an incidental DVA found on imaging and misidentified as an AVM.

Epidemiology

1. DVAs are found in some 2.6% of autopsies.[8–10]
2. A review of 7,266 brain MRIs found a frequency of DVAs of 0.7%.[11]

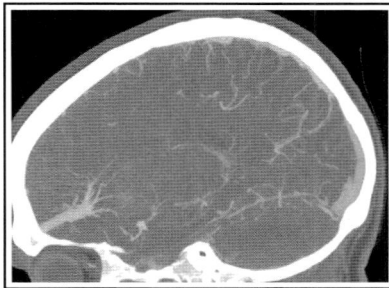

Fig. 16.1 Frontal lobe venous angioma in a sagittal CT angiogram reconstruction. It has the typical stellate network of veins converging on a single collecting vein.

M.R. Harrigan, J.P. Deveikis, *Handbook of Cerebrovascular Disease and Neurointerventional Technique*, DOI 10.1007/978-1-61779-946-4_16,
© Springer Science+Business Media New York 2013

Aetiology

DVAs are thought to be congenital and result from a failure of normal embryogenesis.[12,13]

Imaging

1. Typical appearance on MRI and CTA: radial pattern, the so-called caput medusa, which converges on an enlarged central trunk.[14]
2. Seen only during the venous phase on angiography.
3. About two thirds are in a supratentorial location and one third are in the cerebellum and brainstem.[11]
4. Often found in close proximity to a cavernous malformation.
5. Of all patients found to have a venous angioma on MRI, 18% had an associated cavernous malformation.[11]

Natural History and Presentation

1. A prospective study with 298 patient-years of observation found a symptomatic haemorrhage rate of 0.34% per year.[15]
2. In *every case* in which there was a haemorrhage associated with the venous angioma, a cavernoma was present.[11]
3. Rarely, spontaneous thrombosis of a very large venous angioma may cause extensive venous infarction or haemorrhage.[16]

Arterialized Venous Malformations

A rare condition associated with DVAs is the so-called arterialized venous malformation (aka venous-predominant AVM, or atypical DVA).[17] These consist of a typical appearing DVA that is associated with arteriovenous shunting. On angiography they show no AVM nidus, but have a homogeneous arterial blush with early appearance of the medullary veins in the DVA.[17–19] (Fig. 16.2) On MR, the typical spoke-wheel appearance of a DVA is seen.[20] These lesions are quite rare, making it difficult to characterize the natural history. The largest series[17] includes 15 patients: 6 lesions were asymptomatic, 8 caused haemorrhage, and 1 caused seizures without haemorrhage. After surgical excision, there were 2 post-op haemorrhages, highlighting the inherent danger in trying to remove a DVA.

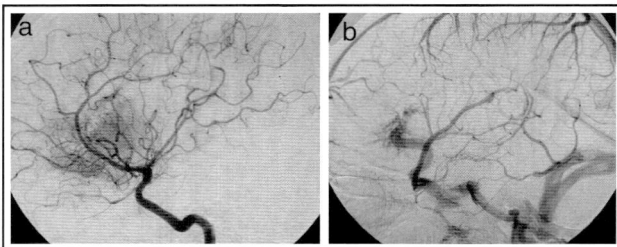

Fig. 16.2 Angio-pathologic correlation! Arterialized developmental venous anomaly. Lateral right internal carotid arteriogram. Early arterial phase (**a**) shows prominent blush in the frontal region, but no shunting. Venous phase (**b**) shows typical DVA draining that area.

Management

1. Most DVAs are incidental findings and do not require treatment or follow-up imaging.
2. During surgery for evacuation of a haemorrhage or resection of a cavernous malformation, it is critical to preserve the associated venous angioma, particularly in the brainstem.
3. Removal of a venous angioma may cause a venous infarction.

Global Gem
Pierre Lasjaunias (1948–2008) was a pioneering Parisian neuroradiologist and neurointerventionalist who was notable for exploring the venous side of cerebrovascular development and disorders, among many other accomplishments. He was probably most famous, along with Alex Berenstein and Karel ter Brugge, for the five-volume epic text *Surgical Neuroangiography*, and for his work in the understanding and management of vein of Galen malformations. Discussion of food, wine, and cerebrovascular disease is much more impressive with a French accent.

Venous Anomalies in Vein of Galen Malformations
1. Vein of Galen Malformations are an arteriovenous shunt into the wall of a dilated vein of Galen. (see Chap. 14)
2. This "vein of Galen" may actually be a fetal median prosencephalic vein of Markowski, which is normally present between 7 and 12 weeks gestation.[1] This is a subarachnoid venous structure that usually drains not into the straight sinus, but into a more cranially directed falcine sinus which then empties into the superior sagittal sinus.
3. Approximately half of all vein of Galen malformations show no filling of the straight sinus.[1]
4. Due to the high flow shunts associated with the fistula, on angiography, deep veins (e.g. internal cerebral veins and basal vein of Rosenthal) are usually not seen draining into the vein of Galen in this condition. This was used historically as a justification for doing transvenous embolization of the venous pouch in vein of Galen malformations.
5. *Au contraire, mon ami.* There are increasing reports indicating visualization of normal deep veins draining into the prosencephalic vein after curative transarterial embolization of the fistula.[5]
6. This deep venous drainage that may not be visible angiographically may explain the relatively poor clinical outcomes achieved with transvenous embolization or open surgical treatment of vein of Galen malformations.[6]

16.2. Sinus Pericranii

Sinus pericranii is a rare venous condition that consists of a large communication between an intracranial venous sinus and an anomalous extracranial venous channel.[21] The extracranial component is a soft, fluctuant scalp mass that is compressible and enlarges in a dependent position or with Valsalva maneuver.[21,22] A young boy with this finding was described by Percival Potts in 1760.[22] The condition was called sinus pericranii by Stromeyer in 1850.[23] Other terms applied to the lesion included *fistula osteovasculare* and *varix sprius circumscriptus venae diploica frontalis.*[24]

Epidemiology

1. Prevalence: Rare. As of 1994 only 100 cases reported in world's literature.[25]
   a. 80% present before age 40[26]
   b. Sometimes associated with trauma.

c. Male–female incidence similar, although post-traumatic varieties more common in males.[27,28]
d. Most are in midline, although rarely, lateral sinus pericranii are found.[26,29,30]
e. Location: 40% frontal, 34% parietal, 23% occipital, 4% temporal.[31]
f. The venous connection trough the skull may be low-flow or high-flow, with 13 of 31 reported cases classified as high-flow.[32]

Aetiology

1. Congenital
   a. Developmental venous anomalies are associated with sinus pericranii.[33]
   b. *Blue rubber bleb naevus syndrome* (multiple compressible cutaneous naevi associated with gastrointestinal nevi and subcutaneous venous malformations) has been seen with sinus pericranii.[34,35]
   c. It is thought that endothelial lining of the vascular spaces indicates a congenital origin of the lesion.[29,36]
2. Traumatic
   a. Trauma to the head with or without a fracture over the dural venous sinus and creation of an extracranial blood space can create sinus pericranii.[37,38]
   b. Histologically, post-traumatic lesions have a connective tissue pseudo-endothelial lining.[39]
3. Other acquired causes
   a. Erosion of Pacchionian granulations.[25]
   b. Raised intracranial pressure.[25]
   c. Venous sinus thrombosis.[40]
   d. After infection in the bone.[24]
   e. A special category is sinus pericranii associated with craniosynostosis. These lesions can spontaneously resolve after surgical repair of the craniosynostosis. The term, "squeezed-out sinus syndrome" is used in this case.[41]

Natural History and Presentation

1. Most present as an unexplained painless, soft, fluctuant swelling on the head, possibly with associated blue discoloration of the overlying skin.
2. Headaches may be a presenting symptom.[27,29]
3. Less common symptoms are nausea, vomiting and vertigo.[27]
4. Rarely bradycardia,[42] hearing loss,[22] or seizures[43] may be associated, but it is uncertain whether there is a causal relationship with the sinus pericranii.
5. Spontaneous partial thrombosis can occur, causing a painful non-compressible mass.[44]
6. Rarely, spontaneous involution of sinus pericranii can occur.[45]

Imaging

1. CT without contrast can show the slightly hyperdense venous malformation and bone windowing can reveal the bony defect through which the communication to the sinus passes.[22]
2. MR studies show flow voids in the subgaleal anomalous veins on T2 images with enhancement of the slow-flowing veins on post-contrast T1 images.[22,46]
3. The lesions can be seen during the venous phase of cerebral angiography, although oblique angles may be necessary to best demonstrate the connection to the intracranial sinus.[43]
4. 3D angiography is particularly helpful to allow optimal visualization of the transcranial connection and the associated bony opening.[26]
5. Percutaneous puncture of the subgaleal venous channel with contrast injection can also show the connection to the venous sinuses.[26]

Management

1. Some advocate aggressive management due to a risk of life-threatening complications after trauma, such as bleeding, infection and air embolism.[43,47]
   a. Patients with sinus pericranii should be counseled to avoid being stabbed, shot, or bludgeoned to avoid those complications.
   b. In reality, most lesions are treated for purely cosmetic reasons.
2. Surgical options include craniectomy with division of the bridging vein and cranioplasty, but there have been reports of serious bleeding from dural sinus lacerations.[31]
   a. Small communications with the dural sinus can be treated by occluding them with bone wax.[48]
3. Percutaneous sclerotherapy of the extracranial venous anomaly may be done for cosmetic reasons, but this is not often curative and transient sixth nerve palsy with this technique has been reported.[44]
4. Transvenous embolization with nBCA of the connecting transcranial vein can effectively treat the lesion.[48]
   a. Percutaneous puncture and injection of Onyx into the transcranial connection has also been described.[26]
5. *Caveat*: When angiography shows that there dominant flow of the intracranial veins preferentially via the sinus pericranii, it is best to treat the lesion conservatively.[21]

16.3.   Venous Malformations

Venous malformations are low-flow congenital vascular anomalies that frequently involve the skin, subcutaneous fat and/or muscle. Especially in the head and neck, they can produce such profound deformity that they can cause serious psychological and social problems for the patient.[49] In addition to cosmesis, they can also have functional implications in the orbit and around the airway. They have often been indiscriminately grouped together with various vascular lesions under the term "vascular birth marks," and are frequently misdiagnosed as haemangiomas (Table 16.1).

Epidemiology

1. Prevalence: Approximately 1–4% of population.[50,51]
2. Incidence: 1–2 per 10,000 births.[52]

Table 16.1 Superficial venous malformations vs. capillary (infantile) haemangiomas[a]

	Venous malformations	**Capillary haemangiomas**
Definition[319]	Low-flow vascular malformation.	Benign vascular neoplasm.
Symptom onset[319]	At birth	Soon after birth
Growth pattern[54]	Slow growth throughout life. May have growth spurts at puberty, pregnancy	Rapid proliferative phase in early infancy, followed by phase of involution after 12 months of age.
Margins[54]	Poorly defined	Usually well defined
Histology[56,319]	Flat endothelium forming dysplastic vessels. Does not proliferate *in vitro*.	Densely packed endothelial cells in clusters. Proliferates *in vitro*.
Treatment[54]	Surgery, sclerotherapy, conservative therapy.	Steroids propranolol, surgery, conservative therapy.

[a]These lesions are often confused, but they are distinct lesions

3. Male–female incidence similar.[51]
4. Left-sided lesions are much more common than right.[53]
5. Location: Often seen in the head and neck, including the tongue, the parotid region, the orbit, as well as virtually anywhere in the body.[54]

Pathophysiology

1. These are congenital anomalies that are present at birth.
    a. Fully 70% of orbital venous and venolymphatic malformations have associated intracranial vascular anomalies, most commonly DVAs.[53]
    b. Many are sporadic, but there are autosomal dominant familial forms that have been mapped to chromosome 9p.[55]
2. Histologically the malformation consists of numerous, disorganized vascular channels.[56]
    a. There may be various combinations of venous channels, lymphatic channels, or a mixture of the two.[56]
3. The anomalous vessels dilate, causing local swelling. These can partially thrombose, causing venous outlet obstruction and dilating the remaining vascular spaces even further.
4. Perivascular lymphocytic infiltrates suggests inflammation, also a mechanism contributing to symptomatic swelling and pain.[56]

Syndromes Associated with Venous Malformations

1. Klippel-Trenaunay syndrome.
    a. Definition: triad of limb hypertrophy, venous and lymphatic malformation of the limb, and a port-wine skin nevus.[57,58]
    b. Although case reports have suggested an association between Klippel-Trenaunay syndrome and spinal arteriovenous malformations, this association does not appear to be valid.[59]
    c. There has been a case combining features of KTS, Sturge Weber, and phakomatosis pigmantovascularis, suggesting that these entities may be part of a spectrum of disease.[60]
2. Autosomal dominant familial venous malformations
    a. Multiple cutaneous and mucosal venous malformations seen in several kindred.[55,61]
3. *Blue rubber bleb naevus syndrome*
    a. A rare inherited condition with multiple raised cutaneous and gastrointestinal tract venous lesions.[35]

Natural History and Presentation

1. Venous malformations are frequently noted at birth and appear as an area of soft tissue swelling. Often with associated bluish discoloration of the skin and sometime with visible abnormal venous spaces.
    a. The lesion is non-pulsitile. A thrill or bruit would suggest an arteriovenous malformation.
    b. Swelling worsens when the lesion is in a dependent position, during Valsalva maneuver, or during crying.
2. These lesions tend to slowly progress as the child ages, with rapid enlargement during puberty, pregnancy,[62,63] after local trauma, or after systemic infection.
3. The lesions tend to involve muscles and can cause pain and limitation of movement related to the muscle.
4. Venous malformations that involve skin or mucosa can cause bleeding.[64]
5. Lesions near the mouth or pharynx can cause difficulty swallowing.
6. Those near the airway can cause dangerous difficulty breathing.
7. Lingual and other oral lesions can cause bleeding in children when they suckle.
8. Orbital venous malformations can cause proptosis, diplopia, and can impair vision, especially if the lesion bleeds.[63,65]
    a. 64% of orbital venous malformations enlarged during a 4-year follow-up.[66]
    b. 40% of patients with orbital lesions progress to vision loss.[67]

Imaging

1. The appearance of venous malformations on CT without contrast can be indistinct and confusing. Calcification is common. Contrast-enhanced studies confirm the vascular nature of the lesion.[56]
2. MRI is the imaging modality of choice, and shows the lesion to have high T2 signal with intervening septations.[68–70] Contrast enhancement will distinguish venous malformations from lymphatic malformations.[70,71]
3. The malformations typically spread across tissue planes with poorly defined margins.[72]
4. Catheter angiography is *not needed*, since, at best, it may only show irregular venous structures very late in the venous phase.
5. Direct needle puncture of the lesion with contrast injection shows very abnormal vascular spaces.[73]

Management

1. Surgical excision
   a. Surgical excision rapidly removes the bulk of the lesion and is the primary treatment of these malformations.[73]
   b. Post-operative recurrence is not uncommon, especially with extensive lesions.[74]
2. Conservative therapy
   a. Analgesics and anti-inflammatory medications as well as selective use of compressive dressings or clothing can ameliorate some symptoms of venous malformations.
   b. Lesions that are small and minimally symptomatic can easily be treated conservatively.
   c. Many of these measures can be used to complement more invasive therapy.
3. Sclerotherapy
   a. Technique: percutaneous puncture of the abnormal venous channels and injection of a sclerosing agent:
      i. Ethanol (most commonly used), OK-432, Ethibloc, or bleomycin.[75]
   b. 70% of patients treated with ethanol sclerotherapy are improved or cured.[76]
   c. Complications of ethanol include skin ulceration in 13% and blistering in as many as 50%.[76]
   d. Complications may be lowered by placing a second needle in the vascular space to decompress it as the ethanol is injected.[77]
   e. Ethanol doses of over 1 ml/kg risk complications of pulmonary hypertension and shock.[78]
   f. Series comparing ethanol to bleomycin as the sclerosing agent show slightly less efficacy with bleomycin but considerably lower complication rates.[79]
4. Neodynium-YAG laser therapy
   a. Application of high-intensity light either percutaneously or by direct intralesional insertion of a probe has been used for venous malformations.[80,81]
   b. Laser therapy can treat the tiny intradermal vessels that may be difficult to treat with other forms of therapy.[82]

16.4.   Venous Stenosis

Recognition of venous stenosis and its association with various disease processes is an emerging field with only a few isolated cases reports or very small series, and limited understanding of the significance of venous disease.

Idiopathic Intracranial Hypertension

Idiopathic intracranial hypertension (IIH) (a.k.a psuedotumour cerebri, benign intracranial hypertension) is a potentially disabling condition producing symptoms of increased intracranial pressure, with absence of an underlying mass lesion to explain the symptoms.

The Dandy criteria for diagnosis include[83]
1. CSF pressure >25 cm H_2O
2. No localizing neurological signs (except abducens palsy)
3. Normal CSF composition, and
4. Normal to small ventricles on pneumoencephalography.

Since the CT and MRI imaging became available, amendments to the Dandy criteria include imaging to exclude obstructive hydrocephalus,[84] and venous thrombosis as causes of the increased intracranial pressure.[85] Small series of patients with signs of IIH and imaging evidence of dural venous sinus stenosis has prompted some to propose a causal relationship between venous stenosis and IIH.[86]

Statistics

1. Incidence: 0.9 case per 100,000 population in Iowa, Louisiana, and Minnesota.[87,88]
   a. 2.2 cases per 100,000 in Libya.[89]
2. Most commonly: obese women of childbearing age.
   a. 7.9–21.4 cases per 100,000 in obese women.[87–89]
   b. For patients weighing 38% over ideal female-to-male ratio 8:1.[87]
3. Interestingly, males with IIH are less likely to be obese but are more prone to having vision loss.[90,91]
4. IIH in younger children is less associated with obesity or with permanent vision loss.[92]

Aetiology

Idiopathic intracranial hypertension by definition has no known cause, but there are several theories. In fact, whenever a convincing aetiology for the symptom complex is finally found, the term *idiopathic* intracranial hypertension no longer applies.
1. Cerebrospinal fluid malabsorption
   a. This concept was first promulgated by Heinrich Quincke in the nineteenth century.[93]
   b. Recent publications continue to promote abnormal CSF dynamics as the aetiology of IIH.[94]
   c. This theory has prompted the development of and is supported by positive outcomes from CSF diversion techniques including repeated therapeutic lumbar punctures and ventriculo-peritoneal shunting.
   d. Skeptics argue that there is no evidence of ventricular dilatation in IIH, whereas other conditions manifesting abnormal CSF production or absorption usually are associated with imaging evidence of hydrocephalus.[95]
2. Cerebral blood flow dysregulation
   a. Elevated cerebral blood flow[96,97] and cerebral blood volume[98] has been seen in patients with IIH.
   b. One wonders why acetazolamide would help in these patients since that drug increases cerebral blood flow.
   c. Decreased cerebral blood flow seen in some patients correlates with the presence of venous outflow obstruction, and the disease in this subgroup of patients has been called secondary intracranial hypertension (SIH).[97]
3. Causes of venous outflow obstruction
   a. Increased intra-abdominal pressure
      i. Animal models show a direct correlation between intracranial pressure and intra-abdominal pressure.[99]
      ii. Increased abdominal pressure in obese IIH patients may be transmitted to the intracranial venous system.
      iii. Small series show transient symptom relief in obese IIH patients when an external device was used to lower abdominal pressure.[100]
      iv. Skeptics say this theory does not explain the female predominance in IIH and that hormones may have a role as well.[101]

b. Venous sinus stenosis
  i. Given the role of dural venous sinuses in the removal of cerebrospinal fluid from the intracranial compartment, and the observation of elevated venous pressures on intracranial venography in 10 out of 10 patients with pseudotumour, Karahalios and coworkers proposed that venous hypertension may be the final common pathway for production of elevated CSF pressure.[86]
  ii. An MRV study showed significant bilateral venous sinus stenoses in 27 of 29 IIH patients compared to 4 of 59 matched control subjects.[102]
  iii. A contrary opinion is that increased intracranial pressure causes venous stenosis.[103] A small series[104] and several case reports[105,106] have shown resolution of venous sinus stenosis after normalization of CSF pressure by lumbar puncture.
  iv. An interesting study showed coupling of CSF and superior sagittal sinus pressure, suggesting the potential for a vicious cycle, in which high CSF pressure raises venous pressure, which creates a further worsening of CSF pressure.[107]
  v. On the other hand, in a study of nine patients with IIH and venous sinus stenosis, the stenosis persisted even after normalization of CSF pressure, medically and by lumbar puncture.[108]
4. IIH mimics: Any medical condition that can raise CSF pressure can cause symptoms similar to IIH. See reviews of IIH diagnosis from Friedman and Jacobson[85] as well as Wall.[109]

Natural History and Presentation

1. Symptoms of headache, blurred vision, occasionally tinnitus or diplopia.[85]
  a. Headache frequently unrelenting.
2. Elevated CSF pressure is present; one study showed pressure 18–45 cm H_2O at baseline with spikes up to 70 cm H_2O.[110]
3. Papilloedema is common.
4. The incidence of significant visual impairment is 22–96%.[87,111]

Imaging

By definition, idiopathic intracranial hypertension is a diagnosis of exclusion, and imaging should be done to exclude other causes of increased intracranial pressure such as tumors, vascular malformations, inflammatory processes, and venous sinus thrombosis.

1. CT studies typically showed small ("slit-like") ventricles.[95]
2. High-resolution brain and orbital MR frequently shows flattening of the globes, an enlarged optic nerve sheath containing CSF, protrusion and enhancement of the optic nerve head, kinking or tortuosity of the optic nerves, empty sella syndrome, and narrowing of Meckel's cave.[112,113]

Management

a. Traditional therapy includes medical therapy with analgesics, corticosteroids, acetazolamide, cerebrospinal fluid diversion with periodic lumbar puncture or ventriculoperitoneal shunting, and optic nerve sheath decompression to relieve pressure on the nerve.[114]
b. Weight loss can be helpful
  i. Bariatric surgery can resolve symptoms of IIH in severely obese patients.[115]
c. Stenting has commonly been used in the treatment of benign intracranial hypertension, or pseudotumour cerebri, caused by dural sinus stenosis.[116–123]
d. Although there are no prospective randomized trials of surgical intervention, a systematic review found improved or resolved visual deficits in 38% of patients after VP shunting, 44% of patients after lumboperitoneal

shunting, 47% of patients after venous stenting, and 80% of eyes after optic nerve fenestration.[124]

e. More recently, a series of 52 patients stented showed a 100% success rate of improving signs and symptoms of papilloedema and headache.[125] There were six recurrences requiring additional stent placement, but no complications.

Venous Tinnitus

1. Continuous "whooshing" sound accentuated in systole and is heard by the patient and may even be audible to the examiner.[126]
2. Venous tinnitus frequently appears as neck bruit, as opposed to a venous hum, which can be heard in half of normal individuals and even more commonly in pregnant women.[127]
3. Tends to be on the side of the dominant internal jugular vein, which is usually on the right.[128-130]
4. Features supporting a venous aetiology in patients with tinnitus include increased prominence of the sound when the patient is recumbent and compressing the contralateral jugular vein, as well as dampening of the sound by compressing the ipsilateral jugular.
5. Causes:
    a. Systemic hyperdynamic states[126,131,132]
        i. Anemia[133]
        ii. Pregnancy
        iii. Thyrotoxicosis
    b. Increased intracranial pressure
        i. Any condition with increased intracranial pressure[134]
        ii. Idiopathic intracracranial hypertension.[135,136]
        iii. Pneumocephalus.[137]
    c. Venous abnormalities
        i. High-riding and enlarged jugular bulbs.[128,130,131]
        ii. Transverse sinus stenosis.[116,138]
    d. Some cases are idiopathic
6. Treatment
    a. Tinnitus related to systemic disease usually improves after treatment of the underlying condition.
    b. Similarly, resolution of the increased intracranial pressure can improve the tinnitus.
    c. Since compression of the affected jugular vein improves tinnitus, jugular vein ligation has been advocated.[126,131,139]
        i. However, recurrent tinnitus after jugular ligation as been reported.[131,140]
        ii. What's worse is that intracranial venous hypertension can occur after ligation.[141] This chapter illustrates many of the bad things that can happen due to venous obstruction.
    d. Stenting of transverse sinus stenosis can treat the tinnitus and does not impair venous outflow.[116]
    e. Stenting is preferable to jugular ligation and should be considered in patients with classic venous tinnitus ipsilateral to a significant stenosis confirmed on direct retrograde venography (see Chap. 12).
    f. Similarly, some patients with a sigmoid diverticulum, or "venous aneurysm" may be successfully treated by stent placement with, or without associated coiling of the aneurysmal area.[142,143]

Venous Stenosis and Arteriovenous Fistulas and Malformations

Venous structures play an important role in cerebral arteriovenous fistulas and arteriovenous malformations (see Chap. 15). There is increasing recognition of the role of venous structures in the development these lesions and their evolution over time.
1. Venous occlusive disease is a factor in development of arteriovenous fistulas.
    a. Venous occlusive disease has been shown to play a role in development of dural arteriovenous fistulas in animal models.[144-146]
    b. Venous hypertension appears to be the main factor require for fistula development, since thrombosis without venous hypertension is not sufficient.[145]

c. Genetic thrombophyllic abnormalities are seen more commonly in patients with dural arteriovenous fistulae than in the general public.[147]
d. There are reports of *de novo* dural arteriovenous fistula formation in the setting of venous hypertension and sinus thrombosis.[148–151]
e. A new dural-pial arteriovenous malformation developed 29 months after superior sagittal sinus and transverse sinus thrombosis.[152]

2. Venous occlusive disease can contribute to increased risk of haemorrhage and/or worsening symptoms from intracranial AVMs.
   a. Venous occlusive disease can redirect flow in dural arteriovenous fistula toward cortical veins and that can affect symptomatology.[153]
   b. Computer modeling of brain AVMs shows impairment of venous drainage increases the risk of haemorrhage.[154]
   c. Stenting of stenotic venous sinuses seems to help patients with dural arteriovenous fistulas with cortical venous hypertension.[155,156]
   d. Three out of four cases of transverse or sigmoid sinus dural AVF's were completely cured by stenting after partial transarterial embolization, and some even without adjunctive embolization.[157]

3. High-flow venopathy
   a. Venous stenosis is seen in patients with cerebral AVMs and is thought to be related to intimal hypertrophy related to high flow.[158,159]
   b. Development of severe venous sinus stenosis developed during a 5 year follow-up of an arteriovenous malformation containing a high-flow fistula.[160]

Venous Stenosis and Its Relationship (or Lack Thereof) to Multiple Sclerosis

The notion that multiple sclerosis (MS) may be related to venous stenosis has received considerable attention since 2008. It is also very controversial.[161] The concept of chronic cerebrospinal venous insufficiency (CCSVI) holds that insufficient intracranial venous outflow leads to a build-up of cerebral venous pressure and the changes associated with multiple sclerosis. The leading proponent of this theory is Paolo Zamboni, an Italian vascular surgeon.

1. Chronic cerebrospinal venous insufficiency (CCSVI)
   a. Zamboni and colleagues[162] proposed venous flow criteria for the diagnosis of CCSVI based on color Doppler criteria:
      i. Reflux in internal jugular and vertebral veins in sitting and supine position.
      ii. Reflux in deep cerebral veins.
      iii. Visible jugular vein stenosis on B-mode images
      iv. No flow in jugular or vertebral veins.
      v. If the cross-sectional area in the jugular becomes greater in upright than the supine position.
   b. Using these Doppler criteria, patients with multiple sclerosis in Zamboni's studies showed significantly more of these criteria compared to controls, suggesting that the demyelinating disease is causally related to venous abnormalities.
   c. Using susceptibility-weighted MRI imaging, a study of 16 multiple sclerosis patients showed greater iron deposition compared to 8 control patients, and this was interpreted to be evidence supporting CCSVI's deleterious effects on the brain parenchyma.[163]
   d. The same group proceeded to an open label trial of venous angioplasty, with no control group.[164] Of a total of 65 patients treated, the 35 relapsing remitting patients showed significant improvements in relapse free rates, fewer enhancing lesions on MRI and improved quality of life measures. Less improvement was seen in secondary progressive and primary progressive patients. Restenosis at the angioplasty site occurred in 47% of patients.

2. The carnival of publicity concerning CCSVI
   a. A recent Google search for CCSVI reveals over one million possible sites. Many are posts to multiple sclerosis patient forums, informational sites (including www.ccsvi.org where the logo states "Opening veins, opening minds.") and also doctors, hospitals and clinics advertising and offering the procedure.
   b. The popular media have reported on the topic. Many of the web sites and media reports use Zamboni's term "liberation procedure" when referring to the venous angioplasty.

c. This simple solution to a complex disease appeals to patients and especially those that are suspicious of the motives of the neurologists and multiple sclerosis researchers.[165]
d. This procedure costs many thousands of dollars and is not covered by insurance in the United States.

3. Evidence against CCSVI
   a. A larger series evaluating the prevalence of CCSVI characteristics among multiple sclerosis patients showed lower prevalence than earlier studies (56%) compared to 43% in other neurological disorders, prompting the authors to conclude that CCSVI does not have a causative role in MS.[166]
   b. Several other studies did not find the predicted venous occlusive disease in MS patients.[167–170]
   c. Patients treated with "the liberation procedure" were still on standard immunomodulation therapy and had a remitting and relapsing form of the disease.[164] It would not be surprising to see improvement in symptoms over time in this population.[171]
   d. The angioplasty procedures are not without risk. Jugular venous thrombosis has been reported following the "liberation procedure".[172]
   e. The CCSVI criteria are based on Doppler ultrasound imaging, which is operator-dependent.
   f. Venous anatomy is extremely variable and extracranial veins are easily compressed and distorted.
   g. On a theoretical basis, Khan and coworkers[173] took issue to the reasoning behind CCSVI according to the following arguments:
      i. MS is more common in young women, and chronic venous disease is not.
      ii. All the well-known epidemiological associations with MS including geography, ethnicity, vitamin D levels, etc. are not related to venous outflow insufficiency.
      iii. As shown elsewhere in this chapter, venous occlusive disease causes haemorrhagic infarction, edema, and increased intracranial pressure, which are not signs of MS.
      iv. Venous occlusive disease would be expected to progress over time, yet the natural course of MS trails off over time.
      v. Immune disorders elsewhere in the body do not have a venous basis.
      vi. Transient global amnesia has been associated with jugular venous reflux, but does not appear to be associated with MS.
      vii. A model that should confirm the association of MS with venous disease is the radical neck dissections performed for cancer treatment. The jugular veins are occluded and secondary occurrence of MS in this setting has not been observed.

4. Recommendations
   a. Multiple sclerosis patients should undergo venous angioplasty procedures only in well-designed clinical trials.

16.5. Cerebral Venous Thrombosis

Cerebral venous thrombosis (CVT) can occur in the form of cortical venous thrombosis, venous sinus thrombosis, deep venous thrombosis, jugular venous thrombosis, or various combinations of the above.

Epidemiology

1. Annual incidence
   a. Cerebral Venous Thrombosis in adults: 3–4 per million.[174]
   b. More common in children: 7 per million.[174]
2. Represents less than 1% of stroke.[175]

Aetiology

1. A hypercoagulable state is present in 31% of cases.[176]
2. Predisposing factors
    a. Factor V Leiden mutation[177]
    b. Oral contraceptive use[177,178]
    c. Complicated pregnancy[179]
    d. Uncomplicated pregnancy.[180]
    e. Mastoiditis and otitis media[181]
    f. Central nervous system infection[175]
    g. History of cancer[182,183]
    h. Thalidomide use in multiple myeloma.[184]
    i. Tamoxifen use.[185]
    j. Erythropoietin use.[186]
    k. Phytoestrogens.[187]
    l. Post-operative thrombosis.[188,189]
    m. Spontaneous intracranial hypotension.[190–192]
    n. Placement of a lumbar drain.[192]
    o. Ulcerative colitis.[193]
    p. High-altitude.[194]
    q. Bone compression of the sinus in neonates.[195]

Genetics

A comprehensive meta-analysis that evaluated 1,183 CVT cases and 5,189 controls in 26 studies revealed associations with genes involved in the clotting cascade:[196]
    a. Factor V Leiden/G1691A: Pooled odds ratio (OR) 2.40 (95% CI 1.75–3.3 $p < 0.00001$) CVT cases attributable to this polymorphism 6.8%.
    b. Prothrombin/G20210A: Pooled OR 5.43 (95% CI 3.88–7.74 $p < 0.00001$) CVT cases attributable: 14.2%.
    c. Metylene tetrafolate reductase/C677T: Pooled OR 1.83 (95% CI 0.88–3.80 $p < 0.09$) CVT cases attributable: 17.9%.
    d. Associated risk of CVT with these genes is greater in adults than children.
    e. A non-significant increased association with venous compared to arterial ischemia.

Imaging

1. General concepts
    a. May see generalized brain edema or more focal edema that is not in a typical arterial territory. Territories involved:
        i. Sagittal sinus thrombosis: Parasagittal cortex *bilaterally*.
        ii. Transverse sinus thrombosis: Ipsilateral temporal and occipital lobes, and even the ipsilateral cerebellar hemisphere.
        iii. Deep cerebral venous thrombus: Bithalamic region oedema.
        iv. Cortical vein thrombosis: More localized cortical oedema.
    b. As the impairment of blood flow progresses to venous infarction, further oedema and haemorrhagic transformation may occur.[197]
    c. Subdural and subarachnoid bleeding may be present as well.[198–200]
2. CT
    a. Non-contrast CT may show hyperdense clot in the thrombosed vein or sinus.
    b. CT angiography can be timed to optimize visualization of the venous sinuses (CT venography)
    c. CT venography is less prone to artifact compared with MR venography
3. MR
    a. T2 and FLAIR sequences show oedema.
    b. T1 may show high signal clot in venous structures and bleeding in the brain
    c. Susceptibility-weighted imaging (gradient echo or T2*) is very sensitive in detecting haemorrhage.

4. Angiographic findings:
   a. Sluggish arteriovenous transit and congested veins
   b. Absence of flow in thrombosed veins
   c. Filling defects may be seen in partially occluded venous structures but care should be taken to not misinterpret unopacified blood flowing in from arterial territories that were not injected.
   d. Direct catheter venography can confirm the presence of clot, but flow patterns can sometimes simulate solid filling defects (see Chap. 12)

Presentation and Clinical Features

1. Protean manifestations include headaches, decreasing visual acuity, declining cognitive ability, hemiparesis, hemianaesthesia, aphasia, disturbed consciousness, coma, and even death.
2. Cortical or dural sinus thrombosis may also manifest as subarachnoid haemorrhage.[198,199]
3. Delay in diagnosis is common: A study of 91 patients admitted for CVT showed the median time of hospital admission after symptom onset was 4 days, and only 25% were admitted within the first 24 h.[200]
4. When there is a clinical suspicion for CVT, imaging confirms the diagnosis 16.3% of patients.[201]
5. Mortality
   a. Overall mortality 10–13% [175]
   b. 4.3% died acutely and 3.4% within 30 days.[175]
   c. Patients over 65 years old had a 27% chance of death and 22% chance of dependency compared to 7% death and 2% incapacitation in younger adults.[202]
   d. A series of 38 children with CVT had no mortality from the condition.[203]
   e. On the other hand, a study of CVT in neonates showed 5 out of 90 died and a full 61% had a bad outcome.[204]
   f. Factors predicting a higher risk of death include:[175]
      i. Seizures, coma, disturbed consciousness, deep cerebral venous thrombosis, right-sided intraparenchymal bleed, posterior fossa involvement, and progressive focal neurological deficits.
   g. Transtentorial herniation is the most common immediate cause of mortality in the acute phase of the disease.[205]

Management

1) Medical management
   a) Isotonic saline hydration
   b) Aggressive management of intracranial hypertension.
2) Systemic anticoagulation
   a) Anticoagulation does not dissolve the thrombus but prevents propagation of the thrombus and reocclusion as the natural fibrinolytic processes take place.
   b) An early randomized trial of 20 patients and retrospective study demonstrated significantly better outcomes in CVT patients treated with heparin, even in the presence of intracerebral haemorrhage.[206]
   c) A retrospective study of 79 cases of CVT treated with heparin showed a mortality rate of 10% despite anticoagulation[207]
   d) Long term anticoagulation is required, since recurrent CVT or other venous thrombosis may occur 3–6 months later in 5.5–26% of these patients.[208]
   e) A recent prospective, nonrandomized cohort study of 624 patients with CVT found that low-molecular weight heparin had better efficacy and safety than unfractionated heparin for the initial treatment of CVT.[209]
3) European Federation of Neurological Societies recommendations:[210]
   a) Oral anticoagulation for 3 months
   b) Three months oral anticoagulation if CVT due to transient risk factor.
   c) Six to 12 months if idiopathic or mild thrombophilia such as heterozygous factor V Leiden or prothrombin G20210A mutation.
   d) Anticoagulation for an indefinite period for patients with recurrent CVT or with "severe" thrombophilia like prothrombin, protein C or S deficiency, homozygous factor V Leiden, or prothrombin G20210A, antiphospholipid antibodies, or a combination of thrombophilias.

4) Endovascular management
   a) Endovascular treatment is indicated for patients unable to receive anticoagulation and for those who deteriorate despite anticoagulation heparin.
      i) Consider endovascular therapy for patients in high-risk categories including those with seizures, coma, disturbed consciousness, deep cerebral vein thrombosis, posterior fossa involvement, and/or progressive focal deficits.[175]
   b) Thrombolytics can be infused directly into the thrombus via microcatheters placed via a transfemoral venous route.[197,211,212]
   c) Transarterial thrombolytic injections have been done for resolving venous clot for cortical vein thrombosis[213] or deep cerebral vein thrombosis.[214]
   d) Earlier reports describe thrombolytics slowly infused over many hours.[211]
   e) Quicker restoration of flow can be achieved with mechanical clot disruption using curved guidewires, angioplasty balloons,[215] micro-snares,[216] or rheolytic thrombectomy catheters like the AngioJet® catheter (Possis Medical, Minneapolis, MN).[213,217]
   f) Most use tPA or urokinase, but an animal study of abciximab infusion for dural venous sinus thrombosis showed recanalization comparable to tPA with better functional outcome.[218]
   g) Extreme cases of uncontrollable oedema may require decompressive craniectomy and/or barbiturate coma induction.[197]
   h) No randomized, prospective study comparing endovascular treatment with intravenous heparin.
   i) Several non randomized comparisons between endovascular therapy and systemic heparin show that outcomes are no worse with endovascular therapy.[197,219]
5) Surgical management
   a) Extreme cases of uncontrollable oedema may require decompressive craniectomy and/or barbiturate coma induction.[197]
   b) A retrospective study of decompressive craniectomy in 69 patients with CVT[220] showed at 12 month follow-up:
      i) 56.5% had good outcome (mRS 0–2)
      ii) 17.4% had bad outcome (mRS >2)
      iii) 15.9% mortality
         (1) *Three of the nine patients with fixed pupils recovered fully!*
   c) Patients in coma less likely to have good outcome (45% vs. 84%; p=0.003).
   d) Bilateral involvement more likely to have bad outcome (50% vs. 11%; p=0.025)

16.6.   Cavernous Malformations

Cavernous malformations (aka cerebral cavernous malformations, cavernous angiomas, cavernomas, cavernous hemangiomas, cryptic vascular malformations, cryptic vascular malformation, or angiographically occult vascular malformations) are distinctive cerebrovascular abnormalities. They may appear throughout and around the central nervous system, including the brain, spinal cord, cranial nerves, ventricles and orbit.[221,222] Overall, cavernous malformations are thought to account for some 10% of all cerebrovascular malformations. Cavernous malformations occur in two forms: *sporadic* and *familial*. In the sporadic form, the patient usually has only one lesion and there is no family history of the disorder. The familial form is characterized by multiple lesions and a family history of seizures.

Angioma Alliance

The Angioma Alliance is a non-profit organization that has established a DNA/ Tissue Bank and Patient Registry for the use of researchers investigating cerebral and spinal cavernous malformations: www.angiomaalliance.org. Email: Biobank@ AngiomaAlliance.org.

Epidemiology

1. Prevalence
   a. The prevalence of cavernomas in the general population appears to be about 0.5%.
      i. Large autopsy series: frequency of cavernomas was 0.5%[223]
      ii. Frequency of cavernomas on brain MRI: 0.4–0.5%[224,225]
2. Multiple in 50% of cases[226]
3. Sex prevalence is equal[225,227,228]
4. Risk factors
   a. Family history (see below)
   b. Cranial irradiation
      i. Radiation treatment is an established risk factor for the de novo formation of cavernous malformations.
      ii. A review of published reports of radiation-associated cavernomas found:[229]
         1. Most cases are in children (mean age, 11.7 years) although adult cases have been reported.
         2. Majority of lesions occurred in males.
         3. Mean radiation dose: 60.45 Gy.
         4. Mean latency period before detection of the cavernoma: 8.9 years.
         5. Most common presenting symptom was seizures.
         6. Most common reason for radiation treatment, in order of frequency:
            a. Medulloblastoma
            b. Glioma
            c. Acute lymphoblastic lymphoma

Pathophysiology

Cavernous malformations are well circumscribed, lobulated lesions, varying from <1 mm to 9 cm in diameter.[230]

1. Cavernous malformations consist of dilated, thin-walled vascular structures ("caverns") with an endothelial lining and a variable layer of fibrous adventitia. Elastic fibers have been reported[231] but are usually absent. Extensive haemosiderin deposits, indicating previous haemorrhage, and thrombosis may be present.[232] Calcification is present in 11–40% of cases.[231,233]
2. Gross appearance resembles a mulberry.
3. Ultrastructural analysis has demonstrated defects in the tight junctions between endothelial cells that form the blood–brain barrier, which may account for leakage of blood elements into the surrounding brain.[234,235]
4. Cavernoma growth appears to occur by a process of cavern proliferation in the setting of repeated lesional haemorrhages and brittle vascular morphology devoid of mature vessel wall elements.[236–238]
5. *Association with venous angiomas* (see below for a discussion of venous angiomas)
   a. The percentage of patients with a cavernoma who also have an associated venous angioma on MRI: approximately 25%.[239,240]
      • MRI may underestimate the prevalence of associated venous angiomas. In a surgical series of 86 patients undergoing resection of brainstem cavernomas, an associated venous angioma was found in *all* cases.[241]
      • Some authors believe that all cavernomas are associated with a venous angioma, whether or not the venous angioma is visible on imaging or not.[242]
   b. Percentage of patients with a venous angioma on MRI who also have an associated cavernous malformation: 18%.[11]
   c. Direct connections between venous angiomas and cavernous malformations have been found.[243,244]
      • Abnormal haemodynamics within venous angiomas may lead to the formation of cavernous malformations.[7,19,245,246]

- Local venous hypertension within a venous angioma may lead to a reactive process called *haemorrhagic angiogenic proliferation*, contributing to the formation of a cavernous malformation.[19]
  - The occurrence of de novo cavernous malformations after radiation therapy further supports this hypothesis, as vessel changes after radiation therapy occur mostly on the venous side and simulate the histological findings of venous angiomas.[246]
  - The authors have seen a case of extensive dural arteriovenous fistulas with developmental venous anomalies develop *de novo* cavernous malformations over time.

Familial Form

1. Definition of familial cavernous malformation: one or several lesions in at least two members of a family.[247,248]
   a. The presence of three or more lesions is "almost pathognomonic" for the familial form.[249]
2. Familial cases comprise 6–50% of all cavernous malformation cases.[223,226,250,251]
3. Hispanic patients of Mexican descent appear to have the highest incidence of familial cavernomas, although familial forms have been identified in almost every other ethnic group.
4. Familial form patients are most likely to have multiple lesions, and the number of lesions increases with age.[248,252]
   a. Multiple lesions are found in 50–84% of familial form patients.[247,250,253]
   b. The number of lesions per patient depends on the MRI technique (gradient echo imaging has the greatest sensitivity, see below).
      i. Mean number of lesions detected by gradient echo was 20.2 in symptomatic patients and 16.3 in asymptomatic subjects.[248]
5. Familial form lesions are *not* usually associated with a venous angioma.
6. Some 40% of patients with the familial form remain asymptomatic despite the presence of multiple lesions.[247]

Genetics

1. Three genes for cerebral cavernous malformations (CCM) have been identified:
   a. *CCM1* on chromosome 7q.[254–256]
      - The *CCM1* gene is also known as *KRIT1*, which is thought to be involved in arterial development.[257]
      - Mutation of the *CCM1* gene is responsible for nearly all inherited cavernomas among the Hispanic population of the United States.[258,259]
   b. *CCM2* on chromosome 7p.[260]
   c. *CCM3* on chromosome 3q.[260]
2. No differences in clinical presentation have been found for the three different loci.[257]

Imaging

1. MRI
   a. MRI is the imaging modality of choice for the identification and follow-up, being more accurate than both CT and angiography in the detection of cavernous malformations.[250]
   b. Characteristic MRI findings:
      - Both T2 and T1-weighted images typically show discrete areas of mixed signal intensity surrounded by a black rim of diminished signal intensity (looks like *popcorn*). Or, when the lesion is small, a discrete "black dot."
      - *Gradient echo* sequences demonstrate cavernous malformations with greater sensitivity than T1 or T2 images.[261–264]
        - Gradient echo shows haemosiderin staining the best.
      - An associated venous angioma is present on MRI in about 25% of sporadic cases,[239,240] but is not usually seen in familial cases.

- Zabramski and colleagues described 4 categories of lesions in patients with the familial form based on MRI findings:[247]
  - *Type I.* Subacute haemorrhage surrounded by a rim of haemosiderin-stained macrophages and gliotic brain.
    a. T1: Hyperintense core.
    b. T2: Hyper- or hypointense core with surrounding hypointense rim.
  - *Type II.* Loculated areas of haemorrhage and thrombosis of varying age, surrounded by gliotic, haemosiderin-stained brain. Most common finding in patients with cavernomas.[224]
    a. T1: Reticulated mixed signal core.
    b. T2: Reticulated mixed signal core with surrounding hypointense rim.
  - *Type III.* Chronic, resolved haemorrhage with haemosiderin within and around the lesion. Therefore, findings on T2-weighted SE sequences are hypointense, with greater magnification on T2-weighted GE sequences, whereas T1-weighted SE sequences exhibit hypointense to isointense signals.
    a. T1: Iso- or hypointense.
    b. T2: Hypointense with a hypointense rim.
    c. Gradient echo: Hypointense.
  - *Type IV.* Very small lesions, or "telangiectasias."
    a. T1: Poorly seen or not visualized at all.
    b. T2: Poorly seen or not visualized at all.
    c. Gradient echo: Punctate hypointense lesions.
  c. If the diagnosis is uncertain, the presence of an associated venous angioma can help confirm that the lesion is a cavernous malformation.
  d. Other lesions may have an appearance on MRI that is similar to cavernomas:[230] AVMs, calcified neoplasms (e.g.. oligodendrogliomas), infectious, inflammatory and granulomatous lesions, haemorrhagic tumors, and tumors containing melanin or fat.
    - High intensity T1 signal around the lesion is strongly suggestive of cavernoma and can help differentiate from haemorrhagic tumors or other haemorrhages.[265]
2. CT
  a. Focal area of increased density, with or without enhancement.
  b. Calcifications are present in 40% of cases.[266]
3. Angiography
  a. Cavernomas are usually "angio-occult," although venous pooling may be seen in rare cases.[250]

Presentation and Clinical Features

1. Age at presentation
   a. Most patients present in the 3rd and 5th decades of life.[224,233,247,267]
   b. Mean age at presentation in one series was 37.6 years.[224]
   c. Some 25% of patients are <18 years of age.[228,268]
      i. Age at presentation for pediatric patients has a bimodal pattern with peaks at 3 and 11 years of age.[269]
2. The most common presenting symptom of cavernous malformations are seizures, occurring in up to 55% of patients.[224,225,231,250,251,270]
3. Focal neurological deficits are present in 12–45% of patients at presentation.[9,224,225,250,270]
4. Headache may be the only "manifestation" of the lesion in some 25% of patients diagnosed with a cavernoma.[270] A history of chronic headaches is present in 3–52% of patients.[224,225,247,248,270]
5. The clinical manifestations of cavernomas are similar in both the sporadic and familial forms.[263]
6. Pregnancy and cavernomas.
   a. An increase in cavernoma size occurs during pregnancy.[227,271,272]
   b. Anecdotal evidence suggests that pregnancy is associated with the de novo appearance of new lesions,[225,273,274] and may increase the risk of haemorrhage from cavernomas.[225,261,271,273,275,276]

    c. Hormonal stimulation has been hypothesized to have a role in cavernoma growth and haemorrhage.[225,241,271,273,277]

    d. Resection of asymptomatic lesions may be a reasonable option in patients anticipating pregnancy.

Natural History

1. Cavernomas are dynamic lesions and may demonstrate spontaneous enlargement, regression, and de novo formation.[278]
   a. In a prospective MRI volumetric study of patients with cavernous malformations, over a 24 month period, 43% of lesions increased in volume, 35% decreased in volume, and 22% remained stable.[278]
   b. Another prospective study found that the average lesion size decreased by 9.1 mm over mean follow-up period of 16.2 months.[279]
2. Annual symptomatic haemorrhage risk may depend on whether the patient has a previous history of symptomatic haemorrhage:
   a. Annual risk of haemorrhage *without* a prior symptomatic haemorrhage: ~0.5%.[224,225,277,280]
   b. Annual risk of haemorrhage *with* a prior symptomatic haemorrhage: ~4.5%.[261,280]
      • A retrospective Japanese series found an annual haemorrhage rate for patients with a prior haemorrhage of 22.9%.[277]
   c. However, another prospective natural history study found an annual haemorrhage rate of 3.1%, with no difference between patients with or without a previous symptomatic haemorrhage.[251]
3. Symptomatic haemorrhage
   a. Risk factors for symptomatic haemorrhage:
      • Previous haemorrhage.[280]
      • Female sex.[225,251,277]
      • An associated venous angioma.[239,240]
   b. Lesion location does not appear to affect the risk of symptomatic haemorrhage.[280]

Management

Asymptomatic Cavernous Malformations

Asymptomatic lesions are frequently discovered as incidental findings on imaging, or in association with another, symptomatic lesion. Patients with asymptomatic lesions, or a vague complaint such as headaches, can be reassured that the expected natural history is likely to be relatively benign, and do not necessarily require treatment.[222] Surveillance imaging is an option. Alternatively, resection of a surgically accessible asymptomatic lesion may be reasonable if the patient is a good surgical candidate, is relatively young, female, anticipating pregnancy, or has a family history of symptomatic cavernous malformations.[230,281]

Seizures Associated with a Cavernous Malformation

1. Cerebral cavernous malformations are known to be more epileptogenic than other cerebrovascular lesions, presumably because of the deposition of ferric ions resulting from repeated micro-haemorrhages within and around the lesions.[282]
   a. Lesion locations at highest risk for seizures are the cerebral cortex and temporal, frontal, and perilimbic sites.[283]
   b. Cavernomas are nearly twice as likely to be associated with seizures compared to other lesions, such as AVMs and tumors, in similar locations.[230]
2. The annual risk of developing seizures is 0.4–1.51%.[224,277]
3. The need for treatment with anticonvulsant medications is obvious in patients presenting with a first seizure. Although some authors recommend medical therapy as the first-line treatment for patients with seizures attributable to a cavernoma,[283] resection of a cavernoma for treatment of epilepsy can be advantageous for the following reasons:

a. Long-term anticonvulsant therapy carries a cost in terms of side effects, medication expense, and possible effects on neuronal plasticity.
b. There is a hypothesis that resection of an epileptic lesion may prevent further seizures if done before repeated seizures occur and "kindling" develops.
c. Surgery is usually indicated for patients with medically-refractory seizures.

4. A complete seizure work-up, including EEG monitoring, is necessary in all patients anticipating resection of a cavernoma for treatment of a seizure disorder.
   a. A cavernoma seen on imaging is *not* a cause of seizures in some 6% of patients with a cavernoma and epilepsy.[284]

5. Surgical results: About 60–80% of patients are seizure-free after lesion resection, with or without anticonvulsant medications.[285,286]
   a. Seizure outcome after resection of cavernous malformations is better when surrounding haemosiderin-stained brain also is removed.[287]
   b. Predictors for good seizure outcome are age >30 years at the time of surgery, mesiotemporal lesion localization, cavernoma size <1.5 cm, and the absence of secondarily generalized seizures.[286]
   c. Seizure control may be better if resection of epileptogenic cortex is combined with resection of the underlying lesion. A systematic review comparing lesionectomy with the combined procedure found that at 2-year follow-up, patients having the combined surgery were significantly less likely to have persistent seizures.[288]

Symptomatic Haemorrhagic Cavernous Malformations

1. *Definition of symptomatic haemorrhagic cavernous malformation*: Clinical history of *apoplectic haemorrhage* or neurologic symptoms attributable to a cerebral mass lesion, with evidence of *extralesional haemorrhage* on imaging.[230,281]
2. Similar to the situation in patients with multiple intracranial aneurysms and subarachnoid haemorrhage, among patients with multiple cavernomas, the largest lesion is usually symptomatic.[223,247]
3. Surgery should be considered for patients with symptomatic lesions in a surgically accessible location who are acceptable candidates for cranial surgery. Patients who present with a haemorrhagic lesion are at increased risk of subsequent rehaemorrhage.[280]
4. Surgical considerations.
   a. Frameless stereotactic guidance and intraoperative cortical mapping, if eloquent cortex is involved, can be helpful.
   b. Intraoperative ultrasound can also help localize a cavernoma.
   c. Any associated venous angioma should be spared.[7,241,244,289]

Brainstem Cavernous Malformations

1. About 20% of intracranial cavernomas are located in the brainstem,[251] and are most commonly found in the pons, followed in frequency by the midbrain and the medulla.[225,284,290]
2. Selection of surgical candidates. Surgery should be considered for patients that meet at least one of the following criteria:[241] (1) lesion anatomy is favorable for resection; (2) repeated haemorrhages have occurred; and/or (3) significant mass effect is produced by the haemorrhage.
   a. <u>Favorable anatomy</u>. Surgical resection is appropriate only for cases in which the cavernoma, or the cavernoma-associated haemorrhage, has reached the surface of the brainstem. Disruption of even 1 mm of normal brainstem tissue can cause significant morbidity.
      • T1-weighted imaging provides the most accurate indication of the relationship between the cavernoma and the surface of the brainstem. T2-weighted imaging may provide an incorrect measure of the proximity of the lesion to the pial surface due to the ferromagnetic properties of the hemosiderin ring.[291,292]
      • 3D-constructive interference in steady-state (CISS) MRI is useful in demonstrating the thickness of the parenchymal layer over brainstem cavernomas and in clarifying spatial relationships of the lesion to nuclei, tracts, cranial nerves, and vessels.[293]

- Conservative management is recommended for cavernomas or hematomas that do not reach the pial surface.[241,291]
- b. Repeated versus single haemorrhage. Traditionally, surgery on brainstem cavernomas has been recommended for patient having had at least two symptomatic haemorrhages. Some recent reports, however, have advocated surgery after only one haemorrhage, if the anatomy is favorable.[291,294,295] Another recent report did not find a relationship between timing of surgery or number of previous haemorrhages and long-term results.[296]
3. Surgical considerations.
  a. Timing of surgery.
    - Surgery ≥3–5 days after the haemorrhage helps to insure that the clot will be liquefied.[242]
    - Some authors recommend relatively early surgery (e.g., <1 month) after haemorrhage, attributing better outcomes with early surgery to the advantages of operating within a clot cavity and without reactive gliosis.[291,294,295]
  b. Frameless stereotactic guidance and intraoperative monitoring can be helpful.
  c. The optimal surgical approach can be planned in MRI images using the "two-point method".[297] One point is placed in the center of the lesion and the second is placed where the lesion most closely reaches the pial surface. A surgical trajectory is then mapped along a straight line connecting the two points.
  d. Although exophytic lesions are readily apparent during surgery, intrinsic lesions can be identified by haemosiderin staining or a bulge on the surface of the brainstem.
  e. Great care must be taken to preserve any associated developmental venous anomaly that may be encountered.[241]
  f. Postoperative care.
    - The patient may be left intubated for 24 h after surgery and extubated only after adequate cough and gag reflexes are identified.[242]
      1. Tracheostomy and feeding-tube placement may be necessary, and may be removed as the patient recovers lower cranial nerve function.
    - An early postoperative MRI (<48 h) can assess for residual lesion. Imaging-incomplete resection is associated with recurrent haemorrhage.[298]
4. Outcomes
  a. A series of 86 surgically treated patients with brainstem cavernomas found:[241]
    - Complications. The rate of temporary and/or permanent morbidity was 35%; permanent or severe deficits occurred in 12%. Mortality was 8%. A total of 33% had one or more new cranial nerve deficits.
    - Long-term outcome. At a mean follow-up of 35 months, 87% of patients reported that they were better or the same as before surgery. The average GOS score was 4.53.

Radiosurgery for Cavernous Malformations

Inspired by the success of radiosurgery in the treatment of brain AVMs, radiosurgery has been used for the treatment of cavernomas at several centers. A number of single-center series have been published.[299–314] Some reports have shown disappointing results with radiosurgery for cavernomas, particularly when compared to the natural history (with respect to haemorrhage)[294,311] or surgery (for patients with seizures).[299] Furthermore, some evidence indicates that complications after radiosurgery some lesions, particularly brainstem cavernomas, are more significant for cavernomas compared to AVMs.[311,315,316] One author who had advocated radiosurgery for brainstem cavernomas in the past later reversed his position, based on long-term complication rates.[317] In addition, a pathological analysis of cavernomas after radiosurgery did not find histological evidence of vessel occlusion.[318] Radiosurgery for cavernomas remains controversial, and requires further investigation before it becomes an established technique.

References

1. Raybaud CA, Strother CM, Hald JK. Aneurysms of the vein of Galen: embryonic considerations and anatomical features relating to the pathogenesis of the malformation. Neuroradiology. 1989;31:109–28

2. Roberson GH, Kase CS, Wolpow ER. Telangiectases and cavernous angiomas of the brainstem: "cryptic" vascular malformations. Report of a case. Neuroradiology. 1974;8:83–9.

3. McCormick WF. The pathology of vascular ("arteriovenous") malformations. J Neurosurg. 1966;24:807–16.

4. Lasjaunias P, Burrows P, Planet C. Developmental venous anomalies (DVA): the so-called venous angioma. Neurosurg Rev. 1986;9:233–42.

5. Gailloud P, O'Riordan DP, Burger I, Lehmann CU. Confirmation of communication between deep venous drainage and the vein of Galen after treatment of a vein of Galen aneurysmal malformation in an infant presenting with severe pulmonary hypertension. AJNR Am J Neuroradiol. 2006; 27:317–20.

6. Lasjaunias P. Vascular diseases in neonates, infants, and children: interventional neuroradiology management. Berlin: Springer; 1997.

7. Rigamonti D, Spetzler RF, Medina M, Rigamonti K, Geckle DS, Pappas C. Cerebral venous malformations. J Neurosurg. 1990;73:560–4.

8. Sarwar M, McCormick WF. Intracerebral venous angioma. Case report and review. Arch Neurol. 1978;35:323–5.

9. McCormick WF, Hardman JM, Boulter TR. Vascular malformations ("angiomas") of the brain, with special reference to those occurring in the posterior fossa. J Neurosurg. 1968; 28:241–51.

10. Iizuka Y, Kakihara T, Suzuki M, Komura S, Azusawa H. Endovascular remodeling technique for vein of Galen aneurysmal malformations – angiographic confirmation of a connection between the median prosencephalic vein and the deep venous system. J Neurosurg Ped air. 2008;1:75–8.

11. Topper R, Jurgens E, Reul J, Thron A. Clinical significance of intracranial developmental venous anomalies. J Neurol Neurosurg Psychiatry. 1999;67:234–8.

12. Awad IA, Spetzler RF, Hodak JA, Awad CA, Carey R. Incidental subcortical lesions identified on magnetic resonance imaging in the elderly. I. Correlation with age and cerebrovascular risk factors. Stroke. 1986;17:1084–9.

13. Morgan MK, Johnston IH, Sundt Jr TM. Normal perfusion pressure breakthrough complicating surgery for the vein of Galen malformation: report of three cases. Neurosurgery. 1989;24:406–10.

14. Rigamonti D, Spetzler RF, Drayer BP, et al. Appearance of venous malformations on magnetic resonance imaging. J Neurosurg. 1988;69:535–9.

15. McLaughlin MR, Kondziolka D, Flickinger JC, Lunsford S, Lunsford LD. The prospective natural history of cerebral venous malformations. Neurosurgery. 1998;43:195–200.

16. Pereira VM, Geibprasert S, Krings T. et al. Pathomechanisms of symptomatic developmental venous anomalies. Stroke. 2008;39:3201–15.

17. Im SH, Han MH, Kwon BJ, et al. Venous-predominant parenchymal arteriovenous malformation: a rare subtype with a venous drainage pattern mimicking developmental venous anomaly. J Neurosurg. 2008;108:1 42–7.

18. Hirata Y, Matsukado Y, Nagahiro S, Kuratsu J. Intracerebral venous angioma with arterial blood supply: a mixed angioma. Surg Neurol. 1986;25:227–32.

19. Awad IA, Robinson Jr JR, Mohanty S, Estes ML. Mixed vascular malformations of the brain: clinical and pathogenetic considerations. Neurosurgery. 1993;33:179–88; discussion 88.

20. Lee C, Pennington MA, Kenney 3rd CM. MR evaluation of developmental venous anomalies: medullary venous anatomy of venous angiomas. AJNR Am J Neuroradiol. 1996;17: 61–70.

21. Gandolfo C, Krings T, Alvarez H, et al. Sinus pericranii: diagnostic and therapeutic considerations in 15 patients. Neuroradiology. 2007;49:505–14.

22. Sadler LR, Tarr RW, Jungreis CA, Sekhar L. Sinus pericranii: CT and MR findings. J Comput Assist Tomogr. 1990;14: 124–7.

23. Stromeyer L. Ueber sinus pericranii. Dtsch Klin. 1850;2:160–1.

24. Mastin W. Venous blood tumors of the cranium in communication with the intracranial venous circulation, especially the sinuses of the dura mater. JAMA. 1886;7:309–30.

25. Vinas FC, Valenzuela S, Zuleta A. Literature review: sinus pericranii. Neurol Res. 1994;16:471–4.

26. Rangel-Castilla L, Krishna C, Klucznik R, Diaz O. Endovascular embolization with Onyx in the management of sinus pericranii: a case report. Neurosurg Focus. 2009; 27:E13.

27. Ota T, Waga S, Handa H, Nishimura S, Mitani T. Sinus pericranii. J Neurosurg. 1975;42:704–12.

28. Bonioli E, Bellini C, Palmieri A, Fondelli MP, Tortori Donati P. Radiological case of the month. Sinus pericranii. Arch Pediatr Adolesc Med. 1994;148:607–8.

29. Kohshu K, Takahashi S. Two cases of laterally situated sinus pericranii (author's transl). Rinsho Hoshasen. 1981;26: 391–4.

30. Spektor S, Weinberger G, Constantini S, Gomori JM, Beni-Adani L. Giant lateral sinus pericranii. Case report. J Neurosurg. 1998;88:145–7.

31. Buxton N, Vloeberghs M. Sinus pericranii. Report of a case and review of the literature. Pediatr Neurosurg. 1999;30:96–9.

32. Ernemann U, Lowenheim H, Freudenstein D, Koerbel A, Heininger A, Tatagiba M. Hemodynamic evaluation during balloon test occlusion of the sigmoid sinus: clinical and technical considerations. AJNR Am J Neuroradiol. 2005;26: 179–82.

33. Cerqueira L, Reis FC. Sinus pericranii and developmental venous anomalies: a frequent association. Acta Med Port. 1995;8:239–42.

34. Sherry RG, Walker ML, Olds MV. Sinus pericranii and venous angioma in the blue-rubber bleb nevus syndrome. AJNR Am J Neuroradiol. 1984;5:832–4.

35. Gabikian P, Clatterbuck RE, Gailloud P, Rigamonti D. Developmental venous anomalies and sinus pericranii in the blue rubber-bleb nevus syndrome. Case report. J Neurosurg. 2003;99:409–11.

36. Bollar A, Allut AG, Prieto A, Gelabert M, Becerra E. Sinus pericranii: radiological and etiopathological considerations. Case report. J Neurosurg. 1992;77:469–72.

37. Courville CB, Rocovich PM. A contribution to the study of sinus pericranii (Stromeyer); report of case with some comments on pathology of the lesion. Bull Los Angel Neuro Soc. 1946;11:145–58.

38. Kihara S, Koga H, Tabuchi K. Traumatic sinus pericranii. Case report. Neurol Med Chir (Tokyo). 1991;31:982–5.

39. Sawamura Y, Abe H, Sugimoto S, et al. Histological classification and therapeutic problems of sinus pericranii. Neurol Med Chir (Tokyo). 1987;27:762–8.

40. Kurosu A, Wachi A, Bando K, Kumami K, Naito S, Sato K. Craniosynostosis in the presence of a sinus pericranii: case report. Neurosurgery. 1994;34:1090–2; discussion 2–3.

41. Park SC, Kim SK, Cho BK, et al. Sinus pericranii in children: report of 16 patients and preoperative evaluation of surgical risk. J Neurosurg Pediatr. 2009;4:536–42.

42. Anegawa S, Hayashi T, Torigoe R, Nakagawa S, Ogasawara T. Sinus pericranii with severe symptom due to transient disorder of venous return–case report. Neurol Med Chir. 1991;31: 287–9.

43. Inci S, Turgut M, Saygi S, Ozdemir G. Sinus pericranii associated with epilepsy. Turk Neurosurg. 1996;6:21–4.

44. Carpenter JS, Rosen CL, Bailes JE, Gailloud P. Sinus pericranii: clinical and imaging findings in two cases of spontaneous partial thrombosis. AJNR Am J Neuroradiol. 2004;25:121–5.

45. Rozen WM, Joseph S, Lo PA. Spontaneous involution of two sinus pericranii – a unique case and review of the literature. J Clin Neurosci. 2008;15:833–5.

46. Bigot JL, Iacona C, Lepreux A, Dhellemmes P, Motte J, Gomes H. Sinus pericranii: advantages of MR imaging. Pediatr Radiol. 2000;30:710–2.

47. Sheu M, Fauteux G, Chang H, Taylor W, Stopa E, Robinson-Bostom L. Sinus pericranii: dermatologic considerations and literature review. J Am Acad Dermatol. 2002;46:934–41.

48. Brook AL, Gold MM, Farinhas JM, Goodrich JT, Bello JA. Endovascular transvenous embolization of sinus pericranii. Case report. J Neurosurg Pediatr. 2009;3:220–4.

49. Shaw WC. Folklore surrounding facial deformity and the origins of facial prejudice Br J Plast Surg. 1981;34:237–46.

50. Eifert S, Villavicencio JL, Kao TC, Taute BM, Rich NM. Prevalence of deep venous anomalies in congenital vascular malformations of venous predominance. J Vasc Surg. 2000; 31:462–71.

51. Venous malformations. 2008. http://emedicine.medscape.com/article/1296303-overview. Accessed 3 Aug 2011.

52. Puig S, Aref H, Chigot V, Bonin B, Brunelle F. Classification of venous malformations in children and implications for sclerotherapy. Pediatr Radiol. 2003;33:99–103.

53. Bisdorff A, Mulliken JB, Carrico J, Robertson RL, Burrows PE. Intracranial vascular anomalies in patients with periorbital lymphatic and lymphaticovenous malformations. AJNR Am J Neuroradiol. 2007;28:335–41.

54. Donnelly LF, Adams DM, Bisset 3rd GS. Vascular malformations and hemangiomas: a practical approach in a multidisciplinary clinic. AJR Am J Roentgenol. 2000;174:597–608.

55. Boon LM, Mulliken JB, Vikkula M, et al. Assignment of a locus for dominantly inherited venous malformations to chromosome 9p. Hum Mol Genet. 1994;3:1583–7.

56. Chung FM, Smirniotopoulos JG, Specht CS, Schroeder JW, Cube R. From the archives of the AFIP: pediatric orbit tumors and tumorlike lesions: nonosseous lesions of the extraocular orbit. Radiographics. 2007;27:1777–99.

57. Klippel M, Trenaunay P. Du naevus variqueux osteohypertophique. Arch Gen Med. 1900;85:641–72.

58. Servelle M. Klippel and Trenaunay's syndrome. 768 operated cases. Ann Surg. 1985;201:365–73.

59. Alomari AI, Orbach DB, Mulliken JB, et al. Klippel-Trenaunay syndrome and spinal arteriovenous malformations: ar erroneous association. AJNR Am J Neuroradiol. 2010;31:1608–12.

60. Chhajed M, Pandit S, Dhawan N, Jain A. Klippel-Trenaunay and Sturge-Weber overlap syndrome with phakomatosis pigmentovascularis. J Pediatr Neurosci. 2010;5:138–40.

61. Gallione CJ, Pasyk KA, Boon LM, et al. A gene for familial venous malformations maps to chromosome 9p in a second large kindred. J Med Genet. 1995;32:197–9.

62. Bilaniuk LT. Vascular lesions of the orbit in children. Neuroimaging Clin N Am. 2005;15:107–20.

63. Katz SE, Rootman J, Vangveeravong S, Graeb D. Combined venous lymphatic malformations of the orbit (so-called lymphangiomas). Association with noncontiguous intracranial vascular anomalies. Ophthalmology. 1998;105:176–84.

64. Devzikis JP. Percutaneous ethanol sclerotherapy for vascular malformations in the head and neck. Arch Facial Plast Surg. 2005;7:322–5.

65. Forbes G. Vascular lesions in the orbit. Neuroimaging Clin N Am. 1996;6:113–22.

66. Wright JE, Sullivan TJ, Garner A, Wulc AE, Moseley IF. Orbital venous anomalies. Ophthalmology. 1997;104:905–13.

67. Greene AK, Burrows PE, Smith L, Mulliken JB. Periorbital lymphatic malformation: clinical course and management in 42 patients. Plast Reconstr Surg. 2005;115:22–30.

68. Burrows PE, Laor T, Paltiel H, Robertson RL. Diagnostic imaging in the evaluation of vascular birthmarks. Dermatol Clin. 1998;16:455–88.

69. Baker LL, Dillon WP, Hieshima GB, Dowd CF, Frieden IJ. Hemangiomas and vascular malformations of the head and neck: MR characterization. AJNR Am J Neuroradiol. 1993;14:307–14.

70. Meyer JS, Hoffer FA, Barnes PD, Mulliken JB. Biological classification of soft-tissue vascular anomalies: MR correlation AJR Am J Roentgenol. 1991;157:559–64.

71. Barnes PD, Burrows PE, Hoffer FA, Mulliken JB. Hemangiomas and vascular malformations of the head and neck: MR characterization. AJNR Am J Neuroradiol. 1994;15:193–5.

72. Fordham LA. Chung CJ, Donnelly LF. Imaging of congenital vascular and lymphatic anomalies of the head and neck. Neuroimaging Clin N Am. 2000;10:117–36, viii.

73. Marler JJ, Mulliken JB. Current management of hemangiomas and vascular malformations. Clin Plast Surg. 2005;32:99–116, ix.

74. Hill RA, Pho RW, Kuma- VP. Resection of vascular malformations. J Hand Surg Br. 1993;18:17–21.

75. Legiehn GM, Heran MK. Venous malformations: classification, development, diagnosis, and interventional radiologic management. Radiol Clin North Am. 2008 46:545–97, vi.

76. Berenguer E, Burrows PE, Zurakowski D, Mulliken JB. Sclerotherapy of craniofacial venous malformations: complications and results. Plast Reconstr Surg. 1999;104:1–11; discussion 2–5.

77. Puig S, Aref H, Brunelle F. Double-needle sclerotherapy of lymphangiomas and venous angiomas in children: a simple technique to prevent complications. AJR Am J Roentgenol. 2003;180:1399–401.

78. Mason KP, Michna E, Zurakowski D, Koka BV, Burrows PE. Serum ethanol levels in children and adults after ethanol embolization or sclerotherapy for vascular anomalies. Radiology. 2000;217:127–32.

79. Spence J, Krings T, TerBrugge KG, Agid R. Percutaneous treatment of facial venous malformations: a matched comparison of alcohol and bleomycin sclerotherapy. Head Neck. 2011;33:125–30.

80. Werner JA, Lippert BM, Hoffmann P, Rudert H. Nd: YAG laser therapy of voluminous hemangiomas and vascular malformations. Adv Otorhinolaryngol. 1995;49:75–80.

81. Alani HM, Warren RM. Percutaneous photocoagulation of deep vascular lesions using a fiberoptic laser wand. Ann Plast Surg. 1992;29:143–8.

82. Apfelberg DB. Intralesional laser photocoagulation-steroids as an adjunct to surgery for massive hemangiomas and vascular malformations. Ann Plast Surg. 1995;35:144–8; discussion 9.

83. Dandy WE. Intracranial pressure without brain tumor: diagnosis and treatment. Ann Surg. 1937;106:492–513.

84. Smith JL. Whence pseudotumor cerebri? J Clin Neuroophthalmol. 1985;5:55–6.

85. Friedman DI Jacobson DM. Diagnostic criteria for idiopathic intracranial hypertension. Neurology. 2002;59:1492–5.

86. Karahalios DG, Rekate HL, Khayata MH, Apostolides PJ. Elevated intracranial venous pressure as a universal mechanism in pseudotumor cerebri of varying etiologies. Neurology. 1996;46:198–202.

87. Durcan FJ, Corbett JJ, Wall M. The incidence of pseudotumor cerebri. Population studies in Iowa and Louisiana. Arch Neurol. 1988;45:875–7.

88. Radhakrishnan K, Thacker AK, Bohlaga NH, Maloo JC, Gerryo SE. Epidemiology of idiopathic intracranial hypertension: a prospective and case–control study. J Neurol Sci. 1993;116:18–28.

89. Radhakrishnan K, Ahlskog JE, Cross SA, Kurland LT, O'Fallon WM. Idiopathic intracranial hypertension (pseudotumor cerebri). Descriptive epidemiology in Rochester, Minn, 1976 to 1990. Arch Neurol. 1993;50:78–80.

90. Kesler A, Goldhammer Y, Gadoth N. Do men with pseudomotor cerebri share the same characteristics as women? A retrospective review of 141 cases. J Neuroophthalmol. 2001;21:15–7.

91. Bruce BB, Kedar S, Van Stavern GP, et al. Idiopathic intracranial hypertension in men. Neurology. 2009;72:304–9.

92. Kesler A, Fattal-Valevski A. Idiopathic intracranial hypertension in the pediatric population. J Child Neurol. 2002;17:745–8.

93. Johnston I. The historical development of the pseudotumor concept. Neurosurg Focus. 2001;11:E2.

94. Najjar MW, Azzam NI, Khalifa MA. Pseudotumor cerebri: disordered cerebrospinal fluid hydrodynamics with extraaxial CSF collections. Pediatr Neurosurg. 2005;41:212–5.

95. Levine DN. Ventricular size in pseudotumor cerebri and the theory of impaired CSF absorption. J Neurol Sci. 2000;177:85–94.

96. Gross CE, Tranmer BI, Adey G, Kohut J. Increased cerebral blood flow in idiopathic pseudotumour cerebri. Neurol Res. 1990;12:226–30.

97. Bateman GA. Vascular hydraulics associated with idiopathic and secondary intracranial hypertension. AJNR Am J Neuroradiol. 2002;23:1180–6.

98. Mathew NT, Meyer JS, Ott EO. Increased cerebral blood volume in benign intracranial hypertension. Neurology. 1975;25:646–9.

99. Bloomfield GL, Ridings PC, Blocher CR, Marmarou A, Sugerman HJ. A proposed relationship between increased intra-abdominal, intrathoracic, and intracranial pressure. Crit Care Med. 1997;25:496–503.

100. Sugerman HJ, Felton 3rd IW, Sismanis A, et al. Continuous negative abdominal pressure device to treat pseudotumor cerebri. Int J Obes Relat Metab Disord. 2001;25:486–90.

101. Kesler A, Kliper E, Shenkerman G, Stern N. Idiopathic intracranial hypertension is associated with lower body adiposity. Ophthalmology. 2010;117:169–74.

102. Farb RI, Vanek I, Scott JN, et al. Idiopathic intracranial hypertension: the prevalence and morphology of sinovenous stenosis. Neurology. 2003;60:1418–24.

103. Brazis PW. Pseudotumor cerebri. Curr Neurol Neurosci Rep. 2004;4:111–6.

104. Stienen A, Weinzierl M, Ludolph A, Tibussek D, Hausler M. Obstruction of cerebral venous sinus secondary to idiopathic intracranial hypertension. Eur J Neurol. 2008;15:1416–8.

105. Higgins JN, Pickard JD. Lateral sinus stenoses in idiopathic intracranial hypertension resolving after CSF diversion. Neurology. 2004;62:1907–8.

106. De Simone R, Marano E, Fiorillo C, et al. Sudden re-opening of collapsed transverse sinuses and longstanding clinical remission after a single lumbar puncture in a case of idiopathic intracranial hypertension. Pathogenetic implications. Neurol Sci. 2005;25:342–4.

107. Pickard JD, Czosnyka Z, Czosnyka M, Owler B, Higgins JN. Coupling of sagittal sinus pressure and cerebrospinal fluid pressure in idiopathic intracranial hypertension – a preliminary report. Acta Neurochir Suppl. 2008;102:283–5.

108. Bono F, Giliberto C, Mastrandrea C, et al. Transverse sinus stenoses persist after normalization of the CSF pressure in IIH. Neurology. 2005;65:1090–3.

109. Wall M. Idiopathic intracranial hypertension. Neurol Clin. 2010;28:593–617.

110. Sorensen PS, Krogsaa B, Gjerris F. Clinical course and prognosis of pseudotumor cerebri. A prospective study of 24 patients. Acta Neurol Scand. 1988;77:164–72.

111. Radhakrishnan K, Ahlskog JE, Garrity JA, Kurland LT. Idiopathic intracranial hypertension. Mayo Clin Proc. 1994;69:169–80.

112. Degnan AJ, Levy LM. Pseudotumor cerebri: brief review of clinical syndrome and imaging findings. AJNR Am J Neuroradiol. 2011;32:1986–93.

113. Degnan AJ, Levy LM. Narrowing of Meckel's cave and cavernous sinus and enlargement of the optic nerve sheath in Pseudotumor Cerebri. J Comput Assist Tomogr. 2011;35:308–12.

114. Skau M, Brennum J, Gjerris F, Jensen R. What is new about idiopathic intracranial hypertension? An updated review of mechanism and treatment. Cephalalgia. 2006;26:384–99.

115. Sugerman HJ, Felton 3rd WL, Sismanis A, Kellum JM, DeMaria EJ, Sugerman EL. Gastric surgery for pseudotumor cerebri associated with severe obesity. Ann Surg. 1999;229:634–40; discussion 40–2.

116. Marks MP, Dake MD, Steinberg GK, Norbash AM, Lane B. Stent placement for arterial and venous cerebrovascular disease: preliminary experience. Radiology. 1994;191:441–6.

117. Higgins JN, Cousins C, Owler BK, Sarkies N, Pickard JD. Idiopathic intracranial hypertension: 12 cases treated by venous sinus stenting. J Neurol Neurosurg Psychiatry. 2003;74:1662–6.

118. Higgins JN, Owler BK, Cousins C, Pickard JD. Venous sinus stenting for refractory benign intracranial hypertension. Lancet. 2002;359:228–30.

119. Owler BK, Allan R, Parker G, Besser M. Pseudotumour cerebri, CSF rhinorrhoea and the role of venous sinus stenting in treatment. Br J Neurosurg. 2003;17:79–83.

120. Owler BK, Parker G, Halmagyi GM, et al. Pseudotumor cerebri syndrome: venous sinus obstruction and its treatment with stent placement. J Neurosurg. 2003;98:1045–55.

121. Ogungbo B, Roy D, Gholkar A, Mendelow AD. Endovascular stenting of the transverse sinus in a patient presenting with benign intracranial hypertension. Br J Neurosurg. 2003;17:565–8.

122. Metellus P, Levrier O, Fuentes S, et al. Endovascular treatment of benign intracranial hypertension by stent placement in the transverse sinus. Therapeutic and pathophysiological considerations illustrated by a case report. Neurochirurgie. 2005;51:113–20.

123. Bussiere M, Falero R, Nicolle D, Proulx A, Patel V, Pelz D. Unilateral transverse sinus stenting of patients with idiopathic intracranial hypertension. AJNR Am J Neuroradiol. 2010;31:645–50.

124. Feldon SE. Visual outcomes comparing surgical techniques for management of severe idiopathic intracranial hypertension. Neurosurg Focus. 2007;23:E6.

125. Ahmed RM, Wilkinson M, Parker GD, et al. Transverse sinus stenting for idiopathic intracranial hypertension: a review of 52 patients and of model predictions. AJNR Am J Neuroradiol. 2011;32 1408–14.

126. Cary FH. Symptomatic venous hum. Report of a case. N Engl J Med. 1961;264:869–70.

127. Cutforth R, Wiseman J Sutherland RD. The genesis of the cervical venous hum. Am Heart J. 1970;80:488–92.

128. Dichiro G, Fisher RL, Nelson KB. The jugular foramen. J Neurosurg. 1964;21:447–60.

129. George B, Reizine D, Laurian C, Riche MC, Merland JJ. Tinnitus of venous origin. Surgical treatment by the ligation of the jugular vein and lateral sinus jugular vein anastomosis. J Neuroradiol. 1982;10:23–30.

130. Adler JR, Ropper AH. Self-audible venous bruits and high jugular bulb. Arch Neurol. 1986;43:257–9.

131. Buckwalter JA, Sasaki CT, Virapongse C, Kier EL, Bauman N. Pulsatile tinnitus arising from jugular megabulb deformity: a treatment rationale. Laryngoscope. 1983;93:1534–9.

132. Hardison JE, Smith 3rd RB, Crawley IS, Battey LL. Self-heard venous hums. JAMA. 1981;245:1146–7.

133. Cochran Jr JH, Kosmicki PW. Tinnitus as a presenting symptom in pernicious anemia. Ann Otol Rhinol Laryngol. 1979;88:297.

134. Meador KJ, Swift TR. Tinnitus from intracranial hypertension. Neurology. 1984;34:1258–61.

135. Sismanis A, Butts FM Hughes GB. Objective tinnitus in benign intracranial hypertension: an update. Laryngoscope. 1990;100:33–6.

136. Biousse V, Newman NJ. Lessell S. Audible pulsatile tinnitus in idiopathic intracranial hypertension. Neurology. 1998;50:1185–6.

137. Saitoh Y, Takeda N, Yagi R, Oshima K, Kubo T, Yoshimine T. Pneumocephalus causing pulsatile tinnitus. Case illustration. J Neurosurg. 2000;92:505.

138. Dietz RR, Davis WL, Harnsberger HR, Jacobs JM, Blatter DD. MR imaging and MR angiography in the evaluation of pulsatile tinnitus. AJNR Am J Neuroradiol. 1994;15:879–89.

139. Ward PH, Babin R, Calcaterra TC, Konrad HR. Operative treatment of surgical lesions with objective tinnitus. Ann Otol Rhinol Laryngol. 975;84:473–82.

140. Hentzer E. Objective tinnitus of the vascular type. A follow-up study. Acta Otolaryngol. 1968;66:273–81.

141. Lam BL, Schatz NJ, Claser JS, Bowen BC. Pseudotumor cerebri from cranial venous obstruction. Ophthalmology. 1992;99:706–12.

142. Sanchez TG, Murao M. de Medeiros IR, et al. A new therapeutic procedure for treatment of objective venous pulsatile tinnitus. Int Tinnitus J. 2002;8:54–7.

143. Zenteno M, Murillo-Borilla L, Martinez S, et al. Endovascular treatment of a transverse-sigmoid sinus aneurysm presenting as pulsatile tinnitus. Case report. J Neurosurg. 2004;100:120–2.

144. Terada T, Higashida RT, Halbach VV, et al. Development of acquired arteriovenous fistulas in rats due to venous hypertension. J Neurosurg. 1994;80:884–9.

145. Herman JM, Spetzler RF, Bederson JB, Kurbat JM, Zabramski JM. Genesis of a dural arteriovenous malformation in a rat model. J Neurosurg. 1995;83:539–45.

146. Lawton MT, Jacobowitz R, Spetzler RF. Redefined role of angiogenesis in the pathogenesis of dural arteriovenous malformations. J Neurosurg. 1997;87:267–74.

147. Gerlach R, Boehm-Weigert M, Berkefeld J, et al. Thrombophilic risk factors in patients with cranial and spinal dural arteriovenous fistulae. Neurosurgery. 2008;63:693–8; discussion 8–9.

148. Sundt Jr TM, Piepgras DG. The surgical approach to arteriovenous malformations of the lateral and sigmoid dural sinuses. J Neurosurg. 1983;59:32–9.

149. Witt O, Pereira PL, Tillmann W. Severe cerebral venous sinus thrombosis and dural arteriovenous fistula in an infant with protein S deficiency. Childs Nerv Syst. 1999;15:128–30.

150. Kraus JA, Stuper BK, Muller J, et al. Molecular analysis of thrombophilic risk factors in patients with dural arteriovenous fistulas. J Neurol. 2002;249:680–2.

151. Saito A, Takahashi N, Furuno Y, et al. Multiple isolated sinus dural arteriovenous fistulas associated with antithrombin III deficiency – case report. Neurol Med Chir (Tokyo). 2008;48:455–9.

152. Ozawa T, Miyasaka Y, Tanaka R, Kurata A, Fujii K. Dural-pial arteriovenous malformation after sinus thrombosis. Stroke. 1998;29:1721–4.

153. Lasjaunias P, Chiu M, ter Brugge K, Tolia A, Hurth M, Bernstein M. Neurological manifestations of intracranial dural arteriovenous malformations. J Neurosurg. 1986;64:724–30.

154. Hademenos GJ, Massoud TF. Risk of intracranial arteriovenous malformation rupture due to venous drainage impairment. A theoretical analysis. Stroke. 1996;27:1072–83.

155. Murphy KJ, Gailloud P, Venbrux A, Deramond H, Hanley D, Rigamonti D. Endovascular treatment of a grade IV transverse sinus dural arteriovenous fistula by sinus recanalization, angioplasty, and stent placement: technical case report. Neurosurgery. 2000;46:497–500; discussion –1.

156. Troffkin NA, Graham 3rd CB, Berkmen T, Wakhloo AK. Combined transvenous and transarterial embolization of a tentorial-incisural dural arteriovenous malformation followed by primary stent placement in the associated stenotic straight sinus. Case report. J Neurosurg. 2003;99:579–83.

157. Liebig T, Henkes H, Brew S, Miloslavski E, Kirsch M, Kuhne D. Reconstructive treatment of dural arteriovenous fistulas of the transverse and sigmoid sinus: transvenous angioplasty and stent deployment. Neuroradiology. 2005;47:543–51.

158. Tomura N, Hirata K, Watarai J, et al. An occlusion and stenosis of the venous drainage system in cerebral AVMs – angiographical investigation. No To Shinkei. 1993;45:531–6.

159. Challa VR, Moody DM, Brown WR. Vascular malformations of the central nervous system. J Neuropathol Exp Neurol. 1995;54:609–21.

160. Song JK, Patel AB, Duckwiler GR, et al. Adult pial arteriovenous fistula and superior sagittal sinus stenosis: angiographic evidence for high-flow venopathy at an atypical location. Case report. J Neurosurg. 2002:96:792–5.

161. Dorne H, Zaidat OO, Fiorella D, et al. Chronic cerebrospinal venous insufficiency and the doubtful promise of an endovascular treatment for multiple sclerosis. J NeuroIntervent Surg. 2010;2:309–11.

162. Zamboni P, Galeotti R, Menegatti E, et al. Chronic cerebrospinal venous insufficiency in patients with multiple sclerosis. J Neurol Neurosurg Psychiatry. 2009;80:392–9.

163. Zivadinov R, Schirda C, Dwyer MG, et al. Chronic cerebrospinal venous insufficiency and iron deposition on susceptibility-weighted imaging in patients with multiple sclerosis: a pilot case–control study. Int Angiol. 2010;29:158–75.

164. Zamboni P, Galeotti R, Menegatti E, et al. A prospective open-label study of endovascular treatment of chronic cerebrospinal venous insufficiency. J Vasc Surg. 2009;50:1348–58 e1-3.

165. Multiple sclerosis: studies probe role of clogged neck veins. 2011.http://abcnews.go.com/Health/MindMoodNews/multiple-sclerosis-studies-probe-role-clogged-neck-veins/story?id=13374572. Accessed 11 Aug 2011.

166. Zivadinov R, Marr K, Cutter G, et al. Prevalence, sensitivity, and specificity of chronic cerebrospinal venous insufficiency in MS. Neurology. 2011;77:138–44.

167. Sundstrom P, Wahlin A, Ambarki K, Birgander R, Eklund A, Malm J. Venous and cerebrospinal fluid flow in multiple sclerosis: a case–control study. Ann Neurol. 2010;68:255–9.

168. Doepp F, Paul F, Valdueza JM, Schmierer K, Schreiber SJ. No cerebrocervical venous congestion in patients with multiple sclerosis. Ann Neurol. 2010;68:173–83.

169. Yamout E, Herlopian A, Issa Z, et al. Extracranial venous stenosis is an unlikely cause of multiple sclerosis. Mult Scler. 2010;16:1341–8

170. Baracchini C, Perini P, Calabrese M, Causin F, Rinaldi F, Gallo P. No evidence of chronic cerebrospinal venous insufficiency at multiple sclerosis onset. Ann Neurol. 2011;69:90–9.

171. Compston A, Coles A. Multiple sclerosis. Lancet. 2008;372:1502–17.

172. Thapar A, Lane TR, Pandey V, et al. Internal jugular thrombosis post venoplasty for chronic cerebrospinal venous insufficiency. Phlebology. 2011;26:254–6.

173. Khan O, Filippi M, Freedman MS, et al. Chronic cerebrospinal venous insufficiency and multiple sclerosis. Ann Neurol. 2010;67:286–90.

174. Stam J. Thrombosis of the cerebral veins and sinuses. N Engl J Med. 2005;352:1791–8.

175. Ferro JM, Canhao P, Stam J, Bousser MG, Barinagarrementeria F. Prognosis of cerebral vein and dural sinus thrombosis: results of the international study on cerebral vein and dural sinus thrombosis (ISCVT). Stroke. 2004;35:664–70.

176. Maqueda VM, Thijs V. Risk of thromboembolism after cerebral venous thrombosis. Eur J Neurol. 2006;13:302–5.

177. Martinelli I, Sacchi E, Landi G, Taioli E, Duca F, Mannucci PM. High risk of cerebral-vein thrombosis in carriers of a prothrombin gene mutation and in users of oral contraceptives. N Engl J Med. 1998;338:1793–7.

178. de Bruijr SF, Stam J, Koopman MM, Vandenbroucke JP. Case-control study of risk of cerebral sinus thrombosis in oral contraceptive users and in correction of who are carriers of hereditary prothrombotic conditions. The Cerebral Venous Sinus Thrombosis Study Group. BMJ. 1998;316:589–92.

179. Arxer A, Pardina B, Elas I, Ramio L, Villalonga A. Dural sinus thrombosis in a late preeclamptic woman. Can J Anaesth. 2004;51:1050–1.

180. Wysokinska EM, Wysokinski WE, Brown RD, et al. Thrombophilia differences in cerebral venous sinus and lower extremity deep venous thrombosis. Neurology. 2008;70:627–33.

181. Zapanta FE, Chi DH, Faust RA. A unique case of Bezold's abscess associated with multiple dural sinus thromboses. Laryngoscope. 2001; 11:1944–8.

182. Ciccone A, Canhao P, Falcao F, Ferro JM, Sterzi R. Thrombolysis for cerebral vein and dural sinus thrombosis. Cochrane Database Syst Rev. 2004:CD003693.

183. Ferro JM, Lopes MG, Rosas MJ, Fontes J. Delay in hospital admission of patients with cerebral vein and dural sinus thrombosis. Cerebrovasc Dis. 2005;19:152–6.

184. Lenz RA, Saver J. Venous sinus thrombosis in a patient taking thalicamide. Cerebrovasc Dis. 2004;18:175–7.

185. Masjuan J, Pardo J, Callejo JM, Andres MT, Alvarez-Cermenc JC. Tamoxifen: a new risk factor for cerebral sinus thrombosis. Neurology. 2004;62:334–5.

186. Finelli PF, Carley MD. Cerebral venous thrombosis associated with epoetin alfa therapy. Arch Neurol. 2000;57:260–2.

187. Guimaraes J, Azevedo E. Phytoestrogens as a risk factor for cerebral sinus thrombosis. Cerebrovasc Dis. 2005;20:137–8.

188. Nakase H, Shin Y, Nakagawa I, Kimura R, Sakaki T. Clinical features of postoperative cerebral venous infarction. Acta Neurochir (Wien). 2005;147:621–6; discussion 6.

189. Emir M, Ozisik K, Cagli K, Bakuy V, Ozisik P, Sener E. Dural sinus thrombosis after cardiopulmonary bypass. Perfusio . 2004;19:173–5.

190. Berroir S, Grabli D, Heran F. Bakouche P, Bousser MG. Cerebral sinus venous thrombosis in two patients with spontaneous intracranial hypotension. Cerebrovasc Dis. 2004;17:9–12.

191. Yoon KW, Cho MK, Kim YJ, Lee SK. Sinus thrombosis in a patient with intracranial hypotension: a suggested hypothesis of venous stasis. A case report. Interv Neuroradiol. 2011;17 248–51.

192. Miglis MG, Levine DN. Intracranial venous thrombosis after placement of a lumbar drain. Neurocrit Care. 2010;12:83–7.

193. De Cruz P, Lust M, Trost N, Wall A, Gerraty R, Connell WR. Cerebral venous thrombosis associated with ulcerative colitis. Intern Med J. 2008;38:865–7.

194. Skaiaa SC, Stave H. Recurrent sagittal sinus thrombosis occurring at high altitude during expeditions to Cho Oyu. Wilderness Environ Med. 2006;17:132–6.

195. Tan M, Deveber G, Shroff M, et al. Sagittal sinus compression is associated with neonatal cerebral s inovenous thrombosis. Pediatrics. 2011;128:e429–35.

196. Marjot T, Yadav S, Hasan N, Bentley P, Sharma P. Genes associated with adult cerebral venous thrombosis. Stroke. 2011;42:913–8.

197. Smith AG, Cornblath WT, Deveikis JP. Local thrombolytic therapy in deep cerebral venous thrombosis. Neurology. 1997;48:1613–9.

198. Chang R, Friedman DP. Isolated cortical venous thrombosis presenting as subarachnoid hemorrhage: a report of three cases. AJNR Am J Neuroradiol. 2004;25:1676–9.

199. Oppenheim C, Domigo V, Gauvrit JY, et al. Subarachnoid hemorrhage as the initial presentation of dural sinus thrombosis. AJNR Am J Neuroradiol. 2005;26:614–7.

200. Spitzer C, Mull M, Rohde V, Kosinski CM. Non-traumatic cortical subarachnoid haemorrhage: diagnostic work-up and aetiological background. Neuroradiology. 2005;47:525–31.

201. Tanislav C, Siekmann R, Sieweke N, et al. Cerebral vein thrombosis: clinical manifestation and diagnosis. BMC Neurol. 2011;11:69.

202. Ferro JM, Canhao P, Bousser MG, Stam J, Barinagarrementeria F. Cerebral vein and dural sinus thrombosis in elderly patients. Stroke. 2005;36:1927–32.

203. Bonduel M, Sciuccati G, Hepner M, et al. Arterial ischemic stroke and cerebral venous thrombosis in children: a 12-year Argentinean registry. Acta Haematol. 2006;115:180–5.

204. Moharir MD, Shroff M, Pontigon AM, et al. A prospective outcome study of neonatal cerebral sinovenous thrombosis. J Child Neurol. 2011;26:1137–44.

205. Canhao P, Ferro JM, Lindgren AG, Bousser MG, Stam J, Barinagarrementeria F. Causes and predictors of death in cerebral venous thrombosis. Stroke. 2005;36:1720–5.

206. Einhaupl KM, Villringer A, Meister W, et al. Heparin treatment in sinus venous thrombosis. Lancet. 1991;338:597–600.

207. Masuhr F, Mehraein S. Cerebral venous and sinus thrombosis: patients with a fatal outcome during intravenous dose-adjusted heparin treatment. Neurocrit Care. 2004;1:355–61.

208. van Nuenen BF, Munneke M, Bloem BR. Cerebral venous sinus thrombosis: prevention of recurrent thromboembolism. Stroke. 2005;36:1822–3.

209. Coutinho JMMD, Ferro JMMDP, Canhao PMDP, et al. Unfractionated or low-molecular weight heparin for the treatment of cerebral venous thrombosis. Stroke. 2010;41:2575–80.

210. Einhaupl K, Stam J, Bousser MG, et al. EFNS guideline on the treatment of cerebral venous and sinus thrombosis in adult patients. Eur J Neurol. 2010;17:1229–35.

211. Barnwell SL, Higashida RT, Halbach VV, Dowd CF, Hieshima GB. Direct endovascular thrombolytic therapy for dural sinus thrombosis. Neurosurgery. 1991;28:135–42.

212. Horowitz M, Purdy P, Unwin H, et al. Treatment of dural sinus thrombosis using selective catheterization and urokinase. Ann Neurol. 1995;38:58–67.

213. Chow K, Gobin YP, Saver J, Kidwell C, Dong P, Vinuela F. Endovascular treatment of dural sinus thrombosis with rheolytic thrombectomy and intra-arterial thrombolysis. Stroke. 2000;31:1420–5.

214. Liebetrau M, Mayer TE, Bruning R, Opherk C, Hamann GF. Intra-arterial thrombolysis of complete deep cerebral venous thrombosis. Neurology. 2004;63:2–44–5.

215. Chaloupka JC, Mangla S, Huddle DC. Use of mechanical thrombolysis via microballoon percutaneous transluminal angioplasty for the treatment of acute dural sinus thrombosis: case presentation and technical report. Neurosurgery. 1999;45:650–6; discussion 6–7.

216. Philips MF, Bagley LJ, Sinson GP, et al. Endovascular thrombolysis for symptomatic cerebral venous thrombosis. J Neurosurg. 1999;90:65–71.

217. Dowd CF, Malek AM, Phatouros CC, Hemphill 3rd JC. Application of a rheolytic thrombectomy device in the treatment of dural sinus thrombosis: a new technique. AJNR Am J Neuroradiol. 1999;20:568–70.

218. Rottger C, Madlener K, Heil M, et al. Is heparin treatment the optimal management for cerebral venous thrombosis? Effect of abciximab, recombinant tissue plasminogen activator, and enoxaparin in experimentally induced superior sagittal sinus thrombosis. Stroke. 2005;36:841–6.

219. Wasay M, Bakshi R, Kojan S, Bobustuc G, Dubey N, Unwin DH. Nonrandomized comparison of local urokinase thrombolysis versus systemic heparin anticoagulation for superior sagittal sinus thrombosis. Stroke. 2001;32:2310–7.

220. Ferro JM, Crassard I, Coutinho JM, et al. Decompressive surgery in cerebrovenous thrombosis: a multicenter registry and a systematic review of individual patient data. Stroke. 2011;42:2825–31.

221. Herter T, Bennefeld H, Brandt M. Orbital cavernous hemangiomas. Neurosurg Rev. 1988;11:143–7.

222. Raychaudhuri R, Batjer HH, Awad IA. Intracranial cavernous angioma: a practical review of clinical and biological aspects. Surg Neurol. 2005;63:319–28; discussion 28.

223. Otten P, Pizzolato GP, Rilliet B, Berney J. 131 cases of cavernous angioma (cavernomas) of the CNS, discovered by retrospective analysis of 24,535 autopsies. Neurochirurgie. 1989;35(82–3):128–31.

224. Del Curling Jr O, Kelly Jr DL, Elster AD, Craven TE. An analysis of the natural history of cavernous angiomas. J Neurosurg. 1991;75:702–8.

225. Robinson JR, Awad IA, Little JR. Natural history of the cavernous angioma. J Neurosurg. 1991;75:709–14.

226. Rigamonti D, Drayer BP, Johnson PC, Hadley MN, Zabramski J, Spetzler RF. The MRI appearance of cavernous malformations (angiomas). J Neurosurg. 1987;67:518–24.

227. Yamasaki T, Handa H, Yamashita J, et al. Intracranial and orbital cavernous angiomas. A review of 30 cases. J Neurosurg. 1986;64:197–208.

228. Herter T, Brandt M, Szuwart U. Cavernous hemangiomas in children. Childs Nerv Syst. 1988;4:123–7.

229. Nimjee SM, Powers CJ, Bulsara KR. Review of the literature on de novo formation of cavernous malformations of the central nervous system after radiation therapy. Neurosurg Focus. 2006;21:e4.

230. Maraire JN, Awad IA. Intracranial cavernous malformations: lesion behavior and management strategies. Neurosurgery. 1995;37:591–605.

231. Simard JM, Garcia-Bengochea F, Ballinger Jr WE, Mickle JP, Quisling RG. Cavernous angioma: a review of 126 collected and 12 new clinical cases. Neurosurgery. 1986;18:162–72.

232. Zabramski JM, Henn JS, Coons S. Pathology of cerebral vascular malformations. Neurosurg Clin N Am. 1999;10:395–410.

233. Voigt K, Yasargil MG. Cerebral cavernous haemangiomas or cavernomas. Incidence, pathology, localization, diagnosis, clinical features and treatment. Review of the literature and report of an unusual case. Neurochirurgia (Stuttg). 1976;19:59–68.

234. Wong JH, Awad IA, Kim JH. Ultrastructural pathological features of cerebrovascular malformations: a preliminary report. Neurosurgery. 2000;46:1454–9.

235. Clatterbuck RE, Eberhart CG, Crain BJ, Rigamonti D. Ultrastructural and immunocytochemical evidence that an incompetent blood–brain barrier is related to the pathophysiology of cavernous malformations. J Neurol Neurosurg Psychiatry. 2001;71:188–92.

236. Gault J, Sarin H, Awadallah NA, Shenkar R, Awad IA. Pathobiology of human cerebrovascular malformations: basic mechanisms and clinical relevance. Neurosurgery. 2004;55:1–16; discussion –7.

237. Robinson Jr JR, Awad IA, Masaryk TJ, Estes ML. Pathological heterogeneity of angiographically occult vascular malformations of the brain. Neurosurgery. 1993;33:547–54; discussion 54–5.

238. Rothbart D, Awad IA, Lee J, Kim J, Harbaugh R, Criscuolo GR. Expression of angiogenic factors and structural proteins in central nervous system vascular malformations. Neurosurgery. 1996;38:915–24; discussion 24–5.

239. Abdulrauf SI, Kaynar MY, Awad IA. A comparison of the clinical profile of cavernous malformations with and without associated venous malformations. Neurosurgery. 1999; 44:41–6; discussion 6–7.

240. Wurm G, Schnizer M, Fellner FA. Cerebral cavernous malformations associated with venous anomalies: surgical considerations. Neurosurgery. 2005;57:42–58; discussion 42–58.

241. Porter RW, Detwiler PW, Spetzler RF, et al. Cavernous malformations of the brainstem: experience with 100 patients. J Neurosurg. 1999;90:50–8.

242. Porter RW, Detwiler PW, Spetzler RF. Infratentorial cavernous malformations. In: Winn HR, editor. Youmans neurological surgery. Philadelphia: Saunders; 2004. p. 2321–39.

243. Little JR, Awad IA, Jones SC, Ebrahim ZY. Vascular pressures and cortical blood flow in cavernous angioma of the brain. J Neurosurg. 1990;73:555–9.

244. Sasaki O, Tanaka R, Koike T, Koide A, Koizumi T, Ogawa H. Excision of cavernous angioma with preservation of coexisting venous angioma. Case report. J Neurosurg. 1991;75: 461–4.

245. Ciricillo SF, Dillon WP, Fink ME, Edwards MS. Progression of multiple cryptic vascular malformations associated with anomalous venous drainage. Case report. J Neurosurg. 1994;81:477–81.

246. Perrini P, Lanzino G. The association of venous developmental anomalies and cavernous malformations: pathophysiological, diagnostic, and surgical considerations. Neurosurg Focus. 2006;21:e5.

247. Zabramski JM, Wascher TM, Spetzler RF, et al. The natural history of familial cavernous malformations: results of an ongoing study. J Neurosurg. 1994;80:422–32.

248. Brunereau L, Labauge P, Tournier-Lasserve E, Laberge S, Levy C, Houtteville J-P. Familial form of intracranial cavernous angioma: MR imaging findings in 51 families1. Radiology. 2000;214:209–16.

249. Johnson EW, Marchuk DA, Zabramski JM. The genetics of cerebral cavernous malformations. In: Winn HR, editor. Youmans neurological surgery. Philadelphia: Saunders; 2004. p. 2299–304.

250. Rigamonti D, Hadley MN, Drayer BP, et al. Cerebral cavernous malformations. Incidence and familial occurrence. N Engl J Med. 1988;319:343–7.

251. Moriarity JL, Wetzel M, Clatterbuck RE, et al. The natural history of cavernous malformations: a prospective study of 68 patients. Neurosurgery. 1999;44:1166–71; discussion 72–3.

252. Kattapong VJ, Hart BL, Davis LE. Familial cerebral cavernous angiomas: clinical and radiologic studies. Neurology. 1995;45:492–7.

253. Dobyns WB, Michels VV, Groover RV, et al. Familial cavernous malformations of the central nervous system and retina. Ann Neurol. 1987;21:578–83.

254. Marchuk DA, Gallione C, Morrison LA, et al. A locus for cerebral cavernous malformations maps to chromosome 7q in two families. Genomics. 1995;28:311–4.

255. Gunel M, Awad IA, Anson J, Lifton RP. Mapping a gene causing cerebral cavernous malformation to 7q11.2-q21. Proc Natl Acad Sci USA. 1995;92:6620–4.

256. Dubovsky J, Zabramski JM, Kurth J, et al. A gene responsible for cavernous malformations of the brain maps to chromosome 7q. Hum Mol Genet. 1995;4:453–8.

257. Plummer NW, Zawistowski JS, Marchuk DA. Genetics of cerebral cavernous malformations. Curr Neurol Neurosci Rep. 2005;5:391–6.

258. Johnson EW, Iyer LM, Rich SS, et al. Refined localization of the cerebral cavernous malformation gene (CCM1) to a 4-cM interval of chromosome 7q contained in a well-defined YAC contig. Genome Res. 1995;5:368–80.

259. Gunel M, Awad IA, Finberg K, et al. A founder mutation as a cause of cerebral cavernous malformation in Hispanic Americans. N Engl J Med. 1996;334:946–51.

260. Craig HD, Gunel M, Cepeda O, et al. Multilocus linkage identifies two new loci for a mendelian form of stroke, cerebral cavernous malformation, at 7p15-13 and 3q25.2-27. Hum Mol Genet. 1998;7:1851–8.

261. Porter PJ, Willinsky RA, Harper W, Wallace MC. Cerebral cavernous malformations: natural history and prognosis after clinical deterioration with or without hemorrhage. J Neurosurg. 1997;87:190–7.

262. Labauge P, Laberge S, Brunereau L, Levy C, Tournier-Lasserve E. Hereditary cerebral cavernous angiomas: clinical and genetic features in 57 French families. Societe Francaise de Neurochirurgie. Lancet. 1998;352:1892–7.

263. Brunereau L, Leveque C, Bertrand P, et al. Familial form of cerebral cavernous malformations: evaluation of gradient-spin-echo (GRASE) imaging in lesion detection and characterization at 1.5 T. Neuroradiology. 2001;43:973–9.

264. Lehnhardt F-G, von Smekal U, Ruckriem B, et al. Value of gradien-echo magnetic resonance imaging in the diagnosis of familial cerebral cavernous malformation. Arch Neurol. 2005;62: 653–8.

265. Yun TJ, Na DG, Kwon BJ, et al. A T1 hyperintense perilesional signal aids in the differentiation of a cavernous angiom from other hemorrhagic masses. AJNR Am J Neuroradiol. 2008;29:494–500.

266. Houtteville JP. Brain cavernoma: a dynamic lesion. Surg Neurol. 1997;48:610–4.

267. Vaquero J, Leunda G, Martinez R, Bravo G. Cavernomas of the brain. Neurosurgery. 1983;12:208–10.

268. Scott RM, Barnes P, Kupsky W, Adelman LS. Cavernous angiomas of the central nervous system in children. J Neurosurg. 1992;76:38–46.

269. Edwards M, Baumgartner J, Wilson C. Cavernous and other cryptic vascular malformations in the pediatric age group. In: Awad IA, Barrow DL, editors. Cavernous malformations. Park Ridge: AANS; 1993. p. 163–83.

270. Giombini S, Morello G. Cavernous angiomas of the brain. Account of fourteen personal cases and review of the literature. Acta Neurochir (Wien). 1978;40:61–82.

271. Katayama Y, Tsubokawa T, Maeda T, Yamamoto T. Surgical management of cavernous malformations of the third ventricle. J Neurosurg. 1994;80:64–72.

272. Zauberman H, Feinsod M. Orbital hemangioma growth during pregnancy. Acta Ophthalmol (Copenh). 1970;48:929–33.

273. Pozzati E, Acciarri N, Tognetti F, Marliani F, Giangaspero F. Growth, subsequent bleeding, and de novo appearance of cerebral cavernous angiomas. Neurosurgery. 1996;38:662–9; discussion 9–70.

274. Awada A, Watson T, Obeid T. Cavernous angioma presenting as pregnancy-related seizures. Epilepsia. 1997;38:844–6.

275. Aiba T, Koike T, Takeda N, Tanaka R. Intracranial cavernous malformations and skin angiomas associated with middlefossa arachnoid cyst: a report of three cases. Surg Neurol. 1993;43:31–3; discussion 4.

276. Flemming KD, Goodman BP, Meyer FB. Successful brainstem cavernous malformation resection after repeated hemorrhages during pregnancy. Surg Neurol. 2003;60:545–7; discussion 7–8.

277. Aiba T, Tanaka R, Koike T, Kameyama S, Takeda N, Komata T. Natural history of intracranial cavernous malformations. J Neurosurg. 1995;83:56–9.

278. Clatterbuck RE, Moriarity JL, Elmaci I, Lee RR, Breiter SN, Rigamonti D. Dynamic nature of cavernous malformations: a prospective magnetic resonance imaging study with volumetric analysis. J Neurosurg. 2000;93:981–6.

279. Kim DS, Park Y-G, Choi J-U, Chung S-S, Lee K-C. An analysis of the natural history of cavernous malformations. Surg Neurol. 1997;48:9–17.

280. Kondziolka D, Lunsford LD, Kestle JR. The natural history of cerebral cavernous malformations. J Neurosurg. 1995;83:820–4.

281. Vives KP, Gunel M, Awad IA. Surgical management of supratentorial cavernous malformations. In: Winn HR, editor. Youmans neurological surgery. Philadelphia: Saunders; 2004. p. 2305–19.

282. Willmore LJ, Triggs WJ, Gray JD. The role of iron-induced hippocampal peroxidation in acute epileptogenesis. Brain Res. 1986;382:422–6.

283. Awad I, Jabbour P. Cerebral cavernous malformations and epilepsy. Neurosurg Focus. 2006;21:e7.

284. Requena I, Arias M, Lopez-Ibor L, et al. Cavernomas of the central nervous system: clinical and neuroimaging manifestations in 47 patients. J Neurol Neurosurg Psychiatry. 1991;54:590–4.

285. Noto S, Fujii M, Akimura T, et al. Management of patients with cavernous angiomas presenting epileptic seizures. Surg Neurol. 2005;64:495–8.

286. Baumann CR, Acciarri N, Bertalanffy H, et al. Seizure outcome after resection of supratentorial cavernous malformations: a study of 168 patients. Epilepsia. 2007;48:559–63.

287. Baumann CR, Schuknecht B, Lo Russo G, et al. Seizure outcome after resection of cavernous malformations is better when surrounding hemosiderin-stained brain also is removed. Epilepsia. 2006;47:563–6.

288. Weber JP, Silbergeld DL, Winn HR. Surgical resection of epileptogenic cortex associated with structural lesions. Neurosurg Clin N Am. 1993;4:327–36.

289. Rigamonti D, Spetzler RF. The association of venous and cavernous malformations. Report of four cases and discussion of the pathophysiological, diagnostic, and therapeutic implications. Acta Neurochir (Wien). 1988;92:100–5.

290. Lobato RD, Perez C, Rivas JJ, Cordobes F. Clinical, radiological, and pathological spectrum of angiographically occult intracranial vascular malformations. Analysis of 21 cases and review of the literature. J Neurosurg. 1988; 68:518–31.

291. Bruneau M, Bijlenga P, Reverdin A, et al. Early surgery for brainstem cavernomas. Acta Neurochir (Wien). 2006;148: 405–14.

292. Ferroli P, Sinisi M, Franzini A, Giombini S, Solero CL, Broggi G. Brainstem cavernomas: long-term results of microsurgical resection in 52 patients. Neurosurgery. 2005;56:1203–12; discussion 12–4.

293. Zausinger S, Yousry I, Brueckmann H, Schmid-Elsaesser R, Tonn JC. Cavernous malformations of the brainstem: three-dimensional-constructive interference in steady-state magnetic resonance imaging for improvement of surgical approach and clinical results. Neurosurgery. 2006;58: 322–30; discussion –30.

294. Mathiesen T, Edner G, Kihlstrom L. Deep and brainstem cavernomas: a consecutive 8-year series J Neurosurg. 2003;99:31–7.

295. Wang C-C, Liu A, Zhang J-T, Sun B, Zhao Y-L. Surgical management of brain-stem cavernous malformations: report of 137 cases. Surg Neurol. 2003;59:444–54.

296. Samii M, Eghbal R, Carvalho GA, Matthies C. Surgical management of brainstem cavernomas. J Neurosurg. 2001; 95:825–32.

297. Brown AP, Thompson BG, Spetzler RF. The two-point method: evaluating brain stem lesions. BNI Q. 1996; 12:20–4.

298. Kikuta K, Nozaki K, Takahashi JA, Miyamoto S, Kikuchi H, Hashimoto N. Postoperative evaluation of microsurgical resection for cavernous malformations of the brainstem. J Neurosurg. 2004;101:607–12.

299. Shih YH, Pan DH. Management of supratentorial cavernous malformations: craniotomy versus gammaknife radiosurgery. Clin Neurol Neurosurg. 2005;107:108–12.

300. Yoon PH, Kim DI, Jeon P, Ryu YH, Hwang GJ, Park SJ. Cerebral cavernous malformations: serial magnetic resonance imaging findings in patients with and without gamma knife surgery. Neurol Med Chir (Tokyo). 1998; 38(Suppl):255–61.

301. Kida Y, Kobayashi T, Mori Y. Radiosurgery of angiographically occult vascular malformations. Neurosurg Clin N Am. 1999;10:291–303.

302. Seo Y, Fukuoka S, Takanashi M, et al. Gamma knife surgery for angiographically occult vascular malformations. Stereotact Funct Neurosurg. 1995;64 Suppl 1:98–109.

303. Kida Y, Kobayashi T, Tanaka T. Treatment of symptomatic AOVMs with radiosurgery. Acta Neurochir Suppl. 1995;63: 68–72.

304. Alexander 3rd E, Loeffler JS. Radiosurgery for intracranial vascular malformations: techniques, results, and complications. Clin Neurosurg. 1992;39:273–91.

305. Huang Y-C, Tseng C-K, Chang C-N, Wei K-C, Liao C-C, Hsu P-W. LINAC radiosurgery for intracranial cavernous malformation: 10-year experience. Clin Neurol Neurosurg. 2006;108:750–6.

306. Liscak R, Vladyka V, Simonova G, Vymazal J, Novotny Jr J. Gamma knife surgery of brain cavernous hemangiomas. J Neurosurg. 2005;102(Suppl):207–13.

307. Kim MS, Pyo SY, Jeong YG, Lee SI, Jung YT, Sim JH. Gamma knife surgery for intracranial cavernous hemangioma. J Neurosurg. 2005;102(Suppl):102–6.

308. Liu KD, Chung WY, Wu HM, et al. Gamma knife surgery for cavernous hemangiomas: an analysis of 125 patients. J Neurosurg. 2005;102(Suppl):81–6.

309. Hasegawa T, McInerney J, Kondziolka D, Lee JY, Flickinger JC, Lunsford LD. Long-term results after stereotactic radiosurgery for patients with cavernous malformations. Neurosurgery. 2002;50:1190–7; discussion 7–8.

310. Zhang N, Pan L, Wang BJ, Wang EM, Dai JZ, Cai PW. Gamma knife radiosurgery for cavernous hemangiomas. J Neurosurg. 2000;93 Suppl 3:74–7.

311. Pollock BE, Garces YI, Stafford SL, Foote RL, Schomberg PJ, Link MJ. Stereotactic radiosurgery for cavernous malformations. J Neurosurg. 2000;93:987–91.

312. Regis J, Bartolomei F, Kida Y, et al. Radiosurgery for epilepsy associated with cavernous malformation: retrospective study in 49 patients. Neurosurgery. 2000;47:1091–7.

313. Mitchell P, Hodgson TJ, Seaman S, Kemeny AA, Forster DM. Stereotactic radiosurgery and the risk of haemorrhage from cavernous malformations. Br J Neurosurg. 2000;14: 96–100.

314. Kondziolka D, Lunsford LD, Flickinger JC, Kestle JR. Reduction of hemorrhage risk after stereotactic radiosurgery for cavernous malformations. J Neurosurg. 1995;83: 825–31.

315. Chang SD, Levy RP, Adler Jr JR, Martin DP, Krakovitz PR, Steinberg GK. Stereotactic radiosurgery of angiographically occult vascular malformations: 14-year experience. Neurosurgery. 1998;43:213–20; discussion 20–1.

316. Amin-Hanjani S, Ogilvy CS, Candia GJ, Lyons S, Chapman PH. Stereotactic radiosurgery for cavernous malformations: Kjellberg's experience with proton beam therapy in 98 cases at the Harvard Cyclotron. Neurosurgery. 1998;42: 1229–36; discussion 36–8.

317. Coffey RJ. Brainstem cavernomas. J Neurosurg. 2003;99: 1116–7; author reply 7.

318. Gewirtz RJ, Steinberg GK, Crowley R, Levy RP. Pathological changes in surgically resected angiographically occult vascular malformations after radiation. Neurosurgery. 1998;42:738–42; discussion 42–3.

319. Mulliken JB, Glowacki J. Hemangiomas and vascular malformations in infants and children: a classification based on endothelial characteristics. Plast Reconstr Surg. 1982;69: 412–22.

17. Acute Ischaemic Stroke

Agnieszka Anna Ardelt

This chapter focuses on acute ischaemic stroke: mechanisms, risk factors, clinical presentation, diagnostic evaluation, and treatment other than thrombolysis and thrombectomy, which are discussed in Chap. 9. The topics are arranged alphabetically. Ischaemic stroke in paediatric patients is discussed separately in an appendix.

17.1. Acute Ischaemic Stroke: Burden of Disease

In the United States, approximately 795,000 people suffer a stroke annually, and the vast majority of strokes are ischaemic in nature. Over 130,000 people with stroke die each year; only cardiac disease, cancer, and chronic lung diseases result in more deaths than stroke.[1] Stroke leaves survivors with disabilities which have both personal and societal implications: 20–30% will need assistance with activities of daily living or walking, and the majority will be unable to return to work.[2] Estimated cost of stroke in 2010 was $73.7 billion.[1]

17.2. Acute Ischaemic Stroke: Terminology and Differential Diagnosis of Acute Onset Focal Neurologic Dysfunction

Terminology

1. Stroke.
    (a) Focal (or, less frequently, global) neurologic dysfunction of *any* cause.
    (b) Most frequent colloquial use signifies cerebral ischaemia and/or haemorrhage.
    (c) Most common use in *clinical studies* signifies cerebral ischaemia, cerebral haemorrhage, and subarachnoid haemorrhage.
    (d) Sometimes used colloquially to mean cerebral *infarct*.
2. Acute stroke.
    (a) *Apoplectic* onset of focal (or, less frequently, global) neurologic dysfunction of *any* cause.
    (b) Commonly used synonymously with "acute ischaemic stroke," implying that the underlying cause of acute focal neurologic dysfunction is ischaemic.
3. Acute ischaemic stroke.
    (a) Acute, *apoplectic* onset of focal neurologic dysfunction of *ischaemic cause*, i.e., acute cerebral ischaemia due to arterial blockage or narrowing and cessation or diminution of blood flow to an area of brain.
4. Cerebral infarct.
    (a) A localized area of dead tissue, as a consequence of having been deprived of its blood supply.
    (b) The term is usually used in reference to a pathologic specimen or radiologic imaging, where particular features suggest tissue death due to ischaemia.
5. Transient ischaemic attack (TIA).
    (a) See Sect. 17.5.

M.R. Harrigan, J.P. Deveikis, *Handbook of Cerebrovascular Disease and Neurointerventional Technique*, DOI 10.1007/978-1-61779-946-4_17, © Springer Science–Business Media New York 2013

6. Vasculopathy.
   (a) Generic term for disease of blood vessels, regardless of aetiology.
      • If the aetiology is inflammatory, the term *vasculitis* is used.
   (b) Classification by blood vessel size (diameter).
      • Large vessel vasculopathy.
         – Also referred to as *arteriopathy* if the arteries or arterioles are predominantly affected.
         – If the aetiology is inflammatory, the term *arteritis* may be used.
      • Small vessel vasculopathy.
         – Also referred to as *angiopathy* or *microangiopathy*.
         – When referring to cerebral vasculature, terms including *penetrating vessel disease*, *lacunar disease*, *small vessel disease*, or *periventricular white matter disease* are also used.
         – If the aetiology is inflammatory, the term *angiitis* is used.

Differential Diagnosis of Acute Onset Focal Neurologic Dysfunction

Most patients presenting with acute stroke symptoms will be found to have cerebral ischaemia or haemorrhage; however, in one study, of 350 presentations with stroke symptoms, 31% were attributable to *mimics*.[3]

1. Acute cerebral ischaemia.
   (a) Most common aetiology of focal neurologic dysfunction, especially in patients with ischaemic stroke risk factors.
   (b) Approximately 60–70% of all causes of acute focal neurologic dysfunction.
   (c) Whether cerebral *ischaemia* will result in *infarction* depends on the severity and duration of ischaemia; the longer and more severe, the more likely an infarct will ensue.
2. Intracranial haemorrhage
   (a) Approximately 10–15% of all causes of acute focal neurologic dysfunction.
   (b) Usually readily ruled out with noncontrast head CT.
      • Isodense subdural haemorrhages may be difficult, but critical, to diagnose; administering IV tPA could have fatal consequences (Fig. 17.1).
3. Mimics of cerebral ischaemia.
   (a) It is important to efficiently rule out mimics of cerebral ischaemia when evaluating patients with acute focal neurologic deficit who present within the thrombolysis time window; noncontrast head CT and the pattern of deficit on neurologic examination are helpful in ruling in a vascular cause (see Sect. 17.5 and 17.6).
   (b) Frequency of mimics of cerebral ischaemia or haemorrhage.

Frequency of stroke mimics in acute presentations[3]	
Conditions mimicking acute stroke	**Frequency (%)**
Sepsis or metabolic derangement	23.8
Seizure or Todd's paralysis	21.1
Syncope and presyncope	9.2
Cerebral mass lesion	9.2
Vestibular dysfunction	6.4
Confusional state	6.4
Mononeuropathy	5.5
Functional (medically unexplained)	5.5
Dementia	3.7
Migraine	2.8
Spinal cord pathology	2.8
Other	3.6

[a]Transient postictal paralysis, usually resolving within 48 h

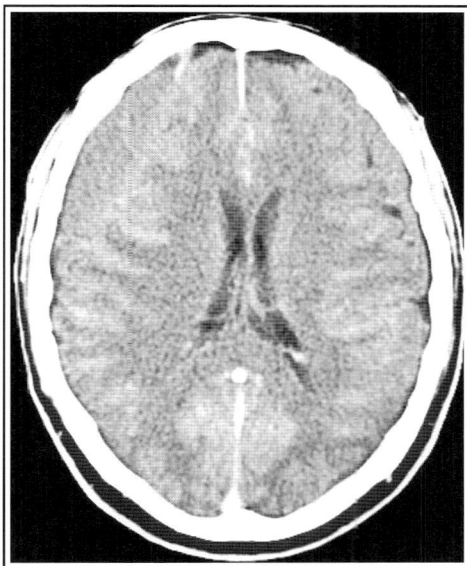

Fig. 17.1 Isodense chronic subdural haematoma. There is a chronic SDH in the *right frontal* region and a smaller one in the *left frontal* area. They blend in with the adjacent brain and are somewhat hard to see. The clinical presentation of a patient with a chronic SDH may mimic an acute ischaemic stroke.

(c) Selected conditions mimicking acute ischaemic and haemorrhagic strokes.

- Sepsis and metabolic derangement.
    - *Sepsis.* Less likely to present with lateralizing signs unless in the setting of *anamnestic* symptoms (recurrent symptoms related to a chronic brain injury) or concomitant intracranial or extracranial artery stenosis resulting in focal hypoperfusion in the setting of hypotension.
    - *Blood glucose abnormalities.* Hypoglycemia (or, rarely, hyperglycemia) can present with global neurologic dysfunction including altered mental status and/or coma, as well as focal neurologic signs and symptoms including hemiplegia (*hypoglycemic hemiplegia*) and/or aphasia.[4]; symptoms resolve quickly with the administration of dextrose; failure to make this diagnosis may lead to permanent neurologic injury.
- Seizure and/or postictal paralysis.
    - Less likely to account for focal symptoms if still present more than 6 h from symptom onset.[3]
    - Seizures may occur *as a result* of acute cerebral ischaemia or haemorrhage: In one study, 8.6% of patients with ischaemic stroke experienced first-ever seizures, and 40% of poststroke seizures occurred within 24 h of ictus;[5] in another study, 7.7% of patients presenting with acute focal neurologic dysfunction had seizure activity at the time of onset and, of those, 55% were found to have cerebral ischaemia.
    - Emergent CT perfusion and angiography,[6] MR perfusion and angiography,[7] carotid and transcranial Doppler (TCD) ultrasound, or conventional angiography may be used to rule

in acute cerebrovascular cause and clarify the diagnosis in patients with acute focal neurologic deficit and seizures at onset.
- The so-called *limb-shaking transient ischaemic attacks* may be especially difficult to clinically differentiate from seizures (see Sect. 17.5).
- Syncope and presyncope.
    - Unlikely to present with true lateralizing signs, unless there is concomitant intracranial or extracranial artery stenosis resulting in focal hypoperfusion in the setting of hypotension.
    - Common reason for referrals to vascular neurologists, despite the fact that cerebrovascular disease is a rare aetiology of true *syncope*, defined as transient, self-limited loss of consciousness.[8]
    - In the rare cases where the cause of syncope is cerebrovascular, vertebrobasilar insufficiency or subclavian steal is usually involved.
- Intracranial space occupying lesion (tumor, abscess, arteriovenous malformation, etc.).
    - May be asymptomatic until reaches a large size, or results in haemorrhage, oedema, or seizure.
    - Usually readily identified with noncontrast head CT.
- Migraine.
    - The relationship of migraines and cerebral ischaemia is complex: migraines (*complicated migraines*) may mimic acute ischaemic stroke; migraines are a risk factor for cerebral ischaemia (see Migraines in Sect. 17.4); and headache can occur in the setting of cerebral ischaemia: up to 32% of patients with cerebral ischaemia complained of headache.[9]
- Psychiatric disease (aka functional, medically unexplained, presentation).
    - Diagnosis of exclusion.
    - Pattern of deficit may be suspicious for non organic aetiology, i.e., exam does not readily suggest a cerebral vascular distribution.
    - The aetiology may be conversion disorder or malingering.
- Spinal cord pathology.
    - Pattern of weakness and sensory deficit may suggest spinal cord localization.
- Cerebral sinus or venous thrombosis.
    - Risk factors include infection, dehydration, oral contraceptive use, coagulopathy, or pregnancy/puerperium.
    - Usually readily identified with noncontrast head CT.
    - Focal neurologic dysfunction is usually due to cerebral oedema, haemorrhage, or seizure.
- Anamnestic syndrome.
    - Recurrence of focal neurologic deficit similar to that seen with prior cerebral injury, in the setting of current systemic derangement, i.e., infection or metabolic derangement, usually in an elderly patient. Not to be confused with *amnesia*, which is loss of memory.
    - Diagnosis of exclusion in patients with previous brain injury.

17.3. Acute Ischaemic Stroke: Mechanisms

Three basic mechanisms can result in cessation or diminution of flow to regions of brain: embolism from a proximal source with occlusion of the downstream artery; local occlusion, usually due to in situ thrombosis, of a proximal or distal artery; or global hypoperfusion. The majority of ischaemic strokes are split between embolic (with 25% cardioembolic) and local occlusion, with global hypoperfusion accounting for the minority. In large vessel disease, all three mechanisms may be involved, e.g., a carotid artery severely stenotic (because of a large atherosclerotic plaque) may cause distal ischaemia from plaque emboli and/or worsening stenosis with distal hypoperfusion due to acute plaque rupture and thrombosis, which may be exacerbated by low cardiac output or relative systemic hypotension. Sometimes one mechanism may predominate at different times in the evolution of cerebrovascular pathology. Detailed discussion of risk factors and conditions associated with ischaemic stroke follows in the subsequent section; some examples of specific conditions discussed in the subsequent section are listed within each mechanistic category below.

1. Embolism.
    (a) Artery-to-artery embolism.
        • Extracranial and intracranial large vessel vasculopathy of any cause.
            – Atherosclerotic (most common).
            – Nonatherosclerotic.
                (a) Dissection or fibromuscular dysplasia.
                (b) Dolichoectasia.
                (c) Vasculitis/arteritis.
                (d) Moya-moya disease/syndrome.
                (e) Vasospasm/vasoconstriction.
        • Aortic arch abnormality of any cause.
            – Atherosclerotic atheroma.
            – Dissection/aneurysm.
            – Connective tissue disease or infection.
    (b) Cardioembolism.
        • Arrhythmia
            – Atrial fibrillation (most common)
        • Valvulopathy
            – Rheumatic heart disease
            – Prosthetic heart valves
            – Endocarditis
                (a) Infectious
                (b) Nonbacterial thrombotic
            – Mitral valve prolapse
        • Cardiomyopathy, dilated
        • Acute MI and ventricular thrombus.
        • Paradoxical embolism
            – Patent foramen ovale
            – Pulmonary AVM
        • Intracardiac lesions
            – Tumors, e.g., atrial myxoma
2. Local occlusion
    (a) Small vessel vasculopathy of any cause.
        • Related to multiple risk factors: hypertension, hyperlipidemia, diabetes mellitus, cigarette smoking, etc. (most common)
        • Cerebral autosomal dominant arteriopathy with subcortical infarcts and leukoencephalopathy (CADASIL)
        • Cerebral angiitis
        • Cerebral amyloid angiopathy
    (b) Abnormalities of coagulation.
        • Malignancy
        • Hormonal
            – Pregnancy and puerperium
            – Oral contraceptives
            – Hormone replacement
        • Genetic coagulopathies
        • Antiphospholipid antibody syndrome
    (c) Abnormalities of platelet function.
        • Heparin-induced thrombocytopaenia
        • Thrombotic thrombocytopaenic purpura
    (d) Hyperviscosity.
        • Sickle cell disease
        • Hyperfibrinogenemia
        • Polycythemia vera
3. Hypoperfusion
    (a) Systemic hypotension of any cause.
    (b) Heart failure/low cardiac output.
    (c) Cardiac arrhythmia or arrest.

17.4. Acute Ischaemic Stroke: Conventional Risk Factors, Predisposing Conditions, and Risk Factor Modification

The approach to the patient with cerebral ischaemia starts with the understanding of the *patient milieu*: the constellation of ischaemic stroke risk factors, some modifiable and some not, which, alone and in combination, confer specific ischaemic stroke risk. The main pathophysiologic theme underlying the conventional risk factors is endothelial injury leading to (1) *atherosclerosis* (discussed in Chap. 18) which manifests as large artery disease (extracranial and intracranial), (2) cerebral *microangiopathy* which manifests as lacunar infarcts and periventricular white matter disease, and (3) coronary artery disease which leads to abnormalities of cardiac function and rhythm. These disease processes predispose to cerebral ischaemia due to embolism, local occlusion, and/or hypoperfusion.

Conventional ischaemic stroke risk factors
Age
Sex
Ethnicity/heredity/genetics
Hypertension
Diabetes mellitus
Hyperlipidemia
Cigarette smoking
Cardiac disease[a]
Atrial fibrillation
Cervical carotid stenosis
Intracranial stenosis
Extracranial vertebral stenosis

[a]Includes cardiomyopathy, myocardial infarction with intraventricular thrombus, intracardiac lesions (tumors), valvular diseases, etc.

In 25–39% of patients the specific cause of ischaemic stroke is not identified: these are referred to as *cryptogenic* strokes. There may be biological or technical reasons for failure to identify the aetiology of ischaemic stroke in specific patients. These include as yet unidentified risk factors and partial diagnostic work-ups or work-ups undertaken too late to identify the cause, e.g., after an intracardiac thrombus had embolized.[10]

It is likely that with further research, additional risk factors for ischaemic stroke will be discovered, accounting for some of the currently cryptogenic events. One exciting emerging area of investigation is the delineation of molecular markers and gene expression profiles that correlate with specific mechanisms of ischaemic stroke. These markers could potentially be developed in the future as clinical tools for determining ischaemic stroke aetiology in specific patients.[11]

Conventional risk factors, constellations of risk factors, as well as uncommon conditions, either emerging or established as ischaemic stroke risk factors, are discussed below in alphabetical order below. American Heart Association (AHA)/American Stroke Association Guidelines for primary and secondary prevention of ischaemic stroke have been updated in 2011 and are good references.[12,13]

Acute Myocardial Infarction (MI) with Left Ventricular (IV) Thrombus

1. Ischaemic stroke risk in MI with LV thrombus
   (a) Up to 12% in patients with MI and LV thrombus, but can be as high as 20% if thrombus is apical.[14]

---

2. Management of stroke risk in MI with LV thrombus
   (a) Primary prevention of ischaemic stroke.
      – Warfarin sodium with INR goal of 2.0–3.0 for 3 months to 1 year may be considered[15]
   (b) Secondary prevention of ischaemic stroke.[14]
      – Warfarin sodium with INR goal of 2.0–3.0 for 3 months to 1 year
      – Concomitant low-dose aspirin should be used in the setting of coronary artery disease.

Age

Age is the strongest risk factor for ischaemic stroke. Incidence of cerebral ischaemia increases with age irrespective of ethnicity and gender: incidence doubles with each decade after age 55.[16]

Alcohol

There is a protective effect of consumption of small amounts of alcohol, and a deleterious effect of consumption of >5 drinks per day, on ischaemic stroke risk in primary[15] and secondary stroke prevention.[14]
1. Potential mechanisms of deleterious effect of alcohol:
   (a) Hypertension, coagulopathy, and cardiac arrhythmias.
2. Potential mechanisms of beneficial effect of alcohol:
   (a) Increase in HDL/LDL ratio and decreased platelet aggregation.

2006 AHA Recommendation[15]
Patients with ischaemic stroke or TIA who consume alcohol should eliminate alcohol consumption or decrease it to no more than 1–2 drinks per day.

Aortic Arch Atheroma

Aortic arch atheromas are found most frequently using transesophageal echocardiography in elderly patients with atherosclerotic disease at other sites.
1. Ischaemic stroke risk with aortic arch atheroma
   (a) Plaques ≥4-mm thick. Associated with high risk of recurrent cerebral ischaemia or death during 2-year follow up; HR 2.12 (95% CI: 1.04–4.32) regardless of anticoagulation or antiplatelet therapy. Risk is further increased if plaques exhibit a complex morphology.[17] Up to 11% ischaemic stroke recurrence at 1 year has been observed in some elderly patients with cryptogenic stroke, despite antiplatelet therapy.[18]
2. Mechanism of ischaemic stroke with aortic arch atheroma: thromboembolism
3. Management of ischaemic stroke risk with aortic arch atheroma
   (a) Best therapy is unknown
      • Antiplatelet therapy, antihypertensive drugs, smoking cessation aids, as well as HMG CoA reductase inhibitors (statins) are routinely prescribed.[19]
   (b) Systemic anticoagulation or dual antiplatelet therapy, most commonly with aspirin and clopidogrel, has been advocated for specific patients (e.g., plaque with a mobile component or free-floating thrombus).[20,21]
      • Randomized therapeutic trials comparing antiplatelet drugs to warfarin are lacking
      • Benefit of dual antiplatelet therapy is offset by risk of haemorrhage (MATCH study).[22]
   (c) Routine aortic atherectomy, aortic filters, or stenting are not currently recommended.[19]

Arrhythmia

The most common and best-studied arrhythmia predisposing to ischaemic stroke through a thromboembolic mechanism is atrial fibrillation (see Atrial fibrillation). Other abnormalities of cardiac rhythm including sick sinus syndrome or tachycardia-bradycardia syndrome may be associated with increased risk ischaemic stroke.[23] Ischaemic stroke prevention in paroxysmal atrial fibrillation and atrial flutter should be approached in the same manner as persistent atrial fibrillation.[24,25]

Atherosclerosis

Atherosclerotic disease can affect both extracranial and intracranial vasculature and is discussed in Chaps. 18 and 19, respectively.

Atrial Fibrillation

Atrial fibrillation is the most common arrhythmia. Thromboembolism may occur as a result of clot formation primarily within the left atrium and left atrial appendage.

1. Predisposing factors[26]
   (a) Heart disease: cardiac ischaemia, valvular heart disease, myocardial dysfunction
   (b) Medical conditions: thyrotoxicosis, pulmonary embolism, sleep apnea, obesity, neurologic emergencies
   (c) Idiopathic, aka lone atrial fibrillation
   (d) Familial
   (e) Perioperative
   (f) Associated with caffeine or alcohol use
2. Prevalence
   (a) Increases with age[27]
      - Age 65: 5% of the population
      - Age 80: 10% of the population
   (b) Causes 15% of ischaemic strokes in the US
      - Age 80: 24% of ischaemic strokes
3. Ischaemic stroke risk
   (a) Nonrheumatic atrial fibrillation *not treated* with antithrombotic therapy[28]
      - Approximate average risk: 5% per year (primary prevention); 12% per year (secondary prevention)[29]
      - Stratification based on patient characteristics: CHADS$_2$ Score

CHADS$_2$ Score for ischaemic stroke risk stratification in atrial fibrillation[28]	
Prognostic factor in atrial fibrillation	CHADS$_2$ score, points
C	Recent congestive heart failure	1
H	Hypertension	1
A	Age$\geq$75	1
D	Diabetes mellitus	1
S$_2$	Previous stroke or transient ischaemic attack	2

CHADS$_2$ score	Ischaemic stroke in atrial fibrillation without antithrombotic therapy (rate per 100 person-years)
0	1.9
1	2.8
2	4.0
3	5.9
4	8.5
5	12.5
6	18.2

4. Management
   (a) Prevention of thromboembolism in persistent or paroxysmal AF
      • Risk reduction and complication rates with antithrombotic therapy[25,29,30]

Risk reduction and complication rates with antithrombotic therapy in atrial fibrillation		
	Aspirin (25–1,300 mg/day)	Warfarin sodium (INR 2–3)
Ischaemic stroke	23% (RRR/year)	65% (RRR/year)
Primary prevention	1.5% (ARR/year)	2.7% (ARR/year) (NNT for 1 year to prevent 1 stroke: 37)
Secondary prevention	2.5% (ARR/year)	8.4% (ARR/year) (NNT for 1 year to prevent 1 stroke: 12)
Complications (intracranial and extracranial haemorrhages)	3.5 per 100 person-years	7.9 per 100 person-years

ARR absolute risk reduction, [b]RRR relative risk reduction compared to placebo, [c]NNT number needed to treat

   • Selection of antithrombotic therapy in patients with atrial fibrillation using the CHADS$_2$ score[12,26]
      – CHADS$_2$=0: aspirin (81–325 mg)
      – CHADS$_2$=1: aspirin or warfarin sodium
      – CHADS$_2$ 2: warfarin sodium with goal INR 2–3
      – If unable to take oral anticoagulants, use aspirin alone
      – If at high risk for ischaemic stroke and oral anticoagulation is to be interrupted, consider bridging with low molecular weight heparin subcutaneously
   • New anticoagulants for atrial fibrillation[31]
      – Rationale for developing alternatives to warfarin
         • Warfarin use requires monitoring of anticoagulation and attention to potential interactions with food and other drugs
         • Anticoagulation intensity may be difficult to control resulting in loss of benefit and increased risk of haemorrhage
      – Classes of compounds and examples of orally available drugs in various stages of development
         • Direct thrombin inhibitors: dabigatran (Pradaxa® in Australia, Europe and USA, Pradax in Canada, Prazaxa in Japan, Boehringer Ingelheim, Ingelheim am Rhein, Germany), ximelagatran (Xanta or Xarta, AstraZenica, London, UK)
         • Factor Xa inhibitors: rivaroxaban, apixaban, betrixaban, edoxaban

- Advantages and disadvantages of both classes of drugs
  - Advantages: fixed dose; no anticoagulation monitoring
  - Disadvantage: no antidote for rapid reversal in the case of bleeding
- Comments on specific drugs
  - Ximelagatran: showed efficacy in AF in two Phase III trials; this drug has been withdrawn due to hepatotoxicity
  - Dabigatran: studied in phase II and phase III trials for AF and showed similar efficacy to warfarin while reducing the rate of haemorrhagic stroke
  - Apixaban: studied in one phase III trial and shown to be superior to warfarin (lower rate of bleeding, mortality, and ischaemic/haemorrhagic stroke, with the biggest effect on haemorrhagic stroke)[32]
  - Rivaroxaban: studied in one recent phase III trial and found to be non-inferior to warfarin; a lower rate of intracranial haemorrhage was noted with rivaroxaban[33]

(b) Rate control
  - Goals
    - Symptomatic relief from tachycardia
    - Prevention of tachycardia-related cardiomyopathy
(c) Other options for selected patients with atrial fibrillation
  - Rhythm control
  - Cardioversion
    - Anticoagulation is required periprocedure
  - Catheter ablation/pacemaker implantation
  - Closure of the left atrial appendage[34]

Atrial Myxoma

The incidence of primary cardiac tumors is 1 in 5,000.[35] Atrial myxoma is the most common primary cardiac tumor in adults and is usually located in the left atrium. There is a 2:1 female predominance; diagnosis is most common between the third and sixth decade; and some cases are familial.[36] Patients with atrial myxoma present with symptoms related to flow obstruction (50–70% of patients), peripheral or central embolization (16–30%), and/or constitutional disturbance (50–58% of patients). Embolization is related to thrombus located on the surface of the myxoma or embolization of tumor fragments. Tumor emboli may subsequently evolve into mass lesions (myxomatous metastasis) or vascular erosion and aneurysm formation may occur. Myxomatous cerebral aneurysms are similar to infectious aneurysms and feature fusiform shape and distal locations.[36] The diagnosis of atrial myxoma can be made on transesophageal echocardiography; treatment centers on surgical resection, which is typically curative.

Birth Control Pills

See Oral contraceptives.

Cerebral Amyloid Angiopathy

Cerebral amyloid angiopathy is characterized by deposition of amyloid β-protein in the walls of cortical and leptomeningeal blood vessels.[37] This condition is associated with dementia and intracerebral haemorrhage, but may manifest with cerebral ischaemia due to microvascular disease. In some patients, pathologic specimens feature amyloid deposits in association with a vascular inflammatory reaction (vasculitis) on brain biopsy, for which immunosuppressive therapy may eventually be an option.[38] There is no specific treatment for cerebral amyloid angiopathy or specific primary or secondary ischaemic stroke prevention strategy.[37]

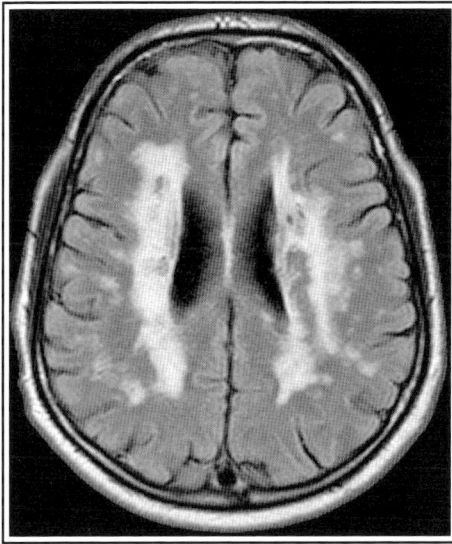

Fig. 17.2 MRI of the brain in a patient with CADASIL. Multiple subcortical infarcts are evident.

Cerebral Autosomal Dominant Arteriopathy with Subcortical Infarcts and Leukoencephalopathy (CADASIL)

CADASIL is a dominantly inherited disorder caused by mutation of the Notch3 gene, resulting in damage to the endothelium of small cerebral arteries and arterioles, i.e., a small vessel vasculopathy.[39] Central nervous system manifestations include ischaemic stroke, migraine, dementia, psychiatric disorders, and seizures. Other organs affected include skin, muscle, heart, liver, GI tract, and peripheral nerves. The diagnosis can be made with genetic testing.[39]

1. Ischaemic stroke and transient ischaemic attack (TIA) in CADASIL
   (a) May occur in up to 85% of affected people, with frequent recurrence.
   (b) Small vessel (lacunar) syndromes predominate, usually beginning in the fourth or fifth decade (Fig. 17.2).
   (c) There is no specific treatment or primary or secondary ischaemic stroke preventative strategy, and while the effect of conventional preventative therapies on stroke recurrence in CADASIL is unknown, control of conventional stroke risk factors is logical; double antiplatelet therapy or systemic anticoagulation is avoided due to intracerebral haemorrhage risk.

Cardiomyopathy

Cardiomyopathy predisposes to thromboembolism by virtue of relative stasis of blood and clot formation within the cardiac apex. Thromboembolism may occur regardless of aetiology of ventricular dysfunction:

1. Relationship of stroke risk to reduction in ejection fraction[40,41]
   (a) Postmyocardial infarction ventricular dysfunction
      • Cumulative risk of stroke (96% of strokes were ischaemic)

Ischaemic stroke risk as a function of ejection fraction[40]	
Ejection fraction (%)	Stroke rate over 5 years after myocardial infarction (%)
<28	8.9
29–35	7.8
>35	4.1

2. Management of ischaemic stroke risk in CM
   (a) Antithrombotic therapy
      • Lack of randomized controlled studies
      • Warfarin with goal of INR 2–3 *may be considered* for patients with severe LV dysfunction for primary prevention[15]
      • *Either* warfarin sodium with goal INR 2–3 *or* anti platelet agents are reasonable for secondary prevention[14]

Cigarette Smoking

See Tobacco, smoked.

Coagulopathy (Aka Thrombophilia)

Venous thrombosis can lead to ischaemic stroke if there is concomitant abnormal right-to-left communication, such as a patent foramen ovale (PFO). Typical conditions increasing the risk of venous thrombosis in the general population are pregnancy, oral contraceptives, nephrotic syndrome, postoperative state, immobility, and malignancy.[42] If the ischaemic stroke is cryptogenic and the patient is <50 years old, the patient is typically screened for genetic coagulopathy, although whether this should be done routinely is controversial.[43] Although a small fraction of the population may indeed harbour genetic disorders of the coagulation pathways which predispose to venous thrombosis, i.e., primary hypercoagulability, caution needs to be exercised in making this diagnosis in the acute phase of ischaemic stroke: acute thrombosis may cause transient hypercoagulability (secondary hypercoagulability), and laboratory tests for coagulation factor levels may be affected. Thus, all tests with the exception of genetic tests (e.g., Factor V Leyden and prothrombin gene mutations) should be performed at least 2 months after the acute stroke phase.[44,45] Additionally, a positive family history and/or personal history suggestive of a clotting disorder antedating the stroke should be sought to increase the pretest probability of primary hypercoagulability.

In summary, rare patients who present with cryptogenic ischaemic stroke may have primary hypercoagulability (up to 4% of patients <50 years old with ischaemic stroke; approximately 1% of all patients with ischaemic stroke).[45] If a patient with primary hypercoagulability and ischaemic stroke shows no evidence of venous thrombosis and a right-to-left shunt (i.e., paradoxical embolism as stroke mechanism), a relationship of the coagulation disorder to arterial thrombosis may be invoked, although this should not preclude screening for conventional ischaemic stroke risk factors.

This section focuses on selected genetic coagulopathies. Additional selected haematologic conditions which are associated with a thrombophilic state are discussed in the sections below on Hyperviscosity, Heparin-Induced Thrombocytopenia, Malignancy, and Sickle Cell Disease.

Prevalence of primary hypercoagulability among patients with ischaemic stroke[44]			
Condition	**Prevalence range (%)**	**Pretest probability (%)**	
		≤50 years old	**All ages**
Hereditary protein C, protein S, and antithrombin III deficiency	0–21	Unknown	Unknown
Hereditary fibrinolytic deficiency (e.g., plasminogen)	0–2.7	Unknown	Unknown
Activated protein C resistance (aka Factor V Leyden mutation)	0–38	11	7
Prothrombin gene mutations	1–12.5	5.7	4.5
Antiphospholipid antibodies			
(a) Anticardiolipin antibody		21	17
(b) Lupus anticoagulant		8	3

1. Prevalence of coagulopathy in ischaemic stroke patients.[44]
2. Clinical factors increasing the pretest probability of coagulopathy in ischaemic stroke patients.
   (a) All disorders: age ≤50, family history of thrombosis, personal history of venous or arterial thrombosis.
   (b) Hereditary protein C, protein S, and antithrombin III deficiency, or fibrinolytic deficiency.
      • Thrombus in atypical location (e.g., upper extremity).
      • Thrombosis during pregnancy/puerperium.
      • Warfarin-induced skin necrosis (protein C or S deficiency).
      • Resistance to heparin (antithrombin III deficiency).
   (c) Activated protein C resistance or prothrombin gene mutation.
      • Cerebral sinus thrombosis.
      • Thrombosis during pregnancy/puerperium.
   (d) Antiphospholipid antibodies.
      • Systemic lupus erythaematosus.
      • Miscarriage.
      • Livedo reticularis (reticulated pattern of purplish discolouration on the skin due to changes in vascular diameter).
      • Idiopathic thrombocytopaenia.
      • Nonbacterial thrombotic endocarditis.
3. Management of patients with ischaemic stroke and coagulopathy.[14]
   (a) All patients should receive a full cerebrovascular evaluation of conventional ischaemic stroke risk factors.
   (b) Established hereditary protein C, protein S, antithrombin III or fibrinolytic deficiency; activated protein C resistance; or prothrombin gene mutation and cryptogenic ischaemic stroke.
      • If deep venous thrombosis is present. Anticoagulation with warfarin sodium to INR 2–3, short or long term, depending on additional patient-specific factors.
      • If deep venous thrombosis is absent. Antiplatelet therapy *or* anticoagulation with warfarin sodium to goal INR 2–3.
      • If there are recurrent thrombotic events on antiplatelet therapy. Anticoagulation with warfarin sodium to goal INR 2–3.
   (c) Established antiphospholipid antibodies and cryptogenic ischaemic stroke.
      • If antiphospholipid antibodies are present, but there are no features of antiphospholipid antibody syndrome (Table 17.1): antiplatelet therapy.
      • If antiphospholipid syndrome is present: anticoagulation with warfarin sodium to INR 2–3.
         – Diagnostic criteria (Sapporo Criteria) for antiphospholipid antibody syndrome.[46]

Table 17.1 Diagnosis of antiphospholipid antibody syndrome (aka Hughes syndrome)

Clinical criteria (one or more required)
Vascular thrombosis: arterial *OR* venous *OR* small vessel thrombosis in any organ
Pregnancy complications: unexplained fetal death after 10 weeks of gestation *OR* premature birth due to pre-eclampsia, eclampsia, or placental insufficiency *OR* three unexplained consecutive spontaneous abortions before 10 weeks of gestation
Laboratory criteria (one or more required)
Anticardiolipin IgG or IgM antibodies detected on two or more occasions separated by at least 6 weeks
Lupus anticoagulant detected on two or more occasions separated by at least 6 weeks

From Ortel.[46], with permission

C-Reactive Protein

High blood levels of C-reactive protein (CRP) and other inflammatory molecules correlate with increased atherosclerosis and risk of coronary disease and ischaemic stroke, although the relationship has been less clear for ischaemic stroke than for coronary disease, and it is uncertain whether CRP is causative or a marker of disease severity.[47] The JUPITER trial was a primary prevention trial in which healthy adult men and women with LDL <130 mg/dL and high sensitivity CRP 2.0 mg/L were randomized to placebo or statin (rosuvastatin, 20 mg daily). There was a 51% reduction in ischaemic stroke rate without effect on haemorrhagic stroke rate: incidence rate of 0.12 and 0.25 per 100 person-years in the statin and placebo cohorts, respectively (HR 0.49; 95% CI, 0.30–0.81; p=0.004).[48] Based on such findings, the 2011 AHA Primary Prevention Guidelines state that treatment of patients with elevated high sensitivity CRP with a statin "might be considered".[13]

Diabetes Mellitus

Diabetes affects 8% of American adults and is a predictor of recurrent ischaemic stroke.[14] Chronically poor glycemic control results in injury to the microvasculature in many organs including the brain, peripheral nerve, retina, and kidney. The microangiopathy in turn causes ischaemic damage. In the brain, manifestations of diabetic microangiopathy include progressive subcortical white matter injury and lacunar ischaemic strokes. Appropriate glycemic control decreases microvascular injury, and is recommended for primary and secondary prevention of ischaemic stroke.[14,15]

1. Diagnosis.

Diagnosis of diabetes mellitus	
	Fasting plasma glucose (mg dL²)
Normal fasting glucose	<100
Impaired fasting glucose	100–126
Diabetes	>126

2. Management.
   (a) Oral hypoglycemic drugs, long- and short-acting insulin, and diabetic diet should be used to achieve glycemic control.
   (b) Glycemic control should be monitored with HbA_1C levels: HbA_1C >7% suggests poor control.
   (c) Concomitant conditions increasing stroke risk, especially hypertension and hyperlipidemia should be aggressively treated in patients with DM.
   (d) Lifestyle changes including weight reduction, decreasing alcohol intake, and smoking cessation should be prescribed for patients with DM.

3. Insulin resistance.
   (a) Relatively common worldwide, affecting perhaps >1 billion people.
   (b) Currently being investigated as a risk factor for vascular disease.[49]

Dissection, Arterial

See Chap. 18.

Dolichoectasia, Arterial

See Chap. 13.

Drug Abuse

Drug abuse can lead to ischaemic stroke through a variety of mechanisms. For example, cocaine use can predispose to acute risk in the form of cerebral vasospasm or chronic risk in the form of hypertensive cerebral vasculopathy (see also Cocaine and Stroke in the section on Vasculitis). Cerebral vasculitis has been associated with amphetamine use. Intravenous drug use of any sort can lead to bacterial endocarditis and embolic stroke risk. Patients who abuse drugs should be counseled as to the risks, encouraged to stop using, and referred to appropriate drug rehabilitation services.

Endocarditis

Endocarditis accounts for less than 1% of thromboembolic ischaemic strokes, and is classified as either bacterial[50] (BE, aka infective) or nonbacterial thrombotic endocarditis (NBTE, aka marantic, or verrucous).[51] Conditions predisposing to BE include valvular abnormalities, catheter-related blood stream infections, intravenous drug use, and immune suppression. BE can occur on native or prosthetic valves, and in the majority of cases either streptococci or staphylococci are involved. NBTE is most often associated with malignancy, disseminated intravascular coagulation, systemic lupus erythaematosus with antiphospholipid syndrome, and primary hypercoagulabilities in the setting of previously normal valves. In these conditions, valvular vegetations are sterile and typically consist of fibrin and platelets. The term *Libman-Sacks endocarditis* usually refers to sterile endocardial lesions in patients with systemic lupus erythaematosus and the antiphospholipid syndrome (see Coagulopathy).
1. Diagnosis of endocarditis.
   (a) Bacterial endocarditis (Table 17.2).
       • Clinical exam findings of systemic embolization.
         – Osler nodes: tender nodules on finger and toe pads, present in 10–25% of patients with BE, but not specific to BE.
         – Janeway lesions: nodular haemorrhages on palms and soles, most likely associated with BE when seen on physical exam.
         – Petechiae and palpable purpura.
         – Splinter haemorrhages: subungal, dark red streaks; may also be seen with trauma.
         – Roth spots: oval retinal haemorrhages with pale centers.
       • New cardiac murmur.
       • Positive blood cultures.
         – See *Culture-negative endocarditis* below.
       • Evidence of vegetations on echocardiography.
         – Transesophageal is more sensitive, but transthoracic may reveal large lesions.
       • Culture-negative endocarditis.
         – Blood cultures may be sterile in up to 5% of cases of bacterial endocarditis diagnosed using strict criteria outlined earlier.
         – Causes of sterile cultures: prior use of antibiotics, right heart endocarditis, slow-growing organisms, fungi, intracellular pathogens, nonbacterial thrombotic endocarditis.[50]

Table 17.2 Modified Duke criteria for diagnosis of bacterial endocarditis

Major criteria
Microorganisms isolated from two separate blood cultures, persistent bacteremia, or a single culture with Coxiella Burnetii
Evidence of endocardial lesion (new valvular regurgitation or positive echocardiogram)
Minor criteria
Predisposition (IV drug use, previous BE, prosthetic heart valve, mitral valve prolapse, etc.)
Fever
Evidence of embolization
Immunologic phenomena (Osler nodes, Janeway lesions, etc.)
Microbiologic findings not meeting major criteria
Definite bacterial endocarditis
2 major criteria *OR* 1 major and 3 minor criteria *OR* 5 minor criteria
Possible bacterial endocarditis
1 major and 1 minor criteria *OR* 3 minor criteria

From Li et al.,[52] with permission

      (b) Nonbacterial thrombotic endocarditis.
- Transesophageal or transthoracic echocardiography showing vegetations.
- Sterile blood cultures.
- Evidence of systemic embolization.
- Underlying primary condition such as cancer or the anti phospho-lipid syndrome.
- Cardiac murmurs infrequent (unlike in bacterial endocarditis).

2. Ischaemic stroke risk in endocarditis.
    (a) Bacterial endocarditis
- Up to 20% of patients have ischaemic stroke and up to 65% may have embolization elsewhere.
- Large vegetations on anterior leaflet of mitral valve are most likely to embolize.
- Cerebral embolization of vegetations containing bacteria can result in cerebral ischaemia, abscess, mycotic aneurysm and arteritis, and haemorrhage (5% of cases).

    (b) Nonbacterial thrombotic endocarditis.
- Systemic (including brain) emboli are present on autopsy in almost half of patients with NBTE.[53]

3. Other complications of endocarditis.
    (a) Bacterial endocarditis.[50]
- Congestive heart failure: up to 50%.
- Glomerulonephritis.
- Annular abscess or cardiac conduction system involvement.
- Mycotic aneurysm or cerebral abscess.

4. Management.
    (a) Bacterial endocarditis.
- Obtain blood cultures.
- Start empiric intravenous antibiotics geared at most likely organisms.
- Tailor antibiotics based on culture sensitivities.
- If valves are prosthetic, continue systemic anticoagulation, unless there is evidence of haemorrhage or the infarct is large, i.e., at risk for haemorrhagic transformation.
- There is *no* role for systemic anticoagulation in case of native valves, and initiation may increase risk of haemorrhagic conversion of cerebral infarcts.
- Surgical management is reserved for cases of valvular insufficiency, heart failure, continued embolization, or persistent bacteremia despite appropriate antibiotic therapy, highly resistant virulent organisms, immediate relapse after completion of therapy, or large vegetations on the mitral valve.

(b) Nonbacterial thrombotic endocarditis.[51]
- Evaluate patient for malignancy, primary hypercoagulability, and the antiphospholipid syndrome and treat primary condition accordingly.
- Unless contraindicated (i.e., in the setting of haemorrhage or moderate-to-large acute cerebral infarcts), systemic anticoagulation should be used.
  - In patients with malignancy, heparins may be more effective than warfarin or other vitamin K antagonists.
  - In patients with primary hypercoagulability or antiphospholipid syndrome, warfarin should be used (see Coagulopathy).
- In cases of large vegetations or destructive valvular lesion, surgical therapy is an option.[54]

Ethnicity (Race)

The effect of ethnicity on ischaemic stroke in the United States has been investigated in large population-based studies such as the Greater Kentucky/Cincinnati Study and the Northern Manhattan Study.[16,55] Americans of African and Hispanic descent exhibit higher ischaemic stroke rates than Caucasions, irrespective of age and gender.

Extracranial Carotid and Vertebral Vasculopathy

See Chap. 18.

Fabry Disease

Fabry disease is an X-linked lysosomal storage disease and a relatively infrequent aetiology of ischaemic stroke. Some patients with Fabry disease develop a cerebral vasculopathy, and up to 4% of young adult patients with cryptogenic stroke may have Fabry disease.[56] Fabry disease is caused by deficiency of α-galactosidase A, which manifests with systemic accumulation of glycosphingolipids, although the mechanism of cerebral vasculopathy is not exactly understood. Fabry disease should be kept in mind when investigating patients with cryptogenic ischaemic stroke: the importance of making this rare diagnosis lies in the availability of disease-modifying therapy.[57]

1. Incidence of Fabry disease.
   (a) 1:55,000 male births.
   (b) Seventy percent of women may be symptomatic: typically milder symptoms and occurring later in life than in men.
2. Disease manifestations of Fabry disease.
   (a) Intermittent paresthesias, especially involving the hands and feet.
   (b) Chronic abdominal complaints, primarily pain.
   (c) Angiokeratomata.
   (d) Renal insufficiency and proteinuria.
   (e) Hypertrophic cardiomyopathy, arrhythmias.
   (f) Cerebral ischaemia, predominantly vertebrobasilar.
3. Diagnostic testing for Fabry disease.
   (a) Males.
      - Pedigree analysis.
      - Plasma or leukocyte α-galactosidosidase A.
   (b) Females.
      - Mutation analysis.
4. Treatment of Fabry disease.
   (a) Enzyme replacement therapy.
      - Agents.
        - Agalsidase alpha is used worldwide, but not approved in the US.
        - Agalsidase beta is approved in the US.

- Treatment effects.
  - Stabilization of cardiac, renal disease.
  - Reversal of cerebrovascular nitric oxide dysfunction.
  - May not be effective in stroke prevention
  (b) Antiplatelet therapy and conventional primary and secondary prevention approaches for ischaemic stroke.[12,56]

Family History of Ischaemic Stroke

Maternal or paternal history of ischaemic stroke is an ischaemic stroke risk factor, increasing risk by up to 30%. Ultimately, this is due to the combination of genetic and environmental (including cultural) influences.[13]

Fibromuscular Dysplasia

See Chap. 18.

Gender

Premenopausal Caucasian females have a lower incidence of ischaemic stroke than males. This difference is lost with advanced age and is affected by ethnicity, e.g., women of African American descent have a higher frequency of cerebral ischaemia than age-matched Caucasian females or males.[16] Outcomes of ischaemic stroke are worse in women than in men, which may relate in part to the older age at which women experience first strokes.[58]

Genetics

In most patients, a predisposition to ischaemic stroke is multifactoral, i.e., a complex interplay of genes relating to intrinsic risk factors like hypertension and diabetes with extrinsic aspects including diet, cigarette smoking, alcohol intake, and physical activity. In general, genetic predispositions to ischaemic stroke can be classified as single gene or polygenic disorders.[39] In the majority of stroke patients, risk is likely polygenic. The unraveling of the genetic complexity has only begun: in several diseases with defined genetic causes, ischaemic stroke is a common manifestation. While family history is useful in identifying patients at risk of stroke, genetic screening for the purposes of primary stroke prevention is currently not recommended.[13] Single gene disorders associated with ischaemic stroke risk are discussed below.

1. Single gene disorders.
   (a) Ischaemic stroke as a recognized manifestation.
     - Cerebral autosomal dominant arteriopathy with subcortical infarcts and leukoencephalopathy (CADASIL) (see CADASIL section).
     - Cerebral autosomal recessive arteriopathy with subcortical infarcts and leukoencephalopathy (CARASIL).
       - Rare; features similar to CADASIL.[59]
     - Fabry disease (see Fabry Disease).
     - Moya-moya Disease (see Chap. 18).
     - Sickle Cell Disease (see Sickle Cell Disease).
   (b) Ischaemic stroke observed occasionally.
     - Ehler-Danlos Type 4.
       - Mutation in collagen type 3 gene.
       - Predisposition to arterial dissection and aneurysm formation (see Chap. 15).
     - Marfan Syndrome.
       - Mutation in fibrillin gene.
       - Associated with aortic dissection and valvular heart disease.

- Neurofibromatosis Type 1.
  - Associated with hypertension and moya-moya syndrome (see Chap. 18).
- Familial Hemiplegic Migraine.
  - Mutation in neuronal voltage-gated calcium channel subunit gene.
- Homocystinuria.
  - Autosomal recessive, cystathione beta-synthase deficiency.
  - Associated with carotid artery disease or dissection.
  - Management is dietary, with pyridoxine supplementation and antiplatelet therapy.
2. Genes currently under investigation.[60]
   (a) Phosphodiesterase 4D gene (PDE 4D).
   - Polymorphisms may be associated with increased ischaemic stroke risk in certain populations.
   - Increased association with large artery ischaemic stroke, but not carotid intima media thickness (see Intima Media Thickness).
   (b) 5-Lipoxygenase-activating protein (ALOX5AP).
   - Polymorphisms may be associated with increased ischaemic stroke risk in certain populations.
   - Associated with atherosclerosis and intima media thickness.
   - New genes with possible links to ischaemic stroke are constantly being added to the list.[61,62]

Another emerging area related to stroke where genetics play a role is response to, and toxicity of, medications commonly used in ischaemic stroke patients such as antiplatelet drugs and anticoagulants, i.e., *pharmacogenetics*. For example, several genes associated with variability of warfarin dosing and clopidogrel resistance have been identified and are undergoing intense study.[63] While expanding knowledge of pharmacogenetics may eventually lead to personalized medicine, i.e., individualized choice, dosing and scheduling of drugs based on one's genetics, this approach is not currently recommended.[13]

Haemoglobinopathy

See Sickle Cell Disease.

Heparin-Induced Thrombocytopaenia (HIT)

There are two forms of HIT: HIT Type I may be nonimmune, occurs within 1–3 days of starting heparin, and is usually self-limited (i.e., platelet counts recover while heparin is continued) and without consequence to the patient; while HIT Type II is a serious, potentially life-threatening immune-mediated disease manifested by thrombocytopaenia and platelet activation, and resulting in thrombosis in 20–50% of patients.[64] The immune reaction in HIT Type II is caused by administration of heparins, either unfractionated or low molecular weight, and the resulting antibodies are directed against platelet factor 4 and heparin. The mere presence of antibodies is not sufficient to make the diagnosis of HIT Type II, as in some patients the existence of antibodies has no clinical consequences (Table 17.3). When used without specifying type, the term HIT usually refers to HIT Type II, and this is how the term will be used in the remainder of this section, unless otherwise specified.
1. Incidence: See Table 17.3.[65]
2. Diagnosis of HIT.
   (a) Heparin exposure: Thrombocytopaenia develops 5–10 days after initiation of heparin therapy, although in patients with recent heparin exposure, thrombocytopaenia may occur within 1 day of re-exposure.
   (b) Otherwise unexplained ≥50% drop in platelet count (or to <150 × 109/L).
   (c) Laboratory diagnosis.
   - Two types of assays: antigen and functional assays.
   - Because neither assay has high sensitivity and specificity, both assays should be used in making the diagnosis.
   - Normalization of platelet count when heparin is discontinued.

Table 17.3 Incidence of antiheparin antibodies and heparin-induced thrombocytopaenia

Patient population/risk	Incidence of heparin antibodies (%)	Incidence of HIT (%)
High risk	14	3–5
Unfractionated heparin in the setting of orthopedic surgery		
Intermediate risk	25–50	1–2
Unfractionated heparin in the setting of cardiac surgery		
Intermediate risk	8–20	0.8–3
Unfractionated heparin in general medical or neurologic patients		
Intermediate risk	2–8	0–0.9
Low molecular weight heparin in medical, neurologic, surgical patients		

3. Thrombosis in HIT.
    (a) Occurs in 20–50% of patients; risk is more than 30 times that of control populations; incidence increases with recent surgery or other causes of increased inflammatory response.
    (b) Venous and arterial thromboses.
        • Most common: pulmonary embolism.
        • Myocardial infarction, ischaemic stroke, extremity infarctions can occur.
        • Venous thromboses are more common in medical and orthopedic patients; arterial thromboses in cardiac surgical or vascular surgical patients.
4. Other, less common, manifestations of HIT.
    (a) Venous limb gangrene, skin necrosis, disseminated intravascular coagulation, and anaphylaxis.
5. Management of HIT.[65]
    (a) Goals of therapy in HIT.
        • Decrease risk of thrombosis by reducing platelet activation and thrombin generation.[65]
    (b) Protocol in suspected HIT.
        • Because it is sometimes difficult to initially differentiate the benign self-limited HIT Type I from HIT Type II, all patients with exposure to heparin and thrombocytopaenia should be suspected of having HIT Type II until ruled out with laboratory testing.
        • All forms of heparin, including unfractionated or low molecular weight injections and heparin central and peripheral line flushes, should be stopped.
        • Laboratory tests for HIT, PTT, INR, and liver function should be obtained.
        • An alternative anticoagulant should be started.
            – Either a direct thrombin inhibitor (e.g., argatroban or lepirudin, or bivalirudin if undergoing percutaneous coronary procedures) or a heparinoid should be used.
            – Warfarin should not be started before full anticoagulation with the alternative agent *and* platelet count recovery due to the possibility of warfarin-induced skin necrosis.
    (c) Protocol in confirmed HIT.
        • All forms of heparin should be stopped: unfractionated or low molecular weight injections and heparin central and peripheral line flushes.
        • Thrombocytopaenia *without* thrombosis.
            – Alternative anticoagulant should be continued until platelet counts recover to patient's baseline or stable plateau.
            – Anticoagulation with an alternative agent or warfarin for a further 4 weeks should be considered, as the risk of thrombosis remains high.

Table 17.4 Ischaemic stroke risk with hormone replacement therapy

Clinical study	Relative risk of ischaemic stroke
Heart and Estrogen/Progestin Study (HERS).[70]	1.18 (NS)
Women Estrogen Stroke Trial (WEST).[71]	1.00
Women's Health Initiative (WHI).[72] (estrogen/progestin arm)	1.44[a]

From Bushnell.[73], with permission
[a]Absolute risk of ischaemic stroke in the treatment cohort is low: 8/10,000 women per year of HRT

- Thrombocytopaenia *with* thrombosis.
  - Alternative anticoagulant should be continued until platelet counts recover to >150 × 109/L.
  - Once platelet count recovers, alternative anticoagulant should be continued during the transition to oral anticoagulation with warfarin until the INR is stably within the goal range.
  - Oral anticoagulation should be continued for 3–6 months.
  - Future exposure to heparin should be avoided.

Hormone Replacement Therapy (HRT)

Estrogens are thought to be beneficial in a variety of conditions, from dementia to sepsis. The incidence of ischaemic stroke is lower in premenopausal women compared to age-matched men, and estrogens were found to be neuroprotective in experimental models of ischaemic stroke.[66–69] Early clinical studies (mostly observational and case controlled) suffered from many shortcomings including variable replacement regimens and resulted in conflicting data on hormone replacement therapy in humans. Although recent randomized, controlled clinical trials of HRT did not show benefit and one revealed higher cardio- and cerebrovascular event rates (Table 17.4), further studies are needed to fully understand the cerebrovascular impact of HRT. Selective estrogen receptor modulators such as tamoxifen, raloxifene, and tibolone do not prevent and may, in fact, increase the rate of ischaemic stroke.[13]

1. Ischaemic stroke risk. See Table 17.4.[73]
2. Factors increasing ischaemic stroke risk: conventional ischaemic stroke risk factors.
3. Current recommendations for prescribing hormone replacement therapy and selective estrogen receptor modulators:
   (a) Hormone replacement therapy is not recommended for routine use in prevention of chronic conditions including ischaemic stroke.[13,74]
   (b) Hormone replacement therapy may be considered for use in specific patients for relief of vasomotor symptoms and vaginal atrophy.[75]
   (c) Selective estrogen receptor modulators should not be prescribed for primary prevention of stroke.[13]

Hyperhomocysteinemia

Plasma homocysteine levels >10 μmol/L correlate with increased risk of ischaemic stroke and coronary ischaemia, but results of studies of vitamin administration to reduce stroke risk have been conflicting.[76] Although the hypothesis that lowering homocysteine reduces ischaemic stroke risk requires further study,[77,78] due to low risk and cost of standard vitamin formulations, it seems reasonable to encourage B-complex vitamin use in patients with hyperhomocysteinemia.[13,14]

Hypertension

Hypertension is one of the major risk factors for ischaemic stroke. Multiple clinical investigations and meta-analyses have shown that controlling hypertension leads to reduction in stroke risk.[14,15]

1. Prevalence of hypertension: estimated >70 million Americans and increasing.
2. Classification of blood pressure (BP) ranges.[79]

Diagnosis of hypertension			
	Systolic BP (mmHg)		Diastolic BP (mmHg)
Normal BP	<120	And	<80
Prehypertension	120–139	Or	81–89
Hypertension, stage 1	140–159	Or	90–99
Hypertension, stage 2	≥160	Or	≥100

3. Stroke (ischaemic and haemorrhagic) risk with hypertension.
   (a) Increases with increasing systolic and diastolic BP.
   (b) Antihypertensive treatment is effective in primary and secondary ischaemic stroke prevention.[80]
      • Stroke (including cerebral haemorrhage), nonfatal stroke, combined vascular events: 20–25% reduction.
   (c) Class effects.[80]
      • β-blockers: no effect on stroke risk.
      • Diuretics: 32% reduction in stroke risk.
      • ACE inhibitors: 26% reduction in all vascular events.
      • Diuretics and ACE inhibitors: 40–45% reduction in stroke, MI, all vascular events.
4. Management of hypertension.
   (a) Antihypertensive medications should be used for primary prevention of ischaemic stroke.[79]
      • General goal BP in patients without concomitant diabetes or renal disease: <140/90 mmHg.
      • Goal in patients with concomitant diabetes or renal disease: <130/80 mmHg.
   (b) Antihypertensive medications should be used for secondary prevention in patients with cerebral infarcts or transient ischaemic attack.[14]
      • Timing.
         – In the hyperacute period after ischaemic stroke, BP is naturally increased.
         – Some data suggests that lower blood pressures during the acute phase after ischaemic stroke are associated with increased morbidity and mortality[81–83], although it is not clear that the lower BP is a cause of worse outcomes or simply a consequence of the stroke. However, it is better established that BP > 180 mmHg is associated with poor outcomes.[84] Avoidance of BP extremes seems to be prudent in acute stroke patients.
            • The decision to start antihypertensive therapy and the class of drugs must be individualized (see Sect. 17.7).[12]
            • Deferral of therapy initiation, or prolongation of the time period over which goal BP are reached, may be appropriate in patients with a BP-dependent neurologic examination or intracranial or extracranial arterial stenosis.
      • Optimal BP.[14]
         – Insufficient data to make absolute, one-size -fits-all recommendation.
         – Goals and timing of therapy must be individualized.
         – Initial reduction of 10/5 mmHg with eventual normalization of BP (<120/80 mmHg) is desired.
      • Preferred agents.[79]
         – Unless contraindicated, thiazide diuretics in combination with ACE inhibitors may be good initial agents in patients with TIA or ischaemic stroke.

- Lifestyle changes.[79]
  - Facilitate BP control.
    (a) Weight loss.
    (b) Diet: low sodium, high potassium and calcium.
    (c) Aerobic exercise regimen.
    (d) Limitation of alcohol intake.

Hypercoagulability

See Coagulopathy.

Hyperviscosity Syndromes

Hyperviscosity is a rare cause of cerebral ischaemia. Haematologic conditions in which increased blood viscosity (but also thrombophilia) may play a role in the pathogenesis of cerebral ischaemia include essential thrombocythemia, polycythemia vera, myeloma, leukemia, thrombotic thrombocytopaenic purpura, and Waldenstrom's macroglobulinemia.[85] Sickle cell disease and other haemoglobinopathies affect blood viscosity during crises, but additional mechanisms are also responsible for ischaemic stroke risk (see Sickle Cell Disease). Many conditions including ischaemic stroke are associated with elevated fibrinogen levels. A recent Cochrane review concluded that there are insufficient data on the use of fibrinogen depleting agents in ischaemic stroke, and further studies are required.[86]

Infections

Infections with specific organisms have been implicated in the pathogenesis of atherosclerosis, although data are sparse on treatment of infections as a means of stroke prevention.[87] Infections have also been implicated in ischaemic stroke risk in children: focal (transient) cerebral vasculopathy in children may be parainfectious (see Sect. 17.9. Appendix 1, Paediatric stroke). Minocycline, an antibiotic, may eventually be proven effective in the treatment of acute ischaemic stroke, although its putative mechanism of action may not related to its antimicrobial activity.[88]

Inflammation

Inflammation plays a role in atherosclerosis, as well as in the pathophysiology of acute and subacute ischaemic stroke. Similar to infections discussed, not enough data are currently available to make recommendations on specific screening and anti-inflammatory treatment regimens in stroke prevention (see also C-Reactive Protein).

Intima Media Thickness

Measurement of carotid artery intima media thickness on ultrasonography is currently under investigation as a marker of atherosclerosis, surrogate vascular endpoint, and predictor of ischaemic stroke risk.[89]

Intracranial Vasculopathy

See Chap. 19.

Lipid Disorders

3-hydroxy-3-methylglutaryl coenzyme A (HMGCoA) reductase inhibitors (statins) have been shown to decrease stroke risk in patients with cardiac disease, in a manner related to the degree of LDL cholesterol lowering.[90] Furthermore, withdrawal of statins in the acute phase of ischaemic stroke results in increased mortality and neurologic disability.[91] The recent Stroke Prevention by Aggressive Reduction in Cholesterol Levels (SPARCL) trial was designed to determine whether atorvastatin at a dose of 80 mg daily prevented strokes in patients with previous stroke (ischaemic or haemorrhagic) or TIA and LDL levels 100–190 mg/dL *without* coronary heart disease.[92]

1. SPARCL study.
   (a) Results, at a median 4.9 years of follow up.

SPARCL study results[92]			
Selected outcomes	Atorvastatin, 80 mg (%)	Placebo (%)	*P* value
Nonfatal or fatal stroke[a]	11.2	13.1	0.03
Stroke or TIA	15.9	20.1	<0.001
Major coronary event	3.4	5.1	0.003
Death	9.1	8.9	NS
Rhabdomyolysis	0.08	0.13	NS
Transaminase elevation >3× normal	2.2	0.5	<0.001

[a]Ischaemic *and* haemorrhagic: 67.4% and 65.9% of strokes were ischaemic in the atorvastatin and placebo groups, respectively; there may be a relationship between statin use and increased risk of cerebral haemorrhage, but further studies are required[93]

2. Management of hyperlipidemia in patients with ischaemic stroke.[14]
   (a) Patients with stroke or transient ischaemic attack who are at very high risk for *cardiovascular* disease (those with established cardiovascular disease and multiple risk factors or poorly controlled risk factors or metabolic syndrome.see later or acute coronary events): goal LDL cholesterol <70 mg dL².
   (b) Other patients with ischaemic stroke or transient ischaemic attack.
      • Patients with coronary disease and hyperlipidemia: statin agents, lifestyle modifications to achieve goal LDL cholesterol <100 mg/dL.
      • Patients with LDL cholesterol 100–190 mg/dL and *no* known coronary disease: atorvastatin 80 mg daily (SPARCL).
      • Patients with HDL cholesterol ≤40 mg/dL: consider niacin or gemfibrozil.
3. Mechanisms of statin benefit beyond lipid lowering.[94]

Mechanisms of statin action in the ischaemic brain
Augmentation of collateral flow[95]
Improvement of endothelial reactivity
Anti-inflammatory and antioxidant activity
Stabilization of atherosclerotic plaques
Stimulation of neural progenitor cells (neurorepair)

4. Additional ischaemic stroke risk factors related to lipid metabolism.[14]
   (a) Lipoprotein a: elevation is associated with increased risk of ischaemic stroke.
      • Treatment with niacin may be considered (although effectiveness as far as stroke risk attenuation is not established) in patients with elevation of lipoprotein a; however, control of other risk factors including glucose and LDL should be achieved as well.[13]
   (b) Apolipoprotein a1 (component of HDL): cardioprotective; low levels may increase risk of developing carotid atherosclerosis.

(c) Apolipoprotein b (component of LDL): high levels may be associated with carotid atherosclerosis.

(d) HDL: low HDL cholesterol is associated with an increased risk of vascular ischaemic events.

Malignancy

Patients with systemic cancer harbour conventional, as well as cancer-specific, risk factors for cerebrovascular disease. The cancer-specific risk factor for stroke is most often hypercoagulability.[96]

1. Prevalence of ischaemic stroke in cancer patients: 0.12% of all admissions to Memorial Sloan–Kettering Cancer Center.
2. Traditional risk factors in patients with cancer.
    (a) Hypertension: 53%.
    (b) Tobacco use: 32%.
    (c) Diabetes mellitus: 19%.
    (d) No identified risk factors other than cancer: 15%.
3. Ischaemic stroke mechanisms in patients with cancer.
    (a) Embolic (54%).
        - Atrial fibrillation.
        - Ventricular thrombus.
        - Bacterial endocarditis.
        - Nonbacterial thrombotic endocarditis.
    (b) Nonembolic (46%).
        - Small vessel disease: 12%.
        - Large vessel disease: 10%.
4. Management of stroke risk in patients with cancer.
    (a) Secondary prevention of stroke: antiplatelet agents, anticoagulation in selected patients, antihypertensive drugs, cholesterol-lowering medications, smoking cessation.
5. Prognosis after ischaemic stroke in patients with cancer.
    (a) Median overall survival: 4.5 months.
    (b) Factors affecting survival.
        - Stroke severity.
        - Mechanism: worst for embolic infarcts.
        - Primary cancer: worst for lung cancer.
        - Presence of metastatic disease.

Metabolic Syndrome

Metabolic Syndrome refers to the clustering of vascular risk factors in certain individuals and includes *hypertriglyceridemia*, *low HDL*, *hypertension*, *abdominal obesity*, and *insulin resistance*. Individuals with metabolic syndrome have an increased risk of ischaemic stroke, and management of its components is recommended.[13,97]

Migraine

The relationship between ischaemic stroke and migraine is complex: migraines may be triggered by cerebral infarction; migraines may cause cerebral infarction (*migrainous infarct*); migraine disorders and conventional ischaemic stroke risk factors may coexist in a patient; and patients may have diseases which predispose both to migraines and ischaemic stroke (see CADASIL and Mitochondrial Diseases).

1. Prevalence of migrainous infarcts.[98]
    (a) 0.5–1.5% of ischaemic strokes overall.
    (b) 10–15% of ischaemic stroke in patients <45 years old.
2. Criteria for diagnosis of migrainous infarct.
    (a) Diagnostic criteria.[99]
        - Patient must have previously met diagnostic criteria for migraine with aura.

- One or more symptoms of focal neurologic dysfunction (aura) developing gradually over more than 4 min, lasting less than 60 min with headache occurring before, after, or simultaneously with aura.
  - Current attack similar to typical attacks, but focal neurologic symptoms not reversible and imaging confirms ischaemic infarction.
  - Diagnostic evaluation rules out other aetiologies of cerebral infarction.
3. Ischaemic stroke risk with migraines.[100]

Ischaemic stroke risk with migraine[100]	
Migraine classification	RR (CI)
Migraine, general	2.16 (1.89–2.48)
Migraine with aura	2.27 (1.61–3.19)
Migraine without aura	1.83 (1.06–3.15)
Female migraineurs <45 years old	2.76 (2.17–3.52)
Migraine with oral contraceptive use	8.72 (5.05–15.05)

4. Cerebral ischaemia in patients with migraines.
   (a) Increased risk of ischaemic stroke.[98]
     - Migrainous infarct: probably too infrequent to account for the entirety of increased risk.
     - Vasoconstrictive drugs used for migraine treatment.
       - Conflicting data on triptans and ergots.
     - Association with other stroke risk factors.
       - Patent foramen ovale: Invoked as a cause of migraines *and* ischaemic strokes largely by virtue of association; this hypothesis is currently being investigated (see Patent Foramen Ovale).
       - Cervical vascular dissection: Migraine is more common in these patients, RR 3.6 (1.5–8.6) with a single, and 6.7 (1.9–24.1) with multiple, dissections; the mechanistic connection between migraine and dissection is unclear.
   (b) Migrainous infarct: The mechanism is unknown, but two have been postulated.
     - Neuronal spreading depression during aura is associated with decreased cerebral blood flow sometimes to levels right at, or slightly below, the ischaemic threshold.
     - Transient cerebral arterial spasm during migraine may result in cerebral hypoperfusion.
5. Management of ischaemic stroke patients with migraines.[98]
   (a) Conventional ischaemic stroke risk factors should be fully investigated in migraineurs before diagnosing a migrainous infarct.
   (b) Risk factors in migraineurs with ischaemic stroke should be modified.
     - Smoking cessation.
     - Control of hypertension.
     - Discontinuation of oral contraceptives.
     - Avoidance of triptans and ergots.

Mitochondrial Diseases, Including MELAS

The mitochondrial disorders are a heterogeneous group of hereditary diseases affecting mitochondrial function. Involvement of the peripheral and central nervous systems is common; onset may be at any time during life. *Stroke-like episodes* have been observed in mitochondrial encephalomyopathy, lactic acidosis, stroke-like episodes (MELAS); myoclonic epilepsy and ragged red fibers (MERFF); and Kearns-Sayre Syndrome. Frequently, episodes occur in close temporal association with migraine. Stroke-like episodes are thought to occur due to energy metabolism exhaustion, rather than a vascular cause, resulting in focal neurological deficits. MRI findings are suggestive of a predominant component of vasogenic, rather than cytotoxic, oedema, and lesions are not in typical vascular territories.

1. Prevalence of mitochondrial disease (estimated prevalence near Madrid, Spain): 5.7 per 100,000 in people >14 years old.[101]
2. Approach to diagnosis of mitochondrial diseases.[102]
   (a) Rule out other more common disorders.
   (b) Evaluation in suspected mitochondrial disorders.
   - History: Determine degree of CNS, PNS, and organ involvement, family history.
   - Blood testing: Lactate, pyruvate, hypothalamic-pituitary axis hormones.
   - CSF: Lactate, pyruvate.
   - Imaging: CT (atrophy, basal ganglia calcifications, white matter hypodensities, largely nonspecific); MRI (most common findings discussed earlier); MR spectroscopy (increased lactate peaks).
   - EEG: No pathognomonic patterns, but seizures have been observed in 40–50% of mitochondrial disorders vi. EMG/NCS: normal, myopathic, or combined features may be seen; neuropathy (usually axonal sensory-motor) can be seen in up to 25% of patients.
   - Muscle/nerve biopsy: May yield pathognomonic features.
   - Brain biopsy: Immunohistochemical evaluation may suggest reduced levels of respiratory chain components; electron microscopy may reveal structurally abnormal mitochondria.
   - DNA testing: Various specific mutations in mitochondrial or nuclear DNA have been identified and can be used to make the diagnosis.
3. Management of mitochondrial disease.[102]
   (a) No specific treatments, aside from some symptomatic therapies based on case reports, are currently available.
   (b) Avoidance of drugs which inhibit the respiratory chain, e.g., valproate, barbiturates, tetracyclines, and phenothiazines, seems prudent.
4. Prognosis in mitochondrial diseases.[102]
   (a) Subclinical disorder may appear during times of mitochondrial stress, e.g., infection.
   (b) Course is usually progressive once disease becomes clinically apparent, with eventual multiorgan involvement and death.
   (c) Death in patients with mitochondrial disease with CNS manifestations is usually in the third decade.[101]

Moya-Moya Disease and Syndrome

See Chap. 18; see also Sickle Cell Disease.

Nutrition

Diets high in sodium may exacerbate hypertension; diets high in carbohydrates may worsen blood glucose control in patients with diabetes; and overeating may lead to obesity (see Obesity). Thus, nutritional counseling should be offered to ischaemic stroke patients, especially those harbouring multiple ischaemic stroke risk factors. Nutritional goals include reduced sodium and increased potassium intake; increased intake of fruits and vegetables; use of low-fat dairy products; and reduced intake of saturated fat.[13]

Obesity

Obesity rates continue to increase in the US: 66.3% of adults are overweight or obese. Obesity is associated with well-established risk factors for ischaemic stroke including hypertension and diabetes, and obese patients have increased stroke mortality. While there are no studies showing that weight reduction is beneficial in reducing stroke risk per se, weight reduction lowers blood pressure and blood glucose.[13,14]

AHA 2006 Recommendation[15]
In patients with ischaemic stroke or TIA, weight reduction to a goal of 18.5–24.9 kg/m² Body Mass Index is recommended.

Obstructive Sleep Apnea

Obstructive sleep apnea is the most common sleep-disordered breathing disorder and is characterized by repetitive episodes of upper airway obstruction during sleep, during which arterial oxygen levels may decrease and carbon dioxide levels may increase. Awakening during these episodes is associated with resumption of respiration and transient elevations in blood pressure. Sleep-disordered breathing and, specifically obstructive sleep apnea, have been increasingly recognized as conditions which coexists with, and may cause or exacerbate, other medical conditions, including hypertension, pulmonary hypertension, diabetes mellitus, and gastroesophageal reflux disease.[103]

Obstructive sleep apnea and stroke are strongly associated, and the disorder is common among patients with acute ischaemic stroke.[104] It may increase stroke risk indirectly by exacerbating systemic hypertension or directly through effects on the cerebral vasculature. It is hypothesized that hypercapnea and hypoxia during apneic episodes may over time affect cerebral vasoreactivity and cause endothelial dysfunction and platelet activation. Whether use of continuous positive airway pressure (CPAP) affects stroke risk, recovery or mortality after stroke is currently under investigation. CPAP should be used cautiously in acute stroke patients, especially in those who are at risk of aspiration.

Oral Contraceptives (OCP)

OCP are associated with increased stroke risk.[73,105] The level of risk at any one time in any one patient may be influenced by: formulation (estrogen or progestin or combination; specific dose and type of estrogen or progestin); duration of use; current vs. remote use; and associated conditions (see later).
1. Stroke risk probably results from OCP-related hypercoagulable state, hypertension, and/or alteration of lipid metabolism.
2. Mechanisms of cerebral ischaemia with OCP.
    (a) Venous thrombosis and embolism.
        • Paradoxical embolism.
        • Cerebral sinus or venous thrombosis.
    (b) Arterial thrombosis.
        Related to hypertension and/or alteration of lipid metabolism.
3. Level of ischaemic stroke risk with OCP use.[105]
    (a) Definitions.
        • High-dose estrogen: ≥50 μg.
        • Low-dose estrogen: <50 μg.
    (b) Role of progestin OCP.
        • Conflicting stroke risk data for estrogen- and progestin-containing OCP.
        • Possibly lower risk with progestin-only OCP compared to estrogen-only or combined OCP.
    (c) Ischaemic stroke rates in women of child-bearing age.
        • Compiled from meta-analyses.

Ischaemic stroke risk with oral contraceptive use[105]	
	Incidence of ischaemic stroke
Women of child-bearing age *without* OCP use	4.4/100,000
Women of child-bearing age using OCP	8.5/100,000 NNH = 1 ischaemic stroke/24,000 women treated with OCP

4. Conditions elevating stroke risk in OCP users include hypertension, cigarette smoking, migraines, and age >35 years old.
5. Prescribing guidelines for OCP.
    (a) Several professional organizations including World Health Organization and the AHA have released OCP-prescribing guidelines.
    (b) The American College of Obstetrics and Gynecology's Practice Bulletin (2006) presents a comprehensive, measured approach to prescribing OCP on a case-by-case basis to women with coexisting medical conditions which elevate stroke risk.[106]

Patent Foramen Ovale (PFO)

The relationship between cardiac septal abnormalities and cerebral ischaemia is controversial. Of septal abnormalities found in adults, PFO is the most common[18], and a higher incidence of PFO in young patients with cryptogenic ischaemic stroke generated the hypothesis that PFO is causal in ischaemic stroke. Recently, PFO was also found to be more prevalent in older (≥55 years old) patients with cryptogenic ischaemic stroke.[107] Unfortunately, many physicians have accepted this hypothesis as a proven fact (guilt by association) and have advocated PFO closure as a means of stroke prevention. However, PFO closure in patients with recurrent ischaemic stroke despite medical therapy is currently under investigation.

1. Prevalence of PFO.[107]
    (a) Normal population: 20–25%.
    (b) 43.9% in patients <55 years old with cryptogenic ischaemic stroke versus 14.3% in those with stroke from a known conventional cause.
    (c) 28.3% in patients ≥55 years old with cryptogenic ischaemic stroke versus 11.9% in those with stroke from a known conventional cause.
2. Potential mechanisms of ischaemic stroke with PFO.
    (a) Deep venous thrombosis and paradoxical embolism.
        • Rarely proven to be the case in clinical practice.
    (b) Local thrombosis nearby or within the PFO with subsequent embolism
        • Possibly increased by presence of atrial septal aneurysm (ASAN) (see Table 17.5).
    (c) Arrhythmia (most likely AF) and subsequent embolism.
        • Possibly increased by presence of ASAN.
3. Ischaemic stroke recurrence with PFO.
    (a) Prospective registry of patients <55 years old with cryptogenic ischaemic stroke, treated primarily with antiplatelet therapy.[108]
4. Management of PFO.[14]
    (a) Antiplatelet therapy for secondary ischaemic stroke prevention.
    (b) Warfarin sodium for patients with concomitant indications for anti coagulation, e.g., documented hypercoagulable state and/or deep venous thrombosis.
    (c) PFO closure may be considered if ischaemic strokes recur despite maximal medical therapy; otherwise PFO closure should be offered only as part of a clinical trial.
5. Results of a prospective multicenter trial (CLOSURE I) of the STARFlex® (NMT Medical, Boston, MA) PFO closure device showed no difference in stroke or TIA at 2 years between patients with PFO treated medically or with PFO closure.[109] There was a significant increase in major vascular complications and atrial fibrillation in the PFO closure group. Several other trials are ongoing.

Table 17.5 Ischaemic stroke recurrence with patent foramen ovale

	Patients with recurrent ischaemic stroke or TIA (%)			
	1 year	2 years	3 years	4 years
No PFO	3.0	4.7	5.2	6.2
PFO	3.7	4.6	5.6	5.6
PFO + ASAN	5.9	8.0	10.3	19.2

From Mas et al.,[108] with permission

Physical Inactivity

Risk of ischaemic stroke is reduced with moderate physical activity, probably due to beneficial effects on blood pressure, weight, and glucose metabolism.

2011AHA Recommendation[13]
In ischaemic stroke patients, at least 30 min of physical activity appropriate for each individual patient 1–3 times per week is recommended.
2008 Physical Activity Guidelines for Americans.[110]
Goals for adults: at least 150 min of moderate, or 75 min of intense, aerobic activity per week.

Pulmonary Arteriovenous Malformation

Pulmonary AVMs are characterized by direct continuity between pulmonary arteries and pulmonary veins.[111] The vast majority of these lesions are congenital, and 47–80% of these occur in the setting of hereditary haemorrhagic telangiectasia (HHT; aka Osler-Weber-Rendu disease, see Chap. 14). HHT is an autosomal dominant disease with variable penetrance. Pulmonary symptoms depend on the degree of right-to-left shunt. 13–55% of patients are asymptomatic; others present with exertional dyspnea, cyanosis, and clubbing. Some patients experience haemoptysis, and other findings associated with HHT are related to the presence of AVMs in other organs and include epistaxis, melena, and neurological manifestations including migraines, seizures, transient ischaemic attacks, cerebral abscess, and ischaemic strokes. One review of 76 patients with pulmonary AVM showed 37% of them presented with transient ischaemic events and 18% had evidence of stroke.[112] The mechanism of cerebral ischaemia and infection is thought to be paradoxical right-to-left embolism across the AVM. Diagnosis of pulmonary AVM is usually made with contrast-enhanced chest CT or pulmonary angiography. TCD performed with agitated saline may detect right-to-left shunt resulting from AVM.[113] Transcatheter occlusion using detachable coils ("embolotherapy" or embolization therapy) is the treatment of choice; surgical resection is reserved for cases that do not respond to embolization or for which embolization is technically inappropriate.[114]

Right-to-Left Shunt

See Patent Foramen Ovale and Pulmonary Arteriovenous Malformation.

Sickle Cell Disease

Sickle cell disease affects approximately 70,000 Americans. There are four common genotypes, with haemoglobin S homozygosity (HbSS) being most frequent in the US.[115] SCD predisposes to both ischaemic (primarily in children) and haemorrhagic (primarily in adults) stroke. By screening MRI and MRA 46% of SS patients had infarction or atrophy and 64% had evidence of vasculopathy.[116] Up to 22% of children experience *silent infarctions*: MRI lesions consistent with infarct which appear without concomitant clinical symptoms and signs.[117]
1. Incidence of ischaemic stroke in sickle cell disease:[118]
    (a) If TCD velocity in distal ICA or proximal MCA $\geq$200 cm s^2 in untreated patient: 10–13% per year.
    (b) Overall, 7–11% of children with HbSS will have a stroke.
2. Mechanisms of ischaemic stroke in SCD.
    (a) Increased blood viscosity and adherence to the endothelium of sickled cells resulting in occlusion of capillaries.
    (b) Chronic activation of coagulation pathways, including platelet activation.
    (c) Depletion of nitric oxide with subsequent endothelial dysfunction.

(d) Progressive obliterative and proliferative vasculopathy.
- May result in moya-moya syndrome (see Chap. 18) characterized by distal internal cerebral artery and proximal middle cerebral artery stenosis/occlusion with ischaemic stroke due to thromboembolism or haemodynamic insufficiency.
- Secondary angiogenesis, usually within the basal ganglia near the ICA trifurcation, may predispose to haemorrhage in adulthood.

3. Primary prevention of ischaemic stroke in SCD.
   (a) Transfusion.
   - Screening with TCD should commence at 2 years of age;[13] distal ICA/proximal MCA TCD velocity ≥200 cm/s predicts ischaemic stroke risk.
   - Benefit: 92% reduction in stroke risk and normalization of TCD velocities.[119]
     - Goal: Reduce proportion of haemoglobin S to <30% and normalize TCD velocities.
   - Risk: May lead to haemosiderosis, venous access difficulty, and other complications.
   (b) Hydroxyurea.
   - Increases proportion of fetal haemoglobin (HbF).
     - HbF does not incorporate into HbS polymer (less sickling).
     - Increasing HbF decreases proportion of HbS, which is protective.
     - Other beneficial effects: Decrease in white blood cell count and blood rheology; enhanced vascular reactivity.
   - Decreases TCD velocities.
   - Decreases stroke risk.[120]
     - Hydroxyurea/phlebotomy: 5.7 strokes per 100 patient-years.
     - Hydroxyurea with transfusion during hydroxyurea titration: 3.6 strokes per 100 patient-years.

4. Secondary prevention of ischaemic stroke.[115]
   (a) Transfusion.
   - Goal: reduce haemoglobin S to <30% of total and increase total haemoglobin to >10 g/dL.
   - Erythrocytapheresis (exchange transfusion) is the treatment of choice acutely.
   - Manual exchange transfusions and simple transfusions may be utilized chronically.
   (b) Hydroxyurea.
   (c) Haematopoietic stem cell transplantation.
   - Currently under investigation.[121]

5. Ischaemic stroke recurrence.
   (a) As high as 23% of patients treated with transfusion.
   - Fifty-seven percent of patients undergoing simple transfusion.
   - Twenty-one percent of patients undergoing exchange transfusion.

Sickle Cell Trait

Sickle cell trait is heterozygosity to the haemoglobin S and is present in over 300 million people worldwide.[122] The gene is thought to confer a beneficial effect on heterozygotes consisting of a relative resistance to malaria. Sporadic reports exist of stroke in young adults[123] and children[124] with no known risk factors other than sickle cell trait. Children with heterozygous sickle cell trait were found to have parenchymal abnormalities on MRI in 10% and vasculopathy manifesting as tortuosity in 19%.[125] The authors of this handbook have seen vasculopathy producing moyamoya syndrome in some patients with sickle cell trait. One study showed sickle cell trait associated with a 15-fold lower risk of ischaemic stroke but 10-fold higher risk of haemorrhagic stroke compared to those without the gene.[126] However, in general it is thought that those heterozygous for the trait have a normal lifespan and there is not sufficient evidence to suggest that the trait alone represents an independent risk factor for stroke.[122]

Sleep-Disordered Breathing

See Obstructive Sleep Apnea.

Spinal Cord Ischaemia

See Chap. 20.

Tobacco

Smoking tobacco-containing cigarettes increases ischaemic stroke risk independently of other risk factors.[14] This risk decreases to baseline 5 years after smoking cessation. The approach to smoking cessation includes counseling and medications: seven medications have been approved for smoking cessation by the FDA: nicotine patch, gum, lozenges, inhaler, and nasal spray; buproprion SR; and varenicline.[127]

Drugs to help stop smoking: Bupropion and varenicline
Varenicline (Chantix™ in the US and Champix® in Europe, Mexico, and Canada; Pfizer, New York, NY) is a partial agonist of the α4β2 subtype of the nicotinic acetylcholine receptor, which has been shown to improve smoking cessation rates.[128,129] Since its introduction in 2006, varenicline has become more popular than bupropion because of its better side effect profile and greater effectiveness (Table 17.6). It is, however, more expensive, and, recently, evaluation of the Adverse Event Reporting Database showed that varenicline was associated with a much higher rate of depression and suicidality than buprion SR.[130]

Standard varenicline dose is 0.5-mg tablets, 1 tablet once a day for 3 days, then 1 tablet twice a day for 4 days, then 2 tablets twice a day for 12 weeks. If smoking cessation has not been achieved it may be continued for another 12 weeks. Side effects are uncommon but may include nausea, headache, flatulence, and insomnia.[131,132] **Bupropion SR** (Zyban®, GlaxoSmithKline, Research Triangle Park, N.C.) has been shown to effectively improve smoking cessation rates[131,133] by its effect on nicotine craving. Standard dose is 150-mg tablets, 1 tablet once a day for 3 days, then 1 tablet twice a day for 7–12 weeks. Higher doses should not be used for smoking cessation. The patient should follow the instructions in the package insert, and quit smoking after being on Zyban for 1 week, to allow a steady-state blood level to be achieved. Common side effects are dry mouth and insomnia, which are usually self-limited. The most common major adverse effect is seizures, particularly in patients with a history of seizures or other conditions which may lower the seizure threshold.

Table 17.6 Varenicline effect in smoking cessation

Abstinence from smoking at 12 months	OR (CI)
Varenicline versus placebo	3.22 (2.43–4.27)
Varenicline versus bupropion	1.66 (1.28–2.16)

From Cahill et al.,[128] with permission

AHA 2006 Recommendation[15]
All smokers with ischaemic stroke should be counseled on smoking cessation, and smoking-cessation aids including nicotine delivery devices, such as gum and patches, and pharmacologic agents should be recommended.

Valvulopathies

Abnormalities of cardiac valves may lead to ischaemic stroke. Mitral valve prolapse is the most common valvulopathy in adults and is thought to be a cause of cerebral embolism in *rare* patients with cryptogenic stroke. Mitral valve prolapse may also predispose to bacterial endocarditis. Mitral annular calcification may be linked with cardiac conduction abnormalities and is thought to be a risk factor for cardioembolism. Prosthetic mechanical valves are extremely thrombogenic and require life-long anticoagulation with warfarin sodium. Rheumatic mitral valve disease and other valvulopathies may be associated with atrial fibrillation, dramatically increasing the risk of cardioembolism.

1. Ischaemic stroke risk with valvulopathies[14]
   (a) Rheumatic mitral valve disease, recurrent embolism: 30–65%, most within 6 months of initial event.
   (b) Mechanical prosthetic heart valves: 4% per year without anticoagulation; 1% per year with anticoagulation.[134]
   (c) Bioprosthetic valves: 1% per year, risk highest within 3 months of valve replacement surgery.[134]
   (d) The risk of stroke with the various valvulopathies has not been well defined.

2. Management of ischaemic stroke risk in patients with valvulopathies.
   (a) Rheumatic heart disease.
     - Primary prevention.[135]
       – With atrial fibrillation: Life-long warfarin therapy, goal INR 2–3.
       – With mitral or tricuspid stenosis and sinus rhythm with enlarged atrium or atrium with clot: Long-term warfarin therapy, goal INR 2–3.
       – Referral for valve repair.
     - Secondary prevention.[14]
       – Long-term warfarin therapy, goal INR 2–3.
       – Addition of ASA, 81 mg per day, to warfarin in cases of recurrent embolism despite proper warfarin anticoagulation.
   (b) Prosthetic heart valves.[14]
     - Modern mechanical valves.
       – Life-long anticoagulation with warfarin, goal INR 2.5–3.5.
       – Addition of ASA, 75–100 mg per day, in to warfarin in cases of thromboembolism despite proper warfarin anticoagulation.
       – A higher INR goal (3–4.5) may be considered for caged ball or disk valves.[134]
     - Bioprosthetic valves.
       – Primary prevention: If mitral bioprosthetic valve, oral anticoagulation to goal INR 2–3 for 3 months after surgery, then ASA 325 mg per day if in sinus rhythm; same approach may be considered for aortic bioprosthetic valves.[134]
       – Secondary prevention: Long-term warfarin therapy, goal INR 2–3.
   (c) Consider antiplatelet therapy in the setting of valvulopathy with TIA or ischaemic stroke.[14]

Vasculitis

The vasculitidies are inflammatory vasculopathies. CNS vasculitis may be associated with a systemic vasculitis; it can be primary, i.e., isolated to the CNS; or it can be related to a connective tissue disease or another systemic disease process.[136,137] Vasculitidies can be classified according to many schemes, including size of predominantly involved blood vessels (small, medium, or large) or type of pathologic process (necrotizing, immune complex-mediated, granulomatous, etc.).

Classification of selected primary systemic vasculitidies[138]		
Vessel size	**Pathophysiology**	**Examples**
Large (aorta, large arteries)	Granulomatous vasculitis	Giant cell arteritis
		Takayasu arteritis
Medium (arteries, arterioles)	Necrotizing arteritis	Polyarteritis nodosa
Small (arterioles, capillaries, venules, veins)	Vascular immune complexes	Lupus vasculitis, rheumatoid vasculitis
	Rare vascular immune complexes	Wegener's granulomatosis, Churg–Strauss syndrome

CNS involvement with vasculitis generally presents with a prolonged and progressive functional decline, encephalopathy, seizures, and cerebral ischaemic and haemorrhagic lesions.[136,137] Although "vasculitis" is often invoked when interpreting cerebral angiograms showing features characteristic of inflammatory vasculopathy, it is important to keep in mind that the diagnosis of CNS vasculitis cannot be made solely on the basis of angiography. Vasculitis is a pathologic diagnosis; and in the absence of a tissue diagnosis, appropriate clinical history, physical exam findings, CSF, and other laboratory values, along with appropriate imaging,[139] are required to make the diagnosis.

1. Systemic vasculitis.
   (a) Giant cell arteritis (aka temporal arteritis, Horton's disease, Hutchinson-Horton disease).
     • Characteristics.
       – Most common primary vasculitis in adults >50 years old.
       – Perivascular inflammation leads to intimal hyperplasia, usually without thrombosis.
       – Largely extracranial involvement, but 20–50% can present with vision loss or ischaemic stroke.[140]
       – Headache is most common symptom; occurs in 65–75% of patients.[141]
       – Scalp tenderness and jaw claudication may occur and are highly suggestive of the diagnosis.
     • Associated findings.
       – Elevated erythrocyte sedimentation rate (ESR); normal ESR may not be meaningful if clinical suspicion is strong.[142]
     • Diagnostic criteria (3 of 5 required).[141]
       – Age of onset 50.
       – New onset or new type of headache.
       – Temporal artery tenderness or attenuated pulsation.
       – Westergren ESR >50 mm/h.
       – Positive temporal artery biopsy.[138]
     • Management.
       – Immune suppression with corticosteroids.
       – Antithrombotic therapy may be considered in patients with ischaemic stroke.[140]
   (b) Takayasu arteritis (aka pulseless disease).
     • Characteristics.
       – Involves aorta and branches, but intracranial involvement may occur.
       – Media and adventitia thickening leads to stenosis and occlusion.
       – Neurologic symptoms are usually transient (TIA), although cerebral infarcts can also occur.[143]
     • Associated findings.
       – Exacerbation of the disease may be associated with elevations in ESR.
     • Diagnostic criteria (3 of 6 required).[144]
       – Age <40 years at onset.
       – Extremity claudication.
       – Decreased brachial artery pulse.
       – 10-mmHg blood pressure difference between arms.
       – Bruit over subclavian artery.
       – Abnormal arteriogram.
     • Management.
       – Immune suppression with corticosteroids.
       – Cyclophosphamide, azathioprine, methotrexate, or others may be necessary.
   (c) Polyarteritis nodosa (PAN).
     • Characteristics.
       – Most common of the necrotizing vasculitidies.
       – Features destruction of the vessel wall and aneurysm formation.
       – Organs involved include brain, nerves, skeletal muscle, heart, and kidney.
       – Microangiopathic brain involvement is more common than medium cerebral vessel vasculitis.[145]

- Associated findings.
  - Hepatitis may be present.
  - Peripheral nerve involvement is usually a mononeuropathy multiplex (scattered, asymmetric involvement of nerves at multiple sites).
- Diagnostic criteria (3 of 10 required).[146]
  - Weight loss ≥4 kg.
  - Livedo reticularis.
  - Testicular tenderness.
  - Myalgias, weakness, leg tenderness.
  - Mono- or polyneuropathy.
  - Diastolic blood pressure >90 mmHg.
  - Elevation of blood urea nitrogen or creatinine.
  - Hepatitis B surface antibody or antigen positive.
  - Arteriogram with visceral artery aneurysms or occlusion.
  - Biopsy showing granulocytes, or granulocytes and monocytes in the artery wall.
- Management.
  - Immune suppression with corticosteroids.
  - Cyclophosphamide, azathioprine, methotrexate, or others may be necessary.

(d) Wegener's granulomatosis (aka necrotizing granulomatosis with polyangiitis).
- Characteristics.
  - Necrotizing vasculitis.
  - Granulomatous infiltration of the respiratory tract and necrotizing glomerulonephritis.
- Associated findings.
  - Presence of circulating antineutrophil-cytoplasmic antibodies (cANCA).
  - Generalized disease: in addition to lung and kidney involvement, manifests with arthritis, palpable purpura, neuropathy, and rarely cerebral infarction (infarcts may be due to nonbacterial thrombotic endocarditis or cerebral vasculitis).[147]
- Diagnostic criteria (2 of 4 required).[148]
  - Oral ulcers or purulent or bloody nasal discharge.
  - Chest X-ray showing nodules, infiltrates, or cavities.
  - Microhematuria or red cell casts in urine.
  - Biopsy with granulomatous inflammation within or around artery or arteriole.
- Management.
  - Immune suppression with corticosteroids.
  - Cyclophosphamide, azathioprine, methotrexate, or others may be necessary.

(e) Churg–Strauss vasculitis (aka allergic granulomatous angiitis).
- Characteristics.
  - Necrotizing vasculitis.
  - Respiratory system involvement.
  - Rare cerebral infarction due to eosinophilic cerebral vasculitis.[149]
- Associated findings.
  - Eosinophilia, pulmonary infiltrates, nasal polyps, skin rash, and GI disturbances.
- Diagnostic criteria (4 of 6 required).[150,151]
  - Asthma.
  - Peripheral eosinophilia >10% of total white blood count.
  - Peripheral neuropathy due to vasculitis.
  - Transient pulmonary infiltrates.
  - Paranasal sinus abnormalities.
  - Biopsy showing eosinophils around blood vessels.
- Management.
  - Immune suppression with corticosteroids.
  - Cyclophosphamide, azathioprine, methotrexate, or others may be necessary.

2. Primary CNS vasculitis (aka CNS angiitis, CNS granulomatous angiitis, primary angiitis of the CNS, isolated angiitis of the CNS).[136, 152, 153]
   (a) Characteristics.
     • Involvement of cortical and leptomeningeal vessels, usually small arteries.
     • Segmental granulomatous angiitis.
     • T-cell mediated process.
   (b) Clinical features.[152]
     • Slight male predominance (4 M:3 F), onset usually in middle age.
     • Presentation typically subacute, evolving over weeks to months with headache, cognitive decline, encephalopathy, seizures, focal neurologic deficits.
   (c) Diagnostic criteria.[152]
     • Definite.
       – Brain biopsy showing perivascular granulomatous infiltrates.
     • Possible.
       – Arteriogram with vascular beading.
       – Neurologic decline for at least 3 months.
       – Increased CSF protein and leukocyte count
         a. Exclusion of other diseases.
     • Brain biopsy: Although cortical and leptomeningeal biopsy may sometimes be negative (due to missing inflammatory foci with the biopsy needle), it is important to perform it, *especially if the patient is declining and cyclophosphamide therapy is being contemplated*, as biopsy may provide an alternate diagnosis such as intravascular lymphoma.
   (d) Management.
     • Immune suppression with corticosteroids; in some cases cyclophosphamide may be necessary.
3. Secondary CNS vasculitis.[136,137]
   (a) Vasculitis associated with CNS infections.
     • Characteristics.
       – Inflammatory exudates around arteries result in fibrosis and constriction or direct vascular infection/invasion results in lumenal stenosis.
     • Selected infections associated with CNS vasculitis.
       – *Meningo*vascular syphilis (aka Heubner's arteritis) involving small and medium-sized vessels.
       – Basilar meningitis with M. tuberculosis or fungi involving the basilar artery and pontine perforators.
       – Bacterial meningitis with involvement of pial vessels.
       – Human immunodeficiency virus (HIV), although the aetiology may be related to a co-existing infectious agent like varicella zoster (see below).
       – Varicella zoster vasculitis.

Varicella Zoster Vasculitis
Reactivation of latent varicella zoster virus (VZV) usually occurs in patients >60 years old and may or may not cause the characteristic dermatomally distributed rash. In immunocompetent hosts, VZV reactivation in the trigeminal ganglia may sometimes be followed several weeks later by ischaemic stroke. Pathologically, cerebral ischaemia is due to a granulomatous-necrotizing vasculitis of cerebral arteries: usually the internal carotid artery, middle cerebral artery, or anterior cerebral artery. In immunocompromised hosts, VZV reactivation may result in a small vessel vasculitis and concomitant encephalitis and/or myelitis.[90] CSF anti-VZV IgG is a sensitive marker of VZV vasculopathy.[159]

     • Diagnosis of CNS vasculitis associated with infections.
       – HIV testing; evaluation of CSF, including white cell count, red cell count, protein glucose, gram stain and culture, specific viral polymerase chain reaction (PCR) tests, anti-VZV IgG antibody, acid-fast stain, India ink fungal stain, cryptococcal antigen, VDRL as well as bacterial, fungal, and

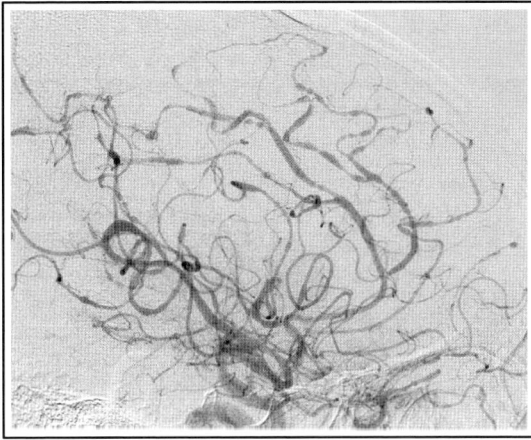

Fig. 17.3 CNS vasculitis. Lateral view of a carotid artery angiogram of a patient with HIV-related CNS vasculitis. Note the widespread characteristic beading of distal arteries that is typical – but nonspecific – for CNS vasculitis. Other conditions (e.g. Call-Fleming syndrome) can look quite similar.

tuberculosis culture. Serum cryptococcal antigen is also a useful test in suspected cryptococcal meningitis. Recently developed interferon gamma release assays have supplemented the tuberculosis diagnostic armamentarium.[154]
- Brain magnetic resonance imaging: cerebral infarction or, less frequently, haemorrhage.
- Cerebral angiography (Fig. 17.3).
- Brain biopsy.
- Management of CNS vasculitis associated with infections.
    - Treatment of underlying infection using appropriate antibiotics at CNS doses.
    - Concomitant corticosteroids.
        (a) Dexamethasone started *prior to* first dose of antibiotic in community-acquired bacterial meningitis improves outcome.[155]
        (b) Steroids used together with antiviral therapy have been used in VZV vasculitis and may be helpful in other similar conditions.[90]
(b) CNS vasculitis associated with connective tissue diseases.
- Characteristics.
    - Inflammatory exudates around arteries result in fibrosis and constriction result in lumenal stenosis.
- Selected connective tissue disorders associated with CNS vasculitis.
    - Systemic lupus erythaematosus (SLE): Autoimmune inflammatory disease which involves multiple organs.

Systemic Lupus Erythaematosus (SLE)
Although cerebral vasculitis is frequently invoked as a cause of cerebral infarction in SLE, it is relatively rare. A seminal study of pathologic specimens from SLE patients showed that true vasculitis with intramural inflammation was present only in 3 of 24 cases.[160] Other, more common, causes of cerebral ischaemia in SLE: noninflammatory cerebral vasculopathy; antiphospholipid antibody syndrome (see Coagulopathy); cerebral microangiopathy due to hypertension; and cardioembolism due to Libman-Sacks endocarditis (see Endocarditis).[161,162]

- Rheumatoid arthritis (RA): A multisystem disorder which can affect the brain by causing a lymphocytic pachymeningitis and arteritis.
- Sjogren's Syndrome: Characterized by keratoconjunctivitis, xerostomia, and a PAN-like vasculitis which may involve multiple organs including the brain; associated with the presence in the blood of Ro (SS-A) and La (SS-B) antibodies, the detection of which can aid with diagnosis.
  - Diagnosis of connective tissue diseases.
    - Clinical and historical evidence of a connective tissue disease.
    - Laboratory evaluation appropriate for suspected condition, including serum rheumatoid factor (RA); SS-A, SS-B antibodies (Sjogren's); antinuclear antibody, anti-DNA antibodies (SLE), and others.
  - Management of connective tissue diseases.
    - Disease specific, usually involving immunosuppression.
- (c) CNS vasculitis associated with drug use.[156]
  - Characteristics.
    - Necrotizing arteritis, similar to PAN.
  - Specific selected agents.
    - Amphetamines: Use may be related to cerebral haemorrhage or ischaemia in the setting of angiographically suggested and histologically proven vasculitis.
    - Cocaine.

Cocaine and Stroke

Cocaine administration by any route predisposes to ischaemic and haemorrhagic strokes. Acute hypertension is thought to be related to haemorrhage especially in the setting of chronic hypertensive vasculopathy or in patients harbouring intracranial aneurysms. Chronic hypertensive vasculopathy, microangiopathy, and acute vasospasm are thought to relate to ischaemic stroke risk. Intravenous use can also predispose to endocarditis. Unlike in cases of amphetamine-related cerebral vasculitis, true cerebral vasculitis in chronic cocaine use has not been frequently demonstrated.[156]

- Heroin and other opioids: Vasculopathy leading to cerebral ischaemia has been observed, although histological proof of an inflammatory aetiology is lacking;[157] endocarditis is another common aetiology of cerebral ischaemia with heroin use.
  - Diagnosis.
    - History, physical exam (needle tracks), urine drug screen.
  - Stroke prevention.
    - Abstinence from drug use.
- (c) CNS vasculitis associated with other selected systemic diseases.[136,137]
  - Behcet's disease: Characterized by oral and genital ulcers, and iritis; the associated vasculitis may involve the brain; treatment is of the underlying disease.[158]
  - Paraneoplastic cerebritis: Perivascular inflammation has sometimes been associated with cerebritis; treatment is of the underlying malignancy.
  - Lymphoma: An associated CNS vasculitis similar to primary CNS vasculitis has been observed; treatment is of the underlying malignancy.

Vasospasm (Aka Vasoconstriction)

The generic term vasoconstriction or vasospasm implies functional contraction of vascular smooth muscle cells. The term implies reversibility, but the length of time during which the vessel is in spasm may be variable, from seconds to days. In neurology, the term *vasospasm* usually refers to the entity observed in patients 7–14 days after aneurysmal subarachnoid haemorrhage. Postsubarachnoid haemorrhage vasospasm is characterized by initial functional arterial contraction resulting in lumenal narrowing, followed by progression to actual structural changes within the arteries: intimal proliferation with progressive lumenal narrowing and, subsequently, necrosis of the tunica media. In a subset of patients, these vascular changes lead to cerebral ischaemia: 5–10% of hospitalized patients with aneurysmal subarachnoid haemorrhage will die from cerebral vasospasm. Subarachnoid haemorrhage and vasospasm are discussed in Chap. 13.

1. Call–Fleming syndrome (aka reversible cerebral constriction, benign cerebral angiopathy, postpartum cerebral angiopathy).[163,164] See also Chap. 13.

   (a) Characteristics.
   - The majority of patients are female; prevalence is low.
   - Presentation is with *thunderclap* headache mimicking subarachnoid haemorrhage; seizures, nausea, vomiting may accompany the headache.
   - Acutely, CT is usually normal and lumbar puncture shows no abnormality; cerebral angiography reveals diffuse arterial lumenal narrowing, sometimes mimicking angiographic findings of vasculitis.

   (b) Associated conditions, possibly precipitating factors.
   - Sympathomimetic and serotonergic drugs.
   - Migraine.
   - Pregnancy/puerperium (aka postpartum cerebral angiopathy).

   (c) Diagnosis

Differentiating Call–Fleming syndrome from CNS Angiitis clinically	
Call–Fleming syndrome	**Primary CNS Angiitis**
Female predominance	Slight male predominance
Sudden onset	Gradual onset
Thunderclap headache	Chronic headaches
Normal sensorium	Altered sensorium
Normal CSF	Abnormal CSF
MRI may be normal[a]	MRI most likely abnormal
Abnormal cerebral angiogram	Cerebral angiogram may be normal
Reversible in 4–12 weeks	Requires prolonged immunosuppressive therapy

[a]In 13 patients, abnormalities included white matter changes (3 patients); infarct (4 patients); subarachnoid haemorrhage (1 patient); and intracranial haemorrhage (2 patients)[164]

   (d) Treatment: No controlled trial data available.
   - In a review of 16 patients, the following therapies were used with very good outcomes.[164]
     – No specific therapy.
     – Calcium channel blockers (usually verapamil).
     – Course of corticosteroids (<6 months).
     – Cytotoxic drugs (minority of patients).
   - Currently, a short course of steroids with or without calcium channel blockers is usually prescribed based on anecdotal experience.[165]
   - If focal neurologic deficits develop: Hypervolemic therapy, haemodynamic augmentation, or balloon angioplasty may be options in select patients.

   (e) Prognosis.
   - In the majority of patients, the course is benign, with resolution of symptoms and angiographic findings over weeks.[164]
   - Ischaemic and haemorrhagic strokes may occur; however, they usually do not result in major disability.

2. Other entities invoked as causes of transient cerebral vascular spasm include: drugs of abuse, direct vascular stimulation during neurosurgical or neuroendovascular procedures, hypertensive emergency, and migraines.

17.5.   Acute Ischaemic Stroke: Clinical Presentation

Cerebral ischaemia (and, thus, neurologic signs and symptoms) may be reversible if the lesion causing decreased cerebral blood flow is treated expeditiously, before brain tissue infarcts. The clinical presentation of acute cerebral ischaemia is variable from patient to patient with respect to the evolution of symptoms over time (temporal classification) as well as specific constellations of symptoms (syndromic classification).

In a recent, prospectively collected database of >2,000 patients with ischaemic stroke, 51% of lesions were located in the middle cerebral artery territory, 13% in typical small vessel territories, 11% in the brainstem, 9% in more than one territory, 7% in the posterior cerebral artery territory, 5% in the anterior cerebral artery territory, and 4% in the cerebellum.[166]

Temporal Classification

Some aspects of the temporal classification of cerebral ischaemia are now obsolete; however, understanding the temporal pattern of symptom evolution is helpful in hypothesizing about the mechanism of cerebral ischaemia and, most importantly, preventing impending or ongoing ischaemia, secondary cerebral injury, and systemic complications of cerebral ischaemia. If a patient experiences a focal neurologic deficit followed by complete remission of symptoms, and the deficit is thought to be ischaemic in nature, i.e., a transient ischaemic attack (TIA), the patient should be *emergently* evaluated, rather than dismissed because he/she experienced *just a TIA*. This kind of patient may have a high stroke risk (see Sect. 17.6). This patient is potentially salvageable once the aetiology of TIA is identified and the underlying lesion treated.

With the emergence of MRI techniques with high sensitivity for cerebral ischaemia, the clinical diagnoses of TIA and acute ischaemic stroke can be readily correlated with imaging. It turns out that many TIA patients have evidence of infarction on DWI imaging in the setting of completely resolved neurologic deficit.[167] Fundamentally, this finding supports the contention that *remitting* and *persisting* deficits in patients, if ischaemic in nature, should be treated equivalently. To reflect this, a clinical term which combines TIA and acute ischaemic stroke has been suggested: *acute ischaemic cerebrovascular syndrome.*[168]

1. Transient ischaemic attack (TIA).
   (a) Acute onset of focal neurologic dysfunction of vascular (ischaemic) origin usually lasting for several minutes and completely remitting.
      - Original definition from 1975 was: "cerebral dysfunction of ischaemic nature lasting no longer than 24 h with a tendency to recur,"[169] but subsequently it became apparent that the majority of TIAs last well under 1 h.[167]
      - New tissue imaging-based definition: transient episode of brain, spinal cord or retinal ischaemia without imaging evidence of infarction.[12]
      - Symptoms occur either because of embolization, local thrombosis, or hypoperfusion and remit because of spontaneous clot lysis and/or increased systemic blood pressure resulting in better cerebral perfusion through collaterals or severely stenotic artery.
      - Differential diagnosis of transient neurologic dysfunction: Cerebral ischaemia, migraine, seizure, postictal paralysis, conversion disorder.
      - Prognosis in TIAs is discussed in Sect. 17.6.
      - Transient global amnesia has sometimes been classified as a TIA, although its aetiology remains a controversial topic.
2. Crescendo TIA.
   (a) Repeated episodes of stereotyped transient focal neurologic dysfunction of ischaemic origin, usually recurring over hours, days, or sometimes weeks.
   (b) Possible mechanism of symptoms and remissions.

Transient Global Amnesia

Transient global amnesia is characterized by sudden onset of anterograde amnesia in association with repetitive questioning such as "where am I?" and "what are we doing?" usually in middle-age individuals. There are no additional neurologic deficits, and the syndrome spontaneously remits, typically in a matter of minutes to hours. In the majority of patients, this syndrome never recurs. Transient global amnesia patients do not have an increased incidence of vascular risk factors, and precipitating events such as sexual intercourse, pain, hot shower, or physical activity have been sometimes documented.[171]

Various hypotheses have been proposed to explain the aetiology of this syndrome, including transient ischaemia, spreading depression, seizures, and venous congestion. The venous congestion mechanism has gained in popularity recently, although it is most likely that the entity has different causes in different subsets of patients.[171–174]

- Repeated embolizations from an unstable proximal (large vessel) plaque with spontaneous clot lysis.
- Repeated bouts of haemodynamic insufficiency in the setting of severely stenotic proximal vessel.
- Repeated local thrombosis and spontaneous lysis in a small, penetrating vessel (see *Lacunar syndromes* section).

3. Reversible ischaemic neurologic deficit (RIND).
   (a) Transient focal neurologic dysfunction of ischaemic origin lasting more than 24 h but resolving completely by 3 weeks.
       - *This term is no longer used in current clinical practice.*

4. Stroke in evolution.
   (a) Progression (worsening) of focal neurologic deficits over hours or days, in the acute period, without return to premorbid baseline or early recovery.
       - Occurs in approximately 30% patients;[170] see Sect. 17.7.

5. Completed stroke.
   (a) Maximal, fixed focal neurologic deficit without remission in the acute period; the deficit may decrease with time and rehabilitation due to synaptic reorganization and other mechanisms of neurorepair.

Syndromic Classification: Large Vessels

Constellations of neurologic signs and symptoms suggest anatomic and vascular localization of a CNS lesion. Vascular supply to the brain is generally stereotyped (see Chap. 1) and, therefore, vascular compromise begets specific patterns of neurologic dysfunction (Fig. 17.4). Specific signs accompanying focal neurologic dysfunction (e.g., carotid bruit or Horner syndrome) may corroborate hypothesized location of a vascular lesion.

Cerebral large vessel syndromes are related mostly to atherosclerotic thromboembolic disease (discussed in Chaps. 18 and 19). Involvement of the most distal branches of the major circulations discussed later may give rise to watershed infarctions, while involvement of the deep, penetrating branches may give rise to small vessel (lacunar) syndromes. The discussion of large vessel and small vessel vascular syndromes is based on *Localization in Clinical Neurology*, by P. W. Brazis, J. C. Masdeu, and J. Biller.[175]

1. Internal carotid artery (ICA).
   (a) General.
       - If Circle of Willis is complete, it gives rise to.
         – Anterior cerebral artery (ACA).
         – Middle cerebral artery (MCA).
         – Anterior choroidal artery.
       - Supplies the majority of the cerebral hemispheres.
       - Occlusion in extracranial (cervical) or intracranial portion is possible.
       - Proximal cervical or intracranial occlusion may be asymptomatic, depending on collateral circulation and rapidity of occlusion.
       - Clinical manifestation of occlusion may be a TIA (may be recurrent), stepwise deficits, progressive deficits, or sudden, fixed deficits.

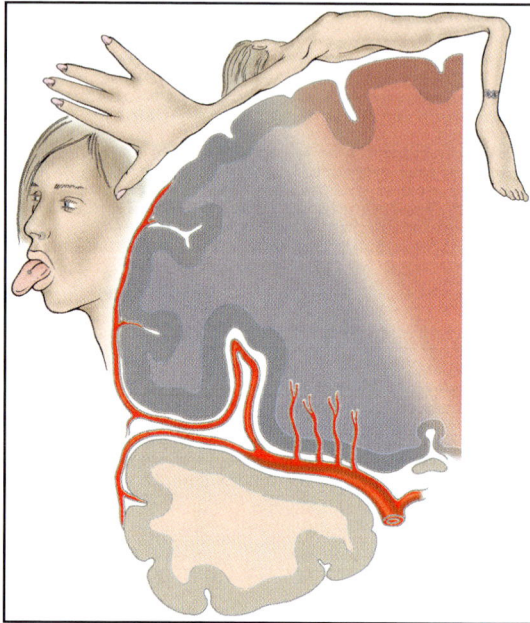

Fig. 17.4 The homunculus. *Pink area* corresponds to the ACA territory; *bluish-gray area* is the MCA territory. Since the lower extremity is functionally represented in cortical tissue perfused by the ACA, infarction of the ACA is likely to result in leg weakness. Similarly, the face and the arm are represented in cortical tissue supplied by the MCA and will be preferentially affected by infarction of the distal MCA.

(b) Clinical ICA syndromes.
- Transient monocular blindness (aka amaurosis fugax).

Transient Monocular Blindness
Acute onset of painless monocular visual loss usually described as a *shade* or *curtain* being drawn or *circumferential* constriction, typically resolving in seconds to minutes. The aetiology is probably an embolism to the ophthalmic artery from a carotid artery plaque, although haemodynamic insufficiency from a high-grade carotid stenosis is also possible.

- Limb-shaking TIA (aka limb-shaking syndrome).

Limb-Shaking TIA
Episodes of rhythmic or arrhythmic involuntary movements of the hand, arm, leg, or any combination thereof. The movements have been described as jerking, twitching, tremulous, trembling, and uncoordinated. There is no *Jacksonian march* (stereotyped spread of dysfunction from the face to the arm and then to the leg or in the opposite direction), and the face is usually not involved. The movements can last for a few minutes and may occur upon arising from a sitting or lying position. The aetiology is thought to be cerebral hypoperfusion of the ACA–MCA watershed region due to a haemodynamically significant proximal carotid artery plaque.[183]

- Variable presentation featuring.
  - MCA syndromes (see later).
  - ACA-MCA Watershed Syndrome (see later).
  - Complete ICA Syndrome combining complete MCA and ACA syndromes.
(c) Findings associated with ICA ischaemic syndromes.
  - Seizures.
    - More likely with involvement of cortical gray matter (e.g., distal or complete MCA syndromes).[176]
    - Seizure rate with ischaemic stroke is approximately 5% across all vascular territories.
  - Carotid bruit.[177,178]
    - Prevalence: 6.4% in men and women >60 years old with systolic hypertension, without previous stroke.
    - General marker of atherosclerosis.
    - Sixty-nine percent of carotid bruits correlate with internal carotid stenosis.
    - Presence of bruit may reflect external carotid turbulence.
    - Absence of bruit is nondiagnostic, e.g., no bruit is evident with complete occlusion.

Horner syndrome
Miosis (small pupil)
Ptosis (eyelid droop)
Forehead anhidrosis[a] (lack of sweating)

[a]Anhidrosis may be absent if the lesion is distal to the carotid bifurcation because interruption of the common or external carotid artery sympathetic fibers is necessary to produce anhidrosis

- Horner Syndrome.
  - Related to a structural lesion of the internal carotid which disrupts the sympathetic fibers traveling alongside it.
  - Dissection or fibromuscular dysplasia of the internal carotid artery may present with Horner Syndrome.
2. Anterior choroidal artery.
  (a) General.
    - Originates from ICA.
    - Supplies posterior limb of the internal capsule, thalamic radiations, optic tract and radiations, and lateral geniculate body.
    - Clinical manifestation of occlusion may be a TIA (may be recurrent), stepwise deficits, progressive deficits, or sudden, fixed deficits (Fig. 17.5).

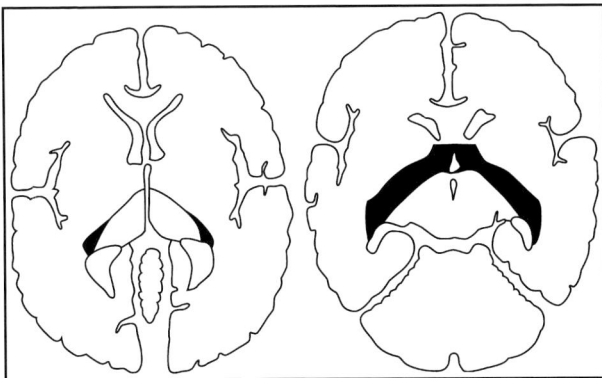

Fig. 17.5 Anterior choroidal artery territory.

(b) Clinical syndromes.

Anterior choroidal artery occlusion	
Involved structure	**Neurologic finding**
Pyramidal tract fibers in the posterior limb of the internal capsule	Contralateral hemiparesis
Superior thalamic radiations in the posterior limb of the internal capsule	Contralateral hemisensory loss
Optic tract, lateral geniculate body, and/or optic radiations	Homonymous hemianopsia or various other visual field deficits

- Unilateral anterior choroidal artery occlusion.
  - Common syndromes: pure motor syndrome, pure sensory syndrome, or ataxic hemiparesis.
  - Rare syndromes: hemineglect or apraxia (if nondominant lesion) or language disturbance (if dominant lesion).
- Bilateral anterior choroidal artery occlusion.
  - Pseudobulbar affect.
  - Mutism, lethargy, neglect.
  - Facial diplegia, bilateral arm and leg weakness/sensory loss.

3. Anterior cerebral artery (ACA).
   (a) General.
   - Arises from the ipsilateral ICA.
   - Sometimes both ACAs arise from one carotid artery or the A1 segment on one side may be hypoplastic.
   - Supplies anterior corpus callosum and parasaggital cortex (Fig. 17.6).
   - Gives rise to the artery of Heubner (aka medial lenticulostriate artery) which supplies anterior limb of the internal capsule.
   - Presentation varies with site of occlusion (proximal vs. distal) and the robustness of Willisian collateral circulation.
   - Clinical manifestation of occlusion may be a TIA (may be recurrent), stepwise deficits, progressive deficits, or sudden, fixed deficits.
   (b) Clinical ACA syndromes.

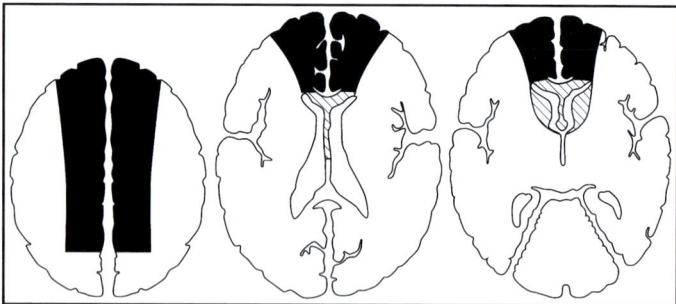

Fig. 17.6 Anterior cerebral artery territory. *Hatched area* corresponds to deep ACA perforators; *solid black areas* indicate the remaining ACA territory.

Anterior cerebral artery occlusion		
Involved ACA branch	Involved structure	Neurologic finding
Hemispheric	Parasaggital motor cortex	Contralateral lower extremity weakness, with possible involvement of the shoulder
Callosal	Anterior corpus callosum	Left arm apraxia[a] (anterior disconnection syndrome); may have contralateral lower extremity sensory loss
Artery of Heubner	Anterior limb of the internal capsule	Contralateral weakness of face and arm without sensory loss

[a]Incapacity to produce purposeful voluntary movement in the absence of sensory or motor deficit

- Additional findings with ACA occlusion.
  - If dominant hemisphere, transcortical motor aphasia (see later).
  - Dysarthria, hypophonia.
  - Abulia (impairment of performance of voluntary actions and/or inability to make decisions), memory impairment, urinary incontinence (especially if bilateral involvement).
  - Transient mild hemiparesis, dysarthria, behavioral deficit (caudate nucleus infarct).
4. Middle Cerebral Artery (MCA) (Fig. 17.7).
   (a) General.
   - The largest branch of the ICA.
   - Supplies majority of cerebral hemispheres and basal ganglia.
   - Most common site of intracranial vascular occlusion: Involved in >50% of all ischaemic strokes.
   - Presentation varies with location of occlusion (stem or proximal MCA vs. superior division vs. inferior division vs. lenticulostriate perforating arteries) and the extent of collateral circulation.
   - Clinical manifestation of occlusion may be a TIA (may be recurrent), stepwise deficits, progressive deficits, or sudden, fixed deficits.

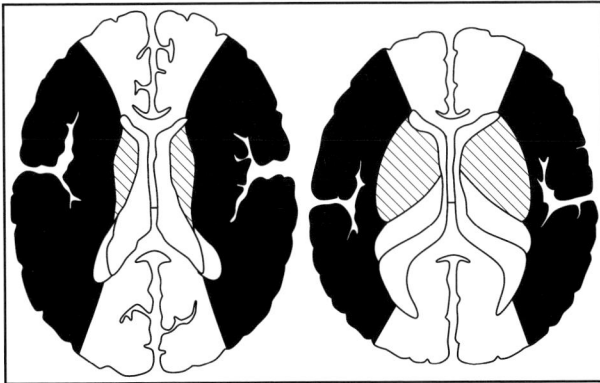

Fig. 17.7 Middle cerebral artery territory. *Hatched area* corresponds to deep MCA perforators (thalamostriates); *solid black areas* indicate the remaining MCA territory.

(b) Clinical MCA syndromes.
- • Complete MCA Syndrome.
  - – Contralateral hemiplegia.
  - – Contralateral hemianesthesia.
  - – Contralateral homonymous hemianopia.
  - – Contralateral visual or sensory neglect.
  - – Gaze deviation and gaze paresis.
  - – "Patient looks at the lesion".
  - – Apraxia.
  - – If dominant hemisphere.
    - (a) Aphasia.[179]

Aphasia classification							
Aphasia type	**Clinical features**						**Lesion location**
	Naming	**Repetition**	**Comprehension**	**Fluency**	**Reading**	**Writing**	
Expressive (Broca)	Poor	Poor	Intact	Poor	Poor	Poor	Frontoparietal operculum
Receptive (Wernicke)	Poor	Poor	Poor	Intact (nonsensical)	Poor	Poor	Inferoposterior perisylvian
Global	Poor	Poor	Poor	Poor	Poor	Poor	Large perisylvian
Conduction	Poor	Poor	Intact	Intact	May be spared	May be spared	Posterior perisylvian
Transcortical sensory	Usually intact	Intact	Poor	Intact (nonsensical)	Poor	Poor	Parietal, temporal, or thalamus
Transcortical motor	Usually intact	Intact	Intact	Poor	May be spared	May be spared	Frontal, striatum

Gerstmann syndrome
Agraphia (inability to write)
Finger agnosia (inability to recognize/name fingers)
Acalculia (inability to calculate)
Right–left confusion

- (b) Gerstmann Syndrome: lesions in the angular and supramarginal gyri
- – If nondominant hemisphere.
  - (a) Anosognosia (ignorance of the presence of disability).
  - (b) Dressing apraxia.
  - (c) Impaired spatial skills.
  - (d) Impaired prosody (intonation).
  - (e) Acute confusional state.
    - • Deep MCA Syndrome: Infarction of territory supplied by lateral lenticulostriate perforating arteries affecting the head of the caudate, anterior limb of the internal capsule, and putamen.
      - – Contralateral hemiparesis (primarily upper extremity).
      - – Aphasia, apraxia, neglect, inattention.
    - • Superficial MCA Syndromes: Infarction of cortical and subcortical regions supplied by distal branches of the MCA with sparing of lenticulostriate perforators; may involve the superficial anterior (superior) territory or superficial posterior (inferior) territory.

Superficial middle cerebral artery syndromes	
Superior (anterior)	**Inferior (posterior)**
Contralateral face and arm weakness and sensory loss	Contralateral homonymous hemianopia
Gaze deviation and gaze paresis: patient "looks at the lesion"	Contralateral visual or sensory neglect
Broca's Aphasia (dominant hemisphere)	Gerstmann syndrome (dominant hemisphere) Wernicke's Aphasia (dominant hemisphere)

- Additional findings in superficial MCA syndromes, especially in nondominant hemisphere: anosognosia, dressing apraxia, impaired spatial skills, impaired prosody, acute confusional state.

5. Posterior Cerebral Artery (PCA) (Fig. 17.8).
   (a) General.
   - Paired PCAs arise from basilar artery bifurcation.
   - Supplies the midbrain, thalamus, and occipital and temporal cortex.
   - Clinical manifestation of occlusion may be a TIA (may be recurrent), stepwise deficits, progressive deficits, or sudden, fixed deficits.
   - Artery of Percheron.
     - Arises from the P1 segment of the PCA.
     - Occlusion results in bilateral thalamic ischaemia and coma.
   (b) Clinical PCA syndromes.
   - Hemispheric PCA branches.
     - Contralateral homonymous hemianopia, sparing the macula.
   - Bilateral involvement of hemispheric PCA branches.
     - Balint Syndrome: bilateral parieto-occipital lesions (including watershed infarcts).

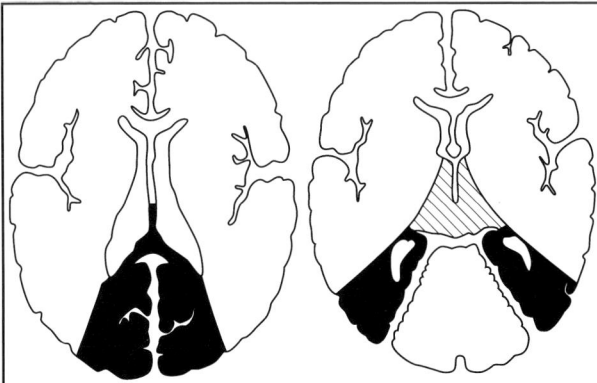

Fig. 17.8 Posterior cerebral artery territory. *Hatched area* corresponds to deep PCA perforators; *solid black areas* indicate the remaining PCA territory.

Balint syndrome
Visual simultanagnosia (inability to recognize the meaning of the whole even though the meaning of the individual parts is understood, also inability to recognize more than one object at a time)
Optic ataxia (impaired visually guided reaching and depth perception)
Gaze apraxia (inability to shift gaze on command)
Decreased visual attention

- Cortical blindness with preserved pupillary reflexes.
- Anton Syndrome (aka denial of blindness): bilateral medial occipital lesions.

Anton syndrome
Cortical blindness
Lack of awareness of blindness
Confabulation about what is "seen"

- Bilateral homonymous hemianopia.
- Visual hallucinations.
- Visual agnosia.
- Color agnosia.
- Prosopagnosia (inability to recognize faces).
- Delirium.
- Confusion.
- Amnesia.
- Callosal PCA branches, dominant hemisphere.
  - Alexia without agraphia (aka pure word blindness): lesion in inferior splenium of the corpus callosum and medial occipital lobe.
  - Color anomia.
  - Object anomia.
  - Contralateral homonymous hemianopia.
- Thalamic branches of the PCA.
  - Pure hemisensory syndrome.
  - Sensorimotor syndrome.
  - Dejerine–Roussy Syndrome.

Dejerine–Roussy Syndrome
Contralateral vasomotor disturbance
Contralateral dysesthesia (thalamic pain)
Contralateral sensory loss
Transient contralateral hemiparesis
Involuntary choreoathetoid or ballistic movements

- Abulia, apathy, disorientation, aphasia if dominant side, alien hand, and neglect if non dominant (anterior thalamus).
- Somnolence, memory loss (paramedian thalamus).
- PCA occlusion can sometimes simulate MCA occlusion; in one series 17.8% of PCA infarcts mimicked MCA infarcts.[180–182]

Posterior cerebral artery occlusion simulating middle cerebral artery occlusion	
Clinical manifestation	**Lesion location**
Contralateral hemiparesis (face, arm > leg)	Cerebral peduncle or posterior limb of the internal capsule
Contralateral hemisensory loss	Ventral posterior thalamic nucleus
Contralateral hemineglect	Centromedian/parafascicular thalamic nuclei
Homonymous hemianopia	Striate cortex or geniculate body
Gaze palsy	Midbrain
Aphasia (if dominant side)	Ventral lateral or pulvinar thalamic nuclei

- Midbrain branches of the PCA: note that the midbrain is also supplied by branches from the BA, SCA, posterior communicating artery, and anterior and posterior choroidal arteries).
  - Weber Syndrome.

Weber syndrome	
Lesion location	**Neurologic findings**
Fascicle of CN III	Ipsilateral pupil-involving CN III palsy
Cerebral peduncle	Contralateral hemiplegia (face-arm-leg)

- Midbrain Syndrome of Foville: Weber Syndrome plus conjugate gaze palsy to the opposite side.
- Benedikt Syndrome.

Benedikt syndrome	
Lesion location	**Neurologic findings**
Red nucleus	Contralateral involuntary movements (tremor, athetosis or chorea)
Fascicle of CN III	Ipsilateral pupil-involving CN III palsy

- Nothnagel syndrome.

Nothnagel syndrome	
Lesion location	**Neurologic findings**
Superior cerebellar peduncle	Contralateral cerebellar ataxia
Fascicle of CN III	Ipsilateral pupil-involving CN III palsy

- Claude syndrome: A combination of Benedikt and Nothnagel Syndromes featuring contralateral asynergia, ataxia, dysmetria, tremor (superior cerebellar peduncle and red nucleus), and ipsilateral pupil-involving CN III palsy (fascicle of CN III).
- Parinaud syndrome (aka dorsal midbrain syndrome, pretectal syndrome, Sylvian aqueduct syndrome, Koeber–Salus–Elsching Syndrome): Most often seen with hydrocephalus or pineal region tumors, but can rarely be observed with infarcts.

Parinaud syndrome
Vertical gaze paralysis
Abnormalities of convergence
Paralysis of accommodation
Convergence–retraction nystagmus
Light-near pupillary dissociation
Lid retraction (aka Collier's sign)
Skew deviation

- Internuclear ophthalmoplegia: May be unilateral or bilateral
- Wall-eyed bilateral internuclear ophthalmoplegia.
- Peduncular hallucinosis: Visual hallucinations, usually very vivid and colorful, involving formed human figures.
- Top of the Basilar Syndrome: Results in variable degree of infarction of the midbrain, thalamus, pons, and temporal and occipital lobes usually secondary to embolus traveling through the basilar, and lodging and/or fragmenting at the PCA origin.

Top of the basilar syndrome
Disturbance of consciousness
Disturbance of memory
Pathologic laughter
Abnormal eye movements including gaze palsies, skew deviation
Pupillary abnormalities
Visual disturbances including Balint and Anton syndromes
Peduncular hallucinosis
Hemi- or quadriparesis and sensory loss

6. Basilar Artery (Fig. 17.9).
   (a) General.
   - Arises from the joining of the two vertebral arteries.
   - Supplies the pons and cerebellum, and bifurcates into the PCAs which supply the midbrain, thalamus, and occipital and temporal cortex.
   - Clinical manifestation of occlusion may be a TIA (may be recurrent), stepwise deficits, progressive deficits, or sudden, fixed deficits.
   - While majority of ischaemic lesions in the brainstem are due to intrinsic perforator (lacunar) disease, BA thrombosis or cardioembolism is one of the most devastating diseases: occlusion of multiple pontine perforating arteries can result in the Locked-in Syndrome in which the patient is awake but unable to move or communicate aside from blinking and vertical eye movements; occlusion of the top of the basilar can result in the Top of the Basilar Syndrome with coma secondary to bilateral thalamic involvement.
   (b) Clinical BA syndromes.
   - Top of the Basilar Syndrome.
   - Penetrating pontine branches.
     - Ventral pontine syndromes: pure motor hemiparesis, dysarthria-clumsy hand, ataxic hemiparesis (see *Lacunar syndromes* section).
     - Paramedian pontine syndromes: variable dysarthria, ataxia, hemiparesis, pseudobulbar palsy (if bilateral involvement).
     - Locked-in syndrome (bilateral ventral pontine infarcts).

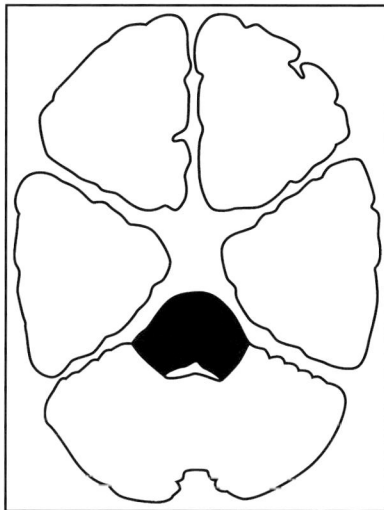

Fig. 17.9 Basilar artery territory.

Locked-in syndrome
Quadriparesis
Aphonia
Paralysis of horizontal eye movements
No disturbance of consciousness
Communication may be possible through vertical eye movements and eye blinking

(c) Other classical pontine syndromes, sometimes observed with infarction.
- • Ventral pons.
  - – Raymond Syndrome: ipsilateral lateral rectus paresis (CN VI fascicles) and contralateral hemiplegia sparing the face (pyramidal tract).
- • Dorsal pons.
  - – Foville syndrome: contralateral hemiplegia (corticospinal tract), ipsilateral peripheral facial palsy (nucleus and/or fascicle of CN VII), and gaze palsy to the lesioned side, i.e., "patient looks away from the lesion" (CN VI and/or paramedian pontine reticular formation.PPRF).
  - – Raymond–Cestan syndrome: ipsilateral ataxia (cerebellum), contralateral sensory loss (spinothalamic tract and medial lemniscus), and sometimes contralateral hemiparesis (corticospinal tract) or paralysis of conjugate gaze toward lesion (PPRF).
- • Lateral pons.
  - – Marie-Foix Syndrome: ipsilateral cerebellar ataxia (cerebellar connections), contralateral hemiparesis (corticospinal tract), contralateral hemisensory loss (spinothalamic tract).

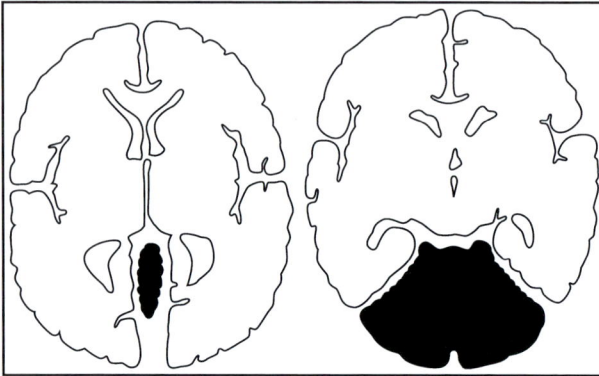

Fig. 17.10 Superior cerebellar artery territory.

7. Superior cerebellar artery (SCA) (Fig. 17.10).
    (a) General.
        • Paired SCAs arise from the distal segment of the basilar artery.
        • Supplies the dorsal surface of the cerebellar hemisphere and vermis, dentate nucleus, middle and superior cerebellar peduncles, and lateral pons.
        • Clinical manifestation of occlusion may be a TIA (may be recurrent), stepwise deficits, progressive deficits, or sudden, fixed deficits.
        • Accounts for 35% of all cerebellar infarcts.
    (b) Clinical SCA syndromes.
        • Dorsal cerebellar infarction.

Superior cerebellar artery syndromes	
Lesion location	**Neurologic findings**
Vestibular nuclei	Vertigo, nausea, vomiting
Medial longitudinal fasciculus and cerebellar connections	Nystagmus
Descending oculosympathetic fibers	Ipsilateral Horner syndrome
Superior cerebellar peduncle and cerebellum	Ipsilateral ataxia and/or intention tremor
Lateral lemniscus	Ipsilateral deafness
Lateral spinothalamic tract	Contralateral trunk and extremity hemisensory loss
Pontine tectum	Contralateral CN IV palsy

8. Anterior inferior cerebellar artery (AICA) (Fig. 17.11).
    (a) General.
        • Paired AICAs arise approximately 1 cm above the basilar artery origin.
        • Supplies anterior surface of cerebellar hemisphere, flocculus, lateral pontomedullary tegmentum.
        • Clinical manifestation of occlusion may be a TIA (may be recurrent), stepwise deficits, progressive deficits, or sudden, fixed deficits.
        • Accounts for 5% of all cerebellar infarcts.

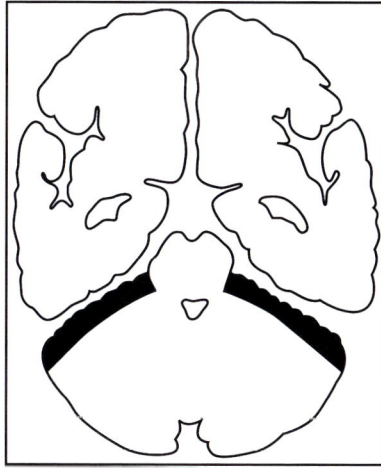

Fig. 17.11 Anterior inferior cerebellar artery territory.

(b) Clinical AICA syndromes.
- Ventral cerebellar infarction.

Anterior inferior cerebellar artery syndromes	
Lesion location	**Neurologic findings**
Trigeminal spinal nucleus and tract	Ipsilateral facial sensory loss
Vestibular nuclei	Vertigo, nausea, vomiting, nystagmus
Lateral pontomedullary tegmentum	Ipsilateral deafness and facial paralysis
Lateral spinothalamic tract	Contralateral trunk and extremity hemisensory loss
Descending oculosympathetic fibers	Ipsilateral Horner syndrome
Middle cerebellar peduncle and cerebellum	Ipsilateral ataxia

9. Posterior Inferior Cerebellar Artery (PICA) (Fig. 17.12).
   (a) General.
      - Arises from intracranial portion of the vertebral artery.
      - Supplies lateral medulla, inferior vermis, inferior cerebellar hemisphere.
      - Clinical manifestation of occlusion may be a TIA (may be recurrent), stepwise deficits, progressive deficits, or sudden, fixed deficits.
      - Accounts for 40% of all cerebellar infarcts.
   (b) Clinical PICA syndromes.
      - Lateral medullary and inferior cerebellar infarction.

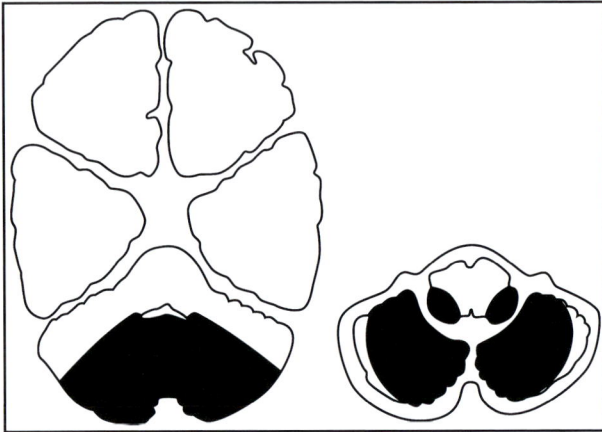

Fig. 17.12 Posterior inferior cerebellar artery territory.

Posterior inferior cerebellar artery syndrome (Lateral Medullary [Wallenberg] syndrome)	
Vestibular nuclei	**Vertigo, nausea, vomiting**
Inferior cerebellar peduncle and cerebellum	Ipsilateral ataxia
Nucleus ambiguous	Dysphagia, dysarthria
Descending oculosympathetic fibers	Ipsilateral Horner Syndrome
Trigeminal spinal nucleus and tract	Ipsilateral facial sensory loss
Spinothalamic tract	Contralateral trunk and extremity hemisensory loss
Dorsal middle medulla	Hiccups
Pons	Diplopia

10. Vertebral Artery.
    (a) General.
        • Clinical manifestation of occlusion may be a TIA (may be recurrent), stepwise deficits, progressive deficits, or sudden, fixed deficit.
    (b) Clinical VA syndromes.
        • Medial Medullary Syndrome (aka Dejerine's Anterior Bulbar Syndrome); note that the medulla is also supplied by the anterior and posterior spinal arteries, PICA, and basilar artery.

Medial medullary syndrome	
Lesion location	**Neurologic findings**
CN XII	Ipsilateral tongue paresis
Pyramid	Contralateral hemiparesis
Medial lemniscus	Contralateral loss of position, vibration sense
Nucleus intercalates	Upbeat nystagmus

11. Watershed territories (border zones).
    (a) General.
        • Definition of watershed: territory supplied by the distal-most branches of the major cerebral circulations. Watershed ischaemic strokes have characteristic appearance on imaging (see Chap. 9, Appendix 1: Primer on imaging in stroke).
        • Mechanism of infarction: haemodynamic, although embolism to the watershed areas, as well as local thrombosis in the setting of decreased flow, is possible.
        • Bilateral or unilateral syndromes are possible: asymmetry results from pre-existing unilateral vasculopathy with stenosis, making the downstream territory more susceptible to hypotension.
    (b) Clinical syndromes.
        • ACA-MCA-PCA watersheds.
            – Bilateral parieto-occipital infarcts with visual field deficits (lower altitudinal), difficulty in visually judging distance, cortical blindness, and/or optic ataxia.
        • ACA-MCA watersheds.
            – Bilateral brachial sensory and motor deficit, sparing lower extremities and shoulders, eventually confined to the hands and forearms, i.e., a variation of the "person in a barrel" syndrome.
        • MCA-PCA watershed.
            – Bilateral parieto-temporal infarcts with difficulties in reading and calculations, cortical blindness, or memory impairment.

Syndromic Classification: Small Vessels

Cerebral small vessel vasculopathy is also referred to as *cerebral microangiopathy*, *penetrating* (or *deep*) *artery disease*, *small vessel disease*, *subcortical white matter disease*, or *lacunar disease*. Long-standing multiple risk factor-related damage to the endothelium of small cerebral arteries results in lipohyalinosis (degeneration of the tunica media and adventitia and subsequent fibrosis). Eventually local thrombosis and occlusion of the vessel may occur, giving rise to an infarct in the territory of the affected small vessel. Another mechanism of local thrombosis is atherosclerotic plaque at arterial branch points, i.e., origins of the penetrating vessels.

A proportion of patients with small vessel ischaemic vasculopathy also harbour cerebral microbleeds and may be at risk for ischaemic and haemorrhagic strokes in the same anatomic distribution, i.e., an *ischaemic-haemorrhagic vasculopathy*. Coexisting ischaemic and haemorrhagic lesions have been observed in cerebral amyloid angiopathy and hypertensive arteriopathy.[184]

1. Lacune.
    (a) Small 0.5–15 mm diameter ischaemic cerebral infarct.
    (b) Territory of small-diameter-penetrating artery to deep brain structures.
    (c) Typical locations, in descending order of frequency.

Locations of lesions causing lacunar syndromes (lacunes)
Putamen
Basis pontis
Thalamus
Posterior limb of internal capsule
Caudate nucleus
Anterior limb of the internal capsule
Subcortical white matter (corona radiata)
Cerebellar white matter
Corpus callosum

2. Lacunar syndromes.

Lacunar syndromes
Pure motor hemiparesis
Pure sensory syndrome
Ataxic hemiparesis
Dysarthria-clumsy hand syndrome

    (a) Pure motor hemiparesis or hemiplegia.
- Unilateral face-arm-leg weakness ± dysarthria.
- Absence of cortical signs.
- Typical lesion locations: internal capsule, corona radiata, basis pontis.

    (b) Pure sensory syndrome.
- Unilateral face-arm-leg numbness ± paresthesias.
- Absence of cortical or motor signs.
- Typical lesion locations.
  - Thalamus (ventroposterolateral nucleus).
  - Corona radiata.
  - Pontine tegmentum (medial lemniscus).
- A small cortical lesion may also cause this syndrome.

    (c) Dysarthria-clumsy hand syndrome.
- Lower extremity weakness, incoordination of the upper and lower extremity, usually no facial weakness.
- Absence of cortical signs.
- Typical lesion locations.
  - Internal capsule.
  - Basis pontis.
- A superficial anterior cerebral artery lesion can also cause this syndrome.

    (d) Ataxic hemiparesis.
- Unilateral facial weakness, tongue deviation, dysarthria, dysphagia, fine motor hand weakness, Babinski sign.
- Absence of cortical signs.
- Typical lesion locations.
  - Basis pontis.
  - Internal capsule.

Clinical Stroke Classification Schemes

Several clinical classification schemas have been developed, primarily for clinical research and quality of care applications. The TOAST Diagnostic Classification is based on the suspected mechanism of cerebral ischaemia and separates patients with ischaemic stroke into five groups: large artery atherosclerosis, cardioembolism, small vessel occlusion (lacunar disease), other determined aetiology, and undetermined aetiology.[185] The Oxfordshire Community Stroke Project Classification assigns the suspected arterial territory based on the clinical syndrome: TAC (total anterior circulation stroke), LAC (lacunar stroke), PAC (partial anterior circulation stroke), and POC (posterior circulation stroke).[186]

17.6.   Acute Ischaemic Stroke: Patient Evaluation

The 2007 AHA Guidelines for the Early Management of Adults with Ischaemic Stroke is a Comprehensive, evidence-based document outlining principles and practical goals for the acute treatment of ischaemic stroke patients.[187] Much of the following discussion, unless otherwise indicated, is based on that reference.

The approach to patients with ischaemic stroke risk consists of: primary prevention; acute assessment and management including intravenous or intraarterial thrombolysis; supportive care including neuroprotection and prevention/treatment of complications during acute presentation; determination of ischaemic stroke aetiology; institution of appropriate secondary prevention; determination of rehabilitation strategy; and commencement of physical and occupational therapy.

Prehospital Assessment of Patients with Acute Cerebral Ischaemia (Stroke or TIA)

The care of the acute stroke patients begins with:
1. Rapid identification of the emergent nature of the complaint by prehospital emergency dispatchers.
2. Appropriate assessment, identification of stroke as a possible cause of the patient's complaint and exam findings, stabilization and management by Emergency Medical Systems providers.
3. Rapid transport to the nearest Emergency Department of an institution that provides acute stroke care.
4. Notification of the receiving institution of the impending arrival of an acute stroke patient in order to rapidly mobilize resources.

In order to facilitate care of acute stroke patients, the Brain Attack Coalition recommended that institutions which have the infrastructure to provide care to uncomplicated stroke patients including thrombolysis with intravenous tPA be designated as Primary Stroke Centers (PSC), and institutions which have the infrastructure for handling complicated cases requiring endovascular procedures, surgical procedures, or intensive care be designated as Comprehensive Stroke Centers (CSC). Admission to PCS and CSC is thought to improve outcomes in patients with stroke.

Selection of TIA Patients for Emergent Cerebrovascular Evaluation

Evaluation of TIA patients, even in the setting of fully resolved deficit, should be expedited and geared toward rapidly identifying aetiology and modifiable, treatable risk factors in order to prevent symptom recurrence.
1. Prognosis during 90 days after emergency department diagnosis of TIA.[188]
   (a) Stroke: 10.5%.
      • 5.3% represented within the first 2 days after TIA.
2. Risk factors associated with stroke recurrence after TIA symptoms.[188]
   (a) Age >60.
   (b) Diabetes mellitus.
   (c) Symptom duration >10 min.
   (d) Weakness.
   (e) Speech impairment.
3. ABCD^2 score for determination of stroke risk within 2 days of TIA.[189]
   (a) Two scores (ABCD and California) had been independently derived to aid in selecting TIA patients with high stroke risk (these patients require emergent cerebrovascular evaluation and treatment, usually necessitating hospital admission).
      • ABCD score predicts risk at 7 days after TIA symptoms.
      • California score predicts risk at 90 days after TIA symptoms.
   (b) ABCD^2, a new, unified score based on the aforementioned aspects, was derived.
      • ABCD^2 score (Age; Blood pressure; Clinical features; Duration; Diabetes).

ABCD² score		
	Clinical feature	**Weight (points)**
A	*Age* 60	1
B	*Blood pressure.* First assessment blood pressure after TIA systolic 140 or diastolic 90 mmHg	1
C	*Clinical features of TIA*	
	Isolated speech impairment	1
	Unilateral weakness	2
D	*Duration of TIA*	
	10–59 min	1
	60 min 10–59 min	2
D²	Diabetes	1

Stroke risk based on the ABCD² score			
ABCD² score	**Stroke risk, 2 days (%)**	**Stroke risk, 7 days (%)**	**Stroke risk, 90 days (%)**
0–3 (low risk)	1.0	1.2	3.1
4–5 (moderate risk)	4.1	5.9	9.8
6–7 (high risk)	8.1	11.7	17.8

Emergency Department Evaluation of Acute Ischaemic Stroke Patients

Patients with acute stroke symptoms should be evaluated *immediately* by individuals trained in the assessment and management of acute stroke patients. The goal is to complete the evaluation, identify candidates for thrombolysis with intravenous tPA, and start treatment within 60 min, i.e., door-to-needle time 60 min.[187]

1. Assess and stabilize the ABCs, obtain vital signs including oxygen saturation.
2. Assess neurologic deficit, perform brief general examination to identify any acute co-morbid conditions.
3. Determine time of symptom onset and whether patient is a candidate for intravenous thrombolysis (see Chap. 9).
4. If not a candidate for intravenous thrombolysis, determine if the patient is a candidate for endovascular rescue therapies (see Chap. 9).
5. Rule out ischaemic stroke mimics: Obtain noncontrast head CT, bedside blood glucose, basic laboratory tests (see later); in a few patients in whom the aetiology of symptoms is not clear or specific nonischaemic conditions are suspected after the initial assessment, perfusion brain imaging, cerebrovascular assessment with ultrasound or angiography, lumbar puncture, or electroencephalogram may be necessary.

General Evaluation of Patients with Cerebral Ischaemia

1. Initial investigation.
   (a) Laboratory testing to rule out metabolic stroke mimics and identify some ischaemic stroke risk factors – this is usually done in the Emergency Department.[187]

Basic laboratory testing in patients with suspected cerebral ischaemia

Laboratory test	...To look for:
All patients	
Chemistry profile	Metabolic derangements
Complete blood count	Infection, polycythemia, thrombotic thrombocytopaenic purpura or heparin-induced thrombocytopaenia
Partial thromboplastin and prothrombin time	Coagulopathy; note that direct thrombin inhibitors or factor Xa inhibitors may not cause abnormalities in routine coagulation tests
Cardiac enzymes	Recent or ongoing myocardial injury
Selected patients:	
Urine and serum toxicology	Drug or alcohol intoxication
Arterial blood gas	Hypercarbia or hypoxia
Hepatic function panel and serum ammonia	Hepatic encephalopathy
Pregnancy test	A bun in the oven

2. Aetiologic investigation.
   (a) Identification of conventional risk factors (usually began in the Emergency Department and continued after hospital admission).

Conventional risk factor evaluation in patients with cerebral ischaemia

Risk factor	Diagnostic approach
Hypertension	Obtain history; physical exam and EKG signs; repeat BP measurements
Diabetes mellitus	Fasting glucose; HbA,C
Hyperlipidemia	Fasting lipid profile
Atrial fibrillation	12-lead EKG; continuous telemetry monitoring; Holter monitor
Myocardial infarction	History; 12-lead EKG; serial cardiac enzyme testing
Smoking (tobacco)	Obtain history; physical exam signs; chest x-ray findings

(b) Evaluation of the extracranial and intracranial vasculature.

Evaluation of extracranial and intracranial vasculature in patients with cerebral Ischaemia

Diagnostic test	PROs and CONs
CT angiography (CTA)	PRO: rapid; usually readily available 24–7; noninvasive; 90% accuracy compared to conventional angiography for internal carotid disease CON: iodinated contrast and radiation (see Chap. 2)
Magnetic resonance angiography (MRA)	PRO: no iodinated contrast; noninvasive; may be used without contrast enhancement CON: lengthy; may not be available 24–7; if performed with contrast, may carry risk of gadolinium-related systemic sclerosis in patients with renal failure (see Chap. 2); turbulence may cause signal drop-out; degree of stenosis may be overestimated
Carotid duplex ultrasound	PRO: rapid; noninvasive CON: operator dependent; compared to conventional angiography, sensitivity and specificity approximately 70%

(continued)

Evaluation of extracranial and intracranial vasculature in patients with cerebral Ischaemia	
Diagnostic test	**PROs and CONs**
Transcranial Doppler ultrasound	PRO: dynamic assessment; can determine direction of collateral flow; rapid; potential for therapeutics; ability to continuously monitor for an extended period in real time; when combined with "bubble" study may detect clinically relevant right-to-left shunts
	CON: operator dependent; may not be able to obtain temporal windows (10–15% of patients); sensitivity lower than conventional angiography.[190]
Conventional angiography	PRO: gold standard; superior resolution; provides collateral vessel assessment
	CON: iodinated contrast and radiation; may not be available 24-7; invasive, carries risk of infarct and other complications (1–2%)

The author of this chapter (AA) prefers contrast-enhanced MRA and ultrasound for the evaluation of the intracranial and extracranial vasculature in patients with acute ischaemic stroke, although she has come to appreciate CT-based imaging more in recent years. The other authors of this handbook (JD and MH) favor CT perfusion and CTA. Both imaging strategies have been shown to provide useful information in a timely manner, and all three authors of this handbook advise the reader to use whichever imaging technology is the most expeditious, reliable, and interpretable in their hands.

(c) Identification of cardiac source of embolism in selected patients.
- Whether echocardiography should be performed in all ischaemic stroke patients or reserved only for those with cryptogenic stroke has been the subject of extensive discussion in the literature.[191–193]

Echocardiography in patients with cerebral ischaemia	
Test	**PRO and CON**
Transthoracic echocardiography	PRO: noninvasive; good ability to image mitral valve and apical region; with "bubble" test, able to detect right-to-left shunts
	CON: poor visualization of aortic arch and atria
Transesophageal echocardiography	PRO: superior ability to assess the aortic arch, valvular vegetations, patent foramen ovale, left atrium and appendage; cost effective
	CON: Invasive; requires sedation (may increase aspiration risk in patients with large infarcts or brainstem infarcts)

- It is the authors' practice to investigate cardiac sources of embolism with TTE with "bubble" test in the majority of patients with cerebral ischaemia. The authors use TEE instead of TTE in young adults and patients with cryptogenic, but suspected to be embolic, cerebral ischaemia. Right-to-left shunts can also be identified using TCD ultrasound[194, 195]

(d) Identification of less common risk factors in patients with cryptogenic stroke.
- Detailed information on less common risk factors and use of specialized diagnostic tests can be found in the Sect. 17.4.

Additional investigations in selected patients with cerebral ischaemia		
Test	**Purpose**	**Comments**
Erythrocyte sedimentation rate	General marker of inflammation	May suggest entities such as giant cell arteritis, other vasculitidies, endocarditis, or systemic infection
Antinuclear antibody	Marker of connective tissue disease	May suggest systemic lupus erythaematosus, Sjogren's syndrome, rheumatoid arthritis, scleroderma, etc.
Rapid plasma reagin	Screening test for syphilis	May suggest meningovascular syphilis

Additional investigations in selected patients with cerebral ischaemia		
Test	Purpose	Comments
Homocysteine	Marker of vascular disease	Although treating elevated homocysteine has not been shown to be protective in stroke prevention, treatment with vitamins is of low risk and cost
Specialized coagulopathy tests	Diagnosis of coagulopathies	See Sect. 17.4, Coagulopathy
Lumbar puncture	Evaluation of infectious, inflammatory, or neoplastic entities	Useful in the diagnostic approach to vasculitis, neoplastic conditions such as lymphoma, and inflammatory conditions such as sarcoid; and for evaluation of subarachnoid haemorrhage
Lower extremity ultrasound	Evaluate for lower extremity thrombus	Useful if a right-to-left shunt is identified and hypercoagulability is suspected

Ischaemic Stroke Evaluation in Young Adults

Although cardioembolism is the most common cause of ischaemic stroke in adults <50 years old, they may still harbour conventional risk factors, and the evaluation should rule these out. Echocardiography (preferably TEE) should be used to investigate the heart, and the cervical and intracranial vasculature should be evaluated for vasculopathy including dissection, moya-moya, and fibromuscular dysplasia. The threshold to evaluate the vasculature with the gold standard, conventional angiography, is generally lower in these patients, especially if no conventional risk factors are identified. In patients with suggestive personal or family history, screening for hypercoagulability and Fabry disease should be performed. See also the Appendix 1: paediatric ischaemic stroke.

17.7.   Acute Ischaemic Stroke: Treatment

The goal of acute treatment of cerebral ischaemia is *rapid reperfusion* in patients who present within the therapeutic window. The overall treatment paradigm for patients with ischaemic stroke consists of:
1. Rapid assessment by a Stroke Team.
2. Acute thrombolysis in selected patients (see Chap. 9).
3. Augmentation of cerebral blood flow and oxygen delivery.
4. Prevention of thrombus extension or re-embolization (i.e., early ischaemic stroke recurrence).
5. Neuroprotection.
6. Prevention and management of neurologic complications.
7. Prevention and management of general medical complications.
8. Secondary stroke prevention.
9. Rehabilitation.

Thrombolysis and Thrombectomy

1. Recommendations and comments.
    a. Intravenous thrombolysis with tPA within 3 h of symptom onset in patients meeting specific criteria (see Chap. 9) was the standard of care until recently when the time window for treatment was extended to 4.5 h based on the ECASS III study.[196] The criteria for 3–4.5 h eligibility are slightly different than for the 0–3 h time window in that they exclude patients >80 years old, those taking oral anticoagulants, those with NIH SS>25, and those with a history of both diabetes and a previous stroke.[197]

b. Intravenous administration of other thrombolytics is considered investigational and should not be offered outside of clinical studies.
c. Endovascular approaches are an option for patients with major ischaemic stroke presenting between 4.5–6 h of symptom onset, and some patients who are within the 0–4.5 h time window but are not candidates for intravenous tPA (see Chap. 9).
d. Approaches to augmentation of intravenous thrombolysis including ultrasonography are currently being investigated in clinical trials.[198]

Augmentation of Cerebral Blood Flow and Oxygen Delivery

Cerebral perfusion is impaired in acute cerebral ischaemia not only due to cessation or decrease in blood flow due to thrombus or embolus, but also due to endothelial dysfunction, increased blood viscosity, increased red blood cell aggregation, decreased red cell deformability, platelet activation, and elevated fibrinogen levels. Cerebral perfusion may be augmented using the following measures.

1. Haemodilution and volume expansion
   (a) Benefits.
       • Improved cerebral blood flow and oxygen delivery.
       • Improved collateral flow to the penumbra.
   (b) Risks.
       • Cardiac and pulmonary adverse events.
   (c) Bottom line for the majority of patients.
       • Not shown to reduce mortality or improve outcome in acute ischaemic stroke.
       • Weight-based maintenance intravenous fluids should be used.
       • Overzealous fluid administration should be avoided.
       • Dehydrated or hypotensive patients may require a greater degree of volume resuscitation.
2. Flat head-of-bed positioning.
   (a) Benefits.
       • Improved collateral flow to the *penumbra* (region of brain in which flow is reduced and metabolic demands are not met but cell death has not yet ensued, i.e., a potentially salvageable area if blood flow is rapidly restored).[199]
   (b) Risks.
       • Respiratory decompensation or aspiration.
   (c) Bottom line for the majority of patients.
       Use acutely unless patient cannot tolerate it due to respiratory dysfunction or high risk of aspiration.
       • Progressively elevate the head on day 2 if the neurologic deficit is stable.
3. Blood pressure (BP) management
   (a) Acute BP management.
       • Transient elevation of BP is extremely common in acute ischaemic stroke.
       • Severe *hypertension* or *hypotension* correlates with worse outcome after ischaemic stroke (see Sect. 17.4, Hypertension).
       • The ideal blood pressure goal in the immediate aftermath of acute ischaemic stroke is not known.
       • Current guidelines allow *permissive hypertension* in the acute stroke period:
         – Lower BP if 220/120 mmHg and no IV t-PA is to be administered.
         – Lower BP if 180/105 and patient received intravenous t-PA (BP must have been lowered to 185/110 *before* treatment with IV t-PA).
         – Lower BP if there is end-organ damage, e.g., myocardial infarction, aortic dissection, pulmonary oedema, etc.
         – Recommended agents: labetalol boluses and/or infusion; nicardipine infusion; sodium nitroprusside infusion if BP elevation is severe or unresponsive to the other agents.

- If BP lowering correlates with worsening of neurologic deficit, therapy should be stopped and BP allowed to rise again.
  - Author's note.
    - Consider lowering BP in patients in whom a large vessel obstruction has been acutely relieved, in order to prevent hyperemia and haemorrhagic conversion of ischaemic lesion.
  (b) Acute *induced* hypertension.
  - Benefits (similar to permissive hypertension).
    - Improved cerebral perfusion to the penumbra.
    - Improved neurologic deficit and outcome.
  - Risks (similar to permissive hypertension).
    - End-organ damage, e.g., myocardial infarction.
    - Worsening of cerebral oedema.
    - Haemorrhagic conversion of ischaemic infarct.
  - Bottom line for the majority of patients.
    - Requires further study.
    - A possible treatment option in special cases in selected patients.
  (c) Chronic BP management.
  - General principles.
    - BP reduction to normal levels reduces risk of recurrent ischaemic stroke (discussed in Sect. 17.4, Hypertension).
    - It is not known exactly how aggressively and when after ictus BP lowering can be safely started.
    - Low-dose antihypertensive medications 1 day after ictus were safe in *mild*-to-*moderate* ischaemic stroke.
  - Author's notes.
    - "One-size-fits-all" approach is probably not appropriate: some patients with haemodynamically significant large vessel lesions which cannot be remedied may require a higher blood pressure in order to perfuse the brain; these patients may still benefit from blood pressure lowering chronically, but in a more gradual fashion.
    - A possible approach to BP lowering: if neurologic deficit is stable and there is no large vessel stenosis, a low-dose ACE inhibitor (unless contraindicated) may be started on day 2 and increased (or a diuretic added) 1 or 2 days later if the neurologic exam remains stable; drugs can then be titrated to achieve normal BP over the next several weeks; patients with haemodynamically significant large vessel stenosis should be approached on a case-by-case basis.
4. HMG CoA reductase inhibitors (statins).
  (a) Improve collateral flow[95] and are currently being investigated as therapy in acute ischaemic stroke.

Prevention of Thrombus Extension or Re-embolization, i.e., Early Ischaemic Stroke Recurrence (Or Why Heparin and Other Blood Thinners Should Be Used Sparingly)

It makes intuitive sense that medications typically utilized chronically to prevent recurrent stroke (secondary stroke prevention), i.e., systemic anticoagulants and antiplatelet drugs, may prevent thrombus extension and/or re-embolization in the acute period of ischaemic stroke. However, at this time, available evidence does not support emergent anticoagulation, loading with antiplatelet agents, double antiplatelet therapy, or the use of intravenous antiplatelet agents in the setting of acute ischaemic stroke.[187]

Anticoagulation and antiplatelet agents are also not proven as adjuncts to intravenous or intra-arterial thrombolysis, and should not be administered within 24 h of thrombolysis.[187] Some experts suggest use of emergent systemic anticoagulation in specific patients, such as those with *minor* infarcts (smaller likelihood of haemorrhagic conversion) and potentially *large territory at risk* in the setting of severe carotid stenosis, atrial fibrillation, free-floating intracardiac or aortic arch thrombus, or basilar thrombosis.[200] Current guidelines, however, reflect the lack of data supporting this practice,[187] and more research is needed on the efficacy and safety of emergent aggressive antiplatelet therapy and acute systemic anticoagulation in selected patients. Fortunately, these questions are currently being addressed in clinical trials.

Global Gem! Global Trends in Clinical Trial Research
Historically, clinical trials have been carried out in relatively wealthy countries in North America and Western Europe. A marked shift has occurred in recent years toward so-called emerging regions, such as Eastern Europe, Latin America and Asia.[201] This is the result of (1) increased research activity in emerging regions, and (2) a decline in clinical research in countries such as the United States and the United Kingdom (Table 17.7). A number of factors are contributing to this trend, including the high cost of clinical trials and stringent regulatory requirements in industrial nations, changing cultural attitudes about human subject research, and economic growth and increasing health care expenditures in developing countries.[202] We are witnessing the gradual decline of western civilization whilst other regions begin to flourish.

Table 17.7   Country trends in participation in biopharmaceutical clinical trials

Rank	Country	Number of sites	Share (%)	ARAGR (%)
1	United States	36,281	48.7	−6.5↓
2	Germany	4,214	5.7	11.7↑
3	France	3,226	4.3	−4.0↓
4	Canada	3,032	4.1	−12.0↓
5	Spain	2,076	2.8	14.9↑
6	Italy	2,039	2.7	8.1↑
7	Japan	2,002	2.7	10.3↑
8	United Kingdom	1,753	2.4	−9.9↓
9	Netherlands	1,394	1.9	2.1↑
10	Poland[a]	1,176	1.6	17.2↑
11	Australia	1,131	1.5	8.1↑
12	Russia[a]	1,084	1.5	33.0↑
13	Belgium	986	1.3	−9.4↓
14	Czech Republic[a]	799	1.1	24.6↑
15	Argentina[a]	757	1.0	26.9↑
16	India[a]	757	1.0	19.6↑
17	Brazil[a]	754	1.0	16.0↑
18	Sweden	739	1.0	−8.6↓
19	Mexico[a]	683	0.9	22.1↑
20	Hungary[a]	622	0.8	22.2↑
21	South Africa[a]	553	0.7	5.5↑
22	Austria	540	0.7	9.6↑
23	China[a]	533	0.7	47.0↑
24	Denmark	492	0.7	9.2↑
25	South Korea[a]	466	0.6	17.9↑

From Thiers et al.[201] Reprinted with permission of Nature Publishing Group
[a]Countries in the emerging regions. ARAGR, average relative annual growth rate. Trial capacity is the number of sites in the country involved in large trials (20 or more sites) divided by the number of large trials in the country. Trial density is the number of recruiting sites on April 12th 2007 divided by the country population in millions

Neuroprotection

Many compounds have been observed in preclinical studies in animals (primarily rodents) to be neuroprotective in acute ischaemic stroke. Disappointingly, most of these compounds have failed in human clinical trials.[203] The reasons for such dismal results are multifactoral, from species differences (rodents vs. humans), to trial design and animal model technical flaws. New strategies for preclinical and clinical testing are needed: one such agent that is currently promising is minocycline.[88] *Presently, however, control of blood glucose and body temperature are the only proven neuroprotective strategies currently available.*

1. Blood glucose management.
   (a) General.[204]
   - Ischaemic stroke patients may be hyperglycemic in the acute period due to underlying diabetes or effects on the hypothalamic-pituitary-adrenal axis, i.e., the *stress response*.
   - Hyperglycemia in the acute period after ischaemic stroke correlates with worse neurologic outcomes (even in patients treated with thrombolysis) and increased morbidity and mortality.[205]
   - Mechanisms of hyperglycemia-related brain injury: proinflammatory effects; anaerobic metabolism with tissue acidosis and free radical formation; blood brain barrier disruption and increased tissue oedema.
   - Hyperglycemia, rather than being causative, may be a marker of larger infarcts and higher disease severity.
   (b) Intensive insulin therapy.
   - Benefit: results in lower mortality and morbidity in ICU patients.
     - Surgical patients, 5 days in the ICU: mortality decreases from 20.2% to 10.6%.[206]
     - Medical patients, 3 days in the ICU: mortality decreases from 52.5% to 43.0%.[207]
   - Mechanisms of benefit: blood glucose lowering and effects independent of blood glucose lowering including vasodilatory, anti-inflammatory, and antioxidant actions.
   - Risk: hypoglycemia-related brain injury, which translates to increased morbidity and mortality in real-world practice.
     - Given the risks associated with intensive insulin therapy, most recent (somewhat controversial) guidelines for general medical and surgical patients suggested blood glucose goals of 140–200 mg/dL.[208]
   (c) Insulin therapy in acute stroke patients.
   - Glucose Insulin in Stroke Trial – United Kingdom (GIST-UK).[209]
     - Insulin infusion for 24 h in acute stroke patients.
     - Failed to prove that lowering blood glucose in hyperglycemic, nondiabetic patients results in improved outcome.
     - Several cautions to conclusions: smaller than planned sample size; mild average blood glucose elevations; BP decrement more pronounced in the study arm; non standardized blood glucose control after the first 24 h
   - Glucose Regulation in Acute Stroke trial (GRASP) trial[210]
     - Showed feasibility and safety of insulin infusion in acute ischaemic stroke patients to achieve glucose control in one of three tiers
     - Hypoglycemia was noted in 30% of patients in the tight control (70–110 mg/dL) group and 4% each in the usual care (70–300 mg/dL) and loose control (70–200 mg/dL) groups
     - This trial was not powered to assess efficacy
   - Bottom line: more randomized, controlled trials of intensive insulin therapy in acute ischaemic stroke are needed.[204]
   (d) Current guidelines for blood glucose control in acute ischaemic stroke.
   - Based on preclinical and observational human data, it is reasonable to propose that patients with ischaemic stroke will benefit from glucose control in the acute period.
   - Suggested goal blood glucose range for patients with acute ischaemic stroke is variable in the literature: some have proposed that blood glucose >140 mg/dL should be treated,[2] while others advocate that treatment should start >180 mg/dL while awaiting results of additional trials.[211]

- Author's notes.
  - The author of this chapter treats blood glucose >160 mg/dL
  - All patients, but especially those with renal failure, low body mass, cachexia, and those who are NPO, should be rigorously monitored for hypoglycemia: Bedside blood glucose measurements should be performed frequently (every 4–6 h for patients not on insulin infusion and every 1 h for patients on insulin infusion), and hypoglycemia should be promptly treated.
  (e) Practical considerations in insulin therapy.
  - Most effective blood glucose control.
    - Insulin infusion (requires ICU admission)
    - Carries risk of hypoglycemia
  - Alternative method in patients with mild hyperglycemia.
    - Early use of scheduled long-acting insulin in addition to sliding scale insulin.
    - Sole reliance on sliding scale insulin is not advised.[212]
2. Temperature management.
  (a) General.
    - Systemic hyperthermia correlates with worse neurologic outcome.[213]
    - Mechanisms of damage: increased metabolic demand, free radical generation, disruption of the blood brain barrier, and potentiation of excitotoxicity.
    - Although no studies in human patients with acute ischaemic brain injury show improved outcomes with treatment of fever, several show worse outcomes with persistent hyperthermia.[214]
    - It makes intuitive sense to seek the aetiology of fever, treat quickly, and maintain normothermia.
  (b) Aetiology of fever in ischaemic stroke patients.

Differential diagnosis of fever in stroke patients
Infection
Urinary tract (especially with indwelling catheter)
Pneumonia (ventilator-associated or aspiration; sometimes may be inflammatory rather than infectious, i.e., *pneumonitis*)
Sinusitis (especially if nasogastric tube is present)
Blood stream (central venous catheter or endocarditis-related)
Ventriculitis/meningitis (especially if intraventricular catheter present; may be aseptic, i.e., chemical, in some cases)
Osteomyelitis (in the setting of decubitus ulcers)
Colitis (e.g., *Clostridium difficile*, especially if history of antibiotic administration)
Cholecystitis, hepatitis, pancreatitis, or peritonitis, etc. (may be inflammatory rather than infectious, especially early in the course)
Abscess
Surgical site infection
Cellulitis
Venous thromboembolism
Deep venous thrombosis
Pulmonary embolism
Drug fever
Transfusion reaction
Gout
Central fever
Diagnosis of exclusion

(c) Induced mild (34°C) hypothermia.
- Protective in hypoxic-ischaemic brain injury in the setting of cardiac arrest.
  - Study 1: Favorable outcome: 75/136 (55%) versus 54/139 (39%), NNT = 6.[215]
  - Study 2: Favorable outcome: 21/43 (49%) versus 9/34 (26%), NNT = 4.[216]
- Can be used as adjunctive therapy to control elevated intracranial pressure.[217]
- Outcome studies in traumatic brain injury and ischaemic stroke are ongoing.
- Risks: cardiac arrhythmia, coagulopathy.
- Guidelines.
  - There are insufficient data to recommend generalized use of induced hypothermia in acute ischaemic stroke patients at this time.[187]

Prevention and Management of Neurologic Complications

1. Neurologic monitoring.
   (a) Treatment with intravenous or intra-arterial thrombolysis usually necessitates observation in a higher acuity setting; some patients with acute cerebral ischaemia who are not candidates for acute thrombolysis may require admission to the ICU for other reasons.

Reasons for ICU admission of stroke patients[218]
Endotracheal intubation – mechanical ventilation
Haemodynamic instability – vasopressor therapy – invasive monitoring
Intensive blood pressure lowering[a]
Marginal[b] neurologic exam – frequent neurologic monitoring
Fluctuating neurologic exam – frequent neurologic monitoring
Acute posterior circulation ischaemia
Large infarct at risk for malignant oedema
After intravenous thrombolysis
After intra-arterial thrombolysis
Increased nursing requirements

[a]In general, blood pressure is not aggressively lowered in the acute period after ischaemic stroke, but exceptions include patients with severe blood pressure elevations, end-organ damage, or status post IV or IA thrombolysis (especially with recanalization)

[b]Marginally responsive patients (GCS 8–9) who may require endotracheal intubation for airway protection or patients with severe dysarthria or dysphagia at high risk of aspiration

(b) Approximately 30% of ischaemic stroke patients worsen clinically during the initial hours to days after ischaemic stroke, and the aetiology of worsening may require specific intervention.[170]
- Early deterioration (≤72 h post ictus): 80.3% from cerebral causes, 19.7% from systemic causes.[219]
- Late deterioration (>72 h): 100% from systemic causes.[219]

Worsening neurologic examination after ischaemic stroke	
Cause	Treatment options
New or ongoing ischaemia	Haemodynamic augmentation; thrombectomy (e.g., mechanical retrieval); augmentation of medical therapy
Cerebral oedema	Endotracheal intubation; osmolar therapy; hemicraniectomy or suboccipital craniotomy
Haemorrhagic conversion	Reversal of coagulopathy (if present); osmolar or surgical therapy if with mass effect
Seizure/status epilepticus	Antiepileptic drug therapy
Concurrent systemic illness	
Urinary tract infection	Antibiotic therapy
Congestive heart failure	Ionotropic therapy
Pneumonia	Antibiotic therapy
Myocardial infarction	Medical and/or interventional therapy
Metabolic abnormality	Correction of abnormality

2. Cerebral oedema and increased intracranial pressure (ICP).
   (a) Incidence of cerebral oedema.
Eight percent of acute ischaemic stroke patients, usually peaking 3–4 days from ictus.
   (b) Characteristics.
      - Cytotoxic oedema, not responsive to corticosteroids.
      - *Malignant* cerebral oedema.
        – May occur as early as 1 day from onset.
        – Usually with complete MCA or ICA infarction, especially if NIH-SS >20; >2/3 MCA territory involved or concomitant ACA or PCA infarct; or DWI lesion >145 mL.
        – May result in brain herniation and death.
      - In cerebellar infarcts, oedema may result in hydrocephalus and brain stem compression.
   (c) Medical management.
- Depends on the rapidity of clinical deterioration and the overall goals of care.
- Mild cerebral oedema without much tissue displacement on head CT or MRI.
   – Serum sodium should be 140–145 mEq L^2.
   – Arterial pCO_2 should be within the normal range, i.e., 35–45 mmHg.
   – Body temperature should be normal.
   Compression of cerebral venous outflow (jugular veins) should be avoided.
   – Head of bed should be elevated at 30° to facilitate venous outflow.
- Severe cerebral oedema.[217]
   – Hyperventilation to pCO_2 goal of 28–35 mmHg is reasonable for the short term while osmolar therapy is being instituted; once other therapies are at goal, pCO_2 should be gently normalized (ideally with concurrent ICP monitoring).
   – Osmolar therapy with hypertonic saline (3% sodium chloride-acetate mix) with initial goal serum sodium of 145–155 mEq L^2; requires central venous access and frequent, usually every 4–6 h, serum sodium monitoring; continuous or bolus therapy can be used.
   – Boluses of mannitol are an alternative therapy.
   – Caution should be exercised in patients requiring haemodialysis: conventional haemodialysis may increase ICP; continuous approaches are preferred.[220]
   – Surgical management (see later).
   – Metabolic suppression with *barbiturates*, *thiopental*, *propofol* or *hypothermia* (temperature goal of 33°C) are options if the patient is not a candidate for surgery.
- Cerebral herniation.[217]

Brain code protocol: treatment of elevated ICP/cerebral herniation	
CSF drainage (if intraventricular catheter, aka external ventricular drain, is present and patent)	Open and/or lower intraventricular catheter to facilitate drainage
Hyperventilation	Open airway
	Hyperventilate: 10–15 rapid bagged breaths; when on ventilator, initial pCO_2 goal 28–35, for no longer than 2–3 h; prolonged hypocapnea results in tachyphylaxis (adaptation); severe degree of hypocapnea may result is decreased cerebral perfusion through cerebral vasoconstriction
	Intubate the trachea (if not already intubated)
Osmolar therapy	Osmolar therapy: mannitol 1 g/kg IV over 15–30 min or 23.4% NaCl[a] IV over 15–30 min
Metabolic suppression	Propofol or thiopental IV injection[b]
Diagnosis	STAT head CT
Surgical management	Neurosurgical evaluation

[a]Available only in specialized Neurointensive Care environments; should be given only through a central venous catheter by a physician familiar with its use; may result in hypotension if given too rapidly

[b]Should only be used in ICU setting by a physician familiar with these agents; if given too rapidly or at too high a dose, serious haemodynamic adverse effects can occur (bradycardia and/or hypotension)

- Can be effectively reversed provided it is recognized early, managed rapidly, and definitively treated.[221]
(d) Surgical management.
  - Medical therapy may only be a temporizing measure, and surgical therapy may be necessary to offer definitive treatment and save the patient's life and neurologic function.
  - Posterior circulation infarction with severe cerebral oedema.
    - Insertion of an intraventricular catheter may relieve acute symptomatic hydrocephalus but will *not* decompress the brain stem.
    - Posterior fossa decompression via suboccipital craniotomy may save the patient's life and minimize injury to the brain stem.
  - Anterior circulation infarction with severe cerebral oedema.

Outcomes at 12 months in malignant middle cerebral artery infarctions[222]		
Modified Rankin scale grade (mRS; see later)	Hemicraniectomy (% of patients)	Medical treatment (% of patients)
2	14	2
3	29	19
4	31	2
5	4	5
6	22	71

- A pooled analysis of three randomized studies of hemi-craniectomy for malignant middle cerebral artery infarction within 48 h of ictus was recently performed.[222]
- Summary of results:
  (a) Significantly fewer deaths with surgery: NNT 2 for survival.
  (b) Significantly fewer survivors with mRS 3 at 12 months with surgery: NNT 4 for the prevention of mRS >3.
  (c) Surgery beneficial in patients *with* and *without* aphasia.

Modified Rankin scale (mRS)	
Grade	Description
0	No deficit
1	No significant disability despite symptoms: able to carry out usual activities
2	Slight disability: unable to carry out all previous activities, but looks after own affairs without assistance
3	Moderate disability: requires help with activities of daily living but able to walk without assistance
4	Moderately severe disability: unable to walk without assistance and unable to attend to bodily needs without assistance
5	Severe disability: bedridden, incontinent, requiring constant nursing care and attention
6	Dead

- Currently, the timing of surgery and patient selection should be individualized, but if decompression is to be performed, it should be done prior to occurrence of irreversible secondary injury.[187,222]

3. Postischaemic stroke seizures.
   (a) Incidence.
   - Two types of poststroke seizures are recognized: *early* (occurring within 14 days of stroke) and *late* (occurring after 14 days).
   - In one study, 5% of patients presenting with stroke (73% with ischaemic stroke) had seizures: 36% were early seizures (25% within the first 24 h); 87% of patients had cortical involvement; 50% had at least one seizure recurrence; recurrence was related to late-onset seizure and occipital location of lesion.[223]
   - Late-onset seizures are more likely to result in epilepsy.[223]
   (b) Management.
   - Prospective data are needed to firmly establish functional effects of poststroke seizures, although worsening neurologic status with repeated seizures has been observed.[176,223]
   - It is unclear whether a single postischaemic stroke seizure requires treatment with antiepileptic drugs (AED), but if patients are treated, control can be achieved with monotherapy in most cases; it is generally agreed that patients with recurrent seizures require treatment with AED.[176]
   - More data are needed regarding appropriate AED for the treatment of poststroke seizures; some agents are neuroprotective in animal studies, but some may impair poststroke recovery and cognition.[176]
   - While no specific AED for use in poststroke epilepsy can be recommended at this time, the most appropriate drug should be used in each individual patient based on the patient milieu, i.e., concurrent medical problems, degree of neurologic disability, and concurrent medications.

Prevention and Management of General Medical Complications

Patients with acute ischaemic stroke, especially the elderly, are at risk for many general medical complications which increase mortality and morbidity and slow neurologic recovery. Some of these complications can be reduced in frequency by early mobilization; however, in some patients who are dependent on collateral flow during the acute phase, upright posture may worsen neurologic status. These patients should be mobilized less rapidly, but should be turned frequently while in bed (to minimize the chance of decubitus ulcers) and treated with prophylaxis against deep venous thrombosis.

1. Infections (especially pneumonia and urinary tract infection).
   (a) Prevention and management.
       - Pneumonia: Early mobilization, pulmonary toilet, early swallowing function assessment; high degree of vigilance for making the diagnosis in the setting of fever; appropriate use of antibiotics; rapid extubation if possible.
       - Urinary tract infection: Whenever possible, indwelling urinary catheters should be avoided or removed as soon as feasible; high degree of vigilance for making the diagnosis in the setting of fever; appropriate use of antibiotics.
2. Deep venous thrombosis (DVT) and pulmonary thromboembolism (PTE).
   (a) Prevalence.
       - Without prophylaxis, DVT can develop in up to 73% of patients with hemiplegia; PTE in up to 20%.[224]
       - With medical prophylaxis, DVT developed in 10–18% of patients with ischaemic stroke who were unable to walk due to lower extremity motor weakness; PTE developed in up to 1%.[225]
   (b) Prevention and management.
       - Mechanical.
         – Use of graduated compression stockings and intermittent pneumatic compression devices decreases the risk of DVT/PTE in a variety of patients, including spinal cord injured and neurosurgical perioperative patients.[226]
       - Medical.
         – Either low molecular weight or unfractionated heparin is generally used.
         – In ischaemic stroke patients, enoxaparin may be more effective at DVT prevention than unfractionated heparin dosed twice daily at no increased risk of major intracranial haemorrhage but increased risk of major extracranial haemorrhage; with enoxaparin, NNT (to prevent one venous thromboembolism) = 13, NNH (to cause one major extracranial haemorrhage) = 173.[225]
       - Combination.
         – Addition of sequential compression devices to subcutaneous heparin prevents more DVT and PTE in stroke patients than heparin alone.[227]
3. Decubitus ulcers (aka pressure sores).[228]
   (a) Prevention and management.
       - Early mobilization in patients who can tolerate upright posture.
       - Frequent turning/repositioning in bed-bound patients.
       - Specialized support surfaces which attenuate pressure on the patient's skin, e.g., special mattresses, mattress overlays, or dynamic support surfaces.
       - Optimization of nutritional status.
       - Treatment of incontinence.
       - Skin care with moisturizer.
4. Falls.
   (a) Prevention and management.
       - Nursing measures to avoid falls.
       - Appropriate use of physical restraints.
       - Prevention and treatment of acute confusional states, maintenance of normal day–night cycle.
5. Dehydration.
   (a) Prevention and management.
       - Hydration and nutrition.
         1. All patients with dysarthria should receive a swallowing evaluation.
         2. Patients in whom swallowing is abnormal may be temporarily fed through a nasogastric tube; some patients may require placement of a percutaneous endoscopic gastrostomy if swallowing function is unlikely to return rapidly.[187]
6. Constipation and fecal impaction.
   (a) Prevention and management.
       - Pharmacologic bowel management regimen.

7. Gastric ulceration (aka stress ulcers).
    (a) Prevention and management.
        • Gastrointestinal prophylaxis with proton pump inhibitors or histamine H_2 receptor blockers is typically utilized in ischaemic stroke patients, especially if they are endotracheally intubated and ventilated.[229] Note that proton pump inhibitors and histamine H_2 receptor blockers are associated with hospital-acquired *C. difficile* infections.[230]
8. Neuropsychiatric disorders.
    (a) Prevention and management.
        • Depression: Occurs in up to 20% patients with stroke and should be managed with antidepressants appropriate for each individual patient.[231]
        • Delirium: Avoidance of CNS-acting medications like benzodiazepines or narcotics; maintenance of normal day-night cycle; high degree of vigilance for making the diagnosis; management with antipsychotic agents if necessary.[232]

Secondary Ischaemic Stroke Prevention

As discussed in this chapter, all patients with acute ischaemic stroke are evaluated to determine stroke aetiology and risk factors for future events. In general, all patients are screened for modifiable conventional risk factors: hypertension, diabetes mellitus, hyperlipidemia, tobacco smoking, cardiac disease, atrial fibrillation, and extracranial and/or intracranial vasculopathy. A summary of general secondary stroke prevention strategies appears later, while risk factor modification is covered in detail in the Sect. 17.4. Extracranial and intracranial atherosclerotic vasculopathy are covered in Chaps. 18 and 19, respectively. Patients in whom conventional risk factors are not identified (i.e., ones with cryptogenic stroke) are usually evaluated further for rare causes of ischaemic stroke. More emphasis on rare causes is placed in adult patients who are <50 years old (see Sect. 17.6, Ischemic stroke in young adults).

Summary of Selected Secondary Ischaemic Stroke Prevention Strategies

1) Antiplatelet therapy
   a) Indicated for noncardioembolic stroke or TIA (see also Chap. 18)
   b) Compared to controls, prevents 36 serious vascular events (non-fatal myocardial infarction, non-fatal stroke, or vascular death) per 1,000 patients during a mean 29 months of treatment.[233]
   c) Current choice of agents: aspirin (50–325 mg/d); or clopidogrel 75 mg/d; or ER dipyridamole 200 mg/aspirin 25 mg twice daily.[12]
   d) Choice of agents should be individualized; e.g., aspirin is less expensive but clopidogrel or dipyridamole/aspirin may provide slightly more risk reduction and different side effects.
   e) *Agents showing promise*: cilostazol and glycoprotein IIb/IIa antagonists.[234]
   f) Combination therapy with aspirin and clopidogrel is not recommended for secondary ischaemic stroke prevention due to lack of efficacy at attenuating stroke rate and severity and increased risk of haemorrhage.[12,235]
   g) Combination therapy with aspirin and clopidogrel may be appropriate in patients with acute coronary syndromes and cardiac and/or cerebrovascular stents.
   h) There is no evidence that increasing the dose of aspirin or changing to another antiplatelet agent is helpful in patients who have an ischaemic event while on antiplatelet therapy, although this is frequently done in actual practice.
   i) Aspirin nonresponsiveness is associated with recurrence of cardio- and cerebrovascular events while on aspirin therapy,[236] but inadequate dosing may play a role.[237]

2) Systemic anticoagulation
   a) Appropriate for patients with cardioembolic stroke risk factors such as atrial fibrillation.
   b) Timing of therapy initiation should be individualized; e.g., anticoagulation may be delayed for 1–2 weeks in the setting of a large infarction, to decrease the risk of haemorrhagic conversion, but may be started earlier in the setting of TIAs or a small infarction.
   c) Not generally recommended for noncardioembolic stroke risk factors, although it may be used in some situations such as arterial dissection or symptom recurrence while on antiplatelet therapy.
3) HMG CoA reductase inhibitors (statins)
   a) Beneficial effects of statins are likely due to mechanisms other than cholesterol lowering.
   b) Statin therapy should not be discontinued in patients presenting with acute ischaemic stroke.
   c) Patients should be warned of side effects and transaminases, creatine kinase, and a lipid panel should be checked prior to and after 1–3 months after therapy initiation.
   d) The appropriate duration of therapy is unknown, but benefits were found after 5 years of therapy.[92]
4) Blood pressure reduction
   a) Hypertension should be treated after the acute phase of stroke.
   b) Choice of agents should be individualized, but ACE inhibitors and diuretics may have particular benefits.
5) Blood glucose management in diabetes
   a) Blood glucose should be tightly controlled using agents appropriate for individual patients.
   b) Efficacy of treatment should be monitored with periodic HbA_1c levels.
6) Smoking cessation
   a) Smoking cessation is not optional in stroke patients.
   b) Comprehensive smoking cessation aids should be used.

A crucial aspect of secondary stroke prevention is education of the patient *and* the patient's family, friends, and caregivers. Education on control of diabetes, hypertension, hyperlipidemia, diet, weight management, and smoking cessation should start in the hospital, because starting patient and caregiver education early is likely to increase medical compliance.

Global Gem! Traditional Chinese Patent Medicine
Traditional Chinese patent medicine consists of herbal medicines used in traditional Chinese medicine. Herbal medicines such as Milk vetch, ma Mailuoning, Ginkgo biloba, Ligustrazine, Danshen agents, Xuesetong, Puerarin, and Acanthopanax have been widely used in China for the treatment of ischaemic stroke for decades.[238] A systematic review of clinical studies of various herbal medicines in this setting, however, found insufficient good quality evidence to make a conclusion about the efficacy of these agents.[239] However, the authors of this review did find enough potential benefit with some of the drugs to justify further randomized trials.

Rehabilitation and Neurorepair

Although more data are needed, it is generally agreed that in order for traditional physical rehabilitation to be effective, it needs to be started early (i.e., during the acute phase in the hospital), be intensive and specific, and last well into the chronic phase.[240] Ongoing investigations in stroke rehabilitation include constraint-induced movement therapy;[241] mechanical aids;[242,243] electrical stimulation;[244] and pharmacologic interventions.[245] Preclinical studies are focusing on stem cell transplantation, as well as pharmacologic enhancement of natural plasticity and stem cell-based neurorepair.[246,247]

17.8.   Acute Ischaemic Stroke: Outcome

Recovery after ischaemic stroke is a dynamic process, but patients generally reach 50% of their maximum recovery within 2 weeks of injury, and 80% of all patients reach their best possible recovery within 4–5 weeks.[240] Factors such as age, sex, medical comorbidities, degree of neurologic (motor and cognitive) disability, as measured by a variety of scales including the Barthel Index (see www.strokecenter.org/professionals/stroke-diagnosis/stroke-assessment-scales/) and the NIH-SS (see Chap. 9), and social factors, affect individual patients' ability to return to work.[248]

17.9.   Appendices

Appendix 1: Paediatric Ischaemic Stroke

Ischaemic stroke trials have typically excluded children, and much of what is currently written about approaches to paediatric stroke patients is based on the standard of care in adults. Mechanistically, what was described for adults more or less holds up in children (29 days to 18 years old), i.e., conditions leading to cerebral embolism and thrombosis may involve the heart, cervical and cerebral arteries, and/or the haematologic system itself, and although the types of specific conditions may be similar, their frequency is different in children. Thus, cerebral vasculopathy from chronic hypertension and atrial fibrillation are uncommon, while congenital heart disease and sickle cell disease are common aetiologies of ischaemic stroke in children. Ischaemic stroke in neonates (<29 days old) are, on the other hand, is more dissimilar: maternal, including placental, diseases and perinatal conditions, including asphyxia and infections, figure prominently.

The approach to paediatric patients with ischaemic stroke risk is similar to what has been discussed in this chapter for adults and consists of: primary prevention; acute assessment and management; supportive care during acute presentation; determination of ischaemic stroke aetiology; institution of appropriate secondary prevention; determination of rehabilitation strategy; and commencement of physical therapy. While the general approach is similar to that in adults, the details are quite different. In acute management, thrombolysis in paediatric acute ischaemic stroke has not been recommended in guidelines primarily because much less is known about its risks and benefits in children, although low level of use of both intravenous and intraarterial thrombolysis has been reported in paediatric patients.[249–251] In the diagnostic evaluation, the determination of appropriate imaging modality in children, perhaps more so than in adults, takes into consideration exposure to ionizing radiation and the need for general anesthesia. And, of course, selection of antithrombotic or anticoagulant medications adheres to paediatric dosing regimens which are typically weight-based, and attention is paid to potential paediatric-specific adverse effects of medications such as Reye's syndrome.[251]

1) Epidemiology
   a) Neonates (<29 days old): 17.8 per 100,000[1]
   b) Children (29 days to 18 years old): range from 1.2–2.4 per 100,000[251,252]
2) Presentation
   a) Neonates: 72% present with seizures, 63% with nonfocal neurological signs.[253]
      i) Median time to diagnosis: 87.9 h from onset.[254]
   b) Children: 22% present with seizures.[255] Associated with seizures: focal deficits, younger age, may have nonconvulsive seizures.[255]
      i) Median time to diagnosis: 24.8 h from onset.[254]
3) Risk factors[1,251,256]
   a) Refer to specific risk factor subsections in the "Acute ischaemic stroke: Conventional risk factors, predisposing conditions, and risk factor modification" section above, as well as other relevant chapters including Chaps. 13, 18, and 19.

b) Neonates
   i) Congenital heart disease
   ii) Coagulopathy
   iii) Maternal risk factors including history of infertility, prolonged rupture of membranes, preeclampsia, chorioamnionitis
   iv) Perinatal infection and asphyxia
c) Children: in up to 30% of cases no risk factor can be identified.[251] Paediatric stroke patients often have more than one risk factor – in one study 52% had multiple risk factors;[256] or a condition may lead to cerebral ischaemia through more than one mechanism, e.g. sickle cell disease with hyperviscosity, arteriopathy, and moya-moya disease
   i) Cardiac disease, 25% of cases: e.g., congenital or acquired heart disease, intracradiac tumors, cardiomyopathy.
   ii) Systemic disease: e.g., sickle cell disease, acute infections, metabolic or mitochondrial disorders, head and neck trauma.
   iii) Cerebral and cervical vasculopathy, 50–80% of cases: e.g., arterial dissection, fibromuscular dysplasia, vasculitis, moya-moya, post-varicella cerebral arteriopathy, focal cerebral arteriopathy of childhood (transient cerebral arteriopathy of childhood).[257,258]
   iv) Hypercoagulable states, 20–50% of cases: e.g., genetic thrombophilias, haemolytic-uremic syndrome, homocystinuria, as well as pregnancy and oral contraceptive use in adolescents.

4) Diagnostic evaluation[251, 259]
   a) Brain tissue imaging
      i) MRI and CT, including perfusion sequences, are available for children as for adults.
      ii) In neonates and young children in whom fontanelles have not closed, ultrasound can be used to assess the brain parenchyma; however, ultrasound is relatively insensitive for detection of ischaemic lesions and evaluation of the posterior fossa.
   b) Vascular imaging (refer also to Sect. 17.6)
      i) MRA may be adequate in most paediatric patients, although it has low sensitivity for distal vasculature.
      ii) Fat-saturated T1 MRI imaging is useful in the evaluation of extracranial vasculature for arteriopathy such as dissection.
      iii) Conventional angiography is reasonable in cases where imaging of smaller cerebral vessel is required or an interventional procedure is anticipated.
      iv) TCD is particularly useful in the monitoring of children with sickle cell disease and screening is recommended starting at 2 years of age.[13]
   c) Cardiac imaging: echocardiogram
   d) Laboratory tests
      i) Thrombophilia screening[259]
      ii) Sickle cell screen
      iii) Additional tests such as prothrombin gene mutation 20210A, activated protein C resistance, Factor V Leiden G1691A mutation, antiphospholipid antibody testing, protein C and S activity, antithrombin III activity, homocysteine level and lipoprotein (a) may be useful.

5) Management[251,260]
   a) Reduce ischaemic stroke recurrence.
      i) Institute appropriate antiplatelet drug or anticoagulate based on results of aetiologic work-up.[261]; employ disease-specific treatments such as transfusion in sickle cell disease and repair of congenital cardiac anomalies.
      ii) Unlike for adults, empiric anticoagulation while evaluating for ischaemic stroke aetiology (if not contraindicated) has been suggested for children because the probability that the ischaemic stroke was due to a condition that will require anticoagulation is higher.
      iii) Antithrombotic medications used in children include aspirin, clopidogrel, warfarin, as well as low molecular weight heparins[262]
   b) Treat seizures: institution of prophylactic antiepileptic medications is generally not recommended.
   c) Maintain supportive care: normothermia, euvolemia, and normoglycemia.

d) Manage blood pressure: although guidelines suggest control of systemic hypertension, specific goals are not proposed.
6) Outcome[1]
    a) Moderate – severe disability: 42%
    b) Recurrence: 10% within 5 years
    c) Mortality: decreased by 19% between 1979 and 1998, but may be still be 3–11%[250]

Appendix 2: Internet Ischaemic Stroke Resources

American Academy of Neurology: http://www.aan.com
American Heart Organization: http://www.americanheart.org
American Stroke Association: http://www.strokeassociation.org
Internet Stroke Center at Washington University: http://www.strokecenter.org
National Stroke Association: http://www.stroke.or

References

1. Lloyd-Jones D, Adams RJ, Brown TM, et al. Executive summary: heart disease and stroke statistics – 2010 update: a report from the American Heart Association. Circulation. 2011;121:948–54.
2. American Heart Association. Heart Disease and Stroke Statistics-2004 Update. Dallas, TX. American Heart Association; 2003, pp. 1–52.
3. Hand PJ, Kwan J, Lindley RI, Dennis MS, Wardlaw JM. Distinguishing between stroke and mimic at the bedside: the brain attack study. Stroke. 2006;37:769–75.
4. Foster JW, Hart RG. Hypoglycemic hemiplegia: two cases and a clinical review. Stroke. 1987;18:944–6.
5. Bladin CF, Alexandrov AV, Bellavance A, et al. Seizures after stroke: a prospective multicenter study. Arch Neurol. 2000;57:1617–22.
6. Sylaja PN, Dzialowski I, Krol A, Roy J, Federico P, Demchuk AM. Role of CT angiography in thrombolysis decision-making for patients with presumed seizure at stroke onset. Stroke. 2006;37:915–7.
7. Selim M, Kumar S, Fink J, Schlaug G, Caplan LR, Linfante I. Seizure at stroke onset: should it be an absolute contraindication to thrombolysis? Cerebrovasc Dis. 2002;14:54–7.
8. Benditt DG, van Dijk JG, Sutton R, et al. Syncope. Curr Probl Cardiol. 2004;29:152–229.
9. Arboix A, Massons J, Oliveres M, Arribas MP, Titus F. Headache in acute cerebrovascular disease: a prospective clinical study in 240 patients. Cephalalgia. 1994;14:37–40.
10. Amarenco P. Underlying pathology of stroke of unknown cause (cryptogenic stroke). Cerebrovasc Dis. 2009;27 Suppl 1:97–103.
11. Sharp FR, Jickling GC, Stamova B, et al. Molecular markers and mechanisms of stroke: RNA studies of blood in animals and humans. J Cereb Blood Flow Metab. 2011;31:1513–31.
12. Furie KL, Kasner SE, Adams RJ, et al. Guidelines for the prevention of stroke in patients with stroke or transient ischemic attack: a guideline for healthcare professionals from the American Heart Association/American Stroke Association. Stroke. 2011;42:227–76.
13. Goldstein LB, Bushnell CD, Adams RJ, et al. Guidelines for the primary prevention of stroke: a guideline for healthcare professionals from the American Heart Association/American Stroke Association. Stroke. 2011;42:517–84.
14. Sacco RL, Adams R, Albers G, et al. Guidelines for prevention of stroke in patients with ischemic stroke or transient ischemic attack: a statement for healthcare professionals from the American Heart Association/American Stroke Association Council on Stroke: co-sponsored by the Council on Cardiovascular Radiology and Intervention: the American Academy of Neurology affirms the value of this guideline. Stroke. 2006;37:577–617.

15. Goldstein LB, Adams R, Alberts MJ, et al. Primary prevention of ischemic stroke: a guideline from the American Heart Association/American Stroke Association Stroke Council: cosponsored by the Atherosclerotic Peripheral Vascular Disease Interdisciplinary Working Group; Cardiovascular Nursing Council; Clinical Cardiology Council; Nutrition, Physical Activity, and Metabolism Council; and the Quality of Care and Outcomes Research Interdisciplinary Working Group: the American Academy of Neurology affirms the value of this guideline. Stroke. 2006;37:1583–633.
16. Kissela B, Schneider A, Kleindorfer D, et al. Stroke in a biracial population: the excess burden of stroke among blacks. Stroke. 2004;35:426–31.
17. Di Tullio MR, Russo C, Jin Z, Sacco RL, Mohr JP, Homma S. Aortic arch plaques and risk of recurrent stroke and death. Circulation. 2009;119:2376–82.
18. Amarenco P. Cryptogenic stroke, aortic arch atheroma, patent foramen ovale, and the risk of stroke. Cerebrovasc Dis. 2005;20 Suppl 2.68–74.
19. Molisse TA, Tunick PA, Kronzon I. Complications of aortic atherosclerosis: atheroemboli and thromboemboli. Curr Treat Options Cardiovasc Med. 2007;9:137–47.
20. Dressler FA, Craig WR, Castello R, Labovitz AJ. Mobile aortic atheroma and systemic emboli: efficacy of anticoagulation and influence of plaque morphology on recurrent stroke. J Am Coll Cardiol. 1998;31:134–8.
21. Ferrari E, Vidal R, Chevallier T, Baudouy M. Atherosclerosis of the thoracic aorta and aortic debris as a marker of poor prognosis: benefit of oral anticoagulants. J Am Coll Cardiol. 1999;33:1317–22.
22. Lutsep HL. MATCH results: implications for the internist. Am J Med. 2006;119:526.e1–7.e1.
23. Orencia AJ, Hammill SC, Whisnant JP. Sinus node dysfunction and ischemic stroke. Heart Dis Stroke. 1994;3:91–4.
24. Scholten MF, Thornton AS, Mekel JM, Koudstaal PJ, Jordaens LJ. Anticoagulation in atrial fibrillation and flutter. Europace. 2005;7:492–9.
25. Hart RG, Pearce LA, Rothbart RM, McAnulty JH, Asinger RW, Halperin JL. Stroke with intermittent atrial fibrillation: incidence and predictors during aspirin therapy. Stroke Prevention in Atrial Fibrillation Investigators. J Am Coll Cardiol. 2000;35:183–7.
26. Medi C, Hankey GJ, Freedman SB. Atrial fibrillation. Med J Aust. 2007;186:197–202.
27. Fang WC, Chen J, Rich MW. Atrial fibrillation in the elderly. Am J Med. 2007;120:481–7.
28. Gage BF, Waterman AD, Shannon W, Boechler M, Rich MW, Radford MJ. Validation of clinical classification schemes for

predicting stroke: results from the National Registry of Atrial Fibrillation. JAMA. 2001;285:2864–70.

29. Hart RG, Benavente O, McBride R, Pearce LA. Antithrombotic therapy to prevent stroke in patients with atrial fibrillation: a meta-analysis. Ann Intern Med. 1999;131:492–501.

30. Petty GW, Brown Jr RD, Whisnant JP, Sicks JD, O'Fallon WM, Wiebers DO. Frequency of major complications of aspirin, warfarin, and intravenous heparin for secondary stroke prevention. A population-based study. Ann Intern Med. 1999;130:14–22.

31. Schirmer SH, Baumhakel M, Neuberger HR, et al. Novel anticoagulants for stroke prevention in atrial fibrillation: current clinical evidence and future developments. J Am Coll Cardiol. 2010;56:2067–76.

32. Granger CB, Alexander JH, McMurray JJ, et al. Apixaban versus warfarin in patients with atrial fibrillation. N Engl J Med. 2011;365:981–92.

33. Patel MR, Mahaffey KW, Garg J, et al. Rivaroxaban versus warfarin in nonvalvular atrial fibrillation. N Engl J Med. 2011;365:883–91.

34. Fuller CJ, Reisman M. Stroke prevention in atrial fibrillation: atrial appendage closure. Curr Cardiol Rep. 2011;13:159–66.

35. Ekinci EI, Donnan GA. Neurological manifestations of cardiac myxoma: a review of the literature and report of cases. Intern Med J. 2004;34:243–9.

36. Lee VH, Connolly HM, Brown Jr RD. Central nervous system manifestations of cardiac myxoma. Arch Neurol. 2007;64:1115–20.

37. Rensink AA, de Waal RM, Kremer B, Verbeek MM. Pathogenesis of cerebral amyloid angiopathy. Brain Res Brain Res Rev. 2003;43:207–23.

38. Kinnecom C, Lev MH, Wendell L, et al. Course of cerebral amyloid angiopathy-related inflammation. Neurology. 2007;68:1411–6.

39. Razvi SS, Bone I. Single gene disorders causing ischaemic stroke. J Neurol. 2006;253:685–700.

40. Loh E, Sutton MS, Wun CC, et al. Ventricular dysfunction and the risk of stroke after myocardial infarction. N Engl J Med. 1997;336:251–7.

41. Pfeffer MA, Braunwald E, Moye LA, et al. Effect of captopril on mortality and morbidity in patients with left ventricular dysfunction after myocardial infarction. Results of the survival and ventricular enlargement trial. The SAVE Investigators. N Engl J Med. 1992;327:669–77.

42. Thomas DP, Roberts HR. Hypercoagulability in venous and arterial thrombosis. Ann Intern Med. 1997;126:638–44.

43. Morris JG, Singh S, Fisher M. Testing for inherited thrombophilias in arterial stroke: can it cause more harm than good? Stroke. 2010;41:2985–90.

44. Bushnell CD, Goldstein LB. Diagnostic testing for coagulopathies in patients with ischemic stroke. Stroke. 2000;31:3067–78.

45. Hart RG, Kanter MC. Hematologic disorders and ischemic stroke. A selective review. Stroke. 1990;21:1111–21.

46. Ortel TL. Thrombosis and the antiphospholipid syndrome. Hematology Am Soc Hematol Educ Program. 2005;2005:462–8.

47. Elkind MS. Inflammation, atherosclerosis, and stroke. Neurologist. 2006;12:140–8.

48. Everett BM, Glynn RJ, MacFadyen JG, Ridker PM. Rosuvastatin in the prevention of stroke among men and women with elevated levels of C-reactive protein: justification for the Use of Statins in Prevention: an Intervention Trial Evaluating Rosuvastatin (JUPITER). Circulation. 2010;121:143–50.

49. Bonora E, Kiechl S, Willeit J, et al. Insulin resistance as estimated by homeostasis model assessment predicts incident symptomatic cardiovascular disease in caucasian subjects from the general population: the Bruneck study. Diabetes Care. 2007;30:318–24.

50. Bashore TM, Cabell C, Fowler Jr V. Update on infective endocarditis. Curr Probl Cardiol. 2006;31:274–352.

51. El-Shami K, Griffiths E, Streiff M. Nonbacterial thrombotic endocarditis in cancer patients: pathogenesis, diagnosis, and treatment. Oncologist. 2007;12:518–23.

52. Li JS, Sexton DJ, Mick N, et al. Proposed modifications to the Duke criteria for the diagnosis of infective endocarditis. Clin Infect Dis. 2000;30(4):633–8.

53. Lopez JA, Ross RS, Fishbein MC, Siegel RJ. Nonbacterial thrombotic endocarditis: a review. Am Heart J. 1987;113:773–84.

54. Rabinstein AA, Giovanelli C, Romano JG, Koch S, Forteza AM, Ricci M. Surgical treatment of nonbacterial thrombotic endocarditis presenting with stroke. J Neurol. 2005;252:352–5.

55. White H, Boden-Albala B, Wang C, et al. Ischemic stroke subtype incidence among whites, blacks, and Hispanics: the Northern Manhattan Study. Circulation. 2005;111:1327–31.

56. Moore DF, Kaneski CR, Askari H, Schiffmann R. The cerebral vasculopathy of Fabry disease. J Neurol Sci. 2007;257:258–63.

57. Clarke JT. Narrative review: fabry disease. Ann Intern Med. 2007;146:425–33.

58. Niewada M, Kobayashi A, Sandercock PA, Kaminski B, Czlonkowska A. Influence of gender on baseline features and clinical outcomes among 17,370 patients with confirmed ischaemic stroke in the international stroke trial. Neuroepidemiology. 2005;24:123–8.

59. Fukutake T. Cerebral autosomal recessive arteriopathy with subcortical infarcts and leukoencephalopathy (CARASIL): from discovery to gene identification. J Stroke Cerebrovasc Dis. 2011;20:85–93.

60. Markus HS, Alberts MJ. Update on genetics of stroke and cerebrovascular disease 2005. Stroke. 2006;37:288–90.

61. Guo JM, Liu AJ, Su DF. Genetics of stroke. Acta Pharmacol Sin. 2010;31:1055–64.

62. Meschia JF, Worrall BB, Rich SS. Genetic susceptibility to ischemic stroke. Nat Rev Neurol. 2011;7:369–78.

63. Donohue MM, Tirschwell DL. Implications of pharmacogenetic testing for patients taking warfarin or clopidogrel. Curr Neurol Neurosci Rep. 2011;11:52–60.

64. Daneschvar HL, Daw H. Heparin-induced thrombocytopenia (an overview). Int J Clin Pract. 2007;61:130–7.

65. Arepally GM, Ortel TL. Clinical practice. Heparin-induced thrombocytopenia. N Engl J Med. 2006;355:809–17.

66. Suzuki S, Brown CM, Wise PM. Mechanisms of neuroprotection by estrogen. Endocrine. 2006;29:209–15.

67. Yang SH, Liu R, Perez EJ, Wang X, Simpkins JW. Estrogens as protectants of the neurovascular unit against ischemic stroke. Curr Drug Targets CNS Neurol Disord. 2005;4:169–77.

68. Merchenthaler I, Dellovade TL, Shughrue PJ. Neuroprotection by estrogen in animal models of global and focal ischemia. Ann N Y Acad Sci. 2003;1007:89–100.

69. Hurn PD, Macrae IM. Estrogen as a neuroprotectant in stroke. J Cereb Blood Flow Metab. 2000;20:631–52.

70. Simon JA, Hsia J, Cauley JA, et al. Postmenopausal hormone therapy and risk of stroke: The Heart and Estrogen-progestin Replacement Study (HERS). Circulation. 2001;103:638–42.

71. Viscoli CM, Brass LM, Kernan WN, Sarrel PM, Suissa S, Horwitz RI. A clinical trial of estrogen-replacement therapy after ischemic stroke. N Engl J Med. 2001;345:1243–9.

72. Rossouw JE, Anderson GL, Prentice RL, et al. Risks and benefits of estrogen plus progestin in healthy postmenopausal women: principal results From the Women's Health Initiative randomized controlled trial. JAMA. 2002;288:321–33.

73. Bushnell CD. Oestrogen and stroke in women: assessment of risk. Lancet Neurol. 2005;4:743–51.

74. U.S. Preventative Services Task Force. Hormone therapy for the prevention of chronic conditions in postmenopausal women: recommendations from the U.S. Preventive Services Task Force. Ann Intern Med. 2005;142: 855–60.

75. American College of Obstetricians and Gynecologists Women's Health Care Physicians. Executive summary. Hormone therapy. Obstet Gynecol. 2004;104:1S–4.

76. Toole JF, Malinow MR, Chambless LE, et al. Lowering homocysteine in patients with ischemic stroke to prevent recurrent stroke, myocardial infarction, and death: the Vitamin Intervention for Stroke Prevention (VISP) randomized controlled trial. JAMA. 2004;291:565–75.

77. Wang X, Qin X, Demirtas H, et al. Efficacy of folic acid supplementation in stroke prevention: a meta-analysis. Lancet. 2007;369:1876–82.

78. Spence JD. Homocysteine-lowering therapy: a role in stroke prevention? Lancet Neurol. 2007;6:830–8.

79. Chobanian AV, Bakris GL, Black HR, et al. Seventh report of the Joint National Committee on Prevention, Detection, Evaluation, and Treatment of High Blood Pressure. Hypertension. 2003;42:1206–52.

80. Rashid P, Leonardi-Bee J, Bath P. Blood pressure reduction and secondary prevention of stroke and other vascular events: a systematic review. Stroke. 2003;34:2741–8.

81. Castillo J, Leira R, García MM, Serena J, Blanco M, Dávalos A. Blood pressure decrease during the acute phase of ischemic stroke is associated with brain injury and poor stroke outcome. Stroke. 2004;35:520–6.

82. Leira R, Millan M, Diez-Tejedor E, et al. Age determines the effects of blood pressure lowering during the acute phase of ischemic stroke: the TICA study. Hypertension. 2009;54:769–74.

83. Sandset EC, Bath PM, Boysen G, et al. The angiotensin-receptor blocker candesartan for treatment of acute stroke (SCAST): a randomised, placebo-controlled, double-blind trial. Lancet. 2011;377:741–50.

84. Ahmed N, Wahlgren N, Brainin M, et al. Relationship of blood pressure, antihypertensive therapy, and outcome in ischemic stroke treated with intravenous thrombolysis. Stroke. 2009;40:2442–9.

85. Arboix A, Besses C. Cerebrovascular disease as the initial clinical presentation of haematological disorders. Eur Neurol. 1997;37:207–11.

86. Liu M, Counsell C, Zhao XL, Wardlaw J. Fibrinogen depleting agents for acute ischaemic stroke. Cochrane Database Syst Rev. 2003:CD000091.

87. Elkind MS, Cole JW. Do common infections cause stroke? Semin Neurol. 2006;26:88–99.

88. Lampl Y, Boaz M, Gilad R, et al. Minocycline treatment in acute stroke: an open-label, evaluator-blinded study. Neurology. 2007;69:1404–10.

89. Touboul PJ, Hennerici MG, Meairs S, et al. Mannheim carotid intima-media thickness consensus (2004–2006). An update on behalf of the Advisory Board of the 3rd and 4th Watching the Risk Symposium, 13th and 15th European Stroke Conferences, Mannheim, Germany, 2004, and Brussels, Belgium, 2006. Cerebrovasc Dis. 2007;23:75–80.

90. Gilden DH, Kleinschmidt-DeMasters BK, LaGuardia JJ, Mahalingam R, Cohrs RJ. Neurologic complications of the reactivation of varicella-zoster virus. N Engl J Med. 2000;342:635–45.

91. Blanco M, Nombela F, Castellanos M, et al. Statin treatment withdrawal in ischemic stroke: a controlled randomized study. Neurology. 2007;69:904–10.

92. Amarenco P, Bogousslavsky J, Callahan 3rd A, et al. High-dose atorvastatin after stroke or transient ischemic attack. N Engl J Med. 2006;355:549–59.

93. Goldstein LB, Low LDL. cholesterol, statins, and brain hemorrhage: should we worry? Neurology. 2007;68:719–20.

94. Cimino M, Gelosa P, Gianella A, Nobili E, Tremoli E, Sironi L. Statins: multiple mechanisms of action in the ischemic brain. Neuroscientist. 2007;13:208–13.

95. Ovbiagele B, Saver JL, Starkman S, et al. Statin enhancement of collateralization in acute stroke. Neurology. 2007;68:2129–31.

96. Cestari DM, Weine DM, Panageas KS, Segal AZ, DeAngelis LM. Stroke in patients with cancer: incidence and etiology. Neurology. 2004;62:2025–30.

97. Bang OY. Intracranial atherosclerotic stroke: specific focus on the metabolic syndrome and inflammation. Curr Atheroscler Rep. 2006;8:330–6.

98. Bousser MG, Welch KM. Relation between migraine and stroke. Lancet Neurol. 2005;4:533–42.

99. Classification and diagnostic criteria for headache disorders, cranial neuralgias and facial pain. Headache Classification Committee of the International Headache Society. Cephalalgia. 1988;8 Suppl 7:1–96.

100. Etminan M, Takkouche B, Isorna FC, Samii A. Risk of ischaemic stroke in people with migraine: systematic review and meta-analysis of observational studies. BMJ. 2005;330:63.

101. Arpa J, Cruz-Martinez A, Campos Y, et al. Prevalence and progression of mitochondrial diseases: a study of 50 patients. Muscle Nerve. 2003;28:690–5.

102. Finsterer J. Central nervous system manifestations of mitochondrial disorders. Acta Neurol Scand. 2006;114:217–38.

103. Collop N. The effect of obstructive sleep apnea on chronic medical disorders. Cleve Clin J Med. 2007;74:72–8.

104. Yaggi H, Mohsenin V. Obstructive sleep apnoea and stroke. Lancet Neurol. 2004;3:333–42.

105. Helms A, Ajayi O, Kittner S. Investigating the link between oral contraceptives and stroke. Pract Neurol. 2007;6:34–40.

106. ACOG Committee on Practice Bulletins-Gynecology. ACOG practice bulletin. No. 73: use of hormonal contraception in women with coexisting medical conditions. Obstet Gynecol. 2006;107:1453–72.

107. Handke M, Harloff A, Olschewski M, Hetzel A, Geibel A. Patent foramen ovale and cryptogenic stroke in older patients. N Engl J Med. 2007;357:2262–8.

108. Mas JL, Arquizan C, Lamy C, et al. Recurrent cerebrovascular events associated with patent foramen ovale, atrial septal aneurysm, or both. N Engl J Med. 2001;345:1740–6.

109. Furlan AJ. A prospective, multicenter, randomized controlled trial to evaluate the safety and efficacy of the Starflex septal closure system versus best medical therapy in patients with a stroke or transient ischemic attack due to presumed paradoxical embolism through a patent foramen ovale. In: American Heart Association. Chicago; 2010.

110. Physical Activity Guidelines Advisory Committee Report, 2008. Washington: US Dept of Health and Human Services; 2008.

111. Khurshid I, Downie GH. Pulmonary arteriovenous malformation. Postgrad Med J. 2002;78:191–7.

112. White Jr RI, Lynch-Nyhan A, Terry P, et al. Pulmonary arteriovenous malformations: techniques and long-term outcome of embolotherapy. Radiology. 1988;169:663–9.

113. Jauss M, Zanette E. Detection of right-to-left shunt with ultrasound contrast agent and transcranial Doppler sonography. Cerebrovasc Dis. 2000;10:490–6.

114. Cottin V, Dupuis-Girod S, Lesca G, Cordier JF. Pulmonary vascular manifestations of hereditary hemorrhagic telangiectasia (rendu-osler disease). Respiration. 2007;74:361–78.

115. Redding-Lallinger R, Knoll C. Sickle cell disease – pathophysiology and treatment. Curr Probl Pediatr Adolesc Health Care. 2002;36:346–76.

116. Steen RG, Xiong X, Langston JW, Helton KJ. Brain injury in children with sickle cell disease: prevalence and etiology. Ann Neurol. 2003;54:564–72.

117. Wang WC. The pathophysiology, prevention, and treatment of stroke in sickle cell disease. Curr Opin Hematol. 2007; 14·191–7.

118. Adams RJ. Big strokes in small persons. Arch Neurol. 2007;64:1567–74.

119. Adams RJ, Brambilla DJ, Granger S, et al. Stroke and conversion to high risk in children screened with transcranial Doppler ultrasound during the STOP study. Blood. 2004; 103:3689–94.

120. Ware RE, Zimmerman SA, Sylvestre PB, et al. Prevention of secondary stroke and resolution of transfusional iron overload in children with sickle cell anemia using hydroxyurea and phlebotomy. J Pediatr. 2004;145: 346–52.

121. Krishnamurti L. Hematopoietic cell transplantation for sickle cell disease: state of the art. Expert Opin Biol Ther. 2007;7:161–72.

122. Tsaras G, Owusu-Ansah A, Boateng FO, Amoateng-Adjepong Y. Complications associated with sickle cell trait: a brief narrative review. Am J Med. 2009;122:507–12.

123. Greenberg J, Massey EW. Cerebral infarction in sickle cell trait. Ann Neurol. 1985;18:354–5.

124. Partington MD, Aronyk KE, Byrd SE. Sickle cell trait and stroke in children. Pediatr Neurosurg. 1994;20:148–51.

125. Steen RG, Hankins GM, Xiong X, et al. Prospective brain imaging evaluation of children with sickle cell trait: initial observations. Radiology. 2003;228:208–15.

126. Lannuzel A, Salmon V, Mevel G, Malpote E, Rabier R, Caparros-Lefebvre D. Epidemiology of stroke in Guadeloupe and role of sickle cell trait. Rev Neurol (Paris). 1999;155:351–6.

127. Fiore MC, Baker TB. Clinical practice. Treating smokers in the health care setting. N Engl J Med. 2011;365:1222–31.

128. Cahill K, Stead LF, Lancaster T. Nicotine receptor partial agonists for smoking cessation. Cochrane Database Syst Rev. 2007:CD006103.

129. Williams KE, Reeves KR, Billing Jr CB, Pennington AM, Gong J. A double-blind study evaluating the long-term safety of varenicline for smoking cessation. Curr Med Res Opin. 2007;23:793–801.

130. Moore TJ, Furberg CD, Glenmullen J, Maltsberger JT, Singh S. Suicidal behavior and depression in smoking cessation treatments. PLoS One. 2011;6:e27016.

131. Haggstram FM, Chatkin JM, Sussenbach-Vaz E, Cesari DH, Fam CF, Fritscher CC. A controlled trial of nortriptyline, sustained-release bupropion and placebo for smoking cessation: preliminary results. Pulm Pharmacol Ther. 2006;19(3):205–9.

132. Administration USFaD. FDA approves novel medication for smoking cessation. 2006. Report No.: http://www.fda.gov/bbs/topics/NEWS/2006/NEW01370.html. Accessed 11 May 2006.

133. Holmes S, Zwar N, Jimenez-Ruiz CA, et al. Bupropion as an aid to smoking cessation: a review of real-life effectiveness. Int J Clin Pract. 2004;58:285–91.

134. Mercadante N. Management of patients with prosthetic heart valves: potential impact of valve site, clinical characteristics, and comorbidity. J Thromb Thrombolysis. 2000;10:29–34.

135. Hardman SM, Cowie MR. Fortnightly review: anticoagulation in heart disease. BMJ. 1999;318:238–44.

136. Kelley RE. CNS vasculitis. Front Biosci. 2004;9:946–55.

137. Younger DS. Vasculitis of the nervous system. Curr Opin Neurol. 2004;17:317–36.

138. Jennette JC, Falk RJ. Nosology of primary vasculitis. Curr Opin Rheumatol. 2007;19:10–6.

139. Kuker W. Cerebral vasculitis: imaging signs revisited. Neuroradiology. 2007;49:471–9.

140. Lee MS, Smith SD, Galor A, Hoffman GS. Antiplatelet and anticoagulant therapy in patients with giant cell arteritis. Arthritis Rheum. 2006;54:3306–9.

141. Melson MR, Weyand CM, Newman NJ, Biousse V. The diagnosis of giant cell arteritis. Rev Neurol Dis. 2007;4:128–42.

142. Salvarani C, Hunder GG. Giant cell arteritis with low erythrocyte sedimentation rate: frequency of occurrence in a population-based study. Arthritis Rheum. 2001;45:140–5.

143. Ringleb PA, Strittmatter EI, Loewer M, et al. Cerebrovascular manifestations of Takayasu arteritis in Europe. Rheumatology (Oxford). 2005;44:1012–5.

144. Arend WP, Michel BA, Bloch DA, et al. The American College of Rheumatology 1990 criteria for the classification of Takayasu arteritis. Arthritis Rheum. 1990;33:1129–34.

145. Reichart MD, Bogousslavsky J, Janzer RC. Early lacunar strokes complicating polyarteritis nodosa: thrombotic microangiopathy. Neurology. 2000;54:883–9.

146. Lightfoot Jr RW, Michel BA, Bloch DA, et al. The American College of Rheumatology 1990 criteria for the classification of polyarteritis nodosa. Arthritis Rheum. 1990;33:1088–93.

147. Lamprecht P, Gross WL. Wegener's granulomatosis. Herz. 2004;29:47–56.

148. Leavitt RY, Fauci AS, Bloch DA, et al. The American College of Rheumatology 1990 criteria for the classification of Wegener's granulomatosis. Arthritis Rheum. 1990;33:1101–7.

149. Kang DW, Kim DE, Yoon BW, Seo JW, Roh JK. Delayed diagnosis: recurrent cerebral infarction associated with Churg-Strauss syndrome. Cerebrovasc Dis. 2001;12:280–1.

150. Keogh KA, Specks U. Churg-Strauss syndrome: clinical presentation, antineutrophil cytoplasmic antibodies, and leukotriene receptor antagonists. Am J Med. 2003;115:284–90.

151. Masi AT, Hunder GG, Lie JT, et al. The American College of Rheumatology 1990 criteria for the classification of Churg-Strauss syndrome (allergic granulomatosis and angiitis). Arthritis Rheum. 1990;33:1094–100.

152. Calabrese LH, Mallek JA. Primary angiitis of the central nervous system. Report of 8 new cases, review of the literature, and proposal for diagnostic criteria. Medicine (Baltimore). 1988;67:20–39.

153. Moore PM. Vasculitis of the central nervous system. Semin Neurol. 1994;14:307–12.

154. Lalvani A, Pareek M. Interferon gamma release assays: principles and practice. Enferm Infecc Microbiol Clin. 2010;28:245–52.

155. de Gans J, van de Beek D. Dexamethasone in adults with bacterial meningitis. N Engl J Med. 2002;347:1549–56.

156. Brust JC. Vasculitis owing to substance abuse. Neurol Clin. 1997;15:945–57.

157. Niehaus L, Meyer BU. Bilateral borderzone brain infarctions in association with heroin abuse. J Neurol Sci. 1998;160:180–2.

158. Serdaroglu P. Behcet's disease and the nervous system. J Neurol. 1998;245:197–205.

159. Nagel MA, Mahalingam R, Cohrs RJ, Gilden D. Virus vasculopathy and stroke: an under-recognized cause and treatment target. Infect Disord Drug Targets. 2010;10:105–11.

160. Johnson RT, Richardson EP. The neurological manifestations of systemic lupus erythematosus. Medicine (Baltimore). 1968;47:337–69.

161. Devinsky O, Petito CK, Alonso DR. Clinical and neuropathological findings in systemic lupus erythematosus: the role of vasculitis, heart emboli, and thrombotic thrombocytopenic purpura. Ann Neurol. 1988;23:380–4.

162. Kitagawa Y, Gotoh F, Koto A, Okayasu H. Stroke in systemic lupus erythematosus. Stroke. 1990;21:1533–9.

163. Call GK, Fleming MC, Sealfon S, Levine H, Kistler JP, Fisher CM. Reversible cerebral segmental vasoconstriction. Stroke. 1988;19:1159–70.

164. Hajj-Ali RA, Furlan A, Abou-Chebel A, Calabrese LH. Benign angiopathy of the central nervous system: cohort of 16 patients with clinical course and long-term followup. Arthritis Rheum. 2002;47:662–9.

165. Calabrese LH. Clinical management issues in vasculitis. Angiographically defined angiitis of the central nervous system: diagnostic and therapeutic dilemmas. Clin Exp Rheumatol. 2003;21:S127–30.

166. Ng YS, Stein J, Ning M, Black-Schaffer RM. Comparison of clinical characteristics and functional outcomes of ischemic stroke in different vascular territories. Stroke. 2007;38:2309–14.

167. Caplan LR. Transient ischemic attack with abnormal diffusion-weighted imaging results: what's in a name? Arch Neurol. 2007;64:1080–2.

168. Kidwell CS, Warach S. Acute ischemic cerebrovascular syndrome: diagnostic criteria. Stroke. 2003;34:2995–8.

169. A classification and outline of cerebrovascular diseases. Neurology. 1958;8:395–434.

170. Ali LK, Saver JL. The ischemic stroke patient who worsens: new assessment and management approaches. Rev Neurol Dis. 2007;4:85–91.

171. Quinette P, Guillery-Girard B, Dayan J, et al. What does transient global amnesia really mean? Review of the literature and thorough study of 142 cases. Brain. 2006;129:1640–58.

172. Bettermann K. Transient global amnesia: the continuing quest for a source. Arch Neurol. 2006;63:1336–8.

173. Roach ES. Transient global amnesia: look at mechanisms not causes. Arch Neurol. 2006;63:1338–9.

174. Menendez Gonzalez M, Rivera MM. Transient global amnesia: increasing evidence of a venous etiology. Arch Neurol. 2006;63:1334–6.

175. Brazis PW, Masdeau JC, Biller J. Localization in clinical neurology. Philadelphia: Lippincott, Williams & Wilkins; 2007.

176. Camilo O, Goldstein LB. Seizures and epilepsy after ischemic stroke. Stroke. 2004;35:1769–75.

177. Murie JA, Sheldon CD, Quin RO. Carotid artery bruit: association with internal carotid stenosis and intraluminal turbulence. Br J Surg. 1984;71:50–2.

178. Shorr RI, Johnson KC, Wan JY, et al. The prognostic significance of asymptomatic carotid bruits in the elderly. J Gen Intern Med. 1998;13:86–90.

179. Hillis AE. Aphasia: progress in the last quarter of a century. Neurology. 2007;69:200–13.

180. Chambers BR, Brooder RJ, Donnan GA. Proximal posterior cerebral artery occlusion simulating middle cerebral artery occlusion. Neurology. 1991;41:385–90.

181. Maulaz AB, Bezerra DC, Bogousslavsky J. Posterior cerebral artery infarction from middle cerebral artery infarction. Arch Neurol. 2005;62:938–41.

182. Hommel M, Besson G, Pollak P, Kahane P, Le Bas JF, Perret J. Hemiplegia in posterior cerebral artery occlusion. Neurology. 1990;40:1496–9.

183. Ali S, Khan MA, Khealani B. Limb-shaking transient ischemic attacks: case report and review of literature. BMC Neurol. 2006;6:5.

184. Gregoire SM, Charidimou A, Gadapa N, et al. Acute ischaemic brain lesions in intracerebral haemorrhage: multicentre cross-sectional magnetic resonance imaging study. Brain. 2011;134:2376–86.

185. Adams Jr HP, Bendixen BH, Kappelle LJ, et al. Classification of subtype of acute ischemic stroke. Definitions for use in a multicenter clinical trial. TOAST. Trial of Org 10172 in Acute Stroke Treatment. Stroke. 1993;24:35–41.

186. Bamford J, Sandercock P, Dennis M, Burn J, Warlow C. Classification and natural history of clinically identifiable subtypes of cerebral infarction. Lancet. 1991;337:1521–6.

187. Adams Jr HP, del Zoppo G, Alberts MJ, et al. Guidelines for the early management of adults with ischemic stroke: a guideline from the American Heart Association/American Stroke Association Stroke Council, Clinical Cardiology Council, Cardiovascular Radiology and Intervention Council, and the Atherosclerotic Peripheral Vascular Disease and Quality of Care Outcomes in Research Interdisciplinary Working Groups: the American Academy of Neurology affirms the value of this guideline as an educational tool for neurologists. Stroke. 2007;38:1655–711.

188. Johnston SC, Gress DR, Browner WS, Sidney S. Short-term prognosis after emergency department diagnosis of TIA. JAMA. 2000;284:2901–6.

189. Johnston SC, Rothwell PM, Nguyen-Huynh MN, et al. Validation and refinement of scores to predict very early stroke risk after transient ischaemic attack. Lancet. 2007;369:283–92.

190. Feldmann E, Wilterdink JL, Kosinski A, et al. The Stroke Outcomes and Neuroimaging of Intracranial Atherosclerosis (SONIA) trial. Neurology. 2007;68:2099–106.

191. Pearson AC, Labovitz AJ, Tatineni S, Gomez CR. Superiority of transesophageal echocardiography in detecting cardiac source of embolism in patients with cerebral ischemia of uncertain etiology. J Am Coll Cardiol. 1991;17:66–72.

192. Rauh R, Fischereder M, Spengel FA. Transesophageal echocardiography in patients with focal cerebral ischemia of unknown cause. Stroke. 1996;27:691–4.

193. McNamara RL, Lima JA, Whelton PK, Powe NR. Echocardiographic identification of cardiovascular sources of emboli to guide clinical management of stroke: a cost-effectiveness analysis. Ann Intern Med. 1997;127:775–87.

194. Angeli S, Del Sette M, Beelke M, Anzola GP, Zanette E. Transcranial Doppler in the diagnosis of cardiac patent foramen ovale. Neurol Sci. 2001;22:353–6.

195. Del Sette M, Dinia L, Rizzi D, Sugo A, Albano B, Gandolfo C. Diagnosis of right-to-left shunt with transcranial Doppler and vertebrobasilar recording. Stroke. 2008;39:2254–6.

196. Hacke W, Kaste M, Bluhmki E, et al. Thrombolysis with alteplase 3 to 4.5 hours after acute ischemic stroke. N Engl J Med. 2008;359:1317–29.

197. Del Zoppo GJ, Saver JL, Jauch EC, Adams Jr HP. Expansion of the time window for treatment of acute ischemic stroke with intravenous tissue plasminogen activator: a science advisory from the American Heart Association/American Stroke Association. Stroke. 2009;40:2945–8.

198. Alexandrov AV, Molina CA, Grotta JC, et al. Ultrasound-enhanced systemic thrombolysis for acute ischemic stroke. N Engl J Med. 2004;351:2170–8.

199. Schwarz S, Georgiadis D, Aschoff A, Schwab S. Effects of body position on intracranial pressure and cerebral perfusion in patients with large hemispheric stroke. Stroke. 2002;33:497–501.

200. Caplan LR. Resolved: Heparin may be useful in selected patients with brain ischemia. Stroke. 2003;34:230–1.

201. Thiers FA, Sinskey AJ, Berndt ER. Trends in the globalization of clinical trials. Nat Rev. 2008;7:13–4.

202. Politis-Virk K. China's clinical trial boom. PharmaFocus Asia Issue 14, 2011 www.languageconnections.com.

203. Faden AI, Stoica B. Neuroprotection: challenges and opportunities. Arch Neurol. 2007;64:794–800.

204. Garg R, Chaudhuri A, Munschauer F, Dandona P. Hyperglycemia, insulin, and acute ischemic stroke: a mechanistic justification for a trial of insulin infusion therapy. Stroke. 2006;37:267–73.

205. Yong M, Kaste M. Dynamic of hyperglycemia as a predictor of stroke outcome in the ECASS-II trial. Stroke. 2008;39:2749–55.

206. van den Berghe G, Wouters P, Weekers F, et al. Intensive insulin therapy in the critically ill patients. N Engl J Med. 2001;345:1359–67.

207. Van den Berghe G, Wilmer A, Hermans G, et al. Intensive insulin therapy in the medical ICU. N Engl J Med. 2006;354:449–61.

208. Qaseem A, Humphrey LL, Chou R, Snow V, Shekelle P. Use of intensive insulin therapy for the management of glycemic control in hospitalized patients: a clinical practice guideline from the American College of Physicians. Ann Intern Med. 2011;154:260–7.

209. Gray CS, Hildreth AJ, Sandercock PA, et al. Glucose-potassium-insulin infusions in the management of post-stroke hyperglycaemia: the UK Glucose Insulin in Stroke Trial (GIST-UK). Lancet Neurol. 2007;6:397–406.

210. Johnston KC, Hall CE, Kissela BM, Bleck TP, Conaway MR. Glucose Regulation in Acute Stroke Patients (GRASP) trial: a randomized pilot trial. Stroke. 2009;40:3804–9.

211. Godoy DA, Di Napoli M, Rabinstein AA. Treating hyperglycemia in neurocritical patients: benefits and perils. Neurocrit Care. 2010;13:425–38.

212. Umpierrez GE, Palacio A, Smiley D. Sliding scale insulin use: myth or insanity? Am J Med. 2007;120:563–7.

213. Zaremba J. Hyperthermia in ischemic stroke. Med Sci Monit. 2004;10:RA148–53.

214. Fernandez A, Schmidt JM, Claassen J, et al. Fever after subarachnoid hemorrhage: risk factors and impact on outcome. Neurology. 2007;68:1013–9.

215. Hypothermia after Cardiac Arrest Study Group. Mild therapeutic hypothermia to improve the neurologic outcome after cardiac arrest. N Engl J Med. 2002;346:549–56.

216. Bernard SA, Gray TW, Buist MD, et al. Treatment of comatose survivors of out-of-hospital cardiac arrest with induced hypothermia. N Engl J Med. 2002;346:557–63.

217. Bhardwaj A, Mirski M, Ulatowski J. Handbook of neurocritical care. Totowa: Humana Press; 2004.

218. Nguyen T, Koroshetz WJ. Intensive care management of ischemic stroke. Curr Neurol Neurosci Rep. 2003;3:32–9.

219. Karepov VG, Gur AY, Bova I, Aronovich BD, Bornstein NM. Stroke-in-evolution: infarct-inherent mechanisms versus systemic causes. Cerebrovasc Dis. 2006;21:42–6.

220. Davenport A. The management of renal failure in patients at risk of cerebral edema/hypoxia. New Horiz. 1995;3:717–24.

221. Qureshi AI, Geocadin RG, Suarez JI, Ulatowski JA. Long-term outcome after medical reversal of transtentorial herniation in patients with supratentorial mass lesions. Crit Care Med. 2000;28:1556–64.

222. Vahedi K, Hofmeijer J, Juettler E, et al. Early decompressive surgery in malignant infarction of the middle cerebral artery: a pooled analysis of three randomised controlled trials. Lancet Neurol. 2007;6:215–22.

223. Berges S, Moulin T, Berger E, et al. Seizures and epilepsy following strokes: recurrence factors. Eur Neurol. 2000;43:3–8.

224. McCarthy ST, Turner J. Low-dose subcutaneous heparin in the prevention of deep-vein thrombosis and pulmonary emboli following acute stroke. Age Ageing. 1986;15:84–8.

225. Sherman DG, Albers GW, Bladin C, et al. The efficacy and safety of enoxaparin versus unfractionated heparin for the prevention of venous thromboembolism after acute ischaemic stroke (PREVAIL Study): an open-label randomised comparison. Lancet. 2007;369:1347–55.

226. Epstein NE. A review of the risks and benefits of differing prophylaxis regimens for the treatment of deep venous thrombosis and pulmonary embolism in neurosurgery. Surg Neurol. 2005;64:295–301; discussion 2.

227. Kamran SI, Downey D, Ruff RL. Pneumatic sequential compression reduces the risk of deep vein thrombosis in stroke patients. Neurology. 1998;50:1683–8.

228. Reddy M, Gill SS, Rochon PA. Preventing pressure ulcers: a systematic review. JAMA. 2006;296:974–84.

229. Martin B. Prevention of gastrointestinal complications in the critically ill patient. AACN Adv Crit Care. 2007;18:158–66.

230. Loo VG, Bourgault AM, Poirier L, et al. Host and pathogen factors for Clostridium difficile infection and colonization. N Engl J Med. 2011;365:1693–703.

231. Chemerinski E, Levine SR. Neuropsychiatric disorders following vascular brain injury. Mt Sinai J Med. 2006;73: 1006–14.

232. Ferro JM, Caeiro L, Verdelho A. Delirium in acute stroke. Curr Opin Neurol. 2002;15:51–5.

233. Antithrombotic Trialists' Collaboration. Collaborative meta-analysis of randomised trials of antiplatelet therapy for prevention of death, myocardial infarction, and stroke in high risk patients. BMJ. 2002;324:71–86.

234. Caplan LR, Fisher M. The endothelium, platelets, and brain ischemia. Rev Neurol Dis. 2007;4:113–21.

235. Connolly SJ, Pogue J, Hart RG, et al. Effect of clopidogrel added to aspirin in patients with atrial fibrillation. N Engl J Med. 2009;360:2066–78.

236. Gengo FM, Rainka M, Robson M, et al. Prevalence of platelet nonresponsiveness to aspirin in patients treated for secondary stroke prophylaxis and in patients with recurrent ischemic events. J Clin Pharmacol. 2008;48:335–43.

237. Chen WH, Cheng X, Lee PY, et al. Aspirin resistance and adverse clinical events in patients with coronary artery disease. Am J Med. 2007;120:631–5.

238. Jin HM. Clinical uses and studies of the mechanism of Dan Shen. J Chin Med. 1978;3:180–3.

239. Wu B, Liu M, Liu H, et al. Meta-analysis of traditional Chinese patent medicine for ischemic stroke. Stroke. 2007;38:1973–9.

240. Kreisel SH, Hennerici MG, Bazner H. Pathophysiology of stroke rehabilitation: the natural course of clinical recovery, use-dependent plasticity and rehabilitative outcome. Cerebrovasc Dis. 2007;23:243–55.

241. Mark VW, Taub E, Morris DM. Neuroplasticity and constraint-induced movement therapy. Eura Medicophys. 2006;42:269–84.

242. O'Malley MK, Ro T, Levin HS. Assessing and inducing neuroplasticity with transcranial magnetic stimulation and robotics for motor function. Arch Phys Med Rehabil. 2006;87:S59–66.

243. Hogan N, Krebs HI, Rohrer B, et al. Motions or muscles? Some behavioral factors underlying robotic assistance of motor recovery. J Rehabil Res Dev. 2006;43:605–18.

244. Sheffler LR, Chae J. Neuromuscular electrical stimulation in neurorehabilitation. Muscle Nerve. 2007;35:562–90.

245. Phillips JP, Devier DJ, Feeney DM. Rehabilitation pharmacology: bridging laboratory work to clinical application. J Head Trauma Rehabil. 2003;18:342–56.

246. Dobkin BH. Behavioral, temporal, and spatial targets for cellular transplants as adjuncts to rehabilitation for stroke. Stroke. 2007;38:832–9.

247. Chen J, Chopp M. Neurorestorative treatment of stroke: cell and pharmacological approaches. NeuroRx. 2006;3: 466–73.

248. Wozniak MA, Kittner SJ. Return to work after ischemic stroke: a methodological review. Neuroepidemiology. 2002; 21: 159–66.

249. Amlie-Lefond C, deVeber G, Chan AK, et al. Use of alteplase in childhood arterial ischaemic stroke: a multicentre, observational, cohort study. Lancet Neurol. 2009;8:530–6.

250. Grunwald IQ, Walter S, Fassbender K, et al. Ischemic stroke in children: new aspects of treatment. J Pediatr. 2011;159:366–70.

251. Roach ES, Golomb MR, Adams R, et al. Management of stroke in infants and children: a scientific statement from a Special Writing Group of the American Heart Association Stroke Council and the Council on Cardiovascular Disease in the Young. Stroke. 2008;39:2644–91.

252. Agrawal N, Johnston SC, Wu YW, Sidney S, Fullerton HJ. Imaging data reveal a higher pediatric stroke incidence than prior US estimates. Stroke. 2009;40:3415–21.

253. Kirton A, Armstrong-Wells J, Chang T, et al. Symptomatic neonatal arterial ischemic stroke: the international pediatric stroke study. Pediatrics. 2011;128:e1402–10.

254. Srinivasan J, Miller SP, Phan TG, Mackay MT. Delayed recognition of initial stroke in children: need for increased awareness. Pediatrics. 2009;124:e227–34.

255. Abend NS, Beslow LA, Smith SE, et al. Seizures as a presenting symptom of acute arterial ischemic stroke in childhood. J Pediatr. 2011;159:479–83.

256. Mackay MT, Wiznitzer M, Benedict SL, Lee KJ, Deveber GA, Ganesan V. Arterial ischemic stroke risk factors: the International Pediatric Stroke Study. Ann Neurol. 2011;69:130–40.

257. Amlie-Lefond C, Bernard TJ, Sebire G, et al. Predictors of cerebral arteriopathy in children with arterial ischemic stroke: results of the International Pediatric Stroke Study. Circulation. 2009;119:1417–23.

258. Steiger HJ, Hanggi D, Assmann B, Turowski B. Cerebral angiopathies as a cause of ischemic stroke in children: differential diagnosis and treatment options. Dtsch Arztebl Int. 2010;107:851–6.

259. Beslow LA, Jordan LC. Pediatric stroke: the importance of cerebral arteriopathy and vascular malformations. Childs Nerv Syst. 2010;26:1263–73.

260. Jordan LC, Hillis AE. Challenges in the diagnosis and treatment of pediatric stroke. Nat Rev Neurol. 2011;7: 199–208.

261. Goldenberg NA, Bernard TJ, Fullerton HJ, Gordon A, deVeber G. Antithrombotic treatments, outcomes, and prognostic factors in acute childhood-onset arterial ischaemic stroke: a multicentre, observational, cohort study. Lancet Neurol. 2009;8:1120–7

262. Amlie-Lefond C, Gill JC. Pharmacology in childhood arterial ischemic stroke. Semin Pediatr Neurol. 2010;17:237–44.

18. Extracranial Cerebrovascular Occlusive Disease

This chapter will discuss extracranial atherosclerotic disease and arterial dissection.

18.1. Atherosclerotic Extracranial Arterial Disease

Large vessel atherosclerotic disease, most commonly extracranial carotid stenosis, accounts for some 15–20% of cerebral ischaemic events.[1,2]

Atherosclerosis

Atherosclerosis is thought to represent an inflammatory response to injury[3] in a hyperlipidemic environment.[4] The fatty streak is believed to precede the development of an atherosclerotic plaque, and is present in infancy.[5] The distinguishing histological feature is the presence of foam cells, lipid-filled macrophages and myointimal smooth muscle cells adjacent to the endothelial layer.[4]

Atherosclerosis Involves Several Stages

1. Atherosclerosis begins with endothelial damage or dysfunction caused by a variety of factors:
   - (a) Elevated or modified low-density lipoprotein[6]
   - (b) Free radicals caused by
     - i. Cigarette smoking
     - ii. Hypertension
     - iii. Diabetes mellitus
   - (c) Genetic alterations
   - (d) Elevated plasma homocysteine levels[7]
   - (e) Infection (associated with atherosclerosis, but not yet shown to *cause* it).
     - i. *Chlamydia pneumoniae*[8]
     - ii. Herpes virus[9]
2. Smooth muscle cells migrate into the lesion and proliferate.[10]
3. The artery wall thickens, and the vessel undergoes gradual compensatory dilation (*remodeling*).
4. Macrophages and lymphocytes are activated and immigrate from the blood, which multiply within the lesion.
   - (a) Activation of mononuclear cells leads to the release of hydrolytic enzymes and cytokines, which can induce further injury and cause focal necrosis.
5. Fibrous tissue accumulates
   - (a) Smooth muscle cells synthesize collagen.
   - (b) Fibrous cap forms over a core of lipid and necrotic tissue.
6. Capacity for compensatory dilation is exceeded and the lesion extends into the lumen of the vessel.
   - (a) Stenosis results.
7. The plaque becomes unstable.
   - (a) The fibrous cap is degraded by metalloproteinases.
   - (b) Rupture of the plaque can occur, followed by thrombosis.

M.R. Harrigan, J.P. Deveikis, *Handbook of Cerebrovascular Disease and Neurointerventional Technique*, DOI 10.1007/978-1-61779-946-4_18, © Springer Science+Business Media New York 2013

Plaque Location

1. Atherosclerotic plaques develop where wall shear stress is reduced, not elevated.[11]
   (a) Metabolic and functional changes influencing an intact endothelium are necessary for plaque formation, rather than endothelial denudation[12]
   (b) Low flow velocity and oscillation also contribute.[13]
   (c) These hemodynamic factors result in delayed clearance of putative blood-borne atherogenic factors.
2. Carotid bifurcation is prone to plaque formation.
   (a) Large area of flow separation and low wall shear stress due to:
      i. Large cross-sectional area of the carotid sinus (twice that of the ICA).
      ii. Branching angle.
   (b) Plaque is largest along the lateral wall of the carotid sinus.
      i. Changing geometric configuration with plaque growth causes hemodynamic changes that favour plaque formation on the side and inner walls.

Statins and Atherosclerosis

1. Statins lower serum cholesterol by inhibition of 3-hydroxy-3-methyglutaryl coenzyme A (HMG-CoA) reductase in the liver.
2. Statins are understood to have a wide array of beneficial effects that are independent of the cholesterol lowering effects.
3. Statins contribute to endothelial function, vascular remodeling, inhibition of vascular inflammation, and possibly also stabilization of atherosclerotic plaques.[14] Statin use also have been found to provide benefits in patients with ischaemic stroke[15–17] subarachnoid haemorrhage,[18] and traumatic brain injury.[19] These cholesterol-independent effects are due mainly to the ability of statins to inhibit isoprenoid synthesis, the products of which are key lipid attachments for intracellular signaling molecules.

Atherosclerosis and Cerebrovascular Disease

Atherosclerosis can cause cerebral ischaemic symptoms via two mechanisms:[20]
1. Hemodynamic compromise due to stenosis.
   (a) Blood flow in a vessel the size of the ICA remains fairly constant until the internal diameter is reduced by approximately 70%.[21]
2. Embolization from an ulcerative plaque.

Carotid Artery Bifurcation Atherosclerotic Disease

PREVALENCE
1. Prevalence of carotid atherosclerosis in the general population: 25%.[22]
   (a) Intimal-medial thickening:
      i. Men: 9.4%, women 11.7%.
   (b) Plaque:
      i. Men 13.3%, women 13.4%.
   (c) Stenotic plaque:
      i. Men 2.7%, women 1.5%.
2. Prevalence of carotid stenosis (≥40%) in the general population: 2–11%.[23–27]

RISK FACTORS FOR CAROTID STENOSIS
1. Advanced age[24,25,27–29]
2. Cigarette smoking[24,25,29,30]
3. Sex:
   (a) Male[24,28,29]
   (b) Female[31]
4. Hypertension[25,26,32–34]
5. Diabetes[35]
6. Coronary artery disease[36]
7. Mitral annulus calcification[37]
8. Peripheral arterial disease[38]

9. Chronic renal failure[39]
10. Total cholesterol[24,29,33]
11. (Inversely) Ratio of high-density lipoprotein cholesterol to total cholesterol[24]
12. Elevated C-reactive protein[40]
13. "Psychological strain"[41]

Carotid Endarterectomy

Carotid endarterectomy (CEA) has an uncommon distinction among surgical procedures in that it has been well studied in randomized clinical trials and has been shown to significantly reduce the risk of stroke in selected patients. It remains the standard of care for most patients. In 2002, some 134,000 CEAs were done in the U.S.[42]

Symptomatic Carotid Stenosis

There have been three major randomized trials comparing CEA to medical therapy for symptomatic stenosis.

NORTH AMERICAN SYMPTOMATIC ENDARTERECTOMY TRIAL (NASCET)
1. 2,885 patients with transient ischaemic attack (TIA) or minor stroke within the previous 120 days who had a 30–99% ipsilateral ICA stenosis were randomized to receive either medical therapy (risk factor modification and aspirin 1,300 mg daily) or medical therapy and CEA.[43]
2. Stenosis was measured on angiography by comparing the residual lumen diameter in the most stenotic portion of the ICA to the lumen diameter of the ICA distal to the stenosis (this method has been used for all randomized trials of CEA except for the ECST).
3. The arm of the trial for patients with ≥70% stenosis was terminated before the end of the study because an interim analysis showed a considerable advantage of surgery.
   (a) For patients with ≥70% stenosis, ipsilateral stroke rate at 2 years was
      i. 26% in the medical group
      ii. 9% in the surgical group ($p < 0.001$),[44]
         1. Absolute risk reduction of 17%
         2. The benefit persisted for at least 8 years[45]
         3. The risk reduction correlated with the degree of stenosis
4. For moderate stenosis (50–69%), the 5-year ipsilateral stroke rate was:
   (a) 22.2% in the medical group
   (b) 15.7% in the surgical group ($p = 0.045$)[45]
      i. Absolute risk reduction of 6.5%.

EUROPEAN CAROTID SURGERY TRIAL (ECST)
1. 3,024 patients with TIA, retinal infarction, or nondisabling stroke within the previous 6 months were randomized to receive either medical therapy (use of aspirin was permitted but not required) or medical therapy and CEA.[46]
2. Stenosis in the ECST was determined on angiography by comparing the residual stenosis at the most stenotic portion of the vessel to the probable original lumen diameter at that site (Fig. 18.1). This method differed from the method used for NASCET; consequently, higher degrees of stenosis were reported in the ECST relative to NASCET angiographic measurements (Table 18.1).
3. The 3-year risk of major stroke or death in patients with ≥80% (approximately ≥60% by the NASCET method):
   (a) 26.5% in the medical group
   (b) 14.9% in the surgical group
      i. Absolute risk reduction for surgery of 11.6%.[51]
      ii. This risk reduction persisted for at least 10 years after surgery.[52]

VETERANS AFFAIRS COOPERATIVE STUDY ON SYMPTOMATIC STENOSIS (VACS)
1. 197 men with symptomatic stenosis were randomized to receive medical therapy, including aspirin (325 mg daily), or medical therapy and CEA.
2. Prematurely terminated when NASCET and ECST data were released.
3. The risk of stroke at an average follow-up of 11.9 months in patients with >50% stenosis:
   (a) 19.4% in the medical group
   (b) 11.7% in the surgical group ($p = 0.011$)
      i. Absolute risk reduction for surgery of 11.7%.[53]

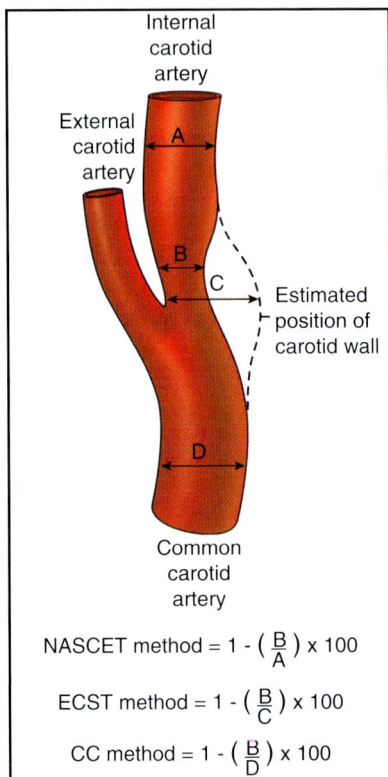

Fig. 18.1 Methods of measurement of carotid stenosis. Methods used by the NASCET and ECST studies. The Common Carotid (CC) method is the most reproducible of all three methods,[47,48] but has not come into wide usage (From Donnan et al.,[49] with permission).

Table 18.1 Carotid stenosis measurement equivalent values

NASCET (%)	ECST and CC (%)
30	58
40	64
50	70
60	76
70	82
80	88
90	94

The following equation was used: ECST and CC method stenosis (%) = $0.6 \times$ NASCET stenosis (%) + 40%. In a comparison of the three methods on 1001 angiograms, the degree of stenosis determined by the ECST method was identical to the degree of stenosis determined by the CC method[50]

4. Benefit of surgery was greater in patients with >70% stenosis,
   (a) Absolute risk reduction of 17.7% ($p = 0.004$).

ANALYSIS OF POOLED DATA
   A meticulous analysis examined the results of the NASCET, ECST, and VACS by remeasuring the degree of stenosis in ECST using the method employed by the two other trials.[54] Data for 6,092 patients, with 35,000 patient-years of follow-up, were pooled. Results were stratified according to degree of stenosis:
1. <30%: CEA increased the risk of ipsilateral stroke.
   (a) Absolute risk *increase*: 2.2% ($p = 0.05$)
2. 30–49%: No effect.
   (a) Absolute risk reduction: 3.2% ($p = 0.06$)
3. 50–69%: Marginal benefit of CEA
   (a) Absolute risk reduction: 4.6% ($p = 0.04$)
4. ≥70% without near occlusion: Highly beneficial
   (a) Absolute risk reduction: 16.0% ($p < 0.001$)
5. Near occlusion :
   (a) Trend toward benefit at 2 years.
       i. Absolute risk reduction: 5.6% ($p = 0.19$)

Global Gem! Carotid Stenosis Measurement
The NASCET method of carotid stenosis measurement has been widely used in North America and other regions since the method was developed, despite evidence that the ECST method has greater reproduceability.[47] The NASCET method was used for the three recent major carotid stenting versus surgery trials.[55–57] The ECST method also continues to be used, but mostly in the United Kingdom and other European countries.[58,59]

   (b) No benefit at 5 years
       i. Absolute risk *increase*: 1.7% ($p = 0.9$)

CLINICAL TRIAL DATA CAVEATS
1. Outcome after CEA strongly depends on risk for perioperative complications. In the NASCET, the 30-day rate of disabling stroke and death after CEA in patients with 70–99% stenosis was 2.1%. In the ECST, the 30-day rate of non-fatal major stroke or death was 7.0%.[51] Complication rates significantly higher than 6% in patients with >70% stenosis can eliminate the benefit of the operation.[60]
2. "Best medical therapy" has evolved since these trials were done, to include combination antiplatelet regimens and lipid-lowering agents.
3. All three trials based measurement of stenosis on catheter angiography; most patient selection for CEA currently is done based on noninvasive imaging, such as duplex ultrasonography, which is less accurate.
4. Not included in the trials were patients with remote symptoms or clinically silent cerebral infarctions identified on imaging.
5. Some 20% of patients with symptomatic 70–99% carotid stenosis subsequently have a stroke related to other causes.[61]

SUBGROUP ANALYSES
1. Ulcerated plaque.
   (a) Natural history. In NASCET, patients in the medical arm with an ulcerated plaque had rates of ipsilateral stroke that increased dramatically with degree of stenosis. The risk of stroke at 24 months by degree of stenosis:[62]
       i. 75%; No ulcer: 21.2%; ulcer: 26.3%
       ii. 85%; No ulcer: 21.3%; ulcer: 43.9%
       iii. 95%; No ulcer: 21.3%; ulcer: 73.2%
   (b) Surgical risk. In NASCET, the perioperative stroke and death rate was 1.5 times higher in the presence of an ulcerated plaque.[63]
2. Hemispheric vs. retinal symptoms. Medically treated patients with hemispheric symptoms are at higher risk of stroke compared to patients with retinal ischaemic events only.
   (a) In NASCET, the relative risk of ipsilateral stroke in patients with 70–99% stenosis and hemispheric symptoms compared to patients with retinal symptoms only was 3.23 (95% CI, 1.47–7.12).[64]
       i. Benefit of surgery included patients whose only symptom was amaurosis fugax, as well as those with hemispheric symptoms.[64]

3. Near occlusion. Defined as a "string sign" on angiography with a very high grade stenosis with reduced caliber of the ICA distal to the stenosis,[65] near occlusion is associated with a lower risk of stroke in medically treated patients.

    (a) In NASCET, patients in the medical arm with near-occlusion had a 1-year stroke risk of 11.1%, which is lower than the 1-year stroke risk for patients with 90–94% stenosis, and approximately equal to the risk for patients with 70–89% stenosis.[66]

        i. Near-occlusion also confers no additional risk of perioperative complications with CEA, compared to other patients with >70% stenosis.

4. Contralateral occlusion. Patients in NASCET with contralateral occlusion were at elevated risk of stroke with both medical therapy and CEA.[67]

    (a) The risk of ipsilateral stroke in medically treated patients with 50–99% stenosis and a contralateral occlusion was more than twice as that of patients without a contralateral occlusion.

    (b) Perioperative risk of stroke or death for patients with 70–99% stenosis:

        i. 14.3% for patients with a contralateral occlusion.

        ii. 4.0% for patients without a contralateral occlusion.

5. Intraluminal thrombus. Angiographic evidence of intraluminal thrombus confers significant risk in both medically and surgically treated patients. In NASCET, 1.8% of patients had intraluminal thrombus. The 30-day rate of any stroke or death for surgical patients was similar to medically treated patients:[68]

    (a) Medical treatment group

        i. With intraluminal thrombus: 10.7%

        ii. Without intraluminal thrombus: 2.2%

    (b) Surgical group

        i. With intraluminal thrombus: 12.0%

        ii. Without intraluminal thrombus: Not reported by Villareal and colleagues. However, for comparison, the 30-day risk of stroke and death rate for all surgical patients in NASCET was 6.5%.[63]

6. Elderly patients. The risk of stroke increases with age.[69] Although the risk of CEA also increases significantly with age (a 36% increase in perioperative risk of stroke or death for patients >75 years),[70] in NASCET, the net benefit of CEA in patients with 50–99% stenosis increased with age.[69]

    (a) Age <65, absolute risk reduction (ARR) 10%

    (b) Age 65–74, ARR 15%

    (c) Age ≥75, ARR 29%

7. Ipsilateral intracranial aneurysms. Forty-eight patients in NASCET had an unruptured intracranial aneurysm ipsilateral to the symptomatic carotid artery.[71]

    (a) Of 25 patients in the surgery group, one patient had a fatal subarachnoid haemorrhage 6 days after CEA.

    (b) There were no haemorrhages among the 23 patients in the medical group.

AMERICAN HEART ASSOCIATION RECOMMENDATION
CEA in symptomatic patients be undertaken by surgeons whose surgical morbidity and mortality rate is <6%.[72]

Asymptomatic Carotid Stenosis

NATURAL HISTORY OF ASYMPTOMATIC CAROTID STENOSIS

Atherosclerotic stenosis of the proximal carotid arteries is common, affecting ~7% of women and >12% of men older than 70 years.[73]

The two largest studies of asymptomatic stenosis were randomized trials of CEA versus medical therapy, the Asymptomatic Carotid Atherosclerosis Study (ACAS)[74] and the Asymptomatic Carotid Surgery Trial (ACST)[75](see below). Both trials found that the annual risk of stroke due to asymptomatic stenosis ≥60% is approximately 2%. However, more recent data indicates that the risk of stroke with asymptomatic stenosis is lower, likely due to improved medical therapy and the expanding use of statins.[76] A recent systematic review found that the risk of stroke in has fallen significantly since the mid-1980s.[77] Studies published in the last decade have reported relatively lower annual ipsilateral stroke rates of 1.3%,[78] 1.2%,[79] 0.6%,[80] and 0.34%.[81] Thus, the earlier landmark trials comparing CEA to medical therapy may be obsolete in terms of risk of stroke with medical therapy. Furthermore, ultrasound examination may be able to identify the patients with asymptomatic stenosis at greatest risk of stroke.[82]

Table 18.2 CEA-8 risk score predicting 30-day risk of stroke or death

Risk factor	CEA-8 risk score points
Female sex	1
Nonwhite race	1
Contralateral stenosis ≥50%	1
Congestive heart failure	1
Coronary artery disease	1
Valvular heart disease	1
Severe disability	2
Quantitative risk category	**Total risk score points**
Low risk (1.4–2.9%)	0–2
Medium risk (5.8%)	3
High risk (8.3%)	≥4

Adapted from Calvillo-King et al.,[83] with permission
Based on a study of 6,553 Medicare patients undergoing CEA for asymptomatic stenosis in New York State.[83] A multivariate logistical regression identified eight independent predictors of stroke or death within 30 days of surgery. The CEA-8 score stratified patients according to risk

OXFORD VASCULAR STUDY
Most recent study of asymptomatic stenosis, the only one to date to include patients enrolled only after the year 2000.[81]
1. Population-based study of 101 patients with stenosis ≥50%, mean follow-up period of 3 years.
2. Average annual rate of ipsilateral stroke was 0.34%.

RISK OF SURGERY FOR ASYMPTOMATIC STENOSIS
The 30-day risk of stroke or death in the major randomized trials of CEA versus medical therapy (ACAS and ACST, see below) were 2.3% and 3.1%, respectively.[74,75] Many patients, however, are not similar to the patients enrolled in these trials. Eight factors have been found to increase the risk of CEA significantly (Table 18.2), and consideration of these factors can guide assessment of risk in patients with asymptomatic stenosis.

AMERICAN HEART ASSOCIATION GUIDELINES
The 2011 Guidelines for the Primary Prevention of Stroke stated, "Prophylactic CEA performed with <3% morbidity and mortality can be useful in highly selected patients with an asymptomatic carotid stenosis (minimum 60% by angiography, 70% by validated Doppler ultrasound)… the benefit of surgery may now be lower than anticipated based on randomized trial results, and the cited 3% threshold for complication rates may be high because of interim advances in medical therapy."[84]

Trials Comparing CEA to Medical Therapy

There have been five randomized trials comparing CEA to medical therapy for asymptomatic carotid stenosis.

ASYMPTOMATIC CAROTID ATHEROSCLEROSIS STUDY (ACAS)
1. 1,662 patients with ≥60% stenosis, defined by either angiography or carotid duplex ultrasonography, were randomized to CEA or medical treatment.[74] All patients received aspirin, 325 mg daily.
2. The study was stopped prematurely when a significant benefit for surgery was found.
3. Aggregate risk over 5 years for ipsilateral stroke and any perioperative stroke or death:
   (a) 11.0% in the medical group
   (b) 5.1% in the surgical group
      i. Aggregate risk reduction of 53% (95% CI, 22–72%).
      ii. Benefit was statistically significant for men but not women.
4. The rate of perioperative stroke and death in the CEA group, 2.3%, was similar to the annual rate of ipsilateral stroke in the medical group (2.2%).
5. No apparent increase in the benefit of CEA with increasing degree of stenosis.

6. Post hoc analysis of patients with contralateral occlusion[85]
   (a) Medically treated patients with a contralateral occlusion were less likely to have a stroke than those patients without a contralateral occlusion. 5-year risk of perioperative and ipsilateral stroke:
      i.   Stroke rate without contralateral occlusion: 11.7%
      ii. Stroke rate with contralateral occlusion: 3.5% ($p = 0.011$)
   (b) CEA may not benefit patients with contralateral carotid occlusion, and may be harmful. Effect on absolute risk of 5-year risk of perioperative and ipsilateral stroke:
      i.   Without contralateral occlusion: 6.7% reduction
      ii. With contralateral occlusion: 2.0 *increase* ($P = 0.047$).

VETERANS ADMINISTRATION COOPERATIVE ASYMPTOMATIC TRIAL
1. 444 men with ≥50% stenosis were randomized to receive medical therapy (recommended: aspirin, 1,300 mg daily) or medical therapy with CEA.[86]
2. After a 4-year follow-up period, the combined incidence of ipsilateral neurologic events:
   (a) 20.6% in the medical group
   (b) 8.0% in the surgical group ($P < 0.001$)
3. The high overall mortality rate of 33%, primarily owing to coronary atherosclerosis, suggests that the study population differed from those in other trials and makes interpretation of these results difficult.[87]

CAROTID ARTERY STENOSIS WITH ASYMPTOMATIC NARROWING: OPERATION VERSUS ASPIRIN (CASANOVA)
1. 410 patients with 50–90% stenosis were randomized to receive CEA and medical therapy or medical therapy only and followed for a mean interval of 42 months.[88] All patients received aspirin, 330 mg, and dipyridamole, 75 mg, three times daily.
2. No significant difference was found in stroke rates in the medical (11.3%) and surgical (10%) groups.
   (a) The small size of the study and the fact that a significant number of crossovers occurred between the groups obscures the importance of the findings.

MAYO ASYMPTOMATIC CAROTID ENDARTERECTOMY TRIAL
1. 158 patients received either medical therapy with aspirin or CEA *without* aspirin.[89] No major strokes or deaths occurred in either group.
2. Rate of myocardial infarction
   (a) 9% in the medical group
   (b) 26% in the surgical group ($p = 0.002$)
3. Study was terminated early owing to the significantly higher number of myocardial infarctions and transient cerebral ischaemic events that occurred in the surgical group, presumably because this group did not receive aspirin.
4. Results underscore the importance of treating patients with cerebrovascular atherosclerosis with antiplatelet agents.

ASYMPTOMATIC CAROTID SURGERY TRIAL (ACST)
1. Largest CEA study completed to date.
2. 3,120 patients with 60–99% stenosis on ultrasound were randomized to receive either *immediate* CEA or indefinite *deferral* of CEA (only 4% per year got CEA in this group).[75] Five-year risk of all strokes
   (a) 11.8% in the deferred group
   (b) 6.4% in the immediate group ($P < 0.0001$).
3. Risk of stroke or death within 30 days of CEA: 3.1%.
4. First study to show a protective effect of CEA in women. Five-year risk of non-perioperative stroke:
   (a) 7.48% in the deferred group
   (b) 3.40% in the immediate group ($p = 0.02$)
5. No apparent increase in benefit with increasing degree of stenosis.

Radiographic Evaluation

1. CEA is only effective when patients are selected appropriately.
2. In the major trials for symptomatic carotid stenosis, patient eligibility was based on angiographic criteria. Thus, radiographic evaluation of carotid stenosis must match the accuracy of catheter angiography.

      (a) In addition, CEA in asymptomatic patients carries a slender risk-benefit ratio, making accurate patient selection essential.
3. Carotid duplex ultrasonography is a useful screening method for detection of 70–99% stenosis.[90]
      (a) Sensitivity 94%
      (b) Specificity 89%
4. Limitations of duplex ultrasonography:
      (a) A significant proportion of CEAs are performed in general practice settings lacking designated, accredited vascular laboratories.[91,92]
      (b) Even accredited, high-volume vascular laboratories may report false-positive results for carotid stenosis ranging from 20% to 41%.[93]
      (c) Duplex scanning cannot image the distal ICA, intracranial vasculature, identify tandem lesions, or accurately distinguish preocclusive disease from total occlusion.[94,95]
      (d) Duplex scanning does not indicate whether the lesion is relatively high in the cervical region, which is information that is important in planning for a CEA.
5. These limitations *necessitate* additional confirmatory studies in the evaluation of patients with carotid stenosis.
      (a) Computed tomography angiography[96] and magnetic resonance angiography[97,98] can be used to confirm the results of carotid duplex imaging with a high degree of accuracy.
      (b) The authors of this handbook prefer to obtain ultrasound studies and a CTA (second choice: MRA) in the evaluation of all patients with carotid stenosis.

Interpretation of Carotid Ultrasound Results

    The term *carotid duplex* refers to a combination of Doppler measurements of velocity and B-mode imaging of the vessel. Carotid stenosis usually begins to cause a change in blood flow velocity when the degree of stenosis exceeds 50% (by NASCET criteria, corresponding to a 70% reduction in cross-sectional area). Flow velocity increases as the severity of stenosis increases (Fig. 18.2). Three validated criteria for measuring stenosis >50% include:[100]
1. Maximum peak systolic velocity (PSV) or Doppler frequency shift
2. B-mode measurements (gray-scale and/or color Doppler) of diameter reduction
3. ICA/CCA PSV ratio
A consensus paper published by the Society of Radiologists in Ultrasound established ultrasound criteria for the diagnosis of ICA stenosis (Table 18.3).[101]

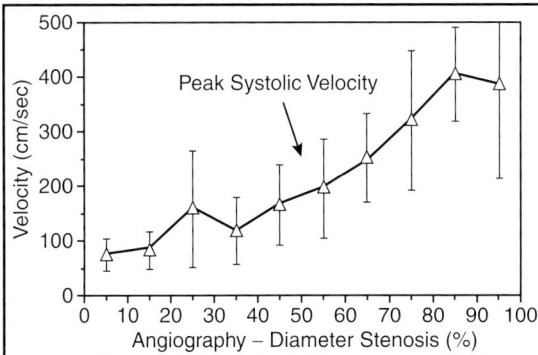

Fig. 18.2 Carotid Doppler velocities and degree of stenosis. Relationship between the mean peak systolic velocity (PSV) and the percentage of stenosis and the percentage of stenosis measured arteriographically. The PSV increases with the increasing severity of stenosis. Error bars show 1 SD about the mean (Reproduced from Grant et al.[99] © 2000 Radiology Society of North America, with permission).

Table 18.3 Consensus panel gray-scale and Doppler ultrasound criteria for diagnosis of ICA stenosis

Degree of stenosis (%)	Primary parameters		Additional parameters	
	ICA PSV (cm/s)	Plaque estimate (%)[a]	ICA/CCA PSV ratio	ICA EDV (cm/s)
Normal	<125	None	<2.0	<40
<50	<125	<50	<2.0	<40
50–69	125–230	≥50	2.0–4.0	40–100
≥70 but less than near occlusion	>230	≥50	>4.0	>100
Near occlusion	High, low, or undetectable	Visible	Variable	Variable
Total occlusion	Undetectable	Visible, no detectable lumen	Not applicable	Not applicable

Reproduced from Grant et al. [101] © 2003 Radiology Society of North America, with permission
[a]Plaque estimate (diameter reduction) with gray-scale and color Doppler ultrasound

1. Primary criteria:
   (a) Parameters (ICA PSV and the presence of plaque on gray-scale and/or color Doppler ultrasound images) that should be used to diagnose and grade ICA stenosis.
2. Additional criteria:
   (a) Additional parameters (ICA/CCA PSV ratio and ICA peak diastolic velocity) that can be used when the ICA PSV may not indicate the actual degree of stenosis due to technical or clinical factors (e.g., tandem lesions, discrepancy between the visual assessment of the plaque and the ICA PSV, elevated CCA velocity, hyperdynamic cardiac state, or low cardiac output).

Recurrent Stenosis After CEA

1. Two forms:
   (a) Early restenosis (<2 years after CEA) is characterized by myointimal cell proliferation. Diffuse thickening of the intima and media results in fibrous hypertrophic scarring throughout the CEA site. Stenosis of this type usually has a smooth, firm, non-ulcerated appearance.
   (b) Late restenosis (>2 years after CEA) is the result of a reaccumulation of atherosclerotic plaque and is typically friable and ulcerated in appearance.
2. Risk of restenosis after CEA:
   (a) Meta-analysis of 29 reports,[102] the risk of recurrent stenosis after CEA:
      i. 10% in the first year
      ii. 3% in the second year
      iii. 3% in the second year
      iv. Long-term risk is about 1% per year
   (b) Risk factors for restenosis:[103]
      i. Diabetes
      ii. Female sex
3. Risk of stroke with recurrent stenosis is unclear.
   (a) Relative risk of stroke in patients with recurrent stenosis compared with that in patients without recurrent stenosis ranged from 0.1 to 10.[102]
   (b) Myointimal hyperplasia leads to a smooth, nonulcerated stenosis without the same potential for ulceration and thromboembolism as atherosclerotic stenosis.
4. Redo-CEA carries a higher risk of complications than primary CEA.
   (a) 30-day perioperative neurological event rate:
      i. 4.8% in reoperation patients
      ii. 0.8% in primary CEA ($p = 0.015$)[104]

(b) Cranial nerve injury:
  i. 17% in reoperation patients
  ii. 5.3% in primary CEA ($p < 0.001$)
      – Although most of these injuries were transient.
5. Treatment of recurrent stenosis should be reserved strictly for patients who are symptomatic.

Medical Management

Medical management of carotid artery disease centers on cholesterol reduction, modification of risk factors, and antiplatelet therapy.

CHOLESTEROL REDUCTION

1. Elevated serum low-density lipoprotein (LDL) cholesterol out of proportion to high-density lipoprotein (HDL) cholesterol is the greatest risk factor for propagation of atherosclerosis.
2. 3-Hydroxy-3-methyl glutaryl coenzyme A (HMG-CoA) reductase inhibitors (statins) have been shown to slow the progression of carotid atherosclerosis[105,106] and reduce the risk of stroke in patients with coronary artery disease.[107]
3. Guidelines for the medical management of hypercholestrolemia have been set forth by the National Institutes of Health (Table 18.4)[108]
4. Patients placed on statins should be informed about and monitored for signs of myopathy, which can affect a small percentage of patients.[109]
5. Lovastatin (Mevacor®, Merck & Co., Inc., Whitehouse Station, NJ)[110]
   (a) Usual recommended starting dose is 20 mg once a day with the evening meal. Recommended dosing range is 10–80 mg/day in single or two divided doses; the maximum recommended dose is 80 mg/day.
   (b) Patients should be advised to report unexplained muscle pain, tenderness, or weakness.

HYPERTENSION

1. Most prevalent risk factor for stroke.[111]
2. Treatment reduces risk of stroke
   (a) An analysis of randomized trials found that a 5–6 mmHg reduction in diastolic blood pressure can reduce the risk of stroke by 42% ($p < 0.0001$).[112]
3. Over-correction of hypertension should be avoided to avert cerebrovascular hemodynamic failure, particularly in patients with hemodynamically significant carotid stenosis or with long-standing untreated hypertension.

CIGARETTE SMOKING

1. In a meta-analysis of 32 studies the relative risk of stroke for smokers was 1.5 (95% CI, 1.4–1.6).[113]
2. A discussion of Zyban[114,115] and other medications to help with smoking cessation is in Chap. 17.

ANTIPLATELET THERAPY

1. Rationale: Symptomatic carotid thromboembolic disease occurs in a high-flow environment, and generally appears with acute plaque rupture and thrombosis[116]
   (a) A characteristic *white clot* – a platelet-rich thombus – forms
   (b) Platelets participate in plaque rupture and thrombosis[117]
   (c) Lipids released by a ruptured plaque activate platelets[118]

Table 18.4 Serum LDL goals according to risk factors[108]

Risk factor(s)	Serum LDL goal
Coronary heart disease (CHD)	<100 mg/dL
Multiple (≤2) risk factors[a]	<130 mg/dL
Zero or one risk factor	<160 mg/dL

Data from Panel NCEPE[108]

[a]Risk factors include cigarette smoking; hypertension (BP ≥140/90 mmHg or on antihypertensive medication); low HDL cholesterol (<40 mg/dL); family history of premature CHD (CHD in male first degree relative <55 years; CHD in female first degree relative <65 years); age (men ≥45 years; women ≥55 years)

2. Aspirin
   (a) Inhibits platelet aggregation by inhibiting cyclo-oxygenase, which produces thromboxane.
   (b) Mayo Asymptomatic Carotid Endarterectomy Study[89]
       i. Terminated early because a significantly higher number of MIs and transient cerebral ischaemic events occurred in the surgical group, presumably due to the absence of aspirin use in the surgical group.
       ii. Underscores the importance of aspirin use in patients with asymptomatic carotid stenosis.
   (c) Appropriate dose of aspirin remains controversial.
       i. Low-dose aspirin (30–283 mg daily) has been shown to reduce the risk of stroke in asymptomatic patients with coronary artery disease[119] and in patients with TIA.[120,121]
       ii. The ASA and Carotid Endarterectomy Trial randomized patients undergoing CEA to receive low doses (81 or 325 mg daily) or high doses (650 or 1,300 mg daily).[122]
           – The combined rate of stroke, myocardial infarction, and death was lower in the low-dose groups than in the high-dose groups at 3 months (6.2 vs 8.4%, $p = 0.03$).
       iii. Conversely, high-dose aspirin (650–1,300 mg daily) may have protective effects that are unrelated to cyclo-oxygenase inhibition.[123]
           – A comparison of studies using doses ≥950 mg daily with those using doses <950 mg daily found a greater reduction in stroke risk in the higher dose studies.[123]
           – Drawback: gastrotoxicity.
3. Clopidogrel
   (a) Inhibits platelet aggregation induced by adenosine diphosphate by inhibiting the platelet adenosine diphosphate receptor.
   (b) Clopidogrel vs. Aspirin in Patients at Risk of Ischaemic Events (CAPRIE) randomized 19,185 patients with vascular disease to receive clopidogrel (75 mg daily) or aspirin (325 mg daily).[124] Annual risk of ischaemic stroke, MI, or vascular death was lower in the clopidogrel group:
       i. Clopidogrel group 5.32%
       ii. Aspirin group 5.83% ($p = 0.043$)
   (c) Management of Atherothrombosis with Clopidogrel in High-Risk Patients with Recent Transient Ischaemic Attack or Ischaemic Stroke (MATCH)[125] randomized 7,599 patients with a recent stroke or TIA to receive wither clopidogrel (75 mg daily) or clopidogrel (75 mg daily) plus low-dose aspirin (75 mg daily). During an 18 month follow-up period, there was:
       i. No significant difference in the rate of ischaemic events (stroke or MI).
       ii. Significant increase in life-threatening haemorrhage in the combination therapy group (2.6% vs. 1.3%) (absolute risk increase 1.3% 95% CI, 0.6–1.9).
4. Dipyridamole
   (a) Inhibits platelet aggregation by inhibiting phosphodiesterase and increasing levels of cyclic adenosine monophosphate.
   (b) The European Stroke Prevention Study-2 (ESPS-2) randomized 6,602 patients with prior stroke or TIA to receive treatment with extended-release dipyridamole (400 mg daily), low-dose aspirin (50 mg daily), the two agents in combination, or placebo.[126] Two-year stroke risk reduction compared to placebo was found to be greatest for the combination regimen:
       i. Risk reduction 37% with combination therapy ($p < 0.001$).
       ii. A post hoc analysis of patients in ESPS-2 at high risk for stroke also found combination therapy to be more effective than low-dose aspirin alone at preventing stroke.[127]
   (c) Available as Aggrenox[®] (aspirin 25 mg/extended release dipyridamole 200 mg) capsules.
   (d) Headaches occur in 38.7% of patients treated with aspirin/dipyridamole combination.[128]
       i. Usually self-limited and decrease in frequency over time.
5. Ticlopidine
   (a) Prevents platelet aggregation by blocking the 5′-diphosphate binding site of the IIa/IIIb receptor, the final common pathway of platelet aggregation.
   (b) The Ticlopidine Aspirin Stroke Study (TASS) randomized 3,069 patients with minor stroke or TIA to receive aspirin 650 mg BID or ticlopine 250 mg BID.[129] The ticlopidine group had a greater reduction in 3-year risk of stroke:

   i. The ticlopine group had a 21% relative risk reduction for stroke compared with aspirin ($p = 0.024$).

  (c) Ticlopidine is associated with an approximately 1–2% incidence of severe neutropenia and >60 cases of ticlopine-associated thrombotic thrombocytopenia purpura (TTP) have been reported.[130]

  (d) Neutrophil counts are required at 2-week intervals for the first 3 months of ticlopine therapy; the drug must be held if the neutrophil count drops below $1,200/mm^3$.

  (e) Ticlopidine is preferred by the authors of this handbook as a second-line agent (in combination with aspirin) in patients undergoing angioplasty and stenting who cannot tolerate clopidogrel.

6. Anticoagulants

  (a) There is no controlled trial data to support the use of warfarin or heparin in patients with either symptomatic or asymptomatic extracranial carotid atherosclerotic disease.

   i. Exception: A short-term course of anticoagulation may be an option when an intraluminal thrombus is present.

7. Antiplatelet Therapy Recommendations:

  (a) Evidence-based guidelines for the prevention of cerebral ischaemic events published by The Seventh ACCP Conference on Antithrombotic and Thrombolytic Therapy:[131]

   i. In patients who have had a noncardiogenic stroke or TIA, the following are all acceptable (Grade IA evidence):

    1. Aspirin 50–325 mg daily, *or*

    2. Combination of aspirin 25 mg and extended-release dipyridamole 200 mg BID, *or*

    3. Clopidogrel 75 mg daily

  (b) The authors' preference is to use aspirin, 325 mg daily for most patients with atherosclerotic carotid disease.

Carotid Angioplasty and Stenting

A Brief History of Carotid Angioplasty and Stenting

  Endovascular treatment of extracranial carotid stenosis has been made possible by developments in endovascular technology for other applications in recent decades. Angioplasty with or without stenting has been established as an alternative to surgical revascularization in patients with coronary artery disease and peripheral vascular disease. Angioplasty for carotid stenosis was first reported in the early 1980s.[132,133] In contrast to CEA, in which the atherosclerotic plaque is removed, angioplasty causes fracture of the plaque and stretching of the media.[134] With angioplasty alone, however, plaque debris may be released into the intracranial circulation; and the resulting irregularity within the plaque can be thrombogenic before remodeling and endothelialization can occur.[135,136] High rates of neurological complications attributable to embolization of plaque fragments were described in the initial reports of carotid angiography.[137,138]

  The development of intravascular stenting was driven by a need for improvement in coronary balloon angioplasty, in which acute occlusion and restenosis after angioplasty are problematic. Following the first report of carotid stenting in 1995,[139] stenting was seen as necessary along with carotid angioplasty to stabilize the plaque and reduce embolization of debris. Angioplasty with stenting has become the endovascular treatment of choice for carotid stenosis.[140] However, angioplasty and stenting alone did not eliminate the problem of embolization. An early trial of CAS vs. CEA was stopped prematurely because of a high rate of stroke in the CAS group.[141] Embolic protection techniques were introduced to prevent embolization during CAS. The first report of an embolic protection technique described a triple coaxial catheter with a latex balloon mounted at the distal end.[142] In recent years, ICA filters and flow-reversal techniques have also been introduced. Presently, filter devices are the most common embolic protection devices. Appropriate sizing of angioplasty balloons has minimized the risk of asystole during CAS, and eliminated the need for routine cardiac pacing. The addition of antiplatelet agents such as clopidogrel and GP IIb/IIIa inhibitors have also served to prevent and treat thromboembolic complications during CAS.[143,144]

  The use of CAS has expanded globally in recent years, driven by a combination of influences, including improvements in technique and devices, the medical device

Table 18.5 Major contemporary randomized trials – CAS versus CEA[a]

Study	Patient population	Country	No. of patients
SAPPHIRE	High risk symptomatic and asymptomatic	US	334
CREST[146]	Symptomatic and asymptomatic	US	2,502
EVA-3S[56,147]	Symptomatic and asymptomatic	France	527
ICSS (aka CAVATAS-2)[148]	Symptomatic	United Kingdom	1,713
SPACE[149]	Symptomatic	Germany, Austria, Switzerland	1,214

[a]Abbreviations: *CREST* Carotid Revascularization Endarterectomy vs. Stent Trial, *EVA-3S* Endarterectomy vs. Angioplasty in Patients With Symptomatic Severe Carotid Stenosis, *ICSS* International Carotid Stenting Study, *CAVATAS* Carotid and Vertebral Transluminal Angioplasty Study, *SPACE* Stent-Protected Percutaneous Angioplasty of the Carotid vs. Endarterectomy

industry, the availability of physicians with endovascular expertise (e.g., interventional cardiologists), increased insurance reimbursement, and a growing popular interest in less invasive treatment. In a study of Medicare claims, the use of CAS was found to have grown four-fold from 1998 to 2007, while the use of CEA declined 31%.[145]

Despite the popularity of CAS, CEA remains the "gold standard" for the treatment of carotid stenosis in selected patients. Four recent major multicenter randomized trials comparing CAS to CEA have been completed (Table 18.5). The Carotid Revascularization Endarterectomy vs. Stent Trial (CREST) was an NIH-sponsored multicenter randomized trial of CEA vs. CAS in non-high-risk patients. CREST originally enrolled only patients with symptomatic stenosis ≥50% by angiography (or >70% by ultrasound); however, in June, 2005, the study protocol was amended to permit enrollment of asymptomatic patients. The first results of CREST were reported in February, 2010. Three major European randomized trials have been completed: SPACE, (Stent-Protected Percutaneous Angioplasty of the Carotid vs. Endarterectomy).[150] EVA-3S (Endarterectomy vs. Angioplasty in Patients with Symptomatic Severe Carotid Stenosis),[56] and the International Carotid Stenting Study (ICSS).[57]

Carotid stenting was approved in the U.S. in August, 2004 by the FDA only for use in patients who are at high risk of adverse events with CEA. In October, 2004, Medicare limited reimbursement for CAS to qualified providers in high-surgical-risk, symptomatic patients or those enrolled in clinical trials. In 2011, the FDA expanded approval of CAS to include patients at regular risk of adverse events with CEA.

Stenting and Angioplasty with Protection in Patients at High Risk for Endarterectomy (SAPPHIRE)

1. 334 patients at high risk for surgery (Table 18.6) with symptomatic stenosis (≥50%) or asymptomatic stenosis (≥80%) were randomized to CEA or CAS. The study was designed to test the hypothesis that CAS is not inferior to CEA. The study was discontinued early because of low enrollment.

Table 18.6 SAPPHIRE criteria for high risk[a]

1. Clinically significant cardiac disease (congestive heart failure, abnormal stress test, or need for open-heart surgery)
2. Severe pulmonary disease
3. Contralateral carotid occlusion
4. Contralateral laryngeal-nerve palsy
5. Previous radical neck surgery or radiation therapy to the neck
6. Recurrent stenosis after endarterectomy
7. Age >80 years

[a]At least one factor required

(a) Primary endpoint (stroke, death, or MI at 30 days plus ipsilateral stroke or death from neurologic causes within 31 days to 1 year):[151]
  i. One year results: Trend toward a lower rate of the primary endpoint in the CAS group:
    1. 4.8% in the CAS group.
    2. 9.8% in the CEA group ($p = 0.09$).
(b) Secondary endpoint (death, stroke, or MI within 30 days or death or ipsilateral stroke between 31 days and 3 years):[152]
  i. Three-year results:
    1. 24.6% in the CAS group.
    2. 26.9% in the CEA group ($p = 0.71$)

Carotid Revascularization Endarterectomy Versus Stent Trial (CREST)

1. 2,502 patients with symptomatic stenosis (>50%) or asymptomatic stenosis (>60%) were randomized to CAS or CEA.[146]
2. Primary endpoint was stroke, myocardial infarction, or death within 30 days of enrollment or any ipsilateral stroke within 4 years after randomization
3. Acculink stents (Abbott, Abbott Park, IL), were used. Accunet embolic protection devices were used in 96.1% of CAS cases.
4. Median follow-up: 2.5 years.
5. The primary endpoint rate was not different between the groups:
   (a) 7.2% in the CAS group
   (b) 6.8% in the CEA group ($p = 0.51$)
6. During the 30-day periprocedural period:
   (a) There was a higher rate of stroke in the stenting group
     i. 4.1% in the CAS group
     ii. 2.3% in the CEA group ($p = 0.01$)
   (b) There was a higher rate of MI in the endarterectomy group
     i. 1.1% in the CAS group
     ii. 2.3% in the CEA group ($p = 0.03$)
7. Effect of age:
   (a) Outcomes (i.e., primary endpont rates) were slightly better after CAS for patients <70 years and better after CEA for patients >70 years.
8. Symptomatics versus asymptomatics: There were no significant differences between CAS and CEA by symptomatic status for the primary end point.[153] However, the periprocedural stroke and death rate was significantly higher for CAS in symptomatic patients:
   (a) Symptomatic patients:
     i. 6.0% in the CAS group
     ii. 3.2% in the CEA group ($p = 0.02$)
   (b) Asymptomatic patients:
     i. 2.5% in the CAS group
     ii. 1.4% in the CEA group ($p = 0.15$)
9. Study results have been somewhat controversial.
   (a) Strengths:
     i. CREST was notable for rigorous training and credentialing of the operators in the study.[154] Indeed, the periprocedural event rates in this study were superior to the results in the other major CAS versus CEA trials, presumably because of this.
     ii. Uniform stenting procedure – with only one stent – with a high rate of embolic protection.
   (b) Weaknesses:
     i. The study had both symptomatic and asymptomatic patients, thus violating the violating the principle of *ceteris paribus* (i.e., the principle of controlling all independent variables in a controlled trial).[155]
     ii. Myocardial infarctions were defined as including cases in which a elevation in cardiac enzymes occurred without EKG changes or chest pain. Thus, relatively minor MIs were counted as adverse events.
     iii. "Silent strokes" (i.e., ischaemic injury as assessed by MRI) were not assessed.

Stent-Supported Percutaneous Angioplasty of the Carotid Versus Endarterectomy (SPACE)[150]

1. 1,214 patients in Germany, Austria, and Switzerland with symptomatic stenosis (≥50%) were randomized to CAS or CEA. The study was designed to test the hypothesis that CAS is not inferior to CEA. The study was stopped prematurely (1,900 patients were planned) because of problems with funding and enrollment.[156]
2. Primary endpoint (ipsilateral ischaemic stroke or death within 30 days):
   (a) 6.92% in the CAS group
   (b) 6.45% in the CEA group ($p = 0.09$)
3. Ipsilateral stroke up to 2 years or any periprocedure stroke or death: *No significant difference.*[55]
   (a) 9.5% in the CAS group
   (b) 8.8% in the CEA group ($p = 0.62$)
4. Effect of age:
   (a) Risk of ipsilateral stroke or death increased significantly with age in the CAS group ($p = 0.001$) but not in the CEA group ($p = 0.534$).[157]
      i. The age with the greatest separation between high-risk and low-risk CAS cases was 68 years. Primary outcome occurred in:
         1. 2.7% who were ≤68 years
         2. 10.8% who were >68 years
5. *SPACE failed to prove noninferiority of carotid-artery stenting compared with carotid endarterectomy for the periprocedural complication rate.*
6. Controversies about SPACE:
   (a) Use of embolic protection devices were not required in this trial, and only 27% of the cases in the CAS group were done with embolic protection devices. However, the 30-day rate of ipsilateral stroke or death in SPACE was 7.3% in CAS cases with embolic protection, compared to 6.7% in those without it.[158]
   (b) The non-inferiority test used by SPACE is different from the analysis used by previous carotid surgery trials, in which the null hypothesis assumed no difference between the two interventions. This may contribute to uncertainty and a perception of ambiguity about the results.[158]

SPACE II[159]

1. Ongoing trial in Europe of patients with asymptomatic stenosis ≥70%. Patients are randomized to CAS, CEA or medical therapy. Planned enrollment: 3,640 patients.
2. Primary endpoint: any stroke or death within 30 days plus ipsilateral stroke within 5 years.

Endarterectomy Versus Angioplasty in Patients with Symptomatic Severe Carotid Stenosis (EVA-3S)[147]

1. A total of 527 patients in France with symptomatic stenosis (≥60%) were randomized to CAS or CEA. Enrollment was stopped prematurely (enrollment of 872 patients was originally planned) for "reasons of safety and futility."
2. Primary endpoint (stroke or death within 30 days after treatment):
   (a) 9.6% in the CAS group
   (b) 3.9% in the CEA group ($p = 0.004$)
3. Ipsilateral stroke or death at 4 years:
   (a) 11.1% in the CAS group
   (b) 6.2% in the CEA group ($p = 0.03$)
      i. The 4 year difference in outcomes was due largely to the higher periprocedural stroke and death rate.
4. Technical factors associated with risk of stroke or death in CAS:[160]
   (a) Risk was higher in patients with ICA-CCA angulation ≥60° and lower in patients with embolic protection
5. Restenosis[161] Duplex exams done at 3-year follow-up, restenosis ≥50%:
   (a) 12.5% in the CAS group
   (b) 5.0% in the CEA group ($p = 0.02$)

6. Controversies about EVA-3S:
   (a) Relatively modest requirements for interventionalists to participate in the study.[156]
   (b) Wide variety of devices used for CAS (any of five different stents and seven different embolic protection devices were permitted).
   (c) Only 85.4% of the CAS group received dual antiplatelet therapy.[56]

International Carotid Stenting Study (ICSS) [57]

1. AKA CAVATAS-2. A total of 1,713 patients with symptomatic stenosis >50% were randomized to CAS or CEA. Enrollment was from 2001 to 2008.
2. Primary outcome results (3-year rate of fatal or disabling stroke in any territory) have not been published yet.
3. Interim analysis (March, 2010) reported 120-day results:
   (a) Stroke, death, or procedural myocardial infarction:
      i. 8.5% in the CAS group
      ii. 5.2% in the CEA group ($p = 0.006$)
4. MRI substudy.[162] A total 231 patients (124 CAS; 107 CEA) had an MRI before and after treatment. New DWI changes, indicating ischaemic injury:
   (a) 50% in the CAS group
   (b) 17% in the CEA group ($p < 0.0001$)
      i. DWI changes occurred despite the use of embolic protection.

Recurrent Stenosis After CAS

1. Global registry[163]
   (a) Restenosis rates of carotid stenting were 2.7%, 2.6%, and 2.4% at 1, 2, and 3 years, respectively.
2. Single-center series, carotid duplex:
   (a) Restenosis (> or =70%), median follow-up 12 months: 3.0%[164]
   (b) Restenosis (> or =80%), median follow-up 16.4 months: 5%[165]
3. Four-center series, carotid duplex. Analysis of 2,172 cases found rates of restenosis (>50%) to be 1%, 2%, and 3.4% after 1, 3, and 5 years, respectively.[166]
4. EVA-3S results:[161]
   (a) Carotid ultrasound follow-up, mean 2.1 years, rate of stenosis ≥5.0%:
      i. 12.5% in the CAS group
      ii. 5.0% in the CEA group ($p = 0.02$)
         1. *Restenosis was not a significant risk factor for recurrent stroke or TIA.*
         2. CAS changes the physiology of atherosclerotic disease. Most strokes attributable to carotid stenosis are embolic; CAS stabilizes the plaque. Therefore, restenosis after CAS may not have the same natural history as native carotid stenosis.

Effect of Embolic Protection on Periprocedural Complication Rates in CAS

Release of embolic material during CAS without embolic protection is common, as demonstrated by transcranial Doppler[167] and post-procedure MRI.[162,168] A variety of embolic protection devices have been introduced for use during CAS (see Chap. 10). No randomized trial has compared CAS with and without embolic protection. A number of series, however, have shown a significant reduction in complication rates with the use of embolic protection devices.

1. The global registry found a periprocedural and death rate of 5.29% in cases without protection, compared to a 2.23% rate with protection.[163]
2. A systematic review of published studies including 2,537 CAS procedures found that the 30-day stroke and death rate in both symptomatic and asymptomatic patients was 1.8% in patients treated with cerebral protection devices compared with 5.5% in patients treated without cerebral protection devices ($p < 0.001$).[169]
   (a) This effect was due to a reduction in both major and minor strokes; the death rates were almost identical.

3. In the French EVA-3S Trial, in which patients are randomized to CEA or CAS with or without embolic protection, the Safety Committee recommended stopping CAS without protection, because the 30-day stroke rate was 3.9 times higher than that of CAS with protection (4/15 versus 5/58).[170]
4. Interestingly, a secondary analysis of the SPACE trial did not find a beneficial effect of embolic protection.[171]

Timing of CEA or CAS After a Stroke

The optimal timing of surgical or endovascular treatment of carotid stenosis after a cerebral ischaemic event is controversial. Surgery within 7 days of a stroke has been found to be a risk factor for complications with CEA.[172] The authors of this handbook prefer to wait for treatment 1–2 weeks after a completed stroke, and to proceed sooner for patients with TIAs only or crescendo TIAs.

Current FDA Approval for CAS

The FDA approved the Rx Acculink Carotid Stent System and cleared the Rx Accunet Embolic Protection System for patients at high risk for adverse events with CEA in August, 2004. The patients must meet the following criteria:[173]
1. Patients with neurological symptoms and ≥50% stenosis of the CCA or ICA by ultrasound or angiogram OR patients without neurological symptoms and ≥80% stenosis of the CCA or ICA AND...
2. The reference vessel diameter measures 4.0–9.0 mm.

Medicare defines "high risk for endarterectomy" as comorbid conditions that include, but are not limited to:[174]
1. Congestive heart failure class III or IV
2. Left ventricular ejection fraction <30%
3. Unstable angina
4. Contralateral carotid occlusion
5. Recent myocardial infarction
6. Previous CEA with recurrent stenosis
7. Prior radiation treatment of the neck; and
8. Other conditions that were used to determine patients at high risk for CEA in prior stenting trials and studies.

Patient Selection: CAS or CEA?

An avalanche of clinical trial data is now available to help guide decision-making in patients with carotid stenosis. Several truths have emerged in the last several years:
1. Asymptomatic stenosis is relatively benign,[78–81] and medical management alone may be the best option. Duplex ultrasonography may be able to identify patients at greatest risk of stroke with asymptomatic stenosis.[82]
2. The risk of stroke is higher with CAS than with CEA, at least in the short term.[57,146,147,175]
3. Patients <70 years do better with CAS than patients >70.[146,176]
4. After the 30-day period, the rate of stroke is similar for both CAS and CEA.[55,146]

Carotid endarterectomy remains the standard of care for the treatment of symptomatic stenosis in appropriate patients. Carotid angioplasty and stenting is probably best reserved for symptomatic patients who are not good candidates for CEA.

Factors that can guide patient selection are summarized in Table 18.7.

Atherosclerotic Carotid Occlusion

Asymptomatic Carotid Occlusion

1. Prevalence
   (a) Prevalence of silent ICA occlusion in the general population age >60 is <1%[177]
2. Prognosis – *excellent*.

Table 18.7 Patient selection for angioplasty and stenting or carotid endarterectomy

Relative indications	Relative contraindications
Carotid angioplasty and stenting	
Age <70 years	Age >70 years
Poor surgical candidate	Elongated aortic arch or otherwise difficult vascular access
Accessible vascular anatomy	High grade carotid stenosis
Focal stenosis	Long region of stenosis
Tandem stenoses	Aortic or femoral artery occlusion
Previous neck surgery	Intolerance to antiplatelet agents
Radiation-induced stenosis	Intolerance to iodinated contrast
High risk for anesthesia complications	Intraluminal thrombus
Carotid endarterectomy	
Age >70 years	Contralateral laryngeal palsy
Few medical conditions	Multiple medical conditions
No previous neck surgery or radiation	Previous neck surgery or radiation
Thin, supple neck	Short, thick neck
Patent, nonstenotic contralateral carotid artery	Contralateral carotid occlusion
Low carotid bifurcation	High carotid bifurcation

(a) Very low risk of ischaemic stroke[178,179]
(b) "The benign course of never-symptomatic carotid occlusion"[180]
    i. Risk of stroke in 30 patients with never-symptomatic carotid occlusion during an average follow-up of 32 months: 3.3%. No strokes occurred in the carotid territory ipsilateral to the occluded artery in these patients.

Symptomatic Carotid Occlusion

1. Incidence
    (a) Annual incidence is 6 per 100,000 persons[181]
2. Prognosis[182,183]
    (a) Overall annual risk of stroke: 5–7%
    (b) Annual risk of stroke ipsilateral to the occluded artery: 2–6%
3. Prognosis depends strongly on *hemodynamic status*.
    (a) Cerebral blood flow in the presence of carotid occlusion is maintained by collateral circulation (e.g., blood flow from the contralateral carotid system via the anterior communicating artery or pial-collaterals on the cortical surface). Some patients with carotid occlusion have little vascular reserve based on collateral circulation (i.e., blood flow in the affected brain region is at or near maximum, and cannot be increased if necessary by autoregulatory dilation of cerebral arterioles). These patients are at elevated risk of stroke. Quantitative assessment of cerebral hemodynamic status in these patients has been best demonstrated by ^{15}O PET measurement of oxygen extraction fraction (OEF) and xenon-CT cerebral blood flow measurement with acetazolamide challenge.
4. ^{15}O PET
    (a) This nuclear medicine technique permits quantitative measurement of CBF, CBV, and OEF.
    (b) Stage 0. Cerebral perfusion pressure (CPP) is normal. OEF shows little regional variation. Moderate reductions in CPP have little effect on cerebral blood flow (CBF) because of autoregulatory compensation.
    (c) Stage I. Chronic, sustained reduction of CPP (e.g., due to ICA occlusion) causes cerebral arterioles to be maximally dilated to maintain adequate CBF. Cerebrovascular reserve is exhausted. PET demonstrates increased cerebral blood volume (CBV) relative to CBF (increased CBV/CBF ratio).

(d) Stage II. Further reduction of CPP leads to a *decrease* in CBF and an *increase* in OEF, to maintain cerebral oxygen metabolism and brain function.
  i. Prospective study of 81 patients with previous stroke or TIA in the territory of an occluded carotid artery.[183] Rate of stroke in average follow-up of 31.5 months:
    – 12 of 39 (30.8%) patients with stage II hemodynamic failure
    – 3 of 42 (7.1%) patients without ($p = 0.004$).
5. Xenon-CT
  (a) Nonradioactive xenon inhalation technique permits quantitative measurement of CBF. Acetazolamide, a carbonic anhydrase inhibitor, causes dilation in cerebral arterioles and an increase in CBF. In regions of the brain with Stage I or Stage II hemodynamic failure, cerebral arterioles are unable to dilate any further in response to acetazolamide, and regional CBF either remains the same after administration of acetazolamide, or decreases as blood flow is diverted from low-flow to high-flow regions.
    i. Prospective study of 68 patients with symptomatic carotid stenosis or occlusion who underwent xenon-CT studies before and after administration of acetazolamide.[184] Patients were classified according to response and followed for a mean of 24 months.
      – Group 2: CBF reduction >5% in at least one vascular territory and baseline flow of 45 cc/100 gm/min or less.
        • 36% rate of stroke (all ipsilateral to side with lowest reserve) ($p = 0.0007$).
      Group 1: all other patients.
        • 4.4% rate of stroke (both strokes occurred contralateral to the side with lowest reserve).

Surgical Options for Cerebral Revascularization in Patients with Carotid Occlusion

1. Direct anastamotic bypass procedures:
  (a) Low flow
    i. e.g., STA-MCA bypass
    ii. The first EC-IC bypass was performed by Yasargil, in Zurich, Switzerland, in 1967.[185]
  (b) High flow
    i. e.g., saphenous vein or radial artery graft
    ii. Can establish up to 3.7-times increase in flow compared to a low-flow bypass[186]
    iii. Excimer laser method is a new technique for high-flow bypass[187]
2. Indirect nonanastomotic bypass procedures:
  (a) Used primarily in younger patients (e.g., Moyamoya Syndrome).
  (b) Examples:
    ii. Temporal muscle grafting (encephalomyosynangiosis); transposition of the STA (encephaloduroarteriosynangiosis).

Extracranial-Intracranial (EC/IC) Bypass Trial

1. 1,377 patients with recent hemisphere stroke, retinal infarction, or TIA and atherosclerotic occlusion or narrowing of the ipsilateral ICA or MCA were randomized to receive either medical care (714 patients, aspirin 325 mg QID) or medical care with STA-MCA bypass (663 patients).[188] Average follow-up was 55.8 months.
  (a) ICA occlusion was the most common angiographic lesion. The percentages of patients with each type of angiographic finding (medical group/surgery group):
    i.   MCA stenosis: 13.0%/14.4%
    ii. MCA occlusion: 11.1%/12.1%
    iii. ICA stenosis (above C2): 16.7%/15.4%
    iv. ICA occlusion: 59.%/58.1%
2. 30-day surgical results:
  (a) Mortality 0.6%
  (b) Major stroke rate 2.5%

3. Postoperative patency rate 96%.
4. Results:
    (a) Overall stroke rate (i.e., total number of patients having a fatal or nonfa-tal stroke over a mean follow-up period of 55.8 months):
        i. Medical group: 28.7%
        ii. Surgical group: 30.9%
    (b) Subgroups:
        i. All patients with ICA occlusion:
            – Medical group: 29.1%
            – Surgical group: 31.4%
        ii. ICA occlusion with symptoms between time of angiogram and randomization:
            – Medical group: 34.7%
            – Surgical group: 45.7%
        iii. ICA stenosis (≥70%):
            – Medical group: 36.1%
            – Surgical group: 37.7%
        iv. MCA stenosis (≥70%):
            – Medical group: 23.7%
            – Surgical group: 44.0%
        v. Bilateral ICA occlusion
            – Medical group: 39.5%
            – Surgical group: 45.2%
        vi. MCA occlusion
            – Medical group: 22.8%
            – Surgical group: 20.0%
5. No subgroup was found to benefit from bypass.
    (a) Two groups did significantly worse with surgery:
        i. MCA stenosis (≥70%) ($n = 109$)
        ii. Ischaemic symptoms and occluded ICA ($n = 287$)
6. *This study thus failed to confirm the hypothesis that extracranial-intracranial anastomosis is effective in preventing cerebral ischaemia in patients with athero-sclerotic arterial disease in the carotid and middle cerebral arteries.*
7. Study results have been highly controversial.[189–192]
    (a) Primary limitations and criticisms:
        i. Study did not base patient selection on hemodynamic assessment.
            – Imaging technology since the EC/IC Bypass trial was done has progressed significantly, enabling identification of patients who have symptomatic cerebrovascular hemody-namic failure, and would thus, presumably, benefit the most from bypass surgery.
        ii. Patients with MCA stenosis were included; bypass in this setting can reduce flow through the stenotic vessel, leading to occlusion.[193–195]
        iii. A large number of patients (2,572) received STA-MCA bypass out-side of the trial while the trial was being conducted.
        iv. Multiple sources of bias were present (e.g., observational bias).

Carotid Occlusion Surgery Study (COSS)

1. Trial to evaluate STA-MCA bypass in patients with symptomatic ICA occlusion and ipsilateral increase OEF measured by PET.
2. A total of 372 patients with recent symptoms (≤120 days) were planned to be randomized to surgical or non-surgical treatment.
3. The trial was stopped by the NIH early, in June, 2010. An interim futility analy-sis showed that it was unlikely that a significant difference would be found between the groups if the total enrollment was completed.
4. Total patients randomized: 195 (98 received surgery, 97 no surgery)
5. 30-day graft patency: 98%
6. Mean ipsilateral/contralateral OEF ratio improved from 1.258 to 1.109 in the surgical group.
7. Results[196]
    (a) Ipsilateral stroke rate in 2 years:
        i. Medical group: 22.7%
        ii. Surgical group: 21% ($p = 0.78$)

(b) Ipsilateral stroke rate at 30 days:
    i. Medical group: 2.0%
    ii. Surgical group: 14.4%
8. *This study was the second large-scale randomized trail that failed to find a benefit in terms of stroke recurrence with EC-IC bypass surgery.*
9. STA-MCA bypass may provide a cognitive benefit that is independent of effects on stroke risk.[197] This possibility is being investigated by the ongoing Randomized Evaluation of Carotid Occlusion and Neurocognition (RECON) trial, an ancillary study of COSS.[198]

Extracranial Vertebral Artery Atherosclerotic Disease

Some 20% of cerebral ischaemic events involve the posterior circulation. In the New England Medical Center Posterior Circulation Registry (NEMC-PCR), the extracranial vertebral artery was the most common site of vascular occlusive lesions in patients with vertebrobasilar insufficiency (VBI).[199] In an angiographic series of 4,728 patients with ischaemic stroke, some degree of extracranial stenosis was seen in 18% of cases on the right and 22.3% on the left.[200]

Atherosclerosis is the most common cause of extracranial vertebral artery stenosis; less common causes are arterial dissection, extrinsic compression due to trauma, osteophytes, or fibrous bands, or vasculitis (most commonly giant-cell arteritis)[201] Risk factors for atherosclerotic extracranial vertebral artery disease are identical to those found in patients atherosclerotic carotid artery disease.[199] However, atherosclerotic plaque at the vertebral artery origin is considered to be "smoother" and less prone to ulceration than in the carotid system.[202] Caucasian patients seem to be preferentially affected by atherosclerosis of the extracranial vertebral artery.[203]

Two patterns of symptoms due to extracranial vertebral artery stenosis have been observed:[199,204]
1. Brief and multiple TIAs, consisting of dizziness, loss of balance, and visual disturbances, and sometimes precipitated by changes in position.
2. Sudden-onset stroke, usually involving the PICA-supplied region of the cerebellum or the distal intracranial posterior circulation territory.

The most common mechanism of stroke in these patients is intra-arterial embolism, rather than hemodynamic failure.[204]

Diagnosis

The diagnosis of VBI attributable to extracranial vertebral artery occlusive disease depends on a combination of symptoms and radiographic findings:
1. Symptoms of VBI (*must include at least two of the following symptoms*):[205]
    (a) Motor or sensory symptoms
    (b) Dysarthria
    (c) Imbalance
    (d) Dizziness or vertigo
    (e) Tinnitus
    (f) Alternating paresthesias
    (g) Homonymous hemianopia
    (h) Diplopia
    (i) Other cranial nerve palsies
    (j) Dysphagia
        i. Fewer than 1% of patients with VBI in the NEMC-PCR had only a single presenting symptom or sign.[199]
        ii. "Drop attacks" (sudden loss of postural tone without warning) are rarely attributable to VBI. No patient in the NEMC-PCR had a drop attack as the only symptom.[199,206]
2. ≥50% stenosis of the vertebral artery by CTA, angiography, or MRA.
    (a) The authors of this handbook favour CTA for imaging; CTA has been found to be as accurate as angiography in imaging of vertebral artery stenosis,[207] and CTA has the additional advantage of also imaging extravascular structures.
3. Additional findings can support the diagnosis of symptomatic VBI:
    (a) MRI evidence of ischaemic injury to the posterior circulation (may not be found in patients with minor stroke or TIAs only).
    (b) Hypoplasia or stenosis affecting the contralateral vertebral artery.

Prognosis

The prognosis of symptomatic extracranial vertebral artery stenosis is not well understood. Although a number of reports have suggested a more benign natural history than for symptomatic carotid stenosis, a more recent systematic review found that the risk of stroke or death in patients with VBI appears to be at least as high as it is in patients with symptomatic carotid bifurcation disease, and possibly higher.[208]

MEDICAL THERAPY

Combination antiplatelet regimens (e.g., aspirin and clopidogrel) are emerging as the mainstay of medical therapy for patients with VBI. A combination of aspirin and dypyridamole was shown to significantly reduce the rate of stroke in patients with VBI compared to placebo.[209] Patients with atherosclerosis and hyperlipidemia should also be treated with a lipid-lowering agent.[210] The authors of this handbook prefer to avoid warfarin therapy for patients with atherosclerotic stenosis, for lack of convincing evidence of efficacy and safety.

ANGIOPLASTY AND STENTING

Although surgery for vertebral artery stenosis has been reported[211], endovascular techniques have become the most common approach in patients who remain symptomatic despite medical therapy. No large series or randomized trial data about treatment of extracranial vertebral artery stenosis are yet available.
1. Immediate results
   (a) High rates of technical success (residual stenosis <50%):
       i. 97–>99%[212,213]
       ii. 100%.[214]
   (b) Relatively low rates of procedure-related complications:
       i. 8.8% (all TIAs without permanent neurologic change)[215]
       ii. 3% (one TIA)[215]
       iii. 0%[214]
2. Long term results
   (a) Relatively high rates of restenosis:
       i. 100% of patients with angioplasty alone.[216]
       ii. Angiographic follow-up (mean 16.2 months) in 30 patients:[212]
           – 13 (43%) had restenosis (>50%)
           – No correlation between restenosis and return of symptoms.
       iii. More recent series: 6-month follow-up restenosis rate of 4.5%.[213] The authors attributed the low restenosis rate to slight over-dilatation during angioplasty.
       iv. High rates of recurrent stenosis are presumably due to vessel wall recoil.
3. Stenting of Symptomatic Atherosclerotic Lesions in the Vertebral or Intracranial Arteries (SSYLVIA).[217]
   (a) Nonrandomized trial using the NEUROLINK System (Guidant Corp.) balloon-mounted stent. 18 patients underwent treatment for extracranial vertebral artery stenosis (6 ostia, 12 proximal to the PICA).
   (b) Technical success (residual stenosis <50%) achieved in 17 (94%) patients.
   (c) No periprocedural neurological events.
   (d) 6-month follow-up angiogram was done in 14 (78%) patients.
       i. 6 (43%) of these 14 showed evidence of in-stent restenosis (>50%).
           – 4 of 6 (67%) of patients with ostial lesions had restenosis.
   (e) 2 (11%) of 18 had a stroke corresponding to the vascular distribution of the treated vertebral artery; both were treated for ostial lesions and both had restenosis on angiography.

VERTEBRAL ARTERY STENOSIS STUDIES

Two multicenter studies of symptomatic extracranial vertebral artery stenosis are underway:
1. Vertebrobasilar Flow Evaluation and Risk of Transient Ischaemic Attack and Stroke (VERiTAS). Observational longitudinal study of patients with symptomatic ≥50% of the extracranial or intracranial vertebral artery (http://veritas.neur.uic.edu). Study endpoints include clinical outcomes as well as hemodynamic assessment with quantitative magnetic resonance angiography (QMRA).
2. Vertebral Artery Stenting Trial (VAST). European randomized trial of stenting versus medical management for patients with symptomatic ≥50% vertebral artery stenosis.[218]

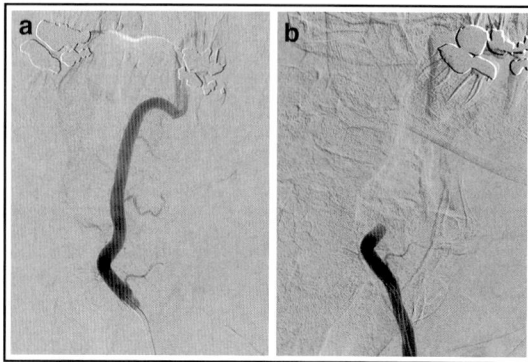

Fig. 18.3 Rotational vertebral artery compression syndrome. Patient with syncope caused by rotation of the neck to the left. The right vertebral artery is hypoplastic. The dominant left vertebral artery is patent in a neutral position (*a*), but the artery is occluded in the mid-cervical region by leftward neck rotation (*b*).

18.2. Rotational Vertebral Artery Occlusion Syndrome

Rotational vertebral artery syndrome (RVAS, aka Bow Hunter Syndrome) consists of symptoms of vertebrobasilar insufficiency caused by rotation of the neck. The most common scenario consists of a patient with a hypoplastic or occluded vertebral artery on one side, a dominant vertebral artery on the other side, and symptoms caused by pinching off of the dominant vertebral artery by rotation of the neck away from the dominant artery.[219] Most reports of RVAS found stenosis at the C1-2 level,[219,220] although the largest published series to date (nine patients) found a significant percentage of cases to involve the subaxial spine.[221]

1. Epidemiology
   (a) Rare
   (b) Patients are more commonly men; average age 61.[221]
2. Pathogenesis
   (a) Usually compression of the dominant vertebral artery by osteophytes or fibrous bands.
      i. Less common causes of compression:
         1. Thyroid cartilage[222]
         2. Herniated cervical disk[223]
         3. Occipital bone anomaly[224]
         4. Dural ring[225]
         5. Anterior scalene muscle[226]
         6. Cervical sympathetic chain[227]
   (b) Most common location of the stenosis is at C1 and/or C2.[221]
   (c) The subaxial spine (usually C4, 5 or 6) is also a relatively common location (Fig. 18.3).[221,228]
   (d) RVAS caused by dissection of the dominant vertebral artery has been reported.[229]
3. Symptoms
   (a) Neck rotation-associated syncope and/or vertigo (most common).[221] Also: ataxia, amaurosis fugax, headache, tinnitus and nystagmus.[230]
4. Diagnosis
   (a) Catheter angiography, with imaging of both vertebral arteries in a neutral and also a neck-rotated position, is standard.
   (b) Neck CTA can provide complementary information to catheter angiography by demonstrating osteophytes, transverse foraminal stenosis and fibrous bands.[231]

5. Management
    (a) Surgical decompression is standard.
        i.   C1-3: posterior (far lateral) approach[221]
        ii. C4 and lower: anterior approach[232,233]
    (b) Cervical fusion may be indicated in cases associated with cervical spondylosis.[234]
6. Prognosis
    (a) Left untreated, RVAS can cause stroke with permanent deficits.[219]
    (b) In recent a series of nine patients, all experienced complete resolution of their symptoms after surgery.[221] A previous review of published cases found an overall success rate with surgery of 85%.[219]

18.3.   Extracranial Arterial Dissection

Carotid Dissection

Spontaneous Internal Carotid Artery Dissection

1. Common cause of stroke in young adults (20%).[235]
    (a) Mean age of patients with stroke due to spontaneous carotid dissection: 44.5 [236]
    (b) 70% of cases are between the ages of 35 and 70.[237]
    (c) No significant gender effect.[237]
    (d) Underlying vasculopathy in 15–20%[238]
        i.   e.g., fibromuscular dysplasia (see below), Marfan's syndrome, Ehlers-Danlos syndrome
    (e) Recent infection is a risk factor:[239]
        i.   e.g., upper respiratory tract, gastrointestinal tract infection
    (f) History of minor trauma may be evident.
        i.   41% have a history of "trivial" trauma[240]
        ii. 24% of cases were associated with chiropractic maneuvers in one series[241]
2. Usually arise from an intimal tear.
    (a) Blood enters the wall of the artery to form an intramural hematoma
        i.   Intramural hematoma is usually located in the tunica media, but may be eccentric, toward the intima or adventitia[242]
             –   Toward intima results in stenosis
             –   Toward adventitia can result in an aneurysmal dilatation.
                 •   The term *pseudoaneurysm* in this setting is misleading, because the aneurysmal wall consists of blood vessel elements.
3. Dissection typically begins 2–3 cm distal to the origin.
    (a) Distal extent is usually limited by the skull base.
4. Cerebral ischaemia can result from:
    (a) Thromboembolism (from platelet aggregation due to disruption of the intima and sludging of blood in low-flow regions, such as in a false lumen).
        i.   *Most common mechanism of stroke following spontaneous carotid dissection.*[236,243]
    (b) Dissection and impairment of blood flow.
        i.   *Less common.*
5. Clinical features:
    (a) Sudden onset of unilateral neck pain (in 82% of patients),[241]) facial pain, and headache.
    (b) Most common physical finding: Horner's syndrome.
        i.   Constricted pupil
        ii. Ptosis
        iii. Unilateral anhydrosis
    (c) Ischaemic symptoms may follow pain symptoms by hours or days.
        i.   Range: a few minutes to 31 days.[244]
        ii. May include retinal ischaemic symptoms, hemispheric TIA, or completed stroke.

6. Radiographic evaluation:
  (a) MRI/MRA accompanied by T1-weighted images with fat saturation is the imaging method of choice.[245]
    i. Fat-suppressed axial T1W images improve detection of the mural hematoma – the so-called *crescent sign*.
  (b) CTA is also a valid option.[246,247]
  (c) Catheter angiography – still the "gold standard."
    i. Can complement MRI by identifying a false lumen, intimal flaps, hemodynamic effects, and collateral circulation.
    ii. Noninvasive imaging is usually adequate.
7. Management:
  (a) *Controversial*.
    i. No randomized trials comparing either anticoagulants to antiplatelet drugs have yet been published.
    ii. A retrospective study of 298 patients receiving either aspirin or anticoagulation for spontaneous carotid dissections found no significant differences in outcomes between the groups.[248]
    iii. The Cervical Artery Dissection in Stroke Study (CADISS) is a randomized trial of anticoagulation versus antiplatelet therapy in patients with carotid and vertebral artery injuries.[249] The trial is currently enrolling in the United Kingdom (www.dissection.co.uk).
  (b) Antithrombotic therapy with either antiplatelet agents or anticoagulation is generally accepted.
  (c) The authors of this handbook follow this protocol:
    i. Screening is done for patients with evidence of dissection (MRA or CTA). A catheter angiogram can be useful to look for intraluminal thrombus.
    ii. Antiplatelet therapy:
      – Aspirin 325 mg daily
    iii. *If there is evidence of an intraluminal thrombus*, or a false lumen or pseudoaneurysm containing thrombus:
      – Treatment with abciximab (an IV loading dose followed by a 12 h infusion) may dissolve the thrombus.
      – If the thrombus is resistant to treatment with abciximab, consider using anticoagulation instead of antiplatelet agents.
        • IV heparin administration to maintain the partial thromboplastin time 50–70 s.
        • Warfarin is begun; heparin is discontinued when the INR is 2.0–3.0.
    iv. The patient is followed with MRA or CTA at 3 and 6 months
      – Once the lesion has recanalized or stabilized:
        • Anticoagulation (if it is being used) and/or clopidogrel is discontinued.
        • Aspirin is continued indefinitely.
  (d) Stenting is an option for patients who remain symptomatic despite antithrombotic therapy[250]
8. Prognosis – *favourable*.
  (a) Recanalization is common.
    i. Occurs in 68–100% of stenotic lesions and 25–43% of occlusions.[251]
      – Resolution of angiographic changes occurs by 3 months in 65% of cases.[252]
    ii. Usually occurs in the first 2 months after the injury but can take up to 6–12 months.[253]
  (b) Recurrence is uncommon.
    i. 4% recurrence rate (mean follow-up 34 months) in one prospective study of spontaneous carotid artery dissections.[254]

Blunt Trauma to the Carotid Artery

1. Uncommon. Incidence among patients with head and neck trauma ranges from 0.67%[255] to 1.03%.[256]
2. Cerebral ischaemia can result from:
  (a) Thromboembolism (see above).
    i. *Most common mechanism of stroke following traumatic carotid dissection*.[257,258]
  (b) Dissection and impairment of blood flow.
    i. *Rare*.

3. Clinical features
    (a) Symptoms may develop hours or weeks after the injury.[259]
    (b) Head and/or neck pain is the most common symptom.
        i. Followed by cerebral or retinal ischaemia.
4. Compared to penetrating injury, blunt carotid injury carries a lower mortality rate but higher stroke rate.[260]
    (a) Mortality: 7%
    (b) Stroke rate: 56%
5. Radiographic evaluation:
    (a) Suggested triggers for evaluation for traumatic carotid dissection:[256]
        i. Cervical spine fracture
        ii. Horner's syndrome
        iii. Le Fort II or III facial fracture
        iv. Skull base fracture involving the carotid canal
        v. Penetrating neck injuries
        vi. Focal neurological deficit not explainable by other causes
    (b) CTA in the evaluation of blunt trauma to the carotid artery.
        i. Can demonstrate other soft tissue and bony injuries.
        ii. Permits examination of the vertebral arteries as well.
        iii. Easy to do.
        iv. However, sensitivity is limited.
            – Comparison of CTA to catheter angiography in patients with blunt carotid artery injury demonstrated a sensitivity of only 47%.[256]
        v. MRI/MRA also has limited sensitivity (50%)[256] and is often problematic in the setting of trauma.
    (c) Angiography is the "gold standard" for diagnosis of arterial injury.
        i. Can also identify intraluminal thrombus, a false lumen, and assess collateral supply to the affected arterial territory.
    (d) Authors of this handbook prefer:
        i. CTA is done as the initial imaging technique.
            – Proceed to catheter angiography if:
                • The CTA indicates a dissection.
                • If the CTA is *negative* and the index of suspicion for an arterial injury is *high* (e.g., there is evidence of neurologic injury attributable to an arterial injury or if there is additional evidence of an arterial injury not seen on CTA).
6. Management.
    (a) *Medical management – Controversial.*
        i. Most agree that some kind of anti-thrombotic therapy is necessary. A nationwide survey found that clinicians are divided between advocates of anticoagulation (42.8%) and antiplatelet therapy (32.5%).[261]
        ii. Anticoagulation
            – Retrospective series have supported the use of systemic anticoagulation with heparin in blunt carotid injury.[262]
            – A logistic regression analysis found heparin therapy to be associated independently with survival ($p < 0.02$) and improvement in neurologic outcome ($p < 0.01$).[255]
            – Biffl et al. recommendations for anticoagulation according to grade of injury (Table 18.8).[263]

Table 18.8 Blunt cerebrovascular injury scale.[263,264]

Injury grade	Description
I	Luminal irregularity or dissection with <25% luminal narrowing
II	Dissection or intramural hematoma with ≥25% narrowing
III	Pseudoaneurysm
IV	Occlusion
V	Transection with free extravasation

- Grade I – may heal without anticoagulation, consider antiplatelet agent.
- Grade II, III, and IV should be treated with systemic anticoagulation.

iii. *However*
- Haemorrhagic complication rates as high as 57% with heparin therapy have been reported.[265]
- A significant percentage of trauma patients are unsuitable for anticoagulation because of bleeding from other sites.
- Most ischaemic strokes appear to occur before diagnosis in patients in centers using CTA screening of blunt trauma patients.[266,267] This observation makes aggressive antithrombotic therapy, particularly in patients with asymptomatic extracranial cerebrovascular injuries, less compelling.

iv. Antiplatelet therapy
- Rationale: disruption of the intima leads to platelet activation and aggregation.
- Bleeding complications were found to be significantly lower for patients treated with aspirin compared to systemic heparinization.[265]

v. The authors of this handbook prefer aspirin 325 mg daily (can be given via NG or as a suppository).
- Systemic anticoagulation (i.e., IV heparin) is reserved for cases in which there is a significant false lumen with stasis and a tangible risk of thromboembolism.

(b) Endovascular intervention
i. Stenting is an option for the treatment of dissections and pseudoaneurysms that continue to enlarge or are symptomatic despite antithrombotic therapy.
- Stent placement lead to resolution of 89% of pseudoaneurysms.[263]
- Risk of thromboembolic complications from endovascular manipulation of an acutely injured vessel is believed to be high.
  - Some authors recommend waiting 7 days before stenting in blunt carotid injury.[268]
- Requires a course of combination antiplatelet therapy
  - Combination antiplatelet therapy may complicate management of other traumatic injuries.

Vertebral Artery Dissection

Spontaneous Vertebral Artery Dissection

1. 67% of cerebellar infarctions in young adults are attributable to vertebral artery dissection.[269]
2. Most patients are in their 30s or 40s.
   (a) 48% of patients have hypertension.[270]
   (b) Associated with FMD (see below), migraine, and oral contraceptives.[271]
   (c) History of sustained hyperextension and rotation in some patients:
      i. *Beauty Parlor Stroke Syndrome.*[272]
      ii. *Bottoms Up Dissection.*[273]
3. The cardinal symptom in patients with vertebral artery dissection is pain, involving the neck, occiput, and shoulder.[270,274]
   (a) Median interval between neck pain an onset of other symptoms is 2 weeks.[275]
   (b) Frequency of VBI symptoms with vertebral artery dissection: 56%.[276]
   (c) After pain, the next most common symptoms are nausea and vertigo.[274]
4. Spontaneous vertebral artery dissections can occur anywhere along the course of the vessel[276]
   (a) Most common location: Distal V1 and proximal V2 region.[274]
   (b) Tend to occur in the dominant vertebral artery.

(c) 36% of patients have dissections at other sites.

(d) 21% have bilateral vertebral artery dissections.[277]

5. Radiographic evaluation

    (a) Catheter angiography is the preferred imaging technique.

    (b) MRI/MRA are not as sensitive for detecting vertebral dissections as for detecting carotid dissections.[278]

        i. Low sensitivity is due to:[279]

           – Inherent asymmetry of the vertebral arteries.

           – Poor delineation of the intramural hematoma against the surrounding soft tissues, and slow flow proximal and distal to the dissection.

           – Enhancement in the vertebral veins may mimic a dissection.

        ii. However, dynamic MRA (i.e., imaging of the vessels in neutral position, then with extension and rotation) can identify areas of impingement by the vertebral arteries by bony or ligamentous structures.[272]

    (c) CTA also has limited sensitivity.

        i. Vertebral artery size and position in the transverse foramina vary markedly in normal young subjects.[280]

           – This variation may make recognition of a dissection difficult.

6. Management

    (a) Same as for spontaneous internal carotid artery dissections (see above).

    (b) The Cervical Artery Dissection in Stroke Study (CADISS) is a randomized trial of anticoagulation versus antiplatelet therapy in patients with carotid and vertebral artery injuries.[249] The trial is currently enrolling in the United Kingdom (www.dissection.co.uk).

7. Prognosis – *favourable*

    (a) Angiographic abnormalities either subside or improve in 76%.[270]

    (b) Recurrence rate is low.[254]

Blunt Trauma to the Vertebral Artery

1. In blunt trauma, vertebral artery injuries are more common than carotid injuries.

    (a) Due to the proximity of the vessel to the bony and ligamental structures of the spine.

2. Blunt vertebral artery injury incidence: 0.53% of all blunt trauma admissions.[264]

3. Vertebral artery injuries were found in 46% of patients with mid-cervical spine fracture or subluxation.[281]

    (a) Conversely, cervical spine injuries were present in 71% of patients with blunt vertebral artery injury.[264]

    (b) Dissections tend to occur where the artery is adjacent to a bony prominence (e.g., C2-2 or at C6 where the vessel enters the foramen transversarium).

4. Incidence of posterior circulation stroke in blunt vertebral artery injury: 24%.[264]

    (a) Symptoms can result from:

        i. Thromboembolism

        ii. Arterial stenosis

        iii. Occlusion

        iv. Aneurysm formation

5. Radiographic evaluation

    (a) Most recommend catheter angiography if the index of suspicion for an arterial injury is high.

        i. Noninvasive imaging accuracy is limited.

           – Comparison of CTA and MRA with cerebral angiography demonstrated sensitivities of 53% (CTA) and 47% (MRA) for vertebral artery injury.[256]

        ii. CTA has limited sensitivity in the evaluation of blunt vertebral artery trauma.

        iii. CTA may not be sensitive for detecting small intimal injuries.[282]

        iv. Vertebral artery size and position in the transverse foramina vary markedly in normal young subjects[280]

           – This variation may make recognition of a dissection difficult

(b) Authors of this handbook prefer:
    i.   CTA is done as the initial imaging technique
        – Proceed to catheter angiography if
            • The CTA indicates a dissection
            • If the CTA is *negative* and the index of suspicion for an arterial injury is *high* (e.g., there is evidence of neurologic injury attributable to an arterial injury or if there is additional evidence of an arterial injury not seen on CTA)

6. Management
  (a) Similar to management of blunt carotid artery injury (see above)
    i.   Systemic anticoagulation has been advocated for blunt vertebral artery injury[264]
    ii. The authors of this handbook prefer:
        – Antiplatelet treatment (aspirin 325 mg daily).
    iii. Endovascular intervention
        – Reserved for patients with active bleeding, symptomatic injuries despite antithrombotic therapy, or an arteriovenous fistula.
        – Usually consists of embolization and occlusion of the vessel[283]
        – Stenting with distal embolic protection has been reported.[284]
  (b) Follow-up imaging is necessary because of the potential for aneurysm or arteriovenous fistula formation[285]
    i.   Authors' preference is to image the affected vessel noninvasively (e.g., CTA) 6 months after the injury.

Penetrating Neck Injury

1. Another kettle of fish.
  (a) Some 36% of patients with penetrating neck injuries have a vascular injury.[286]
  (b) Most discussions of penetrating injury localize the injury to standardized zones in the neck (Fig. 18.4).
2. Mortality is higher but stroke rates are lower with penetrating neck injuries compared to blunt injury[260]
  (a) Overall mortality with penetrating cervical vascular injury: 22%
  (b) Overall stroke rate: 15%
    i.   Zone 1
        – Between cricoid cartilage and clavicles
        – 13% of penetrating neck injuries.[287]

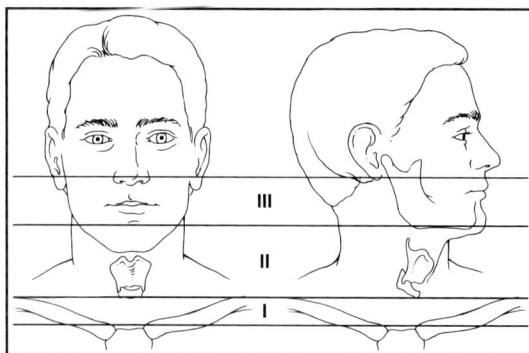

Fig. 18.4 Penetrating neck trauma. Zones of the neck. (1) *Zone I*: Clavicle to cricoid process. (2) *Zone II*: Cricoid process to angle of mandible. (3) *Zone III*: Angle of mandible to skull base.

ii. Zone 2
  - Cricoid cartilage to angle of mandible
  - 67% of injuries.
iii. Zone 3
  - Angle of mandible to skull base
  - 20% of injuries.
3. Radiographic evaluation
  (a) CT/CTA is first-line.[246,288]
    i. Sensitivity of CTA in detecting arterial injury in this setting is high (90–100%).[282,289,290]
    ii. Metal and bone artifact can obscure identification of vascular injuries.
  (b) Angiography
    i. In cases where CTA interpretation is limited or a need for endovascular intervention is anticipated.
    ii. Diagnostic yield is very limited in patients with Zone 2 injuries without physical findings or symptoms of vascular injury.
      - Positive finding in this setting is <1%.[291]
    iii. Some centers use selective angiography according to zone.
      - Zone 1 and zone 3 injuries (symptomatic and asymptomatic) are evaluated with angiography.
        a. These zones are difficult to assess clinically, and surgical access is difficult.
      - Zone 2 injuries are explored surgically if they are symptomatic.
4. Penetrating carotid artery injuries
  (a) Carotid system is involved in 80% of cases.
  (b) ICA occlusion occurs in 36% of cases.[292]
  (c) ICA pseudoaneurysms are found in 33% of cases.[292]
5. Penetrating vertebral artery injuries
  (a) Vertebral arteries are involved in 43% of cases.
  (b) Only some 2.6% of patients have symptoms of transient VBI[286]
6. Management
  (a) Vascular management of penetrating neck injury is in evolution.
  (b) Endovascular management is gaining favour over surgical exploration and repair.[293]
  (c) A number of series have reported favourable results with endovascular management[294–296] (Fig. 18.3).

18.4. Fibromuscular Dysplasia

Fibromuscular dysplasia (FMD) is a nonatherosclerotic, noninflammatory condition that characteristically affects medium-sized arteries (e.g., the internal carotid, vertebral, coronary, and renal arteries). Classification is based on the arterial layer affected.
1. Media
  (a) Medial *fibroplasia*. Most common form; ~80% of FMD cases.
    i. Classic "stack of coins" appearance on angiography (Fig. 18.5).
    ii. Histologically, the media is involved and the intima, internal elastic lamina, and adventitia are spared.
    iii. Associated with Ehlers-Danlos syndrome (type IV).[297]
  (b) Medial *hyperplasia*. <1% of FMD cases.
    i. Smooth muscle cell hyperplasia without fibrosis.
    ii. Smooth tubular stenosis on angiography (Fig. 18.6).
    iii. May be indistinguishable on angiography from intimal fibroplasias.[298]
  (c) Perimedial fibroplasia. ~10–15% of FMD cases.
    i. Characterized by a homogeneous collar of elastic tissue at the junction of the media and adventitia.[299]
    ii. Appears on angiography as a focal stenosis, or, occasionally, multiple stenosis.
    iii. Usually found in girls, age 5–15 years.[299]

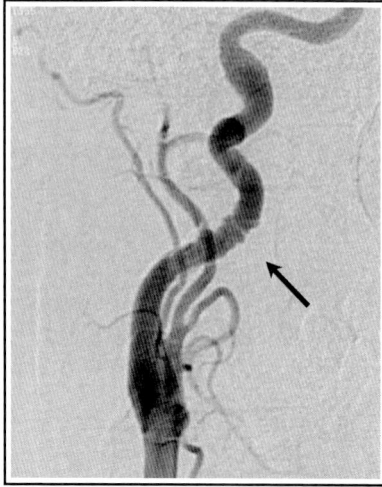

Fig. 18.5 Fibromuscular dysplasia: medial *fibroplasia* variant. Carotid angiogram showing the classic "stack of coins" appearance of the affected part of the ICA (*arrow*).

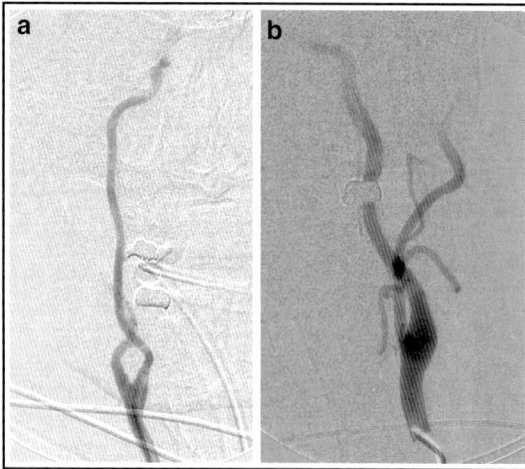

Fig. 18.6 Fibromuscular dysplasia: medial *hyperplasia* variant. Carotid angiogram showing medial hyperplasia causing a long tubular stenosis of the ICA (**a**). The same patient's normal contralateral carotid is shown (**b**) for comparison.

2. Intima.
   (a) Intimal fibroplasia. ~10% of FMD cases.
      i.   May appear on angiography as a focal concentric stenosis, or a long, smooth narrowing
3. Adventitia
   (a) Adventitial hyperplasia. <1% Rarest form of FMD.
      i.   Localized, tubular stenosis on angiography[300]

Pathogenesis of FMD

1. Cause is not yet understood.
2. Risk factors:[299]
   (a) Hypertension
   (b) Cigarette smoking
3. Possible causes:
   (a) Alteration of the vaso vasorum
   (b) Repeated microtrauma
   (c) Hormonal deficiency
   (d) α-antitrypsin deficiency[301]
   (e) Genetic component[302]

Cerebrovascular FMD

1. The extracranial internal carotid and vertebral arteries are affected in 25–30% of cases, and there are associated intracranial aneurysms in 7–50% of cases.[299,303]
   (a) Rarely, FMD may extend intracranially.[304]
2. Usually discovered as an incidental finding during imaging.
3. Bilateral in 85% of cases.[305]
4. Female preponderance (85% of cases).[305]
5. Mean age approximately 50.[299]
6. Typically affects the middle and distal portions of the internal and vertebral arteries, at the level of C1 and C2.
7. Natural history is usually benign.[306-308]
8. Elevated risk of complications during neurointerventional procedures (e.g., dissection, perforation).
9. Cerebrovascular symptoms are uncommon. Symptoms can result from:
   (a) Stenosis or occlusion of the vessel
   (b) Spontaneous dissection
   (c) Platelet aggregation on irregular lumen or dissection.
   (d) Subarachnoid haemorrhage
   (e) Spontaneous vertebro-vertebral arteriovenous fistula[309]
10. Treatment
   (a) Antiplatelet therapy may reduce the risk of thromboembolic events.
   (b) Endovascular treatment has emerged as the primary approach in patients with symptomatic cerebrovascular FMD.[299]
      i.   Angioplasty alone[310,311]
      ii. Angioplasty and stent placement[312]
      iii. Endovascular treatment combined with surgery[313]

References

1. Grau AJ, Weimar C, Buggle F, et al. Risk factors, outcome, and treatment in subtypes of ischemic stroke: the German stroke data bank. Stroke. 2001;32:2559–66.
2. Woo D, Gebel J, Miller R, et al. Incidence rates of first-ever ischemic stroke subtypes among blacks: a population-based study. Stroke. 1999;30:2517–22.
3. Ross R. Atherosclerosis – an inflammatory disease. N Engl J Med. 1999;340:115–26.
4. Schwartz CJ, Valente AJ, Sprague EA, Kelley JL, Nerem RM. The pathogenesis of atherosclerosis: an overview. Clin Cardiol. 1991;14:I1–16.
5. Napoli C, D'Armiento FP, Mancini FP, et al. Fatty streak formation occurs in human fetal aortas and is greatly enhanced by maternal hypercholesterolemia. Intimal accumulation of low density lipoprotein and its oxidation precede monocyte recruitment into early atherosclerotic lesions. J Clin Invest. 1997;100:2680–90.
6. Morel DW, Hessler JR, Chisolm GM. Low density lipoprotein cytotoxicity induced by free radical peroxidation of lipid. J Lipid Res. 1983;24:1070–6.
7. Nehler MR, Taylor Jr LM, Porter JM. Homocysteinemia as a risk factor for atherosclerosis: a review. Cardiovasc Surg. 1997;5:559–67.
8. Espinola-Klein C, Rupprecht H-J, Blankenberg S, et al. Are morphological or functional changes in the carotid artery wall associated with Chlamydia pneumoniae, Helicobacter pylori, Cytomegalovirus, or Herpes simplex virus infection? Stroke. 2000;31:2127–33.
9. Libby P, Egan D, Skarlatos S. Roles of infectious agents in atherosclerosis and restenosis: an assessment of the evidence and need for future research. Circulation. 1997;96:4095–103.
10. Ross R, Glomset JA. Atherosclerosis and the arterial smooth muscle cell: proliferation of smooth muscle is a key event in the genesis of the lesions of atherosclerosis. Science. 1973; 180:1332–9.
11. Zarins CK, Giddens DP, Bharadvaj BK, Sottiurai VS, Mabon RF, Glagov S. Carotid bifurcation atherosclerosis. Quantitative correlation of plaque localization with flow velocity profiles and wall shear stress. Circ Res. 1983;53:502–14.
12. Huo Y, Ley K. Adhesion molecules and atherogenesis. Acta Physiol Scand. 2001;173:35–43.
13. Ku DN, Giddens DP, Zarins CK, Glagov S. Pulsatile flow and atherosclerosis in the human carotid bifurcation. Positive correlation between plaque location and low oscillating shear stress. Arteriosclerosis 1985;5:293–302.
14. Zhou Q, Liao JK. Statins and cardiovascular diseases: from cholesterol lowering to pleiotropy. Curr Pharm Des. 2009;15:467–78.
15. Ford AL, An HD, D'Angelo GP, et al. Preexisting statin use is associated with greater reperfusion in hyperacute ischemic stroke. Stroke. 2011;42:1307–13.
16. Biffi A, Devan WJ, Anderson CD, et al. Statin treatment and functional outcome after ischemic stroke: case–control and meta-analysis. Stroke. 2011;42:1314–9.
17. Ni Chroinin D, Callaly EL, Duggan J, et al. Association between acute statin therapy, survival, and improved functional outcome after ischemic stroke: the North Dublin population stroke study. Stroke. 2011;42:1021–9.
18. Lynch JR, Wang H, McGirt MJ, et al. Simvastatin reduces vasospasm after aneurysmal subarachnoid hemorrhage: results of a pilot randomized clinical trial. Stroke. 2005; 36:2024–6.
19. Wu H, Jiang HP, Lu D, et al. Induction of angiogenesis and modulation of vascular endothelial growth factor receptor-2 by simvastatin after traumatic brain injury. Neurosurgery. 2011;68:1363–71.
20. Julian OC, Dye WS, Javid H, Hunter JA. Ulcerative lesions of the carotid artery bifurcation. Arch Surg. 1963;86:803–9.
21. Moore WS, Malone JM. Effect of flow rate and vessel calibre on critical arterial stenosis. J Surg Res. 1979;26:1–9.
22. Prati P, Vanuzzo D, Casaroli M, et al. Prevalence and determinants of carotid atherosclerosis in a general population. Stroke. 1992;23:1705–11.
23. Colgan MP, Strode GR, Sommer JD, Gibbs JL, Sumner DS. Prevalence of asymptomatic carotid disease: results of duplex scanning in 348 unselected volunteers. J Vasc Surg. 1988; 8:674–8.
24. Fabris F, Zanocchi M, Bo M, et al. Carotid plaque, aging, and risk factors. A study of 457 subjects. Stroke. 1994;25: 1133–40.
25. Fine-Edelstein JS, Wolf PA, O'Leary DH, et al. Precursors of extracranial carotid atherosclerosis in the Framingham study. Neurology. 1994;44:1046–50.
26. Pujia A, Rubba P, Spencer MP. Prevalence of extracranial carotid artery disease detectable by echo-Doppler in an elderly population. Stroke. 1992;23:818–22.
27. Ramsey DE, Miles RD, Lambeth A, Sumner DS. Prevalence of extracranial carotid artery disease: a survey of an asymptomatic population with noninvasive techniques. J Vasc Surg. 1987;5:584–8.
28. Fabris F, Zanocchi M, Bo M, Fonte G, Fiandra U, Poli L. Risk factors for atherosclerosis and aging. Int Angiol. 1994;13: 52–8.
29. Mathiesen EB, Joakimsen O, Bonaa KH. Prevalence of and risk factors associated with carotid artery stenosis: the tromso study. Cerebrovasc Dis. 2001;12:44–51.
30. Mast H, Thompson JLP, Lin IF, et al. Cigarette smoking as a determinant of high-grade carotid artery stenosis in Hispanic, black, and white patients with stroke or transient ischemic attack. Stroke. 1998;29:908–12.
31. Iemolo F, Martiniuk A, Steinman DA, Spence JD. Sex differences in carotid plaque and stenosis. Stroke. 2004;35:477–81.
32. Su T-C, Jeng J-S, Chien K-L, Sung F-C, Hsu H C, Lee Y-T. Hypertension status is the major determinant of carotid atherosclerosis: a community-based study in Taiwan. Stroke. 2001;32:2265–71.
33. Wilson PWF, Hoeg JM, D'Agostino RB, et al. Cumulative effects of high cholesterol levels, high blood pressure, and cigarette smoking on carotid stenosis. N Engl J Med. 1997;337:516–22.
34. Ishizaka N, Ishizaka Y, Toda E, Hashimoto H, Nagai R, Yamakado M. Hypertension is the most common component of metabolic syndrome and the greatest contributor to carotid arteriosclerosis in apparently healthy Japanese individuals. Hypertens Res. 2005;28:27–34.
35. De Angelis M, Scrucca L, Leandri M, et al. Prevalence of carotid stenosis in type 2 diabetic patients asymptomatic for cerebrovascular disease. Diabetes Nutr Metab. 2003;16: 48–55.
36. Kallikazaros IE, Tsioufis CP, Stefanadis CI, Pitsavos CE, Toutouzas PK. Closed relation between carotid and ascending aortic atherosclerosis in cardiac patients. Circulation. 2000;102:263III–8.
37. Adler Y, Koren A, Fink N, et al. Association between mitral annulus calcification and carotid atherosclerotic disease. Stroke. 1998;29:1833–7.
38. Simons PC, Algra A, Eikelboom BC, Grobbee DE, van der Graaf Y. Carotid artery stenosis in patients with peripheral arterial disease: the SMART study. SMART study group. J Vasc Surg. 1999;30:519–25.
39. Oh J, Wunsch R, Turzer M, et al. Advanced coronary and carotid arteriopathy in young adults with childhood-onset chronic renal failure. Circulation. 2002;106:100–5.
40. Blackburn R, Giral P, Bruckert E, et al. Elevated C-reactive protein constitutes an independent predictor of advanced carotid plaques in dyslipidemic subjects. Arterioscler Thromb Vasc Biol. 2001;21:1962–8.
41. Wolff B, Grabe HJ, Volzke H, et al. Relation between psychological strain and carotid atherosclerosis in a general population. Heart. 2005;91:460–4.
42. Association AH. Heart and stroke statistical update – 2005 update. Dallas: Association AH; 2005.
43. Anonymous. Beneficial effect of carotid endarterectomy in symptomatic patients with high-grade carotid stenosis. North American Symptomatic Carotid Endarterectomy Trial Collaborators. N Engl J Med. 1991;325:445–53.

44. Beneficial effect of carotid endarterectomy in symptomatic patients with high-grade carotid stenosis. North American Symptomatic Carotid Endarterectomy Trial Collaborators. N Engl J Med. 1991;325:445–53.

45. Barnett HJ, Taylor DW, Eliasziw M, et al. Benefit of carotid endarterectomy in patients with symptomatic moderate or severe stenosis. North American Symptomatic Carotid Endarterectomy Trial Collaborators. N Engl J Med. 1998;339:1415–25.

46. Anonymous. MRC European Carotid Surgery Trial: interim results for symptomatic patients with severe (70–99%) or with mild (0–29%) carotid stenosis. European Carotid Surgery Trialists' Collaborative Group. Lancet. 1991;337:1235–43.

47. Staikov IN, Arnold M, Mattle HP, et al. Comparison of the ECST, CC, and NASCET grading methods and ultrasound for assessing carotid stenosis. European Carotid Surgery Trial. North American Symptomatic Carotid Endarterectomy Trial. J Neurol. 2000;247:681–6.

48. Rothwell PM, Gibson RJ, Slattery J, Warlow CP. Prognostic value and reproducibility of measurements of carotid stenosis. A comparison of three methods on 1001 angiograms. European Carotid Surgery Trialists' collaborative group. Stroke. 1994;25:2440–4.

49. Donnan GA, Davis SM, Chambers BR, et al. Surgery for prevention of stroke. Lancet. 1996;351:1372–3.

50. Rothwell PM, Gibson RJ, Slattery J, Sellar RJ, Warlow CP. Equivalence of measurements of carotid stenosis. A comparison of three methods on 1001 angiograms. European Carotid Surgery Trialists' Collaborative Group. Stroke. 1994;25:2435–9.

51. Anonymous. Randomised trial of endarterectomy for recently symptomatic carotid stenosis: final results of the MRC European Carotid Surgery Trial (ECST). Lancet. 1998;351:1379–87.

52. Cunningham EJ, Bond R, Mehta Z, Mayberg MR, Warlow CP, Rothwell PM. Long-term durability of carotid endarterectomy for symptomatic stenosis and risk factors for late postoperative stroke. European Carotid Surgery Trialists' Collaborative Group. Stroke. 2002;33:2658–63.

53. Mayberg MR, Wilson SE, Yatsu F, et al. Carotid endarterectomy and prevention of cerebral ischemia in symptomatic carotid stenosis. Veterans Affairs Cooperative Studies Program 309 Trialist Group. JAMA. 1991;266:3289–94.

54. Rothwell PM, Eliasziw M, Gutnikov SA, et al. Analysis of pooled data from the randomised controlled trials of endarterectomy for symptomatic carotid stenosis. Lancet. 2003; 361:107–16.

55. Eckstein HH, Ringleb P, Allenberg JR, et al. Results of the stent-protected angioplasty versus carotid endarterectomy (SPACE) study to treat symptomatic stenoses at 2 years: a multinational, prospective, randomised trial. Lancet Neurol. 2008;7:893–902.

56. Mas J-L, Chatellier G, Beyssen B, et al. Endarterectomy versus stenting in patients with symptomatic severe carotid stenosis. N Engl J Med. 2006;355:1660–71.

57. Ederle J, Dobson J, Featherstone RL, et al. Carotid artery stenting compared with endarterectomy in patients with symptomatic carotid stenosis (International Carotid Stenting Study): an interim analysis of a randomised controlled trial. Lancet. 2010;375:985–97.

58. Nicolaides AN, Kakkos SK, Kyriacou E, et al. Asymptomatic internal carotid artery stenosis and cerebrovascular risk stratification. J Vasc Surg. 2010;52:1486–96e1-5.

59. Saba L, Sanfilippo R, Montisci R, Calleo G, Mallarini G. Carotid artery stenosis quantification: concordance analysis between radiologist and semi-automatic computer software by using Multi-Detector-Row CT angiography. Eur J Radiol. 2011;79:80–4.

60. Biller J, Feinberg WM, Castaldo JE, et al. Guidelines for carotid endarterectomy: a statement for healthcare professionals from a special writing group of the Stroke Council, American Heart Association. Stroke. 1998;29:554–62.

61. Barnett HJ, Gunton RW, Eliasziw M, et al. Causes and severity of ischemic stroke in patients with internal carotid artery stenosis. JAMA. 2000;283:1429–36.

62. Eliasziw M, Streifler JY, Fox AJ, Hachinski VC, Ferguson GG, Barnett HJ. Significance of plaque ulceration in symptomatic patients with high-grade carotid stenosis. North American Symptomatic Carotid Endarterectomy Trial. Stroke. 1994;25:304–8.

63. Ferguson GG, Eliasziw M, Barr HW, et al. The North American Symptomatic Carotid Endarterectomy Trial: surgical results in 1415 patients. Stroke. 1999;30:1751–8.

64. Streifler JY, Eliasziw M, Benavente OR, et al. The risk of stroke in patients with first-ever retinal vs hemispheric transient ischemic attacks and high-grade carotid stenosis. North American Symptomatic Carotid Endarterectomy Trial. Arch Neurol. 1995;52:246–9.

65. Lanzino G, Couture D, Andreoli A, Guterman LR, Hopkins LN. Carotid endarterectomy: can we select surgical candidates at high risk for stroke and low risk for perioperative complications? Neurosurgery. 2001;49:913–23; discussion 23–4.

66. Morgenstern LB, Fox AJ, Sharpe BL, Eliasziw M, Barnett HJ, Grotta JC. The risks and benefits of carotid endarterectomy in patients with near occlusion of the carotid artery. North American Symptomatic Carotid Endarterectomy Trial (NASCET) Group. Neurology. 1997;48:911–5.

67. Gasecki AP, Eliasziw M, Ferguson GG, Hachinski V, Barnett HJ. Long-term prognosis and effect of endarterectomy in patients with symptomatic severe carotid stenosis and contralateral carotid stenosis or occlusion: results from NASCET. North American Symptomatic Carotid Endarterectomy Trial (NASCET) Group. J Neurosurg. 1995;83:778–82.

68. Villarreal J, Silva J, Eliasziw M, et al. Prognosis of patients with intraluminal thrombus in the internal carotid artery (for the North American Symptomatic Carotid Endarterectomy Trial) (Abstract 18). Stroke. 1998;29:276.

69. Alamowitch S, Eliasziw M, Algra A, Meldrum H, Barnett HJ. Risk, causes, and prevention of ischaemic stroke in elderly patients with symptomatic internal-carotid-artery stenosis. North American Symptomatic Carotid Endarterectomy Trial Group. Lancet. 2001;357:1154–60.

70. Rothwell PM, Slattery J, Warlow CP. Clinical and angiographic predictors of stroke and death from carotid endarterectomy: systematic review. BMJ. 1997;315:1571–7.

71. Kappelle LJ, Eliasziw M, Fox AJ, Barnett HJ. Small, unruptured intracranial aneurysms and management of symptomatic carotid artery stenosis. North American Symptomatic Carotid Endarterectomy Trial Group. Neurology. 2000;55:307–9.

72. Moore WS, Barnett HJ, Beebe HG, et al. Guidelines for carotid endarterectomy. A multidisciplinary consensus statement from the ad hoc Committee, American Heart Association. Stroke. 1995;26:188–201.

73. de Weerd M, Greving JP, de Jong AW, Buskens E, Bots ML. Prevalence of asymptomatic carotid artery stenosis according to age and sex: systematic review and metaregression analysis. Stroke. 2009;40:1105–13.

74. Anonymous. Endarterectomy for asymptomatic carotid artery stenosis. Executive Committee for the Asymptomatic Carotid Atherosclerosis Study. JAMA. 1995;273:1421–8.

75. Halliday A, Mansfield A, Marro J, et al. Prevention of disabling and fatal strokes by successful carotid endarterectomy in patients without recent neurological symptoms: randomised controlled trial. Lancet. 2004;363:1491–502.

76. Spence JD, Coates V, Li H, et al. Effects of intensive medical therapy on microemboli and cardiovascular risk in asymptomatic carotid stenosis. Arch Neurol. 2010;67:180–6.

77. Abbott AL. Medical (nonsurgical) intervention alone is now best for prevention of stroke associated with asymptomatic severe carotid stenosis: results of a systematic review and analysis. Stroke. 2009;40:e573–83.

78. Nicolaides AN, Kakkos SK, Griffin M, et al. Severity of asymptomatic carotid stenosis and risk of ipsilateral hemispheric ischaemic events: results from the ACSRS study. Eur J Vasc Endovasc Surg. 2005;30:275–84.

79. Abbott AL, Chambers BR, Stork JL, Levi CR, Bladin CF, Donnan GA. Embolic signals and prediction of ipsilateral stroke or transient ischemic attack in asymptomatic carotid stenosis: a multicenter prospective cohort study. Stroke. 2005;36:1128–33.

80. Goessens BM, Visseren FL, Kappelle LJ, Algra A, van der Graaf Y. Asymptomatic carotid artery stenosis and the risk of new vascular events in patients with manifest arterial disease: the SMART study. Stroke. 2007;38:1470–5.

81. Marquardt L, Geraghty OC, Mehta Z, Rothwell PM. Low risk of ipsilateral stroke in patients with asymptomatic carotid stenosis on best medical treatment: a prospective, population-based study. Stroke. 2010;41:e11–7.

82. Markus HS, King A, Shipley M, et al. Asymptomatic embolisation for prediction of stroke in the Asymptomatic Carotid Emboli Study (ACES): a prospective observational study. Lancet Neurol. 2010;9:663–71.

83. Calvillo-King L, Xuan L, Zhang S, Tuhrim S, Halm EA. Predicting risk of perioperative death and stroke after carotid endarterectomy in asymptomatic patients: derivation and validation of a clinical risk score. Stroke. 2010;41:2786–94.

84. Goldstein LB, Bushnell CD, Adams RJ, et al. Guidelines for the primary prevention of stroke: a guideline for healthcare professionals from the American Heart Association/ American Stroke Association. Stroke. 2011;42:517–84.

85. Baker WH, Howard VJ, Howard G, Toole JF. Effect of contralateral occlusion on long-term efficacy of endarterectomy in the asymptomatic carotid atherosclerosis study (ACAS). ACAS Investigators. Stroke. 2000;31:2330–4.

86. Hobson 2nd RW, Weiss DG, Fields WS, et al. Efficacy of carotid endarterectomy for asymptomatic carotid stenosis. The Veterans Affairs Cooperative Study Group. N Engl J Med. 1993;328:221–7.

87. Tuhrim S, Bederson JB. Patient selection for carotid endarterectomy. In: Tuhrim S, Bederson J, editors. Treatment of carotid disease: a practitioner's manual. Park Ridge: The American Association of Neurological Surgeons; 1998. p. 129–42.

88. Anonymous. Carotid surgery versus medical therapy in asymptomatic carotid stenosis. The CASANOVA Study Group. Stroke. 1991;22:1229–35.

89. Anonymous. Mayo Asymptomatic Carotid Endarterectomy Study Group: results of a randomized controlled trial of carotid endarterectomy for asymptomatic carotid stenosis. Mayo Clin Proc. 1992;67:513–8.

90. Turnipseed WD, Kennell TW, Turski PA, Acher CW, Hoch JR. Combined use of duplex imaging and magnetic resonance angiography for evaluation of patients with symptomatic ipsilateral high-grade carotid stenosis. J Vasc Surg. 1993;17:832–40.

91. Goldstein LB, Bonito AJ, Matchar DB, et al. US national survey of physician practices for the secondary and tertiary prevention of ischemic stroke. Design, service availability, and common practices. Stroke. 1995;26:1607–15.

92. Chassin MR, Brook RH, Park RE, et al. Variations in the use of medical and surgical services by the Medicare population. N Engl J Med. 1986;314:285–90.

93. Qureshi AI, Suri MF, Ali Z, et al. Role of conventional angiography in evaluation of patients with carotid artery stenosis demonstrated by Doppler ultrasound in general practice. Stroke. 2001;32:2287–91.

94. Polak JF, Kalina P, Donaldson MC, O'Leary DH, Whittemore AD, Mannick JA. Carotid endarterectomy: preoperative evaluation of candidates with combined Doppler sonography and MR angiography. Work in progress. Radiology. 1993;186:333–8.

95. Dawson DL, Zierler RE, Strandness Jr DE, Clowes AW, Kohler TR. The role of duplex scanning and arteriography before carotid endarterectomy: a prospective study. J Vasc Surg. 1993;18:673–83.

96. Dillon EH, van Leeuwen MS, Fernandez MA, Eikelboom BC, Mali WP. CT angiography: application to the evaluation of carotid artery stenosis. Radiology. 1993;189:211–9.

97. Lustgarten JH, Solomon RA, Quest DO, Khanjdi AG, Mohr JP. Carotid endarterectomy after noninvasive evaluation by duplex ultrasonography and magnetic resonance angiography. Neurosurgery. 1994;34:612–9.

98. Back MR, Wilson JS, Rushing G, et al. Magnetic resonance angiography is an accurate imaging adjunct to duplex ultrasound scan in patient selection for carotid endarterectomy. J Vasc Surg. 2000;32:429–40.

99. Grant EG, Duerinckx AJ, Baker JD. Ability to use duplex US to quantify internal carotid arterial stenoses: fact or fiction? Radiology. 2000;214:247–52.

100. deBray J, Glatt B. Quantitation of atheromatous stenosis in the extracranial internal carotid artery. Cerebrovasc Dis. 1995;5:414–26.

101. Grant EG, Benson CB, Moneta GL, et al. Carotid artery stenosis: gray-scale and Doppler US diagnosis – society of radiologists in ultrasound consensus conference. Radiology. 2003;229:340–6.

102. Frericks H, Kievit J, van Baalen JM, van Bockel JH. Carotid recurrent stenosis and risk of ipsilateral stroke: a systematic review of the literature. Stroke. 1998;29:244–50.

103. Reina-Gutierrez T, Serrano-Hernando FJ, Sanchez-Hervas L, Ponce A, de Vega Ceniga M, Martin A. Recurrent carotid artery stenosis following endarterectomy: natural history and risk factors. Eur J Vasc Endovasc Surg. 2005;29:334–41.

104. AbuRahma AF, Jennings TG, Wulu JT, Tarakji L, Robinson PA. Redo carotid endarterectomy versus primary carotid endarterectomy. Stroke. 2001;32:2787–92.

105. MacMahon S, Sharpe N, Gamble G, et al. Effects of lowering average of below-average cholesterol levels on the progression of carotid atherosclerosis: results of the LIPID Atherosclerosis Substudy. LIPID Trial Research Group. Circulation. 1998;97:1784–90.

106. Baldassarre D, Veglia F, Gobbi C, et al. Intima-media thickness after pravastatin stabilizes also in patients with moderate to no reduction in LDL-cholesterol levels: the carotid atherosclerosis Italian ultrasound study. Atherosclerosis. 2000;151:575–83.

107. Blauw GJ, Lagaay AM, Smelt AH, Westendorp RG. Stroke, statins, and cholesterol. A meta-analysis of randomized, placebo-controlled, double-blind trials with HMG-CoA reductase inhibitors. Stroke. 1997;28:946–50.

108. National Heart Lung and Blood Institute. Third report of the expert panel on detection, evaluation, and treatment of high blood cholesterol in adults (Adult Treatment Panel III). 2004; http://www.nhlbi.nih.gov/guidelines/cholesterol/index.htm. Accessed May 27, 2012.

109. Pasternak RC, Smith Jr SC, Bairey-Merz CN, et al. ACC/AHA/NHLBI clinical advisory on the use and safety of statins. Stroke. 2002;33:2337–41.

110. Merck & Co. I. Package insert: Mevacor® (Lovastatin). Whitehouse Station: Merck & Co. I; 2002.

111. Sacco RL, Wolf PA, Gorelick PB. Risk factors and their management for stroke prevention: outlook for 1999 and beyond. Neurology. 1999;53:S15–24.

112. Collins R, Peto R, MacMahon S, et al. Blood pressure, stroke, and coronary heart disease. Part 2, short-term reductions in blood pressure: overview of randomised drug trials in their epidemiological context. Lancet. 1990;335:827–38.

113. Shinton R, Beevers G. Meta-analysis of relation between cigarette smoking and stroke. BMJ. 1989;298:789–94.

114. Dale LC, Hurt RD, Hays JT. Drug therapy to aid in smoking cessation. Tips on maximizing patients' chances for success. Postgrad Med. 1998;104(75–8):83–4.

115. Anczak JD, Nogler II RA. Tobacco cessation in primary care: maximizing intervention strategies. Clin Med Res. 2003;1:201–16.

116. Steffen CM, Gray-Weale AC, Byrne KE, Lusby RJ. Carotid artery atheroma: ultrasound appearance in symptomatic and asymptomatic vessels. Aust N Z J Surg. 1989;59:529–34.

117. Ruggeri ZM. Mechanisms of shear-induced platelet adhesion and aggregation. Thromb Haemost. 1993;70:119–23.

118. Siess W, Zangl KJ, Essler M, et al. Lysophosphatidic acid mediates the rapid activation of platelets and endothelial cells by mildly oxidized low density lipoprotein and accumulates in human atherosclerotic lesions. PNAS. 1999;96:6931–6.

119. Anonymous. Randomised trial of intravenous streptokinase, oral aspirin, both, or neither among 17,185 cases of suspected acute myocardial infarction: ISIS-2. ISIS-2 (Second International Study of Infarct Survival) Collaborative Group. Lancet. 1988;2:349–60.

120. Anonymous. A comparison of two doses of aspirin (30 mg vs. 283 mg a day) in patients after a transient ischemic attack or minor ischemic stroke. The Dutch TIA Trial Study Group. N Eng J Med. 1991;325:1261–6.

121. Anonymous. Swedish Aspirin Low-Dose Trial (SALT) of 75 mg aspirin as secondary prophylaxis after cerebrovascular ischaemic events. The SALT Collaborative Group. Lancet. 1991;338:1345–9.

122. Taylor DW, Barnett HJ, Haynes RB, et al. Low-dose and high-dose acetylsalicylic acid for patients undergoing carotid endarterectomy: a randomised controlled trial. ASA and Carotid Endarterectomy (ACE) Trial Collaborators. Lancet. 1999;353:2179–84.

EXTRACRANIAL CEREBROVASCULAR OCCLUSIVE DISEASE

123. Dyken ML, Barnett HJ, Easton JD, et al. Low-dose aspirin and stroke "It ain't necessarily so". Stroke. 1992;23:1395–9.

124. A randomised, blinded, trial of clopidogrel versus aspirin in patients at risk of ischaemic events (CAPRIE). CAPRIE Steering Committee. Lancet. 1996;348:1329–39.

125. Diener HC, Bogousslavsky J, Brass LM, et al. Aspirin and clopidogrel compared with clopidogrel alone after recent ischaemic stroke or transient ischaemic attack in high-risk patients (MATCH): randomised, double-blind, placebo-controlled trial. Lancet. 2004;364:331–7.

126. Diener HC, Cunha L, Forbes C, Sivenius J, Smets P, Lowenthal A. European stroke prevention study. 2. Dipyridamole and acetylsalicylic acid in the secondary prevention of stroke. J Neurol Sci. 1996;143:1–13.

127. Sacco RL, Sivenius J, Diener HC. Efficacy of aspirin plus extended-release dipyridamole in preventing recurrent stroke in high-risk populations. Arch Neurol. 2005;62: 403–8.

128. Lipton RB, Bigal ME, Kolodner KB, et al. Acetaminophen in the treatment of headaches associated with dipyridamole-aspirin combination. Neurology. 2004;63:1099–101.

129. Hass WK, Easton JD, Adams Jr HP, et al. A randomized trial comparing ticlopidine hydrochloride with aspirin for the prevention of stroke in high-risk patients. Ticlopidine Aspirin Stroke Study Group. N Engl J Med. 1989;321: 501–7.

130. Bennett CL, Weinberg PD, Rozenberg-Ben-Dror K, Yarnold PR, Kwaan HC, Green D. Thrombotic thrombocytopenic purpura associated with ticlopidine. A review of 60 cases. Ann Intern Med. 1998;128:541–4.

131. Albers GW, Amarenco P, Easton JD, Sacco RL, Teal P. Antithrombotic and thrombolytic therapy for ischemic stroke: the Seventh ACCP Conference on Antithrombotic and Thrombolytic Therapy. Chest. 2004;126:483S–512.

132. Kerber CW, Cromwell LD, Loehden OL. Catheter dilatation of proximal carotid stenosis during distal bifurcation endarterectomy. AJNR Am J Neuroradiol. 1980;1:348–9.

133. Bockenheimer SA, Mathias K. Percutaneous transluminal angioplasty in arteriosclerotic internal carotid artery stenosis. AJNR Am J Neuroradiol. 1983;4:791–2.

134. Castaneda-Zuniga WR, Formanek A, Tadavarthy M, et al. The mechanism of balloon angioplasty. Radiology. 1980; 135:565–71.

135. Block PC, Fallon JT, Elmer D. Experimental angioplasty: lessons from the laboratory. AJR Am J Roentgenol. 1980; 135:907–12.

136. Zollikofer CL, Salomonowitz E, Sibley R, et al. Transluminal angioplasty evaluated by electron microscopy. Radiology. 1984;153:369–74.

137. Bergeron P, Chambran P, Hartung O, Bianca S. Cervical carotid artery stenosis: which technique, balloon angioplasty or surgery? J Cardiovasc Surg (Torino). 1996;37:73–5.

138. Bergeron P, Chambran P, Benichou H, Alessandri C. Recurrent carotid disease: will stents be an alternative to surgery? J Endovasc Surg. 1996;3:76–9.

139. Shawl FA. Emergency percutaneous carotid stenting during stroke. Lancet. 1995;346:1223.

140. Yadav JS, Roubin GS, Iyer S, et al. Elective stenting of the extracranial carotid arteries. Circulation. 1997;95:376–81.

141. Naylor AR, Bolia A, Abbott RJ, et al. Randomized study of carotid angioplasty and stenting versus carotid endarterectomy: a stopped trial. J Vasc Surg. 1998;28:326–34.

142. Theron J, Courtheoux P, Alachkar F, Bouvard G, Maiza D. New triple coaxial catheter system for carotid angioplasty with cerebral protection. AJNR Am J Neuroradiol. 1990;11:869–77.

143. Tong FC, Cloft HJ, Joseph GJ, Samuels OB, Dion JE. Abciximab rescue in acute carotid stent thrombosis. AJNR Am J Neuroradiol. 2000;21:1750–2.

144. Yadav JS. Management practices in carotid stenting. Cerebrovasc Dis. 2001;11 Suppl 2:18–22.

145. Goodney PP, Travis LL, Malenka D, et al. Regional variation in carotid artery stenting and endarterectomy in the Medicare population. Circ Cardiovasc Qual Outcomes. 2010;3:15–24.

146. Brott TG, Hobson 2nd RW, Howard G, et al. Stenting versus endarterectomy for treatment of carotid-artery stenosis. N Engl J Med. 2010;363:11–23.

147. Mas JL, Trinquart L, Leys D, et al. Endarterectomy versus angioplasty in patients with symptomatic severe carotid stenosis (EVA-3S) trial: results up to 4 years from a randomised, multicentre trial. Lancet Neurol. 2008;7:885–92.

148. Bonati LH, Dobson J, Algra A, et al. Short-term outcome after stenting versus endarterectomy for symptomatic carotid stenosis: a preplanned meta-analysis of individual patient data. Lancet. 2010;376:1062–73.

149. Ringleb PA, Kunze A, Allenberg JR, et al. The stent-supported percutaneous angioplasty of the carotid artery vs. endarterectomy trial. Cerebrovasc Dis. 2004;18:66–8.

150. Ringleb PA, Allenberg J, Bruckmann H, et al. 30 day results from the SPACE trial of stent-protected angioplasty versus carotid endarterectomy in symptomatic patients: a randomised non-inferiority trial. Lancet. 2006;368:1239–47.

151. Yadav JS, Wholey MH, Kuntz RE, et al. Protected carotid-artery stenting versus endarterectomy in high-risk patients. N Engl J Med. 2004;351:1493–501.

152. Gurm HS, Yadav JS, Fayad P, et al. Long-term results of carotid stenting versus endarterectomy in high-risk patients. N Engl J Med. 2008;358:1572–9.

153. Silver FL, Mackey A, Clark WM, et al. Safety of stenting and endarterectomy by symptomatic status in the carotid revascularization endarterectomy versus stenting trial (CREST). Stroke. 2011;42:675–80.

154. Hopkins LN, Roubin GS, Chakhtoura EY, et al. The carotid revascularization endarterectomy versus stenting trial: credentialing of interventionalists and final results of lead in phase. J Stroke Cerebrovasc Dis. 2010;19:153–62.

155. Barnett HJ, Pelz DM, Lownie SP. Reflections by contrarians on the post-CREST evaluation of carotid stenting for stroke prevention. Int J Stroke. 2010;5:455–6.

156. Theiss W, Langhoff R, Schulte KL. SPACE and EVA-3S: two failed studies? Vasa. 2007;36:77–9.

157. Stingele R, Berger J, Alfke K, et al. Clinical and angiographic risk factors for stroke and death within 30 days after carotid endarterectomy and stent-protected angioplasty: a subanalysis of the SPACE study. Lancet Neurol. 2008;7: 216–22.

158. Naylor AR. SPACE: not the final frontier. Lancet. 2006;368:1215–6.

159. Reiff T, Stingele R, Eckstein HH, et al. Stent-protected angioplasty in asymptomatic carotid artery stenosis vs. endarterectomy: SPACE2 – a three-arm randomised-controlled clinical trial. Int J Stroke. 2009;4:294–9.

160. Naggara O, Touze E, Beyssen B, et al. Anatomical and technical factors associated with stroke or death during carotid angioplasty and stenting: results from the endarterectomy versus angioplasty in patients with symptomatic severe carotid stenosis (EVA-3S) trial and systematic review. Stroke. 2011;42:380–8.

161. Arquizan C, Trinquart L, Touboul PJ, et al. Restenosis is more frequent after carotid stenting than after endarterectomy: the EVA-3S study. Stroke. 2011;42:1015–20.

162. Bonati LH, Jongen LM, Haller S, et al. New ischaemic brain lesions on MRI after stenting or endarterectomy for symptomatic carotid stenosis: a substudy of the international carotid stenting study (ICSS). Lancet Neurol. 2010;9:353–62.

163. Wholey MH, Al-Mubarek N, Wholey MH. Updated review of the global carotid artery stent registry. Catheter Cardiovasc Interv. 2003;60:259–66.

164. Willfort-Ehringer A, Ahmadi R, Gschwandtner ME, Haumer M, Lang W, Minar E. Single-center experience with carotid stent restenosis. J Endovasc Ther. 2002;9: 299–307.

165. Levy EI, Hanel RA, Lau T, et al. Frequency and management of recurrent stenosis after carotid artery stent implantation. J Neurosurg. 2005;102:29–37.

166. Bosiers M, Peeters P, Deloose K, et al. Does carotid artery stenting work on the long run: 5-year results in high-volume centers (ELOCAS registry). J Cardiovasc Surg (Torino). 2005;46:241–7.

167. Jordan Jr WD, Voellinger DC, Doblar DD, Plyushcheva NP, Fisher WS, McDowell HA. Microemboli detected by transcranial Doppler monitoring in patients during carotid angioplasty versus carotid endarterectomy. Cardiovasc Surg. 1999;7:33–8.

168. van Heesewijk HPM, Vos JA, Louwerse ES, et al. New brain lesions at MR imaging after carotid angioplasty and stent placement. Radiology. 2002;224:361–5.

169. Kastrup A, Groschel K, Krapf H, Brehm BR, Dichgans J, Schulz JB. Early outcome of carotid angioplasty and stenting with and without cerebral protection devices: a systematic review of the literature. Stroke. 2003;34:813–9.

170. Carotid angioplasty and stenting with and without cerebral protection: clinical alert from the endarterectomy versus angioplasty in patients with symptomatic severe carotid stenosis (EVA-3S) trial. Stroke. 2004;35:18e–20.

171. Jansen O, Fiehler J, Hartmann M, Bruckmann H. Protection or nonprotection in carotid stent angioplasty: the influence of interventional techniques on outcome data from the SPACE trial. Stroke. 2009;40:841–6.

172. Sundt T. Occlusive cerebrovascular disease. Philadelphia: W.D. Saunders; 1987. p. 226–30.

173. Department of Health and Human Services. US FDA. Acculink carotid stent system and RX Acculink carotid stent system. Approval letter.2004. http://www.accessdata. fda.gov/scripts/cdrh/cfdocs/cftopic/pma/pma. cfm?num=p040012. Accessed May 26, 2012.

174. DHHS. CMS Manual System. Pub 100-3 Medicare National Coverage Determinations. Change Request 5660. Transmittal 77. September 12, 2007 www.cms.hhs.gov/ Transmittals/downloads/R77NCD.pdf.

175. Meier P, Knapp G, Tamhane U, Chaturvedi S, Gurm HS. Short term and intermediate term comparison of endartectomy versus stenting for carotid artery stenosis: systematic review and meta-analysis of randomised controlled clinical trials. BMJ. 2010;340:c467.

176. Bonati LH, Fraedrich G. Age modifies the relative risk of stenting versus endarterectomy for symptomatic carotid stenosis – a pooled analysis of EVA-3S, SPACE and ICSS. Eur J Vasc Endovasc Surg. 2011;41:153–8.

177. Pierce GE, Keushkerian SM, Hermreck AS, Iliopoulos JI, Thomas JH. The risk of stroke with occlusion of the internal carotid artery. J Vasc Surg. 1989;9:74–80.

178. Vernieri F, Pasqualetti P, Passarelli F, Rossini PM, Silvestrini M. Outcome of carotid artery occlusion is predicted by cerebrovascular reactivity. Stroke. 1999;30:593–8.

179. Bornstein NM, Norris JW. Benign outcome of carotid occlusion. Neurology. 1989;39:6–8.

180. Powers WJ, Derdeyn CP, Fritsch SM, et al. Benign prognosis of never-symptomatic carotid occlusion. Neurology. 2000;54:878–82.

181. Flaherty ML, Flemming KD, McClelland R, Jorgensen NW, Brown Jr RD. Population-based study of symptomatic internal carotid artery occlusion: incidence and long-term follow-up. Stroke. 2004;35:e349–52.

182. Klijn CJ, Kappelle LJ, Tulleken CA, van Gijn J. Symptomatic carotid artery occlusion. A reappraisal of hemodynamic factors. Stroke. 1997;28:2084–93.

183. Grubb Jr RL, Derdeyn CP, Fritsch SM, et al. Importance of hemodynamic factors in the prognosis of symptomatic carotid occlusion. JAMA. 1998;280:1055–60.

184. Yonas H, Smith HA, Durham SR, Pentheny SL, Johnson DW. Increased stroke risk predicted by compromised cerebral blood flow reactivity. J Neurosurg. 1993;79:483–9.

185. Yasargil M. Anastomosis between the superficial temporal artery and a branch of the middle cerebral artery. In: Yasargil M, editor. Microsurgery applied to neuros-surgery. Stuttgart: Georg Thieme; 1969. p. 105–15.

186. van der Zwan A, Tulleken CA, Hillen B. Flow quantification of the non-occlusive excimer laser-assisted EC-IC bypass. Acta Neurochir (Wien). 2001;143:647–54.

187. Klijn CJM, Kappelle LJ, van der Zwan A, van Gijn J, Tulleken CAF. Excimer laser-assisted high-flow extracranial/intracranial bypass in patients with symptomatic carotid artery occlusion at high risk of recurrent cerebral ischemia: safety and long-term outcome. Stroke. 2002;33:2451–8.

188. Failure of extracranial-intracranial arterial bypass to reduce the risk of ischemic stroke. Results of an international randomized trial. The EC/IC Bypass Study Group. N Engl J Med. 1985;313:1191–200.

189. Ausman JI, Diaz FG. Critique of the extracranial-intracranial bypass study. Surg Neurol. 1986;26:218–21.

190. Awad IA, Spetzler RF. Extracranial-intracranial bypass surgery: a critical analysis in light of the international cooperative study. Neurosurgery. 1986;19:655–64.

191. Day AL, Rhoton Jr AL, Little JR. The extracranial-intracranial bypass study. Surg Neurol. 1986;26:222–6.

192. Goldring S, Zervas N, Langfitt T T. The extracranial-intracranial bypass study. A report of the committee appointed by the American Association of Neurological Surgeons to examine the study. N Engl J Med. 1987;316:817–20.

193. Furlan AJ, Little JR, Dohn DF. Arterial occlusion following anastomosis of the superficial temporal artery to middle cerebral artery. Stroke. 1980;11:91–5.

194. Gumerlock MK, Ono H, Neuwelt EA. Can a patent extracranial-intracranial bypass provoke the conversion of an intracranial arterial stenosis to a symptomatic occlusion? Neurosurgery. 1983;12:391–400.

195. Awad I, Furlan AJ, Little JR. Changes in intracranial stenotic lesions after extracranial-intracranial bypass surgery. J Neurosurg. 1984;60:771–6.

196. Powers WJ. Extracranial-intracranial bypass surgery for stroke prevention in hemodynamic cerebral ischemia. The carotid occlusion surgery study randomized trial. JAMA. 2011;306:1983–92.

197. Marshall RS, Lazar R. Pumps, aqueducts, and drought management: vascular physiology in vascular cognitive impairment. Stroke. 2011;42:221–6.

198. Grubb Jr RL, Powers WJ, Derdeyn CP, Adams Jr HP, Clarke WR. The carotid occlusion surgery study. Neurosurg Focus. 2003;14:e9.

199. Caplan L. Posterior circulation ischemia: then, now, and tomorrow: the Thomas Willis lecture – 2000. Stroke. 2000;31:2011–23.

200. Hass WK, Fields WS, North RR, Kircheff II, Chase NE, Bauer RB. Joint study of extracranial arterial occlusion. II. Arteriography, techniques, sites, and complications. JAMA. 1968;203:961–8.

201. Cloud GC, Markus HS. Diagnosis and management of vertebral artery stenosis. QJM. 2003;96:27–54.

202. Caplan L. Stroke: a clinical approach. 3rd ed. Stoneham: Butterworth-Heinemann; 2000.

203. Caplan LR, Gorelick PB, Hier DB. Race, sex and occlusive cerebrovascular disease: a review. Stroke. 1986;17:648–55.

204. Wityk RJ, Chang HM, Rosengart A, et al. Proximal extracranial vertebral artery disease in the New England Medical Center Posterior Circulation Registry. Arch Neurol. 1998;55:470–8.

205. Charbel F, Guppy K, Carney A, Ausman J. Extracranial vertebral artery disease. In: Winn H, editor. Youmans neurological surgery. 5th ed. Philadelphia: Saunders; 2004. p. 1691–714.

206. Caplan LR, Wityk RJ, Glass TA, et al. New England Medical Center Posterior Circulation registry. Ann Neurol. 2004;56:389–98.

207. Farres MT, Grabenwoger F, Magometschnig H, Trattnig S, Heimberger K, Lammer J. Spiral CT angiography: study of stenoses and calcification at the origin of the vertebral artery. Neuroradiology. 1996;38:738–43.

208. Flossmann E, Rothwell PM. Prognosis of vertebrobasilar transient ischaemic attack and minor stroke. Brain. 2003; 126:1940–54.

209. Sivenius J, Riekkinen PJ, Smets P, Laakso M, Lowenthal A. The European stroke prevention study (ESPS): results by arterial distribution. Ann Neurol. 1991;29:596–600.

210. Grundy SM, Cleeman JI, Merz CN, et al. Implications of recent clinical trials for the National Cholesterol Education Program Adult Treatment Panel III Guidelines. J Am Coll Cardiol. 2004;44:720–32.

211. Berguer R, Flynn LM, Kline RA, Caplan L. Surgical reconstruction of the extracranial vertebral artery: management and outcome. J Vasc Surg. 2000;31:9–18.

212. Albuquerque FC, Fiorella D, Han P, Spetzler RF, McDougall CG. A reappraisal of angioplasty and stenting for the treatment of vertebral origin stenosis. Neurosurgery. 2003; 53:607–14; discussion 14–6.

213. Hatano T, Tsukahara T, Miyakoshi A, Arai D, Yamaguchi S, Murakami M. Stent placement for atherosclerotic stenosis of the vertebral artery ostium: angiographic and clinical outcomes in 117 consecutive patients. Neurosurgery. 2011;68:108–16.

214. Ko YG, Park S, Kim JY, et al. Percutaneous interventional treatment of extracranial vertebral artery stenosis with coronary stents. Yonsei Med J. 2004;45:629–34.
215. Jenkins JS, White CJ, Ramee SR, et al. Vertebral artery stenting. Catheter Cardiovasc Interv. 2001;54:1–5.
216. Cloud GC, Crawley F, Clifton A, McCabe DJH, Brown MM, Markus HS. Vertebral artery origin angioplasty and primary stenting: safety and restenosis rates in a prospective series. J Neurol Neurosurg Psychiatry. 2003;74:586–90.
217. The SSI. Stenting of symptomatic atherosclerotic lesions in the vertebral or intracranial arteries (SSYLVIA): study results. Stroke. 2004;35:1388–92.
218. Compter A, van der Worp H, Schonewille W, et al. VAST: vertebral artery stenting trial. Protocol for a randomised safety and feasibility trial. Trials. 2008;9:65.
219. Kuether TA, Nesbit GM, Clark WM, Barnwell SL. Rotational vertebral artery occlusion: a mechanism of vertebrobasilar insufficiency. Neurosurgery. 1997;41:427–32; discussion 32–3.
220. Dumas JL, Salama J, Dreyfus P, Thoreux P, Goldlust D, Chevrel JP. Magnetic resonance angiographic analysis of atlanto-axial rotation: anatomic bases of compression of the vertebral arteries. Surg Radiol Anat. 1996;18:303–13.
221. Lu DC, Zador Z, Mummaneni PV, Lawton MT. Rotational vertebral artery occlusion-series of 9 cases. Neurosurgery. 2010;67:1066–72.
222. Dabus G, Gerstle RJ, Parsons M, et al. Rotational vertebrobasilar insufficiency due to dynamic compression of the dominant vertebral artery by the thyroid cartilage and occlusion of the contralateral vertebral artery at C1-2 level. J Neuroimaging. 2008;18:184–7.
223. Nemecek AN, Newell DW, Goodkin R. Transient rotational compression of the vertebral artery caused by herniated cervical disc. Case report. J Neurosurg. 2003;98:80–3.
224. Tominaga T, Takahashi T, Shimizu H, Yoshimoto T. Rotational vertebral artery occlusion from occipital bone anomaly: a rare cause of embolic stroke. Case report. J Neurosurg. 2002;97:1456–9.
225. Akar Z, Kafadar AM, Tanriover N, et al. Rotational compression of the vertebral artery at the point of dural penetration. J Neurosurg. 2000;93:300–3.
226. Sell JJ, Rael JR, Orrison WW. Rotational vertebrobasilar insufficiency as a component of thoracic outlet syndrome resulting in transient blindness. Case report. J Neurosurg. 1994;81:617–9.
227. Fujimoto S, Terai Y, Itoh T. Rotational stenosis of the first segment of the vertebral artery through compression by the cervical sympathetic chain – case report. Neurol Med Chir (Tokyo). 1988;28:1020–3.
228. Miele VJ, France JC, Rosen CL. Subaxial positional vertebral artery occlusion corrected by decompression and fusion. Spine (Phila Pa 1976). 2008;33:E366–70.
229. Wakayama K, Murakami M, Suzuki M, Ono S, Shimizu N. Ischemic symptoms induced by occlusion of the unilateral vertebral artery with head rotation together with contralateral vertebral artery dissection – case report. J Neurol Sci. 2005;236:87–90.
230. Strupp M, Planck JH, Arbusow V, Steiger HJ, Bruckmann H, Brandt T. Rotational vertebral artery occlusion syndrome with vertigo due to "labyrinthine excitation". Neurology. 2000;54:1376–9.
231. Bacquey F, Hamon M, Coskun O, et al. Rotational vertebrobasilar insufficiency secondary to a fibrous band of the longus colli muscle: value of CT spiral angiography diagnosis. J Radiol. 2002;83:979–82.
232. Bakay L, Leslie EV. Surgical treatment of vertebral artery insufficiency caused by cervical spondylosis. J Neurosurg. 1965;23:596–602.
233. Nagashima C. Surgical treatment of vertebral artery insufficiency caused by cervical spondylosis. J Neurosurg. 1970;32:512–21.
234. Smith DR, Vanderark GD, Kempe LG. Cervical spondylosis causing vertebrobasilar insufficiency: a surgical treatment. J Neurol Neurosurg Psychiatry. 1971;34:388–92.
235. Bogousslavsky J, Regli F. Ischemic stroke in adults younger than 30 years of age. Cause and prognosis. Arch Neurol. 1987;44:479–82.

236. Milhaud D, de Freitas GR, van Melle G, Bogousslavsky J. Occlusion due to carotid artery dissection: a more severe disease than previously suggested. Arch Neurol. 2002;59:557–61.
237. Schievink WI, Mokri B, Whisnant JP. Internal carotid artery dissection in a community. Rochester, Minnesota, 1987–1992. Stroke. 1993;24:1678–80.
238. Harbaugh RE. Carotid artery dissection, fibromuscular dysplasia, and other disorders of the carotid artery. In: Bederson J, Tuhrim S, editors. Treatment of carotid disease: a practitioner's manual. Park Ridge: The American Association of Neurological Surgeons; 1998. p. 211–28.
239. Guillon B, Berthet K, Benslamia L, Bertrand M, Bousser M-G, Tzourio C. Infection and the risk of spontaneous cervical artery dissection: a case-control study. Stroke. 2003;34:79e–81.
240. Sturzenegger M. Spontaneous internal carotid artery dissection: early diagnosis and management in 44 patients. J Neurol. 1995;242:231–8.
241. Norris JW, Beletsky V, Nadareishvili Z, Brandt T, Grond-Ginsbach C. "Spontaneous" cervical arterial dissection * response. Stroke. 2002;33:1945–6.
242. Schievink WI. Spontaneous dissection of the carotid and vertebral arteries. N Engl J Med. 2001;344:898–906.
243. Benninger DH, Georgiadis D, Kremer C, Studer A, Nedeltchev K, Baumgartner RW. Mechanism of ischemic infarct in spontaneous carotid dissection. Stroke. 2004;35:482–5.
244. Biousse V, D'Anglejan-Chatillon J, Touboul PJ, Amarenco P, Bousser MG. Time course of symptoms in extracranial carotid artery dissections. A series of 80 patients. Stroke. 1995;26:235–9.
245. Gelal FM, Kitis O, Calli C, Yunten N, Vidinli BD, Uygur M. Craniocervical artery dissection: diagnosis and follow-up with MR imaging and MR angiography. Med Sci Monit. 2004;10:MT109–16.
246. Nunez Jr DB, Torres-Leon M, Munera F. Vascular injuries of the neck and thoracic inlet: helical CT-angiographic correlation. Radiographics. 2004;24:1087–98.
247. Stuhlfaut JW, Barest G, Sakai O, Lucey B, Soto JA. Impact of MDCT angiography on the use of catheter angiography for the assessment of cervical arterial injury after blunt or penetrating trauma. Am J Roentgenol. 2005;185:1063–8.
248. Georgiadis D, Arnold M, von Buedingen HC, et al. Aspirin vs anticoagulation in carotid artery dissection: a study of 298 patients. Neurology. 2009;72:1810–5.
249. Anonymous. Antiplatelet therapy vs. anticoagulation in cervical artery dissection: rationale and design of the cervical artery dissection in stroke study (CADISS). Int J Stroke. 2007;2:292–6.
250. Cohen JE, Leker RR, Gotkine M, Gomori M, Ben-Hur T. Emergent stenting to treat patients with carotid artery dissection: clinically and radiologically directed therapeutic decision making. Stroke. 2003;34:254e–7.
251. Zetterling M, Carlstrom C, Konrad P. Internal carotid artery dissection. Acta Neurol Scand. 2000;101:1–7.
252. Ast G, Woimant F, Georges B, Laurian C, Haguenau M. Spontaneous dissection of the internal carotid artery in 68 patients. Eur J Med. 1993;2:466–72.
253. Steinke W, Rautenberg W, Schwartz A, Hennerici M. Noninvasive monitoring of internal carotid artery dissection. Stroke. 1994;25:998–1005.
254. Bassetti C, Carruzzo A, Sturzenegger M, Tuncdogan E. Recurrence of cervical artery dissection: a prospective study of 81 patients. Stroke. 1996;27:1804–7.
255. Fabian TC, Patton Jr JH, Croce MA, Minard G, Kudsk KA, Pritchard FE. Blunt carotid injury. Importance of early diagnosis and anticoagulant therapy. Ann Surg. 1996;223:513–22; discussion 22–5.
256. Miller PR, Fabian TC, Croce MA, et al. Prospective screening for blunt cerebrovascular injuries: analysis of diagnostic modalities and outcomes. Ann Surg. 2002;236:386–93; discussion 93–5.
257. Mokri B, Piepgras DG, Houser OW. Traumatic dissections of the extracranial internal carotid artery. J Neurosurg. 1988;68:189–97.
258. Lucas C, Moulin T, Deplanque D, Tatu L, Chavot D. Stroke patterns of internal carotid artery dissection in 40 patients. Stroke. 1998;29:2646–8.

259. Li MS, Smith BM, Espinosa J, Brown RA, Richardson P, Ford R. Nonpenetrating trauma to the carotid artery: seven cases and a literature review. J Trauma. 1994;36:265–72.

260. Ramadan F, Rutledge R, Oller D, Howell P, Baker C, Keagy B. Carotid artery trauma: a review of contemporary trauma center experiences. J Vasc Surg. 1995;21:46–55; discussion 6.

261. Harrigan MR, Weinberg JA, Peaks YS, et al. Management of blunt extracranial traumatic cerebrovascular injury: a multidisciplinary survey of current practice. WJES. 2011; 6:11.

262. Parikh AA, Luchette FA, Valente JF, et al. Blunt carotid artery injuries. J Am Coll Surg. 1997;185:80–6.

263. Biffl WL, Moore EE, Offner PJ, Brega KE, Franciose RJ, Burch JM. Blunt carotid arterial injuries: implications of a new grading scale. J Trauma. 1999;47:845–53.

264. Biffl WL, Moore EE, Elliott JP, et al. The devastating potential of blunt vertebral arterial injuries. Ann Surg. 2000;231:672–81.

265. Wahl WL, Brandt MM, Thompson BG, Taheri PA, Greenfield LJ. Antiplatelet therapy: an alternative to heparin for blunt carotid injury. J Trauma. 2002;52:896–901.

266. Mayberry JC, Brown CV, Mullins RJ, Velmahos GC. Blunt carotid artery injury: the futility of aggressive screening and diagnosis. Arch Surg. 2004;139:609–12; discussion 12–3.

267. Stein DM, Boswell S, Sliker CW, Lui FY, Scalea TM. Blunt cerebrovascular injuries: does treatment always matter? J Trauma. 2009;66:132–43; discussion 43–4.

268. Biffl WL, Moore EE, Ray C, Elliott JP. Emergent stenting of acute blunt carotid artery injuries: a cautionary note. J Trauma. 2001;50:969–71.

269. Barinagarrementeria F, Amaya LE, Cantu C. Causes and mechanisms of cerebellar infarction in young patients. Stroke. 1997;28:2400–4.

270. Mokri B, Houser OW, Sandok BA, Piepgras DG. Spontaneous dissections of the vertebral arteries. Neurology. 1988;38:880–5.

271. Leys D, Lesoin F, Pruvo JP, Gozet G, Jomin M, Petit H. Bilateral spontaneous dissection of extracranial vertebral arteries. J Neurol. 1987;234:237–40.

272. Weintraub MI. Beauty parlor stroke syndrome: report of five cases. JAMA. 1993;269:2085–6.

273. Trosch RM, Hasbani M, Brass LM. "Bottoms up" dissection. N Engl J Med. 1989;320:1564–5.

274. Bartels E. Dissection of the extracranial vertebral artery: clinical findings and early noninvasive diagnosis in 24 patients. J Neuroimaging. 2006;16:24–33.

275. Silbert PL, Mokri B, Schievink WI. Headache and neck pain in spontaneous internal carotid and vertebral artery dissections. Neurology. 1995;45:1517–22.

276. Provenzale JM, Morgenlander JC, Gress D. Spontaneous vertebral dissection: clinical, conventional angiographic, CT, and MR findings. J Comput Assist Tomogr. 1996;20: 185–93.

277. Lalwani AK, Dowd CF, Halbach VV. Grading venous restrictive disease in patients with Dural arteriovenous fistulas of the transverse/sigmoid sinus. J Neurosurg. 1993;79:11–5.

278. Levy C, Laissy JP, Raveau V, et al. Carotid and vertebral artery dissections: three-dimensional time-of- flight MR angiography and MR imaging versus conventional angiography. Radiology. 1994;190:97–103.

279. Mascalchi M, Bianchi MC, Mangiafico S, et al. MRI and MR angiography of vertebral artery dissection. Neuroradiology. 1997;39:329–40.

280. Sanelli PC, Tong S, Gonzalez RG, Eskey CJ. Normal variation of vertebral artery on CT angiography and its implications for diagnosis of acquired pathology. J Comput Assist Tomogr. 2002;26:462–70.

281. Willis BK, Greene F, Orrison WW, Benzel EC. The incidence of vertebral artery injury after midcervical spine fracture or subluxation. Neurosurgery. 1994;34:435–41; discussion 41–2.

282. Hollingworth W, Nathens AB, Kanne JP, et al. The diagnostic accuracy of computed tomography angiography for traumatic or atherosclerotic lesions of the carotid and vertebral arteries: a systematic review. Eur J Radiol. 2003;48:88–102.

283. Demetriades D, Theodorou D, Asensio J, et al. Management options in vertebral artery injuries. Br J Surg. 1996;83:83–6.

284. Cohen JE, Gomori JM, Umansky F. Endovascular management of symptomatic vertebral artery dissection achieved using stent angioplasty and emboli protection device. Neurol Res. 2003;25:418–22.

285. Nakagawa K, Touho H, Morisako T, et al. Long-term follow-up study of unruptured vertebral artery dissection: clinical outcomes and serial angiographic findings. J Neurosurg. 2000;93:19–25.

286. LeBlang SD, Nunez Jr DB. Noninvasive imaging of cervical vascular injuries. Am J Roentgenol. 2000;174:1269–78.

287. Biffl WL, Moore EE, Rehse DH, Offner PJ, Franciose RJ, Burch JM. Selective management of penetrating neck trauma based on cervical level of injury. Am J Surg. 1997;174:678–82.

288. Munera F, Soto JA, Palacio DM, et al. Penetrating neck injuries: helical CT angiography for initial evaluation. Radiology. 2002;224:366–72.

289. LeBlang S, Nunez Jr D, Rivas L, Falcone S, Pogson S. Helical computed tomographic angiography in penetrating neck trauma. Emerg Radiol. 1997;4:200–6.

290. Munera F, Soto JA, Palacio D, Velez SM, Medina E. Diagnosis of arterial injuries caused by penetrating trauma to the neck: comparison of helical CT angiography and conventional angiography. Radiology. 2000;216:356–62.

291. Menawat SS, Dennis JW, Laneve LM, Frykberg ER. Are arteriograms necessary in penetrating zone II neck injuries? J Vasc Surg. 1992;16:397–400; discussion 1.

292. Kuehne JP, Weaver FA, Papanicolaou G, Yellin AE. Penetrating trauma of the internal carotid artery. Arch Surg. 1996;131:942–7.

293. Thompson EC, Porter JM, Fernandez LG. Penetrating neck trauma: an overview of management. J Oral Maxillofac Surg. 2002;60:918–23.

294. Higashida RT, Halbach VV, Tsai FY, et al. Interventional neurovascular treatment of traumatic carotid and vertebral artery lesions: results in 234 cases. AJR Am J Roentgenol. 1989;153:577–82.

295. Sclafani AP, Sclafani SJ. Angiography and transcatheter arterial embolization of vascular injuries of the face and neck. Laryngoscope. 1996;106:168–73.

296. Albuquerque FC, Javedan SP, McDougall CG. Endovascular management of penetrating vertebral artery injuries. J Trauma. 2002;53:574–80.

297. Schievink WI, Limburg M. Angiographic abnormalities mimicking fibromuscular dysplasia in a patient with Ehlers-Danlos syndrome, type IV. Neurosurgery. 1989;25:482–3.

298. Kincaid OW, Davis GD, Hallermann FJ, Hunt JC. Fibromuscular dysplasia of the renal arteries. Arteriographic features, classification, and observations on natural history of the disease. Am J Roentgenol Radium Ther Nucl Med. 1968;104:271–82.

299. Slovut DP, Olin JW. Fibromuscular dysplasia. N Engl J Med. 2004;350:1862–71.

300. McCormack LJ, Poutasse EF, Meaney TF, Noto Jr TJ, Dustan HP. A pathologic-arteriographic correlation of renal arterial disease. Am Heart J. 1966;72:188–98.

301. Schievink WI, Meyer FB, Parisi JE, Wijdicks EF. Fibromuscular dysplasia of the internal carotid artery associated with alpha1-antitrypsin deficiency. Neurosurgery. 1998;43:229–33; discussion 33–4.

302. Pannier-Moreau I, Grimbert P, Fiquet-Kempf B, et al. Possible familial origin of multifocal renal artery fibromuscular dysplasia. J Hypertens. 1997;15:1797–801.

303. Cloft HJ, Kallmes DF, Kallmes MH, Goldstein JH, Jensen ME, Dion JE. Prevalence of cerebral aneurysms in patients with fibromuscular dysplasia: a reassessment. J Neurosurg. 1998;88:436–40.

304. Spengos K, Vassilopoulou S, Tsivgoulis G, Papadopoulou M, Vassilopoulos D. An uncommon variant of fibromuscular dysplasia. J Neuroimaging. 2008;18:90–2.

305. Tan AK, Venketasubramanian N, Tan CB, Lee SH, Tjia TL. Ischaemic stroke from cerebral embolism in cephalic fibromuscular dysplasia. Ann Acad Med Singapore. 1995;24:891–4.

306. Stewart MT, Moritz MW, Smith 3rd RB, Fulenwider JT, Perdue GD. The natural history of carotid fibromuscular dysplasia. J Vasc Surg. 1986;3:305–10.

307. Wells RP, Smith RR. Fibromuscular dysplasia of the internal carotid artery: a long term follow-up. Neurosurgery. 1982;10:39–43.
308. Wesen CA, Elliott BM. Fibromuscular dysplasia of the carotid arteries. Am J Surg. 1986;151:448–51.
309. Bahar S, Chiras J, Carpena JP, Meder JF, Bories J. Spontaneous vertebro-vertebral arterio-venous fistula associated with fibro-muscular dysplasia. Report of two cases. Neuroradiology. 1984;26:45–9.
310. Welch EL, Lemkin JA, Geary JE. Gruntzig balloon dilation for fibromuscular dysplasia of the internal carotid arteries. N Y State J Med. 1985;85:115–7.
311. Tsai FY, Matovich V, Hieshima G, et al. Percutaneous transluminal angioplasty of the carotid artery. AJNR Am J Neuroradiol. 1986;7:349–58.
312. Finsterer J, Strassegger J, Haymerle A, Hagmuller G. Bilateral stenting of symptomatic and asymptomatic internal carotid artery stenosis due to fibromuscular dysplasia. J Neurol Neurosurg Psychiatry. 2000;69:683–6.
313. Manninen HI, Koivisto T, Saari T, et al. Dissecting aneurysms of all four cervicocranial arteries in fibromuscular dysplasia: treatment with self-expanding endovascular stents, coil embolization, and surgical ligation. AJNR Am J Neuroradiol. 1997;18:1216–20.

19. Intracranial Cerebrovascular Occlusive Disease

This chapter will discuss intracranial arterial stenosis and occlusion due to atherosclerosis and moyamoya syndrome.

19.1. Atherosclerotic Intracranial Arterial Disease

Prevalence and Risk Factors

Approximately 8–10% of ischaemic strokes are attributable to intracranial atherosclerosis.[1,2] In the USA, it is estimated that 40,000 60,000 new strokes per year are due to intracranial atherosclerosis.[3]

Distribution of symptomatic intracranial stenosis by location:
1) Internal carotid – 20.3%
2) MCA – 33.9%
3) Vertebral artery – 19.6%
4) Basilar artery – 20.3%
5) Multiple arteries – 5.9%
   a) Percentages are taken from the patients randomized to aspirin in WASID.[4]

Risk Factors

1) Black, Asian, or Hispanic ethnicity[5]
   a) Black patients with TIA or stroke are more likely than white patients to have intracranial stenosis, whereas whites are more likely to have extracranial carotid atherosclerotic stenosis.[1]
      i) In a comparison of white and black patients with symptomatic posterior circulation disease, black patients had more lesions of the distal basilar artery, more high-grade lesions of intracranial branch vessels, and more symptomatic intracranial branch disease. Race was found to be the only factor increasing the risk of intracranial posterior circulation occlusive disease.[6]
   b) Asian patients have a higher proportion of MCA stenosis compared with Caucasian and black patients.[7]
      i) Intracranial stenosis is responsible for stroke in up to 33% of Chinese patients.[8]
   c) A TCD study of healthy volunteers found a greater mismatch between cortical metabolic demand and cerebral blood flow in Asians compared to whites.[9] This racial difference in neurovascular coupling may be a factor in the difference in rates of intracranial stenosis between the two groups.
2) Hypertension is present in up to 75% of patients.[10] Diabetes, coronary artery disease, cigarette smoking, and hypercholesterolemia, and peripheral arterial occlusive disease are also strongly associated.
3) Patients *without* carotid bifurcation disease are more likely to demonstrate progression of intracranial stenosis compared with patients with it.[11]
4) Cannabis use. Pot smoking has been linked to multifocal intracranial stenosis and ischaemic stroke in young people.[12]

M.R. Harrigan, J.P. Deveikis, *Handbook of Cerebrovascular Disease and Neurointerventional Technique*, DOI 10.1007/978-1-61779-946-4_19, © Springer Science+Business Media New York 2013

5) *Metabolic syndrome* is present in about 50% of patients with symptomatic intracranial atherosclerotic disease and is associated with a substantially higher risk of major vascular events.
   a) Metabolic syndrome is a cluster of interrelated risk factors that together increase an individual's risk of cardiovascular disease.[13] The syndrome consists of four main categories of metabolic abnormalities: atherogenic dyslipidemia (elevated triglycerides and decreased high-density lipoproteins), increased blood pressure, elevated plasma glucose, and a pro-thrombotic state. Some 24% of US adults have metabolic syndrome.[14]

Global Gem! Intracranial Stenosis
It is well established that intracranial arterial stenosis is more prevalent among Asian and African people compared to whites. Based on racial and ethnic patterns, intracranial stenosis may be the most important cause of ischaemic stroke in the world.

Aetiology of Symptoms

Ischaemic symptoms due to intracranial stenosis are believed to arise from the following:
1) Hypoperfusion[15,16]
2) Thrombosis at the site of stenosis due to plaque rupture, haemorrhage within the plaque, or occlusive growth of the plaque[17,18]
3) Thromboembolism distal to the stenosis
4) Occlusion of small perforating arteries at the site of the plaque[7,19]

Natural History

Intracranial stenoses are dynamic lesions that may demonstrate both progression and regression on serial imaging.[11,20]
1) In a study of patients with intracranial stenosis undergoing repeat angiography at an average interval of 26.7 months, 40% of lesions were stable, 20% regressed, and 40% progressed.[11]
2) Stenosis progression, as detected by TCD, is an independent predictor of stroke recurrence.[21]
3) *Extracranial-intracranial (EC-IC) bypass surgery appears to promote progression of the lesion and occlusion of MCA in patients with nonoccluded MCA stenosis.*[20]
Asymptomatic intracranial stenosis is generally believed to be benign. In a series of 50 patients with asymptomatic MCA stenosis followed for a mean of 351 days, no patient had an ischaemic stroke in the corresponding territory.[10]
The best studies of the natural history of *symptomatic* stenosis have been from several prospective studies of medical therapy. Estimates of the overall annual ipsilateral stroke risk in patients with intracranial stenosis from prospective studies range from 2.3 to nearly 13%.[4,7,21–24] The most definitive study so far is the prospective WASID trial, which found a first-year risk of ischaemic stroke in the pertinent vascular territory of 11–12%.[4]
The natural history of intracranial stenosis is somewhat dependent on the location of the lesion. Although a systematic review found no differences in recurrent ipsilateral stroke risk, overall mortality was found to be the lowest for patients with MCA stenosis.[25]
1) Mean overall annual mortality:[25]
   a) MCA stenosis: 6.8%
   b) Vertebrobasilar stenosis: 11.6%
   c) Intracranial ICA stenosis: 12.4%

EC/IC Bypass Study

The subset of patients in the EC/IC Bypass Study with MCA stenosis randomized to medical therapy had an annual ipsilateral ischaemic stroke rate of 7.8% per year.[7] The EC/IC Bypass Study is discussed in detail in Chap. 18.

Warfarin Versus Aspirin for Symptomatic Intracranial Disease (WASID) Studies

The WASID studies evaluated two medical management strategies in the treatment of patients with symptomatic intracranial stenosis. Two separate studies were done. The first study was retrospective and suggested that warfarin is superior to aspirin.[26] The second study was a prospective, multicenter, double-blinded randomized trial. Warfarin was associated with significantly higher rates of adverse events and did not provide a benefit over aspirin.[4]

WASID RETROSPECTIVE STUDY

The retrospective study examined 151 patients with symptomatic intracranial atherosclerotic stenosis evaluated by angiography at seven centers between 1985 and 1991.[26] Treatment consisted of either warfarin or aspirin and was determined at the treating physician's discretion. The mean follow-up period was 14.7 months in the warfarin group and 19.3 months in the aspirin group. The annualized rate of stroke was 3.6% in the warfarin group and 10.4% in the aspirin group ($p = 0.01$), suggesting that warfarin is superior to aspirin in the treatment of patients with symptomatic intracranial stenosis. These findings lead to the organization of the prospective WASID trial.

WASID PROSPECTIVE TRIAL

A total of 569 patients with TIA or stroke attributable to angiographically verified 50–99% stenosis of a major intracranial artery (Fig. 19.1) were randomized to receive warfarin (target INR, 2.0–3.0) or aspirin (1,300 mg per day).[4] Enrollment was stopped prematurely (enrollment of 806 patients was originally planned) because of a significantly higher rate of haemorrhage in the warfarin group. The median time from qualifying event to randomization was 17 days, and the mean follow-up period was 1.8 years.

1) The primary end point of ischaemic stroke, brain haemorrhage, or death from vascular causes other than stroke:
   a) 21.8% in the warfarin group
   b) 22.1% in the aspirin group ($p = 0.83$)

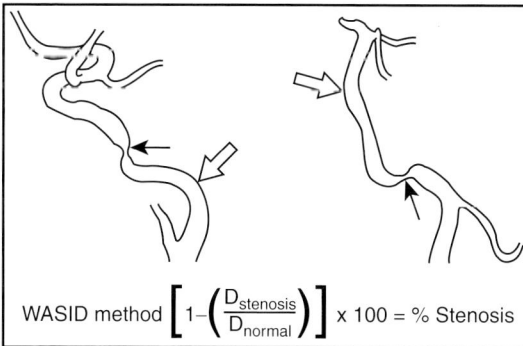

$$\text{WASID method} \left[1 - \left(\frac{D_{stenosis}}{D_{normal}} \right) \right] \times 100 = \% \text{ Stenosis}$$

Fig. 19.1 WASID technique for measuring intracranial stenosis. The equation used for determining percent stenosis of a major intracranial artery in WASID.[228] $D_{stenosis}$ = the diameter of the artery at the site of the most severe degree of stenosis and D_{normal} = the diameter of the proximal normal artery. D_{normal} is selected according to the following criteria: (1) First choice (*left*): The diameter of the proximal part of the artery at its widest, nontortuous, normal segment is selected. Stenotic region (*arrow*); reference area (D_{normal}) (*open arrow*). (2) Second choice (*right*): If the lesion is at the origin of the vessel, or if the proximal artery is diseased (e.g., proximal basilar artery stenosis or M1 segment origin stenosis), the diameter of the distal portion of the artery at its widest, parallel, nontortuous normal segment is used. Stenotic region (*arrow*); reference area (D_{normal}) (*open arrow*). (3) Third choice: If the entire intracranial artery was diseased, the most distal, parallel, nontortuous normal segment of the feeding artery is measured.

2) Rate of death:
   a) 9.7% in the warfarin group
   b) 4.3% in the aspirin group ($p = 0.02$)
3) Major haemorrhage
   a) 8.3% in the warfarin group
   b) 3.2% in the aspirin group ($p = 0.01$)
4) Myocardial infarction or sudden death:
   a) 7.3% in the warfarin group
   b) 2.9% in the aspirin group ($p = 0.02$)
5) Rate of death from vascular causes:
   a) 5.9% in the warfarin group
   b) 3.2% in the aspirin group ($p = 0.16$)
6) Rate of death from nonvascular causes
   a) 3.8% in the warfarin group
   b) 1.1% in the aspirin group ($p = 0.05$)

The risk of ischaemic stroke in the territory of the stenotic artery at 1 year in patients treated with aspirin was 12%, and in patients treated with warfarin the risk was 11% ($p = 0.31$). Because of the high adverse event rates for patients treated with warfarin, and lack of therapeutic benefit of warfarin over aspirin for prevention of ischaemic stroke caused by intracranial stenosis, the WASID investigators concluded that aspirin should be used in preference to warfarin for patients with intracranial arterial stenosis.

WASID PROSPECTIVE TRIAL SUBGROUP ANALYSES

An analysis of selected subgroups of patients in the WASID trial found no advantage of warfarin over aspirin for preventing the primary end point of ischaemic stroke, brain haemorrhage, or vascular death.[27] A statistically significant benefit was associated with warfarin in patients with symptomatic basilar artery stenosis in terms of the primary end point (ischaemic stroke, brain haemorrhage, or death from vascular causes other than stroke). However, the sample size and wide confidence intervals of this finding diminished the credibility of this finding. Furthermore, there was no difference in the rates of ischaemic stroke in the territory of the symptomatic basilar artery between treatment group, and no benefit was found in patients with symptomatic intracranial vertebral artery stenosis. The WASID investigators concluded that warfarin demonstrated no convincing benefit in patients with basilar artery stenosis.

WASID PREDICTORS OF ISCHAEMIC STROKE IN THE TERRITORY OF A SYMPTOMATIC

INTRACRANIAL STENOSIS

The majority of strokes (73%) in WASID patients were in the territory of the stenotic artery.[28] The risk of stroke in the territory of the stenotic artery was greatest in patients with the following characteristics:
1) Severe ($\geq$70%) stenosis ($p = 0.0025$).
2) Patients enrolled early ($\leq$17 days) ($p = 0.028$).
3) There was a statistical trend toward an increased risk for women ($p = 0.051$)
4) Location of stenosis, type of qualifying event, and prior use of antithrombotic medications *were not* associated with increased risk.

GESICA STUDY

The GESICA Study (Groupe d'Etude des Sténoses Intra-Crâniennes Athéromateuses symptomatiques) was a prospective, multicenter nonrandomized study in France.[24] A total of 102 patients with symptoms attributable to intracranial stenosis $\geq$50% indicated by either angiography or ultrasonography were enrolled. *Optimal medical therapy* was left to the discretion of the local investigators. The mean follow-up period was 23.4 months.
1) The annualized risk of a cerebrovascular event (TIA or stroke) in the territory of the affected artery was 19.2%.
   a) Annualized risk of TIA: 12.6%.
   b) Annualized risk of stroke: 7.0%

Medical Treatment of Symptomatic Intracranial Stenosis

Medical management of symptomatic intracranial stenosis consists of antiplatelet therapy, strategies to treat hyperlipidaemia, and aggressive control of medical risk factors, such as diabetes, hypertension, and cigarette smoking. Medical therapy of patients with cerebral ischaemia is discussed in detail in Chap. 17: *Acute Ischaemic Stroke*. The authors of this handbook favor the following regimen for patients with symptomatic intracranial stenosis:

1) Aggrenox™ (Boehinger Ingelheim Pharmaceuticals, Inc.)
   a) Aspirin (25 mg) plus extended-release dipyridamole (200 mg) PO BID has been found in a randomized trial to reduce risk of recurrent stroke.[29]
2) Atorvastatin (Lipitor®, Pfizer, Inc.)
   a) High-dose atorvastatin (80-mg PO QD) was found in a randomized trial to reduce the risk of recurrent stroke.[30]
   b) Note: Myalgia is a common side effect; myopathy and rhabdomyolysis occur in <0.01% of patients. Blood work including serum creatinine, creatine kinase (CK), and liver function tests should be done prior to starting the drug and at 3 months on the drug.
3) Antihypertensive agents, as needed.
4) Tight control of serum glucose, for diabetic patients.
5) Smoking cessation.

Intracranial Angioplasty and Stenting

Intracranial angioplasty with or without stenting is beginning to emerge as an acceptable treatment in very selected patients. However, the efficacy of the technique is difficult to assess from the existing literature due to (1) rapidly evolving technology; (2) a wide variety of techniques reported in the literature; and (3) a paucity of prospective data, and the complete absence of randomized trial data. Most single-center series have reported on angioplasty alone,[31–35] or angioplasty and stenting with balloon-mounted coronary stents.[34,36] Angioplasty without stenting is associated with a significant risk of restenosis,[31] which has lead to interest in angioplasty with stenting. Balloon-mounted coronary stents, however, are limited by the low flexibility of coronary stent system, the high inflation pressures needed to deploy balloon-mounted stents in fragile intracranial vessels, and the risk of shearing the stent from the balloon while navigating to the target lesion.[37] The best studies of intracranial angioplasty and stenting are the *SSYLVIA*[38] and *Wingspan*[37] studies, both of which were prospective, nonrandomized studies using devices specifically designed for the treatment of intracranial stenosis.

A Cochrane systematic review of 79 publications of intracranial angioplasty with or without stenting found the following:[33]

1) Overall perioperative stroke rate of 7.9%
2) Perioperative death rate of 3.4%
3) Perioperative rate of stroke or death of 9.5%

Stenting of Symptomatic Atherosclerotic Lesions in the Vertebral or Intracranial Arteries (SSYLVIA)

The SSYLVIA trial was a multicenter, nonrandomized, prospective feasibility study of the Neurolink® intracranial stent system (a product of the Guidant Corporation, which is now part of Boston Scientific) for treatment of vertebral or intracranial artery stenosis.[38] The Neurolink stent is a balloon-mounted device. A total of 43 patients with symptomatic intracranial stenosis and 18 patients with extracranial vertebral artery stenosis were enrolled.

1) Successful stent placement was achieved in 95% of cases.
2) Thirty-day periprocedural stroke rate: 6.6%. No deaths occurred. Two strokes occurred during the procedure.
3) At 6-month angiographic follow-up, restenosis of >50% occurred in 32.4% of intracranial vessels and 42.9% of extracranial vertebral arteries.
   a) 39% of the recurrent stenoses were symptomatic.
4) Strokes in the distribution of the target lesion occurring after 30 days but by 12 months were seen in 7.3% of patients.

Based upon this study, the FDA granted a humanitarian device exemption to treat patients with significant intracranial and extracranial atherosclerotic disease by balloon angioplasty and stent placement. The manufacturer is not currently marketing the Neurolink device, in favor of the Wingspan® system.

Wingspan Study

The Wingspan™ Stent System with Gateway™ PTA Balloon Catheter (Stryker, Fremont, CA) was designed for the treatment of intracranial atherosclerotic stenosis. Prestent dilation of the lesion is done with the angioplasty balloon, and the stent, a self-expanding nitinol device, is then deployed. The device received an FDA humanitarian device exemption in August 2005 (http://www.fda.gov/cdrh/mda/docs/h050001.html). The Wingspan Study was a prospective, multicenter nonrandomized study of the devices in medically refractory patients with recurrent symptoms attributable to in intracranial stenosis ≥50% in a vessel 2.5–4.5 mm in diameter.[37] A total of 45 patients were enrolled. The mean initial degree of stenosis was 77.9%, and the mean lesion length was 7.2 mm.
1) The stent was successfully deployed in 97.8% of cases.
   a) Procedural adverse events were reported in 27% of patients but none resulted in permanent sequelae.
2) The degree of stenosis was reduced from a baseline of 74.9–31.9% after stenting.
3) The 30-day composite stroke/death rate was 4.5%.
4) Clinical follow-up at 6 months:
   a) Ipsilateral stroke/death rate: 7.0%
   b) Incidence of all strokes: 9.7%
   c) All-cause mortality: 2.3%
5) Angiographic follow-up at 6 months:
   a) Mean degree of stenosis: 28%.
   b) Three patients (6.8%) showed restenosis >50%; all were asymptomatic.
In contrast to SSYLVIA, which reported a rate of restenosis >50% of 32.4% at 6 months, the mean degree of stenosis at 6 months in the Wingspan Study was not significantly different from the degree of stenosis immediately after the procedure.

Other Notable Studies

MORI 1998

Mori et al. reported on angioplasty without stenting in 42 patients with intracranial stenosis >70% stenosis.[32,40] The risk of recurrent stenosis was strongly associated with lesion length and complexity:

	Lesion length and geometry	Rate of restenosis at 3 months
Type A	≤5 mm, concentric or moderately eccentric	0
Type B	5–10 mm, extremely eccentric or totally occluded	30.8%
Type C	>10 mm, >90% angulation, or totally occluded	66.7%

MARKS 2006

Report of 120 patients with intracranial stenosis ≥50% who were treated with angioplasty without stenting.[35] A total of 116 patients were available for a mean follow-up time of 42.3 months.
(a) Degree of stenosis was reduced by angioplasty from a mean of 82.2–36.0%.
(b) Combined 30-day periprocedural stroke and death rate was 5.8%.
(c) Annual postprocedure stroke rate was 3.2% in the territory of treatment and annual overall stroke rate was 4.4%.

SYSTEMATIC REVIEW COMPARING ANGIOPLASTY ALONE TO ANGIOPLASTY AND STENTING

A systematic review of 69 studies of angioplasty alone and 36 studies of angioplasty with stent placement:[41]
1) Technical success
   a) Angioplasty alone: 79.8%
   b) Angioplasty and stenting: 95% (P<0.0001)

2) Pooled incidence of 1-year stroke and/or death
   a) Angioplasty alone: 19.7%
   b) Angioplasty and stenting: 14.2% (P = 0.009)
3) Pooled restenosis rate
   a) Angioplasty alone: 14.2%
   b) Angioplasty and stenting: 11.1% (P = 0.04)

The authors concluded that angioplasty and stenting may be superior to angioplasty alone in this setting.

Position Statement on Intracranial Angioplasty and Stenting for Cerebral Atherosclerosis by the ASITN, SIR, and ASNR[3]

1) For symptomatic patients with >50% intracranial stenosis, who have failed medical therapy, balloon angioplasty with or without stenting should be considered.
2) Patients who have an asymptomatic intracranial arterial stenosis should first be counseled regarding optimizing medical therapy. There is insufficient evidence to make definitive recommendations regarding endovascular therapy in asymptomatic patients with severe intracranial atherosclerosis. They should be counseled regarding the nature and extent of their disease, monitored for new neurological symptoms, and have periodic noninvasive imaging at regular intervals of 6–12 months (MRA or CTA) initially, and then by cerebral angiography if warranted. At a minimum, optimal prophylactic medical therapy should be instituted, which might include antiplatelet and/or statin therapy.
3) Continued evaluation and improvements in both pharmacological and catheter-based therapies are needed to reduce the stroke burden from intracranial atherosclerosis.

Note: *ASITN* American Society of Interventional and Therapeutic Neuroradiology, *SIR* Society of Interventional Radiology, *ASNR* American Society of Neuroradiology

Stenting Versus Aggressive Medical Management for Preventing Recurrent Stroke in Intracranial Stenosis (SAMMPRIS)

Four hundred and fifty one patients with symptomatic 70–99% stenosis of a major intracranial artery were randomized to either aggressive medical management alone (n = 227) or aggressive medical management plus Wingspan angioplasty and stenting (n = 224).[42] Enrollment was stopped prematurely (764 patients were planned) because an interim analysis showed significantly better results for the medical management-only group. Mean follow-up was 11.9 months.

1) One year primary end point rate (stroke or death within 30 days after enrollment or stenting, or stroke in the territory of the qualifying artery beyond 30 days):
   a) 20.0% in the stenting group
   b) 12.2% in the medical management-only group (p = 0.009)
2) 30-day rate of stroke or death:
   a) 14.7% in the stenting group
   b) 5.8% in the medical management-only group (p = 0.002)
3) 30-day rate of symptomatic intracranial haemorrhage:
   a) 4.5% in the stenting group
   b) 0% in the medical management-only group
4) Medical management was identical in both groups and consisted of aspirin 325 mg per day and clopidogrel 75 mg per day for 90 days after enrollment; blood pressure management (target systolic blood pressure <140 mmHg, <130 mmHg in patients with diabetes); hyperlipidemia (target LDL <70 mg/dL); and help with compliance and management of diet, smoking, weight reduction, and exercise with a lifestyle modification program. Medications provided by the study include aspirin, clopidogrel, one drug from each major class of antihypertensive agents, and rosuvastatin.

5) SAMMPRIS controversies
   a) The initial results were a surprise for many people. Like any major study showing unexpected results, there has been a fair bit of controversy over the study findings and their applicability to clinical practice. This debate will likely rage for years. Here are some of the arguments made in the debate about the SAMMPRIS results:
      i) The aggressive medical management of patients in SAMMPRIS does not resemble real-world medical management of patients with intracranial stenosis.
      ii) The adverse event rate in the stenting arm was unacceptably high.
      iii) The results of SAMMPRIS may lend support to the use of angioplasty alone, rather than angioplasty and stenting, for intracranial stenosis.
         (1) Although angioplasty alone may be safer than angioplasty and stenting, a study comparing angioplasty alone to medical management has not yet been published. A systematic review found angioplasty and stenting to be superior to angioplasty alone.[41]
      iv) The results of SAMMPRIS show that the FDA Humanitarian Device Exemption process needs to be reviewed.

Phase III Study of PHAROS™ Vitesse™ Neurovascular Stent System Compared to Best Medical Therapy for the Treatment of Ischaemic Disease (VISSIT)

Industry-sponsored randomized trial of intracranial angioplasty and stenting using the PHAROS™ Vitesse™ (Codman Neurovascular, San Jose, CA) balloon-expandable stent versus medical therapy.[43] Entrance criteria are similar to SAMMPRIS. This study was discontinued in early 2012.

19.2.   Moyamoya Disease and Moyamoya Syndrome

Moyamoya disease (aka spontaneous occlusion of the circle of Willis) is a nonatherosclerotic progressive steno-occlusive arteriopathy that most frequently affects the intracranial ICAs and proximal segments of the MCAs and ACAs. It may rarely also involve the posterior circulation. Spontaneous occlusion of the major intracranial arteries is typically accompanied by the appearance of a tuft of fine collateral vessels at the base of the brain. *Moyamoya* is a Japanese word meaning *puff of smoke*, or *ambiguous*, which are descriptions not only of the tuft of collaterals but also the obscure aetiology of the syndrome, which remains unelucidated.[44] The term moyamoya *disease* is reserved for those cases in which the intracranial vascular changes are primary and truly idiopathic, whereas moyamoya *syndrome* (aka secondary moyamoya, moyamoya phenomenon, syndromic moyamoya, quasi-moyamoya, or moyamoya-like vascular changes) is used with the intracranial vascular changes that occur in association with another condition, such as cranial radiation or neurofibromatosis type 1.[45]

Epidemiology

Ethnicity plays a major role. Japan and South Korea appear to have the highest concentrations of patients with moyamoya disease.
1) Japan:
   a) Approximately 3,900 patients in Japan were treated for moyamoya in 1994.[46]
   b) Prevalence rate of 3.16 and annual incidence of 0.35 per 100,000.
      i) Approximately 100 new cases are identified each year.[47]
   c) Male to female ratio: 1:1.8.

d) Peak ages are 10–14 years and 40s.
   i) Age at onset is <10 years in 47.8% of the patients; some develop the disease at the age of 25–49 years.
   ii) Bony carotid canal hypoplasia has been found in Japanese patients with adult-onset moyamoya disease, suggesting that the pathological process begins early in life in all patients.[48]
2) South Korea:
   a) Female predominance and bimodal age distribution pattern are similar to those seen in Japanese patients. The incidence of adult moyamoya disease in South Korea is 20% higher than that in Japanese patients, and the incidence of familial moyamoya syndrome is only 1.8%.[49]
3) China:
   a) Data on moyamoya in China is very limited. Two reports indicate the following:
   b) More common in males and the average age of onset is higher, compared with Japanese patients.[50,51]
   c) One report has attributed the majority of cases (53%) in China to leptospiral arteritis, and found that 81.4% of patients with moyamoya syndrome have positive leptospiral test results.[50]
4) North America:
   a) The overall incidence of moyamoya syndrome in California and Washington is 0.086 per 100,000.[52]
      i) Male to female ratio: 1:2.15
   b) Incidence per 100,000 is highest among Asian Americans and lowest among Hispanics:
      i) Asian Americans: 0.28
      ii) African Americans 0.13
      iii) Whites: 0.06
      iv) Hispanics: 0.03
   c) Median age of onset is as follows:
      i) Asian Americans: 36
      ii) African Americans: 18
      iii) Whites: 32
      iv) Hispanics: 21
   d) Sickle cell disease likely accounts for the relatively high incidence and low age of onset among African Americans; when patients with sickle cell disease were excluded, the incidence among African Americans was similar to that in whites.
   e) The prevalence of moyamoya disease in Hawaii appears to be higher than in the rest of the USA.[53]
5) Europe:
   a) A survey of European centers lead to an estimate of the incidence of moyamoya to be about 1/10 the incidence in Japan.[54]
   b) A slightly higher incidence in Eastern Europe has been hypothesized to be due to the Mongolian invasion of Europe, which may have spread the genetic predisposition for moyamoya disease.[55]

Pathophysiology

The primary lesion in moyamoya disease is progressive fibrocellular thickening of the intima.[56–58] The intima acquires an onion-like appearance, consisting of fibrocellular materials, but without lipids or calcification as is seen in atherosclerosis.[59] The internal elastic lamina is also abnormal, becoming infolded, tortuous, redundant, and fragmented.[60] The media is thinned, with a diminished number of smooth muscle cells.[58] No inflammatory changes are seen. Intimal thickening has also been found in the superficial temporal arteries of patients with moyamoya.[61] Histological analysis has shown thrombotic lesions in the affected intracranial vessels in 54% of cases.[62]

The secondary lesions in moyamoya syndrome are dilated, tortuous thalamostriate and lenticulostriate arteries at the base of the brain. These vessels do not appear to be normal collateral vessels that would be expected to develop in response to chronic occlusion of major arteries. They exhibit thinned and fragmented internal elastic laminae, medial fibrosis, microaneurysms, and areas of rupture.[56] Stenosis of these vessels, due to fibrous intimal thickening and thrombosis, is seen in 50% of cases.[56]

The aetiology of moyamoya disease is unknown. Several mechanisms have been implicated:
1) Primary defect in smooth muscle cells.
   a) Deoxyribonucleic acid synthesis experiments involving cultured smooth muscle cells from moyamoya patients indicate that the cells are less responsive to their normal mitogens. This suggests that there be a derangement in the vessel wall repair mechanism that leads to long-term proliferation of cells and progressive occlusion of the vessel lumen.[63]
2) Role of angiogenic factors.
   a) Basic fibroblast growth factor (bFGF). Elevated levels of bFGF have been found in the CSF,[64,65] superficial temporal artery,[66] and in the affected ICA.[67] of patients with moyamoya disease. Basic FGF is a potent angiogenic factor. It is not clear whether elevation of bFGF is a primary event in the pathogenesis of moyamoya, or an epiphenomenon in response to chronic ischaemia. Interestingly, elevated CSF bFGF correlates with the degree of angiogenesis seen with indirect revascularization procedures in patients with moyamoya disease.[65,68]
   b) Elevated expression of transforming growth factor beta 1 has been found in cultured smooth muscle cells and in serum from patients with moyamoya disease.[69]
   c) Hepatocyte growth factor, an angiogenic factor, is elevated in CSF and intracranial arteries in patients with moyamoya disease.[70]
3) Alteration in metaloproteinase gene expression.
   a) An association analysis of tissue inhibitor of metalloproteinase 2 in 17q25 showed that a polymorphism in the promoter region was markedly associated with familial moyamoya disease.[71]
4) Excessive prostaglandin synthesis.
   a) Cultured smooth muscle cells from moyamoya patients produce excess amounts of prostaglandin E(2) in response to stimulation with interleukin-1 beta.[72] This may increase vascular permeability and exposure of the vessels to blood constituents, leading to intimal thickening.
5) Epstein-Barr virus (EBV) infection.
   a) Antibody titers of EBV are significantly elevated in patients with moyamoya disease,[73] raising the possibility that EBV infection may be involved.

Diagnosis of Moyamoya Disease

The Ministry of Health and Welfare in Japan has established guidelines for the diagnosis of moyamoya disease.[74] The diagnosis may be made by catheter angiography or MRI and MRA. Cases are defined as either definite or probable, depending on which criteria are satisfied.

Diagnostic Criteria

1) Cerebral angiography should demonstrate the following findings:
   a) Stenosis or occlusion at the terminal portion of the ICA and/or the proximal portion of the ACA and/or MCA.
   b) Abnormal vascular networks in the vicinity of the occlusive or stenotic lesions.
   c) These findings should be present bilaterally.
2) When MRI and MRA clearly demonstrate all of the findings listed later, catheter angiography is not mandatory.
   a) Stenosis or occlusion at the terminal portion of the ICA and at the proximal portion of the ACA and MCA.
   b) An abnormal vascular network in the basal ganglia on MRA. An abnormal vascular network can be diagnosed on MRI when >2 apparent flow voids are seen in one side of the basal ganglia.
   c) (a) and (b) are seen bilaterally.
3) Exclude other causes. Because the aetiology of the disease is unknown, associated cerebrovascular diseases or conditions should be excluded. These include, but are not limited to the following:

a) Arteriosclerosis
b) Autoimmune disease
c) Meningitis
d) Brain neoplasm
e) Down syndrome
f) Neurofibromatosis type 1
g) Head trauma
h) Cranial irradiation
4) Pathological findings that can be helpful in the diagnosis are as follows:
  a) Intimal thickening that causes stenosis or occlusion of the lumen is observed in and around the terminal portion of the internal carotid artery. Lipids deposition is occasionally seen in the proliferating intima.
  b) Arteries of the circle of Willis often show stenosis or occlusion associated with fibrocellular thickening of the intima, waving of the internal elastic lamina, and attenuation of the media.
  c) Numerous small arteries (perforating and anastomotic branches) are observed around the circle of Willis.
  d) Reticular conglomerates of small vessels are often seen in the pia mater.

Diagnosis

1) *Definite case*: Either all criteria in (1) or all criteria in (2) and (3) are fulfilled. In children, however, a case that fulfills (1), (a) and (b) or (2), (a) and (b) on one side and demonstrates narrowing at the terminal portion of the internal carotid artery on the opposite side is also considered to be a definite case.
2) *Probable case*: Either: (1), (a) and (b) or (2), (a) and (b) and (3) are fulfilled (i.e., unilateral involvement).

Evaluation

CT

Significant abnormal findings on CT are present in 92% of cases.[75] These include cortical atrophy, ventricular dilatation, and irregular, multiple or bilateral lucent areas in the cortex, white matter, and central gray matter.

Angiography

Although a diagnosis of moyamoya disease may be made with MRI and MRA alone,[74] the authors of this handbook recommend catheter angiography in most young patients and all adults suspected of having moyamoya disease or moyamoya syndrome. Angiography in children with moyamoya disease is not associated with a higher rate of complications compared with angiography in children without moyamoya.[76] Angiography is the best imaging technique to distinguish high-grade stenosis from occlusion, identify intracranial aneurysms, and assess collateral circulation. Importantly, angiography is critical for planning surgical procedures; for instance, angiography can best demonstrate transdural collateral vessels that should be preserved during revascularization procedures.

1) Angiographic staging of moyamoya disease is summarized in Table 19.1. Stage 4 is the most common stage at presentation. Angiographic stage is usually more advanced in more elderly patients.[77]
2) Stenosis or occlusion of the intracranial ICA and/or the A1 and M1 segments are seen in all cases.
3) Stenosis or occlusion of the PCA is seen in 43% of cases.[78]
4) Involvement of the ECA is usually not seen,[79] although stenosis of branches of the ECA was reported in 20% of cases in one series.[80]
5) Abnormal moyamoya vessels may be seen in several locations.
  a) Basal ganglia – branches of the circle of Willis
  b) Ethmoidal region – branches of the ICA and ophthalmic artery[81]

Table 19.1 Angiographic stages of moyamoya disease

Stage	Angiographic findings
1	Stenosis of the supraclinoid ICA. Usually bilateral. No other abnormalities.
2	Initiation of moyamoya vessels at the base of brain.
3	Intensification of moyamoya vessels. Increased stenosis or occlusion of the ICA, MCA, or ACA.
4	Complete occlusion of the ICA with some reduction in moyamoya vessels. First appearance of collaterals from ECA branches. Most common stage at presentation.
5	Further reduction of moyamoya vessels with increased collateralization from ECA.
6	Complete absence of major intracranial arteries and moyamoya vessels. Uncommon.

From Suzuki and Takaku.,[229] with permission

    c) Cerebral hemispheres (i.e., *vault moyamoya*) – branches of the anterior falx, middle meningeal, occipital, tentorial, and superficial temporal arteries[82]
    d) Posterior choroidal, thalamogeniculate, and other thalamoperforating arteries[83]
6) The extensive development of basal moyamoya is a sign of severe haemodynamic impairment in adult patients with ischaemic moyamoya disease.[84]
7) Moyamoya vessels may recede after surgical revascularization.[85]
8) Intracranial aneurysms are present in about 10% of cases.[86–89] They are attributable to abnormal haemodynamic patterns, or for those that arise from moyamoya vessels, abnormal vessel architecture. Aneurysms are found in three locations:[90]
    a) Circle of Willis, mostly in the posterior circulation: 60% of cases.
    b) Peripheral cerebral arteries, such as the anterior or posterior choroidal arteries: 20%.
    c) Abnormal moyamoya vessels: 20%.
9) Persistent primitive arteries have been observed in both moyamoya disease and moyamoya syndrome at higher frequencies that in the general population.[91]

MRI

1) MRI findings in moyamoya disease:[92–95]
    a) Stenosis or occlusion of the distal ICA or proximal ACA and MCA
    b) Signal voids in the basal ganglia
    c) Marked leptomeningeal enhancement on postcontrast images
    d) Evidence of infarction, atrophy, and ventriculomegaly
    e) Haemorrhage
2) Compared with conventional angiography, the sensitivity and specificity of MRI plus MRA in the diagnosis of moyamoya disease is 92% and 100%, respectively.[92]
    a) Basal cerebral moyamoya vessels were depicted on MRI in 92% of cases and on MRA in 81% of cases[92]
3) In a series of 30 patients with moyamoya disease, all showed clear evidence on MRI of bilateral stenosis or occlusion of the supraclinoid ICA and proximal ACAs and MCAs.[93] Parenchymal lesions were apparent on MRI in 80% of cases. White matter infarctions are the most frequent parenchymal lesions and are seen in 73% of cases.
4) *Ivy sign*: Marked diffuse leptomeningeal enhancement on postcontrast T1-weighted and FLAIR images.[95–97] Considered to represent the fine vascular network over the pial surface.

Cerebral Blood Flow Studies

    CBF imaging techniques for moyamoya patients include PET,[98] xenon CT,[99,100] Xe,[101–103] and SPECT[104,105] Regional CBF in patients with moyamoya is characteristically diminished in the frontal and temporal lobes, and elevated in the posterior circulation territory (cerebellum and occipital lobes), and in central brain structures that are involved with basal moyamoya vessels. The degree of haemodynamic stress in patients with moyamoya disease varies greatly between patients.[106] CBF studies can help predict the risk of stroke[99] and the success of revascularization surgery.[107]

EEG

EEG findings are nonspecific in adults with moyamoya. Although EEG used to be a screening tool for children suspected of having moyamoya disease, it is currently considered to be somewhat obsolete for this purpose.[90] Characteristic EEF findings may be observed in children with moyamoya disease. These include the following:[108]
1) Low-amplitude slow waves, aka hemispheric posterior slowing or centrotemporal slowing.
2) Sleep spindle depression.
3) *Rebuildup phenomenon*: Hyperventilation characteristically causes a buildup of slow waves that resolves within 20–60 s after hyperventilation. In 70% of cases, buildup of slow waves appears after the original buildup had returned to baseline. Rebuildup of slow waves has been localized to the deep cortical sulci in regions of haemodynamic failure.[109] This phenomenon disappears after surgery for moyamoya,[110] and is not observed in adults with moyamoya.[108]

Clinical Features of Moyamoya Disease

The classic description of moyamoya disease separates the *juvenile form* from the *adult form*. This corresponds to the bimodal age distribution – with a higher peak around 5 years of age and a lower peak during the fourth and fifth decades – and the observation that younger patients tend to present with ischaemic symptoms and adult patients often present with haemorrhage. This distinction is appropriate for patients with moyamoya *disease*. Growing evidence suggests that the clinical expression of moyamoya syndrome, particularly in North American and European patients, is fundamentally different, in that ischaemia seems to be the most common presenting symptom, regardless of age.[88–90] The clinical features of moyamoya syndrome are discussed separately below.
1) Juvenile form:
    a) Initial signs and symptoms on admission:[111]
        i)   Motor deficit: 81.5%
        ii) Headache: 27.2%
        iii) Mental retardation: 19.8%
        iv) Speech disturbance: 17.3%
        v)   Sensory disturbance: 16.0%
        vi) Seizure: 6.2%
        vii) Involuntary movement: 6.2%
    b) Neurological symptoms are often precipitated by hyperventilating during activities such as crying or blowing.[44]
    c) Intracranial haemorrhage and aneurysms are rare.[44]
    d) Mental retardation has been described in >50% of cases, and the onset of ischaemic symptoms in patients <5-years old is associated with progressive mental retardation.[112]
    e) Symptoms in children often stabilize over time, as collateral circulation develops and an age-dependent decrease in CBF demand by the brain occurs.[44]
2) Adult form:
    a) Intracranial haemorrhage is the presenting event in >60% of cases.[88]
        i)   Bleeding may arise from the following:[113]
            (1) Abnormal vascular networks
            (2) Intracranial aneurysms
        ii) About 1/3 of patients presenting with haemorrhage will have another haemorrhage within days to years of the initial event.[88]
        iii) Intraventricular haemorrhage is the most common form of haemorrhage, present in 69% of patients presenting with haemorrhage.[114]
        iv) Mortality in the acute phase is 2.4% with infarction and 16.4% with haemorrhage.[90]

v) Risk of rehaemorrhage: In a series of 42 patients with haemorrhagic moyamoya disease followed for a mean of 80.6 months, the average annual rebleeding rate was 7.09% per person.[114] After rebleeding, the rate of good recovery fell from 45.5% to 21.4% and the mortality rate rose from 6.8% to 28.6%.

b) Long-term clinical outcome:
   i) Overall, some 75% of the patients in Japan with moyamoya disease have normal activities of daily life or working ability, even prior to treatment.[46]

3) *Unilateral disease* (aka *probable* moyamoya disease): There is some evidence that unilateral moyamoya disease is distinct from typical bilateral moyamoya disease.
   a) Progression to bilateral disease:
      i) In an analysis of 180 cases of unilateral disease in Japan, only 7% developed into the definite type in an average follow-up period of 6.6 years.[49]
      ii) In a South Korean study, 2 of 7 unilateral cases (28.5%) progressed to bilateral involvement in a mean follow-up period of 5.4 years.[115]
      iii) In a North American study of 18 patients with unilateral disease (defined as no, equivocal, or mild involvement of the contralateral side), progression to bilateral disease was seen in seven patients (38.9%) at a mean follow-up of 12.7 months.[116]
         (1) The presence of mild or equivocal contralateral disease was an important predictor of progression; although 75% of patients with mild or equivocal contralateral findings progressed, only 10% of patients with no initial contralateral findings progressed.
   b) Unilateral disease appears to be more common among adults than among children.[117]
   c) Familial occurrence is less common in patients with unilateral disease.[118,119]
   d) CSF levels of bFGF are lower in patients with unilateral disease compared with patients with definite moyamoya disease.[118]

4) *Asymptomatic moyamoya disease*: A prospective study followed 40 patients with asymptomatic moyamoya disease at 12 centers in Japan for a mean period of 43.7 months.[77] Six of these patients underwent surgical revascularization.
   a) On initial evaluation, 20% of patients had radiographic evidence of infarction and 40% exhibited disturbed cerebral haemodynamics.
   b) The annual risk for any stroke was 3.2%. Of 34 patients treated without surgery, 7 had a neurologic event during the follow-up period, 3 had a TIA, 1 had an ischaemic stroke, and 3 had haemorrhage.
   c) No cerebrovascular event occurred in the six patients who underwent surgical revascularization.

Familial Moyamoya Disease

1) Definition of familial moyamoya disease: when at least one first-degree relative is affected.[120]
   a) Compared to the general population, first- or second-degree relatives of patients with moyamoya disease have a 30- to 40-fold risk of having the disease.[121]
2) Approximately 10% of moyamoya disease cases are familial.[46,122–124]
   a) A family history of moyamoya is present in about 1.8% of Korean patients[49]
3) Mean age of onset (11.8 years) is significantly lower compared with that in sporadic moyamoya disease (30 years).[120]
4) Greater female preponderance compared with sporadic moyamoya disease
   a) Male:female ratio is (1:5)[120] or 1:3.3.[121]
5) Mode of inheritance is autosomal dominant with incomplete penetrance.[125]
6) Familial moyamoya has been linked to chromosomes 3p24.2–p26, 6q25, 8q23, 12p12, and 17a25.[126–129]
7) Familial moyamoya disease is associated with
   a) Systemic lupus erythematosus.[130]
   b) Basilar apex aneurysms.[131]
8) Screening with MRA has been recommended for family members of patients with moyamoya disease.[132]

Conditions Associated with Moyamoya Syndrome

A large number of systemic conditions and other factors have been associated with moyamoya. The presence of one of these factors in a patient with moyamoya-type radiographic findings may indicate that the patient has moyamoya *syndrome*, rather than the *disease*, particularly if the patient is not Asian. Caution must be used in interpreting these associations, because many of them are based only on case reports. Among non-Asian patients with moyamoya syndrome, Down syndrome, sickle cell disease, and a history of cranial irradiation are the most established associated factors.

1) Autoimmune disorders
    a) Graves disease[133,134]
    b) Sjögren syndrome[135,136]
    c) Primary antiphospholipid syndrome[137,138]
    d) Systemic lupus erythematosus[100,130,136]
2) Infections
    a) Pneumococcal meningitis[139]
    b) Tuberculosis[140,141]
    c) Leptospirosis[50]
    d) Congenital human immunodeficiency virus infection[142]
3) Hematological disorders
    a) Sickle cell disease[50,143]
    b) Aplastic anemia[144]
    c) Fanconi anemia[145,146]
    d) Hereditary spherocytosis[147]
    e) Thalassemia[148]
    f) Haemophilia A[149]
    g) Thrombocytopenic purpura[150]
    h) Haemolytic anemia[151]
    i) Essential thrombocytopenia[152]
    j) Acute lymphoblastic anemia[153]
    k) Protein C or S deficiency[154–157]
    l) Hageman factor (Factor XII) deficiency[158]
4) Metabolic disorders
    a) Hyperlipoproteinemia type 2A[159]
    b) Glycogen storage disease type 1[160]
    c) Pseudoxanthoma elasticum[161]
    d) Hyperthyroidism[162]
    e) Impaired NADH-CoQ reductase activity
    f) Hyperhomocysteinemia[163]
5) Genetic syndromes
    a) Down syndrome[52,164]
    b) Neurofibromatosis type I[52,165]
    c) Apert syndrome[166]
    d) Turner syndrome[167]
    e) Williams syndrome[168]
    f) Tuberous sclerosis[169]
    g) Osteogenesis imperfecta[170]
    h) Noonan syndrome[171,172]
    i) Costello syndrome[173]
    j) Alagille syndrome[174,175]
    k) Smith-Magenis syndrome[176]
    l) Trisomy 12p syndrome[177]
6) Connective tissue or collagen vascular syndromes
    a) Fibromuscular dysplasia[178]
    b) Polycystic kidney disease[179]
    c) Marfan syndrome[180]
    d) CREST syndrome[181]
7) Neoplasms
    a) Craniopharyngioma[182]
    b) Pituitary adenoma[183]
    c) Brainstem glioma[184]
    d) Wilm's tumor[185]
8) Medications and recreational drugs
    a) Oral contraceptives[186]
    b) Cocaine[187,188]

9) Radiation
    a) Cranial irradiation[189–191]
10) Other disorders and factors
    a) Atherosclerosis[192]
    b) Behcet's disease[193]
    c) Morning glory syndrome[194]
    d) Brain AVM[195,196] (see Chap. 14)
    e) Cerebral arterial dolichoectasia[197]
    f) Persistent primitive arteries[91,198]
    g) Renovascular hypertension[199,200]
    h) Phakomatosis pigmentovascularis type IIIb[201]
    i) Pulmonary sarcoidosis[202]
    j) Heterotopic ossification[203]
    k) Congenital heart disease[204]
    l) Head injury[205]
    m) Hirschsprung disease[206]
    n) Peripheral vascular occlusive disease[207]

Clinical Features of Moyamoya Disease and Syndrome in North American Patients

The manifestations of moyamoya disease appear to be fundamentally different in North American (and European) patients compared with Japanese and Korean patients.[89,90] Cerebral ischaemia and not haemorrhage appears to be the most common presentation in adults in North America and Europe.[88,89] In addition, moyamoya syndrome seems to be more common than the disease in North America,[208] whereas the reverse is true in Japan.[90] Conditions associated with moyamoya syndrome, therefore, play a greater role in the clinical features of affected American and European patients. Two publications from centers in the USA have shed light on these issues:

1) *Chiu 1998*: Series of 35 patients from Houston, TX with moyamoya disease. Mean age was 32 years (range: 6–59). Thirty-two patients had definite moyamoya disease and three had probable disease. Only two patients were of Asian descent. The male to female ratio was 1:2.5. The mean follow-up period was 40 months after diagnosis.
    a) Ischaemic stroke or TIA was the initial symptom in both adults and children, occurring on presentation in 75% of patients overall. Of the adult patients, 88% presented with ischaemic symptoms and 11.5% presented with haemorrhage. The crude stroke recurrence rate was 10.3% per year.
        i) The stroke recurrence risk was highest in the first year after diagnosis (18%) and decreased to 5% per year thereafter.
    b) IVH was the most common form of haemorrhage, occurring in 83% of patients presenting with intracranial haemorrhage.
    c) Twenty patients underwent surgical revascularization, including indirect and direct procedures.
    d) The 5-year risk of ipsilateral stroke after indirect revascularization was 15%, compared with 20% for medical treatment and 22% overall for surgery.
2) *Hallemeier et al.*:[209] Series of 34 adults with definite or probable moyamoya disease. Patients included both those with bilateral ($n = 22$) and unilateral ($n = 12$) disease. Only two patients were of Asian descent. Patients were excluded from this study if they had another disease that may have been responsible for the vasculopathy. Median age was 42 (range 20–79). The median follow-up period was 5.1 years.
    a) Ischaemia was the initial symptom in 24 (70.6%) of patients. Seven (20.6%) presented with haemorrhage and three were asymptomatic.
        i) In the medically treated patients, the 5-year risk of recurrent ipsilateral stroke was 65% after the initial symptom.
            (1) Patients with bilateral involvement presenting with ischaemic symptoms were at the highest risk of subsequent stroke: 5-year risk of stroke with medical management was 82%.
            (2) Of the seven patients presenting with haemorrhage, none had a subsequent haemorrhage and only one experienced an ischaemic stroke.
    b) None of the asymptomatic patients had a stroke.

3) Fourteen patients underwent surgical revascularization procedures.
   a) In patients treated with surgery, the 5-year risk of perioperative or subsequent ipsilateral stroke or death was 17%.

Management

Medical Management

No medical regimen has been proven to be effective in moyamoya patients. Long-term anticoagulation is not recommended because of the risk of haemorrhagic stroke.[89] Antiplatelet therapy may be useful, given the relatively high frequency of thrombosis noted in pathology reports.[56,62] The authors of this handbook favor aspirin, 325-mg PO QD for most patients with moyamoya syndrome or disease and ischaemic symptoms.

Surgical Management

An array of surgical revascularization techniques has been introduced for patients with moyamoya disease. The first procedure, cervical sympathectomy, which was done to decrease vasomotor tone, was found to be ineffective in the long term.[210] Direct bypass procedures consist of direct anastomoses between the extracranial and intracranial circulations (EC-IC bypass) and can be subdivided into high-flow (e.g., saphenous vein graft anastomosis) or low-flow (e.g., STA-MCA bypass) techniques. Indirect procedures were developed because of the difficulty in doing direct bypass procedures in children, and involve the placement of the STA or vascular tissue, such as the temporalis muscle, dura, or omentum directly on the surface of the brain to promote collateral formation.

INDICATIONS FOR SURGICAL REVASCULARIZATION
No randomized trial of bypass surgery for moyamoya has been completed yet. The Ministry of Health and Welfare in Japan has published guidelines for the use of bypass surgery for patients with moyamoya disease.[74]
1) Ischaemic disease: Bypass surgery is indicated for patients with the following symptoms:
   a) Repeated clinical symptoms due to apparent cerebral ischaemia
   b) Decreased regional cerebral blood flow, vascular response and perfusion reserve, based on the findings of a cerebral circulation and metabolism study
2) Haemorrhagic disease: The benefits of bypass surgery for the prevention of rebleeding are unclear.

SURGICAL TECHNIQUES
1) Direct revascularization
   a) Low-flow bypass
   b) STA-MCA bypass
      i) The first STA-MCA bypass for moyamoya disease was done by Yasargil in 1972.[211]
   c) Occipital artery bypass
      i) For patients with a small STA, occipital artery (OA)-MCA bypass[212] or OA-PCA anastomoses[213] are alternatives.
   d) High-flow bypass
      i) Vein graft bypass[214]
2) Indirect revascularization: An exhaustive listing of published indirect procedures are available in Matsushima.[44] The most commonly used procedures include the following:[215]
   a) Encephalo-myo-synangiosis (EMS): A temporalis muscle flap is applied directly to the surface of the brain.
   b) Encephalo-duro-arterio-synangiosis (EDAS): The STA is sutured to the open dura.
   c) Encephalo-duro-arterio-myo-synangiosis (EDAMS): Temporalis muscle and the STA are applied to the surface of the brain.
3) Combined direct and indirect revascularization:
   a) STA-MCA with EMS
   b) STA-MCA with EDAMS

4) Selection of surgical technique:
    a) The younger the patient, the more likely indirect revascularization will be successful.[216] With advancing age, the ability to develop collaterals eclines, presumably because of declining angiogenic or arteriogenic factor availability or responsiveness.[65,68]
        i) In a report of indirect procedures done in adults with moyamoya disease, patients aged 20–29 had good results – similar to paediatric patients – but patients aged >30 had moderate or poor indirect revascularization results.[216] Patients of age >40 had the worst angiographic results from indirect procedures, leading the authors to conclude that direct procedures (or combined procedures) should be the main treatment option for patients of age >40.
    b) Synangiosis procedures work best when there is some degree of haemodynamic stress, as demonstrated by CBF imaging (e.g., PET, or xenon CT or SPECT with acetazolamide challenge).[107]
    c) Elevated CSF bFGF levels may predict the extent of angiogenesis to be expected with indirect revascularization.[65]
    d) Patients with spontaneous transdural collateral vessels (*vault collaterals*) should not be considered for synangiosis.[89]
5) Surgical results
    a) Paediatric moyamoya disease: A review of 57 studies of revascularization surgery for paediatric moyamoya found the following:[215]
        i) Indirect procedures are the most commonly reported (73% of cases) and combined direct and indirect was next (23%).
        ii) In 87% of cases the patients were reported to derive symptomatic benefit.
        iii) Overall rates of perioperative stroke and reversible deficit were 4.4% and 6.1%, respectively.
    b) Adult ischaemic moyamoya: Several series have reported clinical improvement in most adults undergoing revascularization procedures.[89,104,209,216,217]
        i) Two North American retrospective series have reported a benefit with revascularization:
            (1) Chiu et al.:[89] The 5-year risk of ipsilateral stroke after indirect revascularization was 15%, compared with 20% for medical treatment.
            (2) Hallemeier et al.:[209] The 5-year risk of perioperative or subsequent ipsilateral stroke or death for surgical patients was 17%, compared with 65% for patients not having surgery.
    c) *Cheiro-oral syndrome*
        i) Cheiro-oral syndrome consists of sensory disturbances around the corner of the mouth and the hand without significant motor impairment.[218] Transient cheiro-oral syndrome occurs in 22.9% of patients undergoing bypass surgery for moyamoya disease.[219] This may occur because of a transient reduction in flow through lenticulostriate vessels after surgery.
6) Haemorrhagic moyamoya disease. The value of revascularization in preventing rehaemorrahge in patients with haemorrhagic moyamoya disease is not clear. Several reports have not found a benefit.[114,217,220]
    a) Revascularization has been reported to decrease haemodynamic stress and lead to the obliteration of peripheral intracranial aneurysms.[221]

Intracranial Angioplasty

Several cases of intracranial angioplasty with or without stenting for ischaemic moyamoya disease have been reported.[45,222,223] However, in a report of five patients undergoing endovascular treatment of moyamoya disease, all five had recurrent symptoms after initial treatment.[224] The authors concluded that angioplasty and stenting does not appear to be a durable treatment for moyamoya disease.

Pregnancy and Moyamoya

A review of 30 reported cases of patients with moyamoya disease and pregnancy found that good outcomes were achieved for both mother and child in all but one case.[225] The one poor outcome occurred in a woman with haemorrhagic moyamoya disease.

The authors concluded that pregnancy can be managed successfully in patients with moyamoya disease. Furthermore, they surmised that the presence of moyamoya disease should not determine the method of delivery, as successful deliveries have been obtained with both vaginal delivery and cesarean section.

"Moyamoya-Like Syndrome"

There is a congenital disorder of cerebral vessels that has little to do with moyamoya, but has been called "moyamoya-like syndrome" in several papers.[226,227] The condition is characterized by markedly dysplastic, dolichoectatic petrous internal carotid arteries, peculiarly straight intracranial vessels with abnormal branching patterns, a history of patent ductus arteriosus treated soon after birth, and dilated pupils from iris hypoplasia. There can be stenosis of the middle cerebral arteries.[226] It is a fascinating anomaly with strikingly similar clinical and angiographic findings in all the reports, although the aetiology is unknown.

References

1. Wityk RJ, Lehman D, Klag M, Coresh J, Ahn H, Litt B. Race and sex differences in the distribution of cerebral atherosclerosis. Stroke. 1996;27:1974–80.
2. Sacco RL, Roberts JK, Boden-Albala B, et al. Race-ethnicity and determinants of carotid atherosclerosis in a multiethnic population. The Northern Manhattan Stroke Study. Stroke. 1997;28:929–35.
3. Intracranial angioplasty and stenting for cerebral atherosclerosis: a position statement of the American Society of Interventional and Therapeutic Neuroradiology, Society of Interventional Radiology, and the American Society of Neuroradiology. AJNR Am J Neuroradiol. 2005; 26:2323–7.
4. Chimowitz MI, Lynn MJ, Howlett-Smith H, et al. Comparison of warfarin and aspirin for symptomatic intracranial arterial stenosis. N Engl J Med. 2005;352:1305–16.
5. Caplan LR, Gorelick PB, Hier DB. Race, sex and occlusive cerebrovascular disease: a review. Stroke. 1986;17:648–55.
6. Gorelick PB, Caplan LR, Hier DB, et al. Racial differences in the distribution of posterior circulation occlusive disease. Stroke. 1985;16:785–90.
7. Bogousslavsky J, Barnett HJ, Fox AJ, Hachinski VC, Taylor W. Atherosclerotic disease of the middle cerebral artery. Stroke. 1986;17:1112–20.
8. Wong KS, Huang YN, Gao S, Lam WW, Chan YL, Kay R. Intracranial stenosis in Chinese patients with acute stroke. Neurology. 1998;50:812–3.
9. Hao Q, Wong LK, Lin WH, Leung TW, Kaps M, Rosengarten B. Ethnic influences on neurovascular coupling: a pilot study in whites and asians. Stroke. 2010;41:383–4.
10. Kremer C, Schaettin T, Georgiadis D, Baumgartner RW. Prognosis of asymptomatic stenosis of the middle cerebral artery. J Neurol Neurosurg Psychiatry. 2004;75:1300–3.
11. Akins PT, Pilgram TK, Cross 3rd DT, Moran CJ. Natural history of stenosis from intracranial atherosclerosis by serial angiography. Stroke. 1998;29:433–8.
12. Wolff V, Lauer V, Rouyer O, et al. Cannabis use, ischemic stroke, and multifocal intracranial vasoconstriction: a prospective study in 48 consecutive young patients. Stroke. 2011;42:1778–80.
13. Wilson PW. Estimating cardiovascular disease risk and the metabolic syndrome: a Framingham view. Endocrinol Metab Clin North Am. 2004;33:467–81, v.
14. Ford ES, Giles WH, Dietz WH. Prevalence of the metabolic syndrome among US adults: findings from the third National Health and Nutrition Examination Survey. JAMA. 2002;287:356–9.
15. Naritomi H, Sawada T, Kuriyama Y, Kinugawa H, Kaneko T, Takamiya M. Effect of chronic middle cerebral artery stenosis on the local cerebral hemodynamics. Stroke. 1985;16:214–9.
16. Derdeyn CP, Grubb Jr RL, Powers WJ. Cerebral hemodynamic impairment: methods of measurement and association with stroke risk. Neurology. 1999;53:251.
17. Constantinides P. Pathogenesis of cerebral artery thrombosis in man. Arch Pathol. 1967;83:422–8.
18. Craig DR, Meguro K, Watridge C, Robertson JT, Barnett HJ, Fox AJ. Intracranial internal carotid artery stenosis. Stroke. 1982;13:825–8.
19. Caplan LR. Intracranial branch atheromatous disease: a neglected, understudied, and underused concept. Neurology. 1989;39:1246–50.
20. Awad I, Furlan AJ, Little JR. Changes in intracranial stenotic lesions after extracranial-intracranial bypass surgery. J Neurosurg. 1984;60:771–6.
21. Arenillas JF, Molina CA, Montaner J, Abilleira S, Gonzalez-Sanchez MA, Alvarez-Sabin J. Progression and clinical recurrence of symptomatic middle cerebral artery stenosis: a long-term follow-up transcranial Doppler ultrasound study. Stroke. 2001;32:2898–904.
22. Failure of extracranial-intracranial arterial bypass to reduce the risk of ischemic stroke. Results of an international randomized trial. The EC/IC Bypass Study Group. N Engl J Med. 1985; 313:1191–200.
23. Gao S, Wong KS, Hansberg T, Lam WW, Droste DW, Ringelstein EB. Microembolic signal predicts recurrent cerebral ischemic events in acute stroke patients with middle cerebral artery stenosis. Stroke. 2004;35:2832–6.
24. Mazighi M, Tanasescu R, Ducrocq X, et al. Prospective study of symptomatic atherothrombotic intracranial stenoses: the GESICA study. Neurology. 2006;66:1187–91.
25. Komotar RJ, Wilson DA, Mocco J, et al. Natural history of intracranial atherosclerosis: a critical review. Neurosurgery. 2006;58:595–601; discussion 595–601.
26. Chimowitz MI, Kokkinos J, Strong J, et al. The warfarin-aspirin symptomatic intracranial disease study. Neurology. 1995;45: 1488–93.
27. Kasner SE, Lynn MJ, Chimowitz MI, et al. Warfarin vs aspirin for symptomatic intracranial stenosis: subgroup analyses from WASID. Neurology. 2006;67:1275–8.
28. Kasner SE, Chimowitz MI, Lynn MJ, et al. Predictors of ischemic stroke in the territory of a symptomatic intracranial arterial stenosis. Circulation. 2006;113:555–63.
29. Diener HC, Cunha L, Forbes C, Sivenius J, Smets P, Lowenthal A. European Stroke Prevention Study. 2. Dipyridamole and acetylsalicylic acid in the secondary prevention of stroke. J Neurol Sci. 1996;143:1–13.
30. Amarenco P, Bogousslavsky J, Callahan 3rd A, et al. High-dose atorvastatin after stroke or transient ischemic attack. N Engl J Med. 2006;355:549–59.
31. Mori T, Mori K, Fukuoka M, Arisawa M, Honda S. Percutaneous transluminal cerebral angioplasty: serial angiographic follow-up after successful dilatation. Neuroradiology. 1997;39:111–6.
32. Mori T, Fukuoka M, Kazita K, Mori K. Follow-up study after intracranial percutaneous transluminal cerebral balloon angioplasty. AJNR Am J Neuroradiol. 1998;19:1525–33.
33. Gress DR, Smith WS, Dowd CF, Van Halbach V, Finley RJ, Higashida RT. Angioplasty for intracranial symptomatic vertebrobasilar ischemia. Neurosurgery. 2002;51:23–7; discussion 7–9.
34. Wojak JC, Dunlap DC, Hargrave KR, DeAlvare LA, Culbertson HS, Connors 3rd JJ. Intracranial angioplasty and stenting: long-term results from a single center. AJNR Am J Neuroradiol. 2006;27:1882–92.
35. Marks MP, Wojak JC, Al-Ali F, et al. Angioplasty for symptomatic intracranial stenosis: clinical outcome. Stroke. 2006;37:1016–20.
36. Yu W, Smith WS, Singh V, et al. Long-term outcome of endovascular stenting for symptomatic basilar artery stenosis. Neurology. 2005;64:1055–7.
37. Bose A, Hartmann M, Henkes H, et al. A novel, self-expanding, nitinol stent in medically refractory intracranial atherosclerotic stenoses: the Wingspan trial. Stroke. 2007;38:1531–7.
38. The SSI. Stenting of symptomatic atherosclerotic lesions in the vertebral or intracranial arteries (SSYLVIA): study results. Stroke. 2004;35:1388–92.
39. Cruz-Flores S, Diamond A. Angioplasty for intracranial artery stenosis. Cochrane Database Syst Rev. 2006; 3:CD004133.
40. Mori T, Kazita K, Mori K. Cerebral angioplasty and stenting for intracranial vertebral atherosclerotic stenosis. AJNR Am J Neuroradiol. 1999;20:787–9.
41. Siddiq F, Memon MZ, Vazquez G, Safdar A, Qureshi AI. Comparison between primary angioplasty and stent placement for symptomatic intracranial atherosclerotic disease: meta-analysis of case series. Neurosurgery. 2009;65:1024–34.
42. Chimowitz MI, Lynn MJ, Derdeyn CP, et al. Stenting versus aggressive medical therapy for intracranial arterial stenosis. N Engl J Med. 2011;365:993–1003.
43. U.S. National Institutes of Health. VISSIT intracranial stent study for ischemic therapy. ClinicalTrials.gov. 2012 http://clinicaltrials.gov/ct2/show/NCT00816166. Accessed Feb 10, 2012.
44. Matsushima Y. Moyamoya disease. In: Albright L, Pollack I, Adelson D, editors. Principles and practice of pediatric neurosurgery. New York: Thieme Medical Publishers, Inc.; 1999. p. 1053–69.

45. Rodriguez GJ, Kirmani JF, Ezzeddine MA, Qureshi AI. Primary percutaneous transluminal angioplasty for early moyamoya disease. J Neuroimaging. 2007;17:48–53.

46. Wakai K, Tamakoshi A, Ikezaki K, et al. Epidemiological features of moyamoya disease in Japan: findings from a nationwide survey. Clin Neurol Neurosurg. 1997;99 Suppl 2:S1–5.

47. Fukui M. Current state of study on moyamoya disease in Japan. Surg Neurol. 1997;47:138–43.

48. Watanabe A, Omata T, Koizumi H, Nakano S, Takeuchi N, Kinouchi H. Bony carotid canal hypoplasia in patients with moyamoya disease. J Neurosurg Pediatr. 2010;5:591–4.

49. Ikezaki K, Han DH, Dmsci DH, Kawano T, Kinukawa N, Fukui M. A clinical comparison of definite moyamoya disease between South Korea and Japan. Stroke. 1997;28:2513–7.

50. Cheng MK. A review of cerebrovascular surgery in the People's Republic of China. Stroke. 1982;13:249–55.

51. Matsushima Y, Qian L, Aoyagi M. Comparison of moyamoya disease in Japan and moyamoya disease (or syndrome) in the People's Republic of China. Clin Neurol Neurosurg. 1997;99 Suppl 2:S19–22.

52. Uchino K, Johnston SC, Becker KJ, Tirschwell DL. Moyamoya disease in Washington State and California. Neurology. 2005;65:956–8.

53. Graham JF, Matoba A. A survey of moyamoya disease in Hawaii. Clin Neurol Neurosurg. 1997;99:S31–5.

54. Yonekawa Y, Ogata N, Kaku Y, Taub E, Imhof H-G. Moyamoya disease in Europe, past and present status. Clin Neurol Neurosurg. 1997;99:S58–60.

55. Nyary I. Moyamoya disease: the Hungarian experience. In: International symposium on moyamoya disease. Fukuoa, 1996.

56. Yamashita M, Oka K, Tanaka K. Histopathology of the brain vascular network in moyamoya disease. Stroke. 1983;14:50–8.

57. Hosoda Y, Ikeda E, Hirose S. Histopathological studies on spontaneous occlusion of the circle of Willis (cerebrovascular moyamoya disease). Clin Neurol Neurosurg. 1997;99 Suppl 2:S203–8.

58. Takagi Y, Kikuta K, Nozaki K, Hashimoto N. Histological features of middle cerebral arteries from patients treated for Moyamoya disease. Neurol Med Chir (Tokyo). 2007;47:1–4.

59. Takekawa Y, Umezawa T, Ueno Y, Sawada T, Kobayashi M. Pathological and immunohistochemical findings of an autopsy case of adult moyamoya disease. Neuropathology. 2004;24:236–42.

60. Li B, Wang ZC, Sun YL, Hu Y. Ultrastructural study of cerebral arteries in Moyamoya disease. Chin Med J (Engl). 1992;105:923–8.

61. Aoyagi M, Fukai N, Yamamoto M, Nakagawa K, Matsushima Y, Yamamoto K. Early development of intimal thickening in superficial temporal arteries in patients with moyamoya disease. Stroke. 1996;27:1750–4.

62. Ikeda E, Hosoda Y. Distribution of thrombotic lesions in the cerebral arteries in spontaneous occlusion of the circle of Willis: cerebrovascular moyamoya disease. Clin Neuropathol. 1993;12:44–8.

63. Aoyagi M, Fukai N, Sakamoto H, et al. Altered cellular responses to serum mitogens, including platelet-derived growth factor, in cultured smooth muscle cells derived from arteries of patients with moyamoya disease. J Cell Physiol. 1991;147:191–8.

64. Takahashi A, Sawamura Y, Houkin K, Kamiyama H, Abe H. The cerebrospinal fluid in patients with moyamoya disease (spontaneous occlusion of the circle of Willis) contains high level of basic fibroblast growth factor. Neurosci Lett. 1993;160:214–6.

65. Malek AM, Connors S, Robertson RL, Folkman J, Scott RM. Elevation of cerebrospinal fluid levels of basic fibroblast growth factor in moyamoya and central nervous system disorders. Pediatr Neurosurg. 1997;27:182–9.

66. Hoshimaru M, Takahashi JA, Kikuchi H, Nagata I, Hatanaka M. Possible roles of basic fibroblast growth factor in the pathogenesis of moyamoya disease: an immunohistochemical study. J Neurosurg. 1991;75:267–70.

67. Hosoda Y, Hirose S, Kameyama K. Histopathological and immunohistochemical study of growth factor in spontaneous occlusion of the circle of Willis. In: Fukui M, editor. Annual report of the research committee on spontaneous occlusion of the circle of Willis (Moyamoya disease) 1993. Japan: Ministry of Health and Welfare; 1994. p. 25–8.

68. Yoshimoto T, Houkin K, Takahashi A, Abe H. Angiogenic factors in moyamoya disease. Stroke. 1996;27:2160–5.

69. Hojo M, Hoshimaru M, Miyamoto S, et al. Role of transforming growth factor-beta1 in the pathogenesis of moyamoya disease. J Neurosurg. 1998;89:623–9.

70. Nanba R, Kuroda S, Ishikawa T, Houkin K, Iwasaki Y. Increased expression of hepatocyte growth factor in cerebrospinal fluid and intracranial artery in moyamoya disease. Stroke. 2004;35:2837–42.

71. Kang HS, Kim SK, Cho BK, Kim YY, Hwang YS, Wang KC. Single nucleotide polymorphisms of tissue inhibitor of metalloproteinase genes in familial moyamoya disease. Neurosurgery. 2006;58:1074–80; discussion −80.

72. Yamamoto M, Aoyagi M, Fukai N, Matsushima Y, Yamamoto K. Increase in prostaglandin E(2) production by interleukin-1beta in arterial smooth muscle cells derived from patients with moyamoya disease. Circ Res. 1999;85:912–8.

73. Tanigawara T, Yamada H, Sakai N, Andoh T, Deguchi K, Iwamura M. Studies on cytomegalovirus and Epstein-Barr virus infection in moyamoya disease. Clin Neurol Neurosurg. 1997;99 Suppl 2:S225–8.

74. Fukui M. Guidelines for the diagnosis and treatment of spontaneous occlusion of the circle of Willis ('moyamoya' disease). Research Committee on Spontaneous Occlusion of the Circle of Willis (Moyamoya Disease) of the Ministry of Health and Welfare, Japan. Clin Neurol Neurosurg. 1997;99 Suppl 2:S238–40.

75. Handa J, Nakano Y, Okuno T, Komuro H, Hojyo H, Handa H. Computerized tomography in Moyamoya syndrome. Surg Neurol. 1977;7:315–9.

76. Robertson RL, Chavali RV, Robson CD, et al. Neurologic complications of cerebral angiography in childhood moyamoya syndrome. Pediatr Radiol. 1998;28:824–9.

77. Kuroda S, Hashimoto N, Yoshimoto T, Iwasaki Y. Radiological findings, clinical course, and outcome in asymptomatic moyamoya disease: results of multicenter survey in Japan. Stroke. 2007;38:1430–5.

78. Yamada I, Himeno Y, Suzuki S, Matsushima Y. Posterior circulation in moyamoya disease: angiographic study. Radiology. 1995;197:239–46.

79. Komiyama M, Nishikawa M, Yasui T, Kitano S, Sakamoto H, Fu Y. Steno-occlusive changes in the external carotid system in moyamoya disease. Acta Neurochir (Wien). 2000;142:421–4.

80. Hoshimaru M, Kikuchi H. Involvement of the external carotid arteries in moyamoya disease: neuroradiological evaluation of 66 patients. Neurosurgery. 1992;31:398–400.

81. Suzuki J, Kodama N. Cerebrovascular "Moyamoya" disease. 2. Collateral routes to forebrain via ethmoid sinus and superior nasal meatus. Angiology. 1971;22:223–36.

82. Kodama N, Fujiwara S, Horie Y, Kayama T, Suzuki J. Transdural anastomosis in moyamoya disease – vault moyamoy (author's transl). No Shinkei Geka. 1980;8:729–37.

83. Miyamoto S, Kikuchi H, Karasawa J, Nagata I, Ikota T, Takeuchi S. Study of the posterior circulation in moyamoya disease. Clinical and neuroradiological evaluation. J Neurosurg. 1984;61:1032–7.

84. Piao R, Oku N, Kitagawa K, et al. Cerebral hemodynamics and metabolism in adult moyamoya disease: comparison of angiographic collateral circulation. Ann Nucl Med. 2004;18:115–21.

85. Wang MY, Steinberg GK. Rapid and near-complete resolution of moyamoya vessels in a patient with moyamoya disease treated with superficial temporal artery-middle cerebral artery bypass. Pediatr Neurosurg. 1996;24:145–50.

86. Yabumoto M, Funahashi K, Fujii T, Hayashi S, Komai N. Moyamoya disease associated with intracranial aneurysms. Surg Neurol. 1983;20:20–4.

87. Borota L, Marinkovic S, Bajic R, Kovacevic M. Intracranial aneurysms associated with moyamoya disease. Neurol Med Chir (Tokyo). 1996;36:860–4.

88. Yonekawa Y, Kahn N. Moyamoya disease. Adv Neurol. 2003;92:113–8.

89. Chiu D, Shedden P, Bratina P, Grotta JC. Clinical features of moyamoya disease in the United States. Stroke. 1998;29:1347–51.

90. Yonekawa Y, Taub E. Moyamoya disease: status. Neurologist. 1998;1999:13–23.

91. Komiyama M, Nakajima H, Nishikawa M, et al. High incidence of persistent primitive arteries in moyamoya and quasi-moyamoya diseases. Neurol Med Chir (Tokyo). 1999;39:416–20; discussion 20–2.

92. Yamada I, Suzuki S, Matsushima Y. Moyamoya disease: comparison of assessment with MR angiography and MR imaging versus conventional angiography. Radiology. 1995;196:211–8.

93. Yamada I, Suzuki S, Matsushima Y. Moyamoya disease: diagnostic accuracy of MRI. Neuroradiology. 1995;37:356–61.

94. Hasuo K, Mihara F, Matsushima T. MRI and MR angiography in moyamoya disease. J Magn Reson Imaging. 1998;8:762–6.

95. Yoon H-K, Shin H-J, Chang YW. "Ivy sign" in childhood moyamoya disease: depiction on FLAIR and contrast-enhanced T1-weighted MR images. Radiology. 2002;223:384–9.

96. Ohta T, Tanaka H, Kuroiwa T. Diffuse leptomeningeal enhancement, "ivy sign," in magnetic resonance images of moyamoya disease in childhood: case report. Neurosurgery. 1995;37:1009–12.

97. Maeda M, Tsuchida C. "Ivy sign" on fluid-attenuated inversion-recovery images in childhood moyamoya disease. AJNR Am J Neuroradiol. 1999;20:1836–8.

98. Iwama T, Akiyama Y, Morimoto M, Kojima A, Hayashida K. Comparison of positron emission tomography study results of cerebral hemodynamics in patients with bleeding- and ischemic-type moyamoya disease. Neurosurg Focus. 1998;5:e3.

99. McAuley DJ, Poskitt K, Steinbok P. Predicting stroke risk in pediatric moyamoya disease with xenon-enhanced computed tomography. Neurosurgery. 2004;55:327–32; discussion 32–3.

100. El Ramahi KM, Al Rayes HM. Systemic lupus erythematosus associated with moyamoya syndrome. Lupus. 2000;9:632–6.

101. Ogawa A, Nakamura N, Yoshimoto T, Suzuki J. Cerebral blood flow in moyamoya disease. Part 2: autoregulation and CO₂ response. Acta Neurochir (Wien). 1990;105:107–11.

102. Ogawa A, Yoshimoto T, Suzuki J, Sakurai Y. Cerebral blood flow in moyamoya disease. Part 1: correlation with age and regional distribution. Acta Neurochir (Wien). 1990;105:30–4.

103. Kohno K, Oka Y, Kohno S, Ohta S, Kumon Y, Sakaki S. Cerebral blood flow measurement as an indicator for an indirect revascularization procedure for adult patients with moyamoya disease. Neurosurgery. 1998;42:752–7; discussion 7–8.

104. Han DH, Nam DH, Oh CW. Moyamoya disease in adults: characteristics of clinical presentation and outcome after encephalo-duro-arterio-synangiosis. Clin Neurol Neurosurg. 1997;99 Suppl 2:S151–5.

105. Honda M, Ezaki Y, Kitagawa N, Tsutsumi K, Ogawa Y, Nagata I. Quantification of the regional cerebral blood flow and vascular reserve in moyamoya disease using split-dose iodoamphetamine I 123 single-photon emission computed tomography. Surg Neurol. 2006;66.155–9; discussion 9.

106. Nariai T, Matsushima Y, Imae S, et al. Severe haemodynamic stress in selected subtypes of patients with moyamoya disease: a positron emission tomography study. J Neurol Neurosurg Psychiatry. 2005;76:663–9.

107. Nariai T, Suzuki R, Matsushima Y, et al. Surgically induced angiogenesis to compensate for hemodynamic cerebral ischemia. Stroke. 1994;25:1014–21.

108. Kodama N, Aoki Y, Hiraga H, Wada T, Suzuki J. Electroencephalographic findings in children with moyamoya disease. Arch Neurol. 1979;36:16–9.

109. Qiao F, Kuroda S, Kamada K, Houkin K, Iwasaki Y. Source localization of the re-build up phenomenon in pediatric moyamoya disease-a dipole distribution analysis using MEG and SPECT. Childs Nerv Syst. 2003;19:760–4.

110. Kuroda S, Kamiyama H, Isobe M, Houkin K, Abe H, Mitsumori K. Cerebral hemodynamics and "re-build-up" phenomenon on electroencephalogram in children with moyamoya disease. Childs Nerv Syst. 1995;11:214–9.

111. Matsushima Y, Aoyagi M, Niimi Y, Masaoka H, Ohno K. Symptoms and their pattern of progression in childhood moyamoya disease. Brain Dev. 1990;12:784–9.

112. Moritake K, Handa H, Yonekawa Y, Taki W, Okuno T. Follow-up study on the relationship between age at onset of illness and outcome in patients with moyamoya disease. No Shinkei Geka. 1986;14:957–63.

113. Iwama T, Morimoto M, Hashimoto N, Goto Y, Todaka T, Sawada M. Mechanism of intracranial rebleeding in moyamoya disease. Clin Neurol Neurosurg. 1997;99 Suppl 2:S187–90.

114. Kobayashi E, Saeki N, Oishi H, Hirai S, Yamaura A. Long-term natural history of hemorrhagic moyamoya disease in 42 patients. J Neurosurg. 2000;93:976–80.

115. Seol HJ, Wang KC, Kim SK, et al. Unilateral (probable) moyamoya disease: long-term follow-up of seven cases. Childs Nerv Syst. 2006;22:145–50.

116. Kelly ME, Bell-Stephens TE, Marks MP, Do HM, Steinberg GK. Progression of unilateral moyamoya disease: a clinical series. Cerebrovasc Dis. 2006;22:109–15.

117. Ikezaki K, Inamura T, Kawano T, Fukui M. Clinical features of probable moyamoya disease in Japan. Clin Neurol Neurosurg. 1997;99 Suppl 2:S173–7.

118. Houkin K, Abe H, Yoshimoto T, Takahashi A. Is "unilateral" moyamoya disease different from moyamoya disease? J Neurosurg. 1996;85:772–6.

119. Kusaka N, Tamiya T, Adachi Y, et al. Adult unilateral moyamoya disease with familial occurrence in two definite cases: a case report and review of the literature. Neurosurg Rev. 2006;29:82–7.

120. Nanba R, Kuroda S, Tada M, Ishikawa T, Houkin K, Iwasaki Y. Clinical features of familial moyamoya disease. Childs Nerv Syst. 2006;22:258–62.

121. Kanai N. A genetic study of spontaneous occlusion of the circle of Willis (moyamoya disease). J Tokyo Women Med Univ. 1992;62:1227–58.

122. Kitahara T, Ariga N, Yamaura A, Makino H, Maki Y. Familial occurrence of moya-moya disease: report of three Japanese families. J Neurol Neurosurg Psychiatry. 1979;42:208–14.

123. Yamada H, Nakamura S, Kageyama N. Moyamoya disease in monovular twins: case report. J Neurosurg. 1980;53:109–12.

124. Yamauchi T, Houkin K, Tada M, Abe H. Familial occurrence of moyamoya disease. Clin Neurol Neurosurg. 1997;99 Suppl 2:S162–7.

125. Mineharu Y, Takenaka K, Yamakawa H, et al. Inheritance pattern of familial moyamoya disease: autosomal dominant mode and genomic imprinting. J Neurol Neurosurg Psychiatry. 2006;77:1025–9.

126. Ikeda H, Sasaki T, Yoshimoto T, Fukui M, Arinami T. Mapping of a familial moyamoya disease gene to chromosome 3p24.2-p26. Am J Hum Genet. 1999;64:533–7.

127. Yamauchi T, Tada M, Houkin K, et al. Linkage of familial moyamoya disease (spontaneous occlusion of the circle of Willis) to chromosome 17q25. Stroke. 2000;31:930–5.

128. Inoue TK, Ikezaki K, Sasazuki T, Matsushima T, Fukui M. Linkage analysis of moyamoya disease on chromosome 6. J Child Neurol. 2000;15:179–82.

129. Sakurai K, Horiuchi Y, Ikeda H, et al. A novel susceptibility locus for moyamoya disease on chromosome 8q23. J Hum Genet. 2004;49:278–81.

130. Lee CM, Lee SY, Ryu SH, Lee SW, Park KW, Chung WT. Systemic lupus erythematosus associated with familial moyamoya disease. Korean J Intern Med. 2003;18:244–7.

131. Akutsu H, Sonobe M, Sugita K, Nakai Y, Matsumura A. Familial association of basilar bifurcation aneurysm and moyamoya disease – four case reports. Neurol Med Chir (Tokyo). 2003;43:435–8.

132. Houkin K, Tanaka N, Takahashi A, Kamiyama H, Abe H, Kajii N. Familial occurrence of moyamoya disease. Magnetic resonance angiography as a screening test for high-risk subjects. Childs Nerv Syst. 1994;10:421–5.

133. Im SH, Oh CW, Kwon OK, Kim JE, Han DH. Moyamoya disease associated with Graves disease: special considerations regarding clinical significance and management. J Neurosurg. 2005;102:1013–7.

134. Sasaki T, Nogawa S, Amano T. Co-morbidity of moyamoya disease with Graves' disease. Report of three cases and a review of the literature. Intern Med. 2006;45:649–53.

135. Nagahiro S, Mantani A, Yamada K, Ushio Y. Multiple cerebral arterial occlusions in a young patient with Sjogren's syndrome: case report. Neurosurgery. 1996;38:592–5; discussion 5.

136. Matsuki Y, Kawakami M, Ishizuka T, et al. SLE and Sjogren's syndrome associated with unilateral moyamoya vessels in cerebral arteries. Scand J Rheumatol. 1997;26:392–4.

137. Booth F, Yanofsky R, Ross IB, Lawrence P, Oen K. Primary antiphospholipid syndrome with moyamoya-like vascular changes. Pediatr Neurosurg. 1999;31:45–8.

138. Shuja-Ud-Din MA, Ahamed SA, Baidas G, Naeem M. Moyamoya syndrome with primary antiphospholipid syndrome. Med Princ Pract. 2006;15:238–41.

139. Czartoski T, Hallam D, Lacy JM, Chun MR, Becker K. Postinfectious vasculopathy with evolution to moyamoya syndrome. J Neurol Neurosurg Psychiatry. 2005;76:256–9.

140. Mathew NT, Abraham J, Chandy J. Cerebral angiographic features in tuberculous meningitis. Neurology. 1970;20:1015–23.

141. Nakayama Y, Tanaka A, Nagasaka S, Ikui H. Intracerebral hemorrhage in a patient with moyamoya phenomenon caused by tuberculous arteritis: a case report. No Shinkei Geka. 1999;27:751–5.

142. Hsiung GY, Sotero de Menezes M. Moyamoya syndrome in a patient with congenital human immunodeficiency virus infection. J Child Neurol. 1999;14:268–70.

143. Dobson SR, Holden KR, Nietert PJ, et al. Moyamoya syndrome in childhood sickle cell disease: a predictive factor for recurrent cerebrovascular events. Blood. 2002;99:3144–50.

144. Tomura N, Inugami A, Higano S, et al. Cases similar to cerebrovascular moyamoya disease – investigation by angiography and computed tomography. No To Shinkei. 1988;40:905–12.

145. Cohen N, Berant M, Simon J. Moyamoya and Fanconi's anemia. Pediatrics. 1980;65:804–5.

146. Pavlakis SG, Verlander PC, Gould RJ, Strimling BC, Auerbach AD. Fanconi anemia and moyamoya: evidence for an association. Neurology. 1995;45:998–1000.

147. Tokunaga Y, Ohga S, Suita S, Matsushima T, Hara T. Moyamoya syndrome with spherocytosis: effect of splenectomy on strokes. Pediatr Neurol. 2001;25:75–7.

148. Sanefuji M, Ohga S, Kira R, Yoshiura T, Torisu H, Hara T. Moyamoya syndrome in a splenectomized patient with beta-thalassemia intermedia. J Child Neurol. 2006;21:75–7.

149. Matsuda M, Enomoto T, Yanaka K, Nose T. Moyamoya disease associated with hemophilia A. A case report. Pediatr Neurosurg. 2002;36:157–60.

150. Hiyama H, Kusano R, Muragaki Y, Miura N. Moyamoya disease associated with thrombotic thrombocytopenic purpura (TTP). No Shinkei Geka. 1994;22:567–72.

151. Brockmann K, Stolpe S, Fels C, Khan N, Kulozik AE, Pekrun A. Moyamoya syndrome associated with hemolytic anemia due to Hb Alesha. J Pediatr Hematol Oncol. 2005;27: 436–40.

152. Kornblihtt LI, Cocorullo S, Miranda C, Lylyk P, Heller PG, Molinas FC. Moyamoya syndrome in an adolescent with essential thrombocythemia: successful intracranial carotid stent placement. Stroke. 2005;36:E71–3.

153. Kikuchi A, Maeda M, Hanada R, et al. Moyamoya syndrome following childhood acute lymphoblastic leukemia. Pediatr Blood Cancer. 2007;48:268–72.

154. Andeejani AM, Salih MA, Kolawole T, et al. Moyamoya syndrome with congenital angiographic findings and protein C deficiency: review of the literature. J Neurol Sci. 1998;159:11–6.

155. Akgun D, YiLmaz S, Senbil N, Aslan B, Gurer YY. Moyamoya syndrome with protein S deficiency. Eur J Paediatr Neurol. 2000;4:185–8.

156. Kikuta K, Miyamoto S, Kataoka H, et al. An adult case of moyamoya syndrome that developed dural sinus thrombosis associated with protein C deficiency: case report and literature review. Surg Neurol. 2005;63:480–4; discussion 4.

157. Cheong PL, Lee WT, Liu HM, Lin KH. Moyamoya syndrome with inherited proteins C and S deficiency: report of one case. Acta Paediatr Taiwan. 2005;46:31–4.

158. Dhopesh VP, Dunn DP, Schick P. Moyamoya and Hageman factor (Factor XII) deficiency in a black adult. Arch Neurol. 1978;35:396.

159. Likavcan M, Benko J, Papiernikova E, Lindtnerova L. Moyamoya syndrome with hyperlipoproteinemia type IIa. Cesk Neurol Neurochir. 1979;42:49–53.

160. Goutieres F, Bourgeois M, Trioche P, Demelier JF, Odievre M, Labrune P. Moyamoya disease in a child with glycogen storage disease type Ia. Neuropediatrics. 1997;28:133–4.

161. Meyer S, Zanardo L, Kaminski WE, et al. Elastosis perforans serpiginosa-like pseudoxanthoma elasticum in a child with severe Moya disease. Br J Dermatol. 2005; 153:431–4.

162. Squizzato A, Gerdes VE, Brandjes DP, Buller HR, Stam J. Thyroid diseases and cerebrovascular disease. Stroke. 2005;36:2302–10.

163. Cerrato P, Grasso M, Lentini A, et al. Atherosclerotic adult Moya-Moya disease in a patient with hyperhomocysteinaemia. Neurol Sci. 2007;28:45–7.

164. Cramer SC, Robertson RL, Dooling EC, Scott RM. Moyamoya and Down syndrome. Clinical and radiological features. Stroke. 1996;27:2131–5.

165. Kwong KL, Wong YC. Moyamoya disease in a child with neurofibromatosis type-1. J Paediatr Child Health. 1999;35:108–9.

166. Inoue T, Matsushima T, Fujii K, Fukui M, Hasuo K, Matsuo H. Akin moyamoya disease in children. No Shinkei Geka. 1993;21:59–65.

167. Spengos K, Kosmaidou-Aravidou Z, Tsivgoulis G, Vassilopoulou S, Grigori-Kostaraki P, Zis V. Moyamoya syndrome in a Caucasian woman with Turner's syndrome. Eur J Neurol. 2006;13:e7–8.

168. Kawai M, Nishikawa T, Tanaka M, et al. An autopsied case of Williams syndrome complicated by moyamoya disease. Acta Paediatr Jpn. 1993;35:63–7.

169. Imaizumi M, Nukada T, Yoneda S, Takano Y, Hasegawa K, Abe H. Tuberous sclerosis with moyamoya disease. Case report. Med J Osaka Univ. 1978;28:345–53.

170. Albayram S, Kizilkilic O, Yilmaz H, Tuysuz B, Kocer N, Islak C. Abnormalities in the cerebral arterial system in osteogenesis imperfecta. AJNR Am J Neuroradiol. 2003;24:748–50.

171. Ganesan V, Kirkham FJ. Noonan syndrome and moyamoya. Pediatr Neurol. 1997;16:256–8.

172. Yamashita Y, Kusaga A, Koga Y, Nagamitsu S, Matsushi T. Noonan syndrome, moyamoya-like vascular changes, and antiphospholipid syndrome. Pediatr Neurol. 2004;31:364–6.

173. Shiihara T, Kato M, Mitsuhashi Y, Hayasaka K. Costello syndrome showing moyamoya-like vasculopathy. Pediatr Neurol. 2005;32:361–3.

174. Rachmel A, Zeharia A, Neuman-Levin M, Weitz R, Shamir R, Dinari G. Alagille syndrome associated with moyamoya disease. Am J Med Genet. 1989;33:89–91.

175. Emerick KM, Krantz ID, Kamath BM, et al. Intracranial vascular abnormalities in patients with Alagille syndrome. J Pediatr Gastroenterol Nutr. 2005;41:99–107.

176. Girirajan S, Mendoza-Londono R, Vlangos CN, et al. Smith-Magenis syndrome and moyamoya disease in a patient with del(17)(p11.2p13.1). Am J Med Genet A. 2007;143:999–1008.

177. Kim YO, Baek HJ, Woo YJ, Choi YY, Chung TW. Moyamoya syndrome in a child with trisomy 12p syndrome. Pediatr Neurol. 2006;35:442–5.

178. Pilz P, Hartjes HJ. Fibromuscular dysplasia and multiple dissecting aneurysms of intracranial arteries. A further cause of Moyamoya syndrome. Stroke. 1976;7:393–8.

179. Pracyk JB, Massey JM. Moyamoya disease associated with polycystic kidney disease and eosinophilic granuloma. Stroke. 1989;20:1092–4.

180. Terada T, Yokote H, Tsuura M, Nakai K, Ohshima A, Itakura T. Marfan syndrome associated with moyamoya phenomenon and aortic dissection. Acta Neurochir (Wien). 1999;141:663–5.

181. Terajima K, Shimohata T, Watanabe M, et al. Cerebral vasculopathy showing moyamoya-like changes in a patient with CREST syndrome. Eur Neurol. 2001;46:163–5.

182. Lau YL, Milligan DW. Atypical presentation of craniopharyngioma associated with moyamoya disease. J R Soc Med. 1986;79:236–7.

183. Arita K, Uozumi T, Oki S, et al. Moyamoya disease associated with pituitary adenoma – report of two cases. Neurol Med Chir (Tokyo). 1992;32:753–7.

184. Kitano S, Sakamoto H, Fujitani K, Kobayashi Y. Moyamoya disease associated with a brain stem glioma. Childs Nerv Syst. 2000;16:251–5.

185. Watanabe Y, Todani T, Fujii T, Toki A, Uemura S, Koike Y. Wilms' tumor associated with Moyamoya disease: a case report. Z Kinderchir. 1985;40:114–6.

186. Sequeira W, Naseem M, Bouffard DA. An association with birth control pills. Moyamoya. IMJ Ill Med J. 1984;166: 434–6.

187. Schwartz MS, Scott RM. Moyamoya syndrome associated with cocaine abuse. Case report. Neurosurg Focus. 1998;5:e7.
188. Storen EC, Wijdicks EF, Crum BA, Schultz G. Moyamoya-like vasculopathy from cocaine dependency. AJNR Am J Neuroradiol. 2000;21:1008–10.
189. Bitzer M, Topka H. Progressive cerebral occlusive disease after radiation therapy. Stroke. 1995;26:131–6.
190. Desai SS, Paulino AC, Mai WY, Teh BS. Radiation-induced moyamoya syndrome. Int J Radiat Oncol Biol Phys. 2006;65:1222–7.
191. Ullrich NJ, Robertson R, Kinnamon DD, et al. Moyamoya following cranial irradiation for primary brain tumors in children. Neurology. 2007;68:932–8.
192. Steinke W, Tatemichi TK, Mohr JP, Massaro A, Prohovnik I, Solomon RA. Caudate hemorrhage with moyamoya-like vasculopathy from atherosclerotic disease. Stroke. 1992;23:1360–3.
193. Joo SP, Kim TS, Lee JH, et al. Moyamoya disease associated with Behcet's disease. J Clin Neurosci. 2006;13:364–7.
194. Taskintuna I, Oz O, Teke MY, Kocak H, Firat E. Morning glory syndrome: association with moyamoya disease, mid-line cranial defects, central nervous system anomalies, and persistent hyaloid artery remnant. Retina. 2003;23:400–2.
195. Mawad ME, Hilal SK, Michelsen WJ, Stein B, Ganti SR. Occlusive vascular disease associated with cerebral arterio-venous malformations. Radiology. 1984;153:401 8.
196. Nakashima T, Nakayama N, Furuichi M, Kokuzawa J, Murakawa T, Sakai N. Arteriovenous malformation in association with moyamoya disease. Report of two cases. Neurosurg Focus. 1998;5:e6.
197. Yamada K, Hayakawa T, Ushio Y, Mitomo M. Cerebral arterial dolichoectasia associated with moyamoya vessels. Surg Neurol. 1985;23:19–24.
198. Katayama W, Enomoto T, Yanaka K, Nose T. Moyamoya disease associated with persistent primitive hypoglossal artery: report of a case. Pediatr Neurosurg. 2001;35:262–5.
199. Shoskes DA, Novick AC. Surgical treatment of renovascular hypertension in moyamoya disease: case report and review of the literature. J Urol. 1995;153:450–2.
200. Bayrakci B, Topaloglu R, Cila A, Saatci I. Renovascular hypertension and prolonged encephalopathy associated with moyamoya disease. Eur J Pediatr. 1999;158:342.
201. Tsuruta D, Fukai K, Seto M, et al. Phakomatosis pigmentovascularis type IIIb associated with moyamoya disease. Pediatr Dermatol. 1999;16:35–8.
202. Takenaka K, Ito M, Kumagai M, et al. Moyamoya disease associated with pulmonary sarcoidosis – case report. Neurol Med Chir (Tokyo). 1998;38:566–8.
203. Sharma J, Sehgal KV, Harmon RL. Heterotopic ossification in moyamoya disease: a case report. Am J Phys Med Rehabil. 1998;77:455–7.
204. Lutterman J, Scott M, Nass R, Geva T. Moyamoya syndrome associated with congenital heart disease. Pediatrics. 1998;101:57–60.
205. Fernandez-Alvarez E, Pineda M, Royo C, Manzanares R. 'Moya-moya' disease caused by cranial trauma. Brain Dev. 1979;1:133–8.
206. Fukui M, Natori Y, Matsushima T, Ikezaki K. Surgical treatment of diseases akin to Moyamoya disease in children. In: Fukui M, ed. Annual report of the 1995 research committee on spontaneous occlusion of the circle of Willis. Tokyo, Japan; 1996.
207. Goldenberg HJ. 'Moyamoya' associated with peripheral vascular occlusive disease. Arch Dis Child. 1974;49:964–6.
208. Peerless SJ. Risk factors of moyamoya disease in Canada and the USA. Clin Neurol Neurosurg. 1997;99 Suppl 2:S45–8.
209. Hallemeier CL, Rich KM, Grubb Jr RL, et al. Clinical features and outcome in North American adults with moyamoya phenomenon. Stroke. 2006;37:1490–6.
210. Suzuki J, Takaku A, Kodama N, Sato S. An attempt to treat cerebrovascular 'Moyamoya' disease in children. Childs Brain. 1975;1:193–206.
211. Donaghy RM. Neurologic surgery. Surg Gynecol Obstet. 1972;134:269–70.
212. Spetzler R, Chater N. Occipital artery – middle cerebral artery anastomosis for cerebral artery occlusive disease. Surg Neurol. 1974;2:235–8.
213. Ikeda A, Yamamoto I, Sato O, Morota N, Tsuji T, Seguchi T. Revascularization of the calcarine artery in moyamoya disease: OA-cortical PCA anastomosis – case report. Neurol Med Chir (Tokyo). 1991;31:658–61.
214. Ishii R, Koike T, Takeuchi S, Ohsugi S, Tanaka R, Konno K. Anastomosis of the superficial temporal artery to the distal anterior cerebral artery with interposed cephalic vein graft. Case report. J Neurosurg. 1983;58:425–9.
215. Fung LW, Thompson D, Ganesan V. Revascularisation surgery for paediatric moyamoya: a review of the literature. Childs Nerv Syst. 2005;21:358–64.
216. Mizoi K, Kayama T, Yoshimoto T, Nagamine Y. Indirect revascularization for moyamoya disease: is there a beneficial effect for adult patients? Surg Neurol. 1996;45:541–8; discussion 8–9.
217. Choi JU, Seok Kim D, Kim EY, Lee KC. Natural history of Moyamoya disease: comparison of activity of daily living in surgery and non surgery groups. Clin Neurol Neurosurg. 1997;99:S11–8.
218. Sittig O. Klinische Beitrage zur Lehre von der Lokalisation der sensiblen Rindenzentren. Prag Med Wohenschr. 1914;45:548–50.
219. Sasamori T, Kuroda S, Nakayama N, Iwasaki Y. Incidence and pathogenesis of transient cheiro-oral syndrome after surgical revascularization for moyamoya disease. Neurosurgery. 2010;67:1054–60.
220. Yoshida Y, Yoshimoto T, Shirane R, Sakurai Y. Clinical course, surgical management, and long-term outcome of moyamoya patients with rebleeding after an episode of intracerebral hemorrhage: an extensive follow-up study. Stroke. 1999;30:2272–6.
221. Kuroda S, Houkin K, Kamiyama H, Abe H. Effects of surgical revascularization on peripheral artery aneurysms in moyamoya disease: report of three cases. Neurosurgery. 2001;49:463–7; discussion 7–8.
222. Drazin D, Calayag M, Gifford E, Dalfino J, Yamamoto J, Boulos AS. Endovascular treatment for moyamoya disease in a Caucasian twin with angioplasty and Wingspan stent. Clin Neurol Neurosurg. 2009;111:913–7.
223. El-Hakam LM, Volpi J, Mawad M, Clark G. Angioplasty for acute stroke with pediatric moyamoya syndrome. J Child Neurol. 2010;25:1278–83.
224. Khan N, Dodd R, Marks MP, Bell-Stephens T, Vavao J, Steinberg GK. Failure of primary percutaneous angioplasty and stenting in the prevention of ischemia in Moyamoya angiopathy. Cerebrovasc Dis. 2011;31:147–53.
225. Komiyama M, Yasui T, Kitano S, Sakamoto H, Fujitani K, Matsuo S. Moyamoya disease and pregnancy: case report and review of the literature. Neurosurgery. 1998;43:360–8; discussion 8–9.
226. Kato K, Tomura N, Takahashi S, et al. A case of moyamoya-like vessels combined with brain anomaly. Radiat Med. 1999;17:373–7.
227. Khan N, Schinzel A, Shuknecht B, Baumann F, Ostergaard JR, Yonekawa Y. Moyamoya angiopathy with dolichoectatic internal carotid arteries, patent ductus arteriosus and pupillary dysfunction: a new genetic syndrome? Eur Neurol. 2004;51:72–7.
228. Samuels OB, Joseph GJ, Lynn MJ, Smith HA, Chimowitz MI. A standardized method for measuring intracranial arterial stenosis. AJNR Am J Neuroradiol. 2000;21:643–6.
229. Suzuki J, Takaku A. Cerebrovascular "moyamoya" disease. Disease showing abnormal net-like vessels in base of brain. Arch Neurol. 1969;20:288–99.

20. Spinal Vascular Lesions

Several classification schemes for spinal vascular lesions have been described.[1–4] The following four-type system is the most commonly used, with several other spinal vascular lesions added for completeness:

- Type I: Dural arteriovenous fistula (dAVF)
- Type II: Intramedullary arteriovenous malformation (AVM)
- Type III: Juvenile AVM
- Type IV: Intradural perimedullary AVF
- Extradural arteriovenous fistulas
- Spinal cord aneurysms
- Intramedullary cavernous malformations
- Vascular spinal tumours
- Spinal cord ischaemic stroke

Technical aspects of endovascular treatment of spinal vascular lesions are discussed in Chap. 8, Extracranial Embolization.

20.1.   Type I: Dural Arteriovenous Fistula

Type I lesions (aka angioma racemosum, angioma racemosum venosum, intradural dorsal AVF, long dorsal AVF, dorsal extramedullary AVF) consist of an abnormal communication between the radicular artery in the nerve root sleeve and the intradural venous system, causing venous hypertension (Fig. 20.1). They can be subclassified into type I-A and type I-B lesions, depending on whether there is one or more radicular feeding arteries.[5,6]

Epidemiology and Clinical Features

1. Type I dAVFs are the most common spinal vascular lesion, representing approximately 70% of spinal vascular malformations.[7]
2. More common in males (male/female ratio is 5:1)[8,9]
3. Mean age at presentation is 60; range is 28–83 years.[8–10]
4. Mean duration of symptoms prior to diagnosis: 23 months.[8,9,11]
5. The majority of type I lesions are located in the thoracolumbar spine, with T7, 8, and 9 being the most common levels.[12]
   85% of lesions are below T6, and 100% of lesions are below T3[12]
6. *Extradural* dAVFs are uncommon.[13,14] They cause arterialization of the epidural venous system, and produce symptoms by spinal cord compression, venous congestion,[15] or, rarely, by steal of blood flow from the spinal cord.[2]
7. Presentation:
   a. Symptoms are typically progressive and may be exacerbated by physical activity.[11]
   b. Motor symptoms are present in 78–100% of cases.[8,9,11,16]
   c. Upper or motor neurons may be involved; flaccid paresis is about as common as spastic paresis.[17]
   d. Sensory symptoms are present in 69–90% of cases.[9,11,17]
   e. Paraesthesias, and sensory and gait abnormalities are common.
   f. Pain is a complaint in more than half of cases.[9,11,17]
   g. Patients may report worsening of symptoms with exertion (neurogenic claudication) or with certain postural changes.[12]
8. Imaging:
   a. MRI is the screening procedure of choice for spinal dAVFs.[16] Spinal cord hyperintensity on T2-weighted images and postgadolinium enhancement on T1-weighted images are the most common findings.[7,18] Cord signal changes usually extend for six or seven vertebral levels.[7,17]

M.R. Harrigan, J.P. Deveikis, *Handbook of Cerebrovascular Disease and Neurointerventional Technique*, DOI 10.1007/978-1-61779-946-4_20, © Springer Science+Business Media New York 2013

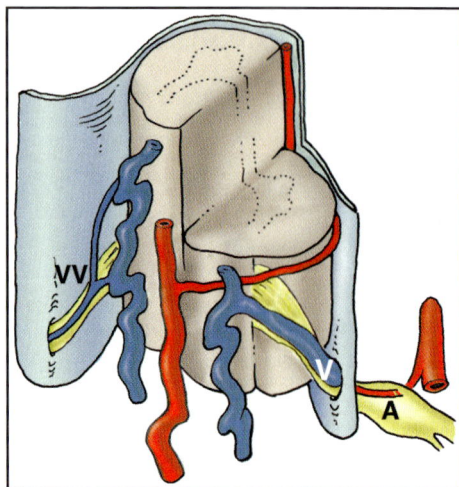

Fig. 20.1 Type I dural arteriovenous fistula (dAVF). There is a direct connection between a radicular artery (*A*) and a radicular vein (*V*) in the dura of the nerve root sleeve. Arterialization of the coronal venous plexus causes engorgement and congestion of the veins. Note that the contralateral radicular vein (*VV*) in this depiction is small; impairment of alternative routes of venous drainage is thought to contribute to the development of venous hypertensive myelopathy.

    i. Cord oedema is seen in up to 74% of cases.[17]
    ii. The coronal venous plexus has a characteristically nodular, shaggy, and tortuous appearance on MRI and MRA.[7]
    iii. Dilated veins on the dorsal surface of the cord can be distinguished from CSF pulsation artifact by a typical salt and pepper appearance on postcontrast T1-weighted images.[17]
    iv. Volumetric myelographic MRI can help localize difficult-to-find spinal dAVFs.[19]
  b. Catheter angiography is the gold standard for the workup of spinal dAVFs.[16]
    i. Selective injection of the thoracic and lumbar spinal arteries should be done first, since the majority of dAVFs are located in those regions.
    ii. When the artery of Adamkiewicz is found, imaging of the venous phase of the angiogram will fail to show normal filling of spinal cord veins in most cases of spinal dAVF.[20] This is evidence of the severe venous hypertension in the cord.
    iii. In some 10% of cases, the sacral arteries are involved.[21,22]
    iv. Rarely, intracranial dural AVFs may drain inferiorly and mimic spinal dural AVFs clinically and on MRI.[22–24]
        With intracranial fistulas draining to spinal cord veins, angiography of the artery of Adamkiewicz may show normal appearance of spinal cord veins in the venous phase.[25] Thus, if a fistula is not found during spinal angiography, angiography of the cerebral vessels should be done.
    v. Dilated, tortuous veins draining a dAVF are characteristic findings, predominantly along the posterior surface of the spinal cord.
    vi. When a fistula is found, the adjacent levels should be imaged as well, because of the possibility of multiple radicular feeding arteries.
    vii. It has been reported that placement of a platinum coil in the major feeding artery can facilitate intraoperative fluoroscopic localization of the fistula.[26]

c. Myelography is very accurate in identifying spinal dAVFs, showing tortuous filling defects in up to 100% of cases.[7,11,27] These abnormal vessels are always located on the dorsal surface of the cord, and may also be present on the ventral surface in some 10% of cases.[11]

Pathophysiology

1. Normal radicular veins have a constriction at the point where the vein passes through the dura, which prevents the transmission of arterial pressure into the valveless coronal venous plexus.[28] Fistulas are usually located at this point or within the nerve root sleeve.[29] The fistula is usually supplied by a meningoradicular branch of a segmental artery, although any artery supplying the dura may be involved.[16] The intrathecal spinal venous system is valveless, and therefore arterial pressure is transmitted via the corresponding radicular vein into the perimedullary and spinal veins, causing venous hypertension, congestion and impairment of the spinal cord and nerve root microcirculation.[30] Direct measurement of the coronal venous pressure during surgery found that the spinal cord venous pressure averages 74% of the simultaneous mean systemic venous pressure.[30]
2. The aetiology of spinal dAVFs is not understood. Interestingly, in contrast to cranial dAVFs, in which venous sinus thrombosis is believed to contribute to the development of those lesions, prothrombotic conditions are not associated with spinal dAVFs.[31]
3. Spinal dAVFs are associated with infection,[32] syringomyelia,[33] spine trauma,[34] and surgery.[35,36]

Management

The natural history of untreated spinal dAVFs is generally thought to be poor. An early series found that 50% of untreated patients became severely disabled (wheelchair-bound) within 3 years of the onset of lower extremity weakness.[37]

Both surgery and endovascular treatment can be effective for treatment of type I lesions. Although surgery appears to be more curative, embolization is less invasive and some authors recommend an attempt at embolization prior to surgery. In a systematic review of 20 published clinical series, 98% of patients treated with surgery were reported to have successful obliteration of their fistulae, compared to only 46% with embolization.[38] Complications were reported in 1.9% of surgical patients and 3.7% of embolization patients.

Extradural dAVFs are treated almost exclusively with embolization of the arterial feeder and rarely require surgery.[2,39]

Surgical Considerations

1. Neurophysiological monitoring with evoked potentials is not necessary, as manipulation of the spinal cord is not required.[21]
2. A two-level hemilaminectomy is done to adequately expose the affected nerve root.
3. The dura is opened in the midline and retracted laterally.
4. The radicular draining vein is exposed where it penetrates the dura and is coagulated and divided.
   Interruption of the radicular vein is an important step for successful cure of the fistula and usually leads to an immediate visible change in venous turgor, and the colour of the arterialized venous plexus may change from red to blue.
5. If the fistula involves a thoracic nerve root, the root may be sacrificed to facilitate dural closure. Obviously, cervical and lumbar nerve roots should be preserved.
6. In cases in which extradural drainage of the fistula is present, the entire fistula including portions of the draining vein should be excised and the intradural and extradural components should be divided to prevent recurrence.[40]
7. Outcomes with surgery:

a. A systematic review of surgical outcomes found that 55% of patients improved after surgery, 34% were stabilized, and 11% worsened.[38] Only 33% of patients showed an improvement in micturition, and 11% worsened.
b. A recent single center series of 154 surgical cases reported complete exclusion of fistula at first attempt in 95% and 96.6% of patients experienced improvement, and 6% worsened.[41]

Endovascular Considerations

1. Case selection: Embolization should be done only when the anatomy of the lesion will permit obliteration of the nidus and proximal part of the vein.
   a. Embolization is feasible in some 75% of cases.[42]
      Barriers to embolization include advanced atherosclerosis, arterial feeders too small to catheterize, and collateralization of the feeding vessel with normal spinal cord vessels.
   b. Embolization is most effective when the glue penetrates the proximal portion of the draining vein; if the glue does not reach the draining vein, the fistula may persist or recanalize. In an endovascular series, the fistula recurred in 68% of cases in which the glue did not reach the draining vein, compared with 50% of cases in which the glue did reach the draining vein.[43]
2. Embolization is particularly useful in patients who are poor candidates for surgery, or in some cases as a temporizing measure, to reduce venous congestion until a definitive surgical procedure can be performed.[44]
3. The embolization agent of choice is N-butyl cyanoacylate.
4. Onyx embolization has also been reported.[45]
5. Partial embolization of the fistula and embolization with particulate agents (e.g., polyvinyl alcohol) should be avoided.[46-49] Failure to permanently obliterate the lesion may lead to recurrence, and further difficulty in later treatment.
6. Reports on long-term outcomes after embolization are lacking. Clinical outcome data on embolization were insufficient for analysis in the systematic review discussed earlier.[38]

The Often Misunderstood Foix–Alajouanine Syndrome

In 1926, Foix and Alajouanine published a 42-page report of two cases of progressive myelopathy.[32] An extensive pathological analysis was carried out, and the authors implicated vascular congestion, as reflected by spinal cord vessel thickening, in the pathological process afflicting both patients. In the decades since this report, numerous authors have included spinal cord venous thrombosis as a central feature of the Foix–Alajouanine Syndrome.[6,44,50-53] Indeed, both authors of this handbook were taught, during their training, that Foix–Alajouanine Syndrome is equivalent to progressive, malignant spinal cord venous thrombosis. In the actual report, however, Foix and Alajouanine emphasized that in their two cases no thrombosis was present.[54] They described vessel wall thickening, without luminal narrowing or obliteration of cord vessels, and excluded the presence of vascular malformations within the cord. The inclusion of thrombosis as a feature of Foix–Alajouanine Syndrome is a myth that has been perpetuated most likely because the original report was written in French. In retrospect, it seems likely that both patients in the original report had progressive myelopathy due to type I dural AVFs,[44] an entity that had not yet been recognized at the time of the publication.[54]

20.2.   Type II: Intramedullary Arteriovenous Malformation

Type II lesions (aka glomus or classic AVM) consist of an AVM within the substance of the spinal cord. The nidus can be classified as compact or diffuse, and they often have multiple feeding vessels arising from the anterior and posterolateral spinal arteries (Fig. 20.2).

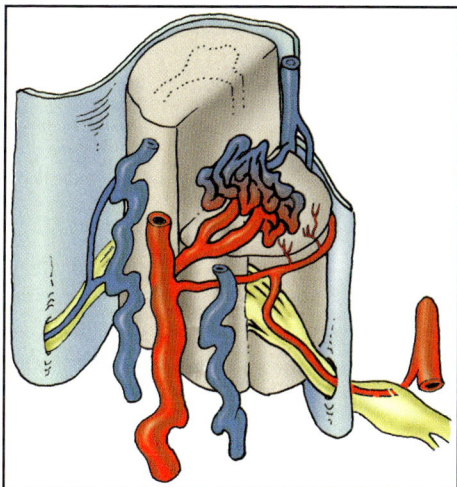

Fig. 20.2 Type II intramedullary AVM. Intramedullary arteriovenous malformation with a compact nidus is illustrated.

Epidemiology and Clinical Features

1. Type II lesions are the second most common kind of spinal vascular lesion, accounting for up to 36–45% of spinal vascular lesions.[3,55]
2. Most commonly present in the third or fourth decade.
   a. Average age at diagnosis is 27[12]
3. Slight male predominance.[39]
4. Associated with neurofibromatosis and the Rendu-Osler-Weber, Klippel-Trenaunay-Weber,[56] and Parkes-Weber syndromes.[57]
5. Aneurysms are present in 20–44% of cases and are associated with haemorrhage.[12,58,59]
6. Spinal cord AVMs are located in the cervical cord in 30% of cases and in the thoracolumbar cord in 70%, which is proportional to the volume of the spinal cord at each segment.[39]
7. Conus AVMs comprise a special category of spinal cord AVMs.[2,60] They are attributed to an abnormality during neurulation and are associated with a tethered cord.[61] Conus AVMs are typically extensive and possess multiple arterial feeders.
8. Presentation:
   a. Symptoms may be acute or progressive, although in most cases the symptoms develop relatively rapidly.[62]
   b. Haemorrhage (intraparenchymal or subarachnoid haemorrhage) is the most common presenting symptom.[12,62,63]
   c. Mortality associated with haemorrhage is 10–20%[64]
   d. Haemorrhage at presentation may be more common among children with cord AVMs compared with adults.[65]
   e. Re-haemorrhage appears to happen at higher rates for spinal cord AVMs compared with brain AVMs, occurring in 10% of patients at 1 month and in 40% within the first year after the initial haemorrhage.[64]
   f. Venous congestion may also produce symptoms in the absence of haemorrhage.[66]
   g. Conus AVMs may present with myelopathy or radiculopathy.

   Supply of conus AVMs can be provided by the artery of Desproges-Goteron (aka the cone artery). This artery may arise from the internal iliac artery or its branches.[67]

9. Imaging:
   a. MRI is highly sensitive and is able to detect all, or nearly all spinal cord AVMs.[51,68,69]
      i. MRI findings include a focal dilatation of the cord around the lesion, an area of low signal around the nidus on T1- and T2-weighted imaging that corresponds to haemosiderin deposition, and multiple flow voids (on axial images) and serpentine structures (on sagittal and coronal images) due to feeding and draining vessels.
      ii. T2 signal change may represent cord oedema due to venous congestion.[66]
      iii. Subacute haemorrhage appears as increased signal on FLAIR and T1-weighted images.
   b. Catheter angiography remains the *gold standard* for the evaluation of spinal cord AVMs.[39] A complete angiogram to characterize all feeding and draining vessels, look for aneurysms, and distinguish the lesion from associated normal vessels is necessary to plan treatment.
      i. Selective injection of numerous arteries is necessary to fully characterize a cord AVM, as feeding vessels may arise from sources as far afield as the occipital, ascending pharyngeal, vertebral, ascending and deep cervical, supreme intercostal, intercostal, lumbar, and the lateral and median sacral arteries.[64]

Management

The natural history of untreated intramedullary AVMs is not clear. Progressive evolution of symptoms, by either worsening myelopathy or subsequent haemorrhages, is reported in 31–71% of patients observed over several years.[12,65,70,71] Because spinal cord AVM anatomy is variable and the risk of potential complications on any procedure involving the cord is relatively high, decision making about the management of these patients is highly individualized. Patients with a cord AVM consisting of a compact, surgically accessible nidus may be good candidates for surgery. Embolization may be a useful adjunct to surgery, or, in some cases, may provide symptomatic relief without necessarily obliterating the lesion. There is a school of thought that holds that partial embolization of spinal cord AVMs, even with impermanent materials (such as PVA) may provide an (impermanent) improvement in symptoms such as pain and myelopathy.[70] The notion that partial treatment of cord AVMs lowers the risk of haemorrhage, which is generally believed not to be the case with intracranial AVMs, is more controversial.

Surgical Considerations

1. Embolization of major feeders prior to surgery can be helpful,[58,72,73] particularly for lesions with multiple feeding vessels, such as conus AVMs.[60]
   Alternatively, intraoperative angiography may be helpful in localizing the lesion during surgery.[74]
2. With *appropriate case selection* (i.e., by operating on patients with a relatively compact, surgically accessible nidus), angiographic obliteration of the lesion can be achieved in up to 94% of cases.[62]
   Surgery for diffuse spinal cord AVMs has been reported. In a series of three cases, the lesion was obliterated in all; neurological outcome improved in one patient and deteriorated slightly to mildly in the other two patients.[75]
3. Surgical approach is via a standard laminotomy. Exposure should extend at least one level above and one level below the lesion. A small myelotomy is done in the posterior median sulcus, and the spinal cord is split between the two posterior columns. Alternatively, a posterolateral myelotomy, done in the dorsal root entry zone between two or more nerve roots, can provide access to lateral lesions.
4. In one series, delayed imaging (mean follow-up, 8.5 years) in patients with no evidence of residual AVM on early postoperative imaging detected new draining veins in 23% of cases.[62]

5. Outcomes with surgery:
   a. As expected, surgical results are better with compact AVMs compared with AVMs with a diffuse nidus.[4]
   b. Surgical series overall clinical results:
      i) Neurologic improvement in 40%,[62] 87%[4]
      ii) Neurologically unchanged 53%,[62] 10%[4]
      iii) Neurologically worsened in 7%,[62] 3%[4]
   c. *Good functional outcome* in 86%[62]
   d. Chronic dysesthetic pain syndromes are common, affecting two-thirds of patients.[62]

Endovascular Considerations

1. Complete obliteration rates with embolization range from 24% to 53%[64,76]
2. Transient complication rates are 10.6–14%[64,76] and permanent complication rates are also 10.6–14%[64,76]
3. Biondi et al. advocate routine yearly spinal angiography and embolization with PVA, regardless of symptoms.[70] Despite frequent lesion revascularization, 63% of patients demonstrated long-term clinical improvement with this strategy. Worsening of symptoms after embolization was observed in 20% of patients.
4. Some authors assert that partial embolization of spinal cord AVMs is protective against haemorrhage, unlike brain AVMs.[39,40]
5. Choice of embolic agent:
   a. The first-line agent for embolization of any cord AVM should be NBCA or Onyx, provided that the microcatheter tip can be placed within the nidus.
   b. If the microcatheter tip can be placed close to the nidus, but beyond angiographically visible normal spinal cord vessels, NBCA is still a good choice.
   c. Particulate embolization should be reserved for cases in which the microcatheter tip is relatively proximal to the lesion. *Flow-directed* embolization with a particulate agent will theoretically carry most of the particles past normal branches and into the nidus. Injection should be done slowly and carefully, without attempting to completely occlude the nidus.
      i. Sizing of the particulate agent is based on the following reasoning: Because the normal anterior spinal artery diameter is 340–1,100 μm and the normal sulcal artery diameter is 60–72 μm, particles with a diameter of 150–250 μm should pass through the anterior spinal artery and into the AVM nidus without entering the normal sulcal arteries.[77,78]
      ii. Although PVA is the particulate agent of choice by some operators, PVA size is highly variable. The authors of this handbook prefer to use 100–300 μm Bead Block™ Microspheres (Terumo Medical Corporation, Somerset, NJ) or 100–300 μm Embosphere® Microspheres (BioSphere Medical, Inc., Rockland, MA).

Radiosurgery

In a preliminary report of stereotactic radiosurgery for intramedullary AVMs, six of seven patients at least 3 years from treatment had a significant reduction in AVM volume, and one patient with a conus lesion was found to have complete angiographic obliteration.[79]

20.3. Type III: Juvenile Arteriovenous Malformation

Type III lesions (aka juvenile, metameric, or extradural-intradural AVM) are complex AVMs that have both intradural and extradural components, and typically involve the spinal cord, vertebra, and paraspinal muscles (Fig. 20.3). The portion of the nidus involving the spinal cord typically has neural tissue within its interstices. They

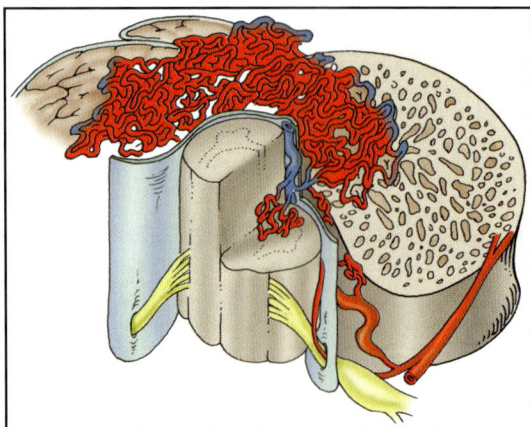

Fig. 20.3 Type III juvenile AVM. Type III lesions characteristically extend across tissue planes from the spinal cord into the adjacent bone and muscle.

are high-flow lesions, and may have a bruit over the lesion. They are extremely rare and may appear as part of Cobb syndrome (see below). Patients are typically children or young adults (thus the term *juvenile*), and present with pain and/or myelopathy. These AVMs typically have multiple feeding vessels arising from diverse locations, such as the vertebral arteries, radicular arteries, and other cervical vessels. Catheter angiography of a juvenile AVM can be somewhat like shining a small flashlight on an elephant in a dark room – only a part of the lesion can be seen with injection of contrast into any particular artery. These lesions are extremely difficult to treat. Although complete lesion resection by staged embolization followed by surgery has been reported,[80,81] fatal complications with this approach have also been reported.[6]

Cobb Syndrome

Cobb syndrome is a rare congenital disorder with a slight male predominance characterized by a combination of vascular skin naevi and a spinal vascular lesion occurring within the same metameres (i.e., the skin lesions are found in the dermatomes corresponding to the spinal levels where the spine lesion is). It was first described by Stanley Cobb, a resident of Harvey Cushing, in a report of a 8-year-old boy who presented with paraplegia.[82] The child had naevi over the 9th to 12th ribs, and at surgery he was found to have an angioma of the thoracic spinal cord. The spinal vascular lesion that occurs as part of Cobb syndrome may be a type III AVM, or a less complex lesion such as a perimedullary AV fistula.[83] Therefore, type III spinal vascular lesions and Cobb syndrome are not exactly synonymous.

20.4. Type IV: Intradural Perimedullary Arteriovenous Fistula

Type IV lesions (aka perimedullary, or ventral intradural AV fistulas) are located on the pial surface of the spinal cord, usually on the anterior or lateral surface (Fig. 20.4). They consist of a fistula between a spinal cord artery or arteries and the coronal venous plexus, and there is often a varix at the artery-to-vein transition site.

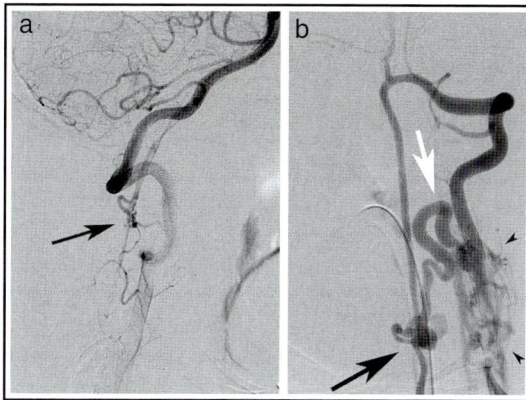

Fig. 20.4 Type IV perimedullary AV fistulas. Lateral view, vertebral artery injection (**a**), showing a small cervical Type A ventral perimedullary AV fistula (*arrow*) fed by several small pedicles arising from the vertebral artery. Frontal view, vertebral artery injection (**b**), showing a large Type C ventral perimedullary AV fistula (*black arrow*), fed by two large arteries, one from superior to the fistula and the other coming from an inferior source. Drainage is into a single vein (*white arrow*), which empties into the spinal venous plexus (*arrow heads*).

Table 20.1 Subtypes of perimedullary AV fistulas

Type	Arterial supply	Venous drainage	Primary mode of treatment
A	Anterior spinal artery only	Ascending	Surgery
B	Anterior and posterolateral spinal arteries	Ascending	Embolization ± surgery
C	Anterior and posterolateral spinal arteries	Dilated segmental veins	Embolization

Type IV lesions account for 13–17% of all spinal vascular lesions.[12,55] They were origi- nally subdivided into type I, II, or III lesions depending on size and complexity;[84] sub- sequent authors have adopted a type A–C system.[2] (Table 20.1). An association with split cord malformation has been reported.[85] Type B and C lesions are associated with Rendu-Osler-Weber and Cobb syndrome.[86]

1. Type A: The least common type IV lesion. Small, single-vessel fistula supplied by the anterior spinal artery, usually located on the anterior surface of the conus or on the upper part of the filum terminale. Venous drainage is slow and is in a rostral direction.
2. Type B: Larger, multiple-vessel fistulae supplied by the anterior and posterolat- eral spinal arteries, usually located on the posterolateral or anterolateral sur- face of the conus. Venous drainage is slow and is in a rostral direction.
3. Type C: The most common type IV lesion (Fig. 20.4). These lesions consist of a single giant fistula supplied by multiple, enlarged feeders from the anterior and posterolateral spinal arteries. They are located on the thoracic cord, or, less com- monly the cervical cord.[55,87] Venous drainage is rapid and into segmental veins.

Clinical Features

1. Patients are relatively young. The average age at presentation is 20–25 years (range 2–42)[55,86]
2. No sex predominance.

3. The location of these lesions along the spinal axis is bimodal, with most occurring at the thoracolumbar junction, particularly at the conus, and, to a lesser extent, in the upper cervical region.[88]
4. Rarely, perimedullary AVFs may develop after spinal cord surgery.[84,89]
5. Presentation:
   a. The majority of patients (91%) present with an asymmetric, slowly progressive myeloradiculopathy of the conus and cauda equina.[55]
   b. An acute onset of symptoms is less common and is usually seen only in patients with type B and C lesions.[55]
   c. Subarachnoid haemorrhage is a presenting feature in 20–40% of cases.[55,86]
6. Imaging:
   a. Type B and C lesions characteristically demonstrate large flow voids on MRI scanning.[86] However, it is important to note that type I lesions may not be apparent on MRI,[90] and myelography or angiography should be done if a type IV-A lesion is suspected but not seen on MRI.
   b. Apparent diffusion coefficient (ADC) values may be reduced, indicating vasogenic oedema, and may normalize after treatment.[91]
   c. CTA diagnosis of type IV-A lesions has been reported.[92]
   d. Catheter angiography is necessary to make a clear diagnosis of a perimedullary fistula and plan therapy.

Management

Because type IV lesions are rare, published series are limited, and firm conclusions about treatment cannot be made. Estimations of the natural history of untreated lesions suggest progression from myelopathy to paraplegia within 5–7 years, and a high incidence of repeated haemorrhage in patients presenting with haemorrhage.[12,55,84,87,88] Most authors recommend prompt diagnosis and treatment of perimedullary fistulae to minimize neurological injury.[12,55,84,87] The objective of treatment should be occlusion of the fistula. The absence of a nidus facilitates surgery;[55] most lesions can be effectively obliterated with either surgery or embolization, or a combination of both.[3,55,86,93,94]
1. Type A: Most authors recommend that subtype A lesions should be treated with surgery, as catheterization of the anterior spinal artery is problematic.[55,84,87,95,96]
2. Type B: Embolization or embolization followed by surgery can occlude the fistula in nearly all cases.[55,87]
3. Type C: Embolization is usually the first-line treatment of type C lesions.[97] Complete occlusion was achieved by embolization alone in 68% of patients with type C lesions.[55]
4. Clinical outcome appears to be somewhat variable, with partial neurological improvement or no change occurring in the majority of patients, and worsening in a small minority of patients.[55,87]

Extradural Arteriovenous Fistula

Spinal extradural AV fistulas (aka epidural AV fistulas, extradural AVMs, or perivertebral AVMs) are rare.[98–103]
1. Classification. The following classification system was recently proposed:[104]
   a. Type A
      Extradural AV fistula with both an arterialized epidural venous plexus and an arterialized vein that pierces the dura, travels intradurally, and drains into the venous plexus that surrounds the spinal cord. This lesion differs from a Type I dural AV fistula in that in a Type A extradural AV fistula the intradural draining vein arises from a extradural venous pouch, whereas in a Type I dural fistula the AV shunt lies within the nerve root sheath and drains directly into an intradural drain.[2,102,104]
   b. Type B1
      Extradural AV fistula that drains only into the Batson plexus with compression of the thecal sac and with myelopathy.
   c. Type B2
      Extradural AV fistula that drains only into the Batson plexus *without* compression of the thecal sac and *without* myelopathy.

2. Imaging
>Type A lesions typically are associated with cord oedema and perimedullary flow voids on MRI.[104] Spinal angiography is necessary for diagnosis.[105] DynaCT (injection of 40 mL of 20% diluted iodinated contrast during 20 s of rotation) provides complementary information to catheter angiography and can help in clarifying the relationships between the fistula and the spinal canal, spinal cord, nerve roots, and surrounding structures.[104]

3. Management
>Options include n-BCA[104] Onyx,[104] or coil embolization[100] and surgical resection.[105]

Spinal Cord Aneurysms

Spinal cord aneurysms are rare. Most are discovered as flow-related lesions associated with an intramedullary AVM, although isolated spinal cord aneurysms do occur.[106–108] and can cause subarachnoid haemorrhage.[108] Spinal aneurysms may explain SAH when no intracranial aneurysm is found; often the patient complains of back or neck pain in addition to and often beginning before the classic headache of SAH. Particularly large aneurysms may present with symptoms of myelopathy or radiculopathy.[106] There appears to be a strong association with developmental vascular anomalies, as metameric angiomatosis was found in 43% of patients in a series of cord aneurysms.[59] Spinal aneurysms are typically fusiform in shape and thus very difficult to treat directly with endovascular techniques.[106] Surgery of spinal cord aneurysms with trapping[106] and wrapping[109] has been reported. Disappearance or a decrease in size of the aneurysm was observed in several patients who underwent treatment of an associated intramedullary AVM.[58] Importantly, even solitary spinal cord aneurysms may spontaneously regress without treatment.[108]

Intramedullary Cavernous Malformation

Cavernous malformations (aka cavernomas) are distributed along the entire neuroaxis and represent 5–12% of all spinal vascular lesions.[110,111] See Chap. 16 for a discussion of intracranial cavernous malformations. Rarely, spinal cavernous malformations may be found in an epidural location.[112] Spinal cavernomas are histologically identical to those in the brain. They are angiographically occult and have a characteristic appearance on MRI.[111] As many as 40% of patients with a spinal cavernoma have similar intracranial lesions.[113] As in the brain, spinal cord cavernomas are frequently associated with a developmental venous anomaly.[109] A systematic review found a female predominance with a peak age at presentation in the forth decade.[114] Symptoms is highly variable and the natural history of symptomatic spinal cavernomas is far from clear. Annual rates of symptomatic rehaemorrhage range from 0%[115] to 66%.[116] Although surgical series report relatively good results,[111,114,117] expectant management of selected patients may also be reasonable.[115] A recent report of long-term results in 80 patients after resection found:[118]

1. Immediately after surgery:
   a. 11% of patients were worse
   b. 83% were the same
   c. 6% improved
2. Perioperative complications occurred in 6% of patients.
3. At mean follow-up of 5 years:
   a. 10% of patients were worse
   b. 68% were the same
   c. 23% were improved
4. Long-term complications, including kyphotic deformity, stenosis and spinal cord tethering, occurred in 14% of patients.

Vascular Spinal Tumours

- Vascular spinal tumors include haemangioma, haemangioblastoma, metastatic tumours, aneurysmal bone cyst, osteoblastoma, angiosarcoma, haemangiopericytoma, angiofibroma, angiolipoma, haemangioendothelioma.
- Indications and technique for endovascular embolization of these lesions is discussed in Chap. 8.

Spinal Cord Infarction

Any part of the central nervous system may suffer ischaemic injury, and this may occur in the spinal cord. Spinal cord ischaemia in the cord is uncommon and may be misdiagnosed as other pathological processes such as transverse myelitis. Cord ischaemia is becoming increasingly recognized due increasing clinical awareness of this condition, especially in association with stent-grafting for aortic aneurysms. Brain ischaemia is discussed in Chap. 17.

Epidemiology and Clinical Features

1. Spinal cord ischaemia is uncommon, representing 1.2% of stroke cases.[119]
2. More common in women.[120–122]
3. Mean age is 56 years (range 19–80) [120]
4. A Norwegian study showed patients with spinal cord infarction were younger, more likely to be female and less likely to have hypertension or cardiac disease than patients with brain infarctions.[122]
5. Presentation:
   a. Some 59% of patients have abrupt onset of back or neck pain at onset of myelopathic symptoms, usually radicular in nature along the distribution of cord injury.[120]
   b. Symptoms develop quickly, within 2 minutes in most cases.[120]
   c. Symptoms develop immediately after a movement in 48% of cases of spontaneous cord infarction.[120] Associated movements include motion of the back, neck, arm or a Valsalva maneuver.
   d. The sudden nature of the ictus and frequent association with pain may mimic symptoms of angina or myocardial infarction.[123,124]
   e. Symptoms occurred a median of 10.6 h post-operatively in spinal cord ischaemia associated with aortic aneurysm therapy.[125]
   f. Symptoms of myelopathy in spontaneous cord ischaemia can be classified according to geographic distribution in the cord:[120]
      i. 37% had anterior spinal artery infarction with:
         Bilateral motor deficit with spinothalamic sensory deficit.
      ii. 15% had anterior unilateral cord infarction with:
         Hemiparesis with contralateral spinothalamic sensory deficit.
      iii. 15% had posterior unilateral cord infarction with:
         Hemiparesis with ipsilateral lemniscal sensory deficit.
      iv. 11% had central cord infarction with:
         Bilateral spinothalamic sensory deficit but no motor deficit.
      v. 7% had posterior spinal artery infarction with:
         Bilateral motor deficit with lemniscal sensory deficit.
      vi. 7% had transverse cord infarction with:
         Bilateral motor deficit and complete sensory deficit.
      vii. 7% had an unclassifiable pattern.
   g. In 1911, Dejerine described the spinal equivalent of transient ischaemic attacks with repeated stereotypical but transient symptoms of myelopathy.[126]
      i. This has been called *spinal claudication of Dejerine*.[127]
      ii. These transient symptoms may portend infarction in the cord with more persistent motor deficits, most commonly occurring in a cervical cord distribution.[120]
      iii. Periodic transient episodes of myelopathy should also raise suspicion of a Type I dAVF.[8]
6. Imaging
   a. High resolution MRI shows acute spinal cord ischaemic lesions in 67% of patients with suspected acute cord ischaemia.[120]
   b. Ischaemic areas appear hyperintense on T2 weighted images.
   c. Associated high T2 signal in the adjacent vertebral body has been touted as a very specific sign of spinal cord infarction.[128,129]
      i. Another study of cord ischaemia unrelated to aortic surgery showed associated vertebral body signal abnormalities to be uncommon.[120]
      ii. Associated vertebral body signal abnormalities were found to be a strong indicator for the presence of underlying aortic disease.[130]

d. MRI may also show disc disease or bone spurs that may be the cause of vascular compromise.[120]
e. Echo-planar diffusion imaging shows early cord ischaemia.[131,132]
f. Line scan diffusion imaging of the spinal cord is less vulnerable to artifact compared to standard MRI.[133,134]

Etiology

1. No apparent cause is found in 74% of spontaneous cord infarction.[120]
2. Post-aorta surgery
   a. Spinal cord infarction has long been known as a potential complication of surgery for aortic aneurysms.[135,136]
   b. The rate of spinal cord ischaemia in one recent series of open surgical repair of ruptured aortic aneurysms was only 1.2%, but half of all patients treated died.[137]
   c. A systematic review comparing open and endovascular therapy for thoracic aortic aneurysms showed significantly lower mortality and lower spinal cord ischaemia with endovascular stent-grafting.[138]
   d. A systematic review of studies totaling 1,895 patients found a 0–12.5% (mean 2.7%) incidence of cord infarction.[121]
   e. A more recent review of elective aortic stent-grafting in 1,038 patients found a similar 3.1% incidence of post-operative paraplegia.[139]
   f. Aortic stent grafting seems to have a slightly higher risk of cerebral ischaemic complications (4.7%) compared with the spinal ischaemic complications (3.1%)[125]
   g. Risk factors for spinal cord ischaemia after aorta surgery:
      i. Pre-existing renal insufficiency.[125]
      ii. Peri-operative mean arterial pressure <70 mmHg[140]
3. Other surgical procedures associated with postoperative spinal cord ischaemia:
   a. Spinal stabilization procedures.[141,142]
   b. Posterior fossa craniotomy.[143–145]
   c. Procedures using epidural anesthesia, especially in the setting of underlying spinal stenosis, atherosclerotic disease, or use of epinephrine in local anesthetic.[141]
   d. Any surgical procedure having severe perioperative hypotension, especially with associated aortic disease.[141]
4. Other aortic procedures associated with cord ischaemia:
   a. Aortic angiography.[146,147]
   b. Bronchial artery embolization for haemoptysis.[148]
   c. Umbilical artery catheterization in newborns.[149]
   d. Intra-aortic balloon-pump usage.[150] Hypotension could also have been a factor.
5. Aortic disease itself can cause spontaneous cord infarction:
   a. Dissections and dissecting aneurysms are a cause of haemorrhagic and non-haemorrhagic cord infarction.[151,152]
6. Vertebral artery dissection can cause cervical cord infarction.[153,154]
7. Prolonged arterial hypotension for any reason, with or without diffuse atherosclerotic disease has been implicated in some cases.[120,155]
8. Fibrocartilagenous emboli
   a. Acute myelopathy after sudden axial spine loading, often in association with Valsalva maneuver.[156,157]
   b. This has been reported in a ballet dancer.[158]
   c. Most cases go without a diagnosis until autopsy, where small fragments of what looks like intervertebral disc are occluding the anterior spinal artery.[159]
   d. Exactly how the disc material finds its way into the arterial system of the cord is unknown.
   e. When acute onset of pain and weakness during an activity producing an axial load on the spine occurs in a young patient with no other risk factors, one can suspect the diagnosis. At a large center, fibrocartilagenous emboli were suspected in 5.5% of spinal infarct patients.[160]
9. Rare inflammatory causes
   a. Bacterial sepsis, pachymeningitis and vasculitis.[161]
   b. Meningitis.[162]

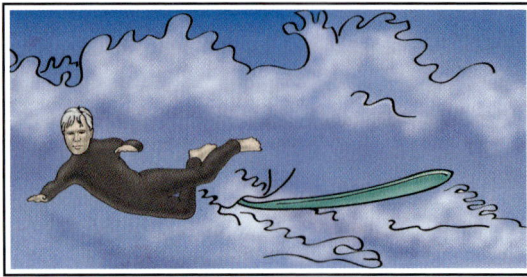

Fig. 20.5 Surfer's myelopathy. This is a depiction of an inexperienced surfer in action. Note the extended back, indicating he is susceptible to spinal cord watershed territory ischaemia.

10. Trauma related cord ischaemia
    a. Major trauma with aortic injury may cause spinal infarction.[163]
    b. Even minor trauma can cause cord ischaemia, especially in children.[164]
    c. Cord ischaemia is postulated in some minor trauma cases as the final pathway resulting in the syndrome of *spinal cord injury without radiographic abnormality* (SCIWORA)[165]
    d. "Surfer's myelopathy" is a syndrome of spinal cord ischaemia from thoracic spine hyperextension in novice surfers (Fig. 20.5)[166,167]
    e. Spinal cord infarction can be associated with acute decompression sickness in divers, and is thought to be due to venous obstruction.[168]
11. Drug-related cord infarction:
    a. A case of cervical cord infarction was associated with the use of sildenafil (Viagra, Pfizer, New York, NY)[169]
    b. Epidural steroid injections, in which the agent is inadvertently injected in arteries supplying the cord.[170–172]
        i. Risk of cord ischaemia may be higher in transforaminal injections.[173]
12. Thrombophilia implicated in cord ischaemia:
    a. G20210A allele of prothrombin gene plus oral birth control pills are associated with cord infarction in a young woman.[174]
    b. G20210A allele alone is associated with acute quadriplegia in a young man.[175]
    c. Essential thrombocythemia is associated with cord ischaemia.[176]

Management

1. Cerebrospinal fluid drainage by placement of a lumbar drain has been advocated.[177,178] Most reports are small series, necessitated by the rarity of spinal cord ischaemia.
    a. Lumbar drains are placed and usually drained to 10 cm H_2O. The theory is that a lower cerebral spinal fluid pressure decreases resistance to spinal cord arterial flow.
    b. An often-quoted study from Safi and colleagues showed a significant reduction in the incidence of cord ischaemia in a consecutive series of patients with aortic aneurysm surgery treated with prophylactic intraoperative distal aortic perfusion and perioperative lumbar drains compared to an earlier series not having these measures.[179]
    c. However, another report of prophylactic lumbar drains placed patients receiving endovascular aortic stent grafts found a 7.4% incidence of cord ischaemia, which was no better than earlier studies without prophylactic drains.[180]
    d. Lumbar drains in the setting of aortic aneurysm repair are associated with a 3.7% rate of catheter-related complications, with no permanent sequelae.[181]

2. Arterial blood pressure augmentation could theoretically improve spinal cord perfusion and has been utilized in patients developing clinical or SSEP evidence of cord ischaemia after aortic stent grafting.[182] Of six patients with signs of cord ischaemia, two resolved completely with blood pressure augmentation alone, another two resolved with both pressure augmentation and lumbar CSF drainage, and another one improved incompletely with both interventions.
3. A small series showed no benefit from steroid therapy.[160]
4. A single case of successful intravenous thrombolytic therapy for a patient with symptoms of spinal cord ischaemia after an abdominal angiographic study was reported.[147] This is insufficient evidence of the efficacy of tPA in this setting.

Outcome

1. A series of 44 patients with cord infarction reported improved motor function in 12 and complete recovery in only one.[183]
2. Another series of spinal cord infarct had a 22% in-hospital mortality, at discharge 57% were wheelchair-bound, 25% ambulatory with assistance, and 17.9% fully ambulatory.[184]
3. Another series had motor recovery in only 20% of anterior spinal occlusive disease.[185]
4. Post-operative cord ischaemia after aortic stent-grafting can have a more favourable outcome with seven of nine affected patients showing complete restoration of function.[125]
5. A large single center study showed 4.5% permanent post-operative cord ischaemia.[186]

References

1. Borden JA, Wu JK, Shucart WA. A proposed classification for spinal and cranial dural arteriovenous fistulous malformations and implications for treatment. J Neurosurg. 1995;82: 166–79.
2. Spetzler RF, Detwiler PW, Riina HA, Porter RW. Modified classification of spinal cord vascular lesions. J Neurosurg. 2002;96:145–56.
3. Bao YH, Ling F. Classification and therapeutic modalities of spinal vascular malformations in 80 patients. Neurosurgery. 1997;40:75–81.
4. Zozulya YP, Slin'ko EL, Al II Q. Spinal arteriovenous malformations: new classification and surgical treatment. Neurosurg Focus. 2006;20:E7.
5. Anson JA, Spetzler RF. Interventional neuroradiology for spinal pathology. Clin Neurosurg. 1992;39:388–417.
6. Ferch RD, Morgan MK, Sears WR. Spinal arteriovenous malformations: a review with case illustrations. J Clin Neurosci. 2001;8:299–304.
7. Gilbertson JR, Miller GM, Goldman MS, Marsh WR. Spinal dural arteriovenous fistulas: MR and myelographic findings. AJNR Am J Neuroradiol. 1995;16:2049–57.
8. Jellema K, Canta LR, Tijssen CC, van Rooij WJ, Koudstaal PJ, van Gijn J. Spinal dural arteriovenous fistulas: clinical features in 80 patients. J Neurol Neurosurg Psychiatry. 2003; 74:1438–40.
9. Van Dijk JM, TerBrugge KG, Willinsky RA, Farb RI, Wallace MC. Multidisciplinary management of spinal dural arteriovenous fistulas: clinical presentation and long-term follow-up in 49 patients. Stroke. 2002;33:1578–83.
10. Thron A. Spinal dural arteriovenous fistulas. Radiologe. 2001;41:955–60.
11. Atkinson JLD, Miller GM, Krauss WE, et al. Clinical and radiographic features of dural arteriovenous fistula, a treatable cause of myelopathy. Mayo Clin Proc. 2001;76:1120–30.
12. Rosenblum B, Oldfield EH, Doppman JL, Di Chiro G. Spinal arteriovenous malformations: a comparison of dural arteriovenous fistulas and intradural AVM's in 81 patients. J Neurosurg. 1987;67:795–802.
13. Heier LA, Lee BC. A dural spinal arteriovenous malformation with epidural venous drainage: a case report. AJNR Am J Neuroradiol. 1987;8:561–3.
14. Arnaud O, Bille F, Pouget J, Serratrice G, Salamon G. Epidural arteriovenous fistula with perimedullary venous drainage: case report. Neuroradiology. 1994;36:490–1.
15. Pirouzmand F, Wallace MC, Willinsky R. Spinal epidural arteriovenous fistula with intramedullary reflux. Case report. J Neurosurg. 1997;87:633–5.
16. Koch C. Spinal dural arteriovenous fistula. Curr Opin Neurol. 2006;19:69–75.
17. Koch C, Kucinski T, Eckert B, Rother J, Zeumer H. Spinal dural arteriovenous fistula: clinical and radiological findings in 54 patients. Rofo. 2003;175:1071–8.
18. Bowen BC, Fraser K, Kochan JP, Pattany PM, Green BA, Quencer RM. Spinal dural arteriovenous fistulas: evaluation with MR angiography. AJNR Am J Neuroradiol. 1995;16:2029–43.
19. Morris JM, Kaufmann TJ, Campeau NG, Cloft HJ, Lanzino G. Volumetric myelographic magnetic resonance imaging to localize difficult-to-find spinal dural arteriovenous fistulas. J Neurosurg Spine. 2011;14:398–404.
20. Willinsky R, Lasjaunias P, Terbrugge K, Hurth M. Angiography in the investigation of spinal dural arteriovenous fistula. A protocol with application of the venous phase. Neuroradiology. 1990;32:114–6.
21. Watson JC, Oldfield EH. The surgical management of spinal dural vascular malformations. Neurosurg Clin N Am. 1999;10:73–87.
22. Partington MD, Rufenacht DA, Marsh WR, Piepgras DG. Cranial and sacral dural arteriovenous fistulas as a cause of myelopathy. J Neurosurg. 1992;76:615–22.
23. Woimant F, Merland JJ, Riche MC, et al. Bulbospinal syndrome related to a meningeal arteriovenous fistula of the lateral sinus draining into spinal cord veins. Rev Neurol (Paris). 1982;138:559–66.
24. Wrobel CJ, Oldfield EH, Di Chiro G, Tarlov EC, Baker RA, Doppman JL. Myelopathy due to intracranial dural arteriovenous fistulas draining intrathecally into spinal medullary veins. Report of three cases. J Neurosurg. 1988;69:934–9.
25. Trop I, Roy D, Raymond J, Roux A, Bourgouin P, Lesage J. Craniocervical dural fistula associated with cervical myelopathy: angiographic demonstration of normal venous drainage of the thoracolumbar cord does not rule out diagnosis. AJNR Am J Neuroradiol. 1998;19:583–6.
26. Britz GW, Lazar D, Eskridge J, Winn HR. Accurate intraoperative localization of spinal dural arteriovenous fistulae with embolization coil: technical note. Neurosurgery. 2004;55:252–4; discussion 254–5.
27. N'Diaye M, Chiras J, Meder JF, Barth MO, Koussa A, Bories J. Water-soluble myelography for the study of dural arteriovenous fistulae of the spine draining in the spinal venous system. J Neuroradiol. 1984;11:327–39.
28. Tadie M, Hemet J, Freger P, Clavier E, Creissard P. Morphological and functional anatomy of spinal cord veins. J Neuroradiol. 1985;12:3–20.
29. Benhaiem N, Poirier J, Hurth M. Arteriovenous fistulae of the meninges draining into the spinal veins. A histological study of 28 cases. Acta Neuropathol (Berl). 1983;62:103–11.
30. Hassler W, Thron A, Grote EH. Hemodynamics of spinal dural arteriovenous fistulas. An intraoperative study. Neurosurg. 1989;70:360–70.
31. Jellema K, Tijssen CC, Fijnheer R, de Groot PG, Koudstaal PJ, van Gijn J. Spinal dural arteriovenous fistulas are not associated with prothrombotic factors. Stroke. 2004;35:2069–71.
32. Foix C, Alajouanine T. Subacute necrotic myelitis, slowly progressive central myelitis with vascular hyperplasia, and slowly ascending, increasingly flaccid amyotrophic paraplegia accompanied by albuminocytologic dissociation (in French). Rev Neurol (Paris). 1926;33:1–42.
33. Finsterer J, Bavinzski G, Ungersbock K. Spinal dural arteriovenous fistula associated with syringomyelia. J Neuroradiol. 2000;27:211–4.
34. Vankan Y, Demaerel P, Heye S, et al. Dural arteriovenous fistula as a late complication of upper cervical spine fracture. Case report. J Neurosurg. 2004;100:382–4.
35. Asakuno K, Kim P, Kawamoto T, Ogino M. Dural arteriovenous fistula and progressive conus medullaris syndrome as complications of lumbar discectomy. Case report. J Neurosurg. 2002;97:375–9.
36. Flannery T, Tan MH, Flynn P, Choudhari KA. Delayed postsurgical development of dural arteriovenous fistula after cervical meningocele repair. Neurol India. 2003;51:390–1.
37. Aminoff MJ, Logue V. The prognosis of patients with spinal vascular malformations. Brain. 1974;97:211–8.
38. Steinmetz MP, Chow MM, Krishnaney AA, et al. Outcome after the treatment of spinal dural arteriovenous fistulae: a contemporary single-institution series and meta-analysis. Neurosurgery. 2004;55:77–87; discussion 87–8.
39. Niimi Y, Berenstein A. Endovascular treatment of spinal vascular malformations. Neurosurg Clin N Am. 1999;10:47–71.
40. Afshar JK, Doppman JL, Oldfield EH. Surgical interruption of intradural draining vein as curative treatment of spinal dural arteriovenous fistulas. J Neurosurg. 1995;82:196–200.
41. Saladino AMD, Atkinson JLDMD, Rabinstein AAMD, et al. Surgical treatment of spinal dural arteriovenous fistulae: a consecutive series of 154 patients. Neurosurgery. 2010;67:1350–8.
42. Song JK, Gobin YP, Duckwiler GR, et al. N-butyl 2-cyanoacrylate embolization of spinal dural arteriovenous fistulae. AJNR Am J Neuroradiol. 2001;22:40–7.
43. Jellema K, Sluzewski M, van Rooij WJ, Tijssen CC, Beute GN. Embolization of spinal dural arteriovenous fistulas: importance of occlusion of the draining vein. J Neurosurg Spine. 2005;2:580–3.
44. Criscuolo GR, Oldfield EH, Doppman JL. Reversible acute and subacute myelopathy in patients with dural arteriovenous fistulas. Foix-Alajouanine syndrome reconsidered. Neurosurg. 1989;70:354–9.

45. Warakaulle DR, Aviv RI, Niemann D, Molyneux AJ, Byrne JV, Teddy P. Embolisation of spinal dural arteriovenous fistulae with Onyx. Neuroradiology. 2003;45:110–2.

46. Niimi Y, Berenstein A, Setton A, Neophytides A. Embolization of spinal dural arteriovenous fistulae: results and follow-up. Neurosurgery. 1997;40:675–82; discussion 682–3.

47. Morgan MK, Marsh WR. Management of spinal dural arteriovenous malformations. J Neurosurg. 1989;70:832–6.

48. Nichols DA, Rufenacht DA, Jack Jr CR, Forbes GS. Embolization of spinal dural arteriovenous fistula with polyvinyl alcohol particles: experience in 14 patients. AJNR Am J Neuroradiol. 1992;13:933–40.

49. McDougall CG, Deshmukh VR, Fiorella DJ, Albuquerque FC, Spetzler RF. Endovascular techniques for vascular malformations of the spinal axis. Neurosurg Clin N Am. 2005;16:395–410, x–xi.

50. Di Chiro G, Wener L. Angiography of the spinal cord. A review of contemporary techniques and applications. J Neurosurg. 1973;39:1–29.

51. Minami S, Sagoh T, Nishimura K, et al. Spinal arteriovenous malformation: MR imaging. Radiology. 1988;169:109–15.

52. Gaensler EH, Jackson Jr DE, Halbach VV. Arteriovenous fistulas of the cervicomedullary junction as a cause of myelopathy: radiographic findings in two cases. AJNR Am J Neuroradiol. 1990;11:518–21.

53. Renowden SA, Molyneux AJ. Case report: spontaneous thrombosis of a spinal dural AVM (Foix-Alajouanine syndrome)–magnetic resonance appearance. Clin Radiol. 1993;47:134–6.

54. Di Chiro G. Foix-Alajouanine syndrome. AJNR Am J Neuroradiol. 1990;11.1286.

55. Mourier KL, Gobin YP, George B, Lot G, Merland JJ. Intradural perimedullary arteriovenous fistulae: results of surgical and endovascular treatment in a series of 35 cases. Neurosurgery. 1993;32:885–91; discussion 891.

56. Djindjian M, Djindjian R, Hurth M, Rey A, Houdart R. Spinal cord arteriovenous malformations and the Klippel-Trenaunay-Weber syndrome. Surg Neurol. 1977;8:229–37.

57. Lasjaunias PL. Spinal arteriovenous shunts. Berlin: Springer; 1997.

58. Biondi A, Merland JJ, Hodes JE, Aymard A, Reizine D. Aneurysms of spinal arteries associated with intramedullary arteriovenous malformations. II. Results of AVM endovascular treatment and hemodynamic considerations. AJNR Am J Neuroradiol. 1992;13:923–31.

59. Biondi A, Merland JJ, Hodes JE, Pruvo JP, Reizine D. Aneurysms of spinal arteries associated with intramedullary arteriovenous malformations. I. Angiographic and clinical aspects. AJNR Am J Neuroradiol. 1992;13:913–22.

60. Gonzalez LF, Spetzler RF. Treatment of spinal vascular malformations: an integrated approach. Clin Neurosurg. 2005;52:192–201.

61. Hurst RW, Bagley LJ, Marcotte P, Schut L, Flamm ES. Spinal cord arteriovenous fistulas involving the conus medullaris: presentation, management, and embryologic considerations. Surg Neurol. 1999;52:95–9.

62. Connolly Jr ES, Zubay GP, McCormick PC, Stein BM. The posterior approach to a series of glomus (Type II) intramedullary spinal cord arteriovenous malformations. Neurosurgery. 1998;42:774–85; discussion 785–6.

63. Tobin WD, Layton DD. The diagnosis and natural history of spinal cord arteriovenous malformations. Mayo Clin Proc. 1976;51:637–46.

64. Berenstein A, Lasjaunias PL. Spine and spinal cord vascular lesions. In: Berenstein A, Lasjaunias PL, editors. Endovascular treatment of spine and spinal cord lesions, Surgical neuroangiography, vol. 5. Berlin: Springer; 1992. p. 1.

65. Riche MC, Modenesi-Freitas J, Djindjian M, Merland JJ. Arteriovenous malformations (AVM) of the spinal cord in children. A review of 38 cases. Neuroradiology. 1982;22:171–80.

66. Kataoka H, Miyamoto S, Nagata I, Ueba T, Hashimoto N. Venous congestion is a major cause of neurological deterioration in spinal arteriovenous malformations. Neurosurgery. 2001;48:1224–9; discussion 1229–30.

67. Tubbs RS, Mortazavi MM, Denardo AJ, Cohen-Gadol AA. Arteriovenous malformation of the conus supplied by the artery of Desproges-Gotteron. J Neurosurg Spine. 2011;14:529–31.

68. Doppman JL, Di Chiro G, Dwyer AJ, Frank JL, Oldfield EH. Magnetic resonance imaging of spinal arteriovenous malformations. J Neurosurg. 1987;66:830–4.

69. Dormont D, Gelbert F, Assouline E, et al. MR imaging of spinal cord arteriovenous malformations at 0.5 T: study of 34 cases. AJNR Am J Neuroradiol. 1988;9:833–8.

70. Biondi A, Merland JJ, Reizine D, et al. Embolization with particles in thoracic intramedullary arteriovenous malformations: long-term angiographic and clinical results. Radiology. 1990;177:651–8.

71. Yasargil MG, Symon L, Teddy PJ. Arteriovenous malformations of the spinal cord. Adv Tech Stand Neurosurg. 1984;11:61–102.

72. Ausman JI, Gold LH, Tadavarthy SM, Amplatz K, Chou SN. Intraparenchymal embolization for obliteration of an intramedullary AVM of the spinal cord. Technical note. J Neurosurg. 1977;47:119–25.

73. Latchaw RE, Harris RD, Chou SN, Gold LH. Combined embolization and operation in the treatment of cervical arteriovenous malformations. Neurosurgery. 1980;6:131–7.

74. Schievink WI, Vishteh AG, McDougall CG, Spetzler RF. Intraoperative spinal angiography. J Neurosurg. 1999;90:48–51.

75. Ohata K, Takami T, El-Naggar A, et al. Posterior approach for cervical intramedullary arteriovenous malformation with diffuse-type nidus. Report of three cases. J Neurosurg. 1999;91:105–11.

76. Rodesch G, Lasjaunias PL, Berenstein A. Embolization of arteriovenous malformations of the spinal cord. In: Valavanis A, editor. Interventional neuroradiology. Berlin: Springer; 1993. p. 135.

77. Horton JA, Latchaw RE, Gold LH, Pang D. Embolization of intramedullary arteriovenous malformations of the spinal cord. AJNR Am J Neuroradiol. 1986;7.113–8.

78. Theron J, Cosgrove R, Melanson D, Ethier R. Spinal arteriovenous malformations: advances in therapeutic embolization. Radiology. 1986;158:163–9.

79. Sinclair J, Chang SD, Gibbs IC, Adler Jr JR. Multisession CyberKnife radiosurgery for intramedullary spinal cord arteriovenous malformations. Neurosurgery. 2006;58:1081–9; discussion1081–9.

80. Spetzler RF, Zabramski JM, Flom RA. Management of juvenile spinal AVM's by embolization and operative excision. Case report. J Neurosurg. 1989;70:628–32.

81. Menku A, Akdemir H, Durak AC, Oktem IS. Successful surgical excision of juvenile-type spinal arteriovenous malformation in two stages following partial embolization. Minim Invasive Neurosurg. 2005;48:57–62.

82. Cobb S. Hemangioma of the spinal cord associated with skin naevi of the same metamer. Ann Surg. 1915;65:641–9.

83. Maramattom BV, Cohen-Gadol AA, Wijdicks EF, Kallmes D. Segmental cutaneous hemangioma and spinal arteriovenous malformation. (Cobb syndrome) Case report and historical perspective. J Neurosurg Spine. 2005;3:249–52.

84. Gueguen B, Merland JJ, Riche MC, Rey A. Vascular malformations of the spinal cord: intrathecal perimedullary arteriovenous fistulas fed by medullary arteries. Neurology. 1987;37:969–79.

85. Vitarbo EA, Sultan A, Wang D, Morcos JJ, Levi AD. Split cord malformation with associated type IV spinal cord perimedullary arteriovenous fistula. Case report. J Neurosurg Spine. 2005;3:400–4.

86. Halbach VV, Higashida RT, Dowd CF, Fraser KW, Edwards MS, Barnwell SL. Treatment of giant intradural (perimedullary) arteriovenous fistulas. Neurosurgery. 1993;33:972–9; discussion 979–80.

87. Hida K, Iwasaki Y, Goto K, Miyasaka K, Abe H. Results of the surgical treatment of perimedullary arteriovenous fistulas with special reference to embolization. J Neurosurg. 1999;90:198–205.

88. Djindjian M, Djindjian R, Rey A, Hurth M, Houdart R. Intradural extramedullary spinal arterio-venous malformations fed by the anterior spinal artery. Surg Neurol. 1977;8:85–93.

89. Barrow DL, Colohan AR, Dawson R. Intradural perimedullary arteriovenous fistulas (type IV spinal cord arteriovenous malformations). J Neurosurg. 1994;81:221–9.

90. Dillon WP, Norman D, Newton TH, Bolla K, Mark A. Intradural spinal cord lesions: Gd-DTPA-enhanced MR imaging. Radiology. 1989;170:229–37.

91. Inoue T, Takahashi T, Shimizu H, Matsumoto Y, Takahashi A, Tominaga T. Congestive myelopathy due to cervical perimedullary arteriovenous fistula evaluated by apparent diffusion coefficient values – case report. Neurol Med Chir (Tokyo). 2006;46:559–62.

92. Lai PH, Weng MJ, Lee KW, Pan HB. Multidetector CT angiography in diagnosing type I and type IVA spinal vascular malformations. AJNR Am J Neuroradiol. 2006;27:813–7.

93. Sure U, Wakat JP, Gatscher S, Becker R, Bien S, Bertalanffy H. Spinal type IV arteriovenous malformations (perimedullary fistulas) in children. Childs Nerv Syst. 2000;16:508–15.

94. Cho KT, Lee DY, Chung CK, Han MH, Kim HJ. Treatment of spinal cord perimedullary arteriovenous fistula: embolization versus surgery. Neurosurgery. 2005;56:232–41; discussion 232–41.

95. Heros RC, Debrun GM, Ojemann RG, Lasjaunias PL, Naessens PJ. Direct spinal arteriovenous fistula: a new type of spinal AVM. Case report. J Neurosurg. 1986;64:134–9.

96. Aminoff MJ, Gutin PH, Norman D. Unusual type of spinal arteriovenous malformation. Neurosurgery. 1988;22:589–91.

97. Ricolfi F, Gobin PY, Aymard A, Brunelle F, Gaston A, Merland JJ. Giant perimedullary arteriovenous fistulas of the spine: clinical and radiologic features and endovascular treatment. AJNR Am J Neuroradiol. 1997;18:677–87.

98. Clarke MJ, Patrick TA, White JB, et al. Spinal extradural arteriovenous malformations with parenchymal drainage: venous drainage variability and implications in clinical manifestations. Neurosurg Focus. 2009;26:E5.

99. Cognard C, Semaan H, Bakchine S, et al. Paraspinal arteriovenous fistula with perimedullary venous drainage. AJNR Am J Neuroradiol. 1995;16:2044–8.

100. Goyal M, Willinsky R, Montanera W, terBrugge K. Paravertebral arteriovenous malformations with epidural drainage: clinical spectrum, imaging features, and results of treatment. AJNR Am J Neuroradiol. 1999;20:749–55.

101. 3rd Hemphill JC, Smith WS, Halbach VV. Neurologic manifestations of spinal epidural arteriovenous malformations. Neurology. 1998;50:817–9.

102. Kim LJ, Spetzler RF. Classification and surgical management of spinal arteriovenous lesions: arteriovenous fistulae and arteriovenous malformations. Neurosurgery. 2006;59:S195–201; discussion S3–13.

103. Silva Jr N, Januel AC, Tall P, Cognard C. Spinal epidural arteriovenous fistulas associated with progressive myelopathy. Report of four cases. J Neurosurg Spine. 2007;6:552–8.

104. Rangel-Castilla L, Holman PJ, Krishna C, Trask TW, Klucznik RP, Diaz OM. Spinal extradural arteriovenous fistulas: a clinical and radiological description of different types and their novel treatment with Onyx. J Neurosurg Spine. 2011;15:541–9.

105. Krings T, Thron AK, Geibprasert S, et al. Endovascular management of spinal vascular malformations. Neurosurg Rev. 2010;33:1–9.

106. el Mahdi MA, Rudwan MA, Khaffaji SM, Jadallah FA. A giant spinal aneurysm with cord and root compression. J Neurol Neurosurg Psychiatry. 1989;52:532–5.

107. Vishteh AG, Brown AP, Spetzler RF. Aneurysm of the intradural artery of Adamkiewicz treated with muslin wrapping: technical case report. Neurosurgery. 1997;40:207–9.

108. Berlis A, Scheufler KM, Schmahl C, Rauer S, Gotz F, Schumacher M. Solitary spinal artery aneurysms as a rare source of spinal subarachnoid hemorrhage: potential etiology and treatment strategy. AJNR Am J Neuroradiol. 2005;26:405–10.

109. Vishteh AG, Sankhla S, Anson JA, Zabramski JM, Spetzler RF. Surgical resection of intramedullary spinal cord cavernous malformations: delayed complications, long-term outcomes, and association with cryptic venous malformations. Neurosurgery. 1997;41:1094–100; discussion 1100–1.

110. Cosgrove GR, Bertrand G, Fontaine S, Robitaille Y, Melanson D. Cavernous angiomas of the spinal cord. J Neurosurg. 1988;68:31–6.

111. Deutsch H, Jallo GI, Faktorovich A, Epstein F. Spinal intramedullary cavernoma: clinical presentation and surgical outcome. J Neurosurg. 2000;93:65–70.

112. Aoyagi N, Kojima K, Kasai H. Review of spinal epidural cavernous hemangioma. Neurol Med Chir (Tokyo). 2003;43:471–5; discussion 476.

113. Cohen-Gadol AA, Jacob JT, Edwards DA, Krauss WE. Coexistence of intracranial and spinal cavernous malformations: a study of prevalence and natural history. J Neurosurg. 2006;104:376–81.

114. Zevgaridis D, Medele RJ, Hamburger C, Steiger HJ, Reulen HJ. Cavernous haemangiomas of the spinal cord. A review of 117 cases. Acta Neurochir (Wien). 1999;141:237–45.

115. Kharkar S, Shuck J, Conway J, Rigamonti D. The natural history of conservatively managed symptomatic intramedullary spinal cord cavernomas. Neurosurgery. 2007;60:865–72; discussion865–72.

116. Sandalcioglu IE, Wiedemayer H, Gasser T, Asgari S, Engelhorn T, Stolke D. Intramedullary spinal cord cavernous malformations: clinical features and risk of hemorrhage. Neurosurg Rev. 2003;26:253–6.

117. Jallo GI, Freed D, Zareck M, Epstein F, Kothbauer KF. Clinical presentation and optimal management for intramedullary cavernous malformations. Neurosurg Focus. 2006;21:e10.

118. Mitha AP, Turner JD, Abla AA, Vishteh AG, Spetzler RF. Outcomes following resection of intramedullary spinal cord cavernous malformations: a 25-year experience. J Neurosurg Spine. 2011;14:605–11.

119. Sandson TA, Friedman JH. Spinal cord infarction. Report of 8 cases and review of the literature. Medicine (Baltimore). 1989;68:282–92.

120. Novy J, Carruzzo A, Maeder P, Bogousslavsky J. Spinal cord ischemia: clinical and imaging patterns, pathogenesis, and outcomes in 27 patients. Arch Neurol. 2006;63:1113–20.

121. Sullivan TM, Sundt 3 rd TM. Complications of thoracic aortic endografts: spinal cord ischemia and stroke. J Vasc Surg. 2006;43(Suppl A):85A–8.

122. Naess H, Romi F. Comparing patients with spinal cord infarction and cerebral infarction: clinical characteristics, and short-term outcome. Vasc Health Risk Manag. 2011;7:497–502.

123. Gross KF. Spinal cord infarction mimicking angina pectoris. Mayo Clin Proc. 2001;76:111.

124. Combarros O, Vadillo A, Gutierrez-Perez R, Berciano J. Cervical spinal cord infarction simulating myocardial infarction. Eur Neurol. 2002;47:185–6.

125. Ullery BW, Cheung AT, Fairman RM, et al. Risk factors, outcomes, and clinical manifestations of spinal cord ischemia following thoracic endovascular aortic repair. J Vasc Surg. 2011;54:677–84.

126. Dejerine J. Claudication Intermittente de la Moelle Epiniere. Presse Med. 1911;19:981–4.

127. Zulch KJ, Kurth-Schumacher R. The pathogenesis of "intermittent spinovascular insufficiency" ("spinal claudication of Dejerine") and other vascular syndromes of the spinal cord. Vasc Surg. 1970;4:116–36.

128. Yuh WT, Marsh 3rd EE, Wang AK, et al. MR imaging of spinal cord and vertebral body infarction. AJNR Am J Neuroradiol. 1992;13:145–54.

129. Faig J, Busse O, Salbeck R. Vertebral body infarction as a confirmatory sign of spinal cord ischemic stroke: report of three cases and review of the literature. Stroke. 1998;29:239–43.

130. Cheng MY, Lyu RK, Chang YJ, et al. Concomitant spinal cord and vertebral body infarction is highly associated with aortic pathology: a clinical and magnetic resonance imaging study. J Neurol. 2009;256:1418–26.

131. Stepper F, Lovblad KO. Anterior spinal artery stroke demonstrated by echo-planar DWI. Eur Radiol. 2001;11:2607–10.

132. Loher TJ, Bassetti CL, Lovblad KO, et al. Diffusion-weighted MRI in acute spinal cord ischaemia. Neuroradiology. 2003;45:557–61.

133. Robertson RL, Maier SE, Mulkern RV, Vajapayam S, Robson CD, Barnes PD. MR line-scan diffusion imaging of the spinal cord in children. AJNR Am J Neuroradiol. 2000;21:1344–8.

134. Bammer R, Herneth AM, Maier SE, et al. Line scan diffusion imaging of the spine. AJNR Am J Neuroradiol. 2003;24:5–12.

135. Skillman JJ, Zervas NT, Weintraub RM, Mayman CI. Paraplegia after resection of aneurysms of the abdominal aorta. N Engl J Med. 1969;281:422–5.

136. Bates T. Paraplegia following resection of abdominal aortic aneurysm. A report of 3 cases. Br J Surg. 1971;58:913–6.

137. Peppelenbosch AG, Vermeulen Windsant IC, Jacobs MJ, Tordoir JH, Schurink GW. Open repair for ruptured abdominal aortic aneurysm and the risk of spinal cord ischemia: review of the literature and risk-factor analysis. Eur J Vasc Endovasc Surg. 2010;40:589–95.

138. Xenos ES, Abedi NN, Davenport DL, et al. Meta-analysis of endovascular vs open repair for traumatic descending thoracic aortic rupture. J Vasc Surg. 2008;48:1343–51.

139. Mustafa ST, Sadat U, Majeed MU, Wong CM, Michaels J, Thomas SM. Endovascular repair of nonruptured thoracic aortic aneurysms: systematic review. Vascular. 2010;18:28–33.

140. Chiesa R, Melissano G, Marrocco-Trischitta MM, Civilini E, Setacci F. Spinal cord ischemia after elective stent-graft repair of the thoracic aorta. J Vasc Surg. 2005;42:11–7.

141. Hobai IA, Bittner EA, Grecu L. Perioperative spinal cord infarction in nonaortic surgery: report of three cases and review of the literature. J Clin Anesth. 2008;20:307–12.

142. Weber P, Vogel T, Bitterling H, Utzschneider S, von Schulze PC, Birkenmaier C. Spinal cord infarction after operative stabilisation of the thoracic spine in a patient with tuberculous spondylodisitis and sickle cell trait. Spine(Phila Pa 1976). 2009;34:E294–7.

143. Rau CS, Liang CL, Lui CC, Lee TC, Lu K. Quadriplegia in a patient who underwent posterior fossa surgery in the prone position. Case report. J Neurosurg. 2002;96:101–3.

144. Morandi X, Riffaud L, Amlashi SF, Brassier G. Extensive spinal cord infarction after posterior fossa surgery in the sitting position: case report. Neurosurgery. 2004;54:1512–5; discussion 1515–6.

145. Martinez-Lage JF, Almagro MJ, Izura V, Serrano C, Ruiz-Espejo AM, Sanchez-Del-Rincon I. Cervical spinal cord infarction after posterior fossa surgery: a case-based update. Childs Nerv Syst. 2009;25:1541–6.

146. Harrington D, Amplatz K. Cholesterol embolization and spinal infarction following aortic catheterization. Am J Roentgenol Radium Ther Nucl Med. 1972;115:171–4.

147. Restrepo L, Guttin JF. Acute spinal cord ischemia during aortography treated with intravenous thrombolytic therapy. Tex Heart Inst J. 2006;33:74–7.

148. Wang GR, Ensor JE, Gupta S, Hicks ME, Tam AL. Bronchial artery embolization for the management of hemoptysis in oncology patients: utility and prognostic factors. J Vasc Interv Radiol. 2009;20:722–9.

149. Brown MS, Phibbs RH. Spinal cord injury in newborns from use of umbilical artery catheters: report of two cases and a review of the literature. J Perinatol. 1988;8:105–10.

150. Singh BM, Fass AE, Pooley RW, Wallach R. Paraplegia associated with intraaortic balloon pump counterpulsation. Stroke. 1983;14:983–6.

151. Scott RW, Sancetta SM. Dissecting aneurysm of aorta with hemorrhagic infarction of the spinal cord and complete paraplegia. Am Heart J. 1949;38:747–57, illust.

152. Hill Jr CS, Vasquez JM. Massive infarction of spinal cord and vertebral boides as a complication of dissecting aneurysm of the aorta. Circulation. 1962;25:997–1000.

153. Weidauer S, Nichtweiss M, Lanfermann H, Zanella FE. Spinal cord infarction: MR imaging and clinical features in 16 cases. Neuroradiology. 2002;44:851–7.

154. Li Y, Jenny D, Bemporad JA, Liew CJ, Castaldo J. Sulcal artery syndrome after vertebral artery dissection. J Stroke Cerebrovasc Dis. 2010;19:333–5.

155. Blumbergs PC, Chin D, Rice JP. Hypotensive central spinal cord infarction: a clinicopathological study of 3 cases of aortic disease. Clin Exp Neurol. 1981;18:36–43.

156. Moorhouse DF, Burke M, Keohane C, Farrell MA. Spinal cord infarction caused by cartilage embolus to the anterior spinal artery. Surg Neurol. 1992;37:448–52.

157. Han JJ, Massagli TL, Jaffe KM. Fibrocartilaginous embolism – an uncommon cause of spinal cord infarction: a case report and review of the literature. Arch Phys Med Rehabil. 2004;85:153–7.

158. Spengos K, Tsivgoulis G, Toulas P, et al. Spinal cord stroke in a ballet dancer. J Neurol Sci. 2006;244:159–61.

159. Tosi L, Rigoli G, Beltramello A. Fibrocartilaginous embolism of the spinal cord: a clinical and pathogenetic reconsideration. J Neurol Neurosurg Psychiatry. 1996;60:55–60.

160. Mateen FJ, Monrad PA, Hunderfund AN, Robertson CE, Sorenson EJ. Clinically suspected fibrocartilaginous embolism: clinical characteristics, treatments, and outcomes. Eur J Neurol. 2011;18:218–25.

161. Mari E, Maraldi C, Grandi E, Gallerani M. Quadriplegia due to pachymeningitis, vasculitis and sepsis in a patient with rheumatoid arthritis: a case report. Eur Rev Med Pharmacol Sci. 2011;15:573–6.

162. Haupt HM, Kurlinski JP, Barnett NK, Epstein M. Infarction of the spinal cord as a complication of pneumococcal meningitis. Case report. J Neurosurg. 1981;55:121–3.

163. Hughes JT. Spinal-cord infarction due to aortic trauma. Br Med J. 1964;2:356.

164. Ahmann PA, Smith SA, Schwartz JF, Clark DB. Spinal cord infarction due to minor trauma in children. Neurology. 1975;25:301–7.

165. Ergun A, Oder W. Pediatric care report of spinal cord injury without radiographic abnormality (SCIWORA): case report and literature review. Spinal Cord. 2003;41:249–53.

166. Thompson TP, Pearce J, Chang G, Madamba J. Surfer's myelopathy. Spine (Phila Pa 1976). 2004;29:E353–6.

167. Lieske J, Cameron B, Drinkwine B, et al. Surfer's myelopathy confirmed by diffusion-weighted magnetic resonance imaging: a case report and literature review. J Comput Assist Tomogr. 2011;35:492–4.

168. Hallenbeck JM, Bove AA, Elliott DH. Mechanisms underlying spinal cord damage in decompression sickness. Neurology. 1975;25:308–16.

169. Walden JE, Castillo M. Sildenafil-induced cervical spinal cord infarction. AJNR Am J Neuroradiol. 2012;33(3):E32–3.

170. Kennedy DJ, Dreyfuss P, Aprill CN, Bogduk N. Paraplegia following image-guided transforaminal lumbar spine epidural steroid injection: two case reports. Pain Med. 2009;10:1389–94.

171. Lyders EM, Morris PP. A case of spinal cord infarction following lumbar transforaminal epidural steroid injection: MR imaging and angiographic findings. AJNR Am J Neuroradiol. 2009;30:1691–3.

172. Popescu A, Lai D, Lu A, Gardner K. Stroke following epidural injections-case report and review of literature. J Neuroimaging. 2011 Epub doi:10.1111/j.1552-6569.2011.00615.x.

173. Glaser SE, Shah RV. Root cause analysis of paraplegia following transforaminal epidural steroid injections: the 'unsafe' triangle. Pain Physician. 2010;13:237–44.

174. Gonzalez-Ordonez AJ, Uria DF, Ferreiro D, et al. Spinal cord infarction and recurrent venous thrombosis in association with estrogens and the 20210A allele of the prothrombin gene. Neurologia. 2001;16:434–8.

175. Sawaya R, Diken Z, Mahfouz R. Acute quadriplegia in a young man secondary to prothrombin G20210A mutation. Spinal Cord. 2011;49:942–3.

176. Faivre A, Bonnel S, Leyral G, Gisserot O, Alla P, Valance J. Essential thrombocythemia presenting as spinal cord infarction. Presse Med. 2009;38:1180–3.

177. Killen DA, Weinstein CL, Reed WA. Reversal of spinal cord ischemia resulting from aortic dissection. J Thorac Cardiovasc Surg. 2000;119:1049–57.

178. Blacker DJ, Wijdicks EF, Ramakrishna G. Resolution of severe paraplegia due to aortic dissection after CSF drainage. Neurology. 2003;61:142–3.

179. Safi HJ, Bartoli S, Hess KR, et al. Neurologic deficit in patients at high risk with thoracoabdominal aortic aneurysms: the role of cerebral spinal fluid drainage and distal aortic perfusion. J Vasc Surg. 1994;20:434–40; discussion 442–3.

180. Greenberg RK, O'Neill S, Walker E, et al. Endovascular repair of thoracic aortic lesions with the Zenith TX1 and TX2 thoracic grafts: intermediate-term results. J Vasc Surg. 2005;41:589–96.

181. Cheung AT, Pochettino A, Guvakov DV, Weiss SJ, Shanmugan S, Bavaria JE. Safety of lumbar drains in thoracic aortic operations performed with extracorporeal circulation. Ann Thorac Surg. 2003;76:1190–6; discussion 1196–7.

182. Cheung AT, Pochettino A, McGarvey ML, et al. Strategies to manage paraplegia risk after endovascular stent repair of descending thoracic aortic aneurysms. Ann Thorac Surg. 2005;80:1280–8; discussion 1288–9.

183. Cheshire WP, Santos CC, Massey EW, Howard Jr JF. Spinal cord infarction: etiology and outcome. Neurology. 1996;47:321–30.

184. Salvador de la Barrera S, Barca-Buyo A, Montoto-Marques A, Ferreiro-Velasco ME, Cidoncha-Dans M, Rodriguez-Sotillo A. Spinal cord infarction: prognosis and recovery in a series of 36 patients. Spinal Cord. 2001;39:520–5.

185. Foo D, Rossier AB. Anterior spinal artery syndrome and its natural history. Paraplegia. 1983;21:1–10.

186. Lee WA, Daniels MJ, Beaver TM, Klodell CT, Raghinaru DE, Hess Jr PJ. Late outcomes of a single-center experience of 400 consecutive thoracic endovascular aortic repairs. Circulation. 2011;123:2938–45.

Index

Page numbers followed by f refer to illustrations; page numbers followed by t refer to tables. The abbreviation "aka" means "also known as."

M.R. Harrigan, J.P. Deveikis, *Handbook of Cerebrovascular Disease
and Neurointerventional Technique*, DOI 10.1007/978-1-61779-946-4,
© Springer Science+Business Media New York 2013

Atherosclerotic extracranial arterial disease
carotid angioplasty and stenting, 759
CREST, 751
embolic protection on
periprocedural complication
rates, 753–754
endarterectomy, high risk for, 754
EVA-3S, 752–753
FDA approval for, 754
history of, 749–750, 750t
ICSS, 753
patient selection, 754, 755t
recurrent stenosis after, 753
SAPPHIRE criteria, 750–751, 750t
SPACE, 752
timing after stroke, 754
carotid artery bifurcation, 738–739
carotid endarterectomy
asymptomatic carotid stenosis,
742–743
to medical therapy, trials, 743–744
symptomatic carotid stenosis, 739–742,
740f, 740t
carotid occlusion
asymptomatic, 754–755
Carotid Occlusion Surgery Study
(COSS), 757–758
cerebral revascularization, surgical
options for, 756
extracranial-intracranial (EC/IC) bypass
trial, 756–757
symptomatic, 755–756
and cerebrovascular disease, 738
medical management, of carotid artery
disease, 747–749, 747t
plaque location, 738
radiographic evaluation
carotid ultrasound results,
interpretation of, 745–746,
745f, 746t
duplex ultrasonography, limitations of,
745
recurrent stenosis, after CEA
forms, 746
redo-CEA, 746–747
risk of, 746
stages, 737
statins and, 738
vertebral artery stenosis
diagnosis, 758
patterns of symptoms, 758
prognosis, 759
Atherosclerotic intracranial arterial disease
aetiology of symptoms, 780
EC/IC bypass study, 780
intracranial angioplasty and stenting,
783–786

medical treatment, 782–783
natural history, 780
prevalence, 779
risk factors, 779–780
WASID studies, 781–782, 781f
Atrial fibrillation, 662–664
Atrial myxoma, 664
Autosomal dominant polycystic kidney disease
(ADPKD), 486–487
AVF. *See* Arteriovenous fistula (AVF)
AV fistulas. *See* Arteriovenous fistula (AVF)
AVM. *See* Arteriovenous malformations
(AVMs)

B

Back-pressure measurement, 245
Bacterial endocarditis, modified Duke
criteria, 670t
Balint syndrome, 702
Balloon
angioplasty, for cerebral vasospasm,
430–433, 431t, 432f, 433t
detachable technique, 291–292
hyperform, 292
for venous test occlusion, 445–447
for venous thrombolysis/thrombectomy,
469
wide-necked aneurysm, 207–209
Balloon-assisted thrombolysis, 471–472
Balloon-expandable stent technique, 324
Balloon-occlusion devices, 409
Balloon test occlusion
blood flow, adjunctive tests
angiography, 245
back-pressure/stump-pressure
measurement, 245
computer simulation, 247
CT perfusion, 246
MR perfusion, 247
positron emission tomography (PET),
246–247
SPECT, 247
transcranial Doppler (TCD), 246
Xenon CT, 246
carotid artery test occlusion, 244
catheter and balloon manipulation,
250–251
complications of
neurological, 248
nonneurological, 248
conditions, for reliability of results,
243–244
devices for
detachable coils, 250
double lumen balloon catheter, 249

intervention phase, 403–404
post-procedure management, 404
tandem stenoses, 402
filter devices, 408–409
flow-reversal device, 409
indications and contraindications
Enderling, 399, 400t
patient preparation
evaluation, 400
pre-procedure preparation, 400–401
stents, 409–410
Carotid blow-out syndrome, 327
Carotid cave, 510
Carotid cavernous fistulas, 296
Carotid dissection
blunt trauma
cerebral ischaemia, 762
cerebrovascular injury scale, 763t
endovascular intervention, 764
medical management, 763–764
radiographic evaluation, 763
spontaneous internal
cause of stroke, in young adults, 761
cerebral ischaemia, 761
clinical features, 761
intimal tear, 761
management, 762
prognosis, 762
radiographic evaluation, 762
Carotid endarterectomy (CEA)
asymptomatic carotid stenosis
ACAS trial, 743–744
ACST, 744
American Heart Association guidelines,
743
CASANOVA, 744
Mayo Asymptomatic Carotid
Endarterectomy Trial, 744
natural history of, 742
Oxford vascular study, 743
risk of surgery, 743
risk score, 743t
Veterans Administration Cooperative
Asymptomatic Trial, 744
vs. CAS, 749, 750t
to medical therapy, trials, 743–744
patient selection, 754, 755t
symptomatic carotid stenosis
American Heart Association
recommendation, 742
clinical trial data caveats, 741
ECST trial, 739
measurement equivalent values, 740t
measurement methods, 740f
NASCET trial, 739
pooled data, analysis of, 741
subgroup analyses
contralateral occlusion, 742
elderly patients, 742

hemispheric *vs.* retinal symptoms,
741
intraluminal thrombus, 742
ipsilateral intracranial aneurysms,
742
near occlusion, 742
ulcerated plaque, 741
VACS trial, 739, 741
Carotid occlusion
asymptomatic, 754–755
measurement, 740f, 741
Carotid Occlusion Surgery Study (COSS),
757–758
cerebral revascularization, surgical options
for, 756
extracranial-intracranial (EC/IC) bypass
trial, 756–757
symptomatic, 755–756
Carotid Revascularization
Endarterectomy Versus Stent
Trial (CREST), 751
Carotid stenosis
and acute ischaemic stroke, 370–372
asymptomatic, 742–743
risk factors for, 738–739
symptomatic, 739–742, 740f, 740t
Carotid-vertebrobasilar anastomoses
persistent hypoglossal artery, 34
persistent otic artery, 34
persistent trigeminal artery, 32–33, 33f
proatlantal intersegmental artery, 34
CAS. *See* Carotid angioplasty and stenting
(CAS)
Catch retriever, 365
Catheter
angiography, aneurysm, 234
angioptic™, 120
angled guide, 270
angled taper, 136f, 136t
and balloon manipulation, 250–251
Cobra, 136f, 136t
double coiling technique, 216–217
Envoy, 270
Foley, placement, 155
guide, 157, 270
care and maintenance, 160–161
head tilt technique, 161f
placement technique, 160
position, 160
selection, 157–158
size, 159
straight/angled, 159–160
technique, 158–159
intermediate technique, 170–172
large-lumen guide, 270
microcatheter technique, 167–168
Mikaelsson, 136f, 136t, 148
navigation, 104, 105f
paediatric, 126

Computed tomography (CT) (*cont'd*)
   blood flow tests, 246
   CBF and CBV, 378–379
      deconvolution method, 380, 381,
         383, 384f
      interpretation of data, 382–384
      in ischemic stroke, 383
      limitations, 382
      maximum slope method, 381, 381f,
         383
      mean transit time (MTT), 380–382
      methods of, 380, 380t
      parameters, 379–380
      time to peak (TTP), 380–382
      validation, 382
Contralateral occlusion, 742, 744
Contrastoma, 368
Contrast-induced nephropathy
   iodinated, 121
   risk factors, 122
   risk reduction technique, 122
Costocervical trunk catheterization, 147
C-reactive protein (CRP), 668
Crescendo TIA, 694–695
CT angiography (CTA), 384, 527
   aneurysm, 234–235
   in blunt trauma evaluation, 763, 766
CT perfusion, 527–528
Cyanoacrylates (aka glue), 317

D

Dandy-Walker complex, 86, 86f
Deconvolution method, CT perfusion, 380,
   381, 383, 384f
Dejerine-Roussy syndrome, 702
Deployus prematurs, 219
Desmetoplase, 345
Detachable balloon technique, 291–292
Detachable coil technique, 195, 282, 293
Detachable embolization, 232–233
Developmental venous anomalies (DVA)
   aetiology, 628
   arterialized venous malformations (AVM),
      628, 628f
   epidemiology, 627
   frontal lobe venous angioma, 627, 627f
   Global Gem, 629
   imaging, 628
   management, 629
   natural history and presentation, 628
   vein, galen malformations, 629
Diffusion-weighted imaging (DWI), 385–387,
   386f
Dipyridamole, 748
Dissecting intracranial aneurysms
   clinical features, 547
   management, 547–548

Dissection, brain AVM embolization, 300
Distal access catheter (DAC), 359, 360, 360f
   selection, 170–171
   triaxial arrangment, 170
Dolichoectatic aneurysms, 548–549
Doppler velocities and degree of stenosis,
   745f
Double aortic arch, 5
Double flushing, 104–105, 439–440
Dual antiplatelet therapy, 164
Duplex ultrasonography, 745
Dural arteriovenous fistula (dAVF)
   anterior fossa
      clinical features, 617
      management, 617–618
   Borden type I, 608
   Borden type II and III, 608
   catheter angiography, 606–607
   cavernous, 463–465
   clinical features, 605, 803–805, 804f
   conservative management, 609
   CTA, 607
   direct carotid-cavernous (CC)
      clinical features, 618–619
      management, 619–620
   Ehlers-Danlos Type IV, 620
   endovascular considerations, 806
   endovascular treatment, 609
   epidemiology, 803–805, 804f
   Foix-Alajouanine syndrome, 806
   formation stages, 603, 604f
   indirect carotid-cavernous (CC) fistulas
      clinical features, 612–613
      management, 613–614
   intracranial, 466–467
   locations, 610, 610f
   management of, 805
   MRI, 607
   natural history, 607
   pathophysiology, 805
      anatomy and classification, 603
      etiology, 603
      three stage hypothesis, 604–605
   pulsatile tinnitus, 606
   radiosurgery, 609
   risk of haemorrhage, 608
   spinal embolization, 337
   superior sagittal sinus, 465–466
      clinical features, 616
      management, 616
   surgery, 609
   surgical considerations, 805–806
   tentorial, 466
      clinical features, 614
      management, 615
   transverse-sigmoid sinus, 465
      clinical features, 610–611
      management, 611–612

E

Echelon™, 315
Eclampsia, 540
Edema
  neurogenic pulmonary, 526
  postembolization, 304
Ehlers-Danlos syndrome (EDS), 487
Ehlers-Danlos Type IV, 620
EKG changes, subarachnoid hemorrhage,
  526
EKOS® Neurowave™ micro-infusion system,
  364–365
Elderly patients
  with aneurysms
    subarachnoid hemorrhage, 542
    unruptured, 541–542
  symptomatic carotid stenosis, 742
Electroencephalography (EEG), 244, 270
  and moyamoya disease, 791
Embolic protection device (EPD), 403–405,
  408, 412, 414–418
  Embolization. *See also* Extracranial
    embolization
  aneurysm, 228–229
    endovascular technique, 190–191
    indications and contraindications, 189
    patient preparation, 189–190
    vascular access phase, 191–192
  aneurysm, detachable, 232–233
  arteriovenous malformations, 585–587,
    587t
  cavernous sinus dAVFs, 613
  complication avoidance
    arterial dissection, 304–305
    AVM rupture, 303–304
    brain AVM embolization, 300
    guide catheter-induced vasospasm, 306
    intracranial tumor embolization, 301
    neurological complications, 300
    non-neurological complications, 300
    postembolization edema/hemorrhage,
      304
    retained microcatheter, 305–306
    thromboembolism, 302–303
    vessel perforation, 301–302
  endovascular technique
    arteriovenous malformation, 295–296
    asleep, 269–270
    awake, 269–270
    bleeding intracranial vessels, 298
    detachable balloon technique, 291–292
    detachable coil technique, 293
    direct carotid cavernous fistulas, 296
    embolization phase, 279
    embolization strategy, 279–280
    ethanol embolization technique, 289

    intracranial dural arteriovenous fistulas,
      296–297
    intracranial tumors, 298–299
    liquid embolics, 280–281
    microcatheter phase, 271, 272t, 273t,
      274–279
    N-BCA embolization technique,
      284–287
    Onyxʳ embolization technique,
      287–289
    particle embolization technique,
      289–290
    particles, 281–283
    pial arteriovenous fistulas, 297
    postprocedure management, 295
    post-traumatic/post surgical fistulas,
      298
    pushable coil technique, 292–293
  silk suture embolization technique, 290–291
    stent-assisted treatment, 293–295
    syringe safety, 279
    vascular access phase, 270–271
    vein of Galen malformation, 297–298
  indications and contraindications, 267–268
  mangement, 300–306
  phase, 279
  pial arteriovenous fistulas, 297
  postprocedure management, 295
  prevention, neurointerventional procedures,
    166
  techniques and devices
    evaluation, 268
    preprocedure preparation, 269
    treatment strategy, 268–269
  transverse-sigmoid sinus dAVFs, 611
Emboshield™, 408
Endarterectomy Versus Angioplasty in Patients
  with Symptomatic Severe
  Carotid Stenosis (EVA-3S),
  752–753
Endovascular treatment
  acute ischaemic stroke
    IA cases, 343
    importance of speed, 343–344
    patient preparation
      evaluation, 345–346
      pre-procedure preparation, 346
    thrombolytic agents
      ancrod, 345
      desmetoplase, 345
      intra arterial, 344t
      prourokinase, 344
      reteplase, 344
      tenecteplase, 344, 345
      urokinase and streptokinase, 344
  carotid artery origin lesions, 414–415
  carotid bifurcation lesions, 401–406
  carotid dissection, blunt trauma, 764

ethanol embolization technique, 321–322
evaluation, 312
head and neck transarterial embolization
  complications of, 329–330
  contraindications, 311
  indications, 311
material selection
  detachable balloons, 318
  detachable fibered coils, 318
  detachable platinum coils, 318
  liquid embolics, 317
  particles, 317
  pushable coils, 318
  sclerosing agents, 317
  silk suture, 317
  stents, 318–319
microcatheter access phase
  flow-directed microcatheter navigation,
    315–316
  irrigation, 315
  microcatheter selection, 314
  microwire selection, 314
  navigation, 315
  preparation, 315
  provocative testing, 316
  steerable microcatheter navigation, 316
n-BCA embolization technique
  glue preparation, 319
  injection technique, 319–320
Onyx® embolization technique, 317
  injection technique, 321
  preparation, 320
particle embolization technique, 322–323
percutaneous procedures
  indications, 330
  n-BCA injection, 332–333
  neurological complications, 333
  non-neurological complications, 334
  sclerotherapy, 330–332
post-procedure management, 324
preprocedure preparation, 312–313
spinal embolization, 334–339
stent-graft placement for active bleeding,
  323–324
syringe safety, 316
treatment strategy, 312
vascular access phase
  guide catheter positioning, 313–314
  guide catheter selection, 313
  systemic anticoagulation, 313
Extradural arteriovenous fistula, 812–813

F

Fabry disease, 671–672
Familial aneurysm, 485–486, 486t
Femoral artery haemorrhage, 368
Fentanyl (Sublimaze®), 103, 156

Fibromuscular dysplasia (FMD), 672
  adventitia, 769
  cerebrovascular, 769
  intima, 769
  medial, 767, 768f
  pathogenesis, 769
Filter devices, 408–409
FilterWire EZ™, 408
Fisher grading system, 521t
Flow diversion, 218, 518
Flow-directed microcatheter, 314–316
Flow-reversal device, 409
Flumazenil (Romazicon®), 103
FMD. *See* Fibromuscular dysplasia (FMD)
Foix-Alajouanine syndrome, 806
Fusiform aneurysms, 548–549

G

Gadolinium and nephrogenic systemic fibrosis,
  388
Gerstmann syndrome, 700
Giant aneurysms
  epidemiology, 545
  evaluation, 545
  management, 546
  natural history, 546
  presentation, 545
Glandular branches, 10
Glidewire®, 250, 257
Glue-in microcatheter, 305
Glucagon, 145
Glycoprotein IIB/IIIA inhibitors, 164, 371
GuardWire®, 249, 250, 252–254, 409
Guide catheters, for embolization, 313–314,
  335–337

H

Haemangioma, capillary, 631
Haemangioma, cavernous, *See* Cavernous
  malformations
Haemoglobinopathy, 673
Haemoglobin S homozygosity (HbSS),
  684–685
Haemorrhage, dural arteriovenous fistula
  (dAVFs), 605
Hagen–Poiseuille equation, 531
Head and neck embolization
  complications of
    avoidance, steps for, 329–330
    neurological, 329
    non-neurological, 329
  disease processes
    arteriovenous fistula (AVF), 325–326
    arteriovenous malformation (AVM), 325
    bleeding tumours, 327

Limb-shaking TIA, 696
Lindegaard ratio, 528
Liquid embolics, 280–281, 461
Locked-in syndrome, 705
Loeys-Dietz syndrome, 488
Lovastatin (Mevacor®), 747
Low-density lipoprotein (LDL) cholesterol, 747t

M

Magnesium infusion, subarachnoid hemorrhage, 530
Magnetic resonance angiography (MRA)
    aneurysm, 235–237
    contrast-enhanced, 388
    gadolinium and nephrogenic systemic fibrosis, 388
    phase contrast, 388
    time of flight, 387–388
Magnetic resonance imaging (MRI)
    acute ischemic stroke, patterns of, 386f
    apparent diffusion coefficient (ADC), 385–387
    arteriovenous malformations, 578
    cerebral infarction, signal characteristics of, 385t
    diffusion-weighted imaging (DWI), 385–387
    hemorrhage, identification of, 388–389, 389t
    and moyamoya disease, 790
    perfusion imaging, 387
Magnetic resonance perfusion, 247
Marfan syndrome, 488
Mayo Asymptomatic Carotid Endarterectomy Study, 744, 748
MCA sign, 378
Mechanical embolectomy, intra-arterial thrombolysis
    Alligator™ Retriever device, 355–356
    intracranial angioplasty, 356
    intracranial stenting, 356–357
    snares
        clot maceration, 355
        clot retrieval, 355
        devices, 355
    suction thrombectomy, 356
Mechanical thrombectomy, devices for, 365–366
Medial medullary syndrome, 708
Mehringer-Hieshima maneuver, 619
Memory testing, 260
    in Wada test, 255
Merci retrieval system, 303
Merci retriever, intra-arterial thrombolysis
    balloon guide catheter, 357, 358f
    devices, 358

distal access catheter (DAC), 359, 360, 360f
    technique, 359–361
Metabolic syndrome, 679
Metaloproteinase gene expression and moyamoya disease, 788
Microballoon catheter technique, 252
Microbleed, 389
Microcatheter, 168–169, 314–316, 353–355, 358, 364
    aneurysm, 202–203
    Echelon™, 167, 272t
    Excelsior®, 167, 272t
    glued-in, 305–306
    Headway®, 272t
    Magic®, 167, 273t
    Marathon™, 273t
    Marksman™, 167, 225, 226
    microwires, 168
    Nautica™, 272t
    phase, embolization, 271, 272t, 273t, 274–279
    Prowler®, 272t
    Rebar®, 272t
    reperfusion, 361–362
    retained, embolization procedures, 305–306
    shape, 168
    steerable, 167–170, 202–203
    Ultraflow™, 167, 273t
Microwire, 314, 315, 353, 361
    Headliner™, 168
    Neuroscout™, 168
    proper technique, 169f
    Synchro®, 168
    Transend™, 168
Midazolam (Versed®), 103, 156
Middle cerebral artery (MCA), 528
    hyperattenuation of M1 segment, 378f
Mikaelsson catheter reconstruction, 148
Mitochondrial encephalomyopathy, lactic acidosis, stroke-like episodes (MELAS), 680–681
Modified Rankin scale (mRS), 724
Montreal test, 255
Moyamoya
    disease
        angiography, 789–790, 790t
        cerebral blood flow studies, 790–791
        clinical features, 791–792, 794–795
        CT, 789
        diagnosis of, 788–789
        EEG, 791
        epidemiology, 786–787
        familial, 792
        intracranial angioplasty, 796
        management, 795–797
        MRI, 790
        pathophysiology, 787–788
        pregnancy and, 796

disease *vs.* syndrome, 681, 786
syndrome
  and arteriovenous malformations
    (AVMs), 574–575
  clinical features of, 794–795
  conditions associated with, 793–795
  management, 795–796
Moyamoya-like syndrome, 796
Myoclonic epilepsy and ragged red fibers
    (MERFF), 680–681

N

Nasal arcade, 17
National Institutes of Health Stroke Scale
    (NIHSS), 389, 390t–391t
N-BCA embolization technique, 319–320
  embolization, 284–287
  percutaneous, 332–333
Neonates, vein of Galen malformations, 593,
    594t
Nephrogenic systemic fibrosis and gadolinium,
    388
Neucrylate™, aneurysm, 204–206
Neuroendovascular suite
  medications, 182t
  organization and essential equipment,
    174–175
  personnel, 180–181
  pharmacologic considerations, 181
  radiation safety, 177–180
  technical specifications, 175–177
Neurofibromatosis type 1, 488
NeuroFlo™ system, perfusion augmentation,
    365–366
Neuroform, 318, 357
  wide-necked aneurysm, 211–214
Neurogenic pulmonary edema, 526
Neurointerventional procedures
  air emboli prevention, 166
  alternative access routes, 162
  antithrombotic therapy
    anticoagulation, 163
    antiplatelet therapy, 163–164
    clopidogrel resistance, 164–166
    platelet function testing, 165–166
  asleep, 156
  awake, 155–156
  contrast agents, 156
  in difficult access cases, 161–162
  error prevention, 153–154
  intervention phase
    devices, 167–168
    imaging technique, 172–173
    intermediate catheter technique,
      170–172
    microcatheter technique, 168–170
  neuroendovascular suite

angiography equipment, 175
medications, 182t
organization and essential equipment,
    174–175
personnel, 180–181
pharmacologic considerations, 181
radiation safety, 177–180
technical specifications, 175–177
postprocedure care, 173
preprocedure preparation, 154
puncture site management, 173
vascular access, 156–161
Neuromeningeal trunk, 10
Neuropsychological testing, 244
Neurovascular anatomy
  aortic arch and great vessels
    anomalies, 4
    branches, 3
    subclavian artery, 4
    variants, 3
  common carotid arteries (CCAs), 5–6
  external carotid artery (ECA)
    anastamoses, 8–9
    ascending pharyngeal artery, 10–13
    branches, 6, 7
    facial artery, 14–17
    internal maxillary artery (IMA),
      21–29
    lingual artery, 14
    occipital artery, 17–19
    origin, 6
    posterior auricular artery, 19–20
    superficial temporal artery, 20–21
    superior thyroid artery, 9–10
    territories, 7
    variants, 7
    ventral and dorsal, 7
NexStent®, 318, 410
Nicardipine, 533
Nimodipine, 528–529, 533
Nitroglycerin, 534
Normal perfusion pressure breakthrough
    syndrome, 304, 582
North American Symptomatic
    Endarterectomy Trial
    (NASCET), 739
Nothnagel syndrome, 703

O

Obstetrical management, subarachnoid
    hemorrhage, 540–541
Obstructive sleep apnea, 682
O'Kelly-Marotta (OKM) grading scale, 503f
One third rule, 377
Onyx®, 317, 320–321
  aneurysm, 203–204
  embolization, 287–289

Ophthalmic segment (C6)
  anatomy, 39, 40f
  ophthalmic artery
    extraorbital group, 42–43
    ocular group, 42
    orbital group, 42
  variants, 43
Oral contraceptives (OCP), 682–683
Oxygen extraction fraction (OEF), 755, 756
Oxytocin, 541

P

Packing density calculation, aneurysm, 207
Papaverine, 534
Paragangioma (aka chemodectoma, glomus tumour), 328
Parinaud syndrome, 703
Parodi anti-emboli system, 409
Particle embolization, 281–283, 289–290, 322–323
Patent foramen ovale (PFO), 683, 683t
Pediatric ischemic stroke, 728–730
Pediatric intracranial aneurysms
  conditions associated with, 538t
  epidemiology and characteristic features, 537–538
  management, 538–539
Paediatric stroke, See Stroke, paediatric
Penetrating neck injury, 766–767
  zones of neck, 766f
Penumbra coil 400™ tips, intracranial aneurysm treatment, 201–202
Penumbra reperfusion system, 470–471
Penumbra System™, intra-arterial thrombolysis
  devices
    guide catheter, 361
    microwire, 361
    reperfusion microcatheters, 361–362
    Separator™, 362
  technique, 362–363
Percutaneous procedures, extracranial embolization
  indications, 330
  n-BCA injection, 332–333
  neurological complications, 333
  non-neurological complications, 334
  sclerotherapy, 330–332
Perfusion-diffusion mismatch, 387
Perimedullary arteriovenous fistula, 338
Perimesencephalic nonaneurysmal subarachnoid hemorrhage (PMSAH), 518–520
Petrous segment (C2)
  branches, 34–35
  caroticotympanic artery, 35

persistent stapedial artery, 35
subsegments, 34
variants, 35
vidian artery (aka artery of pterygoid canal), 35
Pharmacological thrombolysis, 354
Pharmacologic provocative testing
  adjunctive testing, 262
  drug preparation, procedures, 261
  language testing, 260
  memory testing, 260
  pre-embolization, 261
  superselective, 262–263
  syringe safety, 263
  vascular access phase, 262
  Wada test (See Wada test)
Pharos technique, 426–427
Phenox® clot retriever, 365
Pial arteriovenous fistulas, 297
Pipeline, 218–220, 224, 504, 505, 518
Pitchhfork, 63
Platelet function testing, 165–166
Plato™ Microcath, 316
Polyglycolic–polylactic acid (PGLA), 518
Positron emission tomography (PET), 246–247, 755–756
Posterior cerebral artery aneurysms, 514
Posterior inferior cerebellar artery syndrome, 708, 708f
Post-traumatic/post surgical fistulas, embolization, 298
Pravastatin, 529
Precipitated polymer (aka non-adhesive liquid embolic agent), 317
Precise®, 410
Preeclampsia, 540
Pre-embolization provocative testing, 261
Pregnancy and intracranial aneurysms
  evaluation, 539
  subarachnoid hemorrhage
    clinical features, 539
    differential diagnosis, 540
    neurovascular management, 540
    obstetrical management, 540–541
    outcomes, 541
  unruptured, 539
Propofol, for Wada test, 259
Prostaglandin synthesis and moyamoya disease, 788
Protege®, 410
Prourokinase, 344
Provocative testing
  balloon test occlusion, 243–254
  extracranial embolization, 316
  pharmacologic, 254–263
Pseudophlebitic pattern, 607

Pseudoaneurysm, carotid stenting for, 410–411
Pseudoxanthoma elasticum, 488
Pulmonary capillary wedge pressure (PCWP), 531
Pushable coil technique, embolization, 292–293

Q

Qureshi grading system, for acute ischaemic stroke, 349t

R

Radiation safety
    lead apron technique, 179f
    neuroendovascular suite, 177–180
    patient radiation exposure, 177–178
    physiological consideration, 178, 180
    staff radiation exposure, 178
Radiographic evaluation
    atherosclerotic extracranial arterial disease
        carotid ultrasound results, interpretation of, 745–746, 745f, 746t
        duplex ultrasonography, limitations of, 745
    blunt trauma
        carotid dissection, 763
        vertebral artery, 765–766
        penetrating neck injury, 767
        spontaneous vertebral artery dissection, 765
Radiosurgery, in brain AVMs
    advantages and disadvantages, 583
    mechanism of AVM obliteration in, 584
    outcomes, 584
    practical issues, 584–585
    techniques, 583–584
Rebar®, 315
Recurrent stenosis
    after carotid angioplasty and stenting, 753
    after CEA, 746–747
Reocclusion, pharmacological thrombolysis, 354
Retained microcatheter, 305
Retrograde aortic flush, 143–144
Reversible cardiomyopathy, subarachnoid hemorrhage, 526
Reversible ischaemic neurologic deficit (RIND), 695
Reversible vasoconstriction syndrome (Call-Fleming syndrome), 519, 683, 693
Rheolytic catheter, 472–473
Road mapping, 439
Roberts/SC phocomelia syndrome, 488

Rotational vertebral artery occlusion syndrome (RVAS) (aka Bow Hunter syndrome), 760–761
Rubber duckie, 155
Rubicon®, 409

S

SAH. See Subarachnoid hemorrhage (SAH)
SAMMPRIS. See Stenting vs. Aggressive Medical Management for Preventing Recurrent Stroke in Intracranial Stenosis (SAMMPRIS)
Sclerotherapy
    access, 331
    anesthesia, 331
    injection, 331–332
    sclerosing agents, 317, 330–331
Seattle test, 255
Sedation, spinal angiography, 134
Seizures, 300
Seldinger technique, 156
Separator™, 361, 362
Serpentine aneurysm, 548–549
Sheath, 102
    arterial, 135
    femoral artery, 102, 157, 270
Shuttle®, 401
Sickle cell disease, 684–685
Sickle cell trait, 685
Silk, 317, 504–505
    embolization, 290–291
    intracranial aneurysm treatment, 221–224
Single-photon emission computed tomography (SPECT), 247
Sinus pericranii
    aetiology, 630
    epidemiology, 629–630
    imaging, 630
    management, 630
    natural history and presentation, 630
SIR. See Society of Interventional Radiology (SIR)
Skull, venous structures of, 77
SL Flexor®, 401
Snare assisted catheterization, 402, 440f
Snares, mechanical embolectomy, 355
Society of Interventional Radiology (SIR), 785
Sodium methohexital, for Wada test, 259
Softip™ XF guide catheter, 353
Solitaire™, 357, 363
Somatosensory evoked potentials (SSEP), 245
Spetzler-Martin grading system, 581, 581t.
        See also Arteriovenous malformations (AVMs), brain
SpiderFX™, 408

---

neurogenic pulmonary edema, 526
perimesencephalic nonaneurysmal, 518–520
in pregnant patients, 539–541
risk factors
alcohol consumption, 489
atherosclerosis, 490
cigarette smoking, 489
coffee use, 490
hypertension, 489
sexual intercourse, 490
weather and season, 490
serum electrolyte derangements
hypernatremia, 525
hypokalemia, 525
hypomagnesemia, 525
hyponatremia, 524–525
traumatic, 550
vasospasm, 527–534
Subclavian artery origin lesions
endovascular technique
brachial approach, 417–418
femoral artery approach, 416–417
indications, 415
patient preparation, 400–401
Subclavian steal, 415
Submandibular branches, 16
Suction thrombectomy, 356, 371
Superior sagittal sinus dAVFs
clinical features, 616
management, 616
Surfer's myelopathy, 816, 816f
Syphillis, meningovascular (aka Heubner's arteritis), 690
Sylvian dot sign, 378
Syringe safety, 263
embolization, 279
Systemic lupus erythaematosus (SLE), 691
Systolic blood pressure (SBP), 531

T

Tandem stenoses, 402
Telfa™ dressing, 155
Tenecteplase, 344, 345
Tentorial dAVFs
clinical features, 614
management, 615
Terson syndrome, 520
Thrombectomy, for cerebral venous thrombosis
complications, 467–468
indications, 467
procedures, 469–473
technique, 468–469
Thromboembolism, 302–303
aneurysm, 227–228

Thrombolysis, 406
agents, 344–345, 344t, 371
with anterior circulation stroke
absolute contraindications, 346
decision-making, IV/IA thrombolysis, 346–348, 347t
IA thrombolysis, 348, 348t, 349t
indications, 346
IV thrombolysis, 348
relative contraindications, 346
basilar artery occlusion, 369
for cerebral venous thrombosis (CVT)
complications, 467–468
indications, 467
procedures, 469–473
technique, 468–469
Thrombolysis in myocardial infarction (TIMI) scale, 348, 348t
Thryocervical trunk catheterization, 147
Ticlopidine, 748–749
t-PA, intravenous thrombolysis, 350, 366–367
Transarterial n-BCA injection, 461–462
Transarterial Onyx® injection, 462
Transcranial Doppler (TCD) ultrasonography, 246, 350, 528
Transient global amnesia, 695
Transient ischaemic attack (TIA), 694
Transient monocular blindness, 696
Transitional aneurysm, 507
Transvenous embolization
anatomic considerations, 456
arterial access, 459
cavernous dural arteriovenous fistula, 463–465
coil embolization, 460
complications, 456–457
embolic agents, 458–459
extracranial head and neck AVFs, 467
indications, 456
intracranial access, 460
intracranial dAVFs, 466–467
liquid embolic embolization, 461
procedure, 457
spinal AVFs, 467
superior sagittal sinus dAVF, 465–466
tentorial dAVFs, 466
tips on specific disease processes, 463
transarterial n-BCA injection, 461–462
transarterial Onyx® injection, 462
transverse/sigmoid sinus dAVF, 465
vein of Galen aneurysmal malformations, 466
venous access, 459
wires and catheters for, 458
Transvenous stenting
anti-thrombotic medications, 474
complications, 473–474

Transvenous stenting (*cont'd*)
  indications, 473
  postprocedure care, 476
  procedures
    intracranial access, 475
    stent placement, 475–476
  stents for, 475
  technique, 474–475
  venous access, 474
  wires and catheters, 474–475
Transverse-sigmoid sinus dAVFs
  clinical features, 610–611
  management, 611–612
Traumatic aneurysms, 549–550
Traumatic subarachnoid hemorrhage, 550
Treated aneurysm, 235
Trevo™ Stentriever™, 363–364
Tumor, intracranial
  embolization, 301
  hemorrhage, 304
Two-point method, 647

U

UltraFlow™ microcatheter, 353
Ultrasound
  augmentation of IV thrombolysis, 350
  carotid, results, 745–746, 745f, 746t

V

Valvulopathy, 686–687
Varenicline, 686, 686t
Varicella zoster virus (VZV), 690
Vascular access procedures. *See* Embolization
Vascular tumours
  extracranial
    juvenile nasopharyngeal angiofibroma,
      327–328
    Kasabach Merritt syndrome, 328
    paragangioma (aka chemodectoma,
      glomus tumour), 328
  spinal, 339, 813
Vasculitis, 687–692, 691f
Vasospasm, 692–693
  clinical features and diagnosis, 527–528
  endovascular treatment
    access phase, 429–430
    awake *vs.* asleep, 429
    balloon angioplasty, 430–433
    complications, 434
    indications, 429
    intra-arterial pharmacologic treatment,
      434
  frequency and time course, 527
  guide catheter-induced, 306
  ischemic injury, prevention of
    lumbar drainage, 530

magnesium infusion, 530
nimodipine, 528–529
prophylactic hyperdynamic therapy,
  530
statins, 529–530
risk factors, 527
treatment
  angioplasty, 533
  hyperdynamic therapy, 531–532
  intra-arterial pharmacologic treatment,
    533–534
Vein
  angular, 75
  anterior condylar, 76
  anterior pontomesencephalic, 85
  basal vein of Rosenthal, 84
  cervical, 75–77
  coronal venous plexus, 141
  Dandy's, 85
  deep facial, 75
  deep venous system, 82–83, 83f
  diploic, 77
  emissary, 77
  external jugular (EJ), 75
  extracranial, 73–77
    superficial, 74f
  facial, 74f, 75, 76f
  frontal, 73
  of Galen, 84–85
  inferior ophthalmic, 75
  inferior vermian, 85
  infratentorial venous system, 84–85
  internal cerebral, 83–84
  internal jugular (IJ), 75
  labial, 75
  lateral condylar, 76
  lateral mesencephalic, 85
  maxillary, 75
  medial ophthalmic, 75
  medial temporal, 74
  medullary, 82
  meningeal, 77
  occipital, 74
  orbital, 74–75
  petrosal, 85
  pharyngeal, 76
  posterior auricular, 74
  posterior condylar, 76
  posterior mesencephalic, 85
  precentral cerebellar, 84–85
  radicular, 141
  retromandibular, 75
  scalp, 73–74
  spinal radicular, 76
  subependymal, 83
  submental, 75
  suboccipital, 76
  superficial temporal, 74
  superior convexity, 81

superior ophthalmic (SOV), 75
superior vermian, 85
supraorbital, 73
supratentorial cortical, 81–82
supratrochlear, 73
Sylvian, 81
temporo-occipital, 81
tentorial, 85
thyroid, 76
of Trolard, 76
vertebral, 77
Vein of Galen malformation, 85
anatomy, 592
angiographic classification, 591
Bicêtre neonatal evaluation score, 594t
children and adults, 595
clinical features, 592
complications of embolization, 595
embolization, 297–298, 466
embryology, 591
management and outcomes, 593–595
melting brain syndrome, 592
natural history and overall prognosis,
592–593
Venography
indications for, 441
neurological complications, 442
non-neurological complications, 442
suggested wires and catheters for, 442–443
techniques
catheter manipulation, 443
femoral venous access, 443
venogram image evaluation, 443
venous pressure measurements, 443–444
Venous access
anticoagulation, 440–441
catheter navigation, 438–439, 440f
continuous saline infusion, 440
contrast agents, 437
double flushing, 439–440
femoral vein access, 437–438
hand injection, 441
mechanical injection, 441
pre-procedure evaluation, 437
pre-procedure orders, 437
puncture site care, 441
road mapping, 439
sedation/anesthesia, 437
Venous and lymphatic malformation,
superficial, 330
Venous angioma/developmental venous
anomaly (DVA), 85
Venous malformations
autosomal dominant familial, 632
blue rubber bleb naevus syndrome, 632
epidemiology, 631–632
imaging, 633
Klippel-Trenaunay syndrome, 632
management, 633

natural history and presentation, 632
pathophysiology, 632
superficial venous malformations vs.
capillary (infantile)
haemangiomas, 631, 631t
Venous pressure measurements, 443–444
Venous sampling procedures
in acromegaly, 455
cavernous sinus sampling, 451–452
inferior petrosal sinus sampling
catheter manipulation, 449–450
complications, 448
contrast agents, 448
femoral venous access, 449
indications, 447
personnel requirements, 448–449
preprocedure preparations, 448
sedation/analgesia, 449
wires and catheters for, 449
interpretation, 452–455
jugular venous sampling, 452
puncture site management, 452
in suspected ectopic ACTH production,
455
Venous sinuses
angioplasty and stenting, transverse-
sigmoid sinus dAVFs, 612
of Breschet, 81
cavernous, 80–81
inferior group, 80–81
inferior petrosal, 81
inferior sagittal, 79
marginal, 81
occipital, 79
sigmoid, 80
sphenoparietal sinus, 81
straight, 79
superior petrosal, 81
superior sagittal (SSS), 77, 78f, 79
torcular Herophili, 79
transverse, 79
vertebral venous plexus, 81
Venous stenosis
aetiology, 634–635
arteriovenous fistulas and malformations,
636–637
idiopathic intracranial hypertension (IIH),
634
imaging, 635
management, 635–636
multiple sclerosis (MS), 637–638
natural history and presentation, 635
statistics, 634
venous tinnitus, 636
Venous test occlusion
anti-coagulation, 445
catheter manipulation, 446
complications, 444–445
femoral access, 446

French Catheter Scale

Inch	0.039	0.053	0.066	0.079	0.092	0.105	0.118	0.131	0.1441	0.158
mm	1	1.35	1.67	2.0	2.3	2.7	3.0	3.3	3.7	4.0
French	3	4	5	6	7	8	9	10	11	12

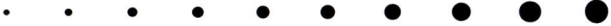

Inch	0.17	0.184	0.197	0.21	0.223	0.236	0.249	0.263	0.288
mm	4.3	4.7	5.0	5.3	5.7	6.0	6.3	6.7	7.3
French	13	14	15	16	17	18	19	20	21

Inch	0.315	0.341	0.367	0.393	0.419	0.445
mm	8.0	8.7	9.3	10.0	10.7	11.3
French	24	26	28	30	32	34

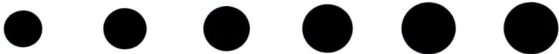

Common Medication Preparations

1) Abciximab (Reopro® Eli Lilly USA, Indianapolis, IN)
   a) Loading dose is 0.25 mg/kg, followed by 125 mcg/kg/min infusion for 12 h.
   b) Reconstitute drug by injecting 5 mL of sterile saline into each bottle containing 10 mg of drug. Most patients require two bottles for the loading dose and one for the infusion. Concentration is 2 mg/mL.
   c) Use 0.22 μm filter to draw the reconstituted drug into a 10 mL syringe.
   d) May be given IV or IA. If giving IV, then use a separate IV for the drug to avoid confusing it with other drugs.
2) Amytal (Amobarbital) for provocative testing
   a) Reconstitute 500 mg powder with 20 mL sterile bacteriostatic-free water.
      i) Mix 5 mL sterile water into vial of Amytal and put it into a 20 mL syringe. Rinse Amytal bottle with additional 5 mL sterile water and add to 20 mL syringe. Add another 10 mL sterile water to the 20 mL syringe. Final concentration is 25 mg/mL. Filter with a 0.22 μm filter prior to injection.
   b) Dose: 1 mL (25 mg) per injection.
3) Lidocaine for IA provocative testing
   a) Use 2% cardiac lidocaine.
   b) Syringe contains 100 mg in 5 mL; buffer this by adding 1 mL of 8.4% USP pediatric sodium bicarbonate injection.
   c) Dose: 1 mL (~20 mg) per injection.
4) Brevital® Sodium (methohexital sodium, JHP Pharmaceuticals, Parsippany, NJ) for Wada tests or provocative testing
   a) Use 500 mg powder bottle; reconstitute by injecting 20 mL sterile water into the bottle then withdraw into a 50 mL syringe. Rinse bottle with 20 mL sterile water and add to 50 mL syringe. Add another 10 mL sterile water to 50 mL syringe and mix thoroughly. Concentration is now 10 mg/mL. Add 1 mL of this solution to 9 mL water for a final concentration of 1 mg/mL
5) Dose: 1–3 mL (1–3 mg) per injection

Printed in the United States of America